OXFORD MEDICAL PUBLICATIONS

Clinical
Neuroimmunology

Clinical Neuroimmunology

Second edition

Edited by
Jack Antel
Gary Birnbaum
Hans-Peter Hartung
Angela Vincent

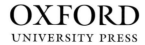

OXFORD

UNIVERSITY PRESS

OXFORD

UNIVERSITY PRESS

Great Clarendon Street, Oxford OX2 6DP

Oxford University Press is a department of the University of Oxford.
It furthers the University's objective of excellence in research, scholarship,
and education by publishing worldwide in

Oxford New York

Auckland Cape Town Dar es Salaam Hong Kong Karachi
Kuala Lumpur Madrid Melbourne Mexico City Nairobi
New Delhi Shanghai Taipei Toronto

With offices in

Argentina Austria Brazil Chile Czech Republic France Greece
Guatemala Hungary Italy Japan South Korea Poland Portugal
Singapore Switzerland Thailand Turkey Ukraine Vietnam

Oxford is a registered trade mark of Oxford University Press
in the UK and in certain other countries

Published in the United States
by Oxford University Press Inc., New York

First Edition published 1998 by Blackwell Science
Second Edition published 2005 by Oxford University Press
Reprinted 2006

A catalogue record for this title is available from the British Library

Library of Congress Cataloging in Publication Data

Clinical neuroimmunology / edited by Jack Antel [et al.]. 2nd ed.
Includes bibliographical references and index.
1. Nervous system–Diseases–Immunological aspects. 2. Neuroimmunology.
[DNLM: 1. Nervous System Diseases–immunology. WL 140C64052005]
RC346.5.C582 2005   616.8'0479–dc22   2005003413
I. Antel, Jack P.

ISBN 0-19-851068-3 (Hbk: alk. paper)
978-0-19-851068-0

10 9 8 7 6 5 4 3 2

Typeset by EXPO Holdings, Malaysia.
Printed in Italy
on acid-free paper

Preface

This second edition of *Clinical Neuroimmunology* is intended to present emerging concepts regarding interactions of the immune and nervous systems under physiologic and disease conditions. In the normal state, the immune system is involved in surveillance of the nervous system and in informing the nervous system of ongoing systemic immune responses. Conversely, the nervous system regulates activity of the immune system. Disease-related issues include how the immune system recognizes and responds to disease or injury within the nervous system and the basis whereby the usually 'immunologically privileged' nervous system becomes a target of immune attack.

The cellular and molecular mediators underlying communication between the immune system and the nervous system continue to be identified. Many of the intersystem active molecules, such as immune system-produced cytokines and nervous system-produced neurotrophins, were initially considered to be active within rather than between specific systems. The nervous system is now known to be capable of producing many of the same molecules used by the immune system for cell–cell signaling. The availability of virtually unlimited amounts of recombinant forms of many of these molecules and of pharmacologic or biologic reagents that can modulate their expression, coupled with novel means to deliver such reagents to a target site, has initiated a new era of therapy for an array of neurologic disorders.

We have complemented our original format, in which the initial chapters of the book presented basic principles regarding the cellular and molecular organization of the immune system, with a chapter on the basic principles of the organization of the nervous system. We hope this provides a stronger foundation for the presentations focused on describing the events involved in promoting immune system interaction with the central and peripheral nervous systems, development of autoimmunity, and strategies for designing immune-directed therapies. We have added chapters on neural regulation of the immune response (psychoneuroimmunology) and immune-mediated protection and repair in the nervous system. These chapters emphasize the diverse interactions of the immune system and the nervous system, a diversity that is dependent on both the nature of the event inducing the interaction and the individual properties of the host.

The second portion of the book presents the application of the above principles in the context of disease or injury of the nervous system, updating the information on the important clinical disorders previously considered and introducing a number of more recently recognized entities. We continue to divide these disorders into those affecting the central nervous system (CNS) and those affecting the peripheral nervous system (PNS). As expected there can be overlapping involvement, and many of the basic pathogenic principles are shared. We present disorders in which current evidence favors immune-mediated mechanisms as being the primary mediators of disease. In our CNS section, we have specifically expanded our presentations related to multiple sclerosis given the new insights and challenges raised by ongoing clinical, pathologic, imaging, immunologic, and therapeutic studies. Our new co-editor Angela Vincent and her colleagues provide new material that implicates the role of antibodies in a wider array of neurologic disorders than previously thought.

We also present neurologic disorders in which an immune response, or lack thereof, contributes to the ultimate disease outcome. The detection of immune system-associated molecules in brain regions affected by Alzheimer's disease and cerebral ischemia raises the possibility of a secondary contribution of immune-mediated mechanisms to the overall tissue injury. Conversely, we add a chapter that addresses the issue of regeneration in the CNS. In cases of neurologic disorders resulting from infection with the retroviruses HTV-l and HTLV-I, and of Lyme disease resulting from infection with the tic-associated spirochete *Borrelia burgdoferi*, the molecular mediators derived from either infiltrating immune cells or endogenous activated glial cells may be the major contributors to tissue injury. Similar considerations would apply to an array of parasitic disorders. Malignant brain tumors represent a situation in which there is usually evidence of an immune response. Although this response seems ineffective in controlling tumor growth, there is hope that a more effective response could be engineered. We also consider the role that the immune response can play in tissue remodeling and regeneration.

The section on PNS-directed disorders focuses on entities in which the immune system is considered a principal mediator. We consider diseases of the peripheral nerves associated with acute and chronic inflammation and with aberrant autoantibodies (dysimmune neuropathies). We consider disorders of the neuromuscular junction in which the role of specific antibodies in disease pathogenesis is firmly established. Finally, we consider the inflammatory disorders of muscle, whose pathologic phenotype implicates immune mechanisms as central disease mediators. As with the CNS, we again take into account how immune response can contribute to remodeling and regeneration of tissues.

The editors feel the continued rapid advances in the field of neuroimmunology as a basic science and clinical discipline justifies the need for an update of the material presented in the first edition. We are grateful to our colleagues for their contributions. We have invited contributions from individuals with diverse backgrounds and insights, hopefully adding to the interest of this book to both basic scientists and clinicians. We are particularly grateful that Byron H. Waksman, whom the editors are honored to consider as a mentor, advisor, and friend, has again provided his personal perspective on the development of the field of neuroimmunology, a field in which he was a major pioneer.

Jack Antel
Gary Birnbaum
Hans-Peter Hartung
Angela Vincent

Contents

List of Contributors

Ayse Altintaş: Istanbul University, Cerrahpasa School of Medicine, Turkey

Jack Antel: Montreal Neurological Institute, Montreal, Canada

Douglas L. Arnold: Montreal Neurological Institute, Montreal, Canada

Rouman Balabanov: Department of Neurology, University of Chicago Hospitals, Chicago, USA

Burkhard Becher: Dartmouth Medical Center, Lebanon, New Hampshire, USA

Gary Birnbaum: Minneapolis Clinic of Neurology, Minnesota, USA

David Brassat: University of California San Francisco, San Francisco, USA

Thomas Calzascia: Departments of Medical Biophysics and Immunology, Ontario Cancer Institute, Toronto, Canada

Iain L. Campbell: Department of Neuropharmacology, The Scripps Research Institute, California, USA

Zografos Caramanos: Magnetic Resonance Spectroscopy Unit and Montreal Neurological Institute, Montreal, Canada

Marinos C. Dalakas: Neuromuscular Diseases Division, National Institute of Neurological Disorders, Bethesda, USA

Josep Dalmau: University of Pennsylvannia, Philadelphia, USA

Samuel David: Centre for Research in Neuroscience, Montreal General Hospital, Montreal, Canada

Nicola De Stefano: NMR Centre and Neurometabolic Unit, University of Siena, Siena, Italy

Pierre-Yves Dietrich: Division of Oncology, University Hospital Geneva, Switzerland

Paula Dore-Duffy: Department of Neurology, Wayne State University, Detroit, USA

Richard M. Evans: Department of Neuroimmunology, GKT School of Medicine, London, UK

Joseph Frank: Experimental Neuroimaging Section, NIH, Bethesda, Maryland, USA

Ralf Gold: Institute for Multiple Sclerosis Research, University of Göttingen, Germany

Edith Gruslin: Institut Armand-Frappier, INRS, Laval, Quebec, Canada

Roger N. Gunn: GlaxoSmithKline, Translational Medicine and Genetics, Greenford, Middlesex, UK

David Hafler: Harvard Medical School Brigham & Women's Hospital, Boston, Massachusetts, USA

John M. Hallenbeck: Stroke Branch, National Institute of Neurological Disorders and Stroke, NIH, Bethesda, Maryland, USA

Hans-Peter Hartung: Heinrich-Heine University, Dusseldorf, Germany

Steven L. Hauser: University of California San Francisco, San Francisco, USA

Bernhard Hemmer: Klinikum der Philipps-Universitat, Marburg, Germany

Reinhard Hohlfeld: Institute for Clinical Neuroimmunology, Unversity of Munich, Munich, Germany

Steven Jacobson: Viral Immunology Section, National Institute of Neurological Disorders, NIH, Bethesda, USA

Hélène Jacomy: Institut Armand-Frappier, INRS, Laval, Quebec, Canada

Sebastian Jander: Heinrich-Heine-University Dusseldorf, Germany

Bernd C. Kieseier: Department of Neurology, University of Dusseldorf, Dusseldorf, Germany

Uwe Koedel: Neurologic Clinic and Institute for Clinical Neuroimmunology, Munich, Germany

Steve Lacroix: Research Center, House CHUL, Laval University, Quebec, Canada

Bethan Lang: Neurosciences Group, John Radcliffe Hospital, Oxford, UK

Norman Latov: Weill Medical College, Cornell University, New York, USA

Robert P. Lisak: Department of Neurology, Wayne State University, Detroit, USA

Catherine Lubetzki: Biologie des Interactions Neurones/Glie, Unité mixte de recherche INSERM U-711; UPMC, Hôpital de la Salpêtrière, Paris, France

Don J. Mahad: Department of Neurosciences, Cleveland, USA

Guido van Marle: University of Calgary, Calgary, Alberta, Canada

Edith G. McGeer: UBC Department of Psychiatry, Vancouver, Canada

Patrick L. McGeer: UBC Department of Psychiatry, Vancouver, Canada

Zurab Nadareishvili: Stroke Branch, National Institute of Neurological Disorders and Stroke, NIH, Bethesda, Maryland, USA

Kevin C. O'Connor: Harvard Medical School, Brigham and Women's Hospital, Boston, Massachusetts, USA

Jorge R. Oksenberg: University of California San Francisco, San Francisco, California, USA

Trevor Owens: Montreal Neurological Institute, Montreal, Quebec, Canada

Andrew R. Pachner: Princeton, New Jersey, USA

H. Walter Pfister: Neurologic Clinic and Institute for Clinical Neuroimmunology, Munich, Germany

John Pollard: Hospital of the University of Pennsylvania, Philadelphia, USA

Christopher Power: Department of Clinical Neuroscience, University of Calgary, Alberta, Canada

Richard M. Ransohoff: Department of Neurosciences, Lerner Research Institute, Cleveland, USA

Susanne Renaud: Weill Medical College, Cornell, New York, USA

Sabahattin Saip: Istanbul University, Cerrahpasa School of Medicine, Turkey

Aksel Siva: Istanbul University, Cerrahpasa School of Medicine, Turkey

Kenneth J. Smith: Department of Neuroimmunology, GKT School of Medicine, London, UK

Andreas Steck: Department of Neurology, University Clinics, Kantonsspital, Basel, Switzerland

Esther M. Sternberg: Neuroendocrine/Immunology, National Institute of Mental Health, NIH, Bethesda, Maryland USA

Guido Stoll: Department of Neurology, Julius-Maximilians-Universität Würzburg, Germany

Olaf Stüve: Department of Neurology, Heinrich Heine-University, Dusseldorf, Germany

Pierre J. Talbot: Institut Armand-Frappier, INRS Laval, Quebec, Canada

Utano Tomaru: Department of Pathology, Hokkaido University, Medical School, Japan

Leonardo Tonelli: Neuroendocrine/Immunology, National Institute of Mental Health, NIH, Bethesda, Maryland USA

Elise H. Tran: Yale University School of Medicine, New Haven, Connecticut, USA

Bruce D. Trapp: Department of Neurosciences, Cleveland, USA

Nicolas de Tribolet: Service de Neurochirurgie, HUG, Geneva, Switzerland

Alex Tselis: Wayne State University, Detroit, Michigan, USA

Jan Verschuuren: Department of Neurology, Leiden University Hospital, Leiden, The Netherlands

Vissia Viglietta: Harvard Medical School Brigham and Women's Hospital, Boston, Massachusetts, USA

Angela Vincent: Neurosciences Group, John Radcliffe Hospital, Oxford, UK

Bryon H. Waksman: Department of Pathology, NYU Medical Center, New York, USA

Paul R. Walker: Division of Oncology, University Hospital Geneva, Switzerland

Jeanette I. Webster: Neuroendocrine/Immunology, National Institute of Mental Health, NIH, Bethesda, Maryland USA

Matthew J. A. Wood: Department of Human Anatomy and Genetics, Oxford, UK

Yoshihisa Yamano: Department of Pathology, Hokkaido University Medical School, Japan

Bernard Zalc: Biologie des Interactions Neurones/Glie, Unité mixte de recherche INSERM U-711; UPMC, Hôpital de la Salpêtrière, Paris, France

1 Introduction to immunology

Gary Birnbaum, Jack Antel, and Hans-Peter Hartung

Any chapter claiming to be an introduction to a field as large and diverse as immunology must, of necessity, be abridged and skewed. Since this text is not intended as one on immunology *per se*, this chapter will deal mainly with those aspects of immunology that have a direct bearing on the diseases discussed in the text. First, we will present a basic overview of the components of the immune system. Secondly, we will discuss how immune responses are regulated. Finally, because autoimmune phenomena play an important role in many of the diseases of the nervous system presented in this book, we will discuss some potential mechanisms for the development of autoimmune responses. A more detailed analysis and review of autoimmune mechanisms and their control is presented in Chapter 2. A Dictionary of Immunologic Terms is presented at the end of the book.

Why an immune system?

The primary role of the mammalian immune system to the protect the organism from external harmful agents, usually infectious but also toxic (Janeway, 1992). In addition, the immune system plays an important role in maintaining antigenic homeostasis in the body by eliminating altered cells perceived to be 'foreign'. To meet these demands the immune system has evolved into two main components, the *innate immune system* and the *adaptive immune system*. The innate immune system evolved to respond immediately to a variety of external agents in a relatively generic or non-clonal fashion. The response does not require immune cell differentiation and maturation and thus occurs very rapidly. It provides the first line of defense to an infectious or toxic agent (Medzhitov and Janeway, 2000). The adaptive immune response evolved to provide responses to particular antigens. This response requires not only recognition of particular antigens but cell selection, differentiation, and proliferation. Thus, initial adaptive immune responses evolve over hours to days. While the two immune systems have different functions, it is now clear that they do not act independently of one another. Indeed, their functions are intertwined with the responses of one system profoundly affecting the responses of the other. Some details of these interactions will be discussed later in this chapter.

The innate immune system

As noted above, the innate immune system has the capacity to respond immediately to infectious and toxic agents. In particular the innate immune system recognizes particular carbohydrate moieties, especially those present on the surfaces of bacteria. These moieties are different from those present on the surfaces of host cells and are recognized by receptors encoded in the germline. Some of these receptors are on cell surfaces, such as Toll-like receptors (Barton and Medzhitov, 2002), and some are soluble. Since they are encoded by non-varying germline genes, the patterns of response of the innate immune system are relatively stereotyped.

Cells of the innate immune system are polymorphonuclear leukocytes (PMLs), macrophages, dendritic cells, natural killer cells (NK cells), and γ/δ T cells. Upon interaction of receptors of the innate immune system with bacterial carbohydrate moieties, macrophages and dendritic cells secrete chemoattractants, including interleukin 2 (IL-2) (Granucci *et al.*, 2003), that result in the accumulation of PMLs and NK cells at the site of injury. These cells in turn become activated and themselves secrete additional chemoattractants, such as cytokines and chemokines, resulting in the further accumulation both of cells of the innate immune system and the adaptive immune system at that site. The spectra of cytokines and chemokines released by the innate immune system at the initial site of tissue injury play an important role in determining the subsequent patterns of response of the adaptive immune system (Dabbagh and Lewis, 2003). In addition, dendritic cells that are activated by interaction with antigens at the site of tissue injury migrate from the site to regional lymph nodes, carrying with them the antigens they absorbed at the site of injury. Once in the lymph nodes, dendritic cells present these antigens to cells of the adaptive immune system, in particular T lymphocytes (Ridge *et al.*, 1998; Banchereau and Steinman, 1998; Lipscomb and Masten, 2002).

The above sequences of events indicate that while mechanisms of response, and cell populations involved in responding, differ greatly between the innate immune system and the adaptive immune system, their interactions are best viewed as a continuum of reactions to infectious or toxic agents.

The adaptive immune system

Cells of the adaptive immune system

Lymphocytes

There are two main categories of lymphocytes, T lymphocytes and B lymphocytes. Both are derived from primary lymphoid tissue such as the bone marrow, spleen, and fetal liver.

T lymphocytes

Mature T lymphocytes are derived from cells called *prothymocytes*. The vast majority of these cells differentiate into T cells in the thymus (Germain, 2002; Palmer, 2003). A much smaller number of such cells differentiate in into T lymphocytes at other sites such as the liver and gut (Rocha *et al.*, 1995) and may subserve different immunologic functions. Here we focus on the thymus. This organ is a combination of ectodermally and mesodermally derived cells such as thymic epithelial cells, macrophages, and interdigitating or dendritic cells (Farr *et al.*, 2002; Petrie, 2002). Two processes occur within the microenvironments created by these cells. The first is the induction of genes leading to the expression of the unique antigen receptor of each T cell as well as other T lymphocyte-specific proteins (such as CD4 and CD8) (Germain, 2002). The second involves a complex process of both negative and positive selection of cells based both on their antigen specificities and on their affinities, or the tightness of their binding, to their antigens. This latter phenomenon is described in greater detail later in this chapter. All T-cell receptors (TCRs) are dimers, composed of either an α chain and a β chain or a γ chain and a δ chain (Royer and Reinherz, 1987; Chan and Mak, 1989; Leiden, 1993). There are also very small subpopulations of T cells composed of two α chains. This population may play a role in certain autoimmune diseases (Komori *et al.*, 1990). Each TCR chain is made up of several different peptides, joined together as a result of genetic recombination. Sets of genes defining these peptides are arranged longitudinally on the chromosome and recombine with one another in a stochastic fashion. The chromosomal segments containing these TCR genes are called the V region, the D region (found only in β chains), the J region, and C (for constant) region. Each region of genes is divided into families, with varying numbers of genes in each family. One of the group of V-region genes will combine with one of the group of D-region genes and these two will then combine with one of the J-region genes. Finally this group of V–D–J genes will combine with one of a limited number of C-region genes. At that point, synthesis of the TCR chain proceeds. Additional diversity of the TCR repertoire results from the addition, during α-chain transcription, of varying numbers of amino acids to the V–J junction (called the N region).

The antigenic specificity of a TCR is determined by the tertiary structure, or complementarity region, of the V–D–(N)–J regions of the chain. No further recombination or diversification of the TCR repertoire occurs once T cells mature. This is in contrast to the situation in B cells where there is continuous somatic mutation of antibody genes during antigenic stimulation and B-cell proliferation. The roles each chain plays in antigen recognition and histocompatibility complex recognition are still being defined, but it is clear that different TCRs can recognize the same antigenic peptide and a single TCR can respond to different peptides. Thus there is a certain 'degeneracy' to the T-cell repertoire (Hemmer *et al.*, 1998; Gran *et al.*, 1999; Bielekova and Martin, 2001; Martin *et al.*, 2001) and one cannot predict antigen specificity on the basis of the amino acid sequence of a TCR alone.

Once the immature T cells in the thymus express TCRs on their cell surfaces they undergo a process of rigorous selection. The selection process involves intrinsically contradictory paradigms. On the one hand, the selection process must eliminate cells that recognize self- or autologous antigens and thus prevent 'horror autotoxicus'. On the other hand cells must have the capability of recognizing peptides in the context of autologous histocompatibility complex proteins. As a result, both negative and positive selection occurs, based on the 'Goldilocks principle'. If the affinity of a a TCR for an antigen is too high that cell is deleted. If the affinity of a a TCR for an antigen is too low, that cell too is deleted. Positive selection occurs in that population of T cells whose TCRs have 'just the right amount' of affinity for antigen and for self- or autologous antigens. Interaction of the TCRs of these cells with endogenous thymic cells results in cell stimulation and the opportunity to emigrate from the thymus. As a result of this highly selective process more than 90% of thymocyte precursors in the thymus die, usually through apoptosis.

In addition to acquisition of TCRs, T cells in the thymus acquire other cell surface proteins. Three of the most important are the CD3 protein complex, CD4, and CD8. These proteins are important in signal transduction, or the transmission of signals from the cell surface to the cell's interior (CD3) and in stabilizing the interaction between TCR and antigen (CD4 and CD8). They are discussed in more detail later in this chapter.

TCRs can be divided into different families based on the amino acid sequences of their V, D, and J regions. The potential diversity is illustrated by the β chains of TCRs, where there are 20 different families of V regions, two different families of D regions, and seven different families of J regions. There are only two C regions. The association of different V, D, and J regions is not entirely random. Rather, certain V, D, and J regions preferentially associate with one another. This is especially notable in T cells expressing γ/δ TCRs. In addition, proportions of T cells bearing receptors coded by the different gene families are not equal but vary from individual to individual and are similar, though not identical, in related individuals (Loveridge *et al.*, 1991; Malhotra *et al.*, 1992). The repertoire of TCR gene expression also varies during the maturation of the immune system and continues to change as an individual ages (Gorczynski *et al.*, 1983).

The antigenic specificity of the TCR is determined by certain key amino acids in the antigen-binding cleft of the TCR in the third complementarity-determining region. The locations of these critical anchor points have been determined for several families of TCRs. In many instances, antigen binding is 'degenerate', in that several different peptides can bind to a TCR (see above). In addition, different TCRs, produced by different genes, can have similar peptide-binding capabilities. In other words, one cannot predict antigen specificity on the bases of gene family expression. In inbred strains of rodents, immune responses to particular antigens involve activation of particular populations of T lymphocytes expressing particular families of V- and J-region genes. The occurrence of restricted, or oligoclonal, TCR utilization in response to antigenic stimulation, especially in response to self-, or autologous antigen stimulation, forms the basis for a potentially important therapeutic approach, namely the elimination of restricted, pathogenic populations of T cells either by immunization with TCR peptides or by administration of monoclonal antibodies directed against TCR proteins recognizing the autoantigens. This approach was successful in the treatment of experimental autoimmune diseases such as experimental autoimmune encephalomyelitis (EAE) (Sakai *et al.*, 1988; Acha-Orbea *et al.*,1988; Kuchroo *et al.*, 1994) and experimental autoimmune myasthenia gravis (Infante *et al.*, 1992; Kraig *et al.*, 1996; Kaul *et al.*, 1997; Standifer *et al.*, 2003). In outbred populations such as in humans, utilization of restricted populations of TCRs in response to antigenic stimulation is not so clear. Some data suggest that persons with presumed autoimmune diseases such as multiple sclerosis (MS) respond to autoantigens such as myelin basic protein (MBP) with a limited number of TCRs (Shimonkevitz *et al.*, 1993; Vandevyver *et al.*, 1995; Qin *et al.*, 1998; Gestri *et al.*, 2001; Jacobsen *et al.* 2002). Other data suggest that the response is heterogeneous, with utilization of large numbers of TCRs (Birnbaum and van Ness, 1992; Heard *et al.* 1999). To date, clinical trials studying whether TCR peptide 'vaccination' or administration of monoclonal antibodies to certain TCRs can modulate the course of MS have not been uniformly successful, though changes in populations of specific populations of T cells have been demonstrated (Wilson *et al.*, 1997; Zipp *et al.*, 1998; Morgan *et al.*, 2001; van der Aa *et al.*, 2003).

B lymphocytes

Immature B lymphocytes originate in primary lymphoid organs (bone marrow, fetal liver) and then migrate to secondary lymphoid organs (spleen, lymph node, gut-associated lymphoid tissues). There they come into contact with antigens, and if their immunoglobulin receptors are able to interact with specific antigens, the immature B cells proliferate and differentiate further. Proliferation and differentiation require both contact with an antigen and a series of additional stimulatory signals. Some antigens are able to stimulate B cells directly (so-called T-cell-independent antigens). An example of such an antigen would be bacterial lipopolysaccharide. Other antigens stimulate B cells only when additional signals are provided to the cell by helper T cells. Such antigens are called T-cell-dependent antigens and include most proteins and peptides.

The unique feature of B cells is their ability to express and secrete antibodies or immunoglobulins. These proteins are heterodimers composed of four peptide chains, that is two light chains (of either the κ or the λ type) and two heavy chains. These chains also arise as a result of genetic recombination. Similar to the phenomenon observed during the maturation of the TCRs, V-region genes are combined with D-region and J-region genes and finally C-region genes to give rise to a final heavy- or light-chain transcript. Diversity is further increased by the addition of non-germline nucleotides onto the ends of recombining genes to give rise to N-residues. However, unlike the situation with TCRs, where the final product is fixed upon maturation of the T cell, antibody genes continually mutate as B cells encounter antigen and proliferate. Certain portions of the V regions of genes, called *hypervariable regions*, are active sites of mutation (Wagner and Neuberger, 1996; Wilson *et al.*, 1998). As a result there is a continually changing repertoire of antibody molecules on the surfaces of B cells as the immune response to a particular antigen or antigens progresses. This continuing evolution of responses also results in changes in the populations of secreted or circulating antibody molecules. Not only are there increases in antibody concentrations with time but the affinities of antibodies for the stimulating antigens continually increase as B cells expressing higher-affinity antibodies on their cell surfaces are selectively activated (Nossal

1992; Wabl *et al.*, 1999; Neuberger *et al.*, 2000; Diaz and Casali, 2002). This 'maturation' of antibodies greatly increases both the efficiency and the specificity of the humoral immune response. There are also changes in the constant or C regions of the heavy chains of the antibody molecules as B cells differentiate. Heavy chains are categorized into five classes, depending on their C regions. They are IgD, IgM, IgA, IgG, and IgE. Most resting B cells and B-cell precursors express IgD and IgM classes of antibodies on their surfaces. After contact with antigen, *class switching* occurs and most B cells will begin to synthesize IgG antibodies. Populations of B cells in secretory organs such as the gut, salivary glands, or lacrimal glands will synthesize and secrete IgA antibodies, whereas B cells in organs such as skin and lung will express IgE antibodies. The antigen specificity of an antibody molecule is determined by the variable or V regions of the heavy and light chains. However, the general biological activity of the antibody molecule (Does it form dimers or pentamers? Does it readily activate the complement cascade? Does it bind to particular cell surface receptors?) is determined by the C region of the heavy chain and does not affect antigen specificity. The determinants of class switching are still not fully defined (Sale *et al.*, 2001; Vercelli, 2002; Zhang, 2003), but cytokines secreted by T cells, as well as co-stimulatory signals provided to these cells in the microenvironment of differentiating B cells, are important, as is the genetic background of the individual.

By virtue of their membrane expressing immunoglobulins, B cells are able to capture and concentrate proteins in an antigen-specific fashion. This enables them to function as highly efficient *antigen-presenting cells* (APCs). That is they have the capacity to bind antigen, internalize it, digest it, and re-express the digested peptides of the protein on their cell surfaces in the context of major histocompatibility complex (MHC) proteins. This is in contrast to other APCs such as macrophages and dendritic cells that capture antigen in a non-antigen-specific fashion. Characteristics and requirements of APCs will be described in more detail later in this chapter.

Natural killer cells (NK cells)

NK cells are bone marrow-derived cells of special lineage. They appear to arise from the same lineage as precursors of T cells and share several characteristics (Kay, 1986; Lanier *et al.*, 1992). They are called *natural* killers because they arise in the absence of any immune challenge and remain relatively unchanged after antigenic stimulation. They are part of the innate immune system. NK cells are able to recognize certain targets and to kill cells, such as tumor cells, bearing these targets. Recent work defined several NK receptors in mice and human (Valiante *et al.*, 1997; Sivakumar *et al.*, 1998). While requirements for antigen recognition are not fully defined, data suggest that expression of MHC Class I proteins (see below) on the cell surface inhibits NK cell activity (Moretta *et al.*, 1994; Valiante *et al.*, 1997; Barao and Ascensao, 1998). Since many neoplastic cells do not display MHC Class I proteins, this may in part explain their susceptibility to NK cell lysis.

Macrophages and dendritic cells (DCs)

Macrophages are bone-marrow-derived cells that have multiple immunological functions. They are not antigen specific in the sense that they do not express receptors on their cell surfaces that are able to recognize individual peptides. However, they do express, especially when activated, cell surface proteins coded for by genes in the MHC. These MHC proteins have grooves into which peptides can fit. The shapes of the grooves are determined certain critical amino acid sites (antigen contact sites) in the α helices and β-pleated sheets of these proteins (Nathenson *et al.*, 1989; Nikolic-Zugic and Carbone, 1991; Appella *et al.*, 1995). Thus, there is a certain specificity in terms of which peptides can nestle into these grooves. However, binding of MHC–peptide–binding grooves is far less discriminatory than the antigen-specific receptors of T and B cells. In addition to expressing MHC proteins, macrophages have the capacity to ingest proteins and digest them via distinct proteolytic pathways. The peptides that result from these digestive processes attach to the binding grooves of newly synthesized MHC proteins and these peptide–MHC complexes are transported to the cell surface. This process of protein ingestion, proteolysis, association of the resulting peptides with MHC proteins, and expression of peptide–MHC complexes on the surface of a cell is called *antigen processing*. It requires metabolic activity, and while it is not unique to macrophages these cells are among the most ubiquitous and efficient cells of the body for this function. In fact, macrophages and DCs are true 'professionals' in this regard, for not only do they process and present peptides to T cells but they also are able to provide essential additional co-stimulatory signals (described below) to T cells, allowing them to proliferate and differentiate when presented with their appropriate antigens. Both macrophages and DCs are also able to secrete biologically active materials called *cytokines*. Again this is especially pronounced when macrophages and DCs are activated. Cytokines are able to modulate T-cell, B-cell, and macrophage function within the microenvironment of the tissue. Important cytokines secreted by macrophages are interleukin 1 (IL-1), tumor necrosis factor alpha (TNF-α), and prostaglandins.

Dendritic cells are pleomorphic populations of cells that originate in the bone marrow and then travel to sites of potential antigen exposure such as the skin, gut, and central nervous system (see Chapter 5). The lineage of these cells continues to be debated but some are closely related to B cells [61] while others may be derived from T cells (Inaba *et al.*, 1990; Fairchild and Austyn, 1990). The morphology of dendritic cells varies with their anatomical location. Characteristically they either have multiple, long processes, or a 'veiled' appearance (Knight *et al.*, 1992). They are concentrated in lymph nodes, having migrated there from areas of recent antigen exposure, such as the skin. They carry the processed antigens from the original site of antigen exposure to regions where contact with circulating lymphocytes is maximized. DCs are highly efficient, professional APCs, and also secrete a variety of cytokines that influence the development of lymphocytes coming into contact with the DCs in the microenvironment of the lymph nodes.

As noted above, DCs reside in areas that are most likely to be exposed to infectious agents or foreign antigens. In the skin, DCs are called Langerhan's cells (Knight *et al.*, 1992). By virtue of their anatomical location, they are often the first cells of the immune system to encounter foreign substances. Following antigen exposure DCs migrate to areas of lymphoid cell differentiation such as the thymus, lymph nodes, and Peyer's patches. In the thymus they play an essential role in T-cell selection. In lymph nodes and Peyer's patches DCs play a central role in stimulating B and T cells, and because they can reside there for extended periods of time, DCs can serve as a reservoir of processed antigens that may be important in maintaining immunologic memory.

Major histocompatibility complex

The MHC is a complex of genes present in humans on chromosome 6. MHC genes are found in all vertebrates and play essential roles not only in the immune system but also in somatic cell differentiation (Honda and Rostami, 1989). A large number of different genes are present in the MHC, many of then not directly involved in immune activities (Cardoso and de Sousa, 2003). However, since there are major differences in MHCs among different geographical and ethnic groups, and since certain MHC phenotypes are associated with autoimmune diseases (Oksenberg *et al.*, 1999), it is possible that these MHC-associated genes play a role in disease susceptibility.

There are three major classes of MHC genes, Class I, Class II, and Class III. There are also a number of minor, or non-classic, MHC genes. Their roles in the immune response are not well defined. Proteins encoded by the Class I and Class II genes are required for antigen recognition by T cells. Class III proteins are part of the complement system and are not directly involved in antigen presentation. The MHC genes are among the most pleomorphic of gene complexes, with large numbers of different alleles in each class. Because of this great polymorphism, it is extremely rare for two individuals, other than identical twins, to have identical MHC alleles.

There are major differences in the patterns of expression of Class I and Class II genes. MHC Class I gene products are expressed on almost all somatic cells of an individual. In contrast, under normal conditions, the products of Class II genes are expressed almost exclusively on the surface of bone-marrow-derived cells such as macrophages, DCs, and B cells. In areas of inflammation, where there are increased concentrations of inflammatory cytokines, such as interferon-γ (IFN-γ) and TNF-α, cells other than those derived from bone marrow can be induced to express MHC Class II proteins. This phenomenon may be important for the development of autoimmune diseases (see below and Chapter 2).

MHC Class I and Class II proteins have peptide-binding grooves into which potential antigens nestle (Apostolopoulos *et al.*, 2001; Gebe *et al.*, 2002). The shapes of these peptide-binding sites vary between Class I and Class II proteins and also between alleles of the different classes. Variations are the result of differences in the primary and secondary sequences of peptide-binding-groove proteins. Peptides lodge within these grooves after the proteins from which they are derived undergo proteolysis. Binding results from a combination of hydrogen bonding and van der Waals interactions between amino acid residues of the peptide and two to three 'anchoring' amino within the MHC groove. Given the allelic variation in Class I and Class II proteins, peptide-binding sites within MHC proteins will differ greatly, resulting in differences in the abilities of different MHC proteins to interact with peptides. If a particular MHC protein groove is unable to bind and present a particular peptide to lymphocytes, that peptide will be 'invisible' to that individual's immune system. This phenomenon in which the nature of the MHC-binding region determines which peptides are recognized by the immune system is called *determinant selection*. Since the characteristic of the peptide-binding grooves of MHC proteins are genetically determined, and since each individual's MHC is different, there will be major differences in the kinds of peptides recognized by different individuals. Such differences are believed to be important in determining susceptibility to autoimmune disease (Oksenberg *et al.*, 1999).

There are important differences in the source of peptides that bind to Class I and Class II grooves. Class I-bound peptides are derived from cytosolic proteins degraded in proteosomes (Apostolopoulos *et al.*, 2001). An example would be proteins synthesized within virally infected cells. In contrast, Class II-bound peptides are derives from exogenous proteins that have undergone endocytosis and proteolysis in endosomes (Gebe *et al.*, 2002). The reasons for these differences in the categories of proteins binding to different MHC proteins are related to the sites of synthesis and assembly of the Class I and Class II molecules as well as the accessory molecules involved in transporting the peptides to the MHC proteins. There also are differences in the sizes of peptides bound within Class I and Class II grooves. Class I binding sites are closed at both ends and peptides of 8 to 10 residues are bound. Class II binding sites are more open, allowing binding of peptides of 10 to 34 amino acid residues.

Requirements for the initiation of an adaptive immune response

TCRs cannot interact with intact proteins. The antigen-binding site of the TCR can only recognize peptides which are 9 to 15 amino acids long. Thus, proteins must undergo antigen processing, a metabolically active process that requires digestion of proteins in the APC. Even that is not sufficient. The peptide must also be nestled in the antigen-binding groove of an MHC molecule. Only this combination of peptide–MHC is recognized by the TCR. This implies at least three things. First, the TCR must have two recognition sites, one for peptide and the other for a non-polymorphic region of the MHC molecule. Since T cells were selected in the thymus on the basis of a modest degree of responsiveness to self-proteins, most T cells respond to peptide presented by their own (autologous) constellation of MHC molecules. In other words, T cells are restricted in their responses to peptides presented by autologous (i.e. self) MHC proteins. Secondly, in the absence of the appropriate MHC molecule, there will be no antigen recognition and thus no immune response. Finally, if there is inappropriate expression of MHC molecules by cells that normally do not express them, inappropriate and possibly pathogenic immune responses may occur.

Still other requirements must be met before a T cell will fully respond to its antigen. There must be stabilization of the TCR–peptide–MHC complex (called *trimolecular complex*) for a sufficient period of time to allow the cascade of transmembrane signaling events engendered by the formation of the complex to activate genes in the nucleus of the T cell. This occurs by interaction of other proteins on the T-cell surface with those of the APC. The major proteins involved in this stabilization are the CD3 protein, present on all T cells, and the CD4 and CD8 proteins present on specific subpopulations of T cells. CD4 proteins interact with MHC Class II molecules. CD8 proteins interact with MHC Class I proteins. T cells that express the CD4 protein (CD4+ cells) recognize antigen presented by Class II molecules. Such cells are usually helper cells because they are involved in the initial stages of an immune response and are required to assist B cells in responding to thymic-dependent antigens. They also are needed to assist in the differentiation of pre-cytolytic T cells into cytolytic or 'killer' T cells. T cells that express the CD8 protein (CD8+ T cells) recognize antigen in the context of MHC Class I molecules and often are cytotoxic cells. Some CD4 cells can also manifest cytotoxicity even though antigen recognition occurred in the context of Class II. T cells that have acquired 'memory' by prior exposure to antigen can be identified by the expression of additional cell surface molecules, with over 150 genes activated in the process of antigen exposure (Holmes *et al.*, 2005).

Yet more requirements must be met before a maximal T-cell response can occur. In addition to interaction of the TCR with the peptide presented in the context of the MHC, and of interaction of either CD4 or CD8 with Class II or Class I respectively, T cells must receive at least one more stimulatory signal. This co-stimulatory signal is provided by 'professional' APCs such as macrophages, DCs, and activated B cells (Khoury and Sayegh, 2004). The T cell receives these co-stimulatory signals via two receptors, CD28 and CTLA-4. The ligands on APCs for these molecules are called B7-1 and B7-2. Different intracellular signal pathways result from the interaction of these receptors and cells expressing them are present in different anatomical locations within lymph nodes. Preferential stimulation of either of these two pathways results in different patterns of T-cell differentiation (see below). If T cells are exposed to a potentially stimulating peptide in the absence of co-stimulation, as occurs when peptide is presented by 'nonprofessional' APCs such as astrocytes, the T cells become unresponsive, or *anergic*. Anergy is a long-lasting state of unresponsiveness in which T cells are unable to produce the cytokine IL-2 which is required for T-cell proliferation. Induction of anergy is one of the major regulatory or controlling mechanisms of the immune system.

The final requirements for T-cell activation require that there be sufficient numbers of trimolecular complexes formed on the surface of the T cell and that they last long enough. Thus the numbers of MHC–peptide complexes available to the T cell must be above a particular threshold, and this is dependent not only on the concentration of antigen at the site of TCR interaction but on the numbers of MHC complexes present on the surface of an APC. If antigen concentrations are too low, or if there are insufficient MHC complexes on the APC's membrane, T cells will not be activated. In addition, since the trimolecular complex is reversible, the formation of the complex must last long enough for sufficient transmembrane signaling to occur. This is dependent in part on the affinity of the TCR for the peptide in the MHC groove and on the interaction of the stabilizing molecules noted above. As trimolecular complexes are formed on the surface of a T cell there is a clustering of these complexes in one region of the T cell and the APC to form what is called an *immunologic synapse* (Kupfer and Kupfer, 2003). If the formation of this synapse lasts long enough, and is of sufficient density, with sufficient co-stimulation, full T-cell activation will occur.

Cytokines

Cytokines are biologically active polypeptides released at sites of inflammation by a variety of cell types, ranging from fibroblasts, to astrocytes, to macrophages, to T cells. Cytokines have a wide variety of effects on the immune system, ranging from activation and recruitment of immune cells, to suppression. Thus, some cytokines are considered *pro-inflammatory*, whereas others are considered *anti-inflammatory*. As expected, cytokines can either synergize with one another or act antagonistically. In many instances, there is a cascade of cytokine secretion within the microenvironment of the responding T cell, such that one cytokine triggers the release of another cytokine. Often, antagonistic cytokines will be released at the same site. Thus, responses of T cells within that microenvironment will be the result of the net effects of these competing molecules. Following secretion of pro-inflammatory cytokines, an additional group of inflammatory mediators called *chemokines* are released (Moser *et al.*, 2004).There are three different groups of chemokines, classified upon the positioning of their cysteine residues (alpha, beta, and gamma). Chemokines function as chemoattractants for lymphocytes but differ in their attractant specificities. Thus, the secretion of different chemokines will result in the recruitment of different lymphocyte subpopulations to the site of inflammation. Receptors for particular chemokines have recently been shown to be sites of entry for HIV into T cells. Since a review of the ever increasing numbers of cytokines is beyond the scope of this chapter, the reader is referred to Moser *et al.* (2004) for a review. One interesting aspect of cytokine biology is that receptors for cytokines exist within the nervous system and thus have the potential to affect the function of the nervous system (Ambrosini and Aloisi, 2004). Details of immune–nervous system interactions are described in greater detail in Chapter 5.

When all necessary TCRs are stimulated, and appropriate signals are transduced into the cytosol of the T cell, the T cell begins to produce a series of cytokines necessary for proliferation. The most important is IL-2. This acts both on the cell producing the cytokine (autocrine function) and on adjacent cells (paracrine function). Other cytokines also are produced and these will vary according to the subtype of T cell. Characterization of T cells based upon their profile of cytokine secretion has become increasingly important, since immune-modulating therapies for such diseases as multiple sclerosis may exert their therapeutic effects by effecting particular subtypes of T cells. In mice, T cells of different subtypes can be clearly distinguished. In humans, the patterns of cytokine secretion by individual T cells is often not as well defined, raising questions about the applicability of rodent models to autoimmune disease to the human state.

CD4+ cells can be separated into two broad categories, defined by the patterns of cytokines they secrete. At one end of the spectrum are Th1 cells. When stimulated, they secrete IFN-γ and IL-2. Th1 cells are involved in delayed-type hypersensitivity (DTH) responses that result in the recruitment of other inflammatory cells to the site of stimulation and the differentiation of CD8+ cells into mature cytotoxic cells. An example of a DTH response mediated by Th1 cells is the tuberculin skin test. Th1 cells have been implicated as effectors in autoimmune diseases in general (Liblau *et al.*, 1995; Romagnani, 1995), and in central nervous system diseases such as EAE and MS in particular (Olsson, 1995*a,b*). At the other end of the spectrum are Th2 cells. They secrete, in addition to IL-2, the cytokines IL-4, IL-5, IL-6, IL-10, and IL-13. Th2 cells and their cytokines are necessary for the stimulation and differentiation of B cells into mature antibody-secreting cells or plasma cells. Th2 cells also secrete a cytokine called transforming growth factor beta (TGF-βΠ. In general, the cytokines produced by Th2 cells have effects antagonistic to those of Th1 cells, thus ameliorating the actions of Th1 cells. Th2 cytokines are being studied as possible therapies for autoimmune diseases such as MS (Johns *et al.*, 1991; Racke *et al.*, 1991, 1993) (see Chapter 8).

The classification of CD4+ cells into discrete Th1 and Th2 subpopulations may be simplistic. More recent data suggest that there is a spectrum of cells between the extremes of Th1 and Th2, with large numbers of cells producing cytokines of both types. This is most notable in humans. The determinants for inducing a particular pattern of cytokine secretion are not fully known, but at least two factors are important. First is the nature of the co-stimulatory signal provided by the APC (i.e. B7-1 versus B7-2). Second is the concentration of other cytokines in the microenvironment of the stimulated cell (Romagnani 1992*a,b*; De Carli *et al.*, 1994). For example, if an uncommitted T cell is stimulated in the presence of IFN-γ, it differentiates into a Th1 cell. If it differentiates in a microenvironment

with an abundance of IL-4, it becomes a Th2 cell. Since cytokines produced by the innate immune system are secreted first in the course of an inflammatory response, the nature of these cytokines is of critical importance in determining the subsequent patterns of adaptive immune responses at that site.

In contrast to TCRs, antibody molecules interact with their specific ligands without the need for antigen processing or presentation. All that is necessary is that the antigenic site of the ligand be exposed to the antibody molecule. Interaction with secreted antibody results in the formation of an antigen–antibody complex and this in turn evokes a wide variety of different biological effects, many of which depend on the heavy-chain class of the antibody bound to the antigen. For example, antibodies with IgM heavy chains tend to form pentamers and these are especially efficient in triggering the complement cascade, activating a series of proteolytic enzymes that create pores in cell membranes, resulting in cell lysis. Many cells, especially macrophages, have cell surface receptors, called *Fc receptors*, that bind to the C regions of antibody molecules. Binding of antibody molecules to Fc receptors on macrophages activates them, resulting in increased phagocytic activity and the secretion of cytokines such as IL-1. Activated macrophages can ingest and destroy antigen–antibody complexes (e.g. on the surface of a harmful bacterium) or can result in the lysis of a cell that has antibody bound to its surface (antibody-dependent cell-mediated lysis (ADCC)). IgE heavy chains bind to Fc receptors on basophils and mast cells, resulting in the release of these cells' granules which contain, among other substances, vasoactive amines such as histamine.

Prior to the release of antibody into the circulation, B cells must be stimulated to secrete antibodies. This can occur in one of two ways. Some antigens have the capacity to stimulate B cells directly. These are called 'T-cell independent antigens'. Examples of such antigens are the polysaccharides. Other antigens require a complex series of T-cell–B-cell interactions as well as the secretion of particular cytokines in order for B cells to be stimulated. These are usually protein antigens and are called 'T-cell-dependent antigens'. Especially important sites of B-cell differentiation to T-cell-dependent antigens are in germinal centers of secondary lymphoid tissue follicles. Such regions contain large numbers of *follicular dendritic cells*, a specialized population of APCs that is particularly efficient in antigen processing and presentation and also has the capacity to retain captured antigens for prolonged periods of time. This results in the continued recruitment, stimulation, and expansion of populations of immunocompetent cells with specificities for the retained antigens. To these antigen-rich regions come a constant stream of T cells as well as B cells of varying specificities, drawn there by chemoattractant cytokines. When a B cell comes into contact with its ligand in a germinal center it does so in a microenvironment consisting of activated T cells, expressing on their cell surfaces ligands for stimulating receptors on B cells (such as CD40), as well as secreted cytokines, such as IL-4 and IL-5, that are necessary for B-cell differentiation. In contrast to T cells, whose TCRs remain immutable during proliferation, the immunoglobulin genes of B cells undergo rapid somatic mutation as the B cells multiply, resulting in the creation of ever-changing repertoires of antibody molecules. B cells expressing antibody molecules of especially high affinity for the antigen are preferentially activated. Over time there is a gradual shift in the fine specificity and affinity of secreted antibodies toward those of greater specificity and higher affinity. In addition, there is a shift in antibody class from IgM antibodies (produced early in the immune response) to IgG antibodies. Different isotypes of IgG antibodies are produced in different cytokine microenvironments. In mice, B cells stimulated in the presence of IL-4 produce antibodies of the IgG1 isotvpe. Those stimulated in the presence of IFN-γ produce IgG2a. Isotypes vary in their abilities to bind to Fc receptors of different cells and in their abilities to activate the complement cascade.

Stimulated B cells differentiate into antibody-secreting factories called plasma cells. These are terminally differentiated cells that die without further proliferation. However, one of the important features of the immune system is its immunologic memory, that is, its capacity to respond quickly to antigens with which it has had previous contact. This trait is the foundation of vaccination therapy. The exact mechanisms for maintaining immunologic memory are not known but it probably results from a combination of phenomena such as retention of antigens in regions of lymphocyte concentration, e.g. germinal centers, the continuous recruitment and expansion of cells specific for a particular antigen, as well as the persistence of committed, but not terminally differentiated, T cells and B cells.

Non-cytokine products of activated lymphocytes

Cells of the immune system can secrete products that have other than immunologic functions. Among the more notable examples are lymphocyte-secreted neurotrophic factors, factors that have the capacity to enhance neuronal survival. One of these is brain-derived neurotrophic factor (BDNF). Such observations are of particular importance in regards to the role of the immune system in presumed autoimmune disease of the nervous system. As described above, it is clear that the immune system is tightly regulated, with opposing responses occurring normally during most immune reactions. As will be described in subsequent chapters, treatments of autoimmune diseases are increasingly being directed at modulating the immune response in such as fashion as to engender shifts in patterns of response from tissue-destructive processes. An example would be in MS, where treatment with the drug glatiramer acetate appears to cause a shift in immune reactivity from a Th1 pattern to a Th2 pattern. However, the finding that cells of the immune system can secrete substances with the capacity to nurture and protect neuronal function additionally changes the paradigm of controlling immune reactivity. Further supporting the concept that neurotrophic factors could play a role in protecting tissues from immune-mediated destruction are the observations that receptors for BDNF are found in the central nervous system in MS, in regions of demyelination (Hohlfeld, 2004). Thus, efforts to prevent tissue destruction by the immune system could, at least theoretically, lead to loss of immune-mediated protective functions. Stimuli necessary for the production neurotrophic factors need to be defined to allow treatments of autoimmune diseases to spare these salubrious functions.

Lymphocyte circulation

One of the essential functions of the immune system is to protect its host from perceived 'foreignness', be it internal or external. While some areas of the organism, such as the skin and mucosal surfaces, are populated by resident populations of immunocompetent cells, other areas do not have such defenses. For immunologic surveillance, they are dependent on the constant recirculation of immunocompetent cells through them. There are two general patterns of lymphocyte circulation. Naive T cells that have yet to encounter their specific ligand continuously circulate to and through lymphoid organs (Butcher and Picker, 1996). Once a T cell encounters its specific antigen and becomes activated it expresses on its cell surface *adhesion molecules* that function as receptors for ligands present on the surfaces of activated endothelial cells. Examples of such receptors are the L-selectin and integrin families of proteins. Activated T cells circulate through both lymphoid organs and non-lymphoid tissues. Not only do they have the capacity to enter non-lymphoid organs, but subpopulations of T cells go to particular organs. For example, T cells expressing γ/δ T-cell receptors preferentially migrate to the gut (Miller *et al.*, 2000). They have this additional capacity because of the expression of particular receptors that come into contact with endothelial cells expressing the appropriate ligands. Tissue specificity of homing is dependent not only on the expression of particular receptors and ligands but also on the sequence of ligand–receptor interactions that the T cell encounters as it literally 'rolls' along activated endothelial cells. An important lymphocyte adhesion molecule is very late antigen-4 (VLA-4), a member of the β1 integrin subfamily. VLA-4 binds to specific ligands, VCAM-1 and the CS-1 fragment of fibronectin expressed by endothelial cells and the extracellular matrix in areas of inflammation. It is this interaction that is mainly responsible for recruitment of lymphocytes (and other white blood cells) to such a site.

Under normal conditions, ligands for adhesion receptors are present only on specialized endothelial cells called *high endothelium* (because of their shape). These are present in the venules of secondary lymphoid tissues

(lymph nodes, spleen, gut-associated lymphoid tissues). Examples of such ligands are vascular cell adhesion molecule (VCAM)-l, intercellular adhesion molecule (ICAM)-1, and P-selectin. Expression of adhesion molecule ligands on the surfaces of endothelial cells results in repeated adhesion of circulating lymphocytes to these cells as they roll along the lumens of capillaries. Once a lymphocyte adheres to an endothelial cell it begins to flatten and secrete a series of proteolytic enzymes called *matrix metalloproteinases*. These dissolve the capillary basement membrane at the site of cell adhesion and allow the lymphocyte to pass through the capillary into the organ stroma. Once inside a secondary lymphoid tissue, lymphocytes are exposed to captured and processed antigens which can lead to further stimulation and expansion. Since endothelial cells in non-lymphoid tissues do not normally express ligands, circulating lymphocytes roll on by. However, endothelial cells in non-lymphoid tissues can become 'activated' and acquire the characteristics of high endothelium; that is, they can express cell surface proteins that are ligands for adhesion molecules on circulating lymphocytes. The stimuli for endothelial cell activation in non-lymphoid organs are multiple, but exposure to cytokines such as IFN-γ and certain chemokines are especially important. Thus, if an endothelial cell is exposed to IFN-γ secreted by a Th1 T cell, it will express proteins able to interact with lymphocyte selectins and integrins. Circulating lymphocytes will adhere to such endothelial cells and begin the process of entering the tissue, analogous to that seen in lymphoid tissues. Once in the organ, lymphocytes will interact with the microenvironment and, ideally, function in their role of protecting the host. Lymphocyte entry into organs is a normal event and is essential to the immune system's role of protecting against infection and cell mutation. However, if lymphocytes specific for autologous antigens are recruited to an organ, their continued stimulation and activation can cause tissue destruction.

While the initial secretion of cytokines almost certainly results from an immunologically specific action, recruitment of circulating lymphocytes into an area of inflammation is not antigen specific. Thus, the overwhelming majority (>95%) of inflammatory cells present at such a site have no specificity for the agent that initiated the immune response. The role of these recruited cells is to amplify an immune response that most likely involved only a limited number of cells and to provide the necessary backup to defend the host. Of course, a key question in the phenomenon of lymphocyte circulation, homing, adhesion, and organ entry is, 'What initiates the primary process?'. That is, what draws the first antigen-specific T cell to the site in question? Perhaps there is tissue destruction, with release of sequestered antigens that are then expressed on the surfaces of endothelial cells, in turn drawing antigen-specific cells to that region. Another important issue, as yet unresolved, is whether there are homing receptors specific for particular organs. While some may exist for certain organs, such as skin, no nervous system-specific ligands have been found. This is especially important if one wishes to prevent the entry of inflammatory cells into organs that are the target of an autoimmune attack such as the brain in persons with MS. Since immune surveillance by circulating lymphocytes is an essential function of the immune system, prevention of lymphocyte adhesion with the use of monoclonal antibodies to adhesion molecules could have serious consequences. Antibodies to homing receptors can prevent the entry of pathogenic lymphocytes into the central nervous systems of animals with EAE and even reverse active disease (Yednock *et al.*, 1992; Kent *et al.*, 1995). Such antibodies are now being studied in human diseases such as MS (see Chapter 3).

The role of genes in immune reactivity

While environmental influences play a major role in shaping the patterns of immune responses to a particular antigen, the genetic background of an individual also plays an critical role in this process. A multitude of different genes are involved. Especially important are the genes encoding for TCRs, the genes of the MHC, genes involved in regulating the secretion of cytokines, and genes associated with proteins involved in antigen processing. For example, individuals of different genetic backgrounds will utilize different families of TCRs in responding to the same antigen (Ben Nun *et al.*, 1991; Boitel *et al.*, 1992; Martin *et al.*, 1992). This has been demonstrated convincingly in inbred strains of mice responding to autoantigens such as MBP (Sakai *et al.*, 1988). In other systems, investigators found that limited or oligoclonal populations of T cells respond to an autoantigen such as MBP (Acha-Orbea *et al.*, 1988; Zamvil *et al.*, 1988). These observations led to a potentially useful treatment approach. By immunization with TCR peptides, or administration of antibodies to the TCRs expressed on these pathogenic T cells, the course of an autoimmune disease such as EAE was ameliorated (Acha-Orbea *et al.*, 1988; Vandenbark *et al.*, 1989). Recent data suggest that persons with autoimmune diseases such as MS utilize certain families of TCRs in their responses to myelin proteins, that is the response, e.g. to MBP, involves oligoclonal CD8+ cells. Certainly, oligoclonal populations of antibodies are present in the central nervous system (CNS) of persons with MS and these remain stable throughout the course of the disease (Buntinx *et al.*, 2002). However, to date, clinical trials in which patients with MS were immunized with TCR peptides believed to be involved in the responses to myelin antigens in the hope of modulating the course of this disease have met with, at best, limited success (Vandenbark *et al.*, 2001). In some experimental animals such as mice, there are strains in which whole families of TCRs are absent. In spite of the polymorphism and flexibility of the immune system, such deletions give rise to a complete lack of responsiveness to particular antigens (Haqqi *et al.*, 1989). While such 'holes' in the repertoire have not been described in humans, they may exist and could play a role in determining susceptibility to autoimmune diseases.

There are major differences in MHC proteins with regard to the molecular configuration of their antigen-binding pockets (Madden 1995; Parker *et al.*, 1995). As a result, a particular peptide may be able to nestle in the antigen-binding groove of one person's MHC molecule but will not 'fit' into the groove of another person's MHC molecule. If peptide binding to MHC does not occur, T-cell immune recognition of the peptide will not occur and no immune response will be evoked. (Sloan-Lancaster and Allen (1996) reviewed this altered peptide ligand concept.) Conversely, recognition of potentially pathogenic peptides may only occur in individuals with particular MHC phenotypes. Such persons may be especially susceptible to autoimmune diseases such as MS. This is discussed in greater detail in Chapter 9. As discussed previously under the MHC heading, the phenomenon whereby the MHC molds the pattern of immune response is called *determinant selection*.

In species such as mice and rats, genetic susceptibility to autoimmune disease is associated with differences in the expression of inflammatory cytokines (Mustafa *et al.*, 1993; de Kozak *et al.*, 1994; Scott *et al.*, 1994; Takacs *et al.*, 1995). For example, susceptibility to EAE is associated with an increased secretion of TNF-α in Lewis rats (Chung *et al.*, 1991). Differences in alleles of genes involved with antigen processing, such as the transporter associated with antigen processing (TAP), are also linked to differences in susceptibility to certain autoimmune diseases (Ploski *et al.*, 1994; Singal *et al.*, 1994; Barron *et al.*, 1995; Gonzalez-Escribano *et al.*, 1995), but not MS (Liblau *et al.* 1993; Bell and Ramachandran, 1995). In addition to genes determining susceptibility there are genes involved in determining severity of disease. Work in this area is relatively new, but is proceeding slowly. Genes implicated in determining the severity of disease in persons with MS are mostly associated with regulating immune responses. The major examples to date are genes encoded within the MHC region. The subject of genetic susceptibility to autoimmune diseases is discussed in greater detail in Chapter 9.

Mechanisms of immune tolerance

The workings of the immune system are, in many ways, paradoxical. For example, great effort is made by the immune system to avoid reactivity to self-antigens, yet responses to self-antigens, in the form of recognition of autologous MHC proteins, is essential for normal T-cell function. Another example is the combination of exquisite antigen specificity of immune system receptors such as TCRs and antibodies that nevertheless allows a certain amount of 'degeneracy' with unrelated peptides binding to and interacting with these receptors if their steric conformations fit into the antigen-binding sites. While the initial triggering of an immune competent cell involves the interaction of its receptor with its ligand peptide, polysaccharide, and lipoglycan, in the process of this response cytokines and chemokines are released that are able to recruit immunocompetent cells to sites of inflammation without regard to their antigen specificity. It is these cells that contribute to an immune and inflammatory reaction by greatly amplifying a response that was initiated by a small number of cells specific for the inciting antigen. The combination of highly specific immune system activation followed by a more generalized, non-antigen-specific recruitment of immunocompetent cells explains both the power of the immune system to respond quickly to a wide variety of antigenic challenges and the potential toxicity that may occur as a result of such a broad-spectrum response. A number of different mechanisms have evolved to prevent that most damaging potential of the immune system, a destructive response to self-antigens. Some of the most important ones related to T-cell regulation are described here:

1. Intrathymic clonal deletion. As noted previously, strong positive and negative selective forces work in the thymus eliminating cells with TCRs that have too high or too low an affinity for self-antigens. If this process is impaired or suppressed during the ontogeny of the immune system, either by exposure to immune-modulating drugs, such as cyclosporine (Sakaguchi and Sakaguchi, 1992; Schuurman *et al.*, 1992), or because of metabolic disturbances, such as deficiencies of certain minerals or vitamins (Revillard and Cozon, 1990), selective processes may be altered, with the result that cells with autoimmune potential are allowed to leave the thymus.

2. Peripheral clonal deletion. Since not all autologous antigens are expressed in the thymus, there must be a means to eliminate such autoreactive cells in the periphery. One mechanism for deletion of potentially harmful T cells occurs when antigen-specific cells are exposed to high doses of antigen (Critchfield *et al.*, 1994, 1995). This results in apoptosis of the stimulated cells, deletion of the pathogenic populations, and recovery from disease, in this case EAE. A similar paradigm of 'clonal exhaustion' and deletion is observed with foreign antigens such as viral proteins (Moskophidis *et al.*, 1993*a,b*).

3. Peripheral clonal unresponsiveness. As described previously, when T cells encounter antigen in the absence of the necessary co-stimulatory signals, the cells become unresponsive or anergic (Kraig *et al.*, 1996). This can occur when antigen is presented by non-professional APCs. Thus, the site of antigen presentation, for example in organs without cells able to provide co-stimulation, is critical to inducing this regulatory phenomenon. However, in the presence of increased concentrations of IL-2, and in the presence of professional APCs, or tissue cells that have acquired professional properties by virtue of exposure to certain cytokines such as IFN-7, anergy can be reversed. This can occur in tissues that are injured or infected. Macrophages and populations of T and B cells with specificity for the antigens of the infectious agent are recruited to that site where they become activated and secrete large amounts of cytokines and other chemoattractants. This results in the non-antigen-specific recruitment of large numbers of additional inflammatory cells to the tissue, some of which may have autoimmune potential but failed to respond because they were anergic. In the cytokine-rich microenvironment of the inflammatory locus, anergy is reversed and previously unresponsive autoimmune cells respond to tissue-specific antigens. These cells then can become self-perpetuating as long as exposure to antigens continues. This sequence of events may explain the association between infections, and traumas such as surgery, with the development or recrudescence of autoimmune processes, and the release of tissue antigens into the circulation.

4. Clonal ignorance. If antigen is 'sequestered' from autoreactive T cells they will not respond. But in some instances, via mechanisms that are not well understood, expression of antigens by cells that are not immunologically competent results in the inactivation of potentially reactive T cells. This was first demonstrated in transgenic mice expressing a viral protein in

pancreatic beta cells (Johnson and Jenkins, 1994). Non-responsiveness was not due to anergy, as vigorous immune responses were obtained when animals were infected with live virus. Activation of cytotoxic CD8+ T cells required the presence of CD4+ T cells, suggesting that lack of responsiveness was the result of deficient T-cell activation separate from the co-stimulation provided by professional APCs.

5. Regulatory networks. As proteins can be potent antigens, it is not unexpected that the proteins of TCRs or antibodies can function as stimulators of immune responses. If responses are directed against the antigen-binding portions of these receptors (the idiotypes), they are called *anti-idiotypic responses* and have the capability of suppressing or augmenting the effects of idiotype-expressing T cells and antibodies (Cerny *et al.*, 1988; Lider *et al.*, 1989; Zaghouani *et al.*, 1989; Offner *et al.*, 1991; Ohashi *et al.*, 1991; Beraud, 1991; Calvanico, 1993; Shoenfeld *et al.*, 1994). Anti-idiotypic responses occur normally, but can also be induced. Induction of anti-idiotypic T-cell responses was used successfully to protect against and modulate the course of EAE (Lider *et al.*, 1988; Offner *et al.*, 1991). Cells and soluble mediators able to suppress immune responses were demonstrated decades ago. The nature of these 'suppressor' cells and mediators is still controversial since suppressor function can be shown in many different experimental paradigms. These data indicate that whether or not a cell or soluble mediator functions as a suppressor depends on its particular immunologic context. For example, a CD4+ Th1 cell may be tissue destructive in one context but that same cell type may be inhibitory in a pathological process in which Th2 cells have a pathological role (such as in parasitic infections). Similarly an antibody may activate complement and cause cytotoxicity yet in a different context that antibody could react with and mask antigenic sites recognized by CD8+ cytotoxic T cells, thus preventing tissue destruction. Markers of suppressor cells, such as CD25 are described (Shevach, 2002), but suppressor function is not limited to cells expressing this marker. Naturally occurring regulatory cells were demonstrated in a transgenic mouse model in which the majority of T cells expressed a receptor for an encephalitogenic epitope of MBP (Lafaille *et al.*, 1994). In the group of mice in which a majority of T cells expressed this receptor, but a portion of 'normal' T cells also existed, few animals became ill with EAE. When animals were manipulated such that 100% of the T cells expressed anti-MBP TCRs, all animals eventually became ill. Thus, even a small population of 'normal', non-autoimmune cells can regulate the responsiveness of autologously reactive lymphocytes. The mechanism of this regulation is not known.

6. Immune deviation. From the previous discussions, it is apparent that the site of antigen expression and presentation is an important variable in determining the pattern of immune responses. For example, exposure of antigen to the immune system via gut-associated lymphoid tissue results in suppression of T-cell-mediated immune responses; that is, the phenomenon of *oral tolerance*. If high doses of antigen are fed, reactive cells become anergic, whereas low doses of ingested antigen result in the induction of anti-inflammatory cytokines by Th2 cells (Keren, 1992; Weiner *et al.*, 1994; Lafaille *et al.*, 1994; Friedman *et al.*, 1994; Mitchison and Sieper, 1995; Staines and Harper, 1995). Inducing changes in patterns of immune responses has therapeutic potential, at least in experimental autoimmune diseases such as EAE (Weiner *et al.*, 1994).

Similar mechanisms to those for T cells exist for the immune regulation of B lymphocytes. Some of these mechanisms are bone marrow clonal deletion, peripheral clonal unresponsiveness, and peripheral clonal deletion. In addition, there are unique, B-cell-specific mechanisms of regulation:

1. Maturational arrest. Normal expression of autoantigens can prevent the maturation of autoreactive B cells. This was demonstrated in B-cell receptor transgenic mice expressing receptors for a cell-membrane-expressed protein (reviewed in Schuurman *et al.* (1992)). Autoreactive precursor B cells were found in the marrow, but no mature cells were detectable in the periphery. When precursor cells were cultured *in vitro*, in the absence of antigen, normal development was noted.

2. Follicular exclusion. Autoreactive B cells, especially those that have captured antigen on their surfaces, are excluded from entering secondary lymphoid follicles. As a result, such cells undergo apoptosis (Cyster *et al.*, 1994; Cyster and Goodnow, 1995). The mechanism for this phenomenon is not known, but exclusion from follicles may also prevent autoreactive B cells from becoming tolerant, and thus may actually promote the development of autoimmune responses.

References

Acha-Orbea, H., Mitchell, D.J., Timmermann, L., Wraith, D.C., Tausch, D.S., Waldor, M.K., *et al.* (1988). Limited heterogeneity of T cell receptors from lymphocytes mediating autoimmune encephalomyelitis allows specific immune intervention. *Cell* 54: 263–273.

Allman, D. and Miller, J.P. (2003). Common lymphoid progenitors, early B-lineage precursors, and IL-7: characterizing the trophic and instructive signals underlying early B cell development. *Immunol Res* 27: 131–140.

Ambrosini, E. and Aloisi, F. (2004). Chemokines and glial cells: a complex network in the central nervous system. *Neurochem Res* 29: 1017–1038.

Apostolopoulos, V., McKenzie, I.F., and Wilson, I.A. (2001). Getting into the groove: unusual features of peptide binding to MHC class I molecules and implications in vaccine design. *Front Biosci* 6: D1311–D1320.

Appella, E., Padlan, E.A., and Hunt, D.F. (1995). Analysis of the structure of naturally processed peptides bound by class I and class II major histocompatibility complex molecules. *EXS* 73: 105–119.

Banchereau, J. and Steinman, R.M. (1998). Dendritic cells and the control of immunity. *Nature* 392: 245–252.

Barao, I. and Ascensao, J.L. (1998). Human natural killer cells. *Arch Immunol Ther Exp (Warsz)* 46: 213–229.

Barron, K.S., Reveille, J.D., Carrington, M., Mann, D.L., and Robinson, M.A. (1995). Susceptibility to Reiter's syndrome is associated with alleles of TAP genes. *Arthritis Rheum* 38: 684–689.

Barton, G.M. and Medzhitov, R. (2002). Toll-like receptors and their ligands. *Curr Top Microbiol Immunol* 270: 81–92.

Bell, R.B. and Ramachandran, S. (1995). The relationship of TAP1 and TAP2 dimorphisms to multiple sclerosis susceptibility. *J Neuroimmunol* 59: 201–204.

Ben Nun, A., Liblau, R.S., Cohen, L., Lehmann, D., Tournier-Lasserve, E., Rosenzweig, A., *et al.* (1991). Restricted T-cell receptor V beta gene usage by myelin basic protein-specific T-cell clones in multiple sclerosis: predominant genes vary in individuals. *Proc Natl Acad Sci USA* 88: 2466–2470.

Beraud, E. (1991). T cell vaccination in autoimmune diseases. *Ann NY Acad Sci* 636: 124–134.

Bielekova, B. and Martin, R. (2001). Antigen-specific immunomodulation via altered peptide ligands. *J Mol Med* 79: 552–565.

Birnbaum, G. and van Ness, B. (1992). Quantitation of T-cell receptor V beta chain expression on lymphocytes from blood, brain, and spinal fluid in patients with multiple sclerosis and other neurological diseases. *Ann Neurol* 32: 24–30.

Boitel, B., Ermonval, M., Panina-Bordignon, P., Mariuzza, R.A., Lanzavecchia, A., and Acuto, O. (1992). Preferential V beta gene usage and lack of junctional sequence conservation among human T cell receptors specific for a tetanus toxin-derived peptide: evidence for a dominant role of a germline-encoded V region in antigen/major histocompatibility complex recognition. *J Exp Med* 175: 765–777.

Buntinx, M., Stinissen, P., Steels, P., Ameloot, M., and Raus, J. (2002). Immune-mediated oligodendrocyte injury in multiple sclerosis: molecular mechanisms and therapeutic interventions. *Crit Rev Immunol* 22: 391–424.

Butcher, E.C. and Picker, L.J. (1996). Lymphocyte homing and homeostasis. *Science* 272: 60–66.

Calvanico, N.J. (1993). The humoral immune response in autoimmunity. *Dermatol Clin* 11: 379–389.

Cardoso, C.S. and de Sousa, M. (2003). HFE, the MHC and hemochromatosis: paradigm for an extended function for MHC class I. *Tissue Antigens* **61**: 263–275.

Cerny, J., Smith, J.S., Webb, C., and Tucker, P.W. (1988). Properties of anti-idiotypic T cell lines propagated with syngeneic B lymphocytes. I. T cells bind intact idiotypes and discriminate between the somatic idiotypic variants in a manner similar to the anti-idiotopic antibodies. *J Immunol* **141**: 3718–3725.

Chan, A. and Mak, T.W. (1989). Genomic organization of the T cell receptor. *Cancer Detect Prev* **14**: 261–267.

Chung, I.Y., Norris, J.G., and Benveniste, E.N. (1991). Differential tumor necrosis factor alpha expression by astrocytes from experimental allergic encephalomyelitis-susceptible and -resistant rat strains. *J Exp Med* **173**: 801–811.

Critchfield, J.M., Racke, M.K., Zuniga-Pflucker, J.C., Cannella, B., Raine, C.S., Goverman, J., et al. (1994). T cell deletion in high antigen dose therapy of autoimmune encephalomyelitis. *Science* **263**: 1139–1143.

Critchfield, J.M., Zuniga-Pflucker, J.C., and Lenardo, M.J. (1995). Parameters controlling the programmed death of mature mouse T lymphocytes in high-dose suppression. *Cell Immunol* **160**: 71–78.

Cyster, J.G. and Goodnow, C.C. (1995). Pertussis toxin inhibits migration of B and T lymphocytes into splenic white pulp cords. *J Exp Med* **182**: 581–586.

Cyster, J.G., Hartley, S.B., and Goodnow, C.C. (1994). Competition for follicular niches excludes self-reactive cells from the recirculating B-cell repertoire. *Nature* **371**: 389–395.

Dabbagh, K. and Lewis, D.B. (2003). Toll-like receptors and T-helper-1/T-helper-2 responses. *Curr Opin Infect Dis* **16**: 199–204.

De Carli, M., D'Elios, M.M., Zancuoghi, G., Romagnani, S., and Del Prete, G. (1994). Human Th1 and Th2 cells: functional properties, regulation of development and role in autoimmunity. *Autoimmunity* **18**: 301–308.

de Kozak, Y., Naud, M.C., Bellot, J., Faure, J.P., and Hicks, D. (1994). Differential tumor necrosis factor expression by resident retinal cells from experimental uveitis-susceptible and -resistant rat strains. *J Neuroimmunol* **55**: 1–9.

Diaz, M. and Casali, P. (2002). Somatic immunoglobulin hypermutation. *Curr Opin Immunol* **14**: 235–240.

Fairchild, P.J. and Austyn, J.M. (1990). Thymic dendritic cells: phenotype and function. *Int Rev Immunol* **6**: 187–196.

Farr, A.G., Dooley, J.L., and Erickson, M. (2002). Organization of thymic medullary epithelial heterogeneity: implications for mechanisms of epithelial differentiation. *Immunol Rev* **189**: 20–27.

Friedman, A., al Sabbagh, A., Santos, L.M., Fishman-Lobell, J., Polanski, M., Das, M.P., et al. (1994). Oral tolerance: a biologically relevant pathway to generate peripheral tolerance against external and self antigens. *Chem Immunol* **58**: 259–290.

Gebe, J.A., Swanson, E., and Kwok, W.W. (2002). HLA class II peptide-binding and autoimmunity. *Tissue Antigens* **59**: 78–87.

Germain, R.N. (2002). T-cell development and the CD4–CD8 lineage decision. *Nat Rev Immunol* **2**: 309–322.

Gestri, D., Baldacci, L., Taiuti, R., Galli, E., Maggi, E., Piccinni, M. P., et al. (2001). Oligoclonal T cell repertoire in cerebrospinal fluid of patients with inflammatory diseases of the nervous system. *J Neurol Neurosurg Psychiatryiat* **70**: 767–772.

Gonzalez-Escribano, M.F., Morales, J., Garcia-Lozano, J.R., Castillo, M.J., Sanchez-Roman, J., Nunez-Roldan, A., et al. (1995). TAP polymorphism in patients with Behcet's disease. *Ann Rheum Dis* **54**: 386–388.

Gorczynski, R.M., Kennedy, M., and MacRae, S. (1983). Alteration in lymphocyte recognition repertoire during aging. II. Changes in the expressed T-cell receptor repertoire in aged mice and the persistence of that change after transplantation to a new differentiative environment. *Cell Immunol* **75**: 226–241.

Gran, B., Hemmer, B., Vergelli, M., McFarland, H.F., and Martin, R. (1999). Molecular mimicry and multiple sclerosis: degenerate T-cell recognition and the induction of autoimmunity. *Ann Neurol* **45**: 559–567.

Granucci, F., Zanoni, I., Feau, S., and Ricciardi-Castagnoli, P. (2003). Dendritic cell regulation of immune responses: a new role for interleukin 2 at the intersection of innate and adaptive immunity. *EMBO J* **22**: 2546–2551.

Haqqi, T.M., Banerjee, S., Jones, W.L., Anderson, G., Behlke, M.A., Loh, D.Y., et al. (1989). Identification of T-cell receptor V beta deletion mutant mouse

strain AU/ssJ (H-2q) which is resistant to collagen-induced arthritis. *Immunogenetics* **29**: 180–185.

Heard, R.N., Teutsch, S.M., Bennetts, B.H., Lee, S.D., Deane, E.M., and Stewart, G.J. (1999). Lack of restriction of T cell receptor beta variable gene usage in cerebrospinal fluid lymphocytes in acute optic neuritis. *J Neurol Neurosurg Psychiatryiat* **67**: 585–590.

Hemmer, B., Pinilla, C., Appel, J., Pascal, J., Houghten, R., and Martin, R. (1998). The use of soluble synthetic peptide combinatorial libraries to determine antigen recognition of T cells. *J Peptide Res* **52**: 338–345.

Hohlfeld, R. (2004). Immunologic factors in primary progressive multiple sclerosis. *Mult Scler* **10**(Suppl. 1): S16–S21.

Holmes, S., He, M., Xu, T., and Lee, P.P. (2005). Memory T cells have gene expression patterns intermediate between naive and effector. *Proc Natl Acad Sci USA* **102**: 5519–5523.

Honda, H. and Rostami, A. (1989). Expression of major histocompatibility complex class I antigens in rat muscle cultures: the possible developmental role in myogenesis. *Proc Natl .Acad Sci USA* **86**: 7007–7011.

Inaba, K., Hosono, M., and Inaba, M. (1990). Thymic dendritic cells and B cells: isolation and function. *Int Rev Immunol* **6**: 117–126.

Infante, A.J., Levcovitz, H., Gordon, V., Wall, K.A., Thompson, P.A., and Krolick, K.A. (1992). Preferential use of a T cell receptor V beta gene by acetylcholine receptor reactive T cells from myasthenia gravis-susceptible mice. *J Immunol* **148**: 3385–3390.

Jacobsen, M., Cepok, S., Quak, E., Happel, M., Gaber, R., Ziegler, A., et al. (2002). Oligoclonal expansion of memory CD8+ T cells in cerebrospinal fluid from multiple sclerosis patients. *Brain* **125**: 538–550.

Janeway, C.A., Jr (1992). The immune system evolved to discriminate infectious nonself from noninfectious self. *Immunol Today* **13**: 11–16.

Johns, L.D., Flanders, K.C., Ranges, G.E., and Sriram, S. (1991). Successful treatment of experimental allergic encephalomyelitis with transforming growth factor-beta 1. *J Immunol* **147**: 1792–1796.

Johnson, J.G. and Jenkins, M.K. (1994). The role of anergy in peripheral T cell unresponsiveness. *Life Sci* **55**: 1767–1780.

Kaul, R., Wu, B., Goluszko, E., Deng, C., Dedhia, V., Nabozny, G.H., et al. (1997). Experimental autoimmune myasthenia gravis in B10.BV8S2 transgenic mice: preferential usage of TCRAV1 gene by lymphocytes responding to acetylcholine receptor. *J Immunol* **158**: 6006–6012.

Kay, N.E. (1986). Natural killer cells. *Crit Rev Clin Lab Sci* **22**: 343–359.

Kent, S.J., Karlik, S.J., Cannon, C., Hines, D.K., Yednock, T.A., Fritz, L.C., et al. (1995). A monoclonal antibody to alpha 4 integrin suppresses and reverses active experimental allergic encephalomyelitis. *J Neuroimmunol* **58**: 1–10.

Keren, D.F. (1992). Antigen processing in the mucosal immune system. *Semin Immunol* **4**: 217–226.

Khoury, S.J. and Sayegh, M.H. (2004). The roles of the new negative T cell costimulatory pathways in regulating autoimmunity. *Immunity* **20**: 529–538.

Knight, S.C., Stagg, A., Hill, S., Fryer, P., and Griffiths, S. (1992). Development and function of dendritic cells in health and disease. *J Invest Dermatol* **99**:33S–38S.

Komori, S., Siegel, R.M., Yui, K., Katsumata, M., and Greene, M.I. (1990). T-cell receptor and autoimmune disease. *Immunol Res* **9**: 245–264.

Kraig, E., Pierce, J.L., Clarkin, K.Z., Standifer, N.E., Currier, P., Wall, K.A., et al. (1996). Restricted T cell receptor repertoire for acetylcholine receptor in murine myasthenia gravis. *J Neuroimmunol* **71**: 87–95.

Kuchroo, V.K., Collins, M., al Sabbagh, A., Sobel, R.A., Whitters, M.J., Zamvil, S.S., et al. (1994).T cell receptor (TCR) usage determines disease susceptibility in experimental autoimmune encephalomyelitis: studies with TCR V beta 8.2 transgenic mice. *J Exp Med* **179**: 1659–1664.

Kupfer, A. and Kupfer, H. (2003). Imaging immune cell interactions and functions: SMACs and the immunological synapse. *Semin Immunol* **15**: 295–300.

Lafaille, J.J., Nagashima, K., Katsuki, M., and Tonegawa, S. (1994). High incidence of spontaneous autoimmune encephalomyelitis in immunodeficient anti-myelin basic protein T cell receptor transgenic mice. *Cell* **78**: 399–408.

Lanier, L.L., Spits, H., and Phillips, J.H. (1992). The developmental relationship between NK cells and T cells. *Immunol Today* **13**: 392–395.

Leiden, J.M. (1993). Transcriptional regulation of T cell receptor genes. *Annu Rev Immunol* **11**: 539–570.

Liblau, R., van Endert, R.M., Sandberg-Wollheim, M., Patel, S.D., Lopez, M.T., Land, S., *et al.* (1993). Antigen processing gene polymorphisms in HLA-DR2 multiple sclerosis. *Neurology* **43**: 1192–1197.

Liblau, R.S., Singer, S.M., and McDevitt, H.O. (1995). Th1 and Th2 CD4+ T cells in the pathogenesis of organ-specific autoimmune diseases. *Immunol Today* **16**: 34–38.

Lider, O., Reshef, T., Beraud, E., Ben Nun, A., and Cohen, I.R. (1988). Anti-idiotypic network induced by T cell vaccination against experimental autoimmune encephalomyelitis. *Science* **239**: 181–183.

Lider, O., Beraud, E., Reshef, T., Friedman, A., and Cohen, I.R. (1989). Vaccination against experimental autoimmune encephalomyelitis using a subencephalitogenic dose of autoimmune effector T cells. (2). Induction of a protective anti-idiotypic response. *J Autoimmun* **2**: 87–99.

Lipscomb, M.F. and Masten, B.J. (2002). Dendritic cells: immune regulators in health and disease. *Physiol Rev* **82**: 97–130.

Loveridge, J.A., Rosenberg, W.M., Kirkwood, T.B., and Bell, J.I. (1991). The genetic contribution to human T-cell receptor repertoire. *Immunology* **74**: 246–250.

Madden, D.R. (1995). The three-dimensional structure of peptide–MHC complexes. *Annu Rev Immunol* **13**: 587–622.

Malhotra, U., Spielman, R., and Concannon, P. (1992). Variability in T cell receptor V beta gene usage in human peripheral blood lymphocytes. Studies of identical twins, siblings, and insulin-dependent diabetes mellitus patients. *J Immunol* **149**: 1802–1808.

Martin, R., Utz, U., Coligan, J.E., Richert, J.R., Flerlage, M., Robinson, E., *et al.* (1992). Diversity in fine specificity and T cell receptor usage of the human CD4+ cytotoxic T cell response specific for the immunodominant myelin basic protein peptide 87–106. *J Immunol* **148**: 1359–1366.

Martin, R., Gran, B., Zhao, Y., Markovic-Plese, S., Bielekova, B., Marques, A., *et al.* (2001). Molecular mimicry and antigen-specific T cell responses in multiple sclerosis and chronic CNS Lyme disease. *J Autoimmun* **16**: 187–192.

Medzhitov, R. and Janeway, C. Jr (2000). Innate immune recognition: mechanisms and pathways. *Immunol Rev* **173**: 89–97.

Miller, C., Roberts, S.J., Ramsburg, E., and Hayday, A.C. (2000). Gamma delta cells in gut infection, immunopathology, and organogenesis. *Springer Semin Immunopathol* **22**: 297–310.

Mitchison, A. and Sieper, J. (1995). Immunological basis of oral tolerance. *Z Rheumatol* **54**: 141–144.

Moretta, L., Ciccone, E., Poggi, A., Mingari, M.C., and Moretta, A. (1994). Ontogeny, specific functions and receptors of human natural killer cells. *Immunol Lett* **40**: 83–88.

Morgan, E.E., Nardo, C.J., Diveley, J.P., Kunin, J., Bartholomew, R.M., Moss, R.B., *et al.* (2001). Vaccination with a CDR2 BV6S2/6S5 peptide in adjuvant induces peptide-specific T-cell responses in patients with multiple sclerosis. *J Neurosci Res* **64**: 298–301.

Moser, B., Wolf, M., Walz, A., and Loetscher, P. (2004). Chemokines: multiple levels of leukocyte migration control. *Trends Immunol* **25**: 75–84.

Moskophidis, D., Laine, E., and Zinkernagel, R.M. (1993a). Peripheral clonal deletion of antiviral memory CD8+ T cells. *Eur J Immunol* **23**: 3306–3311

Moskophidis, D., Lechner, F., Pircher, H., and Zinkernagel, R.M. (1993b). Virus persistence in acutely infected immunocompetent mice by exhaustion of antiviral cytotoxic effector T cells. *Nature* **362**: 758–761.

Mustafa, M., Vingsbo, C., Olsson, T., Ljungdahl, A., Hojeberg, B., and Holmdahl, R. (1993). The major histocompatibility complex influences myelin basic protein 63–88-induced T cell cytokine profile and experimental autoimmune encephalomyelitis. *Eur J Immunol* **23**: 3089–3095.

Nathenson, S.G., Kesari, K., Sheil, J.M., and Ajitkumar, P. (1989). Use of mutants to analyze regions on the H-2Kb molecule for interaction with immune receptors. *Cold Spring Harbor Symp Quant Biol* **54**:521–528.

Neuberger, M.S., Ehrenstein, M.R., Rada, C., Sale, J., Batista, F.D., Williams, G., *et al.* (2000). Memory in the B-cell compartment: antibody affinity maturation. *Phil Trans R Soc Lond B Biol Sci* **355**: 357–360.

Nikolic-Zugic, J. and Carbone, F.R. (1991). Peptide presentation by class-I major histocompatibility complex molecules. *Immunol Res* **10**: 54–65.

Nossal, G.J. (1992). The molecular and cellular basis of affinity maturation in the antibody response. *Cell* **68**: 1–2.

Offner, H., Vainiene, M., Gold, D.P., Morrison, W.J., Wang, R.Y., Hashim, G.A., *et al.* (1991). Protection against experimental encephalomyelitis. Idiotypic autoregulation induced by a nonencephalitogenic T cell clone expressing a cross-reactive T cell receptor V gene. *J Immunol* **146**: 4165–4172.

Ohashi, P.S., Oehen, S., Buerki, K., Pircher, H., Ohashi, C.T., Odermatt, B., *et al.* (1991). Ablation of "tolerance" and induction of diabetes by virus infection in viral antigen transgenic mice. *Cell* **65**: 305–317.

Oksenberg, J.R., Barcellos, L.F., and Hauser, S.L. (1999). Genetic aspects of multiple sclerosis. *Semin Neurol* **19**: 281–288.

Olsson, T. (1995a). Critical influences of the cytokine orchestration on the outcome of myelin antigen-specific T-cell autoimmunity in experimental autoimmune encephalomyelitis and multiple sclerosis. *Immunol Rev* **144**: 245–268.

Olsson, T. (1995b). Cytokine-producing cells in experimental autoimmune encephalomyelitis and multiple sclerosis. *Neurology* **45**: S11–S15.

Palmer, E. (2003). Negative selection—clearing out the bad apples from the T-cell repertoire. *Nat Rev Immunol* **3**: 383–391.

Parker, K.C., Shields, M., DiBrino, M., Brooks, A., and Coligan, J.E. (1995). Peptide binding to MHC class I molecules: implications for antigenic peptide prediction. *Immunol Res* **14**: 34–57.

Petrie, H.T. (2002). Role of thymic organ structure and stromal composition in steady-state postnatal T-cell production. *Immunol Rev* **189**: 8–19.

Ploski, R., Undlien, D.E., Vinje, O., Forre, O., Thorsby, E., and Ronningen, K.S. (1994). Polymorphism of human major histocompatibility complex-encoded transporter associated with antigen processing (TAP) genes and susceptibility to juvenile rheumatoid arthritis. *Hum Immunol* **39**: 54–60.

Qin, Y., Duquette, P., Zhang, Y., Talbot, P., Poole, R., and Antel, J. (1998). Clonal expansion and somatic hypermutation of V(H) genes of B cells from cerebrospinal fluid in multiple sclerosis. *J Clin Invest* **102**: 1045–1050.

Racke, M.K., Dhib-Jalbut, S., Cannella, B., Albert, P.S., Raine, C.S., and McFarlin, D.E. (1991). Prevention and treatment of chronic relapsing experimental allergic encephalomyelitis by transforming growth factor-beta 1. *J Immunol* **146**: 3012–3017.

Racke, M.K., Sriram, S., Carlino, J., Cannella, B., Raine, C.S., and McFarlin, D.E. (1993). Long-term treatment of chronic relapsing experimental allergic encephalomyelitis by transforming growth factor-beta 2. *J Neuroimmunol* **46**: 175–183.

Revillard, J.P. and Cozon, G. (1990). Experimental models and mechanisms of immune deficiencies of nutritional origin. *Food Addit Contam* **7**(Suppl. 1): S82–S86.

Ridge, J.P., Di Rosa, F., and Matzinger, P. (1998). A conditioned dendritic cell can be a temporal bridge between a CD4+ T-helper and a T-killer cell. *Nature* **393**: 474–478.

Rocha, B., Guy-Grand, D., and Vassalli, P. (1995). Extrathymic T cell differentiation. *Curr Opin Immunol* **7**: 235–242.

Romagnani, S. (1992a). Human TH1 and TH2 subsets: regulation of differentiation and role in protection and immunopathology. *Int Arch Allergy Immunol* **98**: 279–285.

Romagnani, S. (1992b). Induction of TH1 and TH2 responses: a key role for the 'natural' immune response? *Immunol Today* **13**: 379–381.

Romagnani, S. (1995). Biology of human TH1 and TH2 cells. *J Clin Immunol* **15**: 121–129.

Royer, H.D. and Reinherz, E.L. (1987). The human T cell receptor for antigen: structure, ontogeny and gene expression. *Behring Inst Mitt* 1–14.

Sakaguchi, N. and Sakaguchi, S. (1992). Causes and mechanism of autoimmune disease: cyclosporin A as a probe for the investigation. *J Invest Dermatol* **98**: 70S–76S.

Sakai, K., Sinha, A.A., Mitchell, D.J., Zamvil, S.S., Rothbard, J.B., McDevitt, H.O., *et al.* (1988). Involvement of distinct murine T-cell receptors in the autoimmune encephalitogenic response to nested epitopes of myelin basic protein. *Proc Natl Acad Sci USA* **85**: 8608–8612.

Sale, J.E., Bemark, M., Williams, G.T., Jolly, C.J., Ehrenstein, M.R., Rada, C., *et al.* (2001). *In vivo* and *in vitro* studies of immunoglobulin gene somatic hypermutation. *Phil Trans R Soc Lond B Biol Sci* **356**: 21–28.

Schuurman, H.J., Van Loveren, H., Rozing, J., and Vos, J.G. (1992). Chemicals trophic for the thymus: risk for immunodeficiency and autoimmunity. *Int J Immunopharmacol* **14**: 369–375.

Scott, B., Liblau, R., Degermann, S., Marconi, L.A., Ogata, L., Caton, A.J., et al. (1994) A role for non-MHC genetic polymorphism in susceptibility to spontaneous autoimmunity. Immunity 1: 73–83.

Shevach, E.M. (2002). CD4+ CD25+ suppressor T cells: more questions than answers. Nat Rev Immunol 2: 389–400.

Shimonkevitz, R., Colburn, C., Burnham, J.A., Murray, R.S., and Kotzin, B.L. (1993). Clonal expansions of activated gamma/delta T cells in recent-onset multiple sclerosis. Proc Natl Acad Sci USA 90: 923–927.

Shoenfeld, Y., Amital, H., Ferrone, S., and Kennedy, R.C. (1994). Anti-idiotypes and their application under autoimmune, neoplastic, and infectious conditions. Int Arch Allergy Immunol 105: 211–223.

Singal, D.P., Ye, M., Qiu, X., and D'Souza, M. (1994). Polymorphisms in the TAP2 gene and their association with rheumatoid arthritis. Clin Exp Rheumatol 12: 29–33.

Sivakumar, P.V., Puzanov, I., Williams, N.S., Bennett, M., and Kumar, V. (1998). Ontogeny and differentiation of murine natural killer cells and their receptors. Curr Top Microbiol Immunol 230: 161–190.

Sloan-Lancaster, J. and Allen, P.M. (1996). Altered peptide ligand-induced partial T cell activation: molecular mechanisms and role in T cell biology. Annu Rev Immunol 14: 1–27.

Staines, N.A. and Harper, N. (1995). Oral tolerance in the control of experimental models of autoimmune disease. Z Rheumatol 54: 145–154.

Standifer, N.E., Kraig, E., and Infante, A.J. (2003). A hierarchy of T cell receptor motifs determines responsiveness to the immunodominant epitope in experimental autoimmune myasthenia gravis. J Neuroimmunol 145: 68–76.

Takacs, K., Douek, D.C., and Altmann, D.M. (1995). Exacerbated autoimmunity associated with a T helper-1 cytokine profile shift in H-2E-transgenic mice. Eur J Immunol 25: 3134–3141.

Valiante, N.M., Lienert, K., Shilling, H.G., Smits, B.J., and Parham, P. (1997). Killer cell receptors: keeping pace with MHC class I evolution. Immunol Rev 155: 155–164.

Vandenbark, A.A., Hashim, G., and Offner, H. (1989). Immunization with a synthetic T-cell receptor V-region peptide protects against experimental autoimmune encephalomyelitis. Nature 341: 541–544.

Vandenbark, A.A., Morgan, E., Bartholomew, R., Bourdette, D., Whitham, R., Carlo, D., et al. (2001). TCR peptide therapy in human autoimmune diseases. Neurochem Res 26: 713–730.

van der Aa, A., Hellings, N., Medaer, R., Gelin, G., Palmers, Y., Raus, J., et al. (2003). T cell vaccination in multiple sclerosis patients with autologous CSF-derived activated T cells: results from a pilot study. Clin Exp Immunol 131: 155–168.

Vandevyver, C., Mertens, N., van den Elsen, P., Medaer, R., Raus, J., and Zhang, J. (1995). Clonal expansion of myelin basic protein-reactive T cells in patients with multiple sclerosis: restricted T cell receptor V gene rearrangements and CDR3 sequence. Eur J Immunol 25: 958–968.

Vercelli, D. (2002). Novel insights into class switch recombination. Curr Opin Allergy Clin Immunol 2: 147–151.

Wabl, M., Cascalho, M., and Steinberg, C. (1999). Hypermutation in antibody affinity maturation. Curr Opin Immunol 11: 186–189.

Wagner, S.D. and Neuberger, M.S. (1996). Somatic hypermutation of immunoglobulin genes. Annu Rev Immunol 14: 441–457.

Weiner, H.L., Friedman, A., Miller, A., Khoury, S.J., al Sabbagh, A., Santos, L., et al. (1994). Oral tolerance: immunologic mechanisms and treatment of animal and human organ-specific autoimmune diseases by oral administration of autoantigens. Annu Rev Immunol 12: 809–837.

Wilson, D.B., Golding, A.B., Smith, R.A., Dafashy, T., Nelson, J., Smith, L., et al. (1997). Results of a phase I clinical trial of a T-cell receptor peptide vaccine in patients with multiple sclerosis. I. Analysis of T-cell receptor utilization in CSF cell populations. J Neuroimmunol 76: 15–28.

Wilson, P., Liu, Y.J., Banchereau, J., Capra, J.D., and Pascual, V. (1998). Amino acid insertions and deletions contribute to diversify the human Ig repertoire. Immunol Rev 162: 143–151.

Yednock, T.A., Cannon, C., Fritz, L.C., Sanchez-Madrid, F., Steinman, L., and Karin, N. (1992). Prevention of experimental autoimmune encephalomyelitis by antibodies against alpha 4 beta 1 integrin. Nature 356: 63–66.

Zaghouani, H., Fidanza, V., and Bona, C.A. (1989). The significance of idiotype-anti-idiotype interactions in the activation of self-reactive clones. Clin Exp Rheumatol 7(Suppl. 3): S19–S25.

Zamvil, S.S., Mitchell, D.J., Lee, N.E., Moore, A.C., Waldor, M.K., Sakai, K., et al. (1988). Predominant expression of a T cell receptor V beta gene subfamily in autoimmune encephalomyelitis. J Exp Med 167: 1586–1596.

Zhang, K. (2003). Accessibility control and machinery of immunoglobulin class switch recombination. J Leukocyte Biol 73: 323–332.

Zipp, F., Kerschensteiner, M., Dornmair, K., Malotka, J., Schmidt, S., Bender, A., et al. (1998). Diversity of the anti-T-cell receptor immune response and its implications for T-cell vaccination therapy of multiple sclerosis. Brain 121: 1395–1407.

2 Principles of autoimmunity

Kevin C. O'Connor, Vissia Viglietta, and David A. Hafler

Introduction

Evading the devastation of the many potential microbial infections is a major role of the immune system. While the immune system evolved in mammals in the presence of existing microbes, the genetic diversity of the immune system, as evidenced by the extreme polymorphism of the major histocompatibility complex (MHC), allows for a multitude of immune responses, both qualitatively and quantitatively. Thus autoimmune diseases, with an 'overactive' immune system, may be regarded as the price we pay as a species to fight off viral infections (alternatively, allergy and asthma may be regarded as the price we pay to fight off parasitic infections). Perhaps multiple sclerosis (MS) should be considered a complex genetic disorder where there is a dissociation between the microbial environment and genetic background of the patient. In this situation, autoreactive T cells become activated by microbial antigens in a genetically susceptible host allowing autoreactive T cells to become pathogenic.

For many years, it was believed that the immune system did not permit the development of autoreactivity, and in fact such an abnormal occurrence was termed *horror autotoxicus*. In the 1950s, several groups conducted convincing experiments revealing for the first time the presence of self-reactive antibodies in autoimmune states (Harrington *et al.*, 1951; Rose and Witebsky, 1956). These findings led to an important tenet of immunology that regarded the elimination or inactivation of self-reactive cells as an essential function of a normal immune system. Since then, a great deal of research has demonstrated that not all self-reactive cells are eliminated or inactivated. We now know that a low level of autoreactivity is physiologic and required for normal immune function in healthy individuals and that it results in no harm to the host. Moreover, T-cell receptor cross-reactivity between microbial antigens and self-antigens appears to be fundamental in the activation of autoreactive T cells. When the systems required to keep this autoreactivity in check fail, presumably in a genetically susceptible host, severe consequences to the host can occur in the form of autoimmune disease.

Autoimmune diseases affect millions of individuals worldwide. In the United States alone, approximately 10 million people are affected (Jacobson *et al.*, 1997). For many of the major autoimmune diseases the incidence is generally higher in females than in males (Whitacre, 2001). Autoimmunity occurs when the adaptive immune system turns on itself and targets self-antigens. In general terms, this is due to the failure of self-tolerance mechanisms. The disease state arises when autoimmunity mediates cell and tissue damage in the absence of any infection or other cause (Davidson and Diamond, 2001; Marrack *et al.*, 2001).

Autoimmune diseases have been divided into two clinical classes: those that are systemic, such as rheumatoid arthritis and systemic lupus erythematosus, in which the targets are primarily synovial components and nuclear antigens, respectively; and those that are considered organ specific, such as, for example, myasthenia gravis, MS and type 1 diabetes, in which the primary targets are the acetylcholine receptor isoforms, myelin proteins, and pancreatic islet cell components, respectively. As the nomenclatures implies, the systemic diseases can affect many organs despite the rather specific targets of the immune response. Organ-specific auto-immune diseases usually present with an effect isolated to one organ. A more recently proposed classification provides more information on the causation of autoimmunity, dividing diseases into those with general dysfunction in the cellular components of the immune system such as B cells and T cells and those with an abnormal response to a self- or foreign antigen (Davidson and Diamond, 2001). Examples of general cellular dysfunction that can manifest in many forms of autoimmune disease include the functional deletion of the Fas protein or its ligand, which are major players in apoptotic mechanisms, resulting in the accumulation of various autoreactive cells (Hildeman *et al.*, 2002). Also, recent data indicate that presentation of self-proteins in the thymus, regulated by the *AIRE* gene, is critical for the deletion of autoreactive T cells. Deletion of this *AIRE* gene results in severe autoimmune diseases in humans and in mouse models (Liston *et al.*, 2003). An example of an antigen-specific disorder is the immune-mediated encephalomyelitis and demyelination that can occur following immunization with the Semple rabies vaccine (Piyasirisilp *et al.*, 1999).

The basic tenets of the adaptive immune response are described elsewhere in this textbook. This chapter will review the determinants that affect the breakdown of tolerance mechanisms leading to autoimmune disease. Where germane, recent findings will be highlighted for illustrative purposes.

Development of the immune system and tolerance

Self-tolerance refers to lack of responsiveness of an individual to its own antigens. Several mechanisms, albeit not entirely understood, have been postulated to explain the tolerant state, they can be broadly classified into two groups: central tolerance and peripheral tolerance. Central tolerance refers to the clonal deletion of self-reactive T and B lymphocytes during their maturation in the central lymphoid organs (thymus for T cells and bone marrow for B cells). Peripheral tolerance concerns those self-reactive cells that escape central tolerance negative selection and can inflict tissue injury unless they are controlled in the peripheral tissues.

T-cell central tolerance

Clonal deletion of developing intrathymic T cells has been investigated extensively. Experiments with transgenic mice provide abundant evidence that T lymphocytes that bear receptors for self-antigens undergo apoptosis within the thymus during the process of T-cell maturation. It has been proposed that many autologous protein antigens are processed and presented by thymic antigen-presenting cells (APC) in association with self-MHC molecules. The developing T cells that express high-affinity receptors for such self-antigens are negatively selected, or deleted, and the peripheral T-cell pool therefore lacks, or is deficient in, self-antigen-reactive cells.

Clonal deletion appears to eliminate only some self-reactive lymphocytes, probably representing the autoreactive lymphocytes with high affinity to self-antigen. Many self-antigens are not present in the thymus or the bone marrow, and hence T or B cells that bear receptors for such autoantigens escape into the periphery. Indeed, B cells that bear receptors for a variety of self-antigens, including thyroglobulin, collagen, and DNA, can be found in the peripheral blood of healthy individuals.

T-cell peripheral tolerance

Several putative mechanisms that deal with these potentially autoreactive T cells are known. They include the following:

1. Clonal deletion. This is a mechanism to prevent uncontrolled T-cell activation during a normal immune response that involves apoptotic death of activated T cells by the Fas–Fas ligand interaction. Lymphocytes and many other cells express Fas (CD95), a member of the tumor necrosis factor (TNF) receptor family. Its expression is up-regulated in antigen-activated T cells. The ligand for Fas (FasL) is expressed chiefly on activated T lymphocytes. The engagement of Fas by FasL, co-expressed on activated T cells, dampens the immune response by inducing apoptosis of activated T cells. In all likelihood, such activation-induced cell death also underlies the peripheral dele-tion of autoreactive T cells. It is believed that those self-antigens that are abundant in peripheral tissues cause repeated and persistent stimula-tion of self-antigen-specific T cells, leading eventually to their elimina-tion via Fas-mediated apoptosis.

2. Clonal anergy. This is a state of unresponsiveness to antigens that is induced by the encounter of T cells with antigens under certain condi-tions. Optimal activation of T cells requires not only antigen recogni-tion (signal 1) but also an additional co-stimulatory signal (signal 2). Co-stimulators such as CD28, present on the T-cell surface, must bind to their ligands CD80 and CD86 (B7-1 and B7-2) on the APC. Presentation of antigen in the absence of this second signal results in a state of functional unresponsiveness. Anergy can be induced not only by the antigen recognition without co-stimulation but also by the inter-action of the ligands B7-1 and B7-2 with inhibitory receptors such as CTLA-4, which results in the delivery of a negative signal. Because co-stimulatory molecules are not expressed or are weakly expressed on most normal tissues, the encounter between autoreactive T cells and their specific self-antigens leads to clonal anergy.

3. Peripheral suppression by T cells. Much interest has recently focused on suppressor T cells that have the ability to inhibit activation and func-tion of other autoreactive T lymphocytes. There is some evidence that the suppression of effector cells in the periphery may be mediated in part by the regulated secretion of cytokines. CD4+ T cells of the Th2 type have been implicated in mediating self-tolerance by regulating the function of pathogenic Th1 type cells. Certainly, cytokines secreted by Th2 cells (e.g. interleukin 4 (IL-4), interleukin 10 (IL-10), and trans-forming growth factor beta (TGF-β)) can down-modulate the Th1 response. TGF-β is capable of suppressing T-cell and B-cell prolifera-tion therefore, T cells that can produce a large amount of this inhibito-ry cytokine are considered suppressors. IL-10 also has inhibitory properties affecting the activation of macrophages and IL-4 and IL-13 (considered Th2 cytokines) regulate the Th1 cytokine interferon-gamma (IFN-γ) preventing it from inducing macrophage activation.

B-cell tolerance

As with T cells, clonal deletion is operative in B cells. The development of transgenic mice facilitated much of the early work describing these mechanisms. Experiments with mice made transgenic for a cell-surface self-antigen indicated that developing B cells that encounter this membrane-bound antigen (multivalent, high avidity) within the bone marrow are deleted (Nemazee and Burki, 1989) or can escape deletion by rearranging and expressing a light chain different from that expressed by the other immunoglobulin allele. The pairing of a different light chain can alter the specificity of the immunoglobulin so that it is no longer autoreactive. This process is termed receptor editing (Gay et al., 1993), essentially giving the developing B cell a second chance of maturation. B cells that interact with a soluble self-antigen in the bone marrow mature and migrate to the peri-phery. However, once in the periphery, these cells are unable to respond to antigen and are termed anergic (Goodnow et al., 1988). Anergic B cells characteristically down-regulate their surface IgM, and their signaling by surface immunoglobulin is greatly diminished (Goodnow, 1996).

Some self-antigens, such as intracellular tissue components, are not pre-sented to developing B cells in the bone marrow. In this case, autoreactive B cells specific for these antigens migrate from the bone marrow to the periphery but are controlled by several mechanisms (Cornall et al., 1995; Goodnow, 1996). To generate a B-cell response in the periphery, activation requires co-stimulation by T cells. Thus, B cells that encounter self-antigens in the periphery but are not provided with T-cell help are eliminated through apoptosis in the lymph nodes or may become anergic. Also, with-in the periphery are subsets of self-reactive T cells that can induce Fas-mediated B-cell apoptosis when the B cell is autoreactive. Finally, autoreactive B cells that arise through somatic mutation in response to a foreign antigen undergo apoptosis when they are bound by large amounts of self-antigen.

Autoimmunity

A general presentation of the determinants of autoimmune disease can be considered interms of three major factors (Fig. 2.1): inheritance, initiation, and dysregulation. The development of autoimmune disease is likely to be due to a variable combination of all factors. *Inheritance* comprises the risk of disease associated with genes that confer susceptibility, including those of the MHC and non-MHC genes. This heading also includes gender, since females have a greater susceptibility than males to most autoimmune diseases. *Initiation* comprises primarily environmental factors. The effects of micro-organisms such as viruses and bacteria have been implicated in molecular mimicry, in which B cells or T cells responding to an infectious agent cross-react with self-antigens or are altered in a manner that helps to break down tolerance. Additional mechanisms initiated by infections include bystander damage, unveiling of hidden self-antigen, and deter-minant spreading. Other initiation factors include agents such as drugs, chemicals, and solar exposure and random events such as genetic errors. *Dysregulation* comprises the malfunction of regulatory mechanisms that influence the immune response. This includes regulatory T cells, the effect of cytokines and chemokines, natural autoantibodies, intracellular signal-ing, and the innate immune system.

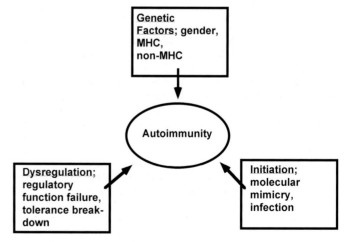

Fig. 2.1 Major factors influencing the development of autoimmunity. It is believed that the development of autoimmunity requires a variable combination of the following factors: genetics, environmental influence, and dysregulation. Different diseases and individuals are expected to have varying contributions from each of the three factors.

Major determinants of autoimmunity

Genetic factors

Genetic predisposition is a major factor in autoimmunity. The concordance rates among monozygotic and dizygotic twins provide clear evidence of the importance of genetics in many autoimmune diseases. For example in multiple sclerosis the concordance rate is 25–40% among monozygotic twins, 1–13% for dizygotic twins, and 6% for non-twin siblings (Kalman and Lublin, 1999). The genes of the MHC play a role in the susceptibility and resistance to autoimmunity. The first evidence for an association between MHC and an autoimmune disease was reported in 1971 (Grumet et al., 1971). Currently, nearly all the major autoimmune diseases have been found to have at least some association with MHC. The association between type 1 diabetes and the MHC class II HLA-DQ beta chain is among the most widely studied. DNA sequencing has revealed that a replacement mutation of the asparagine at position 57 encodes a susceptibility allele (Todd et al., 1987). Several DQB alleles lack the asparagine at this position. Strikingly, approximately 90% of individuals with type 1 diabetes are homozygous for these alleles, whereas the presence of these alleles within the general population approaches 20% (Morel et al., 1988). The inference that the presence of asparagine at position 57 in the DQB allele is protective holds true. A similar pattern is observed in progressive rheumatoid arthritis, with 90% of these patients expressing HLA-DR4 and/or HLA-DR1 (Winchester, 1994). The details regarding the mechanisms by which these HLA genes mediate susceptibility or protection remain to be fully elucidated. The leading concepts addressing protection mechanisms hold that protective alleles play a role in thymic negative selection of potentially autoreactive T cells (Schmidt et al., 1997) and positive selection of other T cells that have suppressive effects (Luhder et al., 1998). Other mechanisms, however, should not be excluded. Susceptibility alleles generally are believed to support the development of pro-inflammatory Th1-type responses, but few additional details are currently considered (McDevitt, 1998).

The strongest genetic association with autoimmunity is related to the MHC genes. MHC genes have the most potent genetic influence on autoimmunity; however, they are not the only genes that affect susceptibility, although the associations of these other genes are, more often than not, weaker than those of MHC (Wanstrat and Wakeland, 2001). Most autoimmune diseases show only a modest association with any single non-MHC locus. However, it is understood that autoimmune susceptibility arises from the combined impact of many common contributing susceptibility genes. Moreover, different combinations of genetic abnormalities (genetic heterogeneity) and the effect of the genetic interaction of one locus on the phenotype of another locus (epsitasis) contribute to the complexity of the inheritance of disease susceptibility.

Isolated human subpopulations limit ethnic heterogeneity, thereby reducing this complexity. Linkage analysis of Scandinavian populations with autoimmune polyglandular syndrome revealed that a mutation in the AIRE gene is responsible for this disease (The Finnish–German APECED Consortium, 1997; Nagamine et al., 1997). The gene, which encodes a putative nuclear protein, is thought to play a role in transcriptional regulation. This is the first report of a single-gene defect that by itself causes a systemic human autoimmune disease and puts it among the few that are localized outside the MHC region. Examples of other non-MHC disease genes reported to be associated with autoimmunity include: microsatellite markers flanking glucokinase that affect susceptibility to diabetes (Rowe et al., 1995); deficiency in the C1q complement component associated with systemic lupus erythematosus (SLE) (Botto et al., 1998; Walport et al., 1998), and several mutations in the CARD15 (NOD2) gene have been associated with Crohn's disease (Hugot et al., 2001; Ogura et al., 2001).

Various autoimmune diseases share common features of immune dysregulation, and whether these genes have anything in common is thus a frequently asked question. The hypothesis has been suggested that susceptibility genes for autoimmunity are shared among various autoimmune diseases. It is too early to conclude that this is the case, there is some evidence to support such a hypothesis. The basic data indicate that susceptibility genes are co-localized in the genome. Furthermore, there is evidence of a higher incidence of autoimmunity within first-degree relatives of probands with multiple sclerosis (Broadley et al., 2000). Also, many autoimmune diseases share pathological and clinical characteristics with other autoimmune diseases (Hafler and Weiner, 1989; Hafler, 2004). Recently, polymorphisms of the cytotoxic T lymphocyte antigen 4 gene (CTLA4), which encodes a vital negative regulatory molecule of the immune system, was shown to be a candidate gene for primary determinants of risk of the common autoimmune disorders (Ueda et al., 2003)

Environmental initiation

In the absence of complete penetrance of spontaneous disease in genetically predisposed individuals, major roles for environmental factors in the development of autoimmune disease must be examined. At best, fewer than 50% of identical twins demonstrate concordance for any known autoimmune disease. An initiating environmental (external) event, such as an infection, may provide a required stimulus in a genetically predisposed individual.

Pathogens may alter immunoreactivity through at least several mechanisms (Marrack et al., 2001). Microbial antigens have the potential to initiate autoimmunity through molecular mimicry, polyclonal activation, or introduction of sequestered antigens. Potentially autoreactive lymphocytes may become activated either by infectious agents or through antigen-non-specific mechanisms. Many products from bacteria and viruses can act as adjuvants, thereby enhancing immune responses to antigens in a non-specific manner. The induction of experimental autoimmune encephalomyelitis (EAE), a model for human multiple sclerosis, requires the use of adjuvant. Furthermore, microbial products such as lipopolysaccharide or bacterial DNA have been shown to hold cytokine-modulating properties that can support, in part, the development of autoimmunity (Segal et al., 1997). Much attention regarding the potential of microbial induction of autoimmunity has been centered on antigen-specific mechanisms, namely molecular mimicry.

Molecular mimicry (Benoist and Mathis, 2001) can occur when an infectious agent and a self-antigen share a structurally similar antigenic determinant. An immune response to such agents may produce tissue-damaging reactions to the cross-reacting self-antigen. For T cells the determinant would be a linear peptide and for B cells the determinant could be linear or conformational. The molecular mimicry theory has gained support, particularly with the acknowledgement that the recognition by the T-cell receptor of the MHC–peptide complex is very degenerate (Wucherpfennig, 2001). Several often-cited examples of molecular mimicry are outlined below, but it is important to point out that it has not yet been accepted as a definitive model for autoimmunity. However, several recently reported experimental lines of evidence lend strong support to the hypothesis that molecular mimicry couples infection with autoimmunity.

1. Lyme arthritis. Lyme arthritis resistant to antibiotic treatment is a chronic inflammatory joint disease that follows infection through the tick-borne spirochete Borrelia burgdorferi. In about 10% of patients with Lyme arthritis, joint inflammation persists after the elimination of the spirochete with antibiotic treatment (Steere et al., 2001). A marked T-cell response to B. burgdorferi outer surface protein A (OspA) often develops during prolonged episodes of arthritis (Trollmo et al., 2001). T-cell-driven molecular mimicry has been proposed as a mechanism for the chronic inflammation. Identification of the initiating bacterial antigen and a cross-reactive autoantigen were reported several years ago (Gross et al., 1998). It was demonstrated that T cells reactive to the B. burgdorferi OspA cross-react with human leukocyte function-associated antigen α1 (hLFA-α1), a self-antigen that is overexpressed in the infected joints.

2. Herpetic stromal keratitis (HSK). HSK can follow ocular infection with herpes simplex virus 1 (HSV-1). There is experimental evidence indicating that the disease may result from a CD4+ T-cell response to a UL6

peptide of HSV-1 that cross-reacts with an unidentified corneal auto-peptide shared with an immunoglobulin isotype (Zhao *et al.*, 1998). As previously mentioned, the molecular mimicry hypothesis is not universally accepted. An additional study of HSK supports the view that autoimmunity, if it is involved, occurs via a bystander activation mechanism rather than via molecular mimicry (Deshpande *et al.*, 2001).

The view that B-cells may be induced to participate in autoimmunity through molecular mimicry mechanisms, although suspected for sometime, has just recently received experimental support.

3. Tropical spastic paraparesis/HTLV-1 associated myelopathy (TSP/HAM). The HTLV-1 virus has been closely associated with multiple sclerosis, and individuals infected by the virus may develop TSP/HAM, a demyelinating disease that imitates multiple sclerosis in many respects, even to the point of the two being indistinguishable. Levin and colleagues established a clear link between viral infection and autoimmunity by demonstrating that immunoglobulin G isolated from patients with HAM/TSP recognize heterogeneous nuclear ribonuclear protein-A1 (hrRNP-A1) (Levin *et al.*, 2002). These antibodies cross-react with the HTLV-1 tax protein, which is an immunodominant antigen associated with neurological disease (Hollsberg *et al.*, 1995). Moreover, these autoantibodies were shown to play a direct role in the inhibition of neuronal firing, indicating their pathogenic potential.

4. Systemic lupus erythematosus (SLE). Demonstrating a link between autoimmune disease pathology and cross-reactivity, Diamond and colleagues identified molecular mimicry between a pentapeptide and double-stranded DNA and the neuronal NR2 glutamate receptor (DeGiorgio *et al.*, 2001). These antibodies are present in some patients with SLE and are positioned as strong contenders for the mediation of some of the central nervous system disturbances in SLE.

Dysregulation

Regulation of the immune response and of tolerance is clearly paramount in keeping autoimmunity in check, and thus disruption of these pathways can lead to autoimmunity. The Fas protein and its ligand FasL are intimately involved in deletion of potentially autoreactive cells through induction of apoptosis. MRL *lpr/lpr* and *gld/gld* mice have disruptions of the Fas protein and its ligand, respectively. These mice spontaneously develop severe systemic autoimmune disease and are commonly used as models for SLE. Mutations associated with Fas have also been described in humans who suffer from autoimmune lymphoproliferative syndrome (ALPS) (Straus *et al.*, 1999).

CD4+CD25+ T cells

Although clonal deletion (negative selection) of self-reactive T cells in the thymus is a major and effective mechanism of immunologic self-tolerance, there is evidence that self-reactive T cells that have escaped thymic selection are present in the peripheral circulation of normal healthy individuals. Those reactive T cells are potentially harmful, but they fail to be activated in the periphery thanks not only to several passive mechanisms of self-tolerance (e.g. ignorance of self-antigen, low avidity of their T-cell receptors, lack of co-stimulation) but also to active suppression mediated by regulatory T cells (Fowell *et al.*, 1991; Sakaguchi *et al.*, 1995; Modigliani *et al.*, 1996; Sakaguchi, 2000; Shevach, 2000). Different types of suppressor cells have been described. One of the most extensively studied is a sub-population of CD4+ T cells that co-express CD25 (interleukin-2 receptor α-chain). In mice, depletion of the CD4+CD25+ population by thymectomy on the third day of life causes organ-specific autoimmune diseases and reconstitution of this population can prevent the development of auto-immunity (Sakaguchi *et al.*, 1985; Sakaguchi, 2000). CD4+CD25+ suppressor cells have also been found in humans (Baecher-Allan *et al.*, 2001) and have the same functional characteristic as those in mice. They are naturally anergic cells capable, upon T-cell receptor stimulation, to suppress proliferation of, and production of IL-2 by, other activated T cells when the two populations are co-cultured (Takahashi *et al.*, 1998; Thornton and Shevach, 1998). The suppression activity is antigen-non-specific, does not require

histocompatibility between the CD4+CD25+ and the stimulated T cells, and appears to be independent of any humoral factors such as cytokines but dependent on cell–cell contact. While further characterization of the CD4+CD25+ T cells is necessary, it is clear that these cells play a key role in maintaining immunologic self-tolerance and that their dysregulation may account for the onset of autoimmune diseases. The recent discovery of methods to evaluate the *in vitro* function of CD4+CD25+ T cells in humans afforded examination of the importance of these regulatory T cells in human immune response and disease. The finding that autoreactive T cells in patients with autoimmune disease are more easily activated compared with those from normal subjects, leads to the hypothesis that either deficient generation or reduced effector function of CD4+CD25+ regulatory T cells play a role in modulating self- and non-self-reactive T cells during normal immune responses. Indeed, recent work by Viglietta *et. al.* (2004) demonstrated a significant decrease in the effector function of CD4+CD25+ regulatory T cells from peripheral blood of patients with MS as compared with healthy donors.

Disruption of other immunoregulatory pathways also can lead to autoimmune disorders. A clear example of this is the defect of the gene encoding for Fas that induces the spontaneous development of a multi-organ autoimmune disorder in MRL *lpr/lpr* mice that is similar in its clinical manifestation to SLE. The same clinical outcome is seen in *gld/gld* mice, in which the disruption occurs in the gene encoding for Fas ligand. It appears clear from this experimental evidence that Fas–FasL interactions are important in the regulation of the immune response through activation-induced cell death of reactive lymphocytes.

A mutation in the Fas gene in humans induces an autoimmune lymphoproliferative syndrome similar to the syndrome that affects mice. Another mechanism of regulation involves CTLA-4: mice deficient for this molecule die a few weeks after birth from a severe lymphoproliferative syndrome with organ infiltration. Remarkably, the gene for CTLA-4 is considered a susceptibility gene in autoimmune diseases such as type 1 diabetes and thyroid disease. The fact that the lack of CTLA-4, CD25, or IL-2 results in autoimmune syndromes indicates that these molecules are involved in the immune regulation by delivering negative signals in the case of the CTLA-4 or because of inadequate activation-induced cell death when IL-2 or CD25 are not present.

Cytokines

Many studies in past years have implicated the equilibrium between the 'pathogenic' and the 'protective' cytokines as a major regulatory mechanism of autoimmunity. Cytokines have long been divided into two main groups: the Th1-type cytokines (IFN-γ, TNF-α, IL-1) that favor inflammation and exacerbate autoimmune diseases and the Th2 cytokines (IL-4, IL-10, TGF-β) that suppress inflammation and promote tolerance. It has been shown that CD4+ T cells derived from non-obese diabetic mice (NOD) that spontaneously develop type 1 diabetes produce more IFN-γ than IL-4 (Rabinovitch, 1994) in response to pancreatic islet antigens. In the EAE mouse model for multiple sclerosis, the antigen response is similarly biased (Liblau *et al.*, 1995). In both models the adoptive transfer of diabetes and EAE with Th1-polarized cells causes accelerated and increased severity of the disease compared with transfer of Th2-polarized cells producing primarily IL-4. The protective function of Th2 cytokines has also been demonstrated since the overexpression of IL-4 in the islets leads to an absence of diabetes in NOD mice (Mueller *et al.*, 1997). It is well understood that the presence of IFN-γ at the site of inflammation results in the activation of macrophages that release other pro-inflammatory cytokines, such as TNF-α and IL-1. Furthermore, IFN-γ up-regulates pro-inflammatory chemokines and accelerates lymphocyte recruitment.

Th2-type cytokines have a prominent suppressive function important to reducing inflammation and inducing tolerance. IL-10 and TGF-β seem to antagonize the activation and expansion of autoreactive T cells through a variety of mechanisms. IL-10 can reduce the efficiency of antigen presentation, inhibiting the expression of IL-12, TNF-α< and co-stimulatory molecules in APC (Moore *et al.*, 2001). IL-10 also prevents the production of pro-inflammatory cytokines and the migration of dendritic cells to lymph nodes. TGF-β can also modulate autoreactive T-cell responses by stopping the maturation of APCs and preventing the differentiation of naïve T cells into effector cells (Th1 or Th2) (Gorelik et al., 2002).

More recent studies have challenged the simplicity of the well-known Th1/Th2 paradigm, proposing that Th1 cytokines, in addition to promoting inflammation and tissue destruction, can also trigger a homeostatic mechanism to suppress inflammation (Cope, 1998). Although it has been shown that the lack of IFN-γ in NOD mice delays the onset of diabetes, it can also cause the development of EAE. Treatment of mice with IFN-γ protects from EAE, probably increasing the rate of apoptosis of the autoreactive lymphocytes in the central nervous system (CNS) (Furlan et al., 2001). In the same way Th2 cytokines not only exert a protective function as subsets of Th2 cells, but also are capable of transferring disease. Myelin-specific Th2 cells generated in vitro are able to cause a non-canonical form of EAE characterized by delayed onset and high morbidity. Antigen-specific Th2 cells, as well as Th1-polarized cells, can induce colitis in immunodeficient recipients and IL-4 treatment can accelerate the disease by increasing the recruitment of inflammatory chemokines and activated T cells (Iqbal et al., 2002). TGF-β can sustain the expansion of CD4+ T cells and favor Th2 responses by inhibiting Th1 responses and may also have a pathogenic role in the development of autoimmune thyroiditis since treatment of mice with antibodies to TGF-β inhibits the disease. IL-10 is capable of promoting recruitment and proliferation of CD8 T cells and of increasing the cytotoxicity of natural killer cells (Moore et al., 2001). Although IL-10, TGF-β, and IL-4 represent valid anti-inflammatory mechanisms and promising tools for the treatment of autoimmunity, they can also have pro-inflammatory functions, depending on the conditions at the site of inflammation determined by the presence of other cytokines and their interactions.

Chemokines

Chemokines are polypeptide effector molecules that mediate the migration of leukocytes participating in an inflammatory response. Thus, they are produced in response to inflammation by activated cells and transfer their signals to specific cell types through the use of a repertoire involving many family members. Many chemokines are secreted and then interact with specific receptors on cells remote from the producing cell. Among other roles, the cytokines participate in autoimmunity and are of particular importance in establishing ectopic lymphoid structures in target organs of autoimmune responses (Godessart and Kunkel, 2001; Karpus, 2001). There are many reports indicating that levels of chemokines and their receptors are altered in the autoimmune disease state. Trafficking of leukocytes into the CNS during the evolution of multiple sclerosis is mediated, in part, by chemokines. In CNS tissue recovered from MS patients, the expression levels of various chemokines and their ligands are elevated. The synovial tissue in rheumatoid arthritis (RA) is characterized by hyperplasia and a cellular infiltrate comprising lymphoid cells. Chemokines have important roles in this process. Elevated levels of chemokines and their receptors are found in the synovial tissue of patients with RA, where they play a role not only in recruitment of the inflammatory cells but also in angiogenesis. The de novo formation of lymphoid tissue, termed lymphoid neogenesis, has been found in chronically inflamed tissue in several autoimmune diseases (Hjelmstrom, 2001). In the synovium of patients with RA, where lymphoid neogenesis is occurring, elevated levels of the chemokine CXCL13 are found only in the synovium in which lymphoid neogenesis was present, suggesting a role for chemokines in the formation of ectopic germinal centers (Shi et al., 2001b).

Natural autoantibodies

Antibodies present in the sera of healthy individuals in the absence of deliberate immunization with any antigen are referred to as natural antibodies. A great majority of natural antibodies react with one or more self-antigens and are termed natural autoantibodies. Natural autoantibodies are present in the serum of normal healthy individuals of all ages (Coutinho et al., 1995). These autoantibodies are directed at many dissimilar self-antigens, such as cytoskeletal proteins, DNA, membrane proteins, and serum pro-

teins. Natural autoantibodies are typically of the IgM isotype but can be IgG or IgA (Kaveri et al., 1998). Their variable domains have not accumulated somatic mutations or undergone affinity maturation. Thus, their V gene segments are usually germline encoded. They are characteristically poly-reactive, binding not only multiple natural antigens but also exogenous antigens. They typically have low affinity for the antigens they bind, with K_a usually less than 10^6 M^{-1} (Kaveri et al., 1998). This is believed to be a major reason why they are not harmful to the host.

The biological significance of natural autoantibodies has not been defined. However, natural autoantibodies may also share a relationship with disease-related autoantibodies, and some evidence supports this notion. Some pathogenic IgG antibodies to DNA react with DNA with high affinity yet are still cross-reactive with other autoantigens (Naparstek et al., 1986). Somatically mutated IgG antibodies to DNA can be encoded by the same variable regions as IgM polyreactive autoantibodies that are germline encoded (Baccala et al., 1989). IgG autoantibodies directed to insulin that were reverted to their germline sequences could still bind insulin, but at lower affinity (Ichiyoshi et al., 1995). Similarly, germline reversion of disease-related antibodies to DNA that react with double-stranded DNA display reactivity toward single-stranded DNA, a frequently observed natural autoantigen (Radic et al., 1993). The detection of natural polyreactive autoantibodies may underlie the contradictory findings regarding the identification of serum autoantibodies in several autoimmune diseases. For example, O'Connor et al. (2003, 2004) used a solution phase radioimmunoassay to examine antibody binding to myelin antigens reported to be present in serum and cerebrospinal fluid (CSF) of patients with MS. With this assay, which measures higher affinity binding, such antibodies were not detected.

Cell signaling

The strength of signal delivered to a T cell during development shapes the repertoire of this immune system compartment. In the thymus, self-antigens generating a strong signal lead to negative selection, whereas weaker signals result in positive selection, thus setting the threshold for peripheral activation. Once in the periphery, self-antigens supply signals to T cells to ensure survival and maintain the repertoire. In the bone marrow newly formed B cells that bear autoreactive receptors and then encounter self-antigen are eliminated, silenced, or re-form themselves through receptor editing. These forms of negative selection have been understood for some time now. What is now becoming clear is that B cells, like T cells, may also require positive selection by self-antigen for maintenance in the periphery (Pillai, 1999). Clearly, the intracellular signaling mechanisms and regulatory elements controlling these events must be precisely tuned to promote the proper result. Defects, imbalance, and abnormalities in this delicate system have the potential to initiate autoimmunity.

Many signaling molecules have been implicated in the development of autoimmunity. Among the best characterized of these is the anti-apoptotic survival protein Bcl-2. Overexpression of Bcl-2, which can result in an excess of B lymphocytes, immunoglobulin-secreting cells, and serum immunoglobulins also results in autoimmunity (Strasser et al., 1991). The B-cell activating factor (BAFF) acts much like Bcl-2, in that it enhances B-cell survival and its overexpression results in autoimmunity. BAFF is found in the literature under several names (Mackay and Browning, 2002). In addition to its demonstrated role in induction of autoimmunity in mouse models, elevated levels of the soluble form of BAFF have been reported in human autoimmune diseases (Zhang et al., 2001).

Another intriguing example includes the finding that the higher incidence of autoimmune disease among females may be related to estrogen. Estrogen may alter the signaling thresholds of apoptotic pathways within B cells (Grimaldi et al., 2002). The net effect of such an alteration is an accumulation of autoreactive B cells in the periphery that would normally be deleted during development.

CD8+ T cells

The role of the CD8+ T cell population in autoimmunity has not, until recently, been appreciated. It is now known that these cells make a significant contribution to tissue damage in autoimmune disorders (Liblau *et al.*, 2002). In the mouse models of diabetes, there is direct evidence that beta-islet cell-specific CD8+ T cells have a pathogenic effect, and in human diseases such as autoimmune diabetes indirect evidence also suggests a role for CD8+ T cells in tissue damage (Vizler *et al.*, 1999). CD8+ T cells infiltrating actively demyelinating MS lesions were examined through sequence analysis. This study revealed that, the majority of infiltrating CD8+ T cells were oligoclonal, suggesting local clonal expansion and perhaps selection by a common antigen specificity (Babbe *et al.*, 2000). In addition, neuronal death directly due to CD8+ T cells has been reported (Medana *et al.*, 2000). This action may contribute to the axonal loss observed in MS. Work by Buckle *et al.* (2003) showed that a significant increase in lymphotoxin secretion from CD8+ T cells was observed in patients with secondary progressive MS as compared with normal controls.

Innate immune system

During infection the adaptive immune system is preceded by the innate (or natural) immune system. Innate immune mechanisms provide the host with a rapid defense and are present in all individuals at all times. The innate immune system is often overlooked in considerations of autoimmunity, but this line of defense can play a role in the development of such a response (Shi *et al.*, 2001*a*). Natural killer (NK) cells are frequently found in the targeted tissue of many autoimmune diseases. However, it appears that, in most instances, they are not directly involved in tissue destruction thorough cell lysis. Several studies have suggested that the role of the NK cell in these situations is regulatory. At this time it not clear if the role of the NK cell promotes or diminishes the autoimmune response.

The γ/δ T-cell population is also found in areas of inflammation related to autoimmunity (Shi *et al.*, 2001*a*). Depletion of γ/δ T cells can lessen the severity of disease in some models of autoimmune disease, but the effect is not observed in others. Thus, the mechanisms by which these cells play a role in autoimmunity is unclear. However, it has been suggested that these cells have MHC Class I inhibitory receptors and therefore play an indirect role in autoimmune induction (Fisch *et al.*, 2000). CD8+ γ/δ T cells from insulin-treated mice suppressed the adoptive transfer of diabetes to non-diabetic mice. These findings revealed a novel mechanism for suppressing cell-mediated autoimmune disease providing further evidence that they posses a regulatory function (Harrison *et al.*, 1996).

Conclusions

Autoimmune disease is the final result of a complex multistep process. Ultimately it occurs as a consequence of breakdown of immune tolerance in genetically susceptible hosts. The major factors affecting autoimmunity include genetics, environment, and dysregulation. The disease state results from a variable combination of each factor. Each of the major autoimmune diseases manifests in variable phenotypes and the clinical and pathological aspects vary within the same disease. An intriguing aspect of this is that the molecular and cellular pathology of the different autoimmune diseases have many striking similarities. Future studies will surely lead to a better understanding of the mechanisms that control autoimmunity and perhaps reveal common mechanisms among them.

References

The Finnish–German APECED Consortium (1997). An autoimmune disease, APECED, caused by mutations in a novel gene featuring two PHD-type zinc-finger domains. *Nat Genet* 17: 399–403.

Babbe, H., Roers, A., Waisman, A., Lassmann, H., Goebels, N., Hohlfeld, R., *et al.* (2000). Clonal expansions of CD8(+) T cells dominate the T cell infiltrate in active multiple sclerosis lesions as shown by micromanipulation and single cell polymerase chain reaction. *J Exp Med* 192: 393–404.

Baccala, R., Quang, T.V., Gilbert, M., Ternynck, T., and Avrameas, S. (1989). Two murine natural polyreactive autoantibodies are encoded by nonmutated germ-line genes. *Proc Natl Acad Sci USA* 86: 4624–4628.

Baecher-Allan, C., Brown, J.A., Freeman, G.J., and Hafler, D.A. (2001). CD4+CD25high regulatory cells in human peripheral blood. *J Immunol* 167: 1245–1253.

Benoist, C. and Mathis, D. (2001) Autoimmunity provoked by infection: how good is the case for T cell epitope mimicry? *Nat Immunol* 2: 797–801.

Botto, M., Dell'Agnola, C., Bygrave, A.E., Thompson, E.M., Cook, H.T., Petry, F., *et al.* (1998). Homozygous C1q deficiency causes glomerulonephritis associated with multiple apoptotic bodies. *Nat Genet* 19: 56–59.

Broadley, S.A., Deans, J., Sawcer, S.J., Clayton, D., and Compston, D.A. (2000). Autoimmune disease in first-degree relatives of patients with multiple sclerosis. A UK survey. *Brain* 123, 1102–1111.

Buckle, G.J., Hollsberg, P., and Hafler, D.A. (2003). Activated CD8+ T cells in secondary progressive MS secrete lymphotoxin. *Neurology* 60: 702–705.

Cope, A.P. (1998). Regulation of autoimmunity by proinflammatory cytokines. *Curr Opin Immunol* 10: 669–676.

Cornall, R.J., Goodnow, C.C., and Cyster, J.G. (1995). The regulation of self-reactive B cells. *Curr Opin Immun* 7: 804–811.

Coutinho, A., Kazatchkine, M.D., and Avrameas, S. (1995). Natural auto-antibodies. *Curr Opin Immun* 7: 812–818.

Davidson, A. and Diamond, B. (2001). Autoimmune diseases. *N Engl J Med* 345: 340–350.

DeGiorgio, L.A., Konstantinov, K.N., Lee, S.C., Hardin, J.A., Volpe, B.T., and Diamond, B. (2001). A subset of lupus anti-DNA antibodies cross-reacts with the NR2 glutamate receptor in systemic lupus erythematosus. *Nat Med* 7: 1189–1193.

Deshpande, S.P., Lee, S., Zheng, M., Song, B., Knipe, D., Kapp, J.A., *et al.* (2001). Herpes simplex virus-induced keratitis: evaluation of the role of molecular mimicry in lesion pathogenesis. *J Virol* 75: 3077–3088.

Fisch, P., Moris, A., Rammensee, H.G., and Handgretinger, R. (2000). Inhibitory MHC class I receptors on gammadelta T cells in tumour immunity and autoimmunity. *Immunol Today* 21: 187–191.

Fowell, D., McKnight, A.J., Powrie, F., Dyke, R., and Mason, D. (1991). Subsets of CD4+ T cells and their roles in the induction and prevention of auto-immunity. *Immunol Rev* 123: 37–64.

Furlan, R., Brambilla, E., Ruffini, F., Poliani, P.L., Bergami, A., Marconi, P.C., *et al.* (2001). Intrathecal delivery of IFN-gamma protects C57BL/6 mice from chronic-progressive experimental autoimmune encephalomyelitis by increasing apoptosis of central nervous system-infiltrating lymphocytes. *J Immunol* 167: 1821–1829.

Gay, D., Saunders, T., Camper, S., and Weigert, M. (1993). Receptor editing: an approach by autoreactive B cells to escape tolerance. *J Exp Med* 177: 999–1008.

Godessart, N. and Kunkel, S.L. (2001). Chemokines in autoimmune disease. *Curr Opin Immunol* 13: 670–675.

Goodnow, C.C. (1996). Balancing immunity and tolerance: deleting and tuning lymphocyte repertoires. *Proc Natl Acad Sci USA* 93: 2264–2271.

Goodnow, C.C., Crosbie, J., Adelstein, S., Lavoie, T.B., Smith-Gill, S.J., Brink, R.A., *et al.* (1988). Altered immunoglobulin expression and functional silencing of self- reactive B lymphocytes in transgenic mice. *Nature* 334: 676–682.

Gorelik, L., Constant, S., and Flavell, R.A. (2002). Mechanism of transforming growth factor beta-induced inhibition of T helper type 1 differentiation. *J Exp Med* 195: 1499–1505.

Grimaldi, C.M., Cleary, J., Dagtas, A.S., Moussai, D., and Diamond, B. (2002). Estrogen alters thresholds for B cell apoptosis and activation. *J Clin Invest* 109: 1625–1633.

Gross, D.M., Forsthuber, T., Tary-Lehmann, M., Etling, C., Ito, K., Nagy, Z.A., *et al.* (1998). Identification of LFA-1 as a candidate autoantigen in treatment-resistant Lyme arthritis. *Science* 281: 703–706.

Grumet, F.C., Coukell, A., Bodmer, J.G., Bodmer, W.F., and McDevitt, H.O. (1971). Histocompatibility (HL-A) antigens associated with systemic lupus erythematosus. A possible genetic predisposition to disease. *N Engl J Med* 285: 193–196.

Hafler, D.A. (2004). Multiple sclerosis. *J Clin Invest* 113: 788–794.

Hafler, D.A. and Weiner, H.L. (1989). MS: a CNS and systemic autoimmune disease. *Immunol Today* 10: 104–107.

Harrington, W.J., Minnich, V., Hollingsworth, J.W., and Moore, C.V. (1951). Demonstration of a thrombocytopenic factor in the blood of patients with thrombocytopenic purpura. *J Lab Clin Med* 115: 636–645.

Harrison, L.C., Dempsey-Collier, M., Kramer, D.R., and Takahashi, K. (1996). Aerosol insulin induces regulatory CD8 gamma delta T cells that prevent murine insulin-dependent diabetes. *J Exp Med* 184: 2167–2174.

Hildeman, D.A., Zhu, Y., Mitchell, T.C., Kappler, J., and Marrack, P. (2002). Molecular mechanisms of activated T cell death *in vivo*. *Curr Opin Immunol* 14: 354–359.

Hjelmstrom, P. (2001). Lymphoid neogenesis: de novo formation of lymphoid tissue in chronic inflammation through expression of homing chemokines. *J Leukocyte Biol* 69: 331–339.

Hollsberg, P., Weber, W.E., Dangond, F., Batra, V., Sette, A., and Hafler, D.A. (1995). Differential activation of proliferation and cytotoxicity in human T-cell lymphotropic virus type I Tax-specific CD8 T cells by an altered peptide ligand. *Proc Natl Acad Sci USA* 92: 4036–4040.

Hugot, J.P., Chamaillard, M., Zouali, H., Lesage, S., Cezard, J.P., Belaiche, J., et al. (2001). Association of NOD2 leucine-rich repeat variants with susceptibility to Crohn's disease. *Nature* 411: 599–603.

Ichiyoshi, Y., Zhou, M., and Casali, P. (1995). A human anti-insulin IgG auto-antibody apparently arises through clonal selection from an insulin-specific "germ-line" natural antibody template. Analysis by V gene segment reassortment and site-directed mutagenesis. *J Immunol* 154: 226–238.

Iqbal, N., Oliver, J.R., Wagner, F.H., Lazenby, A.S., Elson, C.O., and Weaver, C.T. (2002). T helper 1 and T helper 2 cells are pathogenic in an antigen-specific model of colitis. *J Exp Med* 195: 71–184.

Jacobson, D.L., Gange, S.J., Rose, N.R., and Graham, N.M. (1997). Epidemiology and estimated population burden of selected autoimmune diseases in the United States. *Clin Immunol Immunopathol* 84: 223–243.

Kalman, B. and Lublin, F.D. (1999). The genetics of multiple sclerosis. A review. *Biomed Pharmacother* 53: 358–370.

Karpus, W.J. (2001). Chemokines and central nervous system disorders. *J Neurovirol* 7: 493–500.

Kaveri, S.V., Lacroix-Desmazes, S., Mouthon, L., and Kazatchkine, M.D. (1998). Human Natural Autoantibodies: Lessons from physiology and prospects for therapy. *The Immunologist* 6: 227–233.

Levin, M.C., Lee, S.M., Kalume, F., Morcos, Y., Dohan, F.C. Jr, Hasty, K.A., et al. (2002). Autoimmunity due to molecular mimicry as a cause of neurological disease. *Nat Med* 8: 509–513.

Liblau, R.S., Singer, S.M., and McDevitt, H.O. (1995). Th1 and Th2 CD4+ T cells in the pathogenesis of organ-specific autoimmune diseases. *Immunol Today* 16: 34–38.

Liblau, R.S., Wong, F.S., Mars, L.T., and Santamaria, P. (2002). Autoreactive CD8 T cells in organ-specific autoimmunity: emerging targets for therapeutic intervention. *Immunity* 17: 1–6.

Liston, A., Lesage, S., Wilson, J., Peltonen, L., and Goodnow, C.C. (2003). AIRE regulates CHECK negative selection of organ-specific T cells. *Nat Immunol* 4: 350–354.

Luhder, F., Katz, J., Benoist, C., and Mathis, D. (1998). Major histocompatibility complex class II molecules can protect from diabetes by positively selecting T cells with additional specificities. *J Exp Med* 187: 379–387.

Mackay, F. and Browning, J.L. (2002). BAFF: a fundamental survival factor for B cells. *Nat Rev Immunol* 2: 465–475.

Marrack, P., Kappler, J., and Kotzin, B.L. (2001). Autoimmune disease: why and where it occurs. *Nat Med* 7: 899–905.

McDevitt, H.O. (1998). The role of MHC class II molecules in susceptibility and resistance to autoimmunity. *Curr Opin Immunol* 10: 677–681.

Medana, I.M., Gallimore, A., Oxenius, A., Martinic, M.M., Wekerle, H., and Neumann, H. (2000). MHC class I-restricted killing of neurons by virus-specific CD8+ T lymphocytes is effected through the Fas/FasL, but not the perforin pathway. *Eur J Immunol* 30: 3623–3633.

Modigliani, Y., Bandeira, A., and Coutinho, A. (1996). A model for develop-mentally acquired thymus-dependent tolerance to central and peripheral antigens. *Immunol Rev* 149: 155–20.

Moore, K.W., de Waal Malefyt, R., Coffman, R.L., and O'Garra, A. (2001). Interleukin-10 and the interleukin-10 receptor. *Annu Rev Immunol* 19: 683–765.

Morel, P.A., Dorman, J.S., Todd, J.A., McDevitt, H.O., and Trucco, M. (1988). Aspartic acid at position 57 of the HLA-DQ beta chain protects against type I diabetes: a family study. *Proc Natl Acad Sci USA* 85: 8111–8115.

Mueller, R., Bradley, L.M., Krahl, T., and Sarvetnick, N. (1997). Mechanism underlying counterregulation of autoimmune diabetes by IL-4. *Immunity* 7: 411–418.

Nagamine, K., Peterson, P., Scott, H.S., Kudoh, J., Minoshima, S., Heino, M., et al. (1997). Positional cloning of the APECED gene. *Nat Genet* 17: 393–398.

Naparstek, Y., Andre-Schwartz, J., Manser, T., Wysocki, L.J., Breitman, L., Stollar, B.D., et al. (1986). A single germline VH gene segment of normal A/J mice encodes autoantibodies characteristic of systemic lupus erythematosus. 164: 614–626.

Nemazee, D.A. and Burki, K. (1989). Clonal deletion of B lymphocytes in a trans-genic mouse bearing anti-MHC class I antibody genes. *Nature* 337: 562–566.

O'Connor, K.C., Chitnis, T., Griffin, D.E., Piyasirisilp, S., Bar-Or, A., Khoury, S., et al. (2003). Myelin basic protein-reactive autoantibodies in the serum and cerebrospinal fluid of multiple sclerosis patients are characterized by low-affinity interactions. *J Neuroimmunol* 136: 140–148.

O'Connor, K.C., Appel, H., Call, M.E., Chan, J.A., Moore, N.H., Hafler, D.A., et al. (2005). Isolation of autoantibodies recognizing MOG from CNS tissue of patients with MS. Submitted.

Ogura, Y., Bonen, D.K., Inohara, N., Nicolae, D.L., Chen, F.F., Ramos, R., et al. (2001). A frameshift mutation in NOD2 associated with susceptibility to Crohn's disease. *Nature* 411: 603–606.

Pillai, S. (1999). The chosen few? Positive selection and the generation of naive B lymphocytes. *Immunity* 10: 493–502.

Piyasirisilp, S., Hemachudha, T., and Griffin, D.E. (1999). B-cell responses to myelin basic protein and its epitopes in autoimmune encephalomyelitis induced by Semple rabies vaccine. *J Neuroimmunol* 98: 96–104.

Rabinovitch, A. (1994). Immunoregulatory and cytokine imbalances in the pathogenesis of IDDM. Therapeutic intervention by immunostimulation? *Diabetes* 43: 613–621.

Radic, M.Z., Mackle, J., Erikson, J., Mol, C., Anderson, W.F., and Weigert, M. (1993). Residues that mediate DNA binding of autoimmune antibodies *J Immun* 150: 4966–4977.

Rose, N.R. and Witebsky, E. (1956). Studies on organ specificity: V. Changes in the thyroid gland of rabbits following acute immunization with rabbit thyroid extracts *J Immun* 76: 417–423.

Rowe, R.E., Wapelhorst, B., Bell, G.I., Risch, N., Spielman, R.S., and Concannon, P. (1995). Linkage and association between insulin-dependent diabetes mellitus (IDDM). susceptibility and markers near the glucokinase gene on chromosome 7. *Nat Genet* 10: 240–242.

Sakaguchi, S. (2000). Regulatory T cells: key controllers of immunologic self-tolerance. *Cell* 101: 455–458.

Sakaguchi, S., Fukuma, K., Kuribayashi, K., and Masuda, T. (1985). Organ-specific autoimmune diseases induced in mice by elimination of T cell sub-set. I. Evidence for the active participation of T cells in natural self-tolerance: deficit of a T cell subset as a possible cause of autoimmune disease. *J Exp Med* 161: 72–87.

Sakaguchi, S., Sakaguchi, N., Asano, M., Itoh, M., and Toda, M. (1995). Immunologic self-tolerance maintained by activated T cells expressing IL-2 receptor alpha-chains (CD25). Breakdown of a single mechanism of self-tolerance causes various autoimmune diseases. *J Immunol* 155: 1151–1164.

Schmidt, D., Verdaguer, J., Averill, N., and Santamaria, P. (1997). A mechanism for the major histocompatibility complex-linked resistance to autoimmuni-ty. *J Exp Med* 186: 1059–1075.

Segal, B.M., Klinman, D.M., and Shevach, E.M. (1997). Microbial products induce autoimmune disease by an IL-12-dependent pathway. *J Immunol* 158: 5087–5090.

Shevach, E.M. (2000). Regulatory T cells in autoimmunity. *Annu Rev Immunol* 18: 423–449.

Shi, F., Ljunggren, H.G., and Sarvetnick, N. (2001a). Innate immunity and autoimmunity: from self-protection to self-destruction. *Trends Immunol* 22: 97–101.

Shi, K., Hayashida, K., Kaneko, M., Hashimoto, J., Tomita, T., Lipsky, P.E., et al. (2001b). Lymphoid chemokine B cell-attracting chemokine-1 (CXCL13). is expressed in germinal center of ectopic lymphoid follicles within the synovium of chronic arthritis patients. *J Immunol* 166: 650–655.

Steere, A.C., Gross, D., Meyer, A.L., and Huber, B.T. (2001). Autoimmune mechanisms in antibiotic treatment-resistant lyme arthritis. *J Autoimmun* **16**: 263–268.

Strasser, A., Whittingham, S., Vaux, D.L., Bath, M.L., Adams, J.M., Cory, S., *et al.* (1991). Enforced BCL2 expression in B-lymphoid cells prolongs antibody responses and elicits autoimmune disease. *Proc Natl Acad Sci USA* **88**: 8661–8865.

Straus, S.E., Sneller, M., Lenardo, M.J., Puck, J.M., and Strober, W. (1999). An inherited disorder of lymphocyte apoptosis: the autoimmune lymphoproliferative syndrome. *Ann Intern Med* **130**: 591–601.

Takahashi, T., Kuniyasu, Y., Toda, M., Sakaguchi, N., Itoh, M., Iwata, M., *et al.* (1998). Immunologic self-tolerance maintained by CD25+CD4+ naturally anergic and suppressive T cells: induction of autoimmune disease by breaking their anergic/suppressive state. *Int Immunol* **10**: 1969–1980.

Thornton, A.M. and Shevach, E.M. (1998). CD4+CD25+ immunoregulatory T cells suppress polyclonal T cell activation in vitro by inhibiting interleukin 2 production. *J Exp Med* **188**: 287–296.

Todd, J.A., Bell, J.I., and McDevitt, H.O. (1987). HLA-DQ beta gene contributes to susceptibility and resistance to insulin-dependent diabetes mellitus. *Nature* **329**: 599–604.

Trollmo, C., Meyer, A.L., Steere, A.C., Hafler, D.A., and Huber, B.T. (2001). Molecular mimicry in Lyme arthritis demonstrated at the single cell level: LFA-1 alpha L is a partial agonist for outer surface protein A-reactive T cells. *J Immunol* **166**: 5286–5291.

Ueda, H., Howson, J.M., Esposito, L., Heward, J., Snook, H., Chamberlain, G., *et al.* (2003). Association of the T-cell regulatory gene CTLA4 with susceptibility to autoimmune disease. *Nature* **423**: 506–511.

Viglietta, V., Baecher-Allan, C., Weiner, H.L., and Hafler, D.A. (2004). Loss of functional suppression by CD4+CD25+ regulatory T cells in patients with multiple sclerosis. *J Exp Med* **199**: 971–979.

Vizler, C., Bercovici, N., Cornet, A., Cambouris, C., and Liblau, R.S. (1999). Role of autoreactive CD8+ T cells in organ-specific autoimmune diseases: insight from transgenic mouse models. *Immunol Rev* **169**: 81–92.

Walport, M.J., Davies, K.A., and Botto, M. (1998). C1q and systemic lupus erythematosus. *Immunobiology* **199**: 265–285.

Wanstrat, A. and Wakeland, E. (2001). The genetics of complex autoimmune-diseases: non-MHC susceptibility genes. *Nat Immunol* **2**: 802–809.

Whitacre, C.C. (2001). Sex differences in autoimmune disease. *Nat Immunol* **2**: 777–780.

Winchester, R. (1994). The molecular basis of susceptibility to rheumatoid arthritis. *Adv Immunol* **56**: 389–466.

Wucherpfennig, K.W. (2001). Structural basis of molecular mimicry. *J Autoimmun* **16**: 293–302.

Zhang, J., Roschke, V., Baker, K.P., Wang, Z., Alarcon, G.S., Fessler, B.J., *et al.* (2001). Cutting edge: a role for B lymphocyte stimulator in systemic lupus erythematosus. *J Immunol* **166**: 6–10.

Zhao, Z.S., Granucci, F., Yeh, L., Schaffer, P.A., and Cantor, H. (1998). Molecular mimicry by herpes simplex virus-type 1: autoimmune disease after viral infection. *Science* **279**: 1344–1347.

3 Principles of immunotherapy

Bernhard Hemmer, Olaf Stüve, Reinhard Hohlfeld, and Hans-Peter Hartung

Immunotherapy plays an important role in the treatment of a variety of neurological disorders including diseases of the muscles and the central and peripheral nervous system. The aim of this chapter is to give an overview of the rules and general strategies that apply to immunotherapy and to review current and future immunotherapeutic agents that have been used in the treatment of neurological disorders.

Basis of immunotherapy

Overall considerations

Today, a number of drugs are approved for immunotherapy of neurological disorders. Initially, when agents were assessed for their feasibility the primary focus was global immunosuppression. Although these drugs exerted some beneficial effects on several diseases, adverse effects were frequently observed as a consequence of global immunosuppression. With most immunosuppressive agents, potential side-effects often limit the dose and duration of treatment, frequently resulting in suboptimal treatment regimes. Furthermore, several lines of evidence indicate that parts of the immune system are not only involved in the destruction of nervous tissue but that they may participate in protective or regenerative processes (Rep *et al.*, 1996; Weber *et al.*, 1999). Inflammation occurs not only in infectious and autoimmune diseases, but also in ischemic, degenerative, traumatic, and metabolic lesions of the nervous system and muscle (e.g. stroke, Duchenne muscular dystrophy, adrenoleukodystrophy). It now appears that inflammatory events present an (often futile) attempt by the immune system to protect the neuronal tissue (Kerschensteiner *et al.*, 2003). As a consequence, broad-spectrum immunosuppressive treatments may eliminate immunocompetent cells along with the disease-causing offenders. Finally, it became evident in experimental animal models that immunosuppression with leukopenia itself leads to the expansion of autoreactive T cells and the development of autoimmunity (King *et al.*, 2004). Both novel findings may explain why treatment with non-selective immunosuppressive agents often fails to have a convincing clinical benefit.

Both side-effects and possible interference with protective immunity point towards the need for more selective treatment options. These may include selective targeting of defined cell populations (e.g. B cells, T cells, autoantigen-specific T cells), systemic administration (e.g. interleukin-10) and ablation of immune molecules (e.g. tumor-necrosis factor-α (TNF-α), or induction of qualitative changes in the immune response (e.g. T-cell shift from T-helper-1 to T-helper-2). The ultimate goal, however, would be the selective elimination of the disease-conferring cell population or inflammatory mediators.

Selective immune interventions require detailed knowledge of pathogenic disease mechanisms. Since inflammatory cascades still remain largely unknown in most chronic inflammatory neurological disorders, many specific immune intervention strategies are based on hypothetical concepts rather than scientific evidence (Hemmer *et al.*, 2002). It is therefore not surprising that thus far very few of the specific immune intervention strategies have succeeded in clinical trials. This reminds us that our treatment can only become highly specific and effective if we pinpoint the etiology and pathogenetic pathways of the target diseases.

Besides the development of new therapies, combination of approved therapies has become a major issue for therapy (Lublin and Reingold, 1998). It seems intuitive to combine drugs to achieve their beneficial effects through distinct mechanisms. Striking examples for the effectiveness of such strategies have been given by antiviral therapies in HIV infection, immunosuppressive therapies in transplantation, or antineoplastic therapies in cancer. Obviously, the challenge is to select the appropriate agents to be combined. A general problem is the complex immunological network of neuroinflammatory diseases. Since the individual immune mechanisms targeted by specific agents may depend on one another, it is often impossible to predict if combination therapy may result in synergism or antagonism. Controlled clinical trials are required to determine the clinical efficacy and side-effects of such strategies.

With the currently approved agents one of the most important issues has become the optimal timing of treatment initiation. The current view among most experts is that an earlier commencement of therapy will increase the chances of preventing permanent neurological deficits. Arguments against very early treatment include the increased risk of adverse reactions associated with the long-term use of these agents. In this regard there is some evidence that patients with severe clinical impairment have an increased risk of various adverse reactions to immunotherapy. It is also conceivable that, as a consequence of physiologic adjustments, the therapeutic effectiveness may diminish over time if treatment is started early.

There is also the danger of missing the optimal time point to start treatment. Clinical and histopathological evidence suggests that an established, stable chronic deficit cannot be reversed. Therefore, patients with advanced disease, in particular central nervous system (CNS) disease, are not optimal candidates for immunotherapy. Ideally, the degree of immunomodulation and immunosuppression should be adjusted to disease activity during all stages of the disease.

Practical issues

Most immunotherapies that require long-term treatment are sometimes associated with significant side-effects, some of which may be life-threatening. Therefore, the decision to start such a therapy requires careful evaluation of the disease in each individual patient (Fig. 3.1). Before initiating immunotherapy, the treating physician has to review the patient's diagnosis. Only if the diagnosis, or at least the immunological component of the disease, is univocally established should immunotherapy be considered. Next, the patient's clinical status has to be determined to set the objective for the treatment and determine the baseline for follow-up examinations. In parallel, the general medical condition, current medication, and risk factors of the patient need to be reviewed to identify factors that may interfere with the treatment strategy. The physician also needs to evaluate if the patient is likely to comply with regard to the proposed therapy, as well as with all treatment-related examinations and procedures. Usually, the risks of non-compliance outweigh the benefits of treatment, and non-compli-

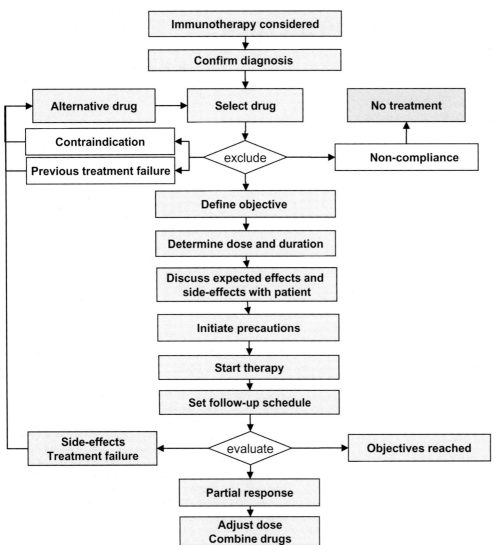

Fig. 3.1 Paradigm on the initiation of immunotherapy.

ance is a contraindication for immunotherapy. If the treating physician eventually decides that immunotherapy would be beneficial to the patient, he or she needs to determine the dose and the duration of the therapy. It is equally important to define for each individual patient when treatment will be discontinued due to lack of efficacy or side-effects. One should recall that most immunotherapies require treatment over a longer period of time, and that there may be a threshold dose required in order to achieve a biological effect. This is important, as a prematurely terminated treatment course may incorrectly be labeled a 'treatment failure'. Another severe consequence of incorrect dosing or inadequate timing may be that a potentially effective therapy will never be used again in an individual patient. Finally, after deciding that the patient may profit from therapy, the treating physician should discuss treatment options with the patient and inform him or her about the expected benefit and possible side-effects. It is also necessary to discuss with the patient which precautions have to be taken (e.g. contraception), and which follow-up examinations are mandatory. The early open discussion with the patient often prevents non-compliance when side-effects emerge or delay in treatment benefits occurs. We usually inform the patient orally, but also provide written documents which contain detailed information about the intended treatment. During a second visit, the patient usually (after discussing additional questions) makes an informed decision. Now, precautions need to be taken as indicated. In women, contraception is a pre-requisite for most immunotherapies. An information sheet or patient passport is issued, which contains all information about

disease, therapy, expected side-effects and routine follow-up examinations. In parallel, all physicians involved, in particular the family physician, have to be informed about the treatment with particular emphasis on the possible side-effects, drug interactions and routine check-ups. It is also helpful to give the patient practical guidelines on measures that have to be taken when or if side-effects occur. All these actions increase the compliance of the patient and reduce the risk of treatment-related events. The effectiveness of any immunomodulatory or immunosuppressive treatment has to be assessed at regular intervals, and as a consequence it should be stopped if ineffectiveness or unacceptable side-effects become evident.

Immunosuppressive and immunomodulatory agents

Glucocorticosteroids

General properties

Glucocorticosteroids (GCS) are the most widely and frequently used immunomodulatory agents. The immunological effects of GCS are mainly mediated through intracellular steroid receptors. The GSC–receptor complex binds glucocorticoid-responsive motifs in nuclear deoxyribonucleic acid (DNA) resulting in down- or up-regulation of a variety of transcripts. Likewise, GCS down-regulate nuclear factor kappa B (NF-κB), a main tran-

Table 3.1 Glucocorticosteroids

Indications	Multiple sclerosis, idiopathic facial palsy, myasthenia gravis (MG), polymyositis, dermatomyositis, chronic inflammatory demyelinating neuropathies (CIDP)
Dosage, duration	Multiple sclerosis: 0.5–1 g methylprednisolone for 5 days, oral taper. Facial palsy: 1 mg/kg prednisolone for 10 days, oral taper. CIDP: 1 mg/kg prednisone per day, at least 1–2 months, then reduction by 10 mg/month. MG: 25 mg prednisone per day, stepwise increase to 50 mg per day, after 1–3 months slow reduction. Myositis: 1 mg/kg prednisone per day, at least 1 month, then slow reduction
Onset of action	Hours (anti-edematous), 1–4 weeks (anti-inflammatory)
Lab. pre-check	Blood sugar, blood cell count, CRP, urine
Exclude	Prior arthroplasty of joint, blood clotting disorders, intra-articular fracture, periarticular infection, juxta-articular, non-arthritic osteoporosis, unstable joint, acute severe infection
Risk–benefit evaluation	Uncontrolled infections, diabetes mellitus, glaucoma, osteoporosis psychosis, inflammatory gastrointestinal disease, cardiac disease (congestive heart failure, hypertension, myocardial infarction), severe renal function disease, hepatic function disease, hyperlipidemia, hypersensitivity to steroids, hyperthyroidism, hypoalbuminemia, acute MG, systemic lupus erythematosus
Co-medication	Protection from peptic ulcer in patients at high risk, low-dose heparin in disabled patients receiving high-dose treatment
Laboratory follow-up	Weeks: serum electrolytes, blood glucose concentrations, prothrombin time, blood pressure. Months to years: occult blood, stool, glucose tolerance test, ophthalmological examinations
Acute effects	Diabetes mellitus, burning, numbness, pain, or tingling at or near injection site, congestive heart failure, generalized allergic reaction, sudden blindness, generalized anaphylaxis, cardiac arrhythmias, flushing of face or cheeks, and seizures
Long-term effects	Cushing's syndrome effects: acne, adrenal suppression, avascular necrosis, cataracts, cutaneous or subcutaneous tissue atrophy, ecchymosis, fluid and sodium retention, glaucoma with possible damage to optic nerves, growth suppression (in children), hypokalemic syndrome), impaired wound healing, increased intracranial pressure, ocular infection, osteoporosis or bone fractures, pancreatitis, peptic ulceration or intestinal perforation, scarring at injection site, steroid myopathy, tendon rupture, and thin, fragile skin

scription factor up-regulated during inflammation. The anti-inflammatory and immunosuppressive effects of GCS are manifold (Gold *et al.*, 2001). Steroids profoundly influence the distribution and trafficking of leukocytes. For example, steroids induce peripheral blood neutrophilia, whereas T cells, monocytes, and eosinophils are depleted from blood. Steroids also influence the properties of T cells and monocytes. Steroids act on the synthesis and secretion of cytokines and immune mediators. Finally, steroids affect microvascular permeability, which may contribute to the effects on leukocyte migration. In addition influencing the number and distribution of immune cells, GCS down-regulate the secretion of several lymphokines, including various interleukins, interferon-gamma (IFN-γ), and TNF-α. The anti-inflammatory effects of GCS include the suppression of the secretion of arachidonic acid metabolites such as prostaglandins and leukotriene, the decrease of capillary dilatation, edema, fibrin deposition, and the blockade of lysosomal enzyme degranulation.

GCS treatment is limited to a short period for some diseases, whereas it is extended over many years for others (Table 3.1). Severe adverse reactions can occur with both treatment strategies, but as a rule are frequently observed with long-term treatment. Specific side-effects, however, depend on the daily dose, dosing frequency, and duration of treatment. When GCS treatment becomes mandatory, particular efforts are necessary to control GCS side-effects while maintaining therapeutic efficacy.

Management of side-effects

Steroid therapy must be managed by qualified clinicians. For some indications it is advisable to hospitalize patients for initiation of steroid therapy. In particular, patients with generalized myasthenia gravis may experience a transient steroid-induced exacerbation of weakness.

The continued administration of GCS carries the risk of side-effects for which patients should be closely monitored. Hypothalamic–pituitary–adrenal axis suppression may occur within a week of systemic therapy. The most important side-effects with long-term treatment are osteoporosis, hypertension, and exacerbation, or precipitation, of diabetes. Obesity, gastrointestinal ulcers, cataracts, and occasional opportunistic infections are also frequently observed. Typical signs of infection may be masked by GCS treatment. Blood pressure, weight, serum electrolytes, and glucose level should be closely followed and adequately treated. Regular slit-lamp examinations (every 6 months) help to detect cataracts early. In patients with a history of ulcer, histamine H_2 receptor antagonists or H^+,K^+-ATPase inhibitors may be necessary to protect the mucosa of the upper gastrointestinal from ulceration and bleeding. To avoid sleeplessness steroids are usually administered in the morning.

GCS-induced osteoporosis is especially problematic in older individuals, particularly those who are estrogen deficient. In order to minimize steroid-induced osteoporosis, the single most effective measure is reduction of dosage or, if possible, the complete discontinuation of the GCS. Calcium supplementation and post-menopausal estrogen repletion are also helpful. The 24-h urine calcium output should be measured after 1–3 months of GCS therapy and oral calcium and vitamin D should be given, based on the level of urinary calcium excretion. Cyclical, oral bisphosphonates prevent GCS-induced loss of bone mineral density in the spine and hip. Potassium replacement is only necessary in patients who develop hypokalemia.

Discontinuation of long-term treatment

Due to the suppression of the hypothalamic–pituitary–adrenal axis dose reduction and eventually discontinuation of therapy requires careful monitoring of the patient. After long-term high-dose therapy, the daily dose is reduced to an equivalent dose of 20 mg prednisone. Then an alternate-day schedule is implemented for at least 1 month. Patients who have been on alternate-day schedules for more than 4 weeks experience fewer difficulties during termination GCS therapy. The dosage is then gradually reduced until the replacement dosage is reached (e.g. 5 mg prednisone) and finally discontinued. It may be helpful to determine plasma cortisol levels before the morning dose, when patients develop symptoms of adrenal insufficiency (e.g. fatigability, weakness, anorexia, nausea and vomiting, weight loss, cutaneous and mucosal pigmentation, hypotension, and occasionally hypoglycemia). A cortisol level of less than 140 nmol/l indicates suppression of the pituitary–adrenal axis and should result in a more cautious tapering of the steroid dose. Following withdrawal of long-term GCS treatment, patients are still vulnerable to diseases requiring higher cortical production such as acute infections, surgery, and trauma. In these instances, patients may require short-term supplementary GCS therapy.

Immunosuppressive and cytotoxic agents
Azathioprine and mycophenolate mofetil
General properties
Azathioprine (AZA) is converted into its metabolite 6-mercaptopurine, which competes with its analog, hypoxanthine, a central component of nucleic acid synthesis interfering with DNA, ribonucleic acid (RNA), and

protein synthesis. AZA acts on proliferating lymphocytes and induces both B- and T-cell lymphopenia, blocking mitogen-driven and antibody responses. Antigen- and mitogen-induced *in vitro* proliferative responses of T cells are less inhibited by AZA than by cytotoxic agents like cyclophosphamide. Probably due to the inhibition of pro-monocyte cell division, AZA also has mild anti-inflammatory properties (El-Azhary, 2003).

AZA is often used as an adjunct to reduce the dose of CGS but may be used alone. It is relatively easy to use but has two major disadvantages; 10% of patients develop an acute idiosyncratic reaction (general malaise, fever, skin reactions, nausea and vomiting) requiring immediate discontinuation. In patients who tolerate AZA therapy, immunosuppressive effects require months of treatment. Therefore, patients have to be followed on treatment for up to 12 months in order to judge treatment efficacy.

Serious side-effects of AZA are only rarely observed. Reversible bone marrow depression with leukopenia, gastrointestinal complications, infections, and transient elevation of liver enzymes are sometimes seen (Weber *et al.*, 1999). The risk of developing malignancies, especially lymphoma, is not certain, but seems to be lower in patients with myasthenia gravis (MG) than in organ transplant recipients. AZA is potentially teratogenic and mutagenic. Although the children of mothers treated with AZA for kidney transplant in one study did not show birth defects, no conclusive data on the actual risk are available. Patients should therefore be strongly advised to use contraceptive measures during treatment and for at least several months after completion of therapy. Up to 10% of patients have a genetically reduced activity of the enzyme thiopurine-5-methyltransferase. In these patients, AZA toxicity is increased. Genetic testing for the defect is possible. An important drug interaction occurs with allopurinol. Inhibition of xanthine oxidase by allopurinol impairs the conversion of azathioprine to 6-thiouric acid, which accumulates and eventually leads to myelosuppression. Therefore concurrent use should be avoided. If allopurinol must be administered, the dose of azathioprine must be reduced to 25% of the regular dose (approximately 0.5 mg/kg body weight) and the white blood count (WBC) should be closely monitored.

Table 3.2 Azathioprine

Indications	Myasthenia gravis, polymyositis, dermatomyositis, (multiple sclerosis)
Dosage, duration	1–3 mg/kg, after objective reached reduction by 0.5 mg/kg every 4 weeks
Onset of action	1–2 months, maximum up to 12 months
Precautions	Carcinogenicity, mutagenicity (animals), reduces reproduction (animals)
Lab. pre-check	Blood cell count, C-reactive protein, urine
Exclude	Pregnancy, breast feeding
Risk-benefit evaluation	Ongoing viral infection (chickenpox, Herpes zoster), gout, hepatic function impairment, pancreatitis, sensitivity to azathioprine, severe xanthine oxidase deficiency, previous cytotoxic drug therapy, and radiation therapy
Co-medication	None
Laboratory follow-up	Complete blood counts (weekly during the first 2 months), later monthly
Side-effects	Leukopenia, loss of appetite, gastrointestinal hypersensitivity reaction (first week of treatment), nausea or vomiting more frequently observed. Infection, megaloblastic anemia, hepatitis or biliary stasis, thrombocytopenia, hepatic veno-occlusive disease, hypersensitivity, pneumonitis, oral and labial sores, hypotension may occasionally occur. Hepatic enzymes may also be elevated, skin rash, bone marrow depression are rarely seen
Drug interactions	Avoid combination with allopurinol (severe myelosuppression)

The use of AZA in MG as a GCS-sparing drug is well established (Richman and Agius, 2003). It is also used in polymyositis, dermatomyositis, and chronic inflammatory demyelinating polyneuropathy (CIDP). AZA reduces relapse rates in multiple sclerosis (MS), but its efficacy in comparison with currently approved drugs is difficult to assess. The studies performed in MS two decades ago did not meet the standards of current treatment trials nor did they involve magnetic resonance imaging (MRI) as a surrogate marker for inflammation. Therefore, AZA is only rarely used as a second-line treatment option in MS.

Mycophenolate mofetil is another immunosuppressive agent acting on DNA metabolism, leading to inhibition of DNA synthesis. In transplantation medicine, mycophenolate mofetil seems more powerful than AZA (Lipsky, 1996). In patients with neuroimmunological disease, including MG, mycophenolate mofetil has been used if AZA was inefficient or not tolerated by the patient (Chaudhry *et al.*, 2001). Its adverse effects include gastrointestinal symptoms, gastrointestinal hemorrhage, hepatotoxicity, and infection. In comparison to AZA, its risk of secondary lymphoma seems to be slightly higher (Lipsky, 1996). The combination of mycophenol mofetil and allopurinol is not problematic.

Management of side-effects

Complete blood counts should be obtained at least weekly during the first 2 months, and monthly thereafter. If the total WBC is reduced to less than 3000 per ml, the medication should be discontinued for a few days, and continued at a lower dose after the WBC returns to more than 3500 per ml. The long-term dose can be adjusted to maintain the WBC around 4000 per ml and lymphocyte counts ranging between 800 and 1000 per μl. However, it is not certain whether the immunosuppressive efficacy of AZA therapy in autoimmune diseases is directly correlated to the WBC or lymphocyte count. In patients receiving AZA and steroids, the total WBC is usually elevated because of steroid-induced neutrophilia. During combined treatment, a WBC of approximately 6000 to 8000 per μl is anticipated. Alternatively, the lymphocyte count, which is less markedly altered by corticosteroids, is monitored. Measuring the mean corpuscular volume (MCV) of red cells, which is usually but not invariably elevated (by up to 15%) during long-term treatment, may be helpful in monitoring patient compliance.

Mild intestinal discomfort is common, but can usually be alleviated by starting treatment with a bedtime dose, taking the drug after meals, and administering the drug in three or more divided doses. If side-effects occur the does may be reduced temporarily. Elevation of liver enzymes up to three times the baseline is also common and may be tolerated since it is usually reversible after the dose has been reduced. A serious gastrointestinal complication is AZA-related pancreatitis. No specific precautions are required for discontinuing AZA treatment.

Immunophilin-binding agents (ciclosporin, sirolimus, and tacrolimus)

Ciclosporin, sirolimus (rapamycin), and tacrolimus (FK506) are immunophilin-binding drugs characterized by inhibition of calcineurin. They prevent transcription of messenger RNAs for key cytokines such as interleukin-2. Ciclosporin targets the immune system more specifically than azathioprine or cyclophosphamide. It targets mainly T lymphocytes; B cells and macrophages are apparently spared. The only appreciable effect of ciclosporin on accessory cells seems to be the disruption of lymphokine-dependent T-lymphocyte/macrophage interactions. Clinical improvement usually begins within 2–4 weeks.

The immunophilin-binding agents very efficiently suppress transplant rejection. Ciclosporin is effective in MG (Tindall *et al.*, 1993) and possibly in MS (The Multiple Sclerosis Study Group, 1990) but has remained a second-line agent, mainly owing to its nephrotoxicity and high cost. It is likely that in the future immunophilin-binding agents will gain more importance in the treatment of neuroimmunological diseases since some of the derivatives seem to have additional neurotrophic effects (Steiner *et al.*, 1997).

Management of side-effects

Major side-effects of ciclosporin include nephrotoxicity and hepatic disorders, but ciclosporin can affect other organs such as the pancreas, CNS, bone, and skeletal muscle. Further adverse reactions include arterial hypertension, tremor, and hirsutism. Most of the adverse effects correlate with the dose and duration of treatment. Optimal dosage is monitored by measuring 'trough drug' levels 12 h after the last dose. A sensitive indicator of nephrotoxicity is the measurement of creatinine clearance. Ciclosporin must be discontinued if idiosyncratic or allergic reactions develop. The risk of late malignancies is not established, but may be similar to that of AZA.

Methotrexate

Methotrexate (MTX) is a chemotherapeutic drug used in oncology and rheumatology. MTX is a structural analog of folic acid acting as a folic acid antagonist, resulting in reduced purine and thymidilate synthesis. Due to its mechanism of action, MTX acts on rapidly dividing cells. MTX is excreted unchanged mainly in the urine within 12 h of administration.

Management of side-effects

Chronic extended use can lead to liver fibrosis and cirrhosis. Further adverse effects include bone marrow suppression, gastrointestinal complications, cystitis, lung fibrosis, alopecia, and cutaneous vasculitis. Concurrent application of folate may reduce the incidence of side-effects without significant reduction in therapeutic efficacy. Non-steroidal anti-inflammatory agents and trimethoprin-sulfamethoxazole can potentiate the toxicity of MTX.

MTX is used as a second-line immunosuppressive treatment for inflammatory myopathies. The use of MTX in advanced MS is controversial. MTX is given orally at a dose from 10 to 20 mg on 1 day each week.

Cyclophosphamide

General properties

Cyclophosphamide (CTX) is an alkylating agent of the nitrogen mustard type. An activated form of cyclophosphamide, phosphoramide mustard, alkylates or binds with many intracellular molecular structures, including nucleic acids. Cytotoxic effects occur because of DNA and RNA cross-linking and inhibition of protein synthesis. It is therefore primarily acting upon rapidly dividing cells from the lymphoid, gastrointestinal, and urothelial systems, the hair follicles, and ovarian and testicular tissue but also on tumor cells. The desired actions (i.e. immunosuppression and decrease of tumor growth) as well as the adverse effects (i.e. leukopenia, hemorrhagic cystitis, amenorrhea, oligospermia, and transient alopecia) are caused by its effect on DNA. CTX acts upon the immune system in a number of different ways including the decrease of T cells of various subclasses and, even more, B-cell numbers and function. Its efficient in lupus nephritis, Wegener's granulomatosis, and various vasculitides. CTX is used in CNS vasculitis and multifocal motor neuropathy (Weiner *et al.*, 1995). It is also used as second-line treatment in progressive MS, although its efficacy has not been established by well-controlled trials.

Management of side-effects

CTX may induce bone marrow suppression and hemorrhagic cystitis. Bladder toxicity can be reduced by a high fluid intake and, during pulse administration of high doses intravenously, by the simultaneous use of a uroprotective agent (mesna). In this connection, even microhematuria is an alarming sign that requires intense investigation to exclude a bladder tumor. CTX has been associated with development of myeloproliferative and lymphoproliferative carcinomas as well as urinary bladder carcinoma (especially in patients who developed hemorrhagic cystitis while receiving CTX) up to several years after administration. The risk of malignancy depends on the cumulative dose, which should not exceed 51 g. Like other cytotoxic agents, CTX is potentially teratogenic and should not be administered during pregnancy, especially in the first trimester. Permanent infertility may occur in both male and female patients. Alopecia may develop with short- and long-term therapy but is mild and reversible after treatment

Table 3.3 Cyclophosphamide

Indications	Multifocal motor neuropathy, vasculitis, (multiple sclerosis, chronic inflammatory demyelinating polyneuropathy)
Dosage, duration	10–15 mg/kg once every 4 weeks, after improvement in 2–3 month intervals. Duration limited by maximum cumulative dose of 50–70 g
Onset of action	Weeks
Lab. pre-check	Serum liver enzymes, bilirubin values, blood urea nitrogen, lactate dehydrogenase (LDH), and creatinine concentrations. Hematocrit or hemoglobin, Differential leukocyte count, platelet count, serum uric acid concentrations. Examination of urine for microscopic hematuria
Precautions	Carcinogenicity, mutagenicity (animals), reduces reproduction (animals)
Exclude	Sensitivity to cyclophosphamide, pregnancy, breast feeding, acute infection, use of other immunosuppressive drugs
Risk–benefit evaluation	Adrenalectomy, bone marrow depression, existing or recent chickenpox or Herpes zoster, gout, urate renal stones, hepatic function impairment, infection, renal function impairment, sensitivity to cyclophosphamide, tumor cell infiltration of bone marrow, previous cytotoxic drug therapy or radiation
Co-medication	Anti-emetic drugs, uroprotective agents
Lab. follow-up	Serum alanine aminotransferase (serum glutamic pyruvic transaminase) and serum aspartate aminotransferase (serum glutamic-oxaloacetic transaminase) levels, bilirubin values, blood urea nitrogen, LDH, creatinine concentration, hematocrit or hemoglobin and differential leukocyte count, platelet count, uric acid concentration, urinary output, urinary specific gravity
Side-effects	Amenorrhea, leukopenia, or infection are frequently observed. After long-term treatment or high-dose treatment cardiotoxicity, including acute myopericarditis, a condition resembling syndrome of inappropriate antidiuretic hormone, hemorrhagic cystitis, hyperuricemia, uric acid nephropathy, non-hemorrhagic cystitis, or nephrotoxicity, pneumonitis or interstitial pulmonary fibrosis may occur. Less frequently anemia, thrombocytopenia, anaphylactic reaction, hemorrhagic colitis, hepatitis hyperglycemia, redness, swelling, or pain at site of injection, stomatitis, darkening of skin and fingernails, loss of appetite, nausea or vomiting, diarrhea or stomach pain, flushing or redness of face, headache, increased sweating, myxedema, skin rash, loss of hair, hemorrhagic cystitis are observed

is stopped. Additional, rarer side-effects include myocardial damage and pulmonary fibrosis. Patients should be informed that during prolonged therapy serious side-effects may develop, and should be instructed to report signs and symptoms immediately.

CTX is given orally at a dose of 1 to 2 mg/kg body weight per day. However, recent studies suggest that intravenous pulse doses (10 to 15 mg/kg) once every 4 weeks have fewer urinary side-effects. After administering CTX, the WBC is closely monitored for 3 weeks. A significant drop in leukocyte count should result in dose reduction. After stabilizing the patient, the pulses may be extended to 3-month intervals for 1–2 years. If possible, therapy with CTX should be limited to 2 or 3 years because of its cumulative toxic and carcinogenic effects. No specific precautions are required for discontinuing CTX treatment.

Mitoxantrone

General properties

Mitoxantrone (MIX) is approved for the treatment of MS. MIX is a synthetic anthracycline derivative that acts on both DNA and RNA synthesis. However, its molecular actions have not been fully understood. The interference with nucleic acid synthesis explains its influence on rapidly dividing and metabolically active cells such as tumor cells and immune cells. Mitoxantrone is given as a single infusion (12 mg/m^2 in 250 ml of 0.9% sodium chloride or 5% dextrose) over 30 min. MIX is effective in progressive MS by reducing relapse rates and disease progression (Hartung *et al.*, 2002). Due to its side-effects it is only approved for patients with secondary progressive, relapsing progressive, and worsening progressive MS (Expanded Disability Status Scale (EDSS) progression >1/year) who do not respond to first-line immunomodulatory therapy (e.g. interferon-beta).

Management of side-effects

To maintain immunosuppression over longer periods, MIX has to be administered every 3 months. In progressive patients with highly aggressive disease, monthly treatment with MIX in combination with GCS may be helpful (Edan *et al.*, 1997). Although the acute toxicity is lower than that seen in patients treated with high-dose cyclophosphamide, MIX, like other anthracycline derivatives, is cardiotoxic. Congestive heart failure and decreased left ventricular ejection fraction have been observed with cumulative doses of 140 mg/m^2 and higher. Patients with pre-existing cardiac problems should therefore not be treated with MIX. In addition, electrocardiogram and echocardiography before initiation of therapy and after 1 year of therapy is mandatory. Patients who were treated with MIX for a tumor, e.g. breast cancer, have an approximately 10-fold higher risk for later development of a secondary hematopoetic malignancy. Besides cardiac

Table 3.4 Mitoxantrone

Indications	Multiple sclerosis
Dosage, duration	12 mg/m^2 of body surface area every 3 months. Duration limited by maximum cumulative dose of 140 mg/m^2 of body surface
Onset of action	1–2 months, maximum 6–12 months
Precautions	Carcinogenicity, mutagenicity (animals), reduces reproduction (animals)
Lab. pre-check	Alanine aminotransferase (ALT), aspartate aminotransferase (AST), lactate dehydrogenase (LDH), bilirubin serum levels, chest X-ray and echocardiography and electrocardiogram (ECG) studies. Hematocrit, hemoglobin, total leukocyte count, serum uric acid concentration
Exclude	Pregnancy, breast feeding, heart disease, bone marrow depression, acute infection, severe hepatic function impairment
Risk–benefit evaluation	Gout, history of urate renal stones
Co-medication	Anti-emetic drugs
Lab. follow-up	ALT, AST, LDH, bilirubin serum levels, hematocrit or hemoglobin and total leukocyte count and, if appropriate, differential and platelet count, serum uric acid concentrations. Cardiological work-up every 12 months
Side-effects	Cough, shortness of breath, gastrointestinal bleeding, leukopenia, infection, stomach pain, stomatitis, mucositis, arrhythmias, congestive heart failure, conjunctivitis, jaundice, renal failure, seizures, thrombocytopenia, allergic reaction, extravasation, local irritation, and phlebitis. Urine may have blue–green color and whites of eyes may have a blue color during treatment. Possibility of hair loss; normal hair growth should return after treatment has ended

problems, adverse reactions include bleeding and nausea and vomiting. Jaundice, infections, renal failure, alopecia, seizures and headaches, cough and dyspnea, and allergic reactions are also sometimes seen. The risks of administration must therefore be carefully weighed against the desired effects. Mainly because of its cumulative cardiotoxicity, the use should be restricted to patients with progressive disease, who should be carefully informed about the potential risks and benefits of this treatment (Ghalie *et al.*, 2002*a,b*).

Since MIX can cause skin necrosis, all precautions have to be taken to avoid paravenous infusion. Anti-emetics (ondansetron or tropisetron) should be co-administered to prevent nausea. The bluish discoloration of urine and of the sclera which occurs within 24 h of administration should be discussed with the patient. Frequent analysis (every other day during the first 2 weeks after therapy and then weekly) of laboratory values including blood counts, liver enzymes, uric acid, and renal laboratory values should be obtained, because myelosuppression occurs within a few days of initiation of therapy. The dose should be reduced by 25% if a significant drop in leukocyte count (<2500 per μl) occurs. Since treatment with MIX is limited to a maximum of 12 applications at standard dose, a dose reduction to 5 mg/m^2 or longer intervals between the applications (e.g. 6 months) should be considered in clinically stable patients. No specific precautions are required for discontinuing MIX treatment.

Immunomodulatory agents

Immunomodulatory agents, in contrast to immunosuppressants, modulate immune functions in a more differentiated manner. For most of these substances the key mechanisms leading to disease amelioration are uncertain. Interferons-beta (IFN-β), glatiramer acetate (GA), and intravenous immunoglobulins (IVIG) play an important role in the treatment of inflammatory disorders of the nervous system.

Interferon-beta

General properties

Interferon-alpha (INF-α) is part of a multigene family, whereas IFN-β and IFN-γ are encoded by single genes. Because IFN-α and IFN-β share components of the same receptor, they are referred to as type I interferons. IFN-γ uses a separate receptor and is referred to as type II interferon. Although the surface receptors are different, IFNs share several components of the intracellular signaling pathways (Darnell *et al.*, 1994; Kohlhuber *et al.*, 1997; Yeh and Chiu, 2000). Type I interferons are produced by most mammalian cells upon stimulation. One important—but not the only—inducer of interferon synthesis by dendritic cells and monocytes is double-stranded RNA, which is produced by most viruses. The release of IFNs has broad biological effects: type I and II interferons increase expression of MHC Class I enhancing recognition of the infected cell by CD8+ T lymphocytes. The expression of MHC Class II molecules is enhanced by IFN-γ on various cell types, but inhibited by IFN-α and IFN-β. In addition, interferons influence several other biological processes. IFN-β up-regulates the expression of the anti-inflammatory cytokine interleukin-10 by several immunocompetent cells (Rudick *et al.*, 1996, 1998; Rep *et al.*, 1996; Weber *et al.*, 1999), and it decreases leukocyte migration across the basement membrane mediated by matrix-degrading enzymes (Leppert *et al.*, 1996; Stuve *et al.*, 1996). Other potential mechanisms include an increase in soluble vascular cell adhesion molecule (VCAM)-1, and the concomitant down-regulation of its corresponding adhesion molecule, very late activated antigen (VLA)-4, on peripheral blood lymphocytes (Calabresi *et al.*, 1997). IFNs also up-regulate the expression of chemokines by numerous cell types, including hematopoietic cells.

Three preparations of recombinant IFN-β have been approved for treatment of MS, IFN-β-1b s.c. (Betaferon, Betaseron), IFN-β-1a s.c. (Rebif), and IFN-β-1a i.m. (Avonex). Interferons were initially introduced for the treatment of MS due to their antiviral effect (reviewed in Jacobs and Johnson (1994)). A pilot trial of systemic recombinant IFN-γ resulted in a sharp increase in clinical exacerbations (Panitch *et al.*, 1987). After systemic

Table 3.5 Interferon-beta

Indications	Multiple sclerosis
Dosage, duration	Interferon-1a intramuscular, 30 µg once a week. Interferon-1a subcutaneously, 22 µg or 44 µg three times per week. Interferon-1b subcutaneously, 0.25 mg every other day. Optimal duration of treatment has not been defined
Onset of action	Within weeks
Precautions	Possible abortifacient activity
Lab. pre-check	Blood chemistry values, including liver function, platelet counts, complete and differential, white blood cell counts
Exclude	Pregnancy (abortive effects), breast feeding, severe depression, especially with suicidal tendency
Risk–benefit evaluation	Depression, sensitivity to natural or recombinant interferon beta, albumin, human USP, or dextrose, children (efficacy has not been established), cardiac disease, liver disease
Co-medication	Non-steroidal antiphlogistics to reduce/prevent flu-like symptoms
Lab. follow-up	Blood chemistry values, including liver function, platelet counts, complete and differential white blood cell counts
Side-effects	Local skin reaction at injection sites, necrotic skin lesions, abdominal pain, headache or migraine, high blood pressure, influenza-like syndrome (chills, fever, increased sweating, malaise, myalgia, palpitations, sinusitis), abnormal vision, breast pain cystitis, dyspnea, lymphadenopathy, pelvic pain, peripheral vascular disorder, tachycardia, weight gain are frequently observed. Amnesia, breast neoplasm, confusion, conjunctivitis, cyst, edema, generalized fibrocystic breast, goiter, hemorrhage, hyperkinesia, hypertonia, mental depression with suicidal ideation, seizure, speech disorder, urinary urgency, weight loss, asthenia, constipation, diarrhea, dizziness, dysmenorrhea or other menstrual disorders, laryngitis, hair loss, anxiety, nervousness, somnolence, vomiting are only rarely observed

treatment with IFN-γ turned out to increase disease activity, the less pro-inflammatory IFN-β was tested and turned out to have beneficial effects in MS (IFNB Multiple Sclerosis Study Group, 1993; PRISMS Study Group, 1998; Jacobs *et al.*, 1996). Most consistent are the reduction of relapses by 30% and the strong decrease of acute CNS inflammation as measured by gadolinium-enhancing MRI lesions. One trial showed that IFN-β seem to affect the course of secondary progressive MS, at least during the active disease phase characterized by defined relapses. The effect in secondary progressive MS without relapses is probably non-existent or negligible, as evidenced by another study. The long-term effects on disease progression have yet to be established. The precise mechanisms of how IFN-β acts in MS remain unknown, and it is conceivable that both antiviral and anti-inflammatory effects may be relevant.

Management of side-effects

Most MS patients experience flu-like symptoms, including fever, myalgia, headache, fatigue, and chills, when the treatment is initiated. The symptoms start 3–6 h after injection and reach their maximum at 24 h but may last several days. The individual pattern and intensity of these symptoms vary greatly from patient to patient and even from injection to injection. The flu-like reactions usually decrease during the first 3 months of treatment. Patients should be advised to start with a reduced dose (half or a quarter of the final dose) and take the injection before bedtime. Co-administration of non-steroidal antiphlogistics (NSAIDs) reduces side-

effects. NSAIDs are routinely used during the initiation phase and may be co-administered during long-term treatment if patients develop side-effects. Many patients experience a transient worsening of pre-existing MS symptoms, especially increased spasticity, which may require adjustment of spasmolytic medications. The most frequently observed laboratory abnormalities are reversible lymphopenia, neutropenia, leukopenia, and raised liver aminotransferase values. Complete blood counts should be obtained each month as well as serum chemistries with liver function tests in the first 3 months, and quarterly thereafter. If significant laboratory changes occur, the dosage should be temporarily reduced or discontinued. Although no evidence for any drug interactions has emerged so far, the concomitant administration of IFN-β and other potentially hepato- or myelotoxic medications should be closely monitored. The incidence and severity of injection site complications depends on the route of administration. Cutaneous reactions range from mild irritation to necrosis. Intramuscular injection causes fewer skin reactions, and so far no necroses have been reported. In contrast, abscess formation is more frequently observed after i.m. injection of IFN-β.

In one study in rhesus monkeys, high doses of IFN-β were not teratogenic to the embryo, but they had a dose-dependent abortive effect. Although it is not known whether IFN-β exerts the same effects in humans, it is generally recommended that interferon therapy should be discontinued before pregnancy. There is consensus among clinicians that IFN therapy should be discontinued during pregnancy and nursing for safety reasons. To lower the risk of a relapse post-partum, one may discuss with the patient an early discontinuation of breast feeding and re-initiating IFN-β therapy as soon as possible. Development of MG, hyper- and hypothyroidism, Raynaud's phenomenon, autoimmune hepatitis, rheumatoid arthritis, and lupus erythematosus have been reported in patients receiving IFN-β treatment. Therefore, other pharmacotherapies should be considered in patients with known autoimmune diseases. Both IFN-β-1b and IFN-β-1a may be associated with a worsening of psoriasis vulgaris. Very rarely, anaphylaxis or shock may occur.

Symptoms of depression are frequent in MS patients. There is evidence that IFN-β increases the prevalence of depression in MS patients. Therefore, patients with severe depression should be adequately clinically assessed, treated, and monitored before initiating IFN-β therapy. If depression and mood disorders appear during therapy with IFN-β they should be treated like all other depressive syndromes. Severe depression may also require shifting the patient to another immunomodulatory therapy.

During therapy with IFN-β patients may develop antibodies that neutralize its biological effects. Such neutralizing antibodies have been observed in MS patients treated with all currently approved drugs (Rudick, 2003). However, i.m. administration seems to induce less frequently neutralizing antibodies than the s.c. applied drugs (Bertolotto *et al.*, 2002). The clinical significance of the neutralizing antibodies is still controversial, although it was demonstrated that they may attenuate or abolish the treatment effect (Sorensen *et al.*, 2003). Whether or not the differences in antibody induction between the three IFN-β preparations affects treatment efficacy has been discussed controversially (Durelli *et al.*, 2002; Panitch *et al.*, 2002). Since neutralizing antibodies develop months after initiation of therapy, long-term studies are necessary to clarify whether a less immunogenic IFN-β preparation provides a clinical benefit for the patient in the long run.

Discontinuation of long-term treatment

IFN-β treatment can be abruptly discontinued. However, patients who had stable disease may develop acute relapses following discontinuing of treatment. In these instances, IFN-β or an alternative treatment should be re-established immediately.

Glatiramer acetate (GA, copolymer-1, COP-1)

Glatiramer acetate (GA, copolymer-1, COP-1) is a synthetic basic random copolymer of the four amino acids L-glutamic acid, L-lysine, L-alanine, and L-tyrosine in a molar residue ratio of 0.14:0.34:0.43:0.1. The polypeptides have an average molecular mass of 4700–11 000 kDa. The polypeptide mix-

Table 3.6 Glatiramer acetate

Indications	Multiple sclerosis
Dosage, duration	Subcutaneously, 20 mg/day. Optimal duration of treatment has not been defined
Onset of action	>1 month
Precautions	Studies on carcinogenicity and mutagenicity are ongoing
Lab. pre-check	None
Exclude	Pregnancy, breast feeding
Risk–benefit evaluation	None
Co-medication	None
Lab. follow-up	None
Side-effects	Side-effects in up to 25% of patients: flushing, chest pain, palpitations, anxiety, dyspnea, constriction of the throat, urticaria, anxiety, arthralgia, chest pain, dyspnea, facial edema, hypertonia, injection-site reactions, lymphadenopathy, neck pain, palpitations, vaginal moniliasis, vasodilatation, agitation, bronchitis, chills, confusion, ecchymosis, edema, flu-like syndrome, infection, laryngismus, migraine, pain, peripheral edema, skin nodules, skin rash, syncope, urinary urgency, urticaria, anorexia, back pain, diarrhea, dysmenorrhea or other menstrual changes, ear pain, hematuria, hypertension, hyperventilation, impotence, nystagmus, oral moniliasis, speech problems, suspicious Papanicolaou test, tachycardia, vertigo, and vision problems

ture resembling the composition of myelin basic protein (MBP) was shown to suppress experimental autoimmune encephalomyelitis (EAE) in various animal models (reviewed in Arnon *et al.* (1996)). Competition with myelin antigens for binding to MHC Class II molecules expressed on antigen-presenting cells (APC) has been proposed as a possible mechanism for how GA suppressed EAE (Arnon *et al.*, 1996; Fridkis-Hareli *et al.*, 1999). Since GA consisting of D-amino acids binds as efficiently to MHC Class II molecules but does not suppress EAE, alternative mechanisms of action are more likely to be responsible for its biological activity. Furthermore, due to the peptidase activity in the blood and at the blood–brain barrier, it is unlikely, that intact COP-1 peptides reach the brain.

Repeated subcutaneous 'immunization' with GA induces a population of GA-reactive T cells (Neuhaus *et al.*, 2000; Gran *et al.*, 2000). These cells are characterized by a T-helper-2 phenotype, raising the possibility that they are regulatory cells suppressing disease-associated T cells. It can be postulated that upon recognition of cross-reactive MBP in the CNS, the GA reactive 'suppressor' T cells are activated (or modulated) to exert their down-regulatory functions. Conversely, systemically circulating MBP-reactive T cells might be altered (e.g. down-regulated, 'tolerized', or shifted in cytokine profile) after cross-activation by GA in the periphery. Indeed, there is some evidence that COP-1 peptides can act as 'altered peptide ligands' (APL) or 'T-cell receptor antagonists' on MBP-specific T cells (Gran *et al.*, 2000). However, GA also exerts effects on a variety of other immune cells, among them dendritic cells and macrophages. More recently, it was shown that GA induces immune cells to produce neurotrophic factors (Ziemssen *et al.*, 2002). In some models of acute or chronic neurodegeneration, GA seems to exert neuroprotective activity, which may be mediated by 'neuroprotective' immune cells.

GA was shown to reduce disease activity and MRI activity in relapsing-remitting MS (Johnson *et al.*, 1995). The therapeutic effect is delayed in comparison with interferons, but seems to reach a similar extent after several months (Johnson *et al.*, 1998). Although a variety of mechanisms for how GA influences disease activity have been proposed, the main mechanisms of how the drug ameliorates EAE and particularly MS still remain uncertain.

Management of side-effects

GA is applied subcutaneously every day. In 25% of patients, chest pain, palpitations, anxiety, dyspnea, constriction of the throat, and urticaria occur at initiation of treatment. GA not infrequently induces local inflammation at injection sites, including swelling of local lymph nodes and lipodystrophy. Severe side-effects, however, are extremely rare. Routine laboratory test are not recommended as long as no side-effects occur. GA therapy can be stopped immediately if severe side-effects occur. However, patients who had stable disease may develop acute relapses following discontinuing of treatment. In these cases, GA or an alternative treatment should be re-established immediately.

Intravenous immunoglobulins

Intravenous immunoglobulins (IVIG) have been widely used for therapy of neuroimmunological diseases (Wiles *et al.*, 2002). The exact mode of action of IVIG is still not completely understood. Several early and long-term effects are considered, such as blockade of Fc receptors, neutralization of circulating antibodies, or increased clearance of immune complexes. Which of these potential mechanisms may play a role in the treatment of neurological disease remains speculative.

IVIG are usually given as a cycle of five consecutive days of 0.4 g/kg body weight in *acute* neuromuscular disorders (like Guillain–Barré syndrome). In *chronic* treatment (like for CIDP or multifocal motor neuropathy (MMN)), IVIG are given in regular intervals, e.g., every 6 weeks (or less or more often, depending on the course) and at these intervals the dose should be adjusted according to the clinical course and individual response. In this manner, the dose of IVIG is 'titrated' to the individual need of the patient.

Management of side-effects

Since IVIG are generated from human sera, transmission of infectious particles (viruses, prions) is theoretically possible. However, the third generation of IVIG preparations seems to be highly safe, at least with respect to transmission of relevant viruses such as HIV, HBV, and HCV. Nevertheless, transmission of infectious particles cannot be completely excluded. If fruc-

Table 3.7 Intravenous immunoglobulins

Indications	Myositis, chronic inflammatory demyelinating polyneuropathy (CIDP), Guillain–Barré syndrome (GBS), myasthenia gravis (MG), multifocal motor neuropathy
Dosage, duration	GBS, MG, severe myositis: 0.4 g/kg body weight for 5 days. Multifocal motor neuropathy: 0.4 g/kg body weight every 4–6 weeks. CIDP: 0.4 g/kg body weight for 5 days, 0.4 g/kg body weight every 4–6 weeks
Onset of action	Within days to a few weeks
Precautions	Possible but extremely low risk of transmitting infectious particles
Lab. pre-check	Serum creatinine, urine output, serum IgA
Exclude	Previous anaphylactic reaction to IVIG (IgA deficiencies)
Risk–benefit evaluation	Impairment of cardiac function in seriously ill patients, diabetes mellitus, renal failure, acute, sensitivity to immune globulins, sensitivity to maltose or sucrose, IgA deficiency (use of IVIG with low amount of IgA)
Co-medication	None
Lab. follow-up	Serum creatinine, urine output in patients with pre-existing renal dysfunction
Side-effects	Dyspnea, tachycardia, arthralgia, backache or pain, headache, malaise, myalgia, nausea, vomiting, chest or hip pain, leg cramps, redness, rash, or pain at injection site. Sometimes burning sensation in head, cyanosis, faintness or lightheadedness, fatigue or wheezing is observed. Anaphylactic reaction or renal failure are rarely seen

tose intolerance or diabetes is known in a patient, a choice may be made from various IVIG preparations with different fructose or glucose contents. Generally, IVIG therapy is well tolerated and considered safe. However, there are reports of mild side-effects in 1–15% of patients treated. In addition, occasional severe side-effects including nephrotoxicity have been reported, which must be closely monitored in patients treated with IVIG (Levy and Pusey, 2000).

Before treatment with IVIG, serum creatinine, urine output, and serum immunoglobulin A (IgA) levels have to be determined. Patients with IgA deficiency (incidence about 1:1000) have a 30% risk of having anti-IgA antibodies, resulting in a higher risk of developing acute fulminant serum sickness. IVIG preparations with low IgA content should be used to minimize reactions in patients with hypogammaglobulinemia and concurrent IgA deficiency or when anti-IgA antibodies are present in a recipient.

In general, a slow infusion rate decreases the risk of developing adverse reactions. If severe side-effects occur, IVIG must be stopped and an alternative treatment considered. If necessary, immunomodulatory treatment with IVIG can be continued through pregnancy. Withdrawal effects have not been observed after discontinuation of IVIG therapy.

Invasive immunomodulatory procedures

Plasmapheresis

In the treatment of autoimmune diseases, plasmapheresis aims to remove circulating autoantibodies and inflammatory mediators (Therapeutics and Technology Assessment Subcommittee, 1996). The response to plasmapheresis can be immediate. Likewise, in MG, early clinical effects of plasmapheresis are occasionally observed in less than 24 h. Such immediate improvement is probably due to the specific removal of antigen-specific pathogenetic antibodies (e.g. anti-acetylcholine-receptor antibodies). Often, the effects of plasmapheresis are more delayed and become obvious after several days. This delayed improvement is best explained by the removal of antibodies that act indirectly (e.g. antibodies which fix complement leading to tissue destruction).

During the 1980s, plasmapheresis (therapeutic plasma exchange) was used in many neuroimmunological disorders, in particular in inflammatory neuropathies. However, IVIG has replaced plasmapheresis due to the better tolerability and more convenient and faster application procedures. However, plasmapheresis still has a therapeutic role in patients who do not adequately respond to IVIG or other treatment options. Recently, plasmapheresis has been used in patients with acute steroid-resistant demyelinating diseases of the CNS. A typical plasmapheresis protocol employs three to five exchanges of 1 to 1.5 plasma volumes per week until the patient shows satisfactory improvement. In chronic diseases plasmapheresis is often followed by immunosuppressive treatment (e.g. CTX, AZA).

Management of side-effects

The complications of plasmapheresis include cardiovascular systemic reactions, electrolyte disturbances, and infections. The removal of clotting factors during plasmapheresis results in impairment of hemostasis for about 24 h. Thrombophlebitis, thromboses, pulmonary embolism, and subacute bacterial endocarditis have been observed. All these complications are more frequent in older patients with multiorgan disease. Bacterial respiratory tract infections are a common problem in myasthenic crisis. Immunoglobulin depletion after plasmapheresis may further decrease resistance to infection. Early administration of appropriate antibiotics and IgG/IgM immunoglobulin substitution is therefore recommended in patients who develop infections during or after plasma exchange therapy. Serious infections may occur after plasma exchange in patients who are severely immunocompromised.

As an alternative to standard plasmapheresis, selective immunoadsorption by tryptophan-linked polyvinylalcohol gels has been introduced. In MG, this procedure is as efficient as plasmapheresis (Yeh and Chiu, 2000). Since there is negligible adsorption of albumin, protein substitution is not required.

Thymectomy

Thymectomy is an invasive treatment that is selectively utilized in MG. Although no controlled clinical trial of thymectomy has been performed in MG, it is widely used in the treatment of this disease (Richman and Agius, 2003). Most reports have not shown any correlation between the severity of myasthenic symptoms before surgery and the timing or degree of improvement after surgery. The time to onset of clinical improvement after thymectomy is variable, ranging from weeks to several years. Most studies report better responses when thymectomy is performed early in the disease but the mechanisms which produce benefit in MG are still unknown (Gronseth and Barohn, 2000). Based on the uncontrolled trials a number of rules have been established for the use of thymectomy in MG; thymoma is generally considered an absolute indication for thymectomy. In all other patients, the best results may be expected in patients between 10 and 40 years of age with relatively recent onset of MG (within 3–5 years). Patients with pure ocular myasthenia are usually excluded from thymectomy unless other therapies have proved unsuccessful or generalized symptoms appear. Patients between 1–5 years or older than 60–65 years are usually not thymectomized, except for thymoma (Lanska, 1990).

The most widely performed surgical approach to the thymus is transsternal. A transcervical approach is not recommended because it does not ensure the removal of ectopic thymic tissue that may be widely distributed in the neck and/or mediastinum. When properly performed, thymectomy has a low mortality rate that is essentially that of anesthesia. However, it should be performed in a center with extensive experience and a neuromuscular consultant available. Perhaps as a consequence of the now absent negative selection of T lymphocytes in the thymus that have a high affinity to self-antigens, the occurrence of various autoimmune disorders has been reported after thymectomy. These include aplastic anemia, systemic lupus erythematosus, and Hashimoto thyroiditis.

Future developments

New therapies

Future immunotherapies are based on our current view of the pathogenesis of immune-mediated disease of the nervous system. Although, the target tissue and the quality of the immune response may vary, general principles apply to all immune-mediated diseases (Fig. 3.2). Based on a genetic predisposition, the immune system matures to a state which provides the basis for the deviant immune response. In conjunction with exogenous factors, most probably infections, immune cells become activated in the peripheral immune network. After acquisition of effector functions and escaping the regulatory immune network, the immune cells are able to migrate to the target tissues. Activation of local resident immune cells (e.g. microglia, macrophages in the CNS) is required to allow infiltrating peripheral immune cells to mediate their effector functions. Following the first hit, a chronic uncontrolled immune response emerges which eventually results in destruction of nerve or muscle tissue.

Based on this paradigm, future therapies may be categorized according to their role in the pathogenic cascade of a specific disease, including genetic predisposition, altered immune maturation, activation of the immune response, migration, and activation of the local immune response. More recently, the possibility of using the immune system to deliver anti-inflammatory molecules or even neuroprotection has been discussed as an additional option.

Altering genetic predisposition and immune cell maturation

Since disease genes and susceptibility genes have not been identified in numerous immune-mediated neurological diseases, global alteration of genetic predisposition or immune cell maturation by bone marrow and hematopoetic stem cell transplantation (SCT) would be the only feasible approach to alter these pathogenetic steps (van Bekkum, 2002; Muraro et al., 2003). Advances in transplantation medicine have made it possible to mobilize, isolate, and successfully transplant autologous hematopoetic stem cells. Prior to transplantation, the immune system of the recipient is ablated by aggressive chemotherapy. In the best and most experienced centers, the

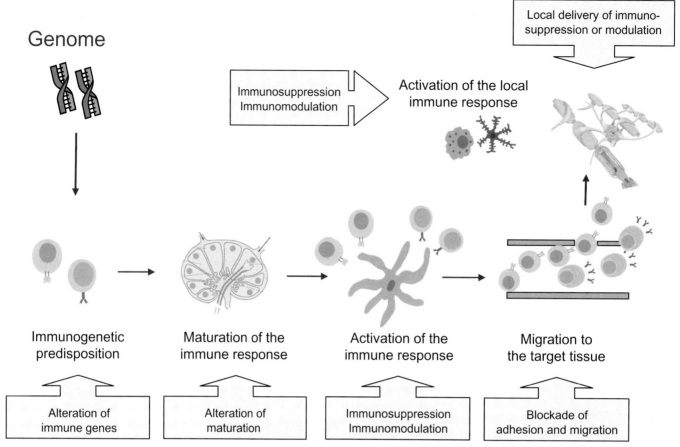

Fig. 3.2 Pathogenetic pathways leading to immune-mediated neurological diseases and possible intervention strategies.

mortality of autologous transplantation is in the range of 5%. Allogeneic transplantation has only been performed in single patients with neuroimmunological diseases and concurrent cancer. Acute lethality of cancer patients with mismatched grafts is in the range of 20–40%. However, the transplantation approach faces not only technical and ethical but also conceptional problems. For example, one report has shown that even after allogenic bone marrow transplant (BMT), MS can exacerbate. This observation may have been due to the fact that despite a complete eradication of encephalitogenic autologous leukocytes, a potential CNS autoantigen persists, and continues to trigger an autoimmune response.

First controlled trials in MS demonstrated that most patients do not progress after therapy, but acute lethality related to therapy ranges between 5 and 10% (Fassas *et al.*, 2002; Burt *et al.*, 2003). SCT and BMT are therefore still considered as experimental procedures and should only be performed within controlled trials (Comi *et al.*, 2000).

Immunosuppression and immunomodulation
During the last decade many new immune therapies have been developed. Besides introducing new immunosuppressive drugs, the aim of most strategies has been a more specific intervention in the immune system. Based in the concept that a pro-inflammatory T-helper-1 response underlies most autoimmune disease of the nervous system, one of the major strategies has been to drive immune responses from a T-helper-1 to a T-helper-2 phenotype, to counteract pro-inflammatory molecules or to selectively inhibit potentially disease-associated immune cells (for details see Chapter 18). Among many others, the most promising drugs that are currently being tested in MS are a humanized anti-interleukin-2 antibody, a B-cell-depleting antibody, and statins (Youssef *et al.*, 2002; Bielekova *et al.*, 2004). All three drugs showed promising results in small pilot trials and are now being tested in large phase II trials in MS (Vollmer *et al.*, 2004). If these drugs succeed in

MS, they may also be promising therapies for other less frequent inflammatory diseases of the nervous system.

Antigen based therapies
Highly selective therapies without global effects on the immune system are considered the optimal choice for immune-intervention therapies in neuroinflammatory diseases. Selective, antigen-specific immunotherapies target the trimolecular complex (TMC) of T-cell stimulation, which is part of the 'immunological synapse'. In principle, each component of the TMC can be targeted. The major histocompatibility (MHC) molecule could be blocked by anti-MHC antibodies or 'blocking peptides'; the antigen (or antigenic peptide) could be applied in such a way that the autoreactive T cells are inhibited rather than stimulated; and the T-cell receptor (TCR) could be targeted with anti-TCR antibodies or by T-cell or TCR peptide vaccination. Although such antigen-selective immunotherapy may seem very promising, it poses a number of special problems. For example, it has been shown that the T-cell response to various candidate CNS autoantigens is much more complex in humans than it is in certain inbred rodent strains (Hemmer *et al.*, 1997). Autoantigens, with a definite pathogenetic role in neuroinflammatory diseases are still largely lacking. Furthermore, there is growing evidence that the autoimmune response is not static but dynamic. For example, the autoimmune response may spread to include new autoantigens over time ('epitope spreading') (Vanderlugt and Miller, 2002). Finally these antigen-based therapies may not only be inefficacious but may also enhance disease activity, as shown for a peptide therapy in MS (Bielekova *et al.*, 2000; Kappos *et al.*, 2000).

Strategies interfering with immune cell migration
Another promising approach is blocking immune cells from migrating into the target tissue. This strategy has also been explored in MS. An anti-

VLA-4 antibody, which blocks migration of immune cells across the blood–brain barrier, has shown prosing results in a phase II trial in MS (Miller *et al.*, 2003). Currently, a large phase III trial is in the process of completion. In parallel, CCR-1, a chemokine receptor, is targeted in another phase II trial. Both drugs may be also promising candidates for the treatment of other neuroinflammatory diseases.

Immune mediated delivery.

Finally, the first experimental strategies have evolved which target the drugs to the local inflammatory environment. These may include specific delivery systems or even immune molecules or cells, which deliver the substances (e.g. neurotrophins, anti-inflammatory drugs) upon recognition of neuronal or myelin antigens (Flugel *et al.*, 2001). Specific delivery may be helpful by enriching the drug at the site of inflammation without generating adverse systemic effects. However, these strategies are currently emerging and are far from clinical application.

Individualized therapy

Besides establishing new treatment strategies and combining approved drugs, individualizing treatment may become an important issue. The technical progress in determining gene polymorphisms, gene transcripts, proteom, and metabolom allows for the monitoring of treatment responses in individual patients. This may eventually identify predictors for treatment responses and side-effects, which may provide a a pharmacotherapy profile for each individual patient. This may provide us with guidelines to select or combine drugs but also with an individual side-effect profile leading to better monitoring of our patients. Overall this may profoundly change our therapeutic strategies in the future.

Acknowledgments

We thank all our MS patients for their continuous support. Bernhard Hemmer is a Heisenberg Fellow of the Deutsche Forschungsgemeinschaft (DFG).

References

Arnon, R., Sela, M., and Teitelbaum, D. (1996). New insights into the mechanism of action of copolymer 1 in experimental allergic encephalomyelitis and multiple sclerosis. *J Neurol* **243**: S8–S13.

Bertolotto, A., Malucchi, S., Sala, A., *et al.* (2002). Differential effects of three interferon betas on neutralising antibodies in patients with multiple sclerosis: a follow up study in an independent laboratory. *J Neurol Neurosurg Psychiatryiat* **73**: 148–153.

Bielekova, B., Goodwin, B., Richert, N., *et al.* (2000). Encephalitogenic potential of the myelin basic protein peptide (amino acids 83–99) in multiple sclerosis: results of a phase II clinical trial with an altered peptide ligand. *Nat Med* **6**: 1167–1175.

Bielekova, B., Richert, N., Howard, T., *et al.* (2004). Humanized anti-CD25 (daclizumab) inhibits disease activity in multiple sclerosis patients failing to respond to interferon beta. *Proc Natl Acad Sci USA* **101**: 8705–8708.

Burt, R.K., Cohen, B A., Russell, E., *et al.* (2003). Hematopoietic stem cell transplantation for progressive multiple sclerosis: failure of a total body irradiation-based conditioning regimen to prevent disease progression in patients with high disability scores. *Blood* **102**: 2373–2378.

Calabresi, P.A., Tranquill, L.R., Dambrosia, J.M., *et al.* (1997). Increases in soluble VCAM-1 correlate with a decrease in MRI lesions in multiple sclerosis treated with interferon beta-1b. *Ann Neurol* **41**: 669–674.

Chaudhry, V., Cornblath, D.R., Griffin, J.W., *et al.* (2001). Mycophenolate mofetil: a safe and promising immunosuppressant in neuromuscular diseases. *Neurology* **56**: 94–96.

Comi, G., Kappos, L., Clanet, M., *et al.* (2000). Guidelines for autologous blood and marrow stem cell transplantation in multiple sclerosis: a consensus report written on behalf of the European Group for Blood and Marrow Transplantation and the European Charcot Foundation. BMT-MS Study Group. *J Neurol* **247**: 376–382.

Darnell, J.E. Jr, Kerr, I.M., and Stark, G.R. (1994) Jak-STAT pathways and transcriptional activation in response to IFNs and other extracellular signaling proteins. *Science* **264**:1415–1421.

Durelli, L., Verdun, E., Barbero, P., *et al.* (2002).Every-other-day interferon beta-1b versus once-weekly interferon beta-1a for multiple sclerosis: results of a 2-year prospective randomised multicentre study (INCOMIN). *Lancet* **359**:1453–1460.

Edan, G., Miller, D., Clanet, M., *et al.* (1997).Therapeutic effect of mitoxantrone combined with methylprednisolone in multiple sclerosis: a randomised multicentre study of active disease using MRI and clinical criteria. *J Neurol Neurosurg Psychiatryiat* **62**: 112–118.

El-Azhary, R.A. (2003). Azathioprine: current status and future considerations. *Int J Dermatol* **42**: 335–341.

Fassas, A., Passweg, J.R., Anagnostopoulos, A., *et al.* (2002). Hematopoietic stem cell transplantation for multiple sclerosis. A retrospective multicenter study. *J Neurol* **249**: 1088–1097.

Flugel, A., Matsumuro, K., Neumann, H., *et al.* (2001). Anti-inflammatory activity of nerve growth factor in experimental autoimmune encephalomyelitis: inhibition of monocyte transendothelial migration. *Eur J Immunol* **31**: 11–22.

Fridkis-Hareli, M., Aharoni, R., Teitelbaum, D., *et al.* (1999). Binding of random copolymers of three amino acids to class II MHC molecules. *Int Immunol* **11**: 635–641.

Ghalie, R.G., Edan, G., Laurent, M., *et al.* (2002*a*). Cardiac adverse effects associated with mitoxantrone (Novantrone) therapy in patients with MS. *Neurology* **59**: 909–913.

Ghalie, R.G., Mauch, E., Edan, G., *et al.* (2002*b*). A study of therapy-related acute leukaemia after mitoxantrone therapy for multiple sclerosis. *Mult Scler* **8**: 441–445.

Gold, R., Buttgereit, F., and Toyka, K. V. (2001). Mechanism of action of glucocorticosteroid hormones: possible implications for therapy of neuroimmunological disorders. *J Neuroimmunol* **117**: 1–8.

Gran, B., Tranquill, L.R., Chen, M., *et al.* (2000). Mechanisms of immunomodulation by glatiramer acetate. *Neurology* **55**: 1704–1714.

Gronseth, G.S. and Barohn, R.J. (2000). Practice parameter: thymectomy for autoimmune myasthenia gravis (an evidence-based review): report of the Quality Standards Subcommittee of the American Academy of Neurology. *Neurology* **55**: 7–15.

Hartung, H.P., Gonsette, R., Konig, N., *et al.* (2002). Mitoxantrone in progressive multiple sclerosis: a placebo-controlled, double-blind, randomised, multicentre trial. *Lancet* **360**: 2018–2025.

Hemmer, B., Vergelli, M., Tranquill, L., *et al.* (1997). Human T-cell response to myelin basic protein peptide (83–99): extensive heterogeneity in antigen recognition, function, and phenotype. *Neurology* **49**: 1116–1126.

Hemmer, B., Archelos, J.J., and Hartung, H.P. (2002). New concepts in the immunopathogenesis of multiple sclerosis. *Nat Rev Neurosci* **3**: 291–301.

IFNB Multiple Sclerosis Study Group (1993). Interferon beta-1b is effective in relapsing–remitting multiple sclerosis. I. Clinical results of a multicenter, randomized, double-blind, placebo-controlled trial. The IFNB Multiple Sclerosis Study Group. *Neurology* **43**: 655–661.

Jacobs, L. and Johnson, K.P. (1994). A brief history of the use of interferons as treatment of multiple sclerosis. *Arch Neurol* **51**: 1245–1252.

Jacobs, L.D., Cookfair, D.L., Rudick, R.A., *et al.* (1996). Intramuscular interferon beta-1a for disease progression in relapsing multiple sclerosis. The Multiple Sclerosis Collaborative Research Group (MSCRG). *Ann Neurol* **39**: 285–294.

Johnson, K.P., Brooks, B.R., Cohen, J.A., *et al.* (1995). Copolymer 1 reduces relapse rate and improves disability in relapsing-remitting multiple sclerosis: results of a phase III multicenter, double-blind placebo-controlled trial. The Copolymer 1 Multiple Sclerosis Study Group. *Neurology* **45**: 1268–1276.

Johnson, K.P., Brooks, B.R., Cohen, J.A., *et al.* (1998). Extended use of glatiramer acetate (Copaxone) is well tolerated and maintains its clinical effect on multiple sclerosis relapse rate and degree of disability. Copolymer 1 Multiple Sclerosis Study Group. *Neurology* **50**: 701–708.

Kappos, L., Comi, G., Panitch, H., *et al.* (2000). Induction of a non-encephalitogenic type 2 T helper-cell autoimmune response in multiple sclerosis after administration of an altered peptide ligand in a placebo-controlled, randomized phase II trial. The Altered Peptide Ligand in Relapsing MS Study

Group. *Nat Med* **6**: 1176–1182.

Kerschensteiner, M., Stadelmann, C., Dechant, G., *et al.* (2003). Neurotrophic cross-talk between the nervous and immune systems: implications for neurological diseases. *Ann Neurol* **53**: 292–304.

King, C., Ilic, A., Koelsch, K., *et al.* (2004). Homeostatic expansion of T cells during immune insufficiency generates autoimmunity. *Cell* **117**: 265–277.

Kohlhuber, F., Rogers, N. C., Watling, D., *et al.* (1997). A JAK1/JAK2 chimera can sustain alpha and gamma interferon responses. *Mol Cell Biol* **17**: 695–706.

Lanska, D.J. (1990). Indications for thymectomy in myasthenia gravis. *Neurology* **40**: 1828–1829.

Leppert, D., Waubant, E., Burk, M.R., *et al.* (1996). Interferon beta-1b inhibits gelatinase secretion and in vitro migration of human T cells: a possible mechanism for treatment efficacy in multiple sclerosis. *Ann Neurol* **40**: 846–852.

Levy, J.B. and Pusey, C.D. (2000). Nephrotoxicity of intravenous immunoglobulin. *Q J Med* **93**: 751–755.

Lipsky, J.J. (1996). Mycophenolate mofetil. *Lancet* **348**: 1357–1359.

Lublin, F.D. and Reingold, S.C. (1998). Combination therapy for treatment of multiple sclerosis. *Ann Neurol* **44**: 7–9.

Miller, D.H., Khan, O.A., Sheremata, W.A., *et al.* (2003). A controlled trial of natalizumab for relapsing multiple sclerosis. *N Engl J Med* **348**: 15–23.

Muraro, P.A., Cassiani, I.R., and Martin, R. (2003). Hematopoietic stem cell transplantation for multiple sclerosis: current status and future challenges. *Curr Opin Neurol* **16**: 299–305.

Neuhaus, O., Farina, C., Yassouridis, A., *et al.* (2000). Multiple sclerosis: comparison of copolymer-1- reactive T cell lines from treated and untreated subjects reveals cytokine shift from T helper 1 to T helper 2 cells. *Proc Natl Acad Sci USA* **97**: 7452–7457.

Panitch, H.S., Hirsch, R.L., Haley, A.S., *et al.* (1987). Exacerbations of multiple sclerosis in patients treated with gamma interferon. *Lancet* **1**: 893–895.

Panitch, H., Goodin, D.S., Francis, G., *et al.* (2002). Randomized, comparative study of interferon beta-1a treatment regimens in MS: the EVIDENCE Trial. *Neurology* **59**: 1496–1506.

PRISMS Study Group (1998). Randomised double-blind placebo-controlled study of interferon beta-1a in relapsing/remitting multiple sclerosis. PRISMS (Prevention of Relapses and Disability by Interferon beta-1a Subcutaneously in Multiple Sclerosis) Study Group. *Lancet* **352**: 1498–1504.

Rep, M.H., Hintzen, R.Q., Polman, C.H., *et al.* (1996). Recombinant interferon-beta blocks proliferation but enhances interleukin-10 secretion by activated human T-cells. *J Neuroimmunol* **67**: 111–118.

Richman, D.P. and Agius, M.A. (2003). Treatment of autoimmune myasthenia gravis. *Neurology* **61**: 1652–1661.

Rudick, R.A. (2003). Biologic impact of interferon antibodies, and complexities in assessing their clinical significance. *Neurology* **61**: S31–S34.

Rudick, R.A., Ransohoff, R.M., Peppler, R., *et al.* (1996). Interferon beta induces interleukin-10 expression: relevance to multiple sclerosis. *Ann Neurol* **40**: 618–627.

Rudick, R.A., Ransohoff, R.M., Lee, J.C., *et al.* (1998). *In vivo* effects of interferon beta-1a on immunosuppressive cytokines in multiple sclerosis. *Neurology* **50**: 1294–1300.

Sorensen, P.S., Ross, C., Clemmesen, K.M., *et al.* (2003). Clinical importance of neutralising antibodies against interferon beta in patients with relapsing-remitting multiple sclerosis. *Lancet* **362**: 1184–1191.

Steiner, J.P., Connolly, M.A., Valentine, H.L., *et al.* (1997). Neurotrophic actions of nonimmunosuppressive analogues of immunosuppressive drugs FK506, rapamycin and cyclosporin A. *Nat Med* **3**: 421–428.

Stuve, O., Dooley, N.P., Uhm, J.H., *et al.* (1996). Interferon beta-1b decreases the migration of T lymphocytes in vitro: effects on matrix metalloproteinase-9. *Ann Neurol* **40**: 853–863.

Therapeutics and Technology Assessment Subcommittee (1996). Assessment of plasmapheresis. Report of the Therapeutics and Technology Assessment Subcommittee of the American Academy of Neurology. *Neurology* **47**: 840–843.

Tindall, R.S., Phillips, J.T., Rollins, J.A., *et al.* (1993). A clinical therapeutic trial of cyclosporine in myasthenia gravis. *Ann NY Acad Sci* **681**: 539–551.

van Bekkum, D.W. (2002). Experimental basis of hematopoietic stem cell transplantation for treatment of autoimmune diseases. *J Leukocyte Biol* **72**: 609–620.

Vanderlugt, C.L. and Miller S.D. (2002). Epitope spreading in immune-mediated diseases: Implications for immunotherapy. *Nat Rev Immunol* **2**: 85–95.

Vollmer, T., Key, L., Durkalski, V., *et al.* (2004). Oral simvastatin treatment in relapsing-remitting multiple sclerosis. *Lancet* **363**: 1607–1608.

Weber, F., Janovskaja, J., Polak, T., *et al.* (1999). Effect of interferon beta on human myelin basic protein-specific T-cell lines: comparison of IFNbeta-1a and IFNbeta-1b. *Neurology* **52**: 1069–1071.

Wiles, C.M., Brown, P., Chapel, H., *et al.* (2002). Intravenous immunoglobulin in neurological disease: a specialist review. *J Neurol Neurosurg Psychiatryiat* **72**: 440–448.

Yeh, J.H. and Chiu, H.C. (2000). Comparison between double-filtration plasmapheresis and immunoadsorption plasmapheresis in the treatment of patients with myasthenia gravis. *J Neurol* **247**: 510–513.

Youssef, S., Stuve, O., Patarroyo, J.C., *et al.* (2002). The HMG-CoA reductase inhibitor, atorvastatin, promotes a Th2 bias and reverses paralysis in central nervous system autoimmune disease. *Nature* **420**: 78–84.

Ziemssen, T., Kumpfel, T., Klinkert, W.E., *et al.* (2002). Glatiramer acetate-specific T-helper 1- and 2-type cell lines produce BDNF: implications for multiple sclerosis therapy. Brain-derived neurotrophic factor. *Brain* **125**: 2381–2391.

4 Organization and development of the central nervous system

Matthew J. A. Wood

The brain serves diverse yet precise functions that are built on neural networks connecting its various parts. Each region of the brain is highly specialized both in its architecture and the specific types of differentiated cells that it contains. The nervous system develops from an epithelial cell sheet, the neural plate, which folds to form the neural tube. This tube is patterned along its length in a region-specific fashion to generate the major early brain regions of spinal cord, hindbrain, midbrain, and forebrain. Within the tube, neural stem cells undergo differentiation into region-specific populations of neurons, for example the principal neurons of the ventral spinal cord (motor neurons), cerebellum (Purkinje neurons), striatum (medium spiny striatal neurons), and hippocampus (pyramidal neurons). In this way, distinct region-specific neural circuits are generated that underpin the functional characteristics of each brain area. Thus the highly complex and specialized structure and function of the developed adult brain has its origins in early embryonic patterning and development of the nervous system.

Introduction

The mammalian nervous system is structurally and functionally complex. It comprises both central and peripheral nervous systems and is divided functionally into somatic and autonomic components. The structural organization of the nervous system is central to its function, arguably more so than for any other organ system. At the heart of the cellular organization of the nervous system is its development. Recent knowledge concerning nervous system stem cells, the regulation of cell diversity, and patterning of the developing brain structure, provides a theoretical framework for understanding higher-level organization in the developed adult brain. Moreover, development does not just take place in the embryo. The system develops throughout life in response to environmental and activity-dependent stimuli. Certain critical parts of the developmental programme are still active in the adult system, for example plasticity at synapses and a limited capacity to generate new central neurons.

The central nervous system (CNS) arises from the neural plate, a cytologically homogeneous group of neuroepithelial cells that form the dorsal surface of the early embryo. The peripheral nervous system arises from neural crest cells generated at the lateral edges of this plate. The neural plate subsequently invaginates and folds along its anteroposterior axis to form a tube, the expanded anterior or rostral end of which forms a series of brain vesicles representing the precursor regions of hindbrain, midbrain, and forebrain. Caudally, the tube forms the spinal cord. These early morphological features of the neural axis, accompanied by position-specific expression of developmental control genes, dictate the overall topographical plan of the CNS and predict its later regional organization. Within each region (spinal cord, hindbrain, midbrain, forebrain), a diversity of neuronal cell types is generated, each with distinct identities in terms of morphology, axon connectivity, synaptic specificity, neurotransmitters, etc. In this way the ordered spatial arrangement of populations of differentiated neurons, essential to the subsequent formation of functional neural circuits, is crucially dependent on successful early regional specification (Wolpert *et al.*, 1998; Jessell and Sanes, 2000; Sadler, 2004).

Formation of the early nervous system— neurulation

In mammalian development, following fertilization and implantation of the blastocyst, cells of the inner cell mass (comprising embryonic stem cells) differentiate into two distinct layers known as the hypoblast and epiblast, forming the *bilaminar germ disc*. This is a prelude to an early embryonic process known as gastrulation, during which this bilaminar disc generates the three embryonic germ layers, *ectoderm*, *mesoderm*, and *endoderm*, of the *trilaminar germ disc*. The development of the nervous system has its origins in this trilaminar disc.

During this very early phase of development the body axes are established, leading to the formation of head and tail structures. This is regulated by signals originating from organizing centres in the primitive streak and node, a structure first identified in *Xenopus* embryos by Spemann and Mangold (1924) as a region with special organizing properties. Within the early embryo an essential early step in neural development is the mapping of a region of ectoderm, called the *neural plate*, as the precursor of the entire nervous system. The process of *neurulation* converts this neural plate into a *neural tube*, which folds and then fuses and closes. The neural tube is subsequently regionalized to form a succession of expansions or vesicles that constitute the embryonic precursors of the major brain regions, *hindbrain*, *midbrain*, and *forebrain*. As neural development continues, a number of transverse constrictions further subdivide the brain into distinct neuronal segments. Thus this very early brain patterning plays an important role in the initiation and formation of region-specific neuronal networks (Weinstein and Hemmati-Brivanlou, 1999).

The generation of cell diversity in the nervous system—neurogenesis

Neurogenesis, the generation of neurons of the nervous system, arises from a population of neuroepithelial stem cells lining the neural tube. Following neurogenesis, newly generated neuron cells migrate towards their final topographical positions within designated neural segments, undergo a functional selection process in which many developing cells die by apoptosis, extend their processes—one of which becomes the functional nerve axon, and finally form synaptic contacts with nerve cells in defined neural networks. The process of neurogenesis also gives rise to the endogenous *glial cell* population of the nervous system, specifically to astrocytes and oligodendrocytes. In the latter stages of development another class of supporting glial cell is also found in the nervous system, the microglial cell. This cell migrates into the developing nervous system from its origins in haematopoietic tissue, and has important immunological properties.

Following studies in *Drosophila* and other organisms, a highly conserved *molecular programme of neurogenesis* is now known to exist. Early work identified a set of neurogenic regulatory genes (with resemblance to similar gene families regulating the development of skeletal muscle, for example), the loss of which results in the generation of excess neurons at the expense of supporting cells. These studies also led to the idea that the selection of the neuronal cell fate depended on intercellular signalling between adjacent cells. Molecular studies showed that these neurogenic genes encode components of this signalling pathway, and include the membrane-associated ligands Delta and Serrate, and their transmembrane receptor, Notch. Activation of Notch signalling biases cells towards non-neural fates whereas inhibition of Notch signalling promotes neuronal differentiation. It is now clear that the Notch signalling pathway is highly conserved and also controls neurogenesis in vertebrates (Lewis, 1996). How is this process of neurogenesis regulated at the transcriptional level? Two classes of transcription factors, the bHLH and LIM-HD transcription factor families, function at different stages of neurogenesis to synchronize neurogenesis with neuronal subtype specification (Allan and Thor, 2003).

Neural stem cells exist not only in the developing nervous system but also in the adult nervous system of all mammalian organisms. Neural stem cells can also be derived from more primitive embryonic stem cells. The precise topographical location of these adult stem cells, the migratory pathways of their progeny, the adult brain regions populated by these new cells, and how these processes are regulated are all currently subjects of intense study. In mammals it is thought that new neurons are added to a restricted number of brain regions, including the olfactory bulb, hippocampus, and possibly other regions. However, it is well known that neurons are added to many brain regions in adult non-mammalian vertebrates. In mammals, neurogenesis in the adult has so far been found to occur in two restricted locations: the subventricular zone of the lateral ventricles, which generates olfactory bulb neurons, and directly in the hippocampus (Cameron and McKay, 1998; Gage, 2000, 2002).

The prevailing model of neural development suggests that the neuronal and glial lineages diverge early, with neural stem cells giving rise to neuron-restricted and glial-restricted progenitor cells. *Glia*, comprising both macroglia and microglia, are the most numerous class of cells in the brain. Microglia have important developmental and phagocytic roles in the brain, whilst macroglia include both oligodendrocytes and astrocytes. Oligodendrocytes are myelin-forming cells that allow the rapid conduction of neuronal impulses along axons and are lost in demyelinating diseases such as multiple sclerosis. Astrocytes are star-shaped cells that provide important structural, metabolic, and trophic support to neurons. They interact with endothelial cells to form the blood–brain barrier, regulate re-uptake of neurotransmitters, maintain extracellular ion homeostasis, and secrete growth factors, cytokines, and components of the extracellular matrix. Astrocytes are further involved in the formation and stabilization of synapses and the modulation of synaptic efficacy. They also underlie the pathological states of reactive gliosis and glial scar formation that accompany brain injury (Doetsch, 2003).

Organization and patterning of the neural tube

The spatial ordering of differentiated populations of neurons within the adult brain, critical to the formation of functional neural circuits, is dependent on correct early regional specification. The early pattern that emerges at the end of gastrulation is progressively refined, resulting in a precise regional organization of neural cell identity. This neural patterning appears to be organized on a pattern resembling a two-dimensional Cartesian grid of positional information. In the 1940s and 1950s, experimental embryological studies suggested that cells in the developing neural tube gain positional identity as a consequence of spatial information derived from the two major neural axes, anteroposterior and dorsoventral. This model suggests that the spatial identity of a cell is determined as a result of exposure to regionally restricted signalling factors operating along these two neural axes. A range of neural cell groups in the developing neural tube, including those of the floor plate and roof plate of the developing spinal cord, and the isthmus of the developing hindbrain, have been identified as key sources of secreted signalling factors that help to establish this regional pattern. Moreover, a relatively small number of families of signalling factors account for many features of regional patterning within the neural tube (Jessell and Sanes, 2000; Tanabe and Jessell, 1996).

As the longitudinal neural tube develops it initially shows three expansions or primary brain vesicles: the *rhombencephalon* or *hindbrain*; the *mesencephalon* or *midbrain*, and the *prosencephalon* or *forebrain*. Subsequently the rhombencephalon divides into metencephalon and myelencephalon, the former giving rise to the pons and cerebellum, while the prosencephalon divides into diencephalon and telencephalon, the latter forming the cerebral hemispheres (Fig. 4.1). During early folding of the neural plate a group of cells emerges at the edge of these neural folds, known as the *neural crest cells*. These are ectodermal in origin and emerge along the anteroposterior length of the neural tube. These cells have migratory properties and give rise to all cells of the peripheral nervous system, including the sensory or dorsal root ganglia, and a range of other cells including melanocytes, and the mesenchyme of the pharyngeal arches, important for craniofacial development.

Spinal cord organization and motor neuron development

The caudal region of the developing neural tube is organized and patterned to form the *spinal cord*. In this region, the inner layer of the neural tube, comprising the differentiating neural stem cells and developing neuroblasts,

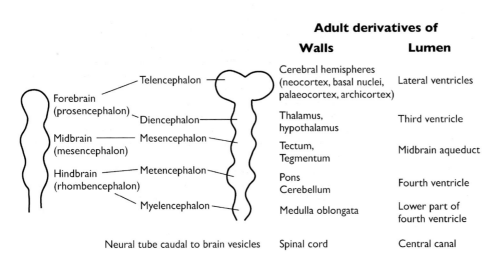

	Adult derivatives of	
	Walls	**Lumen**
Forebrain (prosencephalon) — Telencephalon	Cerebral hemispheres (neocortex, basal nuclei, palaeocortex, archicortex)	Lateral ventricles
Forebrain (prosencephalon) — Diencephalon	Thalamus, hypothalamus	Third ventricle
Midbrain (mesencephalon) — Mesencephalon	Tectum, Tegmentum	Midbrain aqueduct
Hindbrain (rhombencephalon) — Metencephalon	Pons Cerebellum	Fourth ventricle
— Myelencephalon	Medulla oblongata	Lower part of fourth ventricle
Neural tube caudal to brain vesicles	Spinal cord	Central canal

Fig. 4.1 Neural tube and brain vesicles. Schematic illustration of the embryonic brain vesicles showing their relationship to various adult nervous system derivatives. The primary brain vesicles of prosencephalon, mesencephalon, and rhombencephalon give rise to regionally patterned areas of the nervous system as well as distinct components of the ventricular system of the brain.

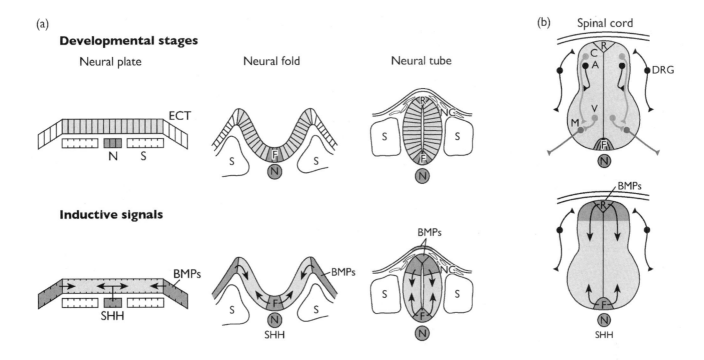

Fig. 4.2 Spinal cord and motor neuron patterning. (a) Stages in the embryonic development of the spinal cord: the neural plate is a columnar epithelium closely related to the notochord (N) and somites (S). The neural tube forms by fusion of the neural folds. Also shown are the sources of ventralizing (Sonic Hedgehog (Shh)) and dorsalizing (BMPs) inductive signals at stages of spinal cord development. (b) Schematic figure showing differentiated spinal cord neurons located at different dorsoventral positions. Subclasses of commissural (C) and association (A) neurons differentiate dorsally, whereas motor neurons (M) and ventral interneurons (V) differentiate ventrally. Dorsal root ganglion (DRG) neurons are generated from neural crest cells. (From Tanabe and Jessell (1996).)

is known as the mantle layer, while the outer layer, containing the emerging axonal processes of theses cells, is known as the marginal layer. Eventually, as a result of myelination of these axon fibres, this layer takes on a white appearance and is called the white matter of the spinal cord. The inner layer of the developing spinal cord, the mantle layer, develops ventral and dorsal expansions resulting from rapid cell proliferation within the neural stem cell layer, to form the *basal* and *alar plates* respectively and a longitudinal groove, the *sulcus limitans*, marking the boundary between the two (Fig. 4.2). The dorsal and ventral midline portions of the neural tube are known as the *roof plate* and *floor plate* respectively. Within the ventral basal plate the developing neural stem cells undergo differentiation into ventral horn motor neurons.

Within the developed spinal cord three major classes of neuronal elements can be defined:

(1) neurons that carry sensory information into the spinal cord (primary afferents, whose cell bodies lie outside the spinal cord in dorsal root ganglia);

(2) neurons whose axons exit the spinal cord to innervate skeletal muscle (somatic motor neurons) or autonomic ganglia (pre-ganglionic autonomic neurons); and

(3) neurons whose axons terminate within the CNS, either locally (interneurons) or at higher levels.

As already outlined, unlike the rest of the CNS, the outer white matter of the spinal cord contains the axons of neurons in parallel to the long axis of the spinal cord itself. Within this, the grey matter, containing the cell bodies of spinal neurons, is organized into two functional regions, the dorsal and

ventral horns, which on the basis of cytoarchitectural characteristics is classically subdivided into layers I through to X (Fig. 4.3) (Shepherd, 1990).

Motor neuron development

Motor neurons are the only CNS neurons that make synaptic contacts on non-neural tissue, i.e. skeletal muscle fibres, and have a precise functional role which is to activate muscle. Motor neuron cell bodies lie within the ventral grey matter of the spinal cord and within certain brainstem cranial nerve nuclei. Motor neurons that innervate a given muscle are aggregated together in circumscribed motor nuclei extending along the anteroposterior axis of the ventral horn of the spinal cord. The process of development of this neuronal population is one of the best characterized in the nervous system at present. In general, the organization of neurons in the developing CNS proceeds along two major schemes first appreciated by Cajal in the late 19th century (Ramon y Cajal, 1894). In some regions of the CNS, such as cerebral cortex and dorsal spinal cord, neurons are organized in a stratified pattern (Rexed, 1952). However, the most prevalent mode of neuronal organization is based on nuclear subdivisions (Ramon y Cajal, 1911), i.e. neurons with similar structures, connectivities, and functional properties are clustered into discrete regions or nuclei. Such nuclear organization of neurons is prominent in the ventral spinal cord.

Two independent signalling systems function to control the regional fate of induced neural cells along the neural axis. One system controls pattern along the anteroposterior axis and sets up regional subdivisions of the neural tube that lead to formation of the forebrain, midbrain, hindbrain, and spinal cord. A second signalling system patterns the neural tube along its dorsoventral axis. Within the developing spinal cord, patterning of the early neural tube along

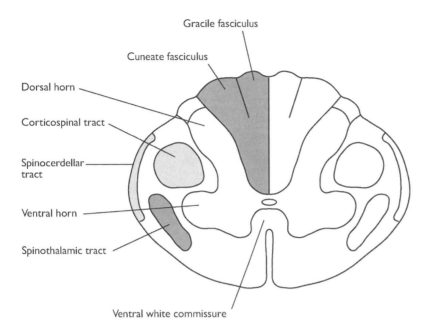

Gracile fasciculus

Cuneate fasciculus

Dorsal horn

Corticospinal tract

Spinocerdellar tract

Ventral horn

Spinothalamic tract

Ventral white commissure

Fig. 4.3 Spinal cord structure. Cross-sectional view of the spinal cord showing the structural arrangement with central grey matter, comprising ventral and dorsal horns, and outer white matter comprising ascending and descending spinal pathways. On the right hand side is indicated the types of motor and/or sensory function compromised as a result of lesions to these pathways

these axes is relatively well understood. It depends on the relative balance of secreted dorsalizing factors of the bone morphogenetic protein (BMP) family, which arise from non-neural ectoderm, and ventralizing factors of the sonic hedgehog (Shh) family, produced by the notochord (a mesodermal derivative and precursor of the axial skeleton of the embryo) and the floor plate. Shh is a member of a family of secreted proteins identified initially by their structural similarity to the *Drosophila* segment polarity gene Hedgehog. Mis-expression of Shh can induce floor plate differentiation *in vivo*, and recombinant Shh can induce floor plate cells and motor neurons in neural plate explants. Shh therefore ventralizes the neural tube; this ventral region then acquires the capacity to form the floor plate and motor neurons (Tanabe and Jessell, 1996).

Following motor neuron differentiation, functional subsets of motor neurons are clustered into groups known as motor columns or pools. Motor pools have been linked to three important features of motor system organization; first, all neurons within a given motor pool have common connectivities, projecting to a single muscle target; second, all receive monosynaptic input from sensory neurons that supply the same muscle target; and third, neurons within a designated motor pool are electrically coupled (Price *et al.*, 2002).

Axon guidance in the spinal cord

Following the specification, differentiation, and patterning of ventral horn motor neurons they extend their axons to ultimately reach their targets on skeletal muscle. The correct navigation of axons to their targets is essential for the formation of functional neuronal circuits. Current models of axon guidance suggest that axons are guided to their synaptic targets by a complex interaction of attractive and repulsive signals. Highly conserved families of guidance molecules including netrins, slits, semaphorins, and ephrins have been discovered in recent years. Such extracellular guidance signals direct developing axons by regulating the cytoskeletal dynamics in the growth cone. As a result of its relatively simple neuronal organization and neural circuitry, the spinal cord has helped to identify the roles of such guidance molecules; for example, attractive signals such as netrin-1 and repulsive signals such as semaphorins and slit are known to regulate the pattern of axonal projections in the spinal cord (Dickson, 2002; Salinas, 2003).

Synaptogenesis and neuromuscular junction development

The brain consists of a vast network of neurons that communicate with each other through specialized cell junctions called synapses. During synap-

togenesis, synapses form, mature, and stabilize and some are also eliminated. Synapses are an absolute requirement for neuronal signalling, and also undergo long-term modifications that are believed to underlie information storage (learning and memory) in the adult brain, known as synaptic plasticity (Cohen-Cory, 2002; Li and Sheng, 2003).

Most of our understanding of synaptogenesis comes from studies of the neuromuscular junction (NMJ), the synapse between motor neurons and skeletal muscle. Biochemical studies have identified the important molecular components of and pathways that establish this synapse. The most important pathway starts with the synthesis and secretion by the pre-synaptic motor nerve terminal of the extracellular matrix protein agrin. Agrin activates a receptor tyrosine kinase on skeletal muscle known as muscle-specific kinase (MuSK) that results in clustering at the developing NMJ of nascent acetylcholine receptors and other critical synaptic proteins. There is also a process of molecular feedback from the post-synaptic structures to the pre-synaptic motor nerve terminal that leads to further pre-synaptic differentiation (Hoch, 2003).

Hindbrain development and the cerebellum

The *rhombencephalon* or *hindbrain* consists of the myelencephalon caudally and the metencephalon; the former giving rise to the medulla and the latter the pons and cerebellum. Both regions, in common with the spinal cord, are characterized by the presence of basal and alar plates, the former giving rise to motor structures and the latter to sensory structures. Each basal plate contains three groups of motor neurons which give rise to a range of cranial nerve structures, while the alar plates comprise groups of sensory structures that give rise to sensory components of cranial nerves.

Along its length, the neural tube develops into different regions by a process known as patterning. One of the regions in which this regionalization or anteroposterior patterning is best understood is the developing hindbrain. During early development, the hindbrain is transiently partitioned into seven transverse neuroepithelial segments called rhombomeres, each of which adopts a distinct set of molecular and cellular properties, restricts local cell mixing, acquires ordered domains of Hox gene expression, and is the forerunner of specific hindbrain structures (Lumsden and Krumlauf, 1996). Not only do rhombomeres give rise to well-defined regions of the adult brain, but their segmental organization is also critical for the development of cranial nerve ganglia and branchiomotor nerves and pathways of neural crest cell migration (Fig. 4.4).

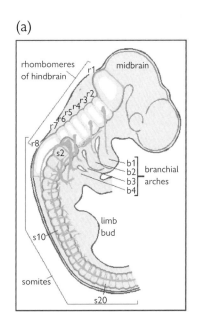

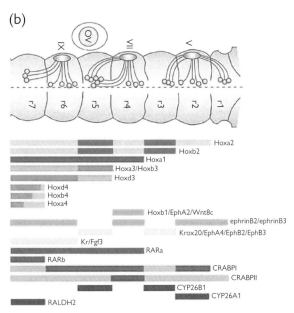

Fig. 4.4 Hindbrain patterning and rhombomeres. (a) The location of the hindbrain and rhombomeres is shown within the developing embryo illustrating their relationship to the developing branchial arches. (b) Map of the hindbrain showing segmentation into seven cell lineage restricted units called rhombomeres which influence subsequent hindbrain patterning. Domains of Hox gene expression are shown and there is a clear spatial distribution of the cranial nerves (V, trigeminal; VII, facial: IX, glossopharyngeal). From Trainor and Krumlauf (2000).

Differential gene expression gives rise to patterning within the developing hindbrain by conferring positional information along its anteroposterior axis, determining the identity of individual rhombomeres, and specifying their derivatives. Evidence shows that the Hox genes themselves, as in other tissues, are responsible for conferring anteroposterior identity of rhombomeric segments. These are the clustered homeobox-containing genes of the Hox family, homologues of the genes that encode parasegment identity in *Drosophila*. The Hox gene expression pattern forms an ordered set of domains along the neural axis, with rhombomere-specific variations in expression levels (Trainor and Krumlauf, 2000).

The cerebellum

The cerebellum represents 10% of the brain's total volume, but contains more than 50% of its neurons. It has undergone enormous elaboration during evolution, and yet strikingly its initial neuronal structure has remained almost invariant during this process. Thus its size rather than its internal circuitry has changed during evolution. It acts as a coordination centre, using sensory inputs from the periphery to fine-tune movement and balance.

It is one of the first structures in the brain to begin to differentiate, developing from the rostral end of the hindbrain near the midbrain junction. The hindbrain is separated from the midbrain by a constriction or isthmus at the mid/hindbrain junction, and is divided into the rostral metencephalon and the caudal myelencephalon. The metencephalon consists of rhombomere 1, which gives rise to the cerebellum and pons, and rhombomere 2. The patterning of the midbrain/hindbrain junction depends on signals from an organizer region in rhombomere 1 near the isthmus. The transcription factors Otx2 and Gbx2 are central to development of this region. Otx2 is expressed in the mesencephalon while Gbx2 is expressed in the metencephalon. Many other genes, including members of the Pax and Hox families, are also involved in patterning this region (Liu and Joyner, 2001; Wang and Zoghbi, 2001).

The cerebellum develops from the dorsal region of the posterior neural tube which gives rise to the midline cerebellar vermis and lateral cerebellar hemispheres. Most cells in the cerebellum arise from the ventricular zone of the neural tube, and migrate laterally to form the deep cerebellar nuclei and *Purkinje cells* of the *cerebellar cortex*. Purkinje cells continue their maturation after birth, projecting to the deep *cerebellar nuclei* and refining the input they receive from the climbing fibres of inferior olivary neurons. Also arising from the ventricular zone is a third population of neurons including the stellate, basket, and Golgi interneurons that can be found in the molecular layer, and which have a modulatory action on the Purkinje cells and cerebellar granule neurons. The latter, unlike the other cell types of the cerebellum, arise from a specialized germinal matrix called the rhombic lip and form the granule cell layer of the cerebellum.

The basic functional operation of the cerebellum involves an interaction between two distinct neuronal elements, those of the cerebellar cortex and those of the deep cerebellar nuclei. The cerebellar cortex (arranged into molecular, Purkinje, and granule cell layers) receives afferent fibres of two types, climbing and mossy fibres (Ramon y Cajal, 1911). Climbing fibres arise from a single brainstem nucleus, the inferior olive. In contrast the mossy fibres have multiple CNS origins, including vestibular nuclei and spinal cord. The deep cerebellar nuclei receive collaterals from these afferent fibres and are the main target of the single output pathway via the axons of Purkinje cells. The basic cerebellar circuit contains only one intrinsic excitatory neuron, the granule cell. This basic circuit is augmented by three types of inhibitory interneurons, the Golgi cells of the granule cell layer, and the basket and stellate cells of the molecular layer (Fig. 4.5).

Midbrain organization and the substantia nigra

In the *mesencephalon* or *midbrain* the basal plates contribute to two groups of motor nuclei giving rise to cranial nerves that control oculomotor functions. Also within the midbrain is located the *substantia nigra*, a neuronal nucleus that is functionally part of the basal ganglia but that comprises the dopaminergic (DA) neurons that degenerate in Parkinson's disease (PD). The substantia nigra is comprised of anatomically distinct regions, the pars compacta and pars reticulata, the former comprising the DA cell population which gives rise to the nigrostriatal pathway in the basal ganglia (see below), that plays an important role in the regulation of neural activity in the striatum (Fig. 4.6).

The mesencephalic DA system is the largest DA system. Although DA cells form a continuous group, they are classically subdivided into three cell groups: A8, A9 and A10. A10 cells are located in the ventral tegmental area (VTA), which is the ventromedial-most region of the midbrain. A9 neurons are located in the substantia nigra, which is continuous medially with the VTA. Most neurons of the A9 group are found in the substantia nigra pars compacta (SNc).

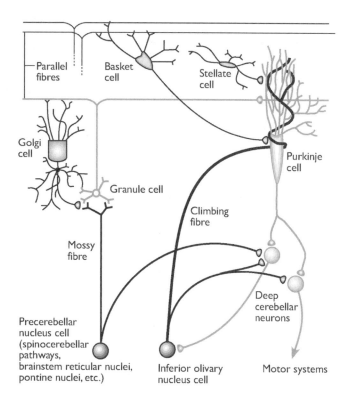

Fig. 4.5 The cerebellum and its circuitry. Schematic diagram showing principal neurons of the cerebellum and their connections. Afferent input to the cerebellum arises from mossy fibres and climbing fibres, the latter originate in the inferior olivary nucleus and form multiple synapses with each Purkinje cell. The axons of cerebellar granule cells also form *en passant* synapses with Purkinje cells. The Purkinje neurons are the primary output neurons of the cerebellar cortex. (From Wang and Zoghbi (2001).)

(a)

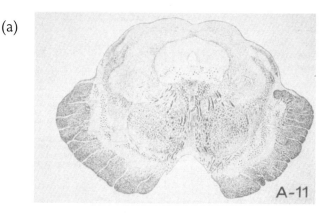

(b)

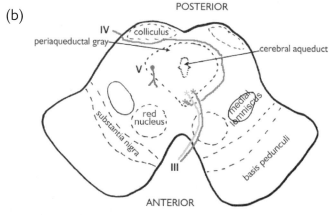

Fig. 4.6 The midbrain. (a) Histological view of the rostral midbrain as revealed by Nissl and myelin stains. (b) Schematic cross-sectional view of the midbrain. Major nuclei are shown, including the substantia nigra and the red nucleus, as are major fibre tracts and cranial nerves (oculomotor, trochlear, and trigeminal).

As a result, the importance of this DA population and also of progress in the development of cell transplantation for PD, much progress has been made in understanding the neurogenesis of this cell population. Recently it has proven possible to recapitulate the cell fate decisions that are made in this region of the midbrain by efficiently generating midbrain DA neurons from embryonic stem cells *in vitro* (Lee *et al.*, 2000). This provides a model system in which this differentiation pathway and the molecular factors involved in regulation of the development of this cell type can be studied further. Moreover, such neurons generated *ex vivo* have been shown to function appropriately in an animal model of PD suggesting that successful molecular and functional programming has been achieved (Kim *et al.*, 2002).

Development and organization of the forebrain

The *prosencephalon* or *forebrain* comprises the telencephalon, that gives rise to the cerebral hemispheres, and the diencephalon. The most caudal part of the diencephalon develops into the pineal body or epithalamus, while the remainder develops into the thalamus and hypothalamus. The vertebrate forebrain is derived from the anterior neural plate, where anteroposterior and dorsoventral patterning mechanisms specify regional identity. Understanding the molecular regulation of these processes will help to elucidate how the major forebrain regions (i.e. the cerebral cortex, basal ganglia, thalamus, and hypothalamus) are formed, and how molecular defects can lead to congenital abnormalities.

Hypothalamus

The hypothalamus, part of the ventral diencephalon, is the major higher centre *regulating autonomic and endocrine activity*. Endocrine regulation is mediated by its intimate relationship to both anterior and posterior parts of the pituitary gland, the former indirectly via the hypothalamic–pituitary portal vascular system, and the latter via direct neuronal connections. The hypothalamus comprises a bilaterally symmetrical collection of *distinct nuclei* within medial and lateral zones, situated on either side of the midline third ventricle in the mammal. Each of these nuclei can be distinguished on the basis of their cellular architecture, neuronal connections, and functional properties (Fig. 4.7).

The hypothalamus and the anterior pituitary gland develop from distinct regions of anterior ectoderm, with classical embryological experiments indicating that development of the anterior pituitary depends on inductive signals from the diencephalon. Most of the hypothalamus appears to arise from the neuroepithelium ventral to the hypothalamic sulcus. Early on periventricular neurosecretory cells become organized into several nuclei including the paraventricular (PVH), supraoptic (SON), arcuate, and periventricular nuclei (PVN). Within the hypothalamus, two separate neurosecretory systems arise. One comprising *magnocellular* neurons projects directly into the posterior part of the pituitary gland, and includes neurons of the PVH and SON that synthesize oxytocin and vasopressin. The other comprises *parvocellular* neurons that synthesize neuropeptides released into the pituitary portal circulation for regulation of the anterior pituitary gland. In addition to the magnocellular neurons, the PVH also contains parvocellular neurons that synthesize corticotrophin-releasing hormone and thyrotrophin-releasing hormone for regulating the ACTH/

(a)

(b)

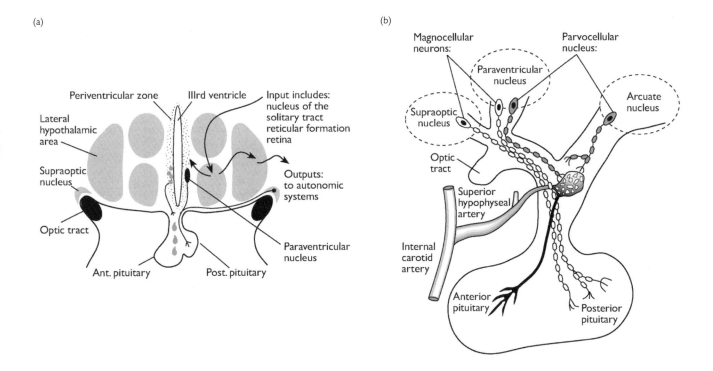

Fig. 4.7 Structure and organization of the hypothalamus. (a) Schematic view in coronal section of the structural organization of the hypothalamus, showing relationships between hypothalamic nuclei in lateral and medial zones and the third ventricle, optic tracts, and pituitary gland. (b) Schematic view of the hypothalamo-pituitary axis illustrating magnocellular neurons located in the supraoptic nucleus and paraventricular nucleus which project their axons directly into the posterior lobe of the pituitary gland. In contrast, parvocelluar neurons, located in several nuclei, including the paraventricular and arcuate nuclei, project their axons to the median eminence, and thence via the pituitary portal circulation into the anterior pituitary gland. (From Andersen and Rosenfeld *Endocrine Rev* **22**: 2–35 (2001).)

adrenal axis and the TSH/thyroid axis, respectively. In the anterior periventricular and arcuate nuclei are parvocellular neurons that provide dopaminergic control of lactotrophs, and somatostatin/growth hormone-releasing hormone control of somatotrophs in the anterior pituitary. Gonadotrophin-releasing hormone neurons originate in the olfactory placode and migrate during embryonic development to reach the pre-optic area of the hypothalamus (Schwanzel-Fukuda and Pfaff, 1989), and regulate synthesis of follicle-stimulating hormone and luteinizing hormone in the anterior pituitary gland and thereby the reproductive system.

The importance of the hypothalamus in interacting with the immune system, and the mechanisms by which the immune system act on hypothalamic function, are discussed in detail in Chapter 7.

Recently, a discrete number of cells in the lateral hypothalamus that contain the neuropeptides orexin A and B (also called hypocretins 1 and 2) have been identified. Absence of orexin seems to be the hallmark of patients with narcolepsy and cataplexy, and loss of the orexin-containing cells has been demonstrated in a few post-mortem studies. Narcolepsy has long been considered to be an autoimmune disease because of the very high association with DQ0602, but how the loss of the orexin-containing neurons occurs and whether the immune system is directly involved, is still unclear (see Taheri *et al.* (2002) for a recent review).

Telencephalon

The *telencephalon* or *rostral forebrain* is the most rostral of the brain vesicles, and gives rise to the primitive cerebral hemispheres. The cavities of these hemispheres comprise the lateral ventricles, the most proximal part of the ventricular system of the developed nervous system. In addition to neocortical and paleocortical regions (such as the hippocampus), the tel-

encephalon also generates subcortical structures, in particular a collection of subcortical nuclei known as the basal ganglia.

The basal ganglia

The basal ganglia consist of a collection of *interconnected subcortical nuclei*, namely, the striatum (caudate nucleus and putamen), subthalamic nucleus, internal and external segments of the globus pallidus, and the substantia nigra (pars compacta and pars reticulata). Together, these nuclei form multiple loops linking the basal ganglia to the cortex, thalamus, and brainstem. The embryonic origin of the striatum is from the ventricular eminences located in the floor of the telencephalic vesicle.

The basal ganglia subserve motor functions that are distinct from those attributed to the pyramidal (corticospinal) tract. The term 'extrapyramidal' emphasizes this distinction and is often used to denote a set of neurological disorders caused by lesions that affect the basal ganglia. Synaptic information travels through the basal ganglia using distinct pathways from the input structure, the striatum, to the output nuclei, the substantia nigra pars reticulata and the globus pallidus internal segment. The activity of the striatal output pathways is influenced by glutamatergic input from the cerebral cortex, DA input from the SNc, and cholinergic interneurons. Since the basal ganglia output nuclei tonically inhibit the motor nuclei of the thalamus, the basal ganglia facilitate motor activity by disinhibiting the thalamus (Fig. 4.8).

A basic circuit for the neostriatum consists of a pathway from cortical areas (neocortex, hippocampus, amygdala) to medium spiny neurones of the striatum that also receive converging synaptic input from midbrain DA neurones. The striatal medium spiny neurones are projection neurones and they form synaptic contacts with output neurones in the globus pallidus

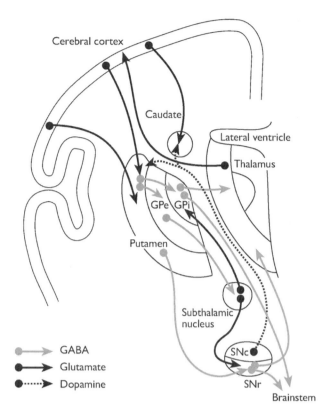

Fig. 4.8 Structure and circuitry of basal ganglia. Anatomical connections of the basal ganglia are shown. Major input nuclei are the caudate nucleus (CN) and putamen, whilst major output nuclei are the globus pallidus, internal segment (GPi) and the substantia nigra pars compacta (SNr). Abbreviations: GABA, gamma-aminobutyric acid; GPe, globus pallidus, external segment; SNc, substantia nigra pars compacta.

and substantia nigra reticulate (SNr). In this way, DA afferents can directly modulate the flow of information from cortical areas through the striatum to areas of the brainstem and to the thalamus (Graybiel, 1995; Smith and Bolam, 1990).

The striatum receives somatotopic cortical input from the frontal, sensory, motor, and parieto-temporal-occipital association areas. Corticostriatal afferents release the excitatory amino acid glutamate. Another major afferent input to the striatum is from neurons in the SNc which synthesize and release DA. The major output nuclei of the basal ganglia, the internal segment of the globus pallidus (GPi) and the SNr, send GABA-containing inhibitory projections to the ventral anterior, ventral lateral, and intralaminar thalamic nuclei. The influence of the basal ganglia circuits on the cortical motor areas is completed by means of the excitatory pathway from the thalamus to the pre-central cortex. The basal ganglia output nuclei (GPi and SNr) are inhibitory to thalamic nuclei and are differentially modulated by GABAergic efferent projects from the striatum. A direct pathway consists of inhibitory striatal efferents which project to the SNr. A parallel indirect pathway projects to the GPi via the external globus pallidus (GPe) and subthalamic nucleus (STN). Activation of the direct pathway results in excitation of thalamocortical circuits and enhancement of cortically initiated movements. Activation of the indirect pathway increases excitatory drive to the subthalamic nucleus and the basal ganglia output nuclei, resulting in inhibition of the thalamocortical circuit. The influence of DA-containing nigrostriatal afferent fibres is to enhance transmission through the direct pathway and suppress transmission through the indirect pathway. The net effect of DA, then, is to enhance positive feedback to the cortical motor areas and facilitate voluntary movements. Deficiency of DA in PD, therefore, inhibits cortically initiated movement.

An important characteristic of the striatum is its patch/matrix compartmental organization. These compartments exhibit different levels of expression of neurotransmitter-related molecules ranging from receptors to second messengers. They also have different input–output connections and different complements of striatal interneurons (Brown *et al.*, 2002). This compartmental segregation into patch and matrix compartments is known to be generated by two waves of neurogenesis, beginning at E12 in the rat. Cells born up to about E17 form the patch compartment, while from E18 until the early post-natal period, a second wave of neurogenesis produces the matrix compartment (Jain *et al.*, 2001).

The hippocampus

The hippocampus is amongst the best characterized cortical brain structures. Together with the adjacent amygdyla, it forms the limbic system. A large body of evidence now indicates that the hippocampus plays a critical role in fundamental aspects of learning and memory (Lynch, 2004). The hippocampus is formed by two interlocking sheets of cortex with a well-defined trilaminar structure. The hippocampus proper comprises four regions designated CA1–CA4 (from the Latin *cornu Ammon*). The *dentate gyrus* (DG), *subiculum*, and the *entorhinal cortex* are included in the more general term hippocampal formation. Both the hippocampus and DG are three-layered cortices, comprising the polymorphic layer, the pyramidal layer, and the molecular layer (Fig. 4.9).

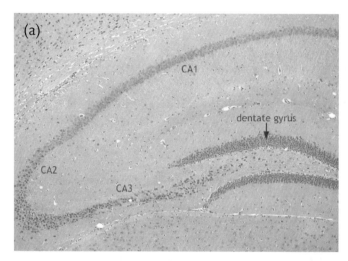

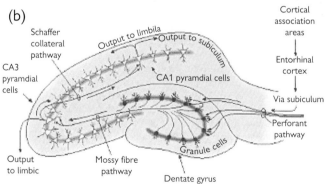

Fig. 4.9 Structure and circuitry of the hippocampus. (a) Histological section of hippocampus viewed in coronal section, to show three regions of the hippocampus proper, CA1, CA2, and CA3 and the dentate gyrus. (b) Schematic illustration of hippocampal circuitry showing three excitatory pathways; the perforant pathway connecting parahippocampal cortex with dentate granule cells, the mossy fibre pathway connecting granule cells to CA3 pyramidal neurons, and the Schaffer collateral pathway connecting CA3 to CA1 pyramidal neurons.

Major hippocampal afferent projections are the entorhino-hippocampal pathway (perforant pathway), the excitatory commissural/associational system, and the septal projection. They terminate in a laminated fashion on target neurons in the DG and CA regions. The perforant pathway is the major input to the hippocampus. The axons of the perforant path arise principally in layers II and III of the entorhinal cortex and these perforate the hippocampal fissure terminating in all parts of the hippocampus. A second input comprises commissural fibres from the contralateral hippocampus, whilst a third significant input originates in the septum. Internally within the hippocampus, fibre systems specifically connect the DG with CA3 (mossy fibres), and CA3 with CA1 (Schaffer collaterals). The mossy fibres are the axons of DG granule cells. They extend from the DG to CA3 pyramidal cells, forming their major input. MF synapses on CA neurons are large aggregations of termini, with multiple transmitter release sites and post-synaptic densities. Multiple granule cells can synapse onto a single CA3 pyramidal cell. This pathway has been studied extensively as a model for the functional roles of kainate receptors in synaptic plasticity. The Schaffer collateral pathway is derived from axons that project from CA3 to the CA1 region of the hippocampus. The axons either come from CA3 neurons in the same hippocampus (ipsilateral) or from contralateral commissural projections. The pathway from CA1 to the subiculum and on to the entorhinal cortex forms the principal output pathway of the hippocampus.

The functional organization of the hippocampus is classically described as a trisynaptic circuit, although current views are more complex (Lawrence and McBain, 2003). The classical pathway comprises perforant path fibres synapsing on granule neurons of the DG, whose mossy fibre axons synapse with pyramidal neurons in the CA3 region. Finally these neurons send Schaffer collaterals to synapse on pyramidal neurons in CA1.

Development and organization of the cerebral cortex

The largest region of the cerebral cortex, the neocortex, is the part of the mammalian brain that has shown the most extensive expansion and specialization during evolution. The neocortex is a six-layered sheet of cells whose cytoarchitecture varies subtly from cortical region to region. Estimates for the human cortex vary between 50 and 100 anatomically distinct areas (Shepherd, 1990). The scheme most commonly used to describe and designate cytoarchitectural differences between cortical regions is that devised by Brodmann in 1908, and in many cases these anatomically distinct regions correspond to important functional differences. The most prominent cellular characteristic of neocortical organization is its lamination. Within this layered structure two basic neuronal cell types predominate, spiny stellate and pyramidal neurons and non-spiny smooth neurons. Within distinct regions of cortex functional groups of neurons are organized into neural circuits within defined cortical columns. Such vertical columns, extending radially from the pial surface, were first identified in somatosensory cortex (Powell and Mountcastle, 1959), but are now known to reflect an underlying organizational principle of neocortex.

Most neocortical neurons, including the projection neurons, are generated within the ventricular and subventricular zones of the lateral ventricle. The first post-mitotic neurons accumulate below the pial surface, forming a layer called the pre-plate. Neurons that are subsequently generated migrate along radial glial processes to form the cortical plate, which splits the pre-plate into a superficial marginal zone and a deep subplate. The cortical plate gradually differentiates in a deep to superficial pattern, forming layers VI to II of the adult neocortex. The cortex also becomes patterned along anteroposterior and mediolateral axes (Bayer and Altman, 1991; Lopez-Bendito and Molnar, 2003).

The idea that the cortical plate is initially patterned in similar ways to the rest of the neural tube has been a recent conceptual breakthrough. Signalling molecules secreted from distinct cortical signalling centres are thought to establish positional information within distinct regions of the cortical plate and regulate regional growth. This now provides a model for

understanding how cortical area maps are established and how such maps may change with activity and experience. Current views suggest that the thalamus and cortex are patterned independently and then interact to generate the final cortical area map (Grove and Fukuchi-Shimogori, 2003; Rubenstein and Beachy, 1998).

Concluding remarks

The nervous system is a complex and highly differentiated structure whose function in the adult is critically dependent on the activities of integrated neural networks. Each specialized adult brain region (for example, ventral spinal cord, cerebellum, basal ganglia, and hippocampus) has arisen via an intricate process of development in which the relatively undifferentiated neural tube, comprising populations of neural stem cells, is patterned along its length in response to anteroposterior and dorsoventral signals to generate the region-specific adult structure. These region-specific processes are relatively well understood in spinal cord and brainstem. An understanding of how these mechanisms operate in other brain regions will help to further elucidate how precise neural networks are established in the developing and adult brain, and how these subserve region-specific brain functions.

References

Allan, D.W. and Thor, S. (2003). Together at last: bHLH and LIM-HD regulators cooperate to specify motor neurons. *Neuron* 38: 675–677.

Bayer, S.A. and Altman, J. (1991). *Neocortical Development*. Raven, New York.

Brown, L.L., Feldman, S.M., Smith, D.M., Cavanaugh, J.R., Ackermann, R.F., and Graybiel, A.M. (2002). Differential metabolic activity in the striosome and matrix compartments of the rat striatum during natural behaviours. *J Neurosci* 22: 305–314.

Cameron, H.A. and McKay, R. (1998). Stem cells and neurogenesis in the adult brain. *Curr Opin Neurobiol* 8: 677–680.

Cohen-Cory, S. (2002). The developing synapse: construction and modulation of synaptic structures and circuits. *Science* 298: 770–776.

Dickson, B.J. (2002). Molecular mechanisms of axon guidance. *Science* 298: 1959–1964.

Doetsch, F. (2003). The glial identity of neural stem cells. *Nat Neurosci* 6: 1127–1134.

Gage, F.H. (2000). Mammalian neural stem cells. *Science* 287: 1433–1438.

Gage, F.H. (2002). Neurogenesis in the adult brain. *J Neurosci* 22: 612–613.

Graybiel, A.M. (1995). The basal ganglia. *Trends Neurosci* 18: 60–62.

Grove, E.A. and Fukuchi-Shimogori, T. (2003). Generating the cerebral cortical area map. *Annu Rev Neurosci* 26: 355–380.

Hoch, W. (2003). Molecular dissection of neuromuscular junction formation. *Trends Neurosci* 26: 335–337.

Jain, M., Armstrong, R.J., Barker, R.A., and Rosser, A.E. (2001). Cellular and molecular aspects of striatal development. *Brain Res Bull* 55: 533–540.

Jessell T.M. and Sanes J.R. (2000). Development. The decade of the developing brain. *Curr Opin Neurobiol* 10: 599–611.

Kim, J.H., Auerbach, J.M., Rodriguez-Gomez, J.A., Velasco, I., Gavin, D., *et al.* (2002). Dopamine neurons derived from embryonic stem cells function in an animal model of Parkinson's disease. *Nature* 418: 50–56.

Lawrence, J.J. and McBain, C.J. (2003). Interneuron diversity series: containing the detonation–feedforward inhibition in the CA3 hippocampus. *Trends Neurosci* 26: 631–640.

Lee, S.H., Lumelsky, N., Studer, L., Auerbach, J.M., and McKay, R.D. (2000). Efficient generation of midbrain and hindbrain neurons from mouse embryonic stem cells. *Nat Biotechnol* 18: 675–679.

Lewis, J. (1996). Neurogenic genes and vertebrate neurogenesis. *Curr Opin Neurobiol* 6: 3–10.

Li, Z. and Sheng, M. (2003). Some assembly required: the development of neuronal synapses. *Nat Rev Mol Cell Biol* 4: 833–841.

Liu, A. and Joyner, A.L. (2001). Early anterior/posterior patterning of the midbrain and cerebellum. *Annu Rev Neurosci* 24: 869–896.

Lopez-Bendito, G. and Molnar, Z. (2003). Thalamocortical development: how are we going to get there? *Nat Rev Neurosci* 4: 276–289.

Lumsden, A. and Krumlauf, R. (1996). Patterning the vertebrate neuraxis. *Science* 274(5290): 1109–1115.

Lynch, M.A. (2004). Long-term potentiation and memory. *Physiol Rev* 84: 87–136.

Powell, T.P.S. and Mountcastle, V.B. (1959). Some aspects of the functional organisation of the cortex of the post-central gyrus of the monkey. *Bull Johns Hopkins Hospital* 105: 133–162.

Price, S.R., De Marco Garcia, N.V., Ranscht, B., and Jessell, T.M. (2002). Regulation of motor neuron pool sorting by differential expression of type II cadherins. *Cell* 109: 205–216.

Ramon y Cajal, S. (1894). La fine structure des centres nerveux. *Proc R Soc Lond* 55: 444–468.

Ramon y Cajal, S. (1911). *Histologie du System Nerveux de l'Homme et des Vertebras*, Vols 1 and 2. A. Maloine, Paris. (Reprinted in 1955 by Consejo Superior de Investigaciones Cientificas, Inst. Ramon y Cajal, Madrid.)

Rexed, B. (1952). The cytoarchitectonic organization of the spinal cord in the cat. *J Comp Neurol* 96: 415–495.

Rubenstein, J.L. and Beachy, P.A. (1998). Patterning of the embryonic forebrain. *Curr Opin Neurobiol* 8: 18–26.

Sadler T.W. (2004). *Langman's Medical Embryology*, 9th edn. Lippincott, Williams and Wilkins, Baltimore, MD.

Salinas, P.C. (2003). The morphogen sonic hedgehog collaborates with netrin-1 to guide axons in the spinal cord. *Trends Neurosci* 26: 641–643.

Schwanzel-Fukuda, M. and Pfaff, D.W. (1989). Origin of luteinizing hormone-releasing hormone neurons. *Nature* 338: 161–164.

Shepherd, G.M. (1990) *The Synaptic Organisation of the Brain*, 3rd edn. Oxford University Press, New York.

Smith, A.D. and Bolam, J.P. (1990). The neural network of the basal ganglia as revealed by the study of synaptic connections of identified neurones. *Trends Neurosci* 13: 259–265.

Spemann, H. and Mangold, H. (1924). Über induktion von Embryonalagen durch Implantation Artfremder Organisatoren. *Roux's Arch Entw Mech* 100: 599.

Taheri, S., Zeitzer, J.M., and Mignot, E. (2002). The role of hypocretins (orexins) in sleep regulation and narcolepsy. *Annu Rev Neurosci* 25: 283–313.

Tanabe, Y. and Jessell, T.M. (1996). Diversity and pattern in the developing spinal cord. *Science* 274: 1115–1123.

Trainor, P.A. and Krumlauf, R. (2000). Patterning the cranial neural crest: hindbrain segmentation and Hox gene plasticity. *Nat Rev Neurosci* 1: 116–124.

Wang, V.Y. and Zoghbi, H.Y. (2001). Genetic regulation of cerebellar development. *Nat Rev Neurosci* 2(7): 484–491.

Weinstein, D.C. and Hemmati-Brivanlou, A. (1999). Neural induction. *Annu Rev Cell Dev Biol* 15: 411–433.

Wolpert L., Beddington, R., Brockes, J., Jessell, T., Lawrence, P., and Meyerowitz, E. (1998). *Principles of Development*. Current Biology/Oxford University Press, Oxford.

5 Immune properties of the central nervous system

Elise H. Tran and Burkhard Becher

Introduction

Antigen presentation is a crucial process in the immune system for the generation of protective T-cell responses against pathogens. This requires antigen-presenting cells (APC) capable of engulfing foreign microorganisms and expressing the antigenic peptides in the major histocompatibility complex (MHC) molecules on the cell surface. CD4 T cells recognize antigens that are associated with the MHC Class II molecules, whereas CD8 T cells bind antigen–MHC Class I complexes. Both naïve CD4 and CD8 T cells become fully activated only when receiving additional co-stimulatory signals from the APC, whereas the activation of T cells that have already been 'primed' or exposed to their antigens may be less dependent on co-stimulation (Croft et al., 1994; Gause et al., 1996). There are 'professional' APC equipped to initiate a primary immune response by the presentation of antigen to naïve T cells, and 'non-professional' APC that can only stimulate a secondary response by the presentation of antigen to primed T cells. Dendritic cells and macrophages of the immune system possess the former ability, whereas B cells and certain stromal cells may engage in secondary T-cell responses (Mellman and Steinman, 2001).

Most tissues of the body contain APC, which can also traffic to the draining lymph nodes for the initiation of T-cell activation. Once activated, T cells leave the lymph nodes and infiltrate and inspect tissues for foreign antigens that are being displayed on resident APC. If T cells are fully activated, they proliferate, differentiate, and acquire an increased sensitivity to antigen on re-stimulation in tissues. Such immune surveillance coordinated by APC and T cells benefits most peripheral tissues, but seems limited in the central nervous system (CNS) where, for instance, allografts were demonstrated to survive longer than those on other tissues (Barker and Billingham, 1977). This immunological privilege of the CNS was attributed to the blood–brain barrier (BBB), which restricts the entry of plasma proteins and components of the immune system such as lymphocytes, antibodies, and complements. Furthermore, the CNS parenchyma was thought to lack resident APC and conventional lymphatic drainage. It was found to produce many anti-inflammatory factors such as transforming growth factor-beta (TGF-β) and vasoactive intestinal peptide, as well as gangliosides and Fas ligands, which inactivate or kill immune cells (Becher et al., 1998; Bechmann et al., 1999; Benveniste, 1998; Gozes et al., 1999; Irani, 1998; Irani et al., 1996; Pender and Rist, 2001; Vitkovic et al., 2001). Thus, the CNS microenvironment was regarded as inefficient for an immune-mediated inflammation, a necessary event to defeat pathogens. In fact, in mice, infection of peripheral tissues with lymphocytic choriomeningitis virus (LCMV) usually induces a massive expansion of virus-specific CD8 T cells, which results in efficient viral clearance and host survival (McGavern et al., 2002). When the virus is inoculated directly to the CNS, however, it causes a lethal disease (McGavern et al., 2002). There is unequivocal evidence that virus-specific T-cell response is implicated in the fatality of LCMV infection in the CNS (Cole et al., 1972; Doherty et al., 1990). Should it be infected, the CNS would appear a defenseless victim, at the mercy of the peripheral immune system to control or end the attack. However, observations that some latent viruses such as JC virus (responsible for the development of progressive multifocal leukoencephalopathy) or varicella zoster (shingles) produces clinical syndromes mainly in immuno-compromised individuals, indicate that some degree of immune surveillance of the CNS is vital to prevent disease development. While the CNS appears to represent an immune priviledged organ, MHC and co-stimulatory molecules are nevertheless strongly up-regulated in CNS infections and in virtually all other CNS pathologies, including ischemia, neoplasm, traumatic nerve injury, and neurodegenerative disorders such as multiple sclerosis (MS), HIV-associated dementia, Alzheimer's, Parkinson's and Creutzfeldt–Jakob disease (An et al., 1996; Dorries, 2001; Graeber et al., 1998; Maehlen et al., 1989; McGeer et al., 1993; O'Keefe et al., 2002; Owens, 2002; Perry, 1998; Piehl and Lidman, 2001). Why and how such immune reactivity occurs in the disturbed CNS remains speculative; such reactivity may reflect an attempt of the CNS to defend and repair itself. For example, CD4 T cells are recruited to sites of myelinated axon injury even when the BBB is not disrupted (Konno et al., 1990; Maehlen et al., 1989) and they may promote regeneration of neurons via secretion of growth factors after *in situ* antigen-specific activation (Hammarberg et al., 2000; Hohlfeld et al., 2000; Kipnis et al., 2002; Moalem et al., 2000; Schwartz, 2001). Nonetheless, immune reactivity in the CNS can become destructive, possibly when critical regulatory mechanisms are lost or inadequate. CD4 T cells are blamed for wrongly attacking CNS myelin in MS through secretion of pro-inflammatory cytokines and activation of cytopathic factors and cytotoxic CD8 T cells (Goebels et al., 2000; Meinl and Hohlfeld, 2002; Steinman et al., 2002). Autoaggressive Th cells even when fully activated only recognize their target A_g in the context of an MHC class II expressing APC. Myelinating cells of the CNS are void of MHC class II molecules. How then is it possible that Th cells attack the CNS? Which cell presents the antigen? It is puzzling how autoimmune inflammation in the brain can be detrimental at one time and beneficial at another. What is special about immunity regulation in the CNS? Recent advances have revealed that the CNS may harbor its own defense system with its own codes and strategies despite sharing certain ammunition and artillery with the peripheral immune system. In this chapter we will focus our discussion on how cells in the CNS compartments outside the parenchyma as well as glial cells within the parenchyma may be the masterminds of CD4 T-cell responses in the brain.

CNS-associated cells: sentinels at the gate of the CNS parenchyma

Compartments in association with the CNS, such as the Virchow–Robin (perivascular) space, the leptomeninges, and the choroid plexus, contain phagocytes that have been identified as macrophages and dendritic cells, based on molecular and functional phenotypes (hereafter referred to as CNS-associated cells) (Fischer and Reichmann, 2001; McMenamin, 1999; Serafini et al., 2000; Williams et al., 2001a). They are continuously replenished by bone marrow-derived (Bechmann et al., 2001; Hickey et al., 1992). Indeed, their normal turnover may be exploited by pathogens, such as lentiviruses, to enable entry into the CNS (Williams et al., 2001b). Under various pathological conditions, these CNS-associated cells can increase in

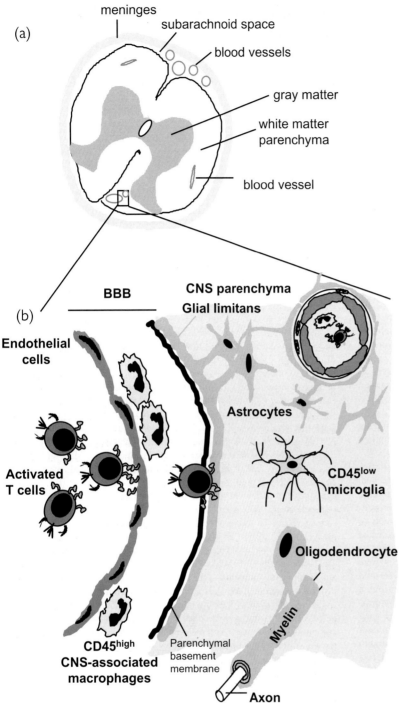

(a)

meninges
subarachnoid space
blood vessels
gray matter
white matter
parenchyma
blood vessel

Fig. 5.1 (a) A schematic representation of a cross-section of the spinal cord. (b) Activated T cells cross the endothelial layer of the blood–brain barrier (BBB) to enter the perivascular space where CD45[high] macrophages and dendritic cells (CNS-associated cells) are located. T cells must further traverse the glial limitans and the parenchymal basement membrane to reach the CNS parenchyma, where astrocytes and CD45[low] microglia are normally kept immunologically quiescent by the vast neuronal network. In experimental autoimmune encephalomyelitis, an animal model for multiple sclerosis, reactivation of infiltrating T cells by resident antigen-presenting cells provokes a cascade of inflammatory events that often result in the destruction of myelin-producing oligodendrocytes and neuronal axons.

(b)

BBB

CNS parenchyma
Glial limitans

Endothelial cells

Astrocytes

Activated T cells

CD45[low] microglia

Oligodendrocyte

CD45[high] CNS-associated macrophages

Parenchymal basement membrane

Myelin

Axon

number transiently or for longer periods (Williams *et al.*, 2001*a*). Like peripheral macrophages, they constitutively express high levels of MHC II, CD11b and the leukocyte common antigen CD45, which distinguish them from the CD45[low] parenchymal microglia (Becher and Antel, 1996; Sedgwick *et al.*, 1991) (Fig. 5.1). Both *in vitro* and *in vivo* studies strongly point to the CNS-associated cells, rather than the microglia, as competent APC (see below). When isolated from adult rodent CNS, these CD45[high] CNS-associated cells were found to activate both naïve and primed CD4 T cells, as efficiently as splenic or lymph node APC, and even more so than CD45[low] parenchymal microglia isolated from the same animals (Carson *et al.*, 1998, 1999; Ford et al., 1996). *In vivo* studies using infectious or autoimmune models also support immune functions of the CNS-associated cells. For

instance, Matyszak and Perry (1998) showed that injection of the pathogen bacille Calmette–Guérin (BCG) to the meninges provokes a typical inflammation and a BCG antigen-specific T-cell response, as seen in the skin after a subcutaneous challenge. By contrast, no such immune response was observed when the pathogen was delivered directly to the CNS parenchyma (Matyszak and Perry, 1998).

In experimental autoimmune encephalomyelitis (EAE), an animal counterpart of MS, an interaction between myelin-reactive CD4 T cells and APC in the CNS is a critical step in the cascade of events leading to the formation of inflammatory lesions (Meinl and Hohlfeld, 2002; Owens and Babcock, 2002; Steinman *et al.*, 2002). Myelin-reactive T cells that have been previously primed in the peripheral lymphoid organs are able to cross the intact BBB, but whether naïve T cells can do so too remains debatable (Brabb *et al.*, 2000; Hickey, 1991). Interestingly, even though naïve myelin-specific T cells may enter the intact CNS, they are kept unresponsive (Brabb *et al.*, 2000) and perhaps remain innocuous until primed myelin-reactive T cells initiate a vigorous inflammatory response. During such an inflammatory response, the BBB breaks down, facilitating the entry of more naïve T cells. But these naïve T cells also require antigen recognition for their activation in the CNS (Krakowski and Owens, 2000). Because of their location and their macrophage/dendritic cell-like behavior, the CNS-associated cells are ideal candidates to present antigen to incoming T cells. These CNS-associated cells may engage in *de novo* processing of myelin antigen for *in situ* activation of primed and naïve T cells (Slavin *et al.*, 2001; Tompkins *et al.*, 2002). They also seem strategically positioned for influencing T-cell trafficking to the CNS parenchyma. When their function is perturbed or absent, lymphocyte migration into the CNS parenchyma is blocked and EAE is prevented (Huitinga *et al.*, 1995; Polfliet *et al.*, 2002; Tran *et al.*, 1998). Recently, we have shown that dendritic cells are the most crucial APC permitting target recognition of invading T cells. In fact, macrophages and mocroglia were not capable of presenting antigen *in vivo* (Greter *et al.* 2005). Furthermore, CNS-associated cells have been shown to be important sources of tumor necrosis factor-alpha (TNF-α), which induces glial production of chemokines, such as TCA3 and MCP, to mediate leukocyte recruitment and initiation of inflammation in the parenchyma (Murphy *et al.*, 2002). Collectively, these *in vivo* studies strongly suggest that compartments associated with the CNS harbor cells capable of initiating both primary and secondary T-cell response locally.

These CNS-associated APC, like certain antigens in the brain, may drain to lymphoid organs to activate naïve T cells. Outflow of the normal brain can escape to the interstitial and cerebrospinal fluids, which follow cranial nerves to drain into nasal lymphatics and cervical lymph nodes or can drain to the spleen via blood. Studies that traced these outflow pathways have revealed that, contrary to the earlier view, both intracranially injected macrophages and antigens drain preferentially to the cervical lymph nodes (Cserr and Knopf, 1992; de Vos *et al.*, 2002). Myelin basic proteins were indeed elevated in the cerebrospinal fluid of patients with relapsing-remitting MS (Lamers *et al.*, 1998) and myelin-ingested APC were also abundant in their cervical lymph nodes (de Vos *et al.*, 2002). In addition, the cervical lymph nodes of marmoset and rhesus monkeys that were immunized with only myelin oligodendrocyte glycoprotein contained an accumulation of APC that had engulfed other myelin antigens, such as myelin basic protein and proteolipid protein (de Vos *et al.*, 2002). These observations indicate that myelin antigens or APC containing them must have drained to the cervical lymph nodes from the inflamed CNS. However, it is unclear whether myelin antigen presentations in the cervical lymph nodes would result in the progression or modulation of immune responses in the CNS. In support of the cervical lymph node implication in disease, encephalitogenic T cells primed in these lymph nodes were found to preferentially target the brain (Lake *et al.*, 1999) and an ablation of the cervical lymph nodes markedly attenuated the cryolesion-enhanced EAE in Lewis rats (Phillips *et al.*, 1997). Although the drainage of CNS-derived antigens into the cervical lymph nodes generates local production of antigen-specific antibodies, it does not provoke a rapid destruction of the CNS (Cserr and Knopf, 1992). Moreover, intracranially injected antigens in normal mice rather evoked a systemic immune deviation that suppresses normal T-cell effector activity (Wenkel *et al.*, 2000). Cervical lymph node cells from the protected mice were able to transfer such suppression to naïve recipients (Wenkel *et al.*, 2000). Also, the cervical lymph nodes but not other lymph nodes have been reported essential in the induction of nasal tolerance (Wolvers *et al.*, 1999). Possibly individual lymph nodes from distinct anatomical sites may possess functional specialization for the defense of the associated organ. For example, CD4+CD25+ regulatory T cells derived from the pancreatic lymph nodes were more potent than those from other peripheral lymph nodes in suppressing the destruction of the pancreas in a murine model of diabetes (Green *et al.*, 2002).

Microglia: sentinels within the CNS parenchyma

Microglia comprise about 10% of the total glial population in the CNS parenchyma (Perry, 1998). The most widely held hypothesis is that early during embryogenesis, myeloid cells from the yolk sac migrate to the CNS and differentiate into microglia (Alliot *et al.*, 1999). Unlike the CNS-associated phagocytes, microglia are not readily repopulated by bone marrow-derived monocytes during adulthood (Becher *et al.*, 2003; Hickey *et al.*, 1992), so may not derive from a common monocytic lineage. Also, the ramified microglia in the normal adult CNS appear more quiescent: phagocytic activity, MHC II and many surface receptors that mediate typical macrophage functions are expressed at lower levels compared with CNS-associated macrophages or other tissue macrophages (Aloisi, 2001).

Regulation of microglial quiescence by neurons

Recent evidence indicates that neurons may keep microglia quiescent in the intact CNS through cell-to-cell interactions, such as the one mediated by CD200. Neurons express on their cell surface CD200, a glycoprotein which interacts with its receptor on microglia (Hoek *et al.*, 2000). In the CNS of CD200-deficient mice, microglia were spontaneously activated as gauged by their enhanced expression of CD11b and CD45 as well as by the loss of their ramified morphology (Hoek *et al.*, 2000). They also mounted a drastically accelerated and increased response after facial nerve transection or EAE induction (Hoek *et al.*, 2000). Another way by which neurons may maintain microglial quiesence is through their electrical activities and release of soluble factors. For example, blockade of neuronal activity by tetrodotoxin or glutamate receptor antagonists facilitates the IFN-γ-mediated induction of MHC II on glial cells that were cultured with neurons (Neumann, 2001). Indeed, neurotransmitters (e.g. norepinephrine, glutamate, vasoactive intestinal peptide) and neurotrophins (e.g. nerve growth factor, brain-derived growth factor, and neurotrophin-3) have all been demonstrated to suppress the expression of MHC II and co-stimulatory molecules, CD40 and CD86, critical in antigen presentation (Neumann, 2001; Wei and Jonakait, 1999). Interestingly, astrocytes have also been reported to inhibit microglial activation, possibly through TGF-β or interleukin (IL)-10 (Aloisi, 2001; Vincent *et al.*, 1997).

Thus, normal physiologically active neurons, together with astrocytes, may coordinately sustain microglial quiescence in the intact CNS parenchyma, thereby limiting the development of inflammatory responses. When neurons are injured, however, microglia rapidly become activated (Aloisi, 2001; Neumann, 2001), probably as a result of both a weakening of neuronal inhibitory signals and the awakening of stimulatory stimuli. During injury, some neurotransmitters, such as substance P, may be released at high amounts to enhance rather than to suppress microglial pro-inflammatory activity (McCluskey and Lampson, 2000). It would appear that microglia may serve as homeostatic sensors with reparative abilities. They become rapidly activated to phagocytose at sites of neuronal damage or degeneration, and increase in numbers, either from proliferation or recruitment, in order to remove debris and promote repair. Nevertheless, when such reactivity is inappropriate or unchecked, as in neurodegenerative disorders, damage to the CNS tissues may be sustained through the release of numerous pro-inflammatory and cytopathic mediators: cytokines (e.g. TNF-α, IL-1, IL-6, IL-12, IL-18), chemokines (e.g. IL-8, MIP, MCP, RANTES), nitric and oxygen free radicals, and prostanoids (e.g. PGD2, PGE2, thromboxane B2). In MS, activated microglia and macrophages are implicated in myelin destruction through antibody- and complement-mediated phagocytosis of myelin as well as free radicals (Smith, 2001).

Microglial activation by external stimuli

The characteristic prompt response of microglia to infectious and inflammatory stimuli relies on constitutive and inducible expression of surface receptors that trigger or amplify both innate and acquired immune responses. The innate immune system distinguishes self-molecules from pathogen-associated non-self structures via pattern-recognition receptors, such as Toll-like receptors (TLR), which are expressed on the cell surface of macrophages and dendritic cells (Medzhitov, 2001). Recognition of pathogens by TLR triggers signaling events that induce the expression of effector molecules, such as cytokines, chemokines, and co-stimulatory molecules, which subsequently control the activation of an antigen-specific CD4 T-cell immune response. Recently, CD4 T cells have been shown to directly respond to stimulation by certain TLRs (Caramalho et al., 2003).

Innate immunity: Toll-like receptors

To date, at least 10 TLRs have been identified in mammals. Each TLR recognizes specific structures of bacteria and viruses. For example, TLR2 recognizes the pathogen-associated molecular patterns (PAMPs) of Gram-positive bacterial cell wall components, whereas TLR4 in association with CD14 binds to lipopolysaccharide (LPS), a cell wall component of the Gram-negative bacteria (Takeuchi et al., 1999). TLR3 and TLR9, on the other hand, are crucial for the recognition of double-stranded viral RNA and bacterial DNA, respectively (Alexopoulou et al., 2001; Hemmi et al., 2000).

Emerging evidence has linked the TLR system to neurodegeneration and neuroprotection (Nguyen et al., 2002). Systemic injection of LPS in rats induces TLR2, TLR4, and CD14 in parenchymal microglia that surround areas devoid of the BBB, such as circumventricular organs, leptomeninges, and choroid plexus (Laflamme and Rivest, 2001; Laflamme et al., 2001). In mice, microglia are the only CNS glial cells that were found to bind fluorescently tagged LPS, and LPS-induced oligodendrocyte death was reduced in mice bearing a loss-of-function mutation in the tlr4 gene (Lehnardt et al., 2002). In the brain of EAE mice, TLR2 and CD14 are up-regulated in microglia and macrophages and were also associated with an increase in NF-κB activity and transcriptional activation of genes encoding numerous pro-inflammatory molecules (Zekki et al., 2002). In culture, human microglia up-regulate CD14 (Becher et al., 1996) and many different TLRs (Bsibsi et al., 2002). Comparisons between microglia derived from control subjects and those with neurodegenerative diseases indicate distinct differences in levels of mRNA encoding the different TLRs in microglia (Bsibsi et al., 2002). The functional significance of microglial TLRs is unclear, but these receptors may endow microglia with the capability of the peripheral APC to mount an innate immune response which may eventually progress to the activation of antigen-specific T-cell responses within the CNS. In fact, murine microglia express TLR9 and can be activated by bacterial CpG-DNA in vitro and in vivo to express MHC II, co-stimulatory molecules, and the cytokines TNF-α and IL-12 (Dalpke et al., 2002). Since IL-12 promotes T helper 1 (Th1) cell differentiation, bacterial DNA containing CpG motifs could not only play an important role during infections of the CNS, but also may trigger and sustain Th1-dominated immunopathologies (Dalpke et al., 2002). Thus, microglial TLRs may be implicated in the development of Th1 or Th2 cells in the CNS. Furthermore, as relapses in MS are often triggered by infections, a clearer understanding of TLR function in the CNS will cast new light on neural immunity, and may possibly open new therapeutic avenues.

Acquired immunity: co-stimulatory molecules and CD4 T cells

During their activation, CD4 Th cells can differentiate into at least two subsets of effector cells: Th1 cells which secrete predominantly IFN-α and TNF-γ, and Th2 cells which secrete IL-4, IL-5 and IL-10. In general, Th1 cells are responsible for eliciting phagocyte-mediated defense against infections and for promoting the differentiation of CD8 T cells into active killer cells, whereas Th2 cells mediate humoral immune responses by stimulating the differentiation of B cells and can down-regulate Th1 responses. As well as their protective roles in host defense, Th1 cells can also mediate organ-specific autoimmunity and have been implicated in the pathogenesis of EAE and MS (Steinman et al., 2002). Conversely, Th2 cells can suppress EAE and MS (Steinman et al., 2002), although they may exacerbate these diseases in immunocompromised hosts (Lafaille et al., 1997). Thus, the final composition of the Th cell response to antigen can determine whether the out-

come of infectious, inflammatory, and autoimmune responses is beneficial or detrimental. Many factors influence the development of Th1 or Th2 cells: for example the cytokines (e.g. IL-12 favors Th1 cells, IL-4 favors Th2 cells), the antigen doses, the co-stimulatory molecules, as well as the types of activated APCs.

Activated microglia up-regulate MHC II and co-stimulatory molecules (e.g. CD40, CD80, CD86), which equip them for antigen presentation to T cells (Aloisi, 2001; Becher et al., 2000b). Also, microglia, like the CNS-associated cells, phagocytose myelin (Li et al., 1993; Slobodov et al., 2001; Williams et al., 1994), indicating that these cells can activate myelin-specific CD4 T cells. Microglia infected with Theiler's murine encephalomyelitis virus have been demonstrated to be activated to efficiently process and present not only endogenous virus epitopes but also exogenous myelin epitopes to CD4 T cells (Olson et al., 2001, 2002). Human microglia, either immediately ex vivo or cultured for several days, have been reported to act as APC, and to induce both primary and secondary proliferative T-cell responses (Becher and Antel, 1996; Becher et al., 2000a). Similar APC potential was also demonstrated for rat microglia isolated from neonatal brains (Frei et al., 1987; Matsumoto et al., 1992), but in these studies with neonatal glial cultures, CNS-associated cells were not separated from microglia and may contribute to T-cell activation. Furthermore, recent reports have raised concern about whether such neonatally derived cells faithfully represent the adult population in vivo. In fact, microglia isolated from adult mice fail to present antigen to naïve antigen-specific CD4 T cells (Havenith et al., 1998), but those that are pre-treated with IFN-γ or isolated from mice with EAE can activate T-cell lines in an antigen- and CD86-dependent manner in vitro (Havenith et al., 1998; Krakowski and Owens, 1997). Nevertheless, adult rodent microglia may not support a typical T-cell activation: T cells become blasts, express activation markers CD25 (IL2 receptor alpha chain) and CD134, and produce the cytokines TNF-α and IFN-γ, in an antigen-specific manner, but do not proliferate (Carson et al., 1998, 1999; Ford et al., 1996; Juedes and Ruddle, 2001). Even when MHC II expression is enhanced by the induction of systemic graft versus host disease, the isolated microglia still do not promote proliferation of T cells, but rather induce the death of these cells through apoptotic mechanisms (Ford et al., 1996). In line with this finding, many T cells in the CNS of rodents with EAE undergo apoptosis within the parenchyma (Bauer et al., 1998; Pender and Rist, 2001), where they are in contact with microglia. It remains unresolved whether microglia actually present antigen to naïve T cells in vivo during an inflammation. It is likely that T-cell activation and expansion are subjected to a tighter regulation in the CNS parenchyma than elsewhere. Indeed, CNS APCs were found to inhibit T-cell proliferation through the release of toxic levels of nitric oxide (Juedes and Ruddle, 2001) and to induce T-cell apoptosis through Fas–Fas ligand interaction (Bonetti et al., 1997; Carson et al., 1999; Ford et al., 1996).

The activation and differentiation of CD4 T cells require MHC II recognition and co-stimulation. Studies using adoptive transfer of primed myelin-reactive CD4 T cells into mice in which APC can no longer deliver a specific co-stimulatory signal have identified CD40, CD80/CD86 (B7) and CD134 (OX40) as important for reactivation of these T cells in the CNS (Chang et al., 1999; Howard and Miller, 2001; Weinberg et al., 1999). The observation that microglia are largely resistant to radiation while CNS-associated cells are radiation sensitive has allowed the generation of radiation bone marrow chimeric mice to further pinpoint the most important source of these co-stimulatory molecules in the CNS. Recent work using such an approach to create bone marrow chimeric mice in which CD40 is deficient only in microglia but is intact in CNS-associated cells has revealed that microglial CD40 is most critical to the reactivation of peripherally primed encephalitogenic T cells for the production of Th1 cytokines and chemokines, the recruitment of leukocytes to the CNS parenchyma, and the progression of EAE (Becher et al., 2001) (Fig. 5.2). Like murine microglia, human microglia can express CD40, and in response to CD40 stimulation produce IL-12 (Aloisi, 2001; Becher et al., 2000a). IL-12 is a 70 kDa heterodimeric, secreted protein consisting of two disulfide-linked subunits, p35 and p40. The p40 subunit can also associate with a different

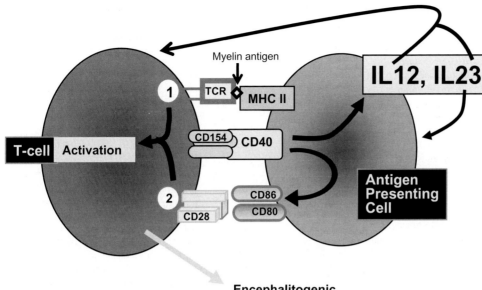

Fig. 5.2 T-cell and CNS antigen-presenting cell (APC) synapse. A CD4 T-cell with an antigen-receptor (TCR) specific for a myelin peptide can recognize its cognate antigen only in the context of an MHC II molecule presented by an APC (signal 1). The T-cell will subsequently up-regulate the expression of CD154 and engage CD40 on the APC. CD40 engagement in turn will induce APC activation/maturation which results in the up-regulation of other co-stimulatory molecules (e.g. CD80/CD86) and an increased density of antigen/MHC II complexes on the surface. Engagement of the co-receptor CD28 provides the T lymphocyte with signal 2, which is required to induce full activation and effector function.

p19 subunit to form IL-23, which has recently been shown to be essential in the activation of the CNS-associated macrophages for autoimmune inflammation in the mouse brain (Cua *et al.*, 2003). This study and others (Becher *et al.*, 2002; Gran *et al.*, 2002; Mendel and Shevach, 2002) have now challenged the view that IL-12 is central in autoimmune inflammation of the CNS. Though both microglia and CNS-associated macrophages can produce IL-23, only macrophages can respond to this cytokine (Cua *et al.*, 2003). Collectively, these observations allow us to speculate that the interplay between microglia and macrophages via IL-23 may regulate CNS inflammation triggered by primed autoimmune CD4 T cells. Infiltrating T cells expressing CD40 ligand (CD154) can stimulate microglial CD40 to up-regulate IL-23. This cytokine in turn can directly act on memory T cells (Frucht, 2002) and activates CNS-associated macrophages to produce critical inflammatory cytokines (e.g. TNF-α and IL-1) and possibly other co-stimulatory molecules (e.g. CD80/CD86 and CD134). In fact, we could recently show that chimeric mice in which IL-23 has been deleted from the CNS compartment are protected from developing EAE. Interestingly, histopathological analysis revealed that the degree of inflammation is comparable to that seen in control mice with severe EAE. We conclude that IL-23 produced by microglia controls T-cell encephalitogenicity without interfering with leukocyte invasion.

CD154 was found to be unexpectedly enhanced on reactive astrocytes in Alzheimer's disease and other brain injuries (Calingasan *et al.*, 2002). Given the paucity of infiltrating T cells in the brain in Alzheimer's disease, interactions between microglial CD40 and astroglial CD154 may therefore promote the production of neurotoxins that mediate neuronal damage (Tan *et al.*, 1999). Paradoxically, CD40 has also been implicated in neuronal development, maintenance, and protection (Tan *et al.*, 2002). A better understanding of the molecular mechanisms regulating the expression of CD40 and its ligand in the CNS will undoubtedly cast new light on functions of these co-stimulatory molecules beyond T-cell activation.

Astrocytes: additional sentinels within the CNS parenchyma

While numerous studies have supported the role of microglia in T-cell activation within the CNS, whether astrocytes, the major glial populations, also play such role is a lively controversy (De Keyser *et al.*, 2003; Dong and Benveniste, 2001). On the one hand, both *in situ* and *in vivo* evidence indicates that astrocytes express high levels of MHC II and co-stimulatory molecules (e.g. CD80, CD86, CD40, ICAM-1 and VCAM-1) upon exposure to IFN-γ (Nikcevich *et al.*, 1997; Vass and Lassmann, 1990; Zeinstra *et al.*, 2003). Interestingly, CD80 and CD86 are differentially regulated on astrocytes during the course of EAE: CD86 is up-regulated at the peak of disease, while CD80 dominates during remission (Issazadeh *et al.*, 1998). Furthermore, astrocytes express elements involved in the MHC II endocytic pathway and are capable of processing native MBP for presentation to myelin-specific T cells *in vitro* (Soos *et al.*, 1998). Myelin-specific T cells that were activated by astrocytes *in vitro* were indeed able to transfer EAE in SJL/J mice (Tan *et al.*, 1998). Although both untreated and IFN-γ-treated astrocytes can initiate secondary T-cell responses, only treated astrocytes activate naïve T cells (Nikcevich *et al.*, 1997). However, many other studies do not support astrocytes as efficient APCs (Aloisi *et al.*, 1999; Cross and Ku, 2000; Matsumoto *et al.*, 1992; Sun *et al.*, 1997). Interestingly, astrocyte-derived soluble factors suppress LPS-induction of co-stimulatory molecules on microglia and macrophages (Hailer *et al.*, 1998), suggesting that astrocytes are not only themselves poor stimulators of CD4 T cells but can also inactivate other APCs.

Unlike microglia, astrocytes may require additional stimuli in combination with IF-γ to provide stronger synergistic activation of their APC function (Williams *et al.*, 1995). Because of their phenotypic and functional heterogeneity (Wilkin *et al.*, 1990), astrocytes may differ in their APC function, and this may add to the controversy. Moreover, strain differences might influence the antigen-presenting potential of astrocytes. Upon *in vitro* stimulation with IFN-γ, astrocytes that were isolated from EAE-susceptible Lewis rats, but not from EAE-resistant Brown Norway rats, expressed higher levels of MHC II and induced proliferation of myelin-specific T-cell lines (Klyushnenkova and Vanguri, 1997). A similar correlation between EAE susceptibility and astroglial MHC II induction was also observed for certain mouse strains (Massa *et al.*, 1987). Surprisingly, microglial MHC II induction does not seem to predispose to EAE susceptibility (Sedgwick *et al.*, 1993).

Conclusion

Activated CD4 T cells that traffic to the CNS first encounter the endothelial cells of the BBB. Such interactions may dampen the responsiveness of these T cells (Bourdoulous *et al.*, 1995; Prat *et al.*, 2000). Those T cells that could cross the endothelial layer would enter the perivascular space or the subarachnoid space of the meninges. There, a rare population of dendritic cells are competent APCs, which allow T-cell entry into the CNS and further dictate the fate of these migrating T cells. In the CNS parenchyma, microglia, and possibly astrocytes, can support secondary T-cell responses. However, these T-cell responses are rather restrictive compared with those in the periphery; microglia activate effector function of T cells but thwart their survival in the brain parenchyma. T cells that arrive in response to a CNS assault can initiate both protective and toxic inflammatory responses. Whether or not the immune responses perpetuate or attenuate disease may depend on the intracellular signaling pathways triggered, for example the balance between Th1 and Th2 cell responses, the ongoing degenerative processes, the brain region, and its susceptibility to the insult. The immune system possesses powerful defense machinery, ensuring the generation of specific, rapid, and protective responses against pathogens, but not without the risk of tissue damage. The CNS appears to have evolved a defense machinery to protect its delicate vital functions from potential 'risky' immune-mediated inflammation. The neuronal microenvironment keeps highly 'immunological' glial cells quiescent. A race between microglia and astrocytes in reacting to any neuronal disturbance is launched to rapidly restore the homeostasis of the brain parenchyma. But in various CNS diseases there may be a deficit or an aberration in such glial defense. The key to therapeutic solutions may reside in how to restore the physiological CNS immunity or how to turn an immune response less 'neurotic'.

References

Alexopoulou, L., Holt, A.C., Medzhitov, R., and Flavell, R.A. (2001). Recognition of double-stranded RNA and activation of NF-kappaB by Toll-like receptor 3. *Nature* 413: 732–738.

Alliot, F., Godin, I., and Pessac, B. (1999). Microglia derive from progenitors, originating from the yolk sac, and which proliferate in the brain. *Brain Res Dev Brain Res* 117: 145–152.

Aloisi, F. (2001). Immune function of microglia. *Glia* 36: 165–179.

Aloisi, F., Ria, F., Columba-Cabezas, S., Hess, H., Penna, G., and Adorini, L. (1999). Relative efficiency of microglia, astrocytes, dendritic cells and B cells in naive CD4+ T cell priming and Th1/Th2 cell restimulation. *Eur J Immunol* 29: 2705–2714.

An, S.F., Ciardi, A., Giometto, B., Scaravilli, T., Gray, F., and Scaravilli, F. (1996). Investigation on the expression of major histocompatibility complex class II and cytokines and detection of HIV-1 DNA within brains of asymptomatic and symptomatic HIV-1-positive patients. *Acta Neuropathol* 91: 494–503.

Barker, C.F. and Billingham, R.E. (1977). Immunologically privileged sites. *Adv Immunol* 25: 1–54.

Bauer, J., Bradl, M., Hickey, W.F., Forss-Petter, S., Breitschopf, H., Linington, C., et al. (1998). T-cell apoptosis in inflammatory brain lesions—destruction of T cells does not depend on antigen recognition. *Am J Pathol* 153: 715–724.

Becher, B. and Antel, J.P. (1996). Comparison of phenotypic and functional properties of immediately *ex vivo* and cultured human adult microglia. *Glia* 18: 1–10.

Becher, B., Fedorowicz, V., and Antel, J.P. (1996). Regulation of CD14 expression on human adult central nervous system- derived microglia. *J Neurosci Res* 45: 375–381.

Becher, B., Barker, P.A., Owens, T., and Antel, J.P. (1998). CD95-CD95L: can the brain learn from the immune system? *Trends Neurosci* 21: 114–117.

Becher, B., Blain, M., and Antel, J.P. (2000a). CD40 engagement stimulates IL-12 p70 production by human microglial cells: basis for Th1 polarization in the CNS. *J Neuroimmunol* 102: 44–50.

Becher, B., Prat, A., and Antel, J.P. (2000b). Brain-immune connection: immunoregulatory properties of CNS-resident cells. *Glia* 29: 293–304.

Becher, B., Durell, B.G., Miga, A.V., Hickey, W.F., and Noelle, R.J. (2001). The clinical course of experimental autoimmune encephalomyelitis and inflammation is controlled by the expression of CD40 within the central nervous system. *J Exp Med* 193: 967–974.

Becher, B., Durell, B.G., and Noelle, R.J. (2002). Experimental autoimmune encephalitis and inflammation in the absence of interleukin-12. *J Clin Invest* 110: 493–497.

Becher, B., Durell, B.G., and Noelle, R.J. (2003). CNS-derived IL-12/23p40 controls encephalitogenicity during the effector phase of experimental autoimmune encephalomyelitis. *J Clin Invest* 112: 1186–1191.

Bechmann, I., Mor, G., Nilsen, J., Eliza, M., Nitsch, R., and Naftolin, F. (1999). FasL (CD95L, Apo1L) is expressed in the normal rat and human brain: evidence for the existence of an immunological brain barrier. *Glia* 27: 62–74.

Bechmann, I., Kwidzinski, E., Kovac, A.D., Simburger, E., Horvath, T., Gimsa, U., et al. (2001). Turnover of rat brain perivascular cells. *Exp Neurol* 168: 242–249.

Benveniste, E. N. (1998). Cytokine actions in the central nervous system. *Cytokine Growth Factor Rev* 9: 259–275.

Bonetti, B., Pohl, J., Gao, Y.L., and Raine, C.S. (1997). Cell death during autoimmune demyelination: effector but not target cells are eliminated by apoptosis. *J Immunol* 159: 5733–5741.

Bourdoulous, S., Beraud, E., Le Page, C., Zamora, A., Ferry, A., Bernard, D., et al. (1995). Anergy induction in encephalitogenic T cells by brain microvessel endothelial cells is inhibited by interleukin-1. *Eur J Immunol* 25: 1176–1183.

Brabb, T., von Dassow, P., Ordonez, N., Schnabel, B., Duke, B., and Goverman, J. (2000). In situ tolerance within the central nervous system as a mechanism for preventing autoimmunity. *J Exp Med* 192: 871–880.

Bsibsi, M., Ravid, R., Gveric, D., and van Noort, J.M. (2002). Broad expression of Toll-like receptors in the human central nervous system. *J Neuropathol Exp Neurol* 61: 1013–1021.

Calingasan, N.Y., Erdely, H.A., and Anthony Altar, C. (2002). Identification of CD40 ligand in Alzheimer's disease and in animal models of Alzheimer's disease and brain injury. *Neurobiol Aging* 23: 31–39.

Caramalho, I., Lopes-Carvalho, T., Ostler, D., Zelenay, S., Haury, M., and Demengeot, J. (2003). Regulatory T cells selectively express Toll-like receptors and are activated by lipopolysaccharide. *J Exp Med* 197: 403–411.

Carson, M.J., Reilly, C.R., Sutcliffe, J.G., and Lo, D. (1998). Mature microglia resemble immature antigen-presenting cells, *Glia* 22: 72–85.

Carson, M.J., Sutcliffe, J.G., and Campbell, I.L. (1999). Microglia stimulate naive T-cell differentiation without stimulating T-cell proliferation. *J Neurosci Res* 55: 127–134.

Chang, T.T., Jabs, C., Sobel, R.A., Kuchroo, V.K., and Sharpe, A.H. (1999). Studies in B7-deficient mice reveal a critical role for B7 costimulation in both induction and effector phases of experimental autoimmune encephalomyelitis. *J Exp Med* 190: 733–740.

Cole, G.A., Nathanson, N., and Prendergast, R.A. (1972). Requirement for theta-bearing cells in lymphocytic choriomeningitis virus-induced central nervous system disease. *Nature* 238: 335–337.

Croft, M., Bradley, L.M., and Swain, S.L. (1994). Naive versus memory CD4 T cell response to antigen. Memory cells are less dependent on accessory cell costimulation and can respond to many antigen-presenting cell types including resting B cells. *J Immunol* 152: 2675–2685.

Cross, A.H., and Ku, G. (2000). Astrocytes and central nervous system endothelial cells do not express B7–1 (CD80) or B7–2 (CD86) immunoreactivity during experimental autoimmune encephalomyelitis. *J Neuroimmunol* 110: 76–82.

Cserr, H.F. and Knopf, P.M. (1992). Cervical lymphatics, the blood-brain barrier and the immunoreactivity of the brain: a new view. *Immunol Today* 13: 507–512.

Cua, D.J., Sherlock, J., Chen, Y., Murphy, C.A., Joyce, B., Seymour, B., et al. (2003). Interleukin-23 rather than interleukin-12 is the critical cytokine for autoimmune inflammation of the brain, *Nature* 421: 744–748.

Dalpke, A.H., Schafer, M.K.H., Frey, M., Zimmermann, S., Tebbe, J., Weihe, E., et al. (2002). Immunostimulatory CpG-DNA activates murine microglia. *J Immunol* 168: 4854–4863.

De Keyser, J., Zeinstra, E., and Frohman, E. (2003). Are astrocytes central players in the pathophysiology of multiple sclerosis? *Arch Neurol* 60: 132–136.

de Vos, A.F., van Meurs, M., Brok, H.P., Boven, L.A., Hintzen, R.Q., van der Valk, P., et al. (2002). Transfer of central nervous system autoantigens and presentation in secondary lymphoid organs. *J Immunol* 169: 5415–5423.

Doherty, P.C., Allan, J.E., Lynch, F., and Ceredig, R. (1990). Dissection of an inflammatory process induced by CD8+ T cells. *Immunol Today* 11: 55–59.

Dong, Y. and Benveniste, E.N. (2001). Immune function of astrocytes. *Glia* 36: 180–190.

Dorries, R. (2001). The role of T-cell-mediated mechanisms in virus infections of the nervous system. *Curr Top Microbiol Immunol* **253**: 219–245.

Fischer, H.G. and Reichmann, G. (2001). Brain dendritic cells and macrophages/microglia in central nervous system inflammation. *J Immunol* **166**: 2717–2726.

Ford, A.L., Foulcher, E., Lemckert, F.A., and Sedgwick, J.D. (1996). Microglia induce CD4 T lymphocyte final effector function and death. *J Exp Med* **184**: 1737–1745.

Frei, K., Siepl, C., Groscurth, P., Bodmer, S., Schwerdel, C., and Fontana, A. (1987). Antigen presentation and tumor cytotoxicity by interferon-gamma-treated microglial cells. *Eur J Immunol* **17**: 1271–1278.

Frucht, D.M. (2002). IL-23: a cytokine that acts on memory T cells. *Sci STKE* **2002**: PE1.

Gause, W.C., Lu, P., Zhou, X.D., Chen, S.J., Madden, K.B., Morris, S.C., *et al.* (1996). H. polygyrus: B7-independence of the secondary type 2 response. *Exp Parasitol* **84**: 264–273.

Goebels, N., Hofstetter, H., Schmidt, S., Brunner, C., Wekerle, H., and Hohlfeld, R. (2000). Repertoire dynamics of autoreactive T cells in multiple sclerosis patients and healthy subjects: epitope spreading versus clonal persistence. *Brain* **123**(3): 508–518.

Gozes, I., Bassan, M., Zamostiano, R., Pinhasov, A., Davidson, A., Giladi, E., *et al.* (1999). A novel signaling molecule for neuropeptide action: activity-dependent neuroprotective protein. *Ann N Y Acad Sci* **897**: 125–135.

Graeber, M.B., Grasbon-Frodl, E., Eitzen, U.V., and Kosel, S. (1998). Neurodegeneration and aging: role of the second genome. *J Neurosci Res* **52**: 1–6.

Gran, B., Zhang, G.X., Yu, S., Li, J., Chen, X.H., Ventura, E.S., *et al.* (2002). IL-12p35-deficient mice are susceptible to experimental autoimmune encephalomyelitis: evidence for redundancy in the IL-12 system in the induction of central nervous system autoimmune demyelination. *J Immunol* **169**: 7104–7110.

Green, E.A., Choi, Y., and Flavell, R.A. (2002). Pancreatic lymph node-derived CD4(+)CD25(+) Treg cells: highly potent regulators of diabetes that require TRANCE-RANK signals. *Immunity* **16**: 183–191.

Greter, M., Heppner, F., Lemos, M.P., Odermatt, B.M., Goebels, N., Laufer, T. *et al.*, (2005) Dendritic cells permit immune invasion of the CNS in an animal model of multiple sclerosis. *Nature Med* **11**: 328–334.

Hailer, N.P., Heppner, F.L., Haas, D., and Nitsch, R. (1998). Astrocytic factors deactivate antigen presenting cells that invade the central nervous system. *Brain Pathol* **8**: 459–474.

Hammarberg, H., Lidman, O., Lundberg, C., Eltayeb, S.Y., Gielen, A.W., Muhallab, S., *et al.* (2000). Neuroprotection by encephalomyelitis: rescue of mechanically injured neurons and neurotrophin production by CNS-infiltrating T and natural killer cells. *J Neurosci* **20**: 5283–5291.

Havenith, C.E.G., Askew, D., and Walker, W.S. (1998). Mouse resident microglia: Isolation and characterization of immunoregulatory properties with naive CD4(+) and CD8(+) T-cells. *Glia* **22**: 348–359.

Hemmi, H., Takeuchi, O., Kawai, T., Kaisho, T., Sato, S., Sanjo, H., *et al.* (2000). A Toll-like receptor recognizes bacterial DNA. *Nature* **408**: 740–745.

Hickey, W.F. (1991). Migration of hematogenous cells through the blood-brain barrier and the initiation of CNS inflammation. *Brain Pathol* **1**: 97–105.

Hickey, W.F., Vass, K., and Lassmann, H. (1992). Bone marrow-derived elements in the central nervous system: an immunohistochemical and ultrastructural survey of rat chimeras. *J Neuropathol Exp Neurol* **51**: 246–256.

Hoek, R.M., Ruuls, S.R., Murphy, C.A., Wright, G.J., Goddard, R., Zurawski, S.M., *et al.* (2000). Down-regulation of the macrophage lineage through interaction with OX2 (CD200). *Science* **290**: 1768–1771.

Hohlfeld, R., Kerschensteiner, M., Stadelmann, C., Lassmann, H., and Wekerle, H. (2000). The neuroprotective effect of inflammation: implications for the therapy of multiple sclerosis. *J Neuroimmunol* **107**: 161–166.

Howard, L.M. and Miller, S.D. (2001). Autoimmune intervention by CD154 blockade prevents T cell retention and effector function in the target organ. *J Immunol* **166**: 1547–1553.

Huitinga, I., Ruuls, S.R., Jung, S., Van Rooijen, N., Hartung, H.P., and Dijkstra, C.D. (1995). Macrophages in T cell line-mediated, demyelinating, and chronic relapsing experimental autoimmune encephalomyelitis in Lewis rats. *Clin Exp Immunol* **100**: 344–351.

Irani, D.N. (1998). Brain-derived gangliosides induce cell cycle arrest in a murine T cell line. *J Neuroimmunol* **87**: 11–16.

Irani, D.N., Lin, K.I., and Griffin, D.E. (1996). Brain-derived gangliosides regulate the cytokine production and proliferation of activated T cells. *J Immunol* **157**: 4333–4340.

Issazadeh, S., Navikas, V., Schaub, M., Sayegh, M., and Khoury, S. (1998). Kinetics of expression of costimulatory molecules and their ligands in murine relapsing experimental autoimmune encephalomyelitis *in vivo*. *J Immunol* **161**: 1104–1112.

Juedes, A.E. and Ruddle, N.H. (2001). Resident and infiltrating central nervous system APCs regulate the emergence and resolution of experimental autoimmune encephalomyelitis. *J Immunol* **166**: 5168–5175.

Kipnis, J., Mizrahi, T., Yoles, E., Ben-Nun, A., Schwartz, M., and Ben-Nur, A. (2002). Myelin specific Th1 cells are necessary for post-traumatic protective autoimmunity. *J Neuroimmunol* **130**: 78–85.

Klyushnenkova, E.N. and Vanguri, P. (1997). Ia expression and antigen presentation by glia: strain and cell type- specific differences among rat astrocytes and microglia. *J Neuroimmunol* **79**: 190–201.

Konno, H., Yamamoto, T., Suzuki, H., Yamamoto, H., Iwasaki, Y., Ohara, Y., *et al.* (1990). Targeting of adoptively transferred experimental allergic encephalitis lesion at the sites of wallerian degeneration. *Acta Neuropathol* **80**: 521–526.

Krakowski, M.L. and Owens, T. (1997). The central nervous system environment controls effector CD4(+) T cell cytokine profile in experimental allergic encephalomyelitis. *Eur J Immunol* **27**: 2840–2847.

Krakowski, M.L. and Owens, T. (2000). Naive T lymphocytes traffic to inflamed central nervous system, but require antigen recognition for activation. *Eur J Immunol* **30**: 1002–1009.

Lafaille, J.J., Keere, F.V., Hsu, A.L., Baron, J.L., Haas, W., Raine, C.S., *et al.* (1997). Myelin basic protein-specific T helper 2 (Th2) cells cause experimental autoimmune encephalomyelitis in immunodeficient hosts rather than protect them from the disease. *J Exp Med* **186**: 307–312.

Laflamme, N. and Rivest, S. (2001). Toll-like receptor 4: the missing link of the cerebral innate immune response triggered by circulating gram-negative bacterial cell wall components. *FASEB J* **15**: 155–163.

Laflamme, N., Soucy, G., and Rivest, S. (2001). Circulating cell wall components derived from gram-negative, not gram-positive, bacteria cause a profound induction of the gene-encoding Toll-like receptor 2 in the CNS. *J Neurochem* **79**: 648–657.

Lake, J., Weller, R.O., Phillips, M.J., and Needham, M. (1999). Lymphocyte targeting of the brain in adoptive transfer cryolesion-EAE. *J Pathol* **187**: 259–265.

Lamers, K.J., de Reus, H.P., and Jongen, P.J. (1998). Myelin basic protein in CSF as indicator of disease activity in multiple sclerosis. *Mult Scler* **4**: 124–126.

Lehnardt, S., Lachance, C., Patrizi, S., Lefebvre, S., Follett, P.L., Jensen, F.E., *et al.* (2002). The toll-like receptor TLR4 is necessary for lipopolysaccharide-induced oligodendrocyte injury in the CNS. *J Neurosci* **22**: 2478–2486.

Li, H., Newcombe, J., Groome, N.P., and Cuzner, M.L. (1993). Characterization and distribution of phagocytic macrophages in multiple sclerosis plaques. *Neuropathol Appl Neurobiol* **19**: 214–223.

Maehlen, J., Olsson, T., Zachau, A., Klareskog, L., and Kristensson, K. (1989). Local enhancement of major histocompatibility complex (MHC) class I and II expression and cell infiltration in experimental allergic encephalomyelitis around axotomized motor neurons. *J Neuroimmunol* **23,**: 125–132.

Massa, P.T., ter Meulen, V., and Fontana, A. (1987). Hyperinducibility of Ia antigen on astrocytes correlates with strain- specific susceptibility to experimental autoimmune encephalomyelitis. *Proc Natl Acad Sci USA* **84**: 4219–4223.

Matsumoto, Y., Ohmori, K., and Fujiwara, M. (1992). Immune regulation by brain cells in the central nervous system: microglia but not astrocytes present myelin basic protein to encephalitogenic T cells under *in vivo*-mimicking conditions. *Immunology* **76**: 209–216.

Matyszak, M.K. and Perry, V.H. (1998). Bacillus Calmette–Guerin sequestered in the brain parenchyma escapes immune recognition. *J Neuroimmunol* **82**: 73–80.

McCluskey, L.P. and Lampson, L.A. (2000). Local neurochemicals and site-specific immune regulation in the CNS. *J Neuropathol Exp Neurol* **59**: 177–187.

McGavern, D.B., Homann, D., and Oldstone, M.B. (2002). T cells in the central nervous system: the delicate balance between viral clearance and disease. *J Infect Dis* **186**(Suppl. 2): S145–S151.

McGeer, P.L., Kawamata, T., Walker, D.G., Akiyama, H., Tooyama, I., and McGeer, E.G. (1993). Microglia in degenerative neurological disease. *Glia* **7**: 84–92.

McMenamin, P.G. (1999). Distribution and phenotype of dendritic cells and resident tissue macrophages in the dura mater, leptomeninges, and choroid plexus of the rat brain as demonstrated in wholemount preparations. *J Comp Neurol* **405**: 553–562.

Medzhitov, R. (2001). Toll-like receptors and innate immunity. *Nat Rev Immunol* **1**: 135–145.

Meinl, E. and Hohlfeld, R. (2002). Immunopathogenesis of multiple sclerosis: MBP and beyond. *Clin Exp Immunol* **128**: 395–397.

Mellman, I. and Steinman, R.M. (2001). Dendritic cells: specialized and regulated antigen processing machines. *Cell* **106**: 255–258.

Mendel, I. and Shevach, E.M. (2002). Differentiated Th1 autoreactive effector cells can induce experimental autoimmune encephalomyelitis in the absence of IL-12 and CD40/CD40L interactions. *J Neuroimmunol* **122**: 65–73.

Moalem, G., Gdalyahu, A., Shani, Y., Otten, U., Lazarovici, P., Cohen, I.R., et al. (2000). Production of neurotrophins by activated T cells: implications for neuroprotective autoimmunity. *J Autoimmun* **15**: 331–345.

Murphy, C.A., Hoek, R.M., Wiekowski, M.T., Lira, S.A., and Sedgwick, J.D. (2002). Interactions between hemopoietically derived TNF and central nervous system-resident glial chemokines underlie initiation of autoimmune inflammation in the brain. *J Immunol* **169**: 7054–7062.

Neumann, H. (2001). Control of glial immune function by neurons. *Glia* **36**: 191–199.

Nguyen, M.D., Julien, J.P., and Rivest, S. (2002). Innate immunity: the missing link in neuroprotection and neurodegeneration? *Nat Rev Neurosci* **3**: 216–227.

Nikcevich, K.M., Gordon, K.B., Tan, L., Hurst, S.D., Kroepfl, J.F., Gardinier, M., et al. (1997). IFN-gamma-activated primary murine astrocytes express B7 costimulatory molecules and prime naive antigen-specific T cells. *J Immunol* **158**: 614–621.

O'Keefe, G.M., Nguyen, V.T., and Benveniste, E.N. (2002). Regulation and function of class II major histocompatibility complex, CD40, and B7 expression in macrophages and microglia: Implications in neurological diseases. *J Neurovirol* **8**: 496–512.

Olson, J.K., Eagar, T.N., and Miller, S.D. (2002). Functional activation of myelin-specific T cells by virus-induced molecular mimicry. *J Immunol* **169**: 2719–2726.

Olson, J.K., Girvin, A.M., and Miller, S.D. (2001). Direct activation of innate and antigen-presenting functions of microglia following infection with Theiler's virus. *J Virol* **75**: 9780–9789.

Owens, T. (2002). Identification of new therapeutic targets for prevention of CNS inflammation. *Expert Opin Ther Targets* **6**: 203–215.

Owens, T. and Babcock, A. (2002). Immune response induction in the central nervous system. *Front Biosci* **7**: d427–d438.

Pender, M.P. and Rist, M.J. (2001). Apoptosis of inflammatory cells in immune control of the nervous system: role of glia. *Glia* **36**: 137–144.

Perry, V.H. (1998). A revised view of the central nervous system microenvironment and major histocompatibility complex class II antigen presentation. *J Neuroimmunol* **90**: 113–121.

Phillips, M.J., Needham, M., and Weller, R.O. (1997). Role of cervical lymph nodes in autoimmune encephalomyelitis in the Lewis rat. *J Pathol* **182**: 457–464.

Piehl, F. and Lidman, O. (2001). Neuroinflammation in the rat–CNS cells and their role in the regulation of immune reactions. *Immunol Rev* **184**: 212–225.

Polfliet, M.M., van de Veerdonk, F., Dopp, E.A., van Kesteren-Hendrikx, E.M., van Rooijen, N., Dijkstra, C.D., et al. (2002). The role of perivascular and meningeal macrophages in experimental allergic encephalomyelitis. *J Neuroimmunol* **122**: 1–8.

Prat, A., Biernacki, K., Becher, B., and Antel, J.P. (2000). B7 expression and antigen presentation by human brain endothelial cells: requirement for proinflammatory cytokines. *J Neuropathol Exp Neurol* **59**: 129–136.

Schwartz, M. (2001). T cell mediated neuroprotection is a physiological response to central nervous system insults. *J Mol Med* **78**: 594–597.

Sedgwick, J.D., Schwender, S., Imrich, H., Dorries, R., Butcher, G.W., and ter Meulen, V. (1991). Isolation and direct characterization of resident microglial cells from the normal and inflamed central nervous system. *Proc Natl Acad Sci USA* **88**: 7438–7442.

Sedgwick, J.D., Schwender, S., Gregersen, R., Dorries, R., and ter Meulen, V. (1993). Resident macrophages (ramified microglia) of the adult brown Norway rat central nervous system are constitutively major histocompatibility complex class II positive. *J Exp Med* **177**: 1145–1152.

Serafini, B., Columba-Cabezas, S., Di rosa, F., and Aloisi, F. (2000). Intracerebral recruitment and maturation of dendritic cells in the onset and progression of experimental autoimmune encephalomyelitis. *Am J Pathol* **157**: 1991–2002.

Slavin, A.J., Soos, J.M., Stuve, O., Patarroyo, J.C., Weiner, H.L., Fontana, A., et al. (2001). Requirement for endocytic antigen processing and influence of invariant chain and H-2M deficiencies in CNS autoimmunity. *J Clin Invest* **108**: 1133–1139.

Slobodov, U., Reichert, F., Mirski, R., and Rotshenker, S. (2001). Distinct inflammatory stimuli induce different patterns of myelin phagocytosis and degradation in recruited macrophages. *Exp Neurol* **167**: 401–409.

Smith, M.E. (2001). Phagocytic properties of microglia in vitro: implications for a role in multiple sclerosis and EAE. *Microsc Res Tech* **54**: 81–94.

Soos, J.M., Morrow, J., Ashley, T.A., Szente, B.E., Bikoff, E.K., and Zamvil, S.S. (1998). Astrocytes express elements of the class II endocytic pathway and process central nervous system autoantigen for presentation to encephalitogenic T cells. *J Immunol* **161**: 5959–5966.

Steinman, L., Martin, R., Bernard, C., Conlon, P., and Oksenberg, J.R. (2002). Multiple sclerosis: deeper understanding of its pathogenesis reveals new targets for therapy. *Annu Rev Neurosci* **25**: 491–505.

Sun, D., Coleclough, C., and Whitaker, J.N. (1997). Nonactivated astrocytes downregulate T cell receptor expression and reduce antigen-specific proliferation and cytokine production of myelin basic protein (MBP)-reactive T cells. *J Neuroimmunol* **78**: 69–78.

Takeuchi, O., Hoshino, K., Kawai, T., Sanjo, H., Takada, H., Ogawa, T., et al. (1999). Differential roles of TLR2 and TLR4 in recognition of Gram-negative and Gram-positive bacterial cell wall components. *Immunity* **11**: 443–451.

Tan, J., Town, T., Paris, D., Mori, T., Suo, Z., Crawford, F., et al. (1999). Microglial activation resulting from CD40-CD40L interaction after beta-amyloid stimulation. *Science* **286**: 2352–2355.

Tan, J., Town, T., Mori, T., Obregon, D., Wu, Y., DelleDonne, A., et al. (2002). CD40 is expressed and functional on neuronal cells. *EMBO J* **21**: 643–652.

Tan, L., Gordon, K.B., Mueller, J. P., Matis, L.A., and Miller, S. D. (1998). Presentation of proteolipid protein epitopes and B7–1-dependent activation of encephalitogenic T cells by IFN-gamma-activated SJL/J astrocytes. *J Immunol* **160**: 4271–4279.

Tompkins, S.M., Padilla, J., Dal Canto, M.C., Ting, J.P., Van Kaer, L., and Miller, S.D. (2002). De novo central nervous system processing of myelin antigen is required for the initiation of experimental autoimmune encephalomyelitis. *J Immunol* **168**: 4173–4183.

Tran, E.H., Hoekstra, K., van Rooijen, N., Dijkstra, C.D., and Owens, T. (1998). Immune invasion of the central nervous system parenchyma and experimental allergic encephalomyelitis, but not leukocyte extravasation from blood, are prevented in macrophage-depleted mice. *J Immunol* **161**: 3767–3775.

Vass, K. and Lassmann, H. (1990). Intrathecal application of interferon gamma. Progressive appearance of MHC antigens within the rat nervous system. *Am J Pathol* **137**: 789–800.

Vincent, V.A., Tilders, F.J., and Van Dam, A.M. (1997). Inhibition of endotoxin-induced nitric oxide synthase production in microglial cells by the presence of astroglial cells: a role for transforming growth factor beta. *Glia* **19**: 190–198.

Vitkovic, L., Maeda, S., and Sternberg, E. (2001). Anti-inflammatory cytokines: expression and action in the brain. *Neuroimmunomodulation* **9**: 295–312.

Wei, R. and Jonakait, G.M. (1999). Neurotrophins and the anti-inflammatory agents interleukin-4 (IL-4), IL- 10, IL-11 and transforming growth factor-beta1 (TGF-beta1) down-regulate T cell costimulatory molecules B7 and CD40 on cultured rat microglia. *J Neuroimmunol* **95**: 8–18.

Weinberg, A.D., Wegmann, K.W., Funatake, C., and Whitham, R.H. (1999). Blocking OX-40/OX-40 ligand interaction in vitro and in vivo leads to decreased T cell function and amelioration of experimental allergic encephalomyelitis. *J Immunol* **162**: 1818–1826.

Wenkel, H., Streilein, J.W., and Young, M.J. (2000). Systemic immune deviation in the brain that does not depend on the integrity of the blood–brain barrier. *J Immunol* **164**: 5125–5131.

Wilkin, G.P., Marriott, D.R., and Cholewinski, A.J. (1990). Astrocyte heterogeneity. *Trends Neurosci* **13**: 43–46.

Williams, K., Ulvestad, E., Waage, A., Antel, J.P., and McLaurin, J. (1994). Activation of adult human derived microglia by myelin phagocytosis *in vitro*. *J Neurosci Res* **38**: 433–443.

Williams, K.C., Dooley, N.P., Ulvestad, E., Waage, A., Blain, M., Yong, V.W., *et al.* (1995). Antigen presentation by human fetal astrocytes with the cooperative effect of microglia or the microglial-derived cytokine IL-1. *J Neurosci* **15**: 1869–1878.

Williams, K., Alvarez, X., and Lackner, A.A. (2001*a*). Central nervous system perivascular cells are immunoregulatory cells that connect the CNS with the peripheral immune system. *Glia* **36**: 156–164.

Williams, K.C., Corey, S., Westmoreland, S.V., Pauley, D., Knight, H., deBakker, C., *et al.* (2001*b*). Perivascular macrophages are the primary cell type productively infected by simian immunodeficiency virus in the brains of macaques: implications for the neuropathogenesis of AIDS. *J Exp Med* **193**: 905–915.

Wolvers, D.A., Coenen-de Roo, C.J., Mebius, R.E., van der Cammen, M.J., Tirion, F., Miltenburg, A.M., *et al.* (1999). Intranasally induced immunological tolerance is determined by characteristics of the draining lymph nodes: studies with OVA and human cartilage gp-39. *J Immunol* **162**: 1994–1998.

Zeinstra, E., Wilczak, N., and De Keyser, J. (2003). Reactive astrocytes in chronic active lesions of multiple sclerosis express co-stimulatory molecules B7–1 and B7–2. *J Neuroimmunol* **135**: 166–171.

Zekki, H., Feinstein, D.L., and Rivest, S. (2002). The clinical course of experimental autoimmune encephalomyelitis is associated with a profound and sustained transcriptional activation of the genes encoding toll-like receptor 2 and CD14 in the mouse CNS. *Brain Pathol* **12**: 308–319.

6 Role of the immune response in tissue damage and repair in the injured spinal cord

Samuel David and Steve Lacroix

Introduction

The immune system has evolved primarily to protect the body from invasion by micro-organisms such as bacteria, viruses, and parasites, and to contribute to repair processes during disease and after injury. Although the immune response to injury in non-central nervous system (CNS) tissue often leads to repair that is desirable, similar responses in the injured mammalian CNS cause gliosis that could be detrimental to the growth of damaged axons and repair of neural circuitry. In addition, these immune responses in the injured CNS have also been implicated in the extensive tissue loss sustained at the site of injury. Despite the evidence that autoimmune responses to self-antigens lead to disease, which most notably in the CNS leads to multiple sclerosis in humans and experimental allergic encephalomyelitis (EAE) in animal models, recent studies suggest that some types of autoimmune responses may be guided to protect the CNS after injury. Other work also indicates that antibody and macrophage responses may also be recruited to promote axon growth and regeneration. These studies appear at a time when other evidence points to the detrimental role of the immune response in neurodegenerative diseases such as Alzheimer's disease and amyotrophic lateral sclerosis (Giulian, 1999; Zhu et al. 2002; Kriz et al., 2002; Wyss-Coray and Mucke, 2002). Can the innate and adaptive arms of the immune response be recruited to favor tissue repair and axon regeneration after spinal cord injury?

One of the consequences of spinal cord injury (SCI) is loss of neural tissue at the site of injury and the damage to axons of long fiber tracts that traverse the length of the cord in both directions. Motor fibers descend from cortical and brainstem neurons, while fibers carrying sensory information from peripheral receptors, such as those in the skin and from sensory neurons in the spinal cord, ascend to neurons in the brainstem, cerebellum, and other regions of the CNS. Damage to these descending and ascending fiber tracts will, therefore, result in loss of motor, sensory, and autonomic functions. Since the CNS environment, unlike that in peripheral nerves, is inhibitory for axon regeneration, damage of axons of the long fiber tracts in the CNS leads to permanent functional deficits.

In this chapter we will focus primarily on SCI. Two aspects of the injury response will be considered: (1) tissue loss and protection at the site of spinal cord lesion and (2) axon damage and regeneration. We will assess the evidence for the involvement of the immune response in the generation of the pathological changes at the site of SCI, as well as its potential for influencing tissue protection and axon regeneration.

Tissue loss and protection

Mechanisms of tissue damage

Two models of SCI are widely used in studies of regeneration and repair: (1) hemisection (dorsal or unilateral hemisections) and (2) contusion injury. The former has been used effectively for many years to study long-distance axon regeneration, while the latter has been the preferred model for studies of trauma-induced tissue loss. Experimental spinal cord contusion injuries in rodents show many histopathological and functional similarities to spinal cord injuries most often sustained in humans. This contusion model has been used to characterize the immediate damage due to mechanical injury, delayed secondary damage resulting in the progressive death of the surrounding neural cells by apoptosis, and the formation of cystic cavities (Noble and Wrathall, 1985; Bresnahan et al., 1991; Behrmann et al., 1992; Reier et al., 1992; Constantini and Young, 1994; Liu et al., 1997).

Results from several studies support the view that the two types of cell death, immediate and secondary cell death, proceed sequentially in the injured spinal cord (Tator and Fehlings, 1991; Tator, 1995; Amar and Levy, 1999). Necrosis is the principal mechanism of cell death at the site of CNS trauma occurring immediately after the injury, whereas apoptosis contributes more to secondary cell loss at later periods. Apoptotic cells are detected from 4 h to at least 3 weeks after spinal cord contusion (Crowe et al., 1997; Liu et al., 1997). Accordingly, the size of the lesion and the extent of cavitation in rats increase progressively over days to weeks following SCI (Steward et al., 1999). While it may be unrealistic to hope to prevent much of the rapid death of neural cells undergoing necrosis due to the direct mechanical effects of the trauma, potential strategies are currently being tested to prevent secondary apoptotic cell death. Although the precise mechanisms of secondary damage are still unclear, it is known that the initial traumatic injury leading to primary cell death is immediately followed by the removal of tissue debris by inflammatory cells. It has been hypothesized that primary cell death and the inflammatory response might both play a role in initiating secondary damage via signals that are still not fully identified.

Among the candidates for mediating secondary toxicity are factors such as calcium, proteases, glutamate, and other excitatory amino acids, to name a few. Over the last few years, however, free radicals, cytokines, and chemokines have received greater attention with regard to their potential contribution as mediators and modulators of secondary CNS degeneration at the site of trauma. Free radicals, cytokines and chemokines are induced in response to various CNS insults and can cause cellular injury and apoptotic cell death both *in vitro* and *in vivo* (Lewen et al., 2000; Allan and Rothwell 2001). Notably, levels of free radicals, cytokines, and chemokines are elevated within spinal cord lesion sites following a time-course that fits well with the timing of secondary cell loss (Hamada et al., 1996b; Bartholdi and Schwab, 1997; McTigue et al., 1998; Streit et al., 1998; Liu et al., 2000; Satake et al., 2000; Xu et al., 2001; Chatzipanteli et al., 2002). Inflammatory cells are the principal source of these factors after CNS trauma. What are some of the roles these inflammatory cells play in CNS trauma, and how can they be manipulated in an attempt to reduce secondary damage and promote neuroprotection?

The influence and consequences of the inflammatory response following SCI is still a matter of intense study. Several reports support a deleterious role of inflammation after CNS injury (Blight, 1985, Giulian et al.; 1993, Popovich et al., 1997; Taoka et al., 1997; Carlson et al., 1998; Popovich et al., 1999). However, other studies have also raised the possibility that inflammatory responses after CNS lesions may have some beneficial effects (David et al., 1990, Rapalino et al., 1998, Hauben et al., 2000; Leon et al., 2000). It is possible that inflammatory cells could participate in both secondary degeneration and tissue protection, depending on their state of activation at various times after the lesion.

Involvement of immune cells and approaches to altering their response

The growing evidence that inflammation makes an important contribution to the orchestration and progression or control of secondary tissue damage has paved the way for studies aimed at blocking or stimulating different aspects of the inflammatory response. A number of approaches have been tested thus far to alter the immune cell response in an attempt to obtain tissue protection after SCI. We will discuss these under the headings of cell-directed and general approaches to modulate the immune response after CNS injury.

Cell-directed approaches to modulate the immune response

Blocking immune cell recruitment

Soon after spinal cord contusion or hemisection, the site of the lesion becomes filled with large numbers of hematogenous inflammatory cells. Neutrophils, lymphocytes, and monocytes are successively chemoattracted to this site and occupy the area of the lesion for limited or prolonged periods of time depending upon the cell type (Dusart and Schwab, 1994; Popovich et al., 1997; Carlson et al., 1998; Schnell et al., 1999a; Ma et al., 2002). These cells release and respond to a multitude of soluble signals and organize an inflammatory response that will lead to phagocytosis of tissue debris and pathogens from the site of injury and ultimately to wound healing. Chemokines and cytokines, in particular, are involved in the attraction of blood-derived inflammatory cells into the CNS parenchyma and their activation (Bell et al., 1996; Schnell et al., 1999b; Asensio and Campbell, 1999). In general, inflammation is thought to proceed when the balance in the levels between pro- and anti-inflammatory cytokines tilts in favor of the former. Inflammatory molecules released in the CNS parenchyma after an injury may participate in both neuropathological and neuroprotective responses. Interestingly, Bethea et al. (1999) showed that interleukin (IL)-10, a potent anti-inflammatory cytokine, reduces spinal cord cavitation and improves functional outcome if provided as a single dose after injury, but worsens the outcome if administered on two occasions 48 h apart after SCI.

Since the pathological changes after SCI are constantly evolving in the early period after injury, the role played by chemokines and cytokines is likely to depend on the time after injury and the levels of these immune modulators. Along these lines, several studies have reported that macrophage inflammatory protein (MIP)-1α, macrophage chemotactic protein (MCP)-1, and tumor necrosis factor-alpha (TNF-α) play a key role in the inflammation and tissue damage that occurs in the CNS in experimental autoimmune encephalomyelitis (EAE) (Karpus et al., 1995; Karpus and Ransohoff, 1998). However, our laboratory has recently shown that MIP-1α, MCP-1, and TNF-α are also key players in lysophosphatidylcholine (LPC)-induced inflammatory responses in the spinal cord that lead to macrophage activation and myelin phagocytosis without causing cell death and tissue damage (Ousman and David, 2001). The differences in these two models may lie in the timing and duration of chemokine/cytokine expression. In the LPC model, the expression of these chemokines and cytokines is limited to a very short period of 1–2 days, while in EAE their expression is prolonged over a period of a week or more (Godiska et al., 1995; Karpus et al., 1995; Glabinski et al., 1997). In addition, in the LPC model, rapid down-regulation of these chemokines and cytokines is accompanied by the expression of anti-inflammatory cytokines such as IL-10 and transforming growth factor-beta (TGF-β) (Ousman and David, 2001). The duration of expression of pro-inflammatory chemokines and cytokines and the coordinated expression of anti-inflammatory molecules are key factors in the development of a safe inflammatory response. Similarly, although a number of chemokines and cytokines have been

implicated in the pathology after SCI based on expression studies (Schnell et al., 1999b; Bartholdi and Schwab, 1997; McTigue et al., 1998; Ghirnikar et al., 2000, 2001), they may exert positive or negative effects depending on the context and time after injury. Inflammatory cells also produce other cytotoxic molecules such as free radicals that could actively participate in secondary degeneration after SCI (Satake et al., 2000; Chatzipanteli et al., 2002). Hydrogen peroxide released after CNS damage can react with ferrous iron to produce highly toxic hydroxyl radicals (Hyslop et al., 1995). The excessive infiltration of immune cells, which contribute to increased levels of pro-inflammatory and cytotoxic molecules, can therefore also lead to cellular damage and tissue destruction after SCI.

Neutrophils

All the evidence points to neutrophils as being one of the first blood-derived inflammatory cells to infiltrate the site of injury after spinal cord contusion or hemisection (Dusart and Schwab, 1994; Carlson et al., 1998; Schnell et al., 1999a). Once activated, most likely through cytokines released by resident CNS cells and/or nearby immune cells that were activated post-traumatically, neutrophils release chemotactic factors such as chemokines which can attract other inflammatory cells to the site of injury and amplify the immune response. Among the well-documented chemokines secreted by the neutrophils are MIP-1α, MIP-1β, and MCPs (Cassatella, 1999; Scapini et al., 2000; Yamashiro et al., 2001), which are all known to recruit granulocytes, lymphocytes, and monocytes into inflammatory sites (Ransohoff and Tani, 1998; Asensio and Campbell, 1999)

A role for activated neutrophils in secondary damage induced after SCI was first suggested several years ago by Means and Anderson (1983). Later, it was shown that neutrophils accumulate in the first few hours following SCI (Blight, 1992; Dusart and Schwab, 1994; Carlson et al., 1998), and that neutrophil infiltration is proportional to the magnitude of the trauma (Xu et al., 1990; Schoettle et al., 1990). Taoka et al. (1997) reported that administration of an antibody against P-selectin, a lectin expressed on the endothelial cell surface after injury, attenuated the accumulation of neutrophils in the injured spinal cord and improved motor functions. Antibodies directed against intercellular cell-adhesion molecule-1 (ICAM-1) also reduced the infiltration of neutrophils into damaged tissue and reduced the motor loss following spinal cord compression in rats (Hamada et al., 1996a). Blocking the interaction between αDβ2 integrin and vascular cell-adhesion molecule-1 (VCAM-1) with an antibody directed against αDβ2 reduced the number of neutrophils at the site of SCI by 43% (Mabon et al., 2000). Lacroix et al. (2002) recently reported that a large number of neutrophils are attracted into the injured spinal cord of rats grafted with fibroblasts releasing a fusion protein consisting of the pro-inflammatory cytokine IL-6 and its alpha receptor which interacts directly with gp130 to transduce the IL-6 signal. This neutrophil influx was associated with increased numbers of macrophages and activated microglia and led to greater tissue damage.

In transgenic mouse models of EAE, increased neutrophil influx was also associated with greater tissue destruction and more severe clinical deficits (Tran et al., 2000). On the other hand, our laboratory has shown that a brief influx of neutrophils into the spinal cord occurring over a period of 6–12 h after LPC injection into the mouse spinal cord is not detrimental and may contribute to the controlled non-destructive inflammatory response seen in this model (Ousman and David, 2000). Taken together, these results suggest that although a limited and brief influx of neutrophils may be required for an effective immune response, excessive neutrophil influx could participate both directly and/or indirectly in secondary tissue destruction after SCI. Neutrophils could accumulate at sites of injury and contribute directly to secondary cell death by secreting cytotoxic factors such as proteases and reactive oxygen species (Harlan, 1987). Alternatively, neutrophils could penetrate the CNS and subsequently trigger the leakage of the blood–brain barrier via the release of inflammatory mediators. This could stimulate circulatory disturbances and cause the migration of more inflammatory cells to sites of trauma and exacerbate tissue damage.

T lymphocytes

T cells are essential cellular components of the adaptive immune response. While normally found in very low numbers in the intact brain and spinal cord, T cells rapidly enter the CNS after an injury (Hirschberg and Schwartz, 1995; Popovich et al., 1997) but their numbers in the injured CNS are lower than in injured peripheral nerve, probably due to elimination via cell death (Moalem et al., 1999b). Activated T cells can protect tissue by directly killing foreign pathogens or by orchestrating the humoral immune response. Such a humoral response will lead to the production of specific antibodies, and ultimately the elimination of foreign cells or pathogens via the induction of the complement cascade. However, T lymphocytes are also implicated in autoimmune disease such as multiple sclerosis (MS) and EAE (Traugott et al., 1983; Zamvil et al., 1985).

Despite the evidence that autoimmune T-cell responses directed against myelin antigens can cause neural damage in EAE (Traugott et al., 1983; Zamvil et al., 1985), it has been proposed in recent years that inducing autoimmunity via manipulation of autoreactive T cells can contribute to neuroprotection after CNS injury (Schwartz, 2001). In the context of SCI, it has been reported that rats with spinal cord contusion injected with myelin basic protein (MBP) reactive T cells show significantly better functional recovery, as measured by the open-field locomotor test of Basso et al. (1995) than rats injected with T cells reactive with ovalbumin (Hauben et al., 2000). Active immunization with MBP was also shown to promote functional recovery (Hauben et al., 2000). Another study reported that rats with spinal cord contusion injury treated with MBP-activated splenocytes derived from other spinal cord injured rats showed better recovery of hindlimb motor skills than control animals treated with splenocytes derived from naïve recipients (Yoles et al., 2001).

It is not yet clear how autoreactive T lymphocytes exert their protective effect in limiting tissue damage at the site of injury. It has been proposed that neurotrophins released by myelin reactive T cells at sites of injury could mediate some of these effects (Kerschensteiner et al., 1999; Moalem et al., 2000). Brain-derived neurotrophic factor (BDNF) delivered via osmotic minipump (10 mg/day) was reported to reduce tissue necrosis and cavity formation, as well as secondary cell death of motor neurons near the lesion site after unilateral spinal cord hemisection in adult rats (Novikova et al., 1996). Effects of other neurotrophins in this regard are not known. Neurotrophins can also be retrogradely transported to the cell soma and enhance the survival of long projecting neurons (Tetzlaff et al., 1994; Tuszynski and Kordower, 1999). Whether T cells release sufficient amounts of neurotrophins for an adequate duration of time under the experimental conditions discussed above to mediate such neuronal protection and prevent cavitation has yet to be demonstrated. Other cell types such as macrophages and activated microglia have also been proposed to participate in the neuroprotective effects mediated by myelin reactive T cells (Butovsky et al., 2001).

One shortcoming of using MPB-reactive T cells is that they induce EAE while seemingly being protective (Moalem et al., 1999a; Hauben et al., 2000). The MBP-reactive T cells that are protective in SCI are T helper 1 (Th1) type T cells, which are also known to underlie the induction of EAE. In an attempt to reduce the probability of inducing EAE, T cells reactive to a potentially non-encephalitogenic cryptic epitope of MBP were tested. Although these T cells were reported to be neuroprotective after optic nerve crush injury, mild EAE paralysis nevertheless occurred in some animals (Moalem et al., 1999a). In other work, Popovich et al. (1996b) showed that SCI sensitized T cells harvested from rat lymph nodes 1 week after a contusion injury can induce EAE-like symptoms when injected into naïve recipients. However, there are no reports of increased incidence of MS in patients with SCI.

More recently, Schwartz and colleagues showed that a Th2 T-cell response that prevents autoimmune responses also leads to neuroprotection (Kipnis et al., 2000; Hauben et al., 2001). They reported that immunization with MBP in incomplete Freund's adjuvant, or treatment with copolymer-1 (Cop-1), a non-pathogenic synthetic compound that mimics MBP, also gives protective responses (Kipnis et al., 2000; Hauben et al., 2001). Cop-1 is currently being tested in the treatment of MS. The treatment protocol used with Cop-1 stimulates a Th2 response, reflected in an increase in IL-10 (Aharoni et al., 2000). Active immunization with Cop-1 or an injection with Cop-1-reactive T cells reduced the death of retinal ganglion cells after a crush injury to the optic nerve (Kipnis et al., 2000). How autoreactive T cells that display a Th1 phenotype capable of producing autoimmune disease might confer neuroprotection to the injured CNS, while in other instances Th2 type T-cell responses that prevent autoimmune disease do the same is not entirely clear at present.

In other work, Jones et al. (2002) reported that transgenic mice in which over 95% of all CD4+ T cells are MBP-reactive had higher intraspinal mRNA levels for pro-inflammatory cytokines, significantly more tissue loss, and impaired motor recovery compared with their littermates after spinal cord trauma. Notably, these transgenic mice also showed significantly less white matter sparing at sites of injury, and T lymphocytes were co-localized with demyelination. However, 95% myelin reactive T cells is far above the percentage that would be encountered normally after CNS damage. After EAE, for example, it is believed that fewer than 10% of the infiltrating T lymphocytes are CNS antigen specific (Cross et al., 1990; Steinman, 1996). Although the study by Jones et al. (2002) point to the potential detrimental effects of MBP-reactive T cells, a potentially protective effect of myelin-reactive T cells at a lower ratio cannot be entirely excluded. Furthermore, there is also the possibility that non-myelin-reactive T lymphocytes, with collaboration from myelin-reactive T cells, could contribute to neuroprotection after CNS injury. In addition, a very short period of T-cell influx into the spinal cord of 6–12 h after LPC injection does not lead to adverse effects, and may be necessary for the subsequent inflammatory changes leading to rapid clearance of myelin damaged by LPC (Ousman and David, 2000). The results presented above clearly highlight some of the uncertainties associated at present with manipulating T cells as a therapy for CNS injury. A better understanding of T-cell function in the context of CNS pathology after traumatic injury is required before such immunotherapies can be safely applied.

Macrophages

Of all the inflammatory cells, macrophages are present in large number at sites of SCI. A high number of macrophages infiltrate the spinal cord 3 days after spinal cord contusion in rats and mice, and their numbers peak between 7 to 28 days after contusion injury (Popovich et al., 1997; Ma et al., 2002). Depleting macrophages lead to tissue sparing in the injured CNS (Giulian and Robertson, 1990; Popovich et al., 1999). Popovich et al. (1999) showed that depletion of blood-derived macrophages using intravenous injections of liposome-encapsulated clodronate decreased cavitation and promoted partial hindlimb recovery after spinal cord contusion. In addition, reduction in the number of macrophages at the site of trauma by blocking αDβ2 integrin with an antibody within 48 h of a clip compression injury of the spinal cord also reduced lesion size and improved locomotor scores (Gris et al., 2004). That macrophages might exacerbate tissue loss after spinal cord trauma remains, however, a subject of some controversy. When appropriately stimulated macrophages are transplanted into the injured optic nerve or spinal cord they do not appear to be detrimental to the tissue but instead promote axon repair (Lazarov-Spiegler et al., 1996, 1998; Prewitt et al., 1997; Rabchevsky and Streit, 1997; Rapalino et al., 1998). Interestingly, macrophages stimulated by incubation in vitro with segments of peripheral nerve but not pieces of optic nerve were capable of phagocytosing myelin as well as stimulating axon regeneration when transplanted into the CNS (Lazarov-Spiegler et al., 1998). Other evidence by Leon et al. (2000) also shows that recruitment and activation of macrophages into the eye induces neuroprotection in the retina and regeneration of retinal ganglion cell axons into the lesioned optic nerve. The effects of macrophages on axon regeneration will be dealt with in more detail in the next section. The apparent discrepancies between the harmful and beneficial effects of macrophages may be due at least in part to the differences in the way they are activated, and the time of their activation or transplantation after injury.

Macrophages may produce a different repertoire of cytokines, trophic factors, free radicals, and other molecules depending on how they are activated or their state of activation. Therefore, it is conceivable that macrophages could support tissue repair under certain conditions but under different conditions could be detrimental for tissue survival and regeneration. This is clearly illustrated in the two models cited earlier, namely the EAE and LPC-induced demyelination models. Macrophages induce tissue destruction at sites of EAE lesions (Huitinga et al., 1990, 1995; Tran et al., 1998), while after LPC injection into the spinal cord the activated macrophages strip axons of their damaged myelin sheaths while leaving the axons and neighboring cells intact (Blakemore et al., 1977; Crang and Blakemore, 1986; Triarhou and Herndon, 1985; Ousman and David, 2000, 2001). Differences in these models may be due to the timing and duration of expression of pro-inflammatory chemokines and cytokines and co-ordinated expression of pro and anti-inflammatory cytokines (Ousman and David, 2001).

A better understanding is needed of how macrophages can be activated to have either tissue protective or tissue damaging properties. Knowledge of the molecular control of such activation and the molecular and functional phenotype of these macrophages is needed if we are to effectively manipulate macrophage function to improve the outcome after SCI or other types of CNS injury.

General approaches to modulate the immune response

Steroid treatment

Anti-inflammatory drugs like methylprednisolone (MP) have been used for several years by physicians to limit the extent of damage after SCI (Young et al., 1994). Although this treatment does not rescue cells directly damaged by the trauma, it is thought to reduce the severity of SCI by reducing secondary cell loss that normally occurs after the initial trauma. Nevertheless, the use of steroids to treat SCI patients remains controversial.

In a multicenter randomized clinical trial in patients with acute SCI, MP was shown to prevent extensive tissue destruction and to enhance neurological recovery when treatment was initiated within 8 h of trauma (Bracken et al., 1990). When treatment was initiated early in experimental models of SCI, MP induced long-term functional recovery as assessed by locomotor tests (Behrmann et al., 1994). However, in clinical trials (George et al., 1995; Gerndt et al., 1997; Nesathurai, 1998; Hurlbert, 2000) and in animal models (Faden et al., 1984; Ross et al., 1993; Haghighi et al., 1998), several other groups have reported a lack of long-term effects of MP on functional recovery after SCI. Takami et al. (2002) reported recently that steroid treatment produced a significant reduction in the volume of damaged tissue in the spinal gray matter without improving axonal sparing or hindlimb locomotor functions after spinal cord contusion. However, sterological analysis by Rabchevsky et al. (2002) indicate that MP treatment had only a marginal effect on lesion volume. They also reported that MP had no effect on the amount of sparing of gray and white matter and failed to improve hindlimb function. If MP has any effect on reducing the lesion volume and cavitation this may be of value, as it would enhance efforts to promote axon regeneration across the lesion.

In addition to any of the possible effects of systemically administered steroids in potentially reducing tissue damage at the site of CNS injury, our laboratory has also studied the effects of topical applications of glucocorticoids on stab wounds to the cerebral cortex in adult rats (Li and David, 1996). This study showed that topically applied steroids produce a remarkable reduction in the astroglial/fibrotic scar and the formation of the glia limitans at the site of cortical stab wounds. This effect is due in part to the influence of the steroids on the proliferation and migration of leptomeningeal cells (Li and David, 1996), which is necessary for the formation of the glia limitans (Sievers et al., 1994). The mechanism of action is analogous to the effects of steroids in reducing keloid formation during wound healing of the skin (William and Mertz, 1978). Therefore, steroids can influence both the level of tissue damage at the site of SCI trauma as well as reduce the development of the astroglial/fibroblastic scar.

Cyclooxygenase-2 inhibitors

Over the last few years it has been suggested that prostaglandins might play a role in inflammation and secondary injury in various tissues and organs. Of particular interest are recent studies showing that blocking the synthesis of prostaglandins using non-steroidal anti-inflammatory drugs prevents neuronal cell death after various types of CNS insults (Patel et al., 1993; Nogawa et al., 1997; Nakayama et al., 1998; Kunz and Oliw, 2001). Significantly higher levels of eicosanoids are present in the cerebrospinal fluid and at the site of lesion after SCI (Mitsuhashi et al., 1994; Nishisho et al., 1996; Tonai et al., 1999). The mRNA and protein levels of cyclooxygenase (COX)-1 and -2, the rate-limiting enzymes for the conversion of arachidonic acid into prostaglandins, are also increased in the injured spinal cord (Resnick et al., 1998; Schwab et al., 2000).

Recent work indicates that COX-2 is involved in inflammation and might be responsible for most of the prostaglandin-mediated cytotoxic effects (Smith and Dewitt, 1996). Interestingly, COX-2 is the predominant COX isoform expressed in the CNS (Lacroix and Rivest, 1998). After an immune insult or treatment with pro-inflammatory cytokines, COX-2 is expressed in monocytes and throughout the brain vasculature (Lacroix and Rivest, 1998; Schiltz and Sawchenko, 2002). Selective COX-2 inhibitors have been tested in neuroprotection studies (Nogawa et al., 1997; Nakayama et al., 1998). Notably, administration of the selective COX-2 inhibitor NS-398 reduced tissue loss, nociceptive behavior, and locomotor deficits after spinal cord contusion in rats (Hains et al., 2001). Although there is a correlation between tissue preservation and the reduction of inflammatory cells at sites of injury, it is possible that blocking the synthesis of prostaglandins might confer neuroprotection by preventing a post-traumatic decrease in spinal cord blood flow and ischemia (Hall and Wolf, 1986). Therefore, there is a need to clarify the mechanism of action of COX-2 inhibitors in the injured spinal cord, optimize the dosage, and define the therapeutic window. Furthermore, based on at least two studies, which suggest that multiple injections of COX inhibitor either have no effect or exacerbate tissue loss and motor deficits after CNS trauma (Guth et al., 1994; Dash et al., 2000), the effects of single versus multiple treatments will need to be compared. One possible explanation for these results could be that COX-2 might have pro-inflammatory effects during the early phase of inflammation but might help resolve the inflammatory response at later stages, as was recently suggested using a model of carrageenan-induced pleurisy (Gilroy et al., 1999).

Investigations using COX-2 knockout mice have also raised important questions that need to be answered. These studies have demonstrated that COX-2 is essential for renal and cardiac homeostasis and the attenuation of the inflammatory reaction in response to several experimental models of inflammation (Morham et al., 1995; Dinchuk et al., 1995; Wallace et al., 1998; Gilroy et al., 1999; Komhoff et al., 2000). Notably, COX-2-deficient mice had a considerably reduced life span compared with wild-type mice (Morham et al., 1995). Other studies have reported that COX-1 can display pro-inflammatory properties, which vary depending on the organ and on the stage of the inflammatory response (Langenbach et al., 1995; Wallace et al., 1998). In the CNS, Schwab et al. (2000, 2001) have recently reported that COX-1 expression is induced in macrophages and activated microglia at the site of cortical stab wounds or SCI. These results suggest that COX-1 could also be involved in inflammatory processes and secondary damage following CNS trauma. A better understanding of the contribution of COX enzymes to the pathology seen after CNS trauma is needed before treatments can be applied safely.

Stimulating axon regeneration

Although axon regeneration does not occur in the damaged adult mammalian CNS, earlier work by David and Aguayo (1981) showed that mature CNS neurons retain the ability to regenerate for long distances if they are provided with an appropriate glial environment. Multiple factors underlie the failure of axon regeneration through CNS tissue. However, work done in the past two decades has revealed that molecules that inhibit axon regeneration play a particularly important role. These inhibitors of axon growth are found in the glial scar and in myelin (David, 1998).

Immune involvement in the formation of the glial scar

Cytokines such as IL-1β, interferon-gamma (IFN-γ), TGF-β, and TNF-α produced by immune cells are known to stimulate astrogliosis and the formation of the glial scar (Yong et al., 1991; Feuerstein et al., 1994; Balasingam et al., 1994; Lagord et al., 2002). Immune cells that enter the site of CNS contusion injury could therefore be sources of these cytokines and contribute to the development of the scar. Furthermore, astrocytes are also capable of secreting chemokines and cytokines such as MCP-1, MIP-1α, IL-1β and TNF-γ (Hurwitz et al., 1995; Guo et al., 1998; Ransohoff and Tani, 1998; Asensio and Campbell, 1999) that can regulate the influx of immune cells into the CNS parenchyma and lead to their activation. Immune cells and astrocytes are therefore capable of signaling each other, and this may have the effect of prolonging the immune cell response locally at the site of CNS injury as well as leading to the glial scar. Blunting the immune response or neutralizing chemokines or cytokines at the site of injury may therefore be one approach to limiting the extent of gliosis.

Reactive astrocytes that form the scar secrete chondroitin sulfate proteoglycans that can inhibit neurite growth in vitro (McKeon et al., 1991) and axon growth in vivo (Davies et al., 1997, 1999). Recent studies have shown that the inhibitory effects of the glial scar can be neutralized with the enzyme chrondroitinase ABC. Unlike other methods to modulate the scar, treatment with this enzyme promotes axon regeneration in the injured brainstem and spinal cord (Moon et al., 2001; Bradbury et al., 2002). As this method does not involve the immune response it will not be dealt with further in this chapter.

Inhibition of axon growth by myelin

In addition to the glial scar, myelin also has very potent neurite and axon growth inhibitory activity (Caroni and Schwab, 1988; David, 1998; Bandtlow and Schwab, 2000). Unlike the glial scar, which forms in response to injury and takes a few days to be fully established, myelin is always present in the CNS and is therefore in a position to immediately exert its inhibitory effects and prevent axon regeneration. Neutralizing the inhibitory effects of myelin on axon growth is therefore one of the prime approaches to foster axon regeneration after SCI. Work done since the late 1980s has revealed that there are several inhibitory activities in myelin, three of which have been identified and characterized. These inhibitors are Nogo-A, myelin-associated glycoprotein (MAG), and the recently identified inhibitor oligodendrocyte myelin glycoprotein (OMgp).

Nogo-A is a splice variant of Nogo, a glycoprotein that belongs to the reticulon family (Chen et al., 2000; GrandPre et al., 2000; Prinjha et al., 2000). It was first identified by Caroni and Schwab (1988) using the monoclonal antibody IN-1. Numerous studies have detailed the ability of this molecule to inhibit axon growth in vitro and in vivo (Huber and Schwab, 2000; Fouad et al., 2001). Two inhibitory domains have been identified in Nogo-A, one of which is a 66-amino-acid region (GrandPre et al., 2000). The receptor to this region (Nogo-66 receptor) has been isolated (Fournier et al., 2001). The neurite growth inhibitory effect of MAG was first described by Mukhopadhyay et al. (1994) and McKerracher et al. (1994). The potent neurite growth inhibitory effects of MAG have also been well characterized (Li et al., 1996; Shibata et al., 1998; David and McKerracher, 1999; Filbin, 2003). Recent evidence indicates that MAG mediates inhibition via the Nogo receptor and competes with Nogo-66 for the same binding site (Domeniconi et al., 2002; Liu et al., 2002). The inhibitor OMgp is a glycosylphosphatidylinositol-linked glycoprotein that like Nogo-A and MAG induces growth cone collapse and inhibits neurite growth. Surprisingly, OMgp also mediates its inhibitory effects on growth cones via the Nogo receptor but interacts with a different binding site from Nogo-66 (Wang et al., 2002).

Neutralizing axon growth inhibitors in myelin

All three axon growth inhibitors in myelin bind to the same receptor on the growth cone to inhibit neurite growth. Recent studies have revealed that neurite growth inhibition induced by myelin substrates is mediated via cAMP and the small GTPase Rho-dependent mechanisms (David and Lacroix, 2003). Axon growth on myelin substrates in vitro can be promoted by increasing intracellular cAMP levels (Ming et al., 1997; Song et al., 1998; Cai et al., 1999, 2001) or inactivating Rho (Lehmann et al., 1999; Winton et al., 2002). These treatments have also been reported to have some effect in promoting axon regeneration in the spinal cord in vivo (Lehmann et al., 1999; Qiu et al., 2002; Neumann et al., 2002; Dergham et al., 2002). Here we will focus attention on two other approaches to neutralize these inhibitors that involve the immune system. One approach is to block the inhibitors with function-blocking antibodies. The other approach is to eliminate or reduce the axon growth inhibitory effects of myelin by rapidly clearing the myelin from areas of the CNS that are damaged and undergoing Wallerian degeneration.

Neutralizing axon growth inhibitors in myelin with antibodies

Use of monoclonal antibodies

The first immunological tool that was used to neutralize axon growth inhibitors in myelin was the monoclonal antibody IN-1 (Caroni and Schwab, 1988). These in vitro studies were soon followed by the in vivo demonstration that delivery of this monoclonal antibody via the transplantation of hybridoma cells into the brain led to long-distance axon regeneration in the injured adult rat spinal cord (Schnell and Schwab, 1990). Schwab's group has shown that this monoclonal antibody is able to promote regeneration of axons in various regions of the adult mammalian CNS (Bandtlow and Schwab, 2000). A large body of evidence now indicates that treatment with this monoclonal antibody leads to regeneration of damaged axons, as well as sprouting of intact fibers from the contralateral tract or adjacent tracts that then reinnervate the denervated targets (Bandtlow and Schwab, 2000; Raineteau and Schwab, 2001; Rainetena et al., 2001). Partially humanized recombinant Fab fragments of the IN-1 antibody delivered by osmotic pump to the site of spinal cord hemisection were also able to promote long-distance axon regeneration (Brosamle et al., 2000). The monoclonal antibody IN-1 recognizes only one of the inhibitors in myelin. This leaves other inhibitors to continue to exert their effect and may explain why only a small proportion of the damaged fibers regenerate after treatment with this antibody. To block all of the inhibitors with the monoclonal antibody approach will require using a cocktail of monoclonal antibodies against each of the inhibitors or their receptor. This will have to be tested in the future. The delivery of monoclonal antibodies is not a method that directly co-opts the immune response to promote regeneration.

Use of a vaccine approach

We have tested a method that has the potential to block multiple axon growth inhibitors in myelin by co-opting the animal's own immune system to generate function-blocking antibodies (Huang et al., 1999). This is essentially a therapeutic vaccine approach using myelin as the immunogen. In an effort to prevent the development of autoimmune disease against myelin antigens, i.e. the generation of EAE, mice were immunized with myelin in incomplete Freund's adjuvant (IFA). EAE is primarily a T-cell-mediated disease. An acute episode of EAE is provoked by a Th1 T-cell response, which produces pro-inflammatory cytokines, while a Th2 response is protective and present during remission. Immunizing mice with myelin or spinal cord homogenates in IFA prevents the development of EAE (Rodriguez et al., 1987; Rodriguez, 1991; O'Neill et al., 1992; Rivero et al., 1997). Such myelin-antigen-induced tolerance and prevention of autoimmune disease may occur via a number of possible mechanisms such as T-cell anergy, reduced responsiveness of antigen-specific T cells, action of suppressor cells and/or switch from Th1 to Th2 cells (Gaur et al., 1992; O'Neill et al., 1992; Weiner et al., 1994; Marusic and Tonegawa, 1997). Immunization with myelin or spinal cord homogenate in IFA also induces the production of antimyelin antibodies (Rodriguez et al., 1987; Rodriguez,

1991; Rivero *et al.*, 1997). One monoclonal antibody generated by such immunizations is capable of inducing remyelination in animal models of demyelination (Rodriguez *et al.*, 1987; Rodriguez, 1991).

The question we addressed is whether immunization with myelin in IFA will result in the generation of antibodies capable of neutralizing the inhibitors in myelin and promote long-distance axon regeneration. One important determinant of the success of this approach is whether the antibodies in the circulation are able to cross the blood–brain barrier. Our work shows that antibodies that are generated are able to block the neurite growth inhibitory effects of myelin. In addition, the antibodies in the circulation were found to cross the blood–brain barrier and bind to myelin in the myelinated tracts adjacent to the lesion that were damaged by the spinal cord hemisection. Other studies have shown that the blood–brain barrier becomes permeable for a distance of 25 mm after spinal cord contusion (Popovich *et al.*, 1996a). Additionally, the blood–brain barrier also becomes leaky in CNS pathways undergoing Wallerian degeneration, probably through mechanisms triggered by activated macrophages (Jensen *et al.*, 1997). In our immunization experiments, the spinal cord lesions that were made were small so as to produce a minimal glial scar. Under these conditions, immunization with myelin resulted in robust axon regeneration for distances of up to 11 mm, which is about a quarter of the length of the mouse spinal cord (Huang *et al.*, 1999). In addition to the antibody-mediated effects, the vaccine approach has also been shown to stimulate increased macrophage activation and myelin clearance (Kuo *et al.*, 2001; Avilés-Trigueros and David, unpublished observations). This effect of the immunization may contribute further to the reduction of the myelin-associated inhibitory activity and the promotion of axon regeneration.

These experiments indicate that, in principle, an immunization strategy could be employed to block myelin-associated inhibitors of axon growth to promote axon regeneration after SCI. Although we were able to prevent EAE in an inbred mouse strain while promoting axon regeneration, it may be difficult to ensure complete protection from an autoimmune response in humans. A safer alternative for the present may be to use a cocktail of purified inhibitors as the immunogen after ensuring that the inhibitory molecules themselves are not encephalitogenic. Our recent studies on SJL/J mice immunized with recombinant Nogo-66 and MAG in alum indicate that some degree of axon regeneration can be stimulated without inducing EAE (Sicotte *et al.*, 2003).

Neutralizing the inhibitory effects of myelin by stimulating rapid myelin phagocytosis

Stimulating myelin phagocytosis may be another way to rid the affected regions of the CNS of the inhibitory effects of myelin and promote axon regeneration. This appears to be the method that peripheral nerves employ to create an environment that is conducive for axon regeneration. Peripheral nerves regenerate robustly, even though peripheral nerve myelin is as inhibitory as CNS myelin (David *et al.*, 1995). This difference in the capacity for regeneration in the CNS and peripheral nerves may be due to differences in the immune response. Immune cells enter damaged peripheral nerves undergoing Wallerian degeneration within 1–3 days after lesion, and phagocytose myelin and axonal debris within 3–10 days (Bruck, 1997). In contrast, immune activation and myelin clearance from CNS regions undergoing Wallerian degeneration is extremely slow, taking several weeks to months in rodents and years in humans (George and Griffin, 1994; Perry *et al.*, 1987; Miklossy and Van der Loos, 1991). As a result, the inhibitors in CNS myelin can continue to exert their inhibitory effects on axon regeneration for prolonged periods of time after injury.

David *et al.* (1990) provided the first direct evidence that activated macrophages can reduce the inhibitory properties of myelinated regions of the CNS. This study showed that myelinated rat optic nerve sections treated with activated macrophages harvested from a cerebral cortical stab wound or peritoneal macrophages activated with muramyl dipeptide were able to convert the inhibitory optic nerve to a permissive substrate for neurite growth. In addition to the ability of macrophages to phagocytose myelin

from damaged areas of the CNS, this *in vitro* study showed that macrophages also secrete molecules capable of neutralizing the inhibitors in myelin. Subsequently, several other groups extended these findings to *in vivo* studies to show that injection of activated macrophages into the adult rat optic nerve or spinal cord results in promotion of axon regeneration after injury (Lazarov-Spiegler *et al.*, 1996, 1998; Prewitt *et al.*, 1997; Rabchevsky and Streit, 1997; Rapalino *et al.*, 1998). It has been suggested that an inhibitory factor in the CNS blocks macrophage recruitment into the injured CNS (Hirschberg and Schwartz, 1995). However, our more recent studies indicated that, under appropriate experimental conditions, hematogenous macrophages can be recruited rapidly into the CNS and activated along with resident microglia to phagocytose myelin from white matter (Ousman and David, 2000, 2001).

An alternative approach to macrophage transplantation is to trigger rapid macrophage influx and activation directly into damaged regions of the CNS or regions undergoing Wallerian degeneration. To achieve this will require the identification of the immune modulators, namely the chemokines and cytokines that regulate rapid myelin clearance from the CNS. This macrophage activation will have to be achieved without provoking a detrimental inflammatory response that leads to secondary tissue damage such as occurs in EAE. In an effort to identify such molecules we utilized the LPC-induced demyelination model in which macrophage activation and myelin clearance occurs without associated damage to axons or neural cells. This work led to the identification of MCP-1, MIP-1α, granulocyte macrophage-colony stimulating factor (GM-CSF), and TNF-α as being key players in regulating the immune response, i.e. T-cell and monocyte/macrophage influx into CNS parenchyma and macrophage activation leading to rapid clearance of damaged myelin without destruction of adjacent cells (Ousman and David, 2001). It will be of interest to know if these or other cytokines (Shamash *et al.*, 2002) and chemokines can enhance Wallerian degeneration in the CNS and if they can be employed to promote rapid clearance of myelin from such areas of the CNS after injury to promote axon regeneration.

Concluding comments

Since the early 1990s we have learned a great deal about the nature of the immune cell response after SCI and the associated changes in chemokines and cytokines. This has led to the testing of a variety of approaches to either block the entry of immune cells into the CNS to reduce tissue damage or the activation of some of these cell types to promote neuroprotective and regenerative effects. As we begin to understand the molecular mechanisms that regulate the activation of these cells toward different phenotypes, and the molecular nature of these phenotypes, we will be able to make sense of the seemly contradictory evidence we now have with regards to the role of macrophages and T cells in SCI. It may then be possible to develop effective approaches to treat SCI by regulating the recruitment and activation of these immune cells.

We can also expect further development of antibody approaches to neutralize axon growth inhibitors. The success of such approaches will require a better understanding of B-cell activation, of adjuvants, and of autoimmune responses and ways to control them. Furthermore, understanding the molecular control of Wallerian degeneration will also permit the development of novel strategies to rapidly clear myelin from areas of the injured CNS and create an environment that is permissive for regeneration.

Acknowledgements

Work in the authors' laboratory was funded by grants from the Canadian Institutes of Health Research (CIHR). SL is a recipient of a postdoctoral fellowship from Fonds de la recherche en santé du Québec (FRSQ). The authors wish to thank Dr Robert Levine for his helpful comment.

References

Aharoni R., Teitelbaum D., Leitner O., Meshorer A., Sela M., and Arnon R. (2000). Specific Th2 cells accumulate in the central nervous system of mice protected against experimental autoimmune encephalomyelitis by copolymer 1. *Proc Natl Acad Sci USA* **97**: 11472–11477.

Allan, S.M. and Rothwell, N.J. (2001). Cytokines and acute neurodegeneration. *Nat Rev Neurosci* **2**: 734–44.

Amar, A.P. and Levy, M.L. (1999). Pathogenesis and pharmacological strategies for mitigating secondary damage in acute spinal cord injury. *Neurosurgery* **44**: 1027–1039 (discussion 1039–1040).

Asensio, V.C. and Campbell, I.L. (1999). Chemokines in the CNS: plurifunctional mediators in diverse states. *Trends Neurosci* **22**: 504–512.

Balasingam, V., Tejada-Berges, T., Wright, E., Bouckova, R., and Yong, V.W. (1994). Reactive astrogliosis in the neonatal mouse brain and its modulation by cytokines. *J Neurosci* **14**: 846–856.

Bandtlow, C.E. and Schwab, M.E. (2000). NI-35/250/nogo-a: a neurite growth inhibitor restricting structural plasticity and regeneration of nerve fibers in the adult vertebrate CNS. *Glia* **29**: 175–181.

Bartholdi, D. and Schwab, M.E. (1997). Expression of pro-inflammatory cytokine and chemokine mRNA upon experimental spinal cord injury in mouse: an *in situ* hybridization study. *Eur J Neurosci* **9**: 1422–1438.

Basso, D.M., Beattie, M.S., and Bresnahan, J.C. (1995). A sensitive and reliable locomotor rating scale for open field testing in rats. *J Neurotrauma* **12**: 1–21.

Behrmann, D.L., Bresnahan, J.C., Beattie, M.S., and Shah, B.R. (1992). Spinal cord injury produced by consistent mechanical displacement of the cord in rats: behavioral and histologic analysis. *J Neurotrauma* **9**: 197–217.

Behrmann, D.L., Bresnahan, J.C., and Beattie, M.S. (1994). Modeling of acute spinal cord injury in the rat: neuroprotection and enhanced recovery with methylprednisolone, U-74006F and YM-14673. *Exp Neurol* **126**: 61–75.

Bell, M.D., Taub, D.D., and Perry, V.H. (1996). Overriding the brain's intrinsic resistance to leukocyte recruitment with intraparenchymal injections of recombinant chemokines. *Neuroscience* **74**: 283–292.

Bethea, J.R., Nagashima, H., Acosta, M.C., *et al.* (1999). Systemically administered interleukin-10 reduces tumor necrosis factor-alpha production and significantly improves functional recovery following traumatic spinal cord injury in rats. *J Neurotrauma* **16**: 851–863.

Blakemore, W.F., Eames, R.A., Smith, K.J., and McDonald, W.I. (1977). Remyelination in the spinal cord of the cat following intraspinal injections of lysolecithin. *J Neurol Sci* **33**: 31–43.

Blight, A.R. (1985). Delayed demyelination and macrophage invasion: a candidate for secondary cell damage in spinal cord injury. *Cent Nerv Syst Trauma* **2**: 299–315.

Blight, A.R. (1992). Macrophages and inflammatory damage in spinal cord injury. *J Neurotrauma* **9**(Suppl. 1): S83–S91.

Bracken, M.B., Shepard, M.J., Collins, W.F., *et al.* (1990). A randomized, controlled trial of methylprednisolone or naloxone in the treatment of acute spinal-cord injury. Results of the Second National Acute Spinal Cord Injury Study [see comments]. *N Engl J Med* **322**: 1405–1411.

Bradbury, E.J., Moon, L.D., Popat, R.J., *et al.* (2002). Chondroitinase ABC promotes functional recovery after spinal cord injury. *Nature* **416**: 636–640.

Bresnahan, J.C., Beattie, M.S., Stokes, B.T., and Conway, K.M. (1991). Three-dimensional computer-assisted analysis of graded contusion lesions in the spinal cord of the rat. *J Neurotrauma* **8**: 91–101.

Brosamle, C., Huber, A.B., Fiedler, M., Skerra, A., and Schwab, M.E. (2000). Regeneration of lesioned corticospinal tract fibers in the adult rat induced by a recombinant, humanized IN-1 antibody fragment. *J Neurosci* **20**: 8061–8068.

Bruck, W. (1997). The role of macrophages in Wallerian degeneration. *Brain Pathol* **7**: 741–752.

Butovsky, O., Hauben, E., and Schwartz, M. (2001). Morphological aspects of spinal cord autoimmune neuroprotection: colocalization of T cells with B7-2 (CD86) and prevention of cyst formation. *FASEB J* **15**: 1065–1067.

Cai, D., Shen, Y., De Bellard, M., Tang, S., and Filbin, M.T. (1999). Prior exposure to neurotrophins blocks inhibition of axonal regeneration by MAG and myelin via a cAMP-dependent mechanism. *Neuron* **22**: 89–101.

Cai, D., Qiu, J., Cao, Z., McAtee, M., Bregman, B.S., and Filbin, M.T. (2001). Neuronal cyclic AMP controls the developmental loss in ability of axons to regenerate. *J Neurosci* **21**: 4731–4739.

Carlson, S.L., Parrish, M.E., Springer, J.E., Doty, K., and Dossett, L. (1998). Acute inflammatory response in spinal cord following impact injury. *Exp Neurol* **151**: 77–88.

Caroni, P. and Schwab, M.E. (1988). Two membrane protein fractions from rat central myelin with inhibitory properties for neurite growth and fibroblast spreading. *J Cell Biol* **106**: 1281–1288.

Cassatella, M.A. (1999). Neutrophil-derived proteins: selling cytokines by the pound. *Adv Immunol* **73**: 369–509.

Chatzipanteli, K., Garcia, R., Marcillo, A.E., Loor, K.E., Kraydieh, S., and Dietrich, W.D. (2002). Temporal and segmental distribution of constitutive and inducible nitric oxide synthases after traumatic spinal cord injury: effect of aminoguanidine treatment. *J Neurotrauma* **19**: 639–651.

Chen, M.S., Huber, A.B., van der Haar, M.E., *et al.* (2000). Nogo-A is a myelin-associated neurite outgrowth inhibitor and an antigen for monoclonal antibody IN-1. *Nature* **403**: 434–439.

Constantini, S. and Young, W. (1994). The effects of methylprednisolone and the ganglioside GM1 on acute spinal cord injury in rats. *J Neurosurg* **80**: 97–111.

Crang, A.J. and Blakemore, W.F. (1986). Observations on Wallerian degeneration in explant cultures of cat sciatic nerve. *J Neurocytol* **15**: 471–482.

Cross, A.H., Cannella, B., Brosnan, C.F., and Raine, C.S. (1990). Homing to central nervous system vasculature by antigen-specific lymphocytes. I. Localization of 14C-labeled cells during acute, chronic, and relapsing experimental allergic encephalomyelitis. *Lab Invest* **63**: 162–170.

Crowe, M.J., Bresnahan, J.C., Shuman, S.L., Masters, J.N., and Beattie, M.S. (1997). Apoptosis and delayed degeneration after spinal cord injury in rats and monkeys. *Nat Med* **3**: 73–76.

Dash, P.K., Mach, S.A., and Moore, A.N. (2000). Regional expression and role of cyclooxygenase-2 following experimental traumatic brain injury. *J Neurotrauma* **17**: 69–81.

David, S. (1998). Axon growth promoting and inhibitory molecules involved in the adult mammalian central nervous system. *Ment Retard Dev Disabil Res Rev* **4**: 171–178.

David, S. and Aguayo, A.J. (1981). Axonal elongation into peripheral nervous system "bridges" after central nervous system injury in adult rats. *Science* **214**: 931–933.

David, S. and Lacroix, S. (2003). Molecular approaches to spinal cord repair. *Ann Rev Neurosci* **26**: 411–440.

David, S. and McKerracher, L. (1999). Inhibition of axon growth by myelin-associated glycoprotein. In: *Nerve Regeneration* (eds. N. Ignoglia and M. Murray), pp. 425–446. Marcel Dekker, New York.

David, S., Bouchard, C., Tsatas, O., and Giftochristos, N. (1990). Macrophages can modify the nonpermissive nature of the adult mammalian central nervous system. *Neuron* **5**: 463–469.

David, S., Braun, P.E., Jackson, D.L., Kottis, V., and McKerracher, L. (1995). Laminin overrides the inhibitory effects of peripheral nervous system and central nervous system myelin-derived inhibitors of neurite growth. *J Neurosci Res* **42**: 594–602.

Davies, S.J., Fitch, M.T., Memberg, S.P., Hall, A.K., Raisman, G., and Silver, J. (1997). Regeneration of adult axons in white matter tracts of the central nervous system. *Nature* **390**: 680–683.

Davies, S.J., Goucher, D.R., Doller, C., and Silver, J. (1999). Robust regeneration of adult sensory axons in degenerating white matter of the adult rat spinal cord. *J Neurosci* **19**: 5810–5822.

Dergham, P., Ellezam, B., Essagian, C., Avedissian, H., Lubell, W.D., and McKerracher, L. (2002). Rho signaling pathway targeted to promote spinal cord repair. *J Neurosci* **22**: 6570–6577.

Dinchuk, J.E., Car, B.D., Focht, R.J., *et al.* (1995). Renal abnormalities and an altered inflammatory response in mice lacking cyclooxygenase II. *Nature* **378**: 406–409.

Domeniconi, M., Cao, Z., Spencer, T., *et al.* (2002). Myelin-associated glycoprotein interacts with the nogo66 receptor to inhibit neurite outgrowth. *Neuron* **35**: 283.

Dusart, I. and Schwab, M.E. (1994). Secondary cell death and the inflammatory reaction after dorsal hemisection of the rat spinal cord. *Eur J Neurosci* **6**: 712–724.

Faden, A.I., Jacobs, T.P., Patrick, D.H., and Smith, M.T. (1984). Megadose corticosteroid therapy following experimental traumatic spinal injury. *J Neurosurg* **60**: 712–717.

Feuerstein, G.Z., Liu, T., and Barone, F.C. (1994). Cytokines, inflammation, and brain injury: role of tumor necrosis factor-alpha. *Cerebrovasc Brain Metab Rev* **6**: 341–360.

Filbin, M.T. (2003). Myelin-associated inhibitors of axonal regeneration in the adult mammalian CNS. *Nature Rev Neurosci* **4**: 703–13.

Fouad, K., Dietz, V., and Schwab, M.E. (2001). Improving axonal growth and functional recovery after experimental spinal cord injury by neutralizing myelin associated inhibitors. *Brain Res Brain Res Rev* **36**: 204–212.

Fournier, A.E., GrandPre, T., and Strittmatter, S.M. (2001). Identification of a receptor mediating Nogo-66 inhibition of axonal regeneration. *Nature* **409**: 341–346.

Gaur, A., Wiers, B., Liu, A., Rothbard, J., and Fathman, C.G. (1992). Amelioration of autoimmune encephalomyelitis by myelin basic protein synthetic peptide-induced anergy. *Science* **258**: 1491–1494.

George, E.R., Scholten, D.J., Buechler, C.M., Jordan-Tibbs, J., Mattice, C., and Albrecht, R.M. (1995). Failure of methylprednisolone to improve the outcome of spinal cord injuries. *Am Surg* **61**: 659–663 (discussion 663–664).

George, R. and Griffin, J.W. (1994). Delayed macrophage responses and myelin clearance during Wallarian degeneration in the central nervous system: the dorsal radiculotomy model. *Exp Neurol* **129**: 225–236.

Gerndt, S.J., Rodriguez, J.L., Pawlik, J.W., *et al.* (1997). Consequences of high-dose steroid therapy for acute spinal cord injury. *J Trauma* **42**: 279–284.

Ghirnikar, R.S., Lee, Y.L., and Eng, L.F. (2000). Chemokine antagonist infusion attenuates cellular infiltration following spinal cord contusion injury in rat. *J Neurosci Res* **59**: 63–73.

Ghirnikar, R.S., Lee, Y.L., and Eng, L.F. (2001). Chemokine antagonist infusion promotes axonal sparing after spinal cord injury in rat. *J Neurosci Res* **64**: 582–589.

Gilroy, D.W., Colville-Nash, P.R., Willis, D., Chivers, J., Paul-Clark, M.J., and Willoughby, D.A. (1999). Inducible cyclooxygenase may have anti-inflammatory properties. *Nat Med* **5**: 698–701.

Giulian, D. (1999). Microglia and the immune pathology of Alzheimer disease. *Am J Hum Genet* **65**: 13–18.

Giulian, D. and Robertson, C. (1990). Inhibition of mononuclear phagocytes reduces ischemic injury in the spinal cord. *Ann Neurol* **27**: 33–42.

Giulian, D., Corpuz, M., Chapman, S., Mansouri, M., and Robertson, C. (1993). Reactive mononuclear phagocytes release neurotoxins after ischemic and traumatic injury to the central nervous system. *J Neurosci Res* **36**: 681–693.

Glabinski, A.R., Tani, M., Strieter, R.M., Tuohy, V.K., and Ransohoff, R.M. (1997). Synchronous synthesis of alpha- and beta-chemokines by cells of diverse lineage in the central nervous system of mice with relapses of chronic experimental autoimmune encephalomyelitis. *Am J Pathol* **150**: 617–630.

Godiska, R., Chantry, D., Dietsch, G.N., and Gray, P.W. (1995). Chemokine expression in murine experimental allergic encephalomyelitis. *J Neuroimmunol* **58**: 167–176.

GrandPre, T., Nakamura, F., Vartanian, T., and Strittmatter, S.M. (2000). Identification of the Nogo inhibitor of axon regeneration as a Reticulon protein. *Nature* **403**: 439–444.

Gris, D., Marsh, D.R., Oatway, M.A., Chen, Y., Hamilton, E.F., Dekaban, G.A., *et al.* (2004). Transient blockade of the CD11d/CD18 integrin reduces secondary damage after spinal cord injury, improving sensory, autonomic, and motor function. *J Neurosci* **24**: 4043–4051.

Guo, H., Jin, Y.X., Ishikawa, M., *et al.* (1998). Regulation of beta-chemokine mRNA expression in adult rat astrocytes by lipopolysaccharide, pro-inflammatory and immunoregulatory cytokines. *Scand J Immunol* **48**: 502–508.

Guth, L., Zhang, Z., DiProspero, N.A., Joubin, K., and Fitch, M.T. (1994). Spinal cord injury in the rat: treatment with bacterial lipopolysaccharide and indomethacin enhances cellular repair and locomotor function. *Exp Neurol* **126**: 76–87.

Haghighi, S.S., Clapper, A., Johnson, G.C., Stevens, A., and Prapaisilp, A. (1998). Effect of 4-aminopyridine and single-dose methylprednisolone on functional recovery after a chronic spinal cord injury. *Spinal Cord* **36**: 6–12.

Hains, B.C., Yucra, J.A., and Hulsebosch, C.E. (2001). Reduction of pathological and behavioral deficits following spinal cord contusion injury with the selective cyclooxygenase-2 inhibitor NS-398. *J Neurotrauma* **18**: 409–23.

Hall, E.D. and Wolf, D.L. (1986). A pharmacological analysis of the patho-physiological mechanisms of posttraumatic spinal cord ischemia. *J Neurosurg* **64**: 951–961.

Hamada, Y., Ikata, T., Katoh, S., *et al.* (1996a). Involvement of an intercellular adhesion molecule 1-dependent pathway in the pathogenesis of secondary changes after spinal cord injury in rats. *J Neurochem* **66**: 1525–1531.

Hamada, Y., Ikata, T., Katoh, S., *et al.* (1996b). Roles of nitric oxide in compression injury of rat spinal cord. *Free Radic Biol Med* **20**: 1–9.

Harlan, J.M. (1987). Consequences of leukocyte-vessel wall interactions in inflammatory and immune reactions. *Semin Thromb Hemost* **13**: 434–444.

Hauben, E., Butovsky, O., Nevo, U., *et al.* (2000). Passive or active immunization with myelin basic protein promotes recovery from spinal cord contusion. *J Neurosci* **20**: 6421–6430.

Hauben, E., Agranov, E., Gothilf, A., *et al.* (2001). Posttraumatic therapeutic vaccination with modified myelin self-antigen prevents complete paralysis while avoiding autoimmune disease. *J Clin Invest* **108**: 591–599.

Hirschberg, D.L. and Schwartz, M. (1995). Macrophage recruitment to acutely injured central nervous system is inhibited by a resident factor: a basis for an immune-brain barrier. *J Neuroimmunol* **61**: 89–96.

Huang, D.W., McKerracher, L., Braun, P.E., and David, S. (1999). A therapeutic vaccine approach to stimulate axon regeneration in the adult mammalian spinal cord. *Neuron* **24**: 639–647.

Huber, A.B. and Schwab, M.E. (2000). Nogo-A, a potent inhibitor of neurite outgrowth and regeneration. *Biol Chem* **381**: 407–419.

Huitinga, I., van Rooijen, N., de Groot, C.J., Uitdehaag, B.M., and Dijkstra, C.D. (1990). Suppression of experimental allergic encephalomyelitis in Lewis rats after elimination of macrophages. *J Exp Med* **172**: 1025–1033.

Huitinga, I., Ruuls, S.R., Jung, S., Van Rooijen, N., Hartung, H.P., and Dijkstra, C.D. (1995). Macrophages in T cell line-mediated, demyelinating, and chronic relapsing experimental autoimmune encephalomyelitis in Lewis rats. *Clin Exp Immunol* **100**: 344–351.

Hurlbert, R.J. (2000). Methylprednisolone for acute spinal cord injury: an inappropriate standard of care. *J Neurosurg* **93**: 1–7.

Hurwitz, A.A., Lyman, W.D., and Berman, J.W. (1995). Tumor necrosis factor alpha and transforming growth factor beta upregulate astrocyte expression of monocyte chemoattractant protein-1. *J Neuroimmunol* **57**: 193–198.

Hyslop, P.A., Zhang, Z., Pearson, D.V., and Phebus, L.A. (1995). Measurement of striatal H_2O_2 by microdialysis following global forebrain ischemia and reperfusion in the rat: correlation with the cytotoxic potential of H_2O_2 *in vitro*. *Brain Res* **671**: 181–186.

Jensen, M.B., Finsen, B., and Zimmer, J. (1997). Morphological and immuno-phenotypic microglial changes in the denervated fascia dentata of adult rats: correlation with blood–brain barrier damage and astroglial reactions. *Exp Neurol* **143**: 103–114.

Jones, T.B., Basso, D.M., Sodhi, A., *et al.* (2002). Pathological CNS autoimmune disease triggered by traumatic spinal cord injury: implications for autoimmune vaccine therapy. *J Neurosci* **22**: 2690–2700.

Karpus, W.J. and Ransohoff, R.M. (1998). Chemokine regulation of experimental autoimmune encephalomyelitis: temporal and spatial expression patterns govern disease pathogenesis. *J Immunol* **161**: 2667–2671.

Karpus, W.J., Lukacs, N.W., McRae, B.L., Strieter, R.M., Kunkel, S.L., and Miller, S.D. (1995). An important role for the chemokine macrophage inflammatory protein-1 alpha in the pathogenesis of the T cell-mediated autoimmune disease, experimental autoimmune encephalomyelitis. *J Immunol* **155**: 5003–5010.

Kerschensteiner, M., Gallmeier, E., Behrens, L., *et al.* (1999). Activated human T cells, B cells, and monocytes produce brain-derived neurotrophic factor in vitro and in inflammatory brain lesions: a neuroprotective role of inflammation? *J Exp Med* **189**: 865–870.

Kipnis, J., Yoles, E., Porat, Z., *et al.* (2000). T cell immunity to copolymer 1 confers neuroprotection on the damaged optic nerve: possible therapy for optic neuropathies. *Proc Natl Acad Sci USA* **97**: 7446–7451.

Komhoff, M., Wang, J.L., Cheng, H.F., *et al.* (2000). Cyclooxygenase-2-selective inhibitors impair glomerulogenesis and renal cortical development. *Kidney Int* 57: 414–422.

Kriz, J., Nguyen, M., and Julien, J.P. (2002). Minocycline slows disease progression in a mouse model of amyotrophic lateral sclerosis. *Neurobiol Dis* 10: 268–278.

Kunz, T. and Oliw, E.H. (2001). The selective cyclooxygenase-2 inhibitor rofecoxib reduces kainate-induced cell death in the rat hippocampus. *Eur J Neurosci* 13: 569–575.

Kuo, D., Ousman, S., Sicotte, M., Tsatas, O., and David, S. (2001). Treatment with a myelin vaccine stimulates rapid T cell and macrophage responses. *Soc Neurosci Abstr* 27: 698.2.

Lacroix, S. and Rivest, S. (1998). Effect of acute systemic inflammatory response and cytokines on the transcription of the genes encoding cyclooxygenase enzymes (COX-1 and COX-2) in the rat brain. *J Neurochem* 70: 452–466.

Lacroix, S., Chang, L., Rose-John, S., and Tuszynski, M.H. (2002). Delivery of Hyper-IL-6 to the injured spinal cord increases neutrophil and macrophage infiltration and inhibits axonal growth. *J Comp Neurol* 454: 213–228.

Lagord, C., Berry, M., and Logan, A. (2002). Expression of TGFβ2 but not TGFβ1 correlates with the deposition of scar tissue in the lesioned spinal cord. *Mol Cell Neurosci* 20: 69–92.

Langenbach, R., Morham, S.G., Tiano, H.F., *et al.* (1995). Prostaglandin synthase 1 gene disruption in mice reduces arachidonic acid-induced inflammation and indomethacin-induced gastric ulceration. *Cell* 83: 483–492.

Lazarov-Spiegler, O., Solomon, A.S., Zeev-Brann, A.B., Hirschberg, D.L., Lavie, V., and Schwartz, M. (1996). Transplantation of activated macrophages overcomes central nervous system regrowth failure. *FASEB J* 10: 1296–1302.

Lazarov-Spiegler, O., Solomon, A.S., and Schwartz, M. (1998). Peripheral nerve-stimulated macrophages simulate a peripheral nerve-like regenerative response in rat transected optic nerve. *Glia* 24: 329–337.

Lehmann, M., Fournier, A., Selles-Navarro, I., *et al.* (1999). Inactivation of Rho signaling pathway promotes CNS axon regeneration. *J Neurosci* 19: 7537–7547.

Leon, S., Yin, Y., Nguyen, J., Irwin, N., and Benowitz, L.I. (2000). Lens injury stimulates axon regeneration in the mature rat optic nerve. *J Neurosci* 20: 4615–4626.

Lewen, A., Matz, P., and Chan, P.H. (2000). Free radical pathways in CNS injury. *J Neurotrauma* 17: 871–890.

Li, M., Shibata, A., Li, C., *et al.* (1996). Myelin-associated glycoprotein inhibits neurite/axon growth and causes growth cone collapse. *J Neurosci Res* 46: 404–414.

Li, M.S. and David, S. (1996). Topical glucocorticoids modulate the lesion interface after cerebral cortical stab wounds in adult rats. *Glia* 18: 306–318.

Liu, B.P., Fournier, A., GrandPre, T., and Strittmatter, S.M. (2002). Myelin-associated glycoprotein as a functional ligand for the Nogo-66 receptor. *Science* 297: 1190–1193.

Liu, D., Ling, X., Wen, J., and Liu, J. (2000). The role of reactive nitrogen species in secondary spinal cord injury: formation of nitric oxide, peroxynitrite, and nitrated protein. *J Neurochem* 75: 2144–2154.

Liu, X.Z., Xu, X.M., Hu, R., *et al.* (1997). Neuronal and glial apoptosis after traumatic spinal cord injury. *J Neurosci* 17: 5395–5406.

Ma, M., Wei, T., Boring, L., Charo, I.F., Ransohoff, R.M., and Jakeman, L.B. (2002). Monocyte recruitment and myelin removal are delayed following spinal cord injury in mice with CCR2 chemokine receptor deletion. *J Neurosci Res* 68: 691–702.

Mabon, P.J., Weaver, L.C., and Dekaban, G.A. (2000). Inhibition of monocyte/macrophage migration to a spinal cord injury site by an antibody to the integrin alphaD: a potential new anti-inflammatory treatment. *Exp Neurol* 166: 52–64.

Marusic, S. and Tonegawa, S. (1997). Tolerance induction and autoimmune encephalomyelitis amelioration after administration of myelin basic protein-derived peptide. *J Exp Med* 186: 507–515.

McKeon, R.J., Schreiber, R.C., Rudge, J.S., and Silver, J. (1991). Reduction of neurite outgrowth in a model of glial scarring following CNS injury is correlated with the expression of inhibitory molecules on reactive astrocytes. *J Neurosci* 11: 3398–3411.

McKerracher, L., David, S., Jackson, D.L., Kottis, V., Dunn, R.J., and Braun, P.E. (1994). Identification of myelin-associated glycoprotein as a major myelin-derived inhibitor of neurite growth. *Neuron* 13: 805–811.

McTigue, D.M., Tani, M., Krivacic, K., *et al.* (1998). Selective chemokine mRNA accumulation in the rat spinal cord after contusion injury. *J Neurosci Res* 53: 368–376.

Means, E.D. and Anderson, D.K. (1983). Neuronophagia by leukocytes in experimental spinal cord injury. *J Neuropathol Exp Neurol* 42: 707–719.

Miklossy, J. and Van der Loos, H. (1991). The long-distance effects of brain lesions: visualization of myelinated pathways in the human brain using polarizing and fluorescence microscopy. *J Neuropathol Exp Neurol* 50: 1–15.

Ming, G.L., Song, H.J., Berninger, B., Holt, C.E., Tessier-Lavigne, M., and Poo, M.M. (1997). cAMP-dependent growth cone guidance by netrin-1. *Neuron* 19: 1225–1235.

Mitsuhashi, T., Ikata, T., Morimoto, K., Tonai, T., and Katoh, S. (1994). Increased production of eicosanoids, TXA2, PGI2 and LTC4 in experimental spinal cord injuries. *Paraplegia* 32: 524–530.

Moalem, G., Leibowitz-Amit, R., Yoles, E., Mor, F., Cohen, I.R., and Schwartz, M. (1999*a*). Autoimmune T cells protect neurons from secondary degeneration after central nervous system axotomy. *Nat Med* 5: 49–55.

Moalem, G., Monsonego, A., Shani, Y., Cohen, I.R., and Schwartz, M. (1999*b*). Differential T cell response in central and peripheral nerve injury: connection with immune privilege. *FASEB J* 13: 1207–1217.

Moalem, G., Gdalyahu, A., Shani, Y., *et al.* (2000). Production of neurotrophins by activated T cells: implications for neuroprotective autoimmunity. *J Autoimmun* 15: 331–345.

Moon, L.D., Asher, R.A., Rhodes, K.E., and Fawcett, J.W. (2001). Regeneration of CNS axons back to their target following treatment of adult rat brain with chondroitinase ABC. *Nat Neurosci* 4: 465–466.

Morham, S.G., Langenbach, R., Loftin, C.D., *et al.* (1995). Prostaglandin synthase 2 gene disruption causes severe renal pathology in the mouse. *Cell* 83: 473–482.

Mukhopadhyay, G., Doherty, P., Walsh, F.S., Crocker, P.R., and Filbin, M.T. (1994). A novel role for myelin-associated glycoprotein as an inhibitor of axonal regeneration. *Neuron* 13: 757–767.

Nakayama, M., Uchimura, K., Zhu, R.L., *et al.* (1998). Cyclooxygenase-2 inhibition prevents delayed death of CA1 hippocampal neurons following global ischemia. *Proc Natl Acad Sci USA* 95: 10954–10959.

Nesathurai, S. (1998). Steroids and spinal cord injury: revisiting the NASCIS 2 and NASCIS 3 trials. *J Trauma* 45: 1088–1093.

Neumann, S., Bradke, F., Tessier-Lavigne, M., and Basbaum, A.I. (2002). Regeneration of sensory axons within the injured spinal cord induced by intraganglionic cAMP elevation. *Neuron* 34: 885–893.

Nishisho, T., Tonai, T., Tamura, Y., and Ikata, T. (1996). Experimental and clinical studies of eicosanoids in cerebrospinal fluid after spinal cord injury. *Neurosurgery* 39: 950–956 (discussion 956–957).

Noble, L.J. and Wrathall, J.R. (1985). Spinal cord contusion in the rat: morphometric analyses of alterations in the spinal cord. *Exp Neurol* 88: 135–149.

Nogawa, S., Zhang, F., Ross, M.E., and Iadecola, C. (1997). Cyclo-oxygenase-2 gene expression in neurons contributes to ischemic brain damage. *J Neurosci* 17: 2746–2755.

Novikova, L., Novikov, L., and Kellerth, J.O. (1996). Brain-derived neurotrophic factor reduces necrotic zone and supports neuronal survivial after spinal cord hemisection in adult rats. *Neurosci Lett* 220: 203–206.

O'Neill, J.K., Baker, D., and Turk, J.L. (1992). Inhibition of chronic relapsing experimental allergic encephalomyelitis in the Biozzi AB/H mouse. *J Neuroimmunol* 41: 177–187.

Ousman, S.S. and David, S. (2000). Lysophosphatidylcholine induces rapid recruitment and activation of macrophages in the adult mouse spinal cord. *Glia* 30: 92–104.

Ousman, S.S. and David, S. (2001). MIP-1alpha, MCP-1, GM-CSF, and TNF-alpha control the immune cell response that mediates rapid phagocytosis of myelin from the adult mouse spinal cord. *J Neurosci* 21: 4649–4656.

Patel, P.M., Drummond, J.C., Sano, T., Cole, D.J., Kalkman, C.J., and Yaksh, T.L. (1993). Effect of ibuprofen on regional eicosanoid production and neuronal injury after forebrain ischemia in rats. *Brain Res* 614: 315–324.

Perry, V.H., Brown, M.C., and Gordon, S. (1987). The macrophage response to central and peripheral nerve injury. A possible role for macrophages in regeneration. *J Exp Med* 165: 1218–1223.

Popovich, P.G., Horner, P.J., Mullin, B.B., and Stokes, B.T. (1996a). A quantitative spatial analysis of the blood-spinal cord barrier. I. Permeability changes after experimental spinal contusion injury. *Exp Neurol* 142: 258–275.

Popovich, P.G., Stokes, B.T., and Whitacre, C.C. (1996b). Concept of auto-immunity following spinal cord injury: possible roles for T lymphocytes in the traumatized central nervous system. *J Neurosci Res* 45: 349–363.

Popovich, P.G., Wei, P., and Stokes, B.T. (1997). Cellular inflammatory response after spinal cord injury in Sprague-Dawley and Lewis rats. *J Comp Neurol* 377: 443–464.

Popovich, P.G., Guan, Z., Wei, P., Huitinga, I., van Rooijen, N., and Stokes, B.T. (1999). Depletion of hematogenous macrophages promotes partial hindlimb recovery and neuroanatomical repair after experimental spinal cord injury. *Exp Neurol* 158: 351–365.

Prewitt, C.M., Niesman, I.R., Kane, C.J., and Houle, J.D. (1997). Activated macrophage/microglial cells can promote the regeneration of sensory axons into the injured spinal cord. *Exp Neurol* 148: 433–443.

Prinjha, R., Moore, S.E., Vinson, M., *et al.* (2000). Inhibitor of neurite outgrowth in humans. *Nature* 403: 383–384.

Qiu, J., Cai, D., Dai, H., *et al.* (2002). Spinal axon regeneration induced by elevation of cyclic AMP. *Neuron* 34: 895–903.

Rabchevsky, A.G. and Streit, W.J. (1997). Grafting of cultured microglial cells into the lesioned spinal cord of adult rats enhances neurite outgrowth. *J Neurosci Res* 47: 34–48.

Rabchevsky, A.G., Fugaccia, I., Sullivan, P.G., Blades, D.A., and Scheff, S.W. (2002). Efficacy of methylprednisolone therapy for the injured rat spinal cord. *J Neurosci Res* 68: 7–18.

Raineteau, O. and Schwab, M.E. (2001). Plasticity of motor systems after incomplete spinal cord injury. *Nature Rev Neurosci* 2: 263–73.

Raineteau, O., Fouad, K., Noth, P., Thallmair, M. and Schwab, M.E. (2001). Functional switch between motor tracts in the presence of the mAb IN-1 in the adult rat. *Proc Natl Acad Sci USA* 98: 6929–34.

Ransohoff, R.M. and Tani, M. (1998). Do chemokines mediate leukocyte recruitment in post-traumatic CNS inflammation? *Trends Neurosci* 21: 154–159.

Rapalino, O., Lazarov-Spiegler, O., Agranov, E., *et al.* (1998). Implantation of stimulated homologous macrophages results in partial recovery of paraplegic rats. *Nat Med* 4: 814–821.

Reier, P.J., Stokes, B.T., Thompson, F.J., and Anderson, D.K. (1992). Fetal cell grafts into resection and contusion/compression injuries of the rat and cat spinal cord. *Exp Neurol* 115: 177–188.

Resnick, D.K., Graham, S.H., Dixon, C.E., and Marion, D.W. (1998). Role of cyclooxygenase 2 in acute spinal cord injury. *J Neurotrauma* 15: 1005–1013.

Rivero, V.E., Maccioni, M., Bucher, A.E., Roth, G.A., and Riera, C.M. (1997). Suppression of experimental autoimmune encephalomyelitis (EAE) by intraperitoneal administration of soluble myelin antigens in Wistar rats. *J Neuroimmunol* 72: 3–10.

Rodriguez, M. (1991). Immunoglobulins stimulate central nervous system remyelination: electron microscopic and morphometric analysis of proliferating cells. *Lab Invest* 64: 358–370.

Rodriguez, M., Lennon, V.A., Benveniste, E.N., and Merrill, J.E. (1987). Remyelination by oligodendrocytes stimulated by antiserum to spinal cord. *J Neuropathol Exp Neurol* 46: 84–95.

Ross, I.B., Tator, C.H., and Theriault, E. (1993). Effect of nimodipine or methyl-prednisolone on recovery from acute experimental spinal cord injury in rats. *Surg Neurol* 40: 461–470.

Satake, K., Matsuyama, Y., Kamiya, M., *et al.* (2000). Nitric oxide via macrophage iNOS induces apoptosis following traumatic spinal cord injury. *Brain Res Mol Brain Res* 85: 114–122.

Scapini, P., Lapinet-Vera, J.A., Gasperini, S., Calzetti, F., Bazzoni, F., and Cassatella, M.A. (2000). The neutrophil as a cellular source of chemokines. *Immunol Rev* 177: 195–203.

Schiltz, J.C. and Sawchenko, P.E. (2002). Distinct brain vascular cell types manifest inducible cyclooxygenase expression as a function of the strength and nature of immune insults. *J Neurosci* 22: 5606–5618.

Schnell, L. and Schwab, M.E. (1990). Axonal regeneration in the rat spinal cord produced by an antibody against myelin-associated neurite growth inhibitors. *Nature* 343: 269–272.

Schnell, L., Fearn, S., Klassen, H., and Schwab, M.E. (1999a). Acute inflammatory responses to mechanical lesions in the CNS: differences between brain and spinal cord. *Eur J Neurosci* 11: 3648–3658.

Schnell, L., Fearn, S., Schwab, M.E., Perry, V.H., and Anthony, D.C. (1999b). Cytokine-induced acute inflammation in the brain and spinal cord. *J Neuropathol Exp Neurol* 58: 245–254.

Schoettle, R.J., Kochanek, P.M., Magargee, M.J., Uhl, M.W., and Nemoto, E.M. (1990). Early polymorphonuclear leukocyte accumulation correlates with the development of posttraumatic cerebral edema in rats. *J Neurotrauma* 7: 207–217.

Schwab, J.M., Brechtel, K., Nguyen, T.D., and Schluesener, H.J. (2000). Persistent accumulation of cyclooxygenase-1 (COX-1) expressing microglia/macrophages and upregulation by endothelium following spinal cord injury. *J Neuroimmunol* 111: 122–130.

Schwab, J.M., Seid, K., and Schluesener, H.J. (2001). Traumatic brain injury induces prolonged accumulation of cyclooxygenase- 1 expressing microglia/brain macrophages in rats. *J Neurotrauma* 18: 881–890.

Schwartz, M. (2001). Protective autoimmunity as a T-cell response to central nervous system trauma: prospects for therapeutic vaccines. *Prog Neurobiol* 65: 489–496.

Shamash, S., Reichert, F., and Rotshenker, S. (2002). The cytokine network of Wallerian degeneration: tumor necrosis factor- alpha, interleukin-1alpha, and interleukin-1beta. *J Neurosci* 22: 3052–3060.

Shibata, A., Wright, M.V., David, S., McKerracher, L., Braun, P.E., and Kater, S.B. (1998). Unique responses of differentiating neuronal growth cones to inhibitory cues presented by oligodendrocytes. *J Cell Biol* 142: 191–202.

Sicotte, M., Tsatas, O., Jeong, S.Y., Cai, C.-H., He, Z., and David, S. (2003). Immunization with myelin or recombinant Nogo-66/MAG in Alum promotes axon regeneration and sprouting after corticospinal tract lesions in the spinal cord. *Mol Cell Neurosci* 23: 251-263.

Sievers, J., Pehlemann, F.W., Gude, S., and Berry, M. (1994). Meningeal cells rganize the superficial glia limitans of the cerebellum and produce components of both the interstitial matrix and basement membrane. *J Neurocytol* 23: 135–149.

Smith, W.L. and Dewitt, D.L. (1996). Prostaglandin endoperoxide H synthases-1 and -2. *Adv Immunol* 62: 167–215.

Song, H., Ming, G., He, Z., *et al.* (1998). Conversion of neuronal growth cone responses from repulsion to attraction by cyclic nucleotides. *Science* 281: 1515–1518.

Steinman, L. (1996). A few autoreactive cells in an autoimmune infiltrate control a vast population of nonspecific cells: a tale of smart bombs and the infantry. *Proc Natl Acad Sci USA* 93: 2253–2256.

Steward, O., Schauwecker, P.E., Guth, L., *et al.* (1999). Genetic approaches to neurotrauma research: opportunities and potential pitfalls of murine models. *Exp Neurol* 157: 19–42.

Streit, W.J., Semple-Rowland, S.L., Hurley, S.D., Miller, R.C., Popovich, P.G., and Stokes, B.T. (1998). Cytokine mRNA profiles in contused spinal cord and axotomized facial nucleus suggest a beneficial role for inflammation and gliosis. *Exp Neurol* 152: 74–87.

Takami, T., Oudega, M., Bethea, J.R., Wood, P.M., Kleitman, N., and Bunge, M.B. (2002). Methylprednisolone and interleukin-10 reduce gray matter damage in the contused Fischer rat thoracic spinal cord but do not improve functional outcome. *J Neurotrauma* 19: 653–666.

Taoka, Y., Okajima, K., Uchiba, M., *et al.* (1997). Role of neutrophils in spinal cord injury in the rat. *Neuroscience* 79: 1177–1182.

Tator, C.H. (1995). Update on the pathophysiology and pathology of acute spinal cord injury. *Brain Pathol* 5: 407–413.

Tator ,C.H. and Fehlings, M.G. (1991). Review of the secondary injury theory of acute spinal cord trauma with emphasis on vascular mechanisms. *J Neurosurg* 75: 15–26.

Tetzlaff, W., Kobayashi, N.R., Giehl, K.M., Tsui, B.J., Cassar, S.L., and Bedard, A.M. (1994). Response of rubrospinal and corticospinal neurons to injury and neurotrophins. *Prog Brain Res* 103: 271–286.

Tonai, T., Taketani, Y., Ueda, N., *et al.* (1999). Possible involvement of interleukin-1 in cyclooxygenase-2 induction after spinal cord injury in rats. *J Neurochem* 72: 302–309.

Tran, E.H., Hoekstra, K., van Rooijen, N., Dijkstra, C.D., and Owens, T. (1998). Immune invasion of the central nervous system parenchyma and experimental allergic encephalomyelitis, but not leukocyte extravasation from blood, are prevented in macrophage-depleted mice. *J Immunol* **161**: 3767–3775.

Tran, E.H., Prince, E.N., and Owens, T. (2000). IFN-gamma shapes immune invasion of the central nervous system via regulation of chemokines. *J Immunol* **164**: 2759–2768.

Traugott, U., Reinherz, E.L., and Raine, C.S. (1983) Multiple sclerosis: distribution of T cell subsets within active chronic lesions. *Science* **219**: 308–310

Triarhou, L.C. and Herndon, R.M. (1985). Effect of macrophage inactivation on the neuropathology of lysolecithin- induced demyelination. *Br J Exp Pathol* **66**: 293–301.

Tuszynski, M.H. and Kordower, J. (1999). *CNS Regeneration: Basic Science and Clinical Advances*. Academic Press, San Diego, CA.

Wallace, J.L., Bak, A., McKnight, W., Asfaha, S., Sharkey, K.A., and MacNaughton, W.K. (1998). Cyclooxygenase 1 contributes to inflammatory responses in rats and mice: implications for gastrointestinal toxicity. *Gastroenterology* **115**: 101–109.

Wang, K.C., Koprivica, V., Kim, J.A., *et al.* (2002). Oligodendrocyte-myelin glycoprotein is a Nogo receptor ligand that inhibits neurite outgrowth. *Nature* **417**: 941–944.

Weiner, H.L., Friedman, A., Miller, A., *et al.* (1994). Oral tolerance: immunologic mechanisms and treatment of animal and human organ-specific autoimmune diseases by oral administration of autoantigens. *Annu Rev Immunol* **12**: 809–837.

William, H.E. and Mertz, P.M. (1978). New method for assessing epidermal wound healing: the effects of triamcinolone acetonide and polyethelene film occulsion. *J Invest Dermatol* **71**: 382–384.

Winton, M.J., Dubreuil, C.I., Lasko, D., Leclerc, N., and McKerracher, L. (2002). Characterization of new cell permeable C3-like proteins that inactivate Rho and stimulate neurite outgrowth on inhibitory substrates. *J Biol Chem* **277**: 32820–32829.

Wyss-Coray, T. and Mucke, L. (2002). Inflammation in neurodegenerative disease-a double-edged sword. *Neuron* **35**: 419.

Xu, J., Kim, G.M., Chen, S., *et al.* (2001). iNOS and nitrotyrosine expression after spinal cord injury. *J Neurotrauma* **18**: 523–532.

Xu, J.A., Hsu, C.Y., Liu, T.H., Hogan, E.L., Perot, P.L. Jr, and Tai, H.H. (1990). Leukotriene B4 release and polymorphonuclear cell infiltration in spinal cord injury. *J Neurochem* **55**: 907–912.

Yamashiro, S., Kamohara, H., Wang, J.M., Yang, D., Gong, W.H., and Yoshimura, T. (2001). Phenotypic and functional change of cytokine-activated neutrophils: inflammatory neutrophils are heterogeneous and enhance adaptive immune responses. *J Leukocyte Biol* **69**: 698–704.

Yoles, E., Hauben, E., Palgi, O., *et al.* (2001). Protective autoimmunity is a physiological response to CNS trauma. *J Neurosci* **21**: 3740–3748.

Yong, V.W., Moumdjian, R., Yong, F.P., *et al.* (1991). Gamma-interferon promotes proliferation of adult human astrocytes in vitro and reactive gliosis in the adult mouse brain *in vivo*. *Proc Natl Acad Sci USA* **88**: 7016–7020.

Young, W., Kume-Kick, J., and Constantini, S. (1994). Glucocorticoid therapy of spinal cord injury. *Ann N Y Acad Sci* **743**: 241–263 (discussion 263–265).

Zamvil, S., Nelson, P., Trotter, J., *et al.* (1985). T-cell specific for myelin-basic protein induce chronic relapsing paralysis and demyelination. *Nature* **317**: 355–358.

Zhu, S., Stavrovskaya, I.G., Drozda, M., *et al.* (2002). Minocycline inhibits cytochrome c release and delays progression of amyotrophic lateral sclerosis in mice. *Nature* **417**: 74–78.

7 Neural immune interactions in inflammatory/autoimmune disease

Jeanette I. Webster, Leonardo Tonelli, and Esther M. Sternberg

Introduction

A large body of work indicates that a bi-directional level of regulation exists between the central nervous system (CNS) and the immune system. These regulatory systems are, in essence, a 'check and balance' system that is critical for health. The CNS regulates the immune system at many levels, through many routes, molecules, and hormones. Thus, both neuroendocrine routes, including the hormones of the hypothalamic–pituitary–adrenal (HPA) axis (J.I. Webster *et al.*, 2002), and neuronal routes, including the sympathetic and parasympathetic nervous system and their neuropeptides and neurotransmitters (Elenkov *et al.*, 2000) are important regulators of the immune system. Conversely, molecules from the immune system, such as cytokines, feed back to the brain to regulate this neuroendocrine system (Rivest, 2001; Haddad *et al.*, 2002). This regulatory system plays an important role in susceptibility and resistance to autoimmune, inflammatory, infectious, and allergic diseases. The immune system responds to a variety of infectious, antigenic, and pro-inflammatory agents in order to protect the host from such attacks. However, a 'shut-off' system is required for this immune response as an uncontrolled immune system can turn upon the host resulting in inflammatory/autoimmune disease. The neuroendocrine system, in particular the HPA axis, provides this regulation through the production of anti-inflammatory and immunosuppressive glucocorticoids produced by the adrenal glands. If this neuroendocrine regulation of the immune system is blunted or ineffective in any way then the immune system is not as tightly regulated as it should be and the host is susceptible to autoimmune/inflammatory disease. Conversely, if this neuroendocrine system is hyperactive then there is too much suppression of the immune system and the host cannot mount an adequate immune response to antigenic or infectious agents and therefore is susceptible to infections.

The neuroendocrine system

Neuroendocrine regulation of the immune system occurs mainly through the HPA axis. Upon stimulation, corticotropin-releasing hormone (CRH) is produced in the paraventricular nucleus (PVN) of the hypothalamus and released into the hypophyseal portal blood supply. In the anterior pituitary gland, CRH stimulates the expression of adrenocorticotropin hormone (ACTH) into the systemic circulation. ACTH then induces the adrenal glands to synthesize and release glucocorticoids. In humans, the endogenous glucocorticoid is cortisol, whereas in the rodent it is corticosterone. Glucocorticoids are the main effector of the HPA axis and it is through the action of these molecules that the HPA axis regulates the immune system (Fig. 7.1).

Glucocorticoids are small lipophilic molecules that elicit their effects though a cytoplasmic receptor, the glucocorticoid receptor (GR) (NR3C1) (Nuclear Receptor Nomenclature Committee, 1999). GR is a member of the nuclear hormone receptor superfamily that also includes the estrogen, mineralocorticoid, progesterone, and thyroid hormone receptors. This family of receptors can essentially be thought of as ligand-dependent transcription factors (Evans, 1988; Adcock, 2000). GR resides in the cytoplasm in the unliganded state in a complex of proteins that includes heat shock proteins and immunophilins. Upon activation by ligand binding, GR dissociates from the protein complex, dimerizes, and translocates to the nucleus where it can either activate or repress transcription of target genes (Aranda and Pascual, 2001). In general, activation of target genes occurs by direct interaction of the GR homodimer with a specific DNA sequence, the glucocorticoid response element (GRE), in the promoter of the target gene. Repression of gene transcription can occur in a similar manner where GR binds to a sequence in the promoter of the gene, a so-called negative GRE (nGRE), e.g. the bovine prolactin gene (Subramaniam *et al.*, 1997). However, GR can also interact with other transcription factors, such as NF-κB and AP-1 to repress their activity (Baldwin, 1996; Ghosh *et al.*, 1998; McKay and Cidlowski, 1999; Adcock, 2000; Karin and Chang, 2001; Herrlich, 2001) (Fig. 7.2).

GR is essential for life. Knockout GR mice die shortly after birth due to lung malfunction (Cole *et al.*, 1995). However, a mouse in which there is a mutation in the D box of GR and in which GR is unable to dimerize is viable (Reichardt *et al.*, 1998). In this mouse, termed the GR$^{dim/dim}$ mouse, normal GR gene activation cannot occur as it requires GR dimerization but GR can still interact with NF-κB and AP-1 (Reichardt *et al.*, 2001). This suggests that it is this GR repression of other signaling pathways that is crucial for life.

Glucocorticoids have been used pharmacologically for many years as anti-inflammatory and immunosuppressive agents. In fact, the Nobel prize was awarded to Kendall, Reichstein and Hench for this in 1950 (Hench *et al.*, 1950). Glucocorticoids function as anti-inflammatory agents by regulating the function of many immune cells and immune-related genes (Barnes, 1998; Adcock, 2000; Webster *et al.*, 2002*a*). Many pro-inflammatory genes encoding cytokines, adhesion molecules, chemoattractants, inflammatory mediators, and other inflammatory molecules are regulated by glucocorticoids (Table 7.1) (for comprehensive reviews see Barnes (1998), Adcock (2000) and J.I. Webster *et al.* (2002)).

Immune system feedback to the brain

To maintain this balance between inflammation and suppression of the immune system, there must be a route of communication between the site of inflammation and glucocorticoid production to the HPA axis. Glucocorticoids negatively feed back to the hippocampus, hypothalamus, and pituitary thereby switching off their own production and preventing over-suppression of the immune system (de Kloet and Reul, 1987; van Haarst *et al.*, 1997; Tanimura and Watts, 2001).

Cytokines, the inflammatory molecules produced at the site of inflammation, also feed back to the brain to stimulate the HPA axis (Rivest, 2001; Haddad *et al.*, 2002). For many years cytokine stimulation of hypothalamic CRH production was not particularly well understood as it was thought that these large molecules could not cross the blood–brain barrier (BBB). However, it has since been shown that cytokines can cross the BBB at certain leaky points, for example at the organum vasculosum lamina terminalis (OVLT) or median eminence, or can in small amounts be actively

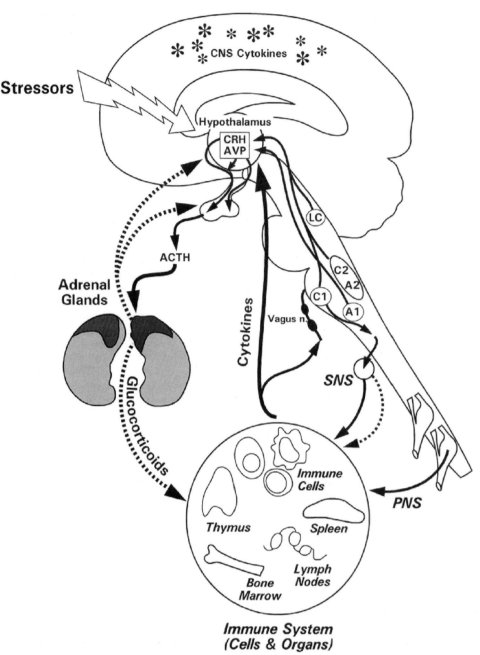

Fig. 7.1 Hypothalamic–pituitary–adrenal (HPA) axis. Schematic diagram showing regulation of the immune system by glucocorticoids and the sympathetic nervous system (SNS) and peripheral nervous system (PNS). Inhibitory loops are shown as a dotted line.

transported across the BBB (Banks *et al.*, 1995). The vagus nerve provides a route though which cytokines can rapidly signal the CNS (Dantzer *et al.*, 2000; Goehler *et al.*, 2000). Additionally, cytokines can activate second messengers, such as nitric oxide and prostaglandins, which bind to receptors on brain endothelial cells and elicit signaling cascades (Elmquist *et al.*, 1997; Gaillard, 1998). In addition, cells of the brain, such as glia, neurons, and macrophages, also express cytokines. These have been shown to play a role both in neuronal cell death (Hopkins and Rothwell, 1995; Benveniste, 1998) and survival (Brenneman *et al.*, 1992) and may have an important role in several neurodegenerative diseases, such as neuroAIDS, Alzheimer's, multiple sclerosis, stroke, and nerve trauma. Although a full understanding of this communication between the CNS and immune systems is important, it will not be the main focus of this chapter and for further information on this regulatory network the review by Mulla and Buckingham (1999) is recommended.

Involvement of the HPA axis in autoimmune/inflammatory disease

Evidence for the involvement of the HPA axis in autoimmune/inflammatory disease is obtained from animal models using inbred strains of rodents, chickens, and from human studies. A blunted HPA axis has been associated with susceptibility to autoimmune/inflammatory disease in Obese strain (OS) chickens (a model for autoimmune thyroiditis) (Wick *et al.*, 1998), certain mouse lupus (SLE) models (Hu *et al.*, 1993; Lechner *et al.*, 1996), and in the inbred rat strain, LEW/N rats (Table 7.2). For a review of these and other animal models of inflammatory diseases see Jafarian-Tehrani and Sternberg (1999) and Tonelli *et al.* (2001).

One animal model, which has been extensively studied by us and by others, is the histocompatible inbred rat strains Lewis (LEW/N) and

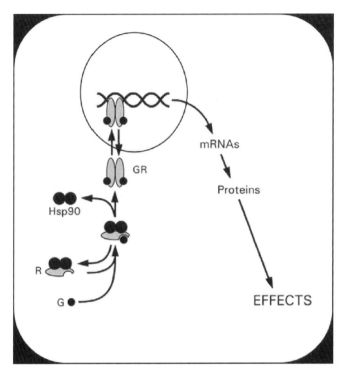

Fig. 7.2 Molecular mechanism of glucocorticoid receptor (GR) action showing direct activation of gene transcription via binding to the glucocorticoid response elements (GREs) of target genes.

Fischer (F344/N). These two strains exhibit differential neuroendocrine responsiveness and differential susceptibility/resistance to autoimmune/ inflammatory disease. The hypo-HPA axis LEW/N rats exhibit a blunted production of CRH, ACTH, and corticosterone upon stimulation of the HPA axis and are highly susceptible to a wide range of autoimmune/ inflammatory diseases in response to a variety of antigenic or pro-inflammatory stimuli whereas the hyperactive HPA axis F344/N rats which exhibit enhanced CRH, ACTH, and corticosterone production upon HPA axis stimulation are relatively resistant to such diseases upon exposure to the same stimuli (Wilder *et al.*, 1982; Sternberg *et al.*, 1989*a,b*; Dhabhar *et al.*, 1993; Moncek *et al.*, 2001). For example, LEW/N rats develop experimental allergic encephalomyelitis (EAE) following immunization with myelin basic protein (Stefferl *et al.*, 1999), arthritis following exposure to heat-killed *Mycobacterium tuberculosis* in adjuvant or streptococcal cell walls, and inflammation following exposure to carrageenan (Sternberg *et al.*, 1989*a,b*; Aksentijevich *et al.*, 1992; Harbuz *et al.*, 1999) whereas F344/N rats do not. In these two rat strains, expression differences of many molecules involved in the HPA axis and glucocorticoid action have been shown, for example hypothalamic CRH (Sternberg *et al.*, 1989*b*), pro-opiomelanocortin (POMC) (Moncek *et al.*, 2001), corticosterone-binding globulin (CBG) (Dhabhar *et al.*, 1993), and GR expression and activation (Dhabhar *et al.*, 1993, 1995; Smith *et al.*, 1994).

Pharmacological intervention studies either blocking these neuro-endocrine and neuronal inputs or reconstituting them, provide more direct evidence than can be obtained in humans of the causal contribution of the nervous and neuroendocrine system to various aspects of immune-mediated diseases. Blockade of the HPA axis by the glucocorticoid receptor antagonist RU486 increased the mortality rates and development of arthritis in F344/N rats following injection of streptococcal cell walls

Table 7.1 Summary of immune-related genes regulated by glucocorticoids

Increase	Decrease
Cytokines: IL-4, IL-10, IL-RI	Cytokines: IL-1, IL-2, IL-3, IL-4, IL-5, IL-6, IL-8, IL-11, IL-13, TNF-α, GM-CSF, IFN-γ
	Chemokines: RANTES, eotaxin, MIPα, MCP-1, MCP-3, CINC/gro
Inflammatory mediators: lipocortin 1 (annexin 1)	Inflammatory mediators: NOS II, iNOS, COX-2, cPLA$_2$
	Adhesion molecules: ICAM-1, ELAM-1, VCAM-1, E-selectin, L-selectin
Receptors: β$_2$-adrenoceptor	Receptors: IL-2R, NK$_1$R, NK$_2$R, IL-4Rα
IκBα	

Table 7.2 Inflammatory/autoimmune diseases correlated with a dysfunctional HPA axis in humans and in some animal models

	Inflammatory/autoimmune disease	Reference
Chicken	Thyroiditis	Wick *et al.* (1998)
Mice	Systemic lupus erythematosus	Lechner *et al.* (1996), Hu *et al.* (1993)
Rat	Arthritis	Sternberg *et al.* (1989*a,b*), Aksentijevich *et al.* (1992), Harbuz *et al.* (1999)
	Experimental allergic encephalomyelitis	Stefferl *et al.* (1999)
	Inflammation	Misiewicz *et al.* (1997)
Human	Rheumatoid arthritis	Cash *et al.* (1992), Chikanza *et al.* (1992), Crofford *et al.* (1992), Eijsbouts and Murphy (1999), Gutierrez *et al.* (1999), Neeck *et al.* (2002)
	Systemic lupus erythematosus	Gutierrez *et al.* (1998), Crofford (2002)
	Sjögren's syndrome	Crofford (2002), Johnson *et al.* (1998)
	Dermatitis	Buske-Kirschbaum *et al.* (1997, 2002, 2003), Buske-Kirschbaum and Hellhammer (2003)
	Fibromyalgia	Crofford (2002), Demitrack (1997), Demitrack and Crofford (1998)
	Chronic fatigue syndrome	Neeck and Crofford (2000), Demitrack *et al.* (1991), Demitrack (1997), Gaab *et al.* (2002), Cleare (2003, 2004), Crofford *et al.* (2004)
	Multiple sclerosis	Wei and Lightman (1997), Michelson *et al.* (1994)
	Inflammatory bowel disease	Straub *et al.* (2002), Niess *et al.* (2002)

Table 7.3 Increased mortality rates following intervention of hypothalamic–pituitary–adrenal (HPA) axis and subsequent survival after glucocorticoid replacement

Infection/disease	HPA axis intervention	Mortality rate	Mortality rate after corticosterone replacement	Reference
Streptococcal cell wall-induced arthritis	Glucocorticoid receptor antagonist RU486	100%	13%	Sternberg et al. (1989a)
Myelin basic protein-induced experimental allergic encephalomyelitis	Adrenalectomy	80%	22%	MacPhee et al. (1989)
Salmonella	Hypophysectomy	100%	5%	Edwards et al. (1991)
Mouse cytomegalovirus	Adrenalectomy	100%	20%	Ruzek et al. (1999)
Shiga toxin	Adrenalectomy	60%	10%	Gomez et al. (2003)

(Sternberg et al., 1989a). Similarly, HPA axis blockade by hypophysectomy increased mortality rates in rats following *Salmonella typhimurium* infection (Edwards et al., 1991), and adrenalectomy increased lethality following mouse cytomegalovirus (MCMV) virus infection (Ruzek et al., 1999), increased mortality from myelin basic protein (MBP)-induced experimental allergic encephalomyelitis (EAE) in LEW/N rats (MacPhee et al., 1989) and increased mortality rates from Shiga toxin (Gomez et al., 2003) (Table 7.3). Thus, these intervention studies provide evidence for the critical importance of an intact HPA axis in protection against septic shock following exposure to a wide range of antigenic, pro-inflammatory, or infectious stimuli.

In such studies, reconstitution of the HPA axis reversed the lethal effects of such antigenic, pro-inflammatory, or infectious stimuli. Arthritis and carrageenan inflammation is attenuated in LEW/N rats by low-dose dexamethasone treatment (Sternberg et al., 1989a) or intracerebroventricular transplantation of F344/N hypothalamic tissue (Misiewicz et al., 1997). Likewise, glucocorticoid replacement protected against lethality from MCMV virus (Ruzek et al., 1999) and MBP-induced EAE (MacPhee et al., 1989) (Table 7.3). Thus, interruption of the HPA axis predisposes to enhanced inflammation and lethality from septic shock, whilst reconstitution attenuates autoimmune/inflammatory disease. These experiments indicate a role for the HPA axis in determining intensity of autoimmune/inflammatory diseases and in protection against septic shock and the lethal effects of such diseases. Furthermore, such pharmacological interventions provide new avenues for treatment of such diseases with agents targeting molecules of the neuroendocrine and nervous systems.

Genetic involvement in autoimmune/inflammatory diseases

Genetic linkage and segregation studies in inbred rodent strains have provided useful insights into the relative contribution of genetic and environmental factors in complex autoimmune/inflammatory diseases. Such studies in inbred strains of rats, whose differential HPA axis responsiveness accounts at least in part for their differential inflammatory susceptibilities, have identified two linkage regions—one definite region on chromosome 10 and one probable region on chromosome 2—that link with inflammatory susceptibility or resistance (Listwak et al., 1999). The large (approximately 16 cM) region between markers GH and R1710 on chromosome 10 that link to inflammatory resistance in F344/N rats appears to be identical to the *Cia5* and *Oia3* linkage regions on chromosome 10 that have been shown to link to models of more complex inflammatory arthritis in other rat intercrosses. Thus, the chromosome 10 linkage region is one of approximately 20 regions on 15 chromosomes that have been shown to link to inflammatory arthritis in rats (Remmers et al., 1996; Furuya et al., 2000; Wilder et al., 2001). It is also syntenic with a region on mouse chromosome 11 and human chromosome 17 that links with other autoimmune diseases in rodents and humans, including EAE in rodents and multiple sclerosis in

humans (Larsen et al., 2000; Nelissen et al., 2000). Consistent with findings in other complex autoimmune inflammatory diseases (Jagodic et al., 2001; Haines et al., 2002), these genetic studies indicate that the genotypic contribution to the inflammatory phenotype is relatively low (approximately 35%), and the environmental variation is relatively high (approximately 65%). Thus the inheritance of this component trait of complex inflammatory arthritis is multigenic and polygenic, i.e. determined by many genes (multigenic), each with small effect (polygenic), and includes a large environmental variation.

The drawback of such genetic studies is that the linkage regions (quantitative trait loci, or QTL) are generally large, as is their environmental variance. While it is possible to narrow down the size of such linkage regions through genetic approaches, such as the use of congenic strains, as have been done in other diseases (Nguyen et al., 2002), the sequencing and further analysis of likely candidate genes found within such linkage regions can also be useful. Thus, several genes present in the rat chromosome 10 linkage region are known to be involved in both inflammation and HPA axis regulation (CRH-R1, ACE, STAT3, STAT5α, and STAT5β) (Listwak et al., 1999; Jafarian-Tehrani et al., 2000). Often, however, even combinations of candidate genes and genetic linkage studies do not identify the gene(s) responsible for the trait. Thus, although in the F1 intercross between LEW/N and F344/N rats, a mutation near one of the active sites of the angiotensin-converting enzyme (ACE) gene was identified that results in a leucine to phenylalanine switch; this mutation was not associated with functional abnormalities in this enzyme, and treatment with ACE inhibitors did not alter the phenotype (Listwak et al., 1999; Jafarian-Tehrani et al., 2000). Furthermore, sequencing of the coding region of the other candidate genes selected from within the chromosome 10 linkage regions, including the CRH-R1 receptor, showed no functional mutations in the coding region, suggesting that structural mutations of these candidate genes alone were not involved in the inflammatory phenotype. This lack of ability to identify an individual gene may be related to the low genotypic contribution to the trait and also to the fact that predisposition may be determined by inheritance of cassettes of genes, or chunks of DNA, rather than inheritance of a single or few genes.

In addition, because of the relatively high environmental contribution to such complex traits, factors that appear to be genetic may actually derive from environmental factors in early development. Thus, maternal–pup interactions during early development are one environmental variable that contribute to differential inflammatory and HPA axis responsiveness in adulthood. Thus, it has long been known that separation of rodent pups from mothers in the first 2 weeks of life results in a long-lived and permanent increase in HPA axis responsiveness (Levine, 1994, 2001; Francis et al., 1999a,b; Francis and Meaney, 1999). Strain differences in maternal behavior exist both in inbred strains and amongst rats of outbred populations (Liu et al., 1997; Francis et al., 1999c). Evidence now supports the notion that such strain-related differences in maternal behavior contribute to the rats' differential HPA axis responsiveness in adult life. Amongst inbred strains, maternal behavior is dramatically higher in LEW/N rats compared with F344/N rats, including more rapid time to retrieval (Gomez-Serrano *et al.*, 2002), with F344/N rats' pup retrieval being virtually non-existent over the entire observation period. Cross-fostering studies in which pups of each strain were cross-fostered to mothers of the opposite strain, with in-fostered pups as controls, showed that strain, gender, and maternal behavior all contribute to adult HPA axis responsiveness, since cross-fostering did not completely overcome HPA axis differences and the effects of cross-fostering differed in male and female pups of each strain (Gomez-Serrano *et al.*, 2001). In contrast, cross-fostering did not affect the inflammatory trait (Gomez-Serrano *et al.*, 2001). The uncoupling between the effects of cross-fostering on HPA axis and inflammatory responsiveness is consistent with the many different factors and multiple different genes that contribute to both these phenotypes. The effects of differential maternal–pup interactions are also consistent with and could account for some of the large environmental variability observed in genetic linkage and segregation studies of these traits. Such contributions of maternal behavior to outbred rodents' adult HPA axis have been related to tissue-specific activation of growth and transcription factors that can permanently alter gene expression by acting at the promoter region of target genes. For example, prevention of DNA methylation in the promoter region of the glucocorticoid receptor during post-natal development leaves the sites unmethylated for enhanced gene expression later in life (Weaver *et al.*, 2001).

Glucocorticoid resistance and exacerbation of human inflammatory disease by disruptions in the HPA axis or glucocorticoid response

There are many levels at which the HPA axis or glucocorticoid response can be disrupted, including the hypothalamus, pituitary, or adrenals, with changes in the expression of CRH, ACTH, or cortisol, respectively, or resulting in changes in the sensitivity of the system to stimuli. HPA axis regulation of immune responses, by the anti-inflammatory immunosuppressive effects of glucocorticoids, occur at the molecular level though the glucocorticoid receptor (GR). There are then many steps involved in the regulation of target genes by cortisol in the target tissue, including entry of the hormone into the cell, binding to GR, dimerization, translocation of GR to the nucleus, and interaction with cofactors and the basal transcription machinery to modulate gene expression. A defective HPA axis or glucocorticoid response could result from interruption of any of these steps, resulting in either reduced glucocorticoid production or glucocorticoid resistance and ultimately leading to enhanced susceptibility to autoimmune/inflammatory diseases. The efficacy of exogenous glucocorticoid therapy in a given disease will be dependent on the specific defect involved. For further information on glucocorticoid resistance syndromes see the recent reviews by Kino and Chrousos (2001) and Kino *et al.* (2002*a*).

It is noteworthy that many autoimmune/inflammatory diseases such as systemic lupus erythematosus (SLE), rheumatoid arthritis, and multiple sclerosis are more predominant in women than in men. Extensive research has investigated the modulation of the immune system by sex hormones, particularly estrogen, and the many interactions between the HPA and hypothalamic–pituitary–gonadal (HPG) axes. Although an important area of research, this subject will not be reviewed here (for further reading see Jansson and Holmdahl (1998) and Crofford *et al.* (1999)).

HPA axis

In patient populations it is difficult to determine precisely where a problem lies within the HPA axis as some of components, e.g. hypothalamic CRH, cannot be directly measured in blood making their analysis virtually impossible. Therefore, as an indirect measure of CRH responsiveness, levels of ACTH and cortisol in peripheral blood are used. Even amongst normal healthy individuals there is considerable variance of HPA axis responsiveness (Petrides *et al.*, 1997; Huizenga *et al.*, 1998*a*). A blunted HPA axis and

resultant low glucocorticoid levels or low glucocorticoid responses have been implicated in a number of inflammatory diseases, such as rheumatoid arthritis (Cash *et al.*, 1992; Chikanza *et al.*, 1992; Crofford *et al.*, 1992; Eijsbouts and Murphy, 1999; Gutierrez *et al.*, 1999; Neeck *et al.*, 2002), SLE (Gutierrez *et al.*, 1998; Crofford *et al.*, 2002), Sjögren's syndrome (Johnson *et al.*, 1998; Crofford, 2002), allergic asthma and atopic skin disease (Buske-Kirschbaum *et al.*, 1997, 2002, 2003; Buske-Kirschbaum and Hellhammer, 2003), chronic fatigue syndrome (CFS) (Demitrack *et al.*, 1991; Demitrack, 1997; Neeck and Crofford, 2000; Gaab *et al.*, 2002; Cleare, 2003, 2004; Crofford *et al.*, 2004), fibromyalgia (Demitrack, 1997; Demitrack and Crofford, 1998; Crofford, 2002; Crofford *et al.*, 2004; Calis *et al.*, 2004), multiple sclerosis (Michelson *et al.*, 1994; Wei and Lightman, 1997) and inflammatory and irritable bowel syndrome (Straub *et al.*, 2002; Niess *et al.*, 2002) (Table 7.2).

Conversely, chronic stress situations, such as those experienced by caregivers of Alzheimer's patients, students taking exams, couples during marital conflict, and Army Rangers undergoing extreme exercise, result in excessive stimulation of the HPA axis and chronically elevated glucocorticoid levels, which have been associated with enhanced susceptibility to viral infection, prolonged wound healing, or decreased antibody production after vaccination (Glaser and Kiecolt-Glaser, 1998; Rozlog *et al.*, 1999; Vedhara *et al.*, 1999; Friedl *et al.*, 2000).

Baseline HPA axis measures can provide evidence for elevated hormonal levels in chronic stress situations; however, they cannot alone provide sufficient evidence for hypo-HPA function. In this situation HPA axis stimulation studies must be performed, for example stimulation using exogenous hormones (ovine CRH, AVP, ACTH) (Demitrack *et al.*, 1991; Michelson *et al.*, 1994), physical stress (exercise) (DeRijk *et al.*, 1996; Gaab *et al.*, 2002), the Trier Social Stress Test (TSST) (a psychosocial stress test involving public speaking and mental arithmetic) (Buske-Kirschbaum *et al.*, 1997, 2002; Gaab *et al.*, 2002), or insulin hypoglycemia (or insulin tolerance test (ITT)) (Gutierrez *et al.*, 1998; Gaab *et al.*, 2002).

Patients with rheumatoid arthritis have been shown to exhibit a hyporesponsive HPA axis in response to IL-6, IL-1, or CRH stimulation and also a loss of the cortisol circadian rhythm (Neeck *et al.*, 1990; Chikanza *et al.*, 1992; Gudbjornsson *et al.*, 1996). In untreated patients, hypersecretion of ACTH without corresponding increase in adrenal production of cortisol has been shown, suggesting a defect in adrenal responsiveness (Hall *et al.*, 1994; Gudbjornsson *et al.*, 1996; Crofford *et al.*, 1997).

Dysfunction of the HPA axis has been associated with both CFS and fibromyalgia. Patients with CFS exhibit reduced free urinary cortisol compared with controls (Poteliakhoff, 1981; Demitrack *et al.*, 1991; Cleare *et al.*, 1995, 2001; Scott and Dinan, 1998; Strickland *et al.*, 1998). However, another study failed to detect any differences in basal urinary cortisol or salivary cortisol compared with controls (Young *et al.*, 1998). Low ACTH and cortisol production in response to ovine CRH but normal basal levels has been described in CFS adults, suggesting a defect at the pituitary or hypothalamus (Demitrack *et al.*, 1991; Demitrack, 1997, 1998; Demitrack and Crofford, 1998). However, no differences in ACTH or cortisol response to human CRH between patients and controls was observed in other studies of CFS patients without depression (Cleare *et al.*, 2001). In another study of CFS patients, also without depression, reduced ACTH responses to ovine CRH HPA axis stimulation was shown (Scott *et al.*, 1998). In yet another study, an increase in insulin-induced ACTH but not cortisol was observed in CFS patients compared with controls (Bearn *et al.*, 1995). In a study using psychological (TSST), physiological (exercise), or pharmacological (insulin hypoglycemia) HPA axis stimulation a dysregulation of the HPA axis at the level of ACTH production was observed. CFS patients were shown to have reduced basal ACTH levels compared with controls and ACTH was unchanged by physiological or pharmacological stimulation, but ACTH responses to pharmacological stimulation (ITT) were reduced (Gaab *et al.*, 2002). In another study of adolescent CFS and control-matched subjects, no differences were observed in basal or CRH-stimulated cortisol and ACTH levels, but a relative resistance to glucocorticoids with regard to T-cell proliferation was observed. This discrepancy in HPA axis responsiveness between these two studies has been attributed to the age of the patients (Kavelaars *et al.*, 2000).

Patients with fibromyalgia also show low 24-h urinary free cortisol and loss of diurnal cortisol secretion (McCain and Tilbe, 1989; Crofford *et al.*, 1994). Abnormal HPA axis responses, including reduced secretion of cortisol but exaggerated ACTH response, to stimulation by ovine CRH has been observed (Crofford *et al.*, 1994). In response to exogenous CRH, insulin-induced hypoglycemia (Griep *et al.*, 1993), or to physical exercise (van Denderen *et al.*, 1992) a blunted cortisol secretion has also been described. However, no differences exist in ACTH response to ovine CRH in fibromyalgia patients or controls, suggesting a deficiency at the level of the adrenal gland (Crofford *et al.*, 1994). In some cases, even higher ACTH response levels have been shown in fibromyalgia patients compared with controls using exogenous CRH or other stimuli of the HPA axis (Griep *et al.*, 1993, 1998).

Dysregulation of the HPA axis has also been associated with multiple sclerosis. A central up-regulation of the HPA axis with some degree of adrenal insensitivity was described in one study. However, a normal stress response was described in these patients (Wei and Lightman, 1997). Previous studies have also shown a relative blunting of ACTH response in AVP stimulation in the context of high basal cortisol in multiple sclerosis patients (Michelson *et al.*, 1994). This association of dysregulation of the HPA axis correlating with activity of multiple sclerosis symptoms has been supported by other studies (Wei and Lightman, 1997; Schumann *et al.*, 2002).

Lower basal HPA axis activity compared with controls as well as hyporesponsiveness of the HPA axis following oCRH stimulation or infusion of CRF has been shown in patients with Sjögren's syndrome. This hyporesponsiveness occurs at the level of the hypothalamus or pituitary as they exhibit a blunted ACTH response (Johnson *et al.*, 1998; Johnson and Moutsopoulos, 2000). An attenuated cortisol response to insulin-induced hypoglycemia compared with controls has also been described in SLE patients (Gutierrez *et al.*, 1998; Rovensky *et al.*, 1998).

Adrenal glands

Dysfunction at the level of the adrenal gland either in the productions of glucocorticoids or other neurotransmitters or in its responsiveness to ACTH stimulation may lead to an impaired HPA axis/glucocorticoid response and autoimmune/inflammatory disease. Isolated glucocorticoid deficiency (IGD), an autosomal recessive disorder characterized by adenocortical but not mineralocorticoid deficiency, has been shown to be due to 17 individual point mutations and frameshifts in the receptor for ACTH (Wu *et al.*, 1998; Tsigos, 1999; Tsigos *et al.*, 2000). Thus, in this situation, the adrenal gland is incapable of sensing the high ACTH levels due to its defective ACTH receptors and therefore the pituitary continues to secrete ACTH due to lack of negative feedback as little or no cortisol is produced. Autoimmune diseases, such as organ-specific autoimmunity and autoimmune-mediated hypothyroidism, have been reported to develop in some patients with IGD (Burke, 1985; Kageyama, 2000). Adrenal insensitivity or a defect in adrenal responsiveness has also been described in rheumatoid arthritis (Hall *et al.*, 1994; Gudbjornsson *et al.*, 1996; Crofford *et al.*, 1997) and multiple sclerosis patients (Wei and Lightman, 1997).

Cortisol-binding globulin (CBG)

The amount of free cortisol available in the blood is limited by CBG. Thus, changes in the expression of this protein or in its binding capacity can also affect the availability of cortisol. The partial or complete resistance to steroids described in some patients with long-standing Crohn's disease has been suggested to be due to the increased expression of CBG, which limits the bioavailability of glucocorticoids (Mingrone *et al.*, 1999). A similar increase in CBG levels has also been described in patients with CFS (Demitrack and Crofford, 1998).

11β-hydroxysteroid dehydrogenase

The enzyme 11β-hydroxysteroid dehydrogenase catalyzes the conversion between active and inactive glucocorticoids (Seckl and Walker, 2001) and therefore changes in this enzyme may cause differences in circulating or tissue glucocorticoid concentrations. In obese men, an impairment in the conversion of inactive cortisone to active cortisol resulting in a drop in plasma cortisol levels was noted, indicating an impairment in the type I 11β-hydroxysteroid dehydrogenase (Rask *et al.*, 2001). A decrease in 11β-hydroxysteroid dehydrogenase mRNA has also shown in ulcerative colitis (Takahasi *et al.*, 1999).

Glucocorticoid receptors

GRα

Differences in the number of glucocorticoid receptors or in their affinity for ligand may also lead to changes in glucocorticoid responses. Familial glucocorticoid resistance is caused by mutations of GR which result in decreased number, stability, or nuclear translocation of receptors or decreased affinity for the ligand. Three different point mutations in the ligand-binding domain of GR, one in the hinge region, and a deletion in the ligand-binding domain, have been identified in families with familial glucocorticoid resistance (for a review see Kino and Chrousos (2001) and Kino *et al.*(2002a)). Recently, a novel C-terminal mutation that interferes with GR-p160 co-activator interactions was described in a French family with familial glucocorticoid resistance (Vottero *et al.*, 2002) and a novel mutation in the DNA-binding domain of GR has been described in a patient with primary cortisol resistance (Ruiz *et al.*, 2001). In patients with lupus nephritis, a phase shift mutation in GR has been described (Jiang *et al.*, 2001). Severe glucocorticoid resistance has also been reported in a heterozygote with a mutation at amino acid 559 (Ile Asn). This mutated receptor cannot translocate to the nucleus and prevents translocation of wild-type GR (Kino *et al.*, 2001). GR polymorphisms can also affect sensitivity to glucocorticoids without causing a mutation in the receptor. A polymorphism in codon 363 of GR has been associated with increased sensitivity to glucocorticoids (Huizenga *et al.*, 1998b); however, five polymorphisms in GR (including the one at codon 363) have been described in a normal population and cannot be correlated with glucocorticoid resistance (Koper *et al.*, 1997).

Some patients with glucocorticoid resistance have no detectable mutation in GR and it is plausible that in these patients other stages of GR function could be impaired (Huizenga *et al.*, 2000). Reduced glucocorticoid receptor numbers have been shown in a subset of steroid-resistant asthmatics (Sher *et al.*, 1994) and in some ulcerative colitis patients with an impaired glucocorticoid response (Raddatz *et al.*, 2004). In other studies, peripheral blood mononuclear cells (PBMCs) either incubated with IL-2 and IL-4 or PBMCs isolated from patients with steroid-resistant asthma showed decreased GR ligand binding (Kam *et al.*, 1993) and in a another subset of steroid-resistant asthmatics reduced GR nuclear translocation and reduced histone acetylation following dexamethasone treatment has been shown (Matthews *et al.*, 2004). The function of GR phosphorylation remains unclear; however, mutation of these GR phosphorylation sites results in reduced GR transactivation and reduced stability of the receptor (Webster *et al.*, 1997). In a study of steroid-insensitive asthma patients, production of IL-2 and IL-4 has been suggested to activate p38 mitogen-activated protein kinase (MAPK), which, in turn, phosphorylates GR and reduces nuclear activity of GR (Irusen *et al.*, 2002). Thus, defects in phosphorylation and in other steps in the pathway leading to gene activation by glucocorticoids could result in glucocorticoid resistance.

Glucocorticoids function as anti-inflammatory molecules through the glucocorticoid receptor by interfering with the pro-inflammatory signaling pathways such as NF-κB and AP-1. In a similar manner NF-κB and AP-1 repress glucocorticoid receptor activity. Thus, changes in this ratio between activation of the glucocorticoid receptor and NF-κB or AP-1 pathways would result in relative sensitivity and resistance to glucocorticoid action. Increased AP-1 activity has been shown in glucocorticoid-resistant asthma (Lane *et al.*, 1998; Adcock *et al.*, 1995) and recently, increased activation of NF-κB has been shown in Crohn's disease patients with glucocorticoid resistance (Bantel *et al.*, 2002).

GRβ

The presence of the proposed dominant negative receptor, GRβ, has been associated with glucocorticoid resistance, both initial and acquired. For example, higher GRβ expression in peripheral blood lymphocytes has been associated with glucocorticoid-resistant asthma (Leung *et al.*, 1997; Hamid *et al.*, 1999; Sousa *et al.*, 2000; Strickland *et al.*, 2001). Increased GRβ expression has been associated with steroid resistance in nocturnal asthma (Kraft *et al.*, 2001) and in fatal asthma (Christodouloplos *et al.*, 2000). In addition, there is increased GRβ expression in mononuclear blood cells of patients with glucocorticoid-resistant ulcerative colitis compared with similar cells from patients with glucocorticoid-sensitive disease (Honda *et al.*, 2000; Orii *et al.*, 2002). Reduced GRα and increased GRβ expression in a patient with generalized glucocorticoid resistance and chronic lymphoid leukemia resulted in decreased GR number and a reduced affinity for dexamethasone (Shahidi *et al.*, 1999) and increased GRβ expression in nasal polyposis disease (Hamilos *et al.*, 2001). A polymorphism at position 3669 in an AUUUA motif in the 3'UTR of exon 9β of the human GRβ gene, which increases the stability of GRβ, has been found to be significantly more prevalent in rheumatoid arthritis than in SLE patients or controls (DeRijk *et al.*, 2001; Schaaf *et al.*, 2002). More recently, another polymorphism at position 2430 in exon 9 has been shown in patients with SLE (Lee *et al.*, 2004). GRβ expression is induced by cytokines (Webster *et al.*, 2001) and therefore during the course of inflammatory disease exacerbation or development of glucocorticoid-resistant states could be caused by cytokine-induced GRβ expression (Leung *et al.*, 1997). Thus, a variety of pre- and post-translational changes in both forms of GR are associated with autoimmune/inflammatory diseases.

Cofactors

Defects in the many cofactors that allow interaction with nuclear hormone receptors, such as GR, and the basal transcriptional machinery could also affect GR functioning. However, to date no mutations in any such cofactors have been found to be associated with glucocorticoid resistance. In a recent study the HIV-1 accessory protein, virion-associated protein (Vpr), has been shown to bind directly to GR and p300/CBP cofactors functioning as an adapter protein between these components and enhancing GR-mediated gene transaction, explaining the glucocorticoid-hypersensitive state associated with HIV-1 infection (Kino *et al.*, 1999, 2002b). In human blood peripheral monocytes, Vpr enhances the endogenous glucocorticoid suppression of IL-12 but not IL-10 (Mirani *et al.*, 2002). Resistance to multiple steroids described in two sisters has also been suggested to be due to a cofactor defect (New *et al.*, 1999).

Transport proteins

The intracellular concentration of the ligand is yet another factor in the process of GR action that can modulate glucocorticoid sensitivity. Although glucocorticoids passively diffuse into cells, evidence exists for an active transport process out of the cells. Increasing evidence from cell systems and animal studies have shown that multidrug resistance (MDR) proteins, members of the ABC family of transporters (Borst and Elferink, 2002), can transport glucocorticoids out of cells (Schinkel *et al.*, 1995; Kralli and Yamamoto, 1996; Medh *et al.*, 1998; Meijer *et al.*, 1998; Webster and Carlstedt-Duke, 2002). Recently, their involvement in glucocorticoid-unresponsive disease states has been investigated and increased expression of the human MDR1 (ABCB1) has been shown in patients with inflammatory bowel disease who have failed medical therapy (Farrell *et al.*, 2000; Farrell and Kelleher, 2003) and also in patients with rheumatoid arthritis (Maillefert *et al.*, 1996; Llorente *et al.*, 2000), SLE (Diaz-Borjon *et al.*, 2000), myasthenia gravis (Richaud-Patin *et al.*, 2004) and immune thrombocytopenic purpura (Ruiz-Soto *et al.*, 2003) but not with steroid-resistant asthma (Montano *et al.*, 1996). These transporter proteins have been shown to be regulated by the novel orphan receptor pregnane X receptor (PXR) (also known as SXR) (Geick *et al.*, 2001; Kast *et al.*, 2002) or by PXR ligands (Kauffmann *et al.*, 2002; Johnson and Klaassen, 2002), which itself is acti-

vated by many ligands including glucocorticoids (Moore and Kliewer, 2000). Thus, this suggests a possible mechanism by which acquired glucocorticoid resistance during long-term therapy might develop. In fact, overexpression of MDR1 in ulcerative colitis patients has been correlated with the dose of glucocorticoids used to treat this inflammatory disease (Hirano *et al.*, 2004).

Implications for novel therapies

Glucocorticoids have been used for many years as anti-inflammatory drugs for the treatment of many autoimmune/inflammatory diseases. However, these studies in rodents and humans shed light on the pathogenesis of autoimmune/inflammatory disease and offer new therapeutic approaches targeted at specific components of these regulatory pathways. One such novel treatment is the use of anticytokine therapy that has been effectively used in the treatment of rheumatoid arthritis (for a review of this therapy see Bresnihan (1999) and Maini and Taylor (2000).

A treatment study with a non-peptide CRH-R1 receptor antagonist (antalarmin) in experimentally induced arthritis showed that although HPA axis responses were inhibited in both LEW/N and F344/N rats treated with this agent, the severity of arthritis was inhibited by 50% in LEW/N rats and unchanged in F344/N rats (E.L. Webster *et al.*, 2002). These findings are counter-intuitive if the only effect of antalarmin were to block the HPA axis. However, it is known that antalarmin also blocks the peripheral pro-inflammatory effects of CRH at sites of inflammation (E.L. Webster *et al.*, 1998, 2002; Elenkov *et al.*, 1999). While there could be many explanations for the uncoupling of the effect of antalarmin on HPA axis responses and arthritis severity, these data are consistent with the hypothesis that inhibition of the peripheral pro-inflammatory effects of CRH in this model had a greater effect on inflammatory outcome than did central inhibition of the glucocorticoid mediated anti-inflammatory effects of the HPA axis.

Conclusion

Taken together these studies in rodents and humans indicate that dysregulation of many components of the HPA axis, other neurohormones, or glucocorticoid receptor action may be associated with enhanced susceptibility to inflammatory/autoimmune diseases, and that both genetic and environmental factors play a role in susceptibility to such diseases. In addition to shedding light on pathogenesis of such illnesses and the role of neuroendocrine factors in regulating immune responses and immune-mediated diseases, such studies also offer new therapeutic approaches targeted at specific components of these regulatory pathways.

Repeated experiments have shown that interruption of the HPA axis through pharmacological or surgical means renders inflammatory resistant hosts susceptible to many aspects of inflammatory/autoimmune diseases (J.I. Webster *et al.*, 2002). Also, in many patient groups an association has been shown between a blunted HPA axis response and autoimmune/inflammatory disease. Therefore, some of the genes that regulate the HPA axis do appear to play a role in the regulation of certain aspects of expression of autoimmune/inflammatory disease, and the degree to which manipulations of different components of the HPA axis affect inflammation will depend on numbers of genes involved, dose, timing, contribution to the overall trait of the component(s) of the HPA axis manipulated, and effects of each of these on specific aspects of the immune or inflammatory response measured.

Future technological approaches promise to allow analyses of the many complex interacting genes and environmental factors that together contribute to overall susceptibility and resistance to autoimmune/inflammatory diseases and differential HPA axis responsiveness. These will include approaches such as expression microarray analysis, validated by real-time RT-PCR, *in situ* hybridization, and immunohistochemical analyses. It is only through integrating all these contributing factors rather than focusing on a single gene or hormone or environmental factor, that the many components leading to individual differences in expression of complex traits such as neuroendocrine responsiveness and inflammatory susceptibility will be identified.

References

Adcock, I.M. (2000). Molecular mechanisms of glucocorticosteroid actions. *Pulm Pharmacol Ther* **13**: 115–126.

Adcock, I.M., Lane, S.J., Brown, C.R., Lee, T.H., and Barnes, P.J. (1995). Abnormal glucocorticoid receptor-activator protein 1 interaction in steroid-resistant asthma. *J Exp Med* **182**: 1951–1958.

Aksentijevich, S., Whitfield, H.J.J., Young, W.S.I., Wilder, R.L., Chrousos, G.P., Gold, P.W., *et al.* (1992). Arthritis-susceptible Lewis rats fail to emerge from the stress hyporesponsive period. *Dev Brain Res* **65**: 115–118.

Aranda, A. and Pascual, A. (2001). Nuclear hormone receptors and gene expression. *Physiol Rev* **81**: 1269–1304.

Baldwin, A.S. Jr (1996). The NF-κB and IκB proteins: new discoveries and insights. *Annu Rev Immunol* **14**: 649–681.

Banks, W.A., Satin, A.J., and Broadwell, R.D. (1995). Passage of cytokines across the blood-brain barrier. *Neuroimmunomodulation* **2**: 241–248.

Bantel, H., Schmitz, M.L., Raible, A., Gregor, M., and Schulze-Osthoff, K. (2002). Critical role of NF-kappaB and stress-activated protein kinases in steroid unresponsiveness. *FASEB J* **16**: 1832–1834.

Barnes, P.J. (1998). Anti-inflammatory actions of glucocorticoids: molecular mechanisms. *Clin Sci* **94**: 557–572.

Bearn, J., Allain, T., Coskeran, P., Munro, N., Butler, J., McGregor, A., et al. (1995). Neuroendocrine responses to D-fenfluramine and insulin-induced hypoglycemia in chronic fatigue syndrome. *Biol Psychiat* **37**: 245–252.

Benveniste, E.N. (1998). Cytokine actions in the central nervous system. *Cytokine Growth Factor Rev* **9**: 259–275.

Borst, P. and Elferink, R.O. (2002). Mammalian ABC transporters in health and disease. *Annu Rev Biochem* **71**: 537–592.

Brenneman, D., Schultzberg, M., Bartfai, T., and Gozes, I. (1992). Cytokine regulation of neuronal cell survival. *J Neurochem* **58**: 454–460.

Bresnihan, B. (1999). Treatment of rheumatoid arthritis with interleukin 1 receptor antagonist. *Ann Rheum Dis* **58**(Suppl. 1): 196–198.

Burke, C.W. (1985). Adrenocortical insufficiency. *Clin Endocrinol Metab* **14**: 947–976.

Buske-Kirschbaum, A. and Hellhammer, D.H. (2003). Endocrine and immune responses to stress in chronic inflammatory skin disorders. *Ann N Y Acad Sci* **992**: 231–240.

Buske-Kirschbaum, A., Jobst, S., Psych, D., Wustman, A., Kirschbaum, C., Rauh, W., *et al.* (1997). Attenuated free cortisol response to psychosocial stress in children with atopic dermatitis. *Psychosom Med* **59**: 419–426.

Buske-Kirschbaum, A., Geiben, A., Hollig, H., Morschhauser, E., and Hellhammer, D. (2002). Altered responsiveness of the hypothalamus–pituitary–adrenal axis and the sympathetic adrenomedullary system to stress in patients with atopic dermatitis. *J Clin Endocrinol Metab* **87**: 4245–4251.

Buske-Kirschbaum, A., von Auer, K., Krieger, S., Weis, S., Rauh, W., and Hellhammer, D. (2003). Blunted cortisol responses to psychosocial stress in asthmatic children: a general feature of atopic disease? *Psychosom Med* **65**: 806–810.

Calis, M., Gokce, C., Ates, F., Ulker, S., Izgi, H.B., Demir, H., *et al.* (2004). Investigation of the hypothalamo-pituitary-adrenal axis (HPA) by 1 microgram ACTH test and metyrapone test in patients with primary fibromyalgia syndrome. *J Endocrinol Invest* **27**: 42–46.

Cash, J.M., Crofford, L.J., Gallucci, W.T., Sternberg, E.M., Gold, P.W., Chrousos, G.P., *et al.* (1992). Pituitary-adrenal axis responsiveness to ovine corticotrophin releasing hormone in patients with rheumatoid arthritis treated with low dose prednisolone. *J Rheumatol* **19**: 1692–1696.

Chikanza, I.C., Petrou, P., Kingsley, G., Chrousos, G.P., and Panayi, G.S. (1992). Defective hypothalamic response to immune and inflammatory stimuli in patients with rheumatoid arthritis. *Arthritis Rheum* **35**: 1281–1288.

Christodoulopoulos, P., Leung, D.Y., Elliott, M.W., Hogg, J.C., Muro, S., Toda, M., *et al.* (2000). Increased number of glucocorticoid receptor-beta-expressing cells in the airways in fatal asthma. *J Allergy Clin Immunol* **106**: 479–484.

Cleare, A.J. (2003). The neuroendocrinology of chronic fatigue syndrome. *Endocr Rev* **24**: 236–252.

Cleare, A.J. (2004). The HPA axis and the genesis of chronic fatigue syndrome. *Trends Endocrinol Metab* **15**: 55–59.

Cleare, A.J., Bearn, J., Allain, T., McGregor, A., Wessely, S., Murray, R.M., *et al.* (1995). Contrasting neuroendocrine responses in depression and chronic fatigue syndrome. *J Affect Disord* **34**: 283–289.

Cleare, A.J., Miell, J., Heap, E., Sookdeo, S., Young, L., Malhi, G.S., *et al.* (2001). Hypothalamo-pituitary-adrenal axis dysfunction in chronic fatigue syndrome, and the effects of low-dose hydrocortisone therapy. *J Clin Endocrinol Metab* **86**: 3545–3554.

Cole, T.J., Blendy, J.A., Monaghan, A.P., Krieglstein, K., Schmid, W., Aguzzi, A., *et al.* (1995). Targeted disruption of the glucocorticoid receptor gene blocks adrenergic chromaffin cell development and severely retards lung maturation. *Genes Dev* **9**: 1608–1621.

Crofford, L.J. (2002). The hypothalamic–pituitary–adrenal axis in the pathogenesis of rheumatic diseases. *Endocrinol Metab Clin North Am* **31**: 1–13.

Crofford, L.J., Sano, H., Karalis, K., Webster, E.L., Goldmuntz, E.A., Chrousos, G.P., *et al.* (1992). Local secretion of corticotropin-releasing hormone in the joints of Lewis rats with inflammatory arthritis. *J Clin Invest* **90**: 2555–2564.

Crofford, L.J., Pillemer, S.R., Kalogeras, K.T., Cash, J.M., Michelson, D., Kling, M.A., *et al.* (1994). Hypothalamic–pituitary–adrenal axis perturbations in patients with fibromyalgia. *Arthritis Rheum* **37**: 1583–1592.

Crofford, L.J., Kalogeras, K.T., Mastorakos, G., Magiakou, M.A., Wells, J., Kanik, K.S., *et al.* (1997). Circadian relationships between interleukin (IL)-6 and hypothalamic-pituitary-adrenal axis hormones: failure of IL-6 to cause sustained hypercortisolism in patients with early untreated rheumatoid arthritis. *J Clin Endocrinol Metab* **82**: 1279–1283.

Crofford, L.J., Jacobson, J., and Young, E. (1999). Modeling the involvement of the hypothalamic-pituitary-adrenal and hypothalamic-pituitary-gonadal axes in autoimmune and stress-related rheumatic syndromes in women. *J Womens Health* **8**: 203–215.

Crofford, L.J., Young, E.A., Engleberg, N.C., Korszun, A., Brucksch, C.B., McClure, L.A., *et al.* (2004). Basal circadian and pulsatile ACTH and cortisol secretion in patients with fibromyalgia and/or chronic fatigue syndrome. *Brain Behav Immun* **18**: 314–325.

Dantzer, R., Konsman, J.P., Bluthe, R.M., and Kelley, K.W. (2000). Neural and humoral pathways of communication from the immune system to the brain: parallel or convergent? *Auton Neurosci* **85**: 60–65.

de Kloet, E.R. and Reul, J.M. (1987). Feedback action and tonic influence of corticosteroids on brain function: A concept arising from the heterogeneity of brain receptor systems. *Psychoneuroendocrinology* **12**: 83–105.

DeRijk, R.H., Petrides, J., Deuster, P., Gold, P.W., and Sternberg, E.M. (1996). Changes in corticosteroid sensitivity of peripheral blood lymphocytes after strenuous exercise in humans. *J Clin Endocrinol Metab* **81**: 228–235.

DeRijk, R.H., Schaaf, M.J., Turner, G., Datson, N.A., Vreugdenhil, E., Cidlowski, J., *et al.* A human glucocorticoid receptor gene variant that increases the stability of the glucocorticoid receptor beta-isoform mRNA is associated with rheumatoid arthritis. *J Rheumatol* **28**: 2383–2388.

Demitrack, M.A. (1997). Neuroendocrine correlates of chronic fatigue syndrome: a brief review. *J Psychiatr Res* **31**: 69–82.

Demitrack, M.A. (1998). Neuroendocrine aspects of chronic fatigue syndrome: a commentary. *Am J Med* **105**: 11S–14S.

Demitrack, M.A. and Crofford, L.J.(1998). Evidence for and pathophysiologic implications of hypothalamic-pituitary-adrenal axis dysregulation in fibromyalgia and chronic fatigue syndrome. *Ann N Y Acad Sci* **840**: 684–697.

Demitrack, M.A., Dale, J.K., Straus, S.E., Laue, L., Listwak, S.J., Kruesi, M.J., *et al.* (1991). Evidence for impaired activation of the hypothalamic-pituitary-adrenal axis in patients with chronic fatigue syndrome. *J Clin Endocrinol Metab* **73**: 1224–1234.

Dhabhar, F.S., McEwen, B.S., and Spencer, R.L. (1993). Stress response, adrenal steroid receptor levels and corticosteroid-binding globulin levels – a comparison between Sprague–Dawley, Fischer 344 and Lewis rats. *Brain Res* **616**: 89–98.

Dhabhar, F.S., Miller, A.H., McEwen, B.S., and Spencer, R.L. (1995). Differential activation of adrenal steroid receptors in neural and immune tissues of Sprague Dawley, Fischer 344, and Lewis rats. *J Neuroimmunol* **56**: 77–90.

Diaz-Borjon, A., Richaud-Patin, Y., Alvarado de la Barrera, C., Jakez-Ocampo, J., Ruiz-Arguelles, A., et al. (2000). Multidrug resistance-1 (MDR-1) in rheumatic autoimmune disorders. Part II: Increased P-glycoprotein activity in lymphocytes from systemic lupus erythematosus patients might affect steroid requirements for disease control. Joint Bone Spine 67: 40–48.

Edwards, C.K.I., Yunger, L.M., Lorence, R.M., Dantzer, R., and Kelley, K.W. (1991). The pituitary gland is required for protection against lethal effects of Salmonella typhimurium. Proc Natl Acad Sci USA 88: 2274–2277.

Eijsbouts, A.M. and Murphy, E.P. (1999). The role of the hypothalamic-pituitary-adrenal axis in rheumatoid arthritis. Baillieres Best Pract Res Clin Rheumatol 13: 599–613.

Elenkov, I.J., Webster, E.L., Torpy, D.J., and Chrousos, G.P. (1999). Stress, corticotropin-releasing hormone, glucocorticoids, and the immune/inflammatory response: acute and chronic effects. Ann N Y Acad Sci 876: 1–11.

Elenkov, I.J., Wilder, R.L., Chrousos, G.P., and Vizi, E.S. (2000). The sympathetic nerve-an integrative interface between two supersystems: the brain and the immune system. Pharmacol Rev 52: 595–638.

Elmquist, J.K., Scammell, T.E., and Saper, C.B. (1997). Mechanisms of CNS response to systemic immune challenge: the febrile response. Trends Neurosci 20: 565–570.

Evans, R.M. (1988). The steroid and thyroid hormone receptor superfamily. Science 240: 889–895.

Farrell, R.J. and Kelleher, D. (2003). Glucocorticoid resistance in inflammatory bowel disease. J Endocrinol 178: 339–346.

Farrell, R.J., Murphy, A., Long, A., Donnelly, S., Cherikuri, A., O'Toole, D., et al. (2000). High multidrug resistance (P-glycoprotein 170) expression in inflammatory bowel disease patients who fail medical therapy. Gastroenterology 118: 279–288.

Francis, D.D. and Meaney, M.J. (1999). Maternal care and the development of stress responses. Curr Opin Neurobiol 9: 128–134.

Francis, D.D., Champagne, F.A., Liu, D., and Meaney, M.J. (1999a). Maternal care, gene expression, and the development of individual differences in stress reactivity. Ann N Y Acad Sci 896: 66–84.

Francis, D.D., Caldji, C., Champagne, F., Plotsky, P.M., and Meaney, M.J. (1999b). The role of corticotropin-releasing factor-norepinephrine systems in mediating the effects of early experience on the development of behavioral and endocrine responses to stress. Biol Psychiatry 46: 1153–1166.

Francis, D., Diorio, J., Liu, D., and Meaney, M.J. (1999c). Nongenomic transmission across generations of maternal behavior and stress responses in the rat. Science 286: 1155–1158.

Friedl, K.E., Moore, R.J., Hoyt, R.W., Marchitelli, L.J., Matinez-Lopez, L.E., and Askew, E.W. (2000). Endocrine markers of semistarvation in healthy lean men in a mulitstressor environment. J Appl Physiol 88: 1820–1830.

Furuya, T., Salstrom, J.L., McCall-Vining, S., Cannon, G.W., Joe, B., Remmers, E.F., et al. (2000). Genetic dissection of a rat model for rheumatoid arthritis: significant gender influences on autosomal modifier loci. Hum Mol Genet 9: 2241–2250.

Gaab, J., Huster, D., Peisen, R., Engert, V., Heitz, V., Schad, T., et al. (2002). Hypothalamic–pituitary–adrenal axis reactivity in chronic fatigue syndrome and health under psychological, physiological, and pharmacological stimulation. Psychosom Med 64: 951–962.

Gaillard, R.C. (1998). Cytokines in the neuroendocrine system. Int Rev Immunol 17: 181–216.

Geick, A., Eichelbaum, M., and Burk, O. (2001). Nuclear receptor response elements mediate induction of intestinal MDR1 by rifampicin. J Biol Chem 276: 14581–14587.

Ghosh, S., May, M.J., and Kopp, E.B. (1998) NF-κB and Rel proteins: evolutionarily conserved mediators of immune responses. Annu Rev Immunol 16: 225–260.

Glaser, R. and Kiecolt-Glaser, J.K. (1998). Stress-associated immune modulation: Relevance to viral infections and chronic fatigue syndrome. Am J Med 105: 35S–42S.

Goehler, L.E., Gaykema, R.P., Hansen, M.K., Anderson, K., Maier, S.F., and Watkins, L.R. (2000). Vagal immune-to-brain communication: a visceral chemosensory pathway. Auton Neurosci 85: 49–59.

Gomez, S.A., Fernandez, G.C., Vanzulli, S., Dran, G., Rubel, C., Berki, T., et al. (2003). Endogenous glucocorticoids attenuate Shiga toxin-2-induced toxicity in a mouse model of haemolytic uraemic syndrome. Clin Exp Immunol 131: 217–224.

Gomez-Serrano, M.A., Tonelli, L., Listwak, A., Sternberg, E., and Riley, A.L. (2001). Effects of cross fostering on open-field behavior, acoustic startle, lipopolysaccharide-induced corticosterone release, and body weight in Lewis and Fischer rats. Behav Genet 31: 427–436.

Gomez-Serrano, M.A., Sternberg, E.M., and Riley, A.L. (2002). Maternal behavior in F344/N and LEW/N rats. Effects on carrageenan-induced inflammatory reactivity and body weight. Physiol Behav 75: 493–505.

Griep, E.N., Boersma, J.W., and de Kloet, E.R. (1993). Altered reactivity of the hypothalamic-pituitary-adrenal axis in the primary fibromyalgia syndrome. J Rheumatol 20: 469–474.

Griep, E.N., Boersma, J.W., Lentjes, E.G., Prins, A.P., van der Korst, J.K., and de Kloet, E.R. (1998). Function of the hypothalamic-pituitary-adrenal axis in patients with fibromyalgia and low back pain. J Rheumatol 25: 1374–1381.

Gudbjornsson, B., Skogseid, B., Oberg, K., Wide, L., and Hallgren, R. (1996). Intact adrenocorticotropic hormone secretion but impaired cortisol response in patients with active rheumatoid arthritis. effect of glucocorticoids. J Rheumatol 23: 596–602.

Gutierrez, M.A., Garcia, M.E., Rodriguez, J.A., Rivero, S., and Jacobelli, S. (1998). Hypothalamic-pituitary-adrenal axis function and prolactin secretion in systemic lupus erythematosus. Lupus 7: 404–408.

Gutierrez, M.A., Garcia, M.E., Rodriguez, J.A., Mardonez, G., Jacobelli, S., and Rivero, S. (1999). Hypothalamic-pituitary-adrenal axis in patients with active rheumatoid arthritis: a controlled study using insulin hypoglycemia stress test and prolactin stimulation. J Rheumatol 26: 277–281.

Haddad, J.J., Saade, N.E., and Safieh-Garabedian, B. (2002). Cytokines and neuro-immune-endocrine interactions: a role for the hypothalamic–pituitary–adrenal revolving axis. J Neuroimmunol 133: 1–19.

Haines, J.L., Bradford, Y., Garcia, M.E., Reed, A.D., Neumeister, E., Pericak-Vance, M.A., et al. (2002). Multiple susceptibility loci for multiple sclerosis. Hum Mol Genet 11: 2251–2256.

Hall, J., Morand, E.F., Medbak, S., Zaman, M., Perry, L., Goulding, N.J., et al. (1994). Abnormal hypothalamic-pituitary-adrenal axis function in rheumatoid arthritis. Effects of nonsteroidal antiinflammatory drugs and water immersion. Arthritis Rheum 37: 1132–1137.

Hamid, Q.A., Wenzel, S.E., Hauk, P.J., Tsicopoulos, A., Wallaert, B., Lafitte, J.-J., et al. (1999). Increased glucocorticoid receptor β in airway cells of glucocorticoid-insensitive asthma. Am J Respir Crit Care Med 159: 1600–1604.

Hamilos, D.L., Leung, D.Y., Muro, S., Kahn, A.M., Hamilos, S.S., Thawley, S.E., et al. (2001). GR beta expression in nasal polyp inflammatory cells and its relationship to the anti-inflammatory effects of intranasal fluticasone. J Allergy Clin Immunol 108: 59–68.

Harbuz, M.S., Rooney, C., Jones, M., and Ingram, C.D. (1999). Hypothalamo-pituitary-adrenal axis responses to lipopolysaccharide in male and female rats with adjuvant-induced arthritis. Brain Behav Immun 13: 335–347.

Hench, P.S., Kendall, E.C., Slocumb, C.H., and Polley, H.F. (1950). Effects of cortisone acetate and primary ACTH on rheumatoid arthritis, rheumatic fever and certain other conditions. Arch Intern Med 85: 545–666.

Herrlich, P. (2001). Cross-talk between glucocorticoid receptor and AP-1. Oncogene 20: 2465–2475.

Hirano, T., Onda, K., Toma, T., Miyaoka, M., Moriyasu, F., and Oka, K. (2004). MDR1 mRNA expressions in peripheral blood mononuclear cells of patients with ulcerative colitis in relation to glucocorticoid administration. J Clin Pharmacol 44: 481–486.

Honda, M., Orii, F., Ayabe, T., Imai, S., Ashida, T., Obara, T., et al. (2000). Expression of glucocorticoid receptor β in lymphocytes of patients with glucocorticoid-resistant ulcerative colitis. Gastroenterology 118: 859–866.

Hopkins, S.J. and Rothwell, N.J. (1995). Cytokines and the nervous system. I: Expression and recognition. Trends Neurosci 18: 83–88.

Hu, Y., Dietrich, H., Herold, M., Heinrich, P.C., and Wick, G. (1993). Disturbed immuno-endocrine communication via the hypothalamo–pituitary–adrenal axis in autoimmune disease. Int Arch Allergy Immunol 102: 232–241.

Huizenga, N.A.T.M., Koper, J.W., de Lange, P., Pols, H.A.P., Stolk, R.P., Grobbee, D.E., et al. (1998a). Interperson variability but intraperson stability of baseline plasma cortisol concentrations, and its relation to feedback sensitivity of the hypothalamo–pituitary–adrenal axis to a low dose of dexamethasone in elderly individuals. *J Clin Endocrinol Metab* **83**: 47–54.

Huizenga, N.A.T.M., Koper, J.W., de Lange, P., Pols, H.A.P., Stolk, R.P., Burger, H., *et al.* (1998*b*). Polymorphism in the glucocorticoid receptor gene may be associated with an increased sensitivity to glucocorticoids *in vivo*. *J Clin Endocrinol Metab* **83**: 144–151.

Huizenga, N.A.T.M., de Lange, P., Koper, J.W., de Herder, W.W., Abs, R., Kasteren, J.H.L.M.V., *et al.* (2000). Five patients with biochemical and/or clinical generalized glucocorticoid resistance without alterations in the glucocorticoid receptor gene. *J Clin Endocrinol Metab* **85**: 2076–2081.

Irusen, E., Matthews, J.G., Takahashi, A., Barnes, P.J., Chung, K.F., and Adcock, I.M. (2002). p38 mitogen-activated protein kinase-induced glucocorticoid receptor phosphorylation reduces its activity: role in steroid-insensitive asthma. *J Allergy Clin Immunol* **109**: 649–657.

Jafarian-Tehrani, M. and Sternberg, E.M. (1999). Animal models of neuro-immune interaction in inflammatory diseases. *J Neuroimmunol* **100**: 13–20.

Jafarian-Tehrani, M., Listwak, S., Barrientos, R.M., Michaud, A., Corvol, P., and Sternberg, E.M. (2000). Exclusion of angiotensin I-converting enzyme as a candidate gene involved in exudative inflammatory resistance in F344/N rats. *Mol Med* **6**: 319–331.

Jagodic, M., Kornek, B., Weissert, R., Lassmann, H., Olsson, T., and Dahlman, I. (2001). Congenic mapping confirms a locus on rat chromosome 10 conferring strong protection against myelin oligodendrocyte glycoprotein-induced experimental autoimmune encephalomyelitis. *Immunogenetics* **53**: 410–415.

Jansson, L. and Holmdahl, R. (1998). Estrogen-mediated immunosuppression in autoimmune diseases. *Inflamm Res* **47**: 290–301.

Jiang, T., Liu, S., Tan, M., Huang, F., Sun, Y., Dong, X., *et al.* (2001). The phase-shift mutation in the glucocorticoid receptor gene: potential etiologic significance of neuroendocrine mechanisms in lupus nephritis. *Clin Chim Acta* **313**: 113–117.

Johnson, D.R. and Klaassen, C.D. (2002). Regulation of rat multidrug resistance protein 2 by classes of prototypical microsomal enzyme inducers that activate distinct transcription pathways. *Toxicol Sci* **67**: 182–189.

Johnson, E.O. and Moutsopoulos, H.M. (2000). Neuroendocrine manifestations in Sjogren's syndrome. Relation to the neurobiology of stress. *Ann N Y Acad Sci* **917**: 797–808.

Johnson, E.O., Vlachoyiannopoulos, P.G., Skopouli, F.N., Tzioufas, A.G., and Moutsopoulos, H.M. (1998). Hypofunction of the stress axis in Sjogren's syndrome. *J Rheumatol* **25**: 1508–1514.

Kageyama, Y. (2000). A case of isolated ACTH deficiency who developed auto-immune-mediated hypothyroidism and impaired water diuresis during glucocorticoid replacement therapy. *Endocr J* **47**: 667–674.

Kam, J.C., Szefler, S.J., Surs, W., Sher, E.R., and Leung, D.Y. (1993). Combination IL-2 and IL-4 reduces glucocorticoid receptor-binding affinity and T cell response to glucocorticoids. *J Immunol* **151**: 3460–3466.

Karin, M. and Chang, L. (2001). AP-1-glucocorticoid receptor crosstalk taken to a higher level. *J Endocrinol* **169**: 447–451.

Kast, H.R., Goodwin, B., Tarr, P.T., Jones, S.A., Anisfeld, A.M., Stoltz, C.M., *et al.* (2002). Regulation of multidrug resistance-associated protein 2 (ABCC2) by the nuclear receptors pregnane X receptor, farnesoid X-activated receptor, and constitutive androstane receptor. *J Biol Chem* **277**: 2908–2915.

Kauffmann, H.M., Pfannschmidt, S., Zoller, H., Benz, A., Vorderstemann, B., Webster, J.I., *et al.* (2002). Influence of redox-active compounds and PXR-activators on human MRP1 and MRP2 gene expression. *Toxicology* **171**: 137–146.

Kavelaars, A., Kuis, W., Knook, L., Sinnema, G., and Heijnen, C.J. (2000). Disturbed neuroendocrine-immune interactions in chronic fatigue syndrome. *J Clin Endocrinol Metab* **85**: 692–696.

Kino, T. and Chrousos, G.P. (2001). Glucocorticoid and mineralocorticoid resistance/hypersensitivity syndromes. *J Endocrinol* **169**: 437–445.

Kino, T., Gragerov, A., Kopp, J.B., Stauber, R.H., Pavlakis, G.N., and Chrousos, G.P. (1999). The HIV-1 virion-associated protein Vpr is a coactivator of the human glucocorticoid receptor. *J Exp Med* **189**: 51–61.

Kino, T., Stauber, R.H., Resau, J.H., Pavlakis, G.N., and Chrousos, G.P. (2001). Pathologic human GR mutant has a transdominant negative effect on the wild-type GR by inhibiting its translocation into the nucleus: importance of the ligand-binding domain for intracellular GR trafficking. *J Clin Endocrinol Metab* **86**: 5600–5608.

Kino, T., Vottero, A., Charmandari, E., and Chrousos, G.P. (2002*a*). Familial/sporadic glucocorticoid resistance syndrome and hypertension. *Ann N Y Acad Sci* **970**: 101–111.

Kino, T., Gragerov, A., Slobodskaya, O., Tsopanomichalou, M., Chrousos, G.P., and Pavlakis, G.N. (2002*b*). Human immunodeficiency virus type 1 (HIV-1) accessory protein Vpr induces transcription of the HIV-1 and gluco-corticoid-responsive promoters by binding directly to p300/CBP coactivators. *J Virol* **76**: 9724–9734.

Koper, J.W., Stolk, R.P., de Lange, P., Huizenga, N.A.T.M., Molijn, G.-J., Pols, H.A.P., *et al.* (1997). Lack of association between five polymorphisms in the human glucocorticoid receptor gene and glucocorticoid resistance. *Hum Genet* **99**: 663–668.

Kraft, M., Hamid, Q., Chrousos, G.P., Martin, R.J., and Leung, D.Y. (2001). Decreased steroid responsiveness at night in nocturnal asthma. Is the macrophage responsible? *Am J Respir Crit Care Med* **163**: 1219–1225.

Kralli, A. and Yamamoto, K.R. (1996). An FK506-sensitive transporter selectively decreases intracellular levels and potency of steroid hormones. *J Biol Chem* **271**: 17152–17156.

Lane, S.J., Adcock, I.M., Richards, D., Hawrylowicz, C., Barnes, P.J., and Lee, T.H. (1998). Corticosteroid-resistant bronchial asthma is associated with increased c-fos expression in monocytes and T lymphocytes. *J Clin Invest* **102**: 2156–2164.

Larsen, F., Oturai, A., Ryder, L.P., Madsen, H.O., Hillert, J., Fredrikson, S., *et al.* (2000). Linkage analysis of a candidate region in Scandinavian sib pairs with multiple sclerosis reveals linkage to chromosome 17q. *Genes Immun* **1**: 456–459.

Lechner, O., Hu, Y., Jafarian-Tehrani, M., Dietrich, H., Schwartz, S., Herold, M., *et al.* (1996). Disturbed immunoendocrine communication via the hypo-thalamo–pituitary–adrenal axis in murine lupus. *Brain Behav Immun* **10**: 337–350.

Lee, Y.M., Fujiwara, J., Munakata, Y., Ishii, T., Sugawara, A., Kaku, M., *et al.* (2004). A mutation of the glucocorticoid receptor gene in patients with systemic lupus erythematosus. *Tohoku J Exp Med* **203**: 69–76.

Leung, D.Y.M., Hamid, Q., Vottero, A., Szefler, S.J., Surs, W., Minshall, E., *et al.* (1997). Association of glucocorticoid insensitivity with increased expression of glucocorticoid receptor β. *J Exp Med* **186**: 1567–1574.

Levine, S. (1994). The ontogeny of the hypothalamic–pituitary–adrenal axis. The influence of maternal factors. *Ann N Y Acad Sci* **746**: 275–288.

Levine, S. (2001). Primary social relationships influence the development of the hypothalamic–pituitary–adrenal axis in the rat. *Physiol Behav* **73**: 255–260.

Listwak, S., Barrientos, R.M., Koike, G., Ghosh, S., Gomez, M., Misiewicz, B., *et al.* (1999). Identification of a novel inflammation-protective locus in the Fischer rat. *Mamm Genome* **10**: 362–365.

Liu, D., Diorio, J., Tannenbaum, B., Caldji, C., Francis, D., Freedman, A., *et al.* (1997). Maternal care, hippocampal glucocorticoid receptors, and hypothalamic–pituitary–adrenal responses to stress. *Science* **277**: 1659–1662.

Llorente, L., Richaud-Patin, Y., Diaz-Borjon, A., Alvarado de la Barrera, C., Jakez-Ocampo, J., de la Fuente, H., *et al.* (2000). Multidrug resistance-1 (MDR-1) in rheumatic autoimmune disorders. Part I: Increased P-glycoprotein activity in lymphocytes from rheumatoid arthritis patients might influence disease outcome. *Joint Bone Spine* **67**: 30–39.

MacPhee, I.A.M., Antoni, F.A., and Mason, D.W. (1989). Spontaneous recovery of rats from experimental allergic encephalomyelitis is dependent on regulation of the immune system by endogenous adrenal corticosteroids. *J Exp Med* **169**: 431–445.

Maillefert, J.F., Maynadie, M., Tebib, J.G., Aho, S., Walker, P., Chatard, C., *et al.* (1996). Expression of the multidrug resistance glycoprotein 170 in the peripheral blood lymphocytes of rheumatoid arthritis patients. The percentage of lymphocytes expressing glycoprotein 170 is increased in patients treated with prednisolone. *Br J Rheumatol* **35**: 430–435.

Maini, R.N. and Taylor, P.C. (2000). Anti-cytokine therapy for rheumatoid arthritis. *Annu Rev Med* **51**: 207–229.

Matthews, J.G., Ito, K., Barnes, P.J., and Adcock, I.M. (2004). Defective gluco-corticoid receptor nuclear translocation and altered histone acetylation patterns in glucocorticoid-resistant patients. *J Allergy Clin Immunol* **113**: 1100–1108.

McCain, G.A. and Tilbe, K.S. (1989). Diurnal hormone variation in fibromyalgia syndrome: a comparison with rheumatoid arthritis. *J Rheumatol Suppl* **19**: 154–157.

McKay, L.I. and Cidlowski, J.A. (1999). Molecular control of immune/inflammatory responses: Interactions between nuclear factor-κβ and steroid receptor-signaling pathways. *Endocr Rev* **20**: 435–459.

Medh, R.D., Lay, R.H., and Schmidt, T.J. (1998). Agonist-specific modulation of glucocorticoid receptor-mediated transcription by immunosuppressants. *Mol Cell Endocrinol* **138**: 11–23.

Meijer, O.C., de Lange. E.C., Breimer, D.D., de Boer, A.G., Workel, J.O., and de Kloet, E.R. (1998). Penetration of dexamethasone into brain glucocorticoid targets is enhanced in mdr1A P-glycoprotein knockout mice. *Endocrinology* **139**: 1789–1793.

Michelson, D., Stone, L., Galliven, E., Magiakou, M.A., Chrousos, G.P., Sternberg, E.M., *et al.* (1994). Multiple sclerosis is associated with alterations in hypothalamic–pituitary–adrenal axis function. *J Clin Endocrinol Metab* **79**: 848–853.

Mingrone, G, DeGaetano, A, Pugeat, M, Capristo, E, Greco, A.V., and Gasbarrini, G. (1999). The steroid resistance of Crohn's disease. *J Invest Med* **47**: 319–325.

Mirani, M., Elenkov, I., Volpi, S., Hiroi, N., Chrousos, G.P., and Kino, T. (2002). HIV-1 protein Vpr suppresses IL-12 production from human monocytes by enhancing glucocorticoid action: potential implications of Vpr coactivator activity for the innate and cellular immunity deficits observed in HIV-1 infection. *J Immunol* **169**: 6361–6368.

Misiewicz, B., Poltorak, M., Raybourne, R.B., Gomez, M., Listwak, S., and Sternberg, E.M. (1997). Intracerebroventricular transplantation of embryonic neuronal tissue from inflammatory resistant into inflammatory susceptible rats suppresses specific components of inflammation. *Exp Neurol* **146**: 305–314.

Moncek, F., Kvetnansky, R., and Jezova, D. (2001). Differential responses to stress stimuli of Lewis and Fischer rats at the pituitary and adrenocortical level. *Endocr Rev* **35**: 35–41.

Montano, E., Schmitz, M., Blaser, K., and Simon, H.U. (1996). P-glycoprotein expression in circulating blood leukocytes of patients with steroid-resistant asthma. *J Investig Allergol Clin Immunol* **6**: 14–21.

Moore, J.T. and Kliewer, S. (2000). Use of the nuclear receptor PXR to predict drug interactions. *Toxicology* **153**: 1–10.

Mulla, A. and Buckingham, J.C. (1999). Regulation of the hypothalamo-pituitary-adrenal axis by cytokines. *Baillieres Best Pract Res Clin Endocrinol Metab* **13**: 503–521.

Neeck, G. and Crofford, L.J. (2000). Neuroendocrine perturbations in fibromyalgia and chronic fatigue syndrome. *Rheum Dis Clin North Am* **26**: 989–1002.

Neeck, G., Federlin, K., Graef, V., Rusch, D., and Schmidt, K.L. (1990). Adrenal secretion of cortisol in patients with rheumatoid arthritis. *J Rheumatol* **17**: 24–29.

Neeck, G., Kluter, A., Dotzlaw, H., and Eggert, M. (2002). Involvement of the glucocorticoid receptor in the pathogenesis of rheumatoid arthritis. *Ann N Y Acad Sci* **966**: 491–495.

Nelissen, I., Fiten, P., Vandenbroeck, K., Hillert, J., Olsson, T., Marrosu, M.G., *et al.* (2000). PECAM1, MPO and PRKAR1A at chromosome 17q21–q24 and susceptibility for multiple sclerosis in Sweden and Sardinia. *J Neuroimmunol* **108**: 153–159.

New, M.I., Nimkarn, S., Brandon, D.D., Cunningham-Rundles, S., Wilson, R.C., Newfield, R.S., *et al.* (1999). Resistance to several steroids in two sisters. *J Clin Endocrinol Metab* **84**: 4454–4464.

Nguyen, C., Limaye, N., and Wakeland, E.K. (2002). Susceptibility genes in the pathogenesis of murine lupus. *Arthritis Res* **4**(Suppl. 3): S255–S263.

Niess, J.H., Monnikes, H., Dignass, A.U., Klapp, B.F., and Arck, P.C. (2002). Review on the influence of stress on immune mediators, neuropeptides and hormones with relevance for inflammatory bowel disease. *Digestion* **65**: 131–140.

Nuclear Receptor Nomenclature Committee (1999). A unified nomenclature system for the nuclear receptor superfamily. *Cell* **97**: 161–163.

Orii, F., Ashida, T., Nomura, M., Maemoto, A., Fujiki, T., Ayabe, T., *et al.* (2002). Quantitative analysis for human glucocorticoid receptor alpha/beta mRNA in IBD. *Biochem Biophys Res Commun* **296**: 1286–1294.

Petrides, J.S., Gold, P.W., Mueller, G.P., Singh, A., Stratakis, C., Chrousos, G.P., *et al.* (1997). Marked differences in functioning of the hypothalamic–pituitary–adrenal axis between groups of men. *J Appl Physiol* **82**: 1979–1988.

Poteliakhoff, A. (1981). Adrenocortical activity and some clinical findings in acute and chronic fatigue. *J Psychosom Res* **25**: 91–95.

Raddatz, D., Middel, P., Bockemuhl, M., Benohr, P., Wissmann, C., Schworer, H., *et al.* (2004). Glucocorticoid receptor expression in inflammatory bowel disease: evidence for a mucosal down-regulation in steroid-unresponsive ulcerative colitis. *Aliment Pharmacol Ther* **19**: 47–61.

Rask, E., Olsson, T., Soderberg, S., Andrew, R., Livingstone, D.E., Johnson, O., *et al.* (2001). Tissue-specific dysregulation of cortisol metabolism in human obesity. *J Clin Endocrinol Metab* **86**: 1418–1421.

Reichardt, H.M., Kaestner, K.H., Tuckermann, J., Kretz, O., Wessely, O., Bock, R., *et al.* (1998). DNA binding of the glucocorticoid receptor is not essential for survival. *Cell* **93**: 531–541.

Reichardt, H.M., Tuckermann, J.P., Gottlicher, M., Vujic, M., Weih, F., Angel, P., *et al.* (2001). Repression of inflammatory responses in the absence of DNA binding by the glucocorticoid receptor. *EMBO J* **20**: 7168–7173.

Remmers, E.F., Longman, R.E., Du, Y., O'Hare, A., Cannon, G.W., Griffiths, M.M., *et al.* (1996). A genome scan localizes five non-MHC loci controlling collagen-induced arthritis in rats. *Nat Genet* **14**: 82–85.

Richaud-Patin, Y., Vega-Boada, F., Vidaller, A., and Llorente, L. (2004). Multidrug resistance-1 (MDR-1) in autoimmune disorders IV. P-glycoprotein overfunction in lymphocytes from myasthenia gravis patients. *Biomed Pharmacother* **58**: 320–324.

Rivest, S. (2001). How circulating cytokines trigger the neural circuits that control the hypothalamic–pituitary–adrenal axis. *Psychoneuroendocrinology* **26**: 761–788.

Rovensky, J., Blazickova, S., Rauova, L., Jezova, D., Koska, J., Lukac, J., *et al.* (1998). The hypothalamic-pituitary response in SLE. Regulation of prolactin, growth hormone and cortisol release. *Lupus* **7**: 409–413.

Rozlog, L.A., Kiecolt-Glaser, J.K., Marucha, P.T., Sheridan, J.F., and Glaser, R. (1999). Stress and immunity: implications for viral disease and wound healing. *J Periodontol* **70**: 786–792.

Ruiz, M., Lind, U., Gafvels, M., Eggertsen, G., Carlstedt-Duke, J., Nilsson, L., *et al.* (2001). Characterization of two novel mutations in the glucocorticoid receptor gene in patients with primary cortisol resistance. *Clin Endocrinol* **55**: 363–371.

Ruiz-Soto, R., Richaud-Patin, Y., Lopez-Karpovitch, X., and Llorente, L. (2003). Multidrug resistance-1 (MDR-1) in autoimmune disorders III: increased P-glycoprotein activity in lymphocytes from immune thrombocytopenic purpura patients. *Exp Hematol* **31**: 483–487.

Ruzek, M.C., Pearce, B.D., Miller, A.H., and Biron, C.A. (1999). Endogenous glucocorticoids protect against cytokine-mediated lethality during viral infection. *J Immunol* **162**: 3527–3533.

Schaaf, M.J. and Cidlowski, J.A. (2002). AUUUA motifs in the 3'UTR of human glucocorticoid receptor alpha and beta mRNA destabilize mRNA and decrease receptor protein expression. *Steroids* **67**: 627–636.

Schinkel, A.H., Wagenaar, E., van Deemter, L., Mol, C.A., and Borst, P. (1995). Absence of the mdr1a P-Glycoprotein in mice affects tissue distribution and pharmacokinetics of dexamethasone, digoxin, and cyclosporin A. *J Clin Invest* **96**: 1698–1705.

Schumann, E.M., Kumpfel, T., Then Bergh, F., Trenkwalder, C., Holsboer, F., and Auer, D.P. (2002). Activity of the hypothalamic-pituitary-adrenal axis in multiple sclerosis: correlations with gadolinium-enhancing lesions and ventricular volume. *Ann Neurol* **51**: 763–767.

Scott, L.V. and Dinan, T.G. (1998). Urinary free cortisol excretion in chronic fatigue syndrome, major depression and in healthy volunteers. *J Affect Disord* **47**: 49–54.

Scott, L.V., Medbak, S., and Dinan, T.G. (1998). Blunted adrenocorticotropin and cortisol responses to corticotropin-releasing hormone stimulation in chronic fatigue syndrome. *Acta Psychiatr Scand* **97**: 450–457.

Seckl, J.R. and Walker, B.R. (2001). Minireview: 11β-hydroxysteroid dehydrogenase type 1-A tissue-specific amplifier of glucocorticoid action. *Endocrinology* **142**: 1371–1376.

Shahidi, H., Vottero, A., Stratakis, C., Taymans, S.E., Karl, M., Longui, C.A., *et al.* (1999). Imbalanced expression of the glucocorticoid receptor isoforms in cultured lymphocytes from a patient with systemic glucocorticoid resistance and chronic lymphocytic leukemia. *Biochem Biophys Res Commun* **254**: 559–565.

Sher, E.R., Leung, D.Y., Surs, W., Kam, J.C., Zieg, G., Kamada, A.K., *et al.* (1994). Steroid-resistant asthma. Cellular mechanisms contributing to inadequate response to glucocorticoid therapy. *J Clin Invest* **93**: 33–39.

Smith, C.C., Omelijaniuk, R.J., Whitfield, H.J.J., Aksentijevich, S., Fellows, M.Q., Zelazowski, E., *et al.* (1994). Differential mineralocorticoid (type I) and glucocorticoid (type II) receptor expression in Lewis and Fischer rats. *Neuroimmunomodulation* **1**: 66–73.

Sousa, A.R., Lane, S.J., Cidlowski, J.A., Staynov, D.Z., and Lee, T.H. (2000). Glucocorticoid resistance in asthma is associated with elevated *in vivo* expression of the glucocorticoid receptor beta-isoform. *J Allergy Clin Immunol* **105**: 943–950.

Stefferl, A., Linington, C., Holsboer, F., and Reul, J.M. (1999). Susceptibility and resistance to experimental allergic encephalomyelitis: relationship with hypothalamic-pituitary-adrenocortical axis responsiveness in the rat. *Endocrinology* **140**: 4932–4938.

Sternberg, E.M., Hill, J.M., Chrousos, G.P., Kamilaris, T., Listwak, S.J., Gold, P.W., *et al.* (1989*a*). Inflammatory mediator-induced hypothalamic-pituitary-adrenal axis activation is defective in streptococcal cell wall arthritis-susceptible Lewis rats. *Proc Natl Acad Sci USA* **86**: 2374–2378.

Sternberg, E.M., Young, W.S.D., Bernardini, R., Calogero, A.E., Chrousos, G.P., Gold, P.W., *et al.* (1989*b*). A central nervous system defect in biosynthesis of corticotropin- releasing hormone is associated with susceptibility to strepto-coccal cell wall-induced arthritis in Lewis rats. *Proc Natl Acad Sci USA* **86**: 4771–4775.

Straub, R.H., Herfarth, H., Falk, W., Andus, T., and Scholmerich, J. (2002). Uncoupling of the sympathetic nervous system and the hypothalamic-pituitary-adrenal axis in inflammatory bowel disease? *J Neuroimmunol* **126**: 116–125.

Strickland, I., Kisich, K., Hauk, P.J., Vottero, A., Chrousos, G.P., Klemm, D.J., *et al.* (2001). High constitutive glucocorticoid receptor b in human neutrophils enables them to reduce their spontaneous rate of cell death in response to corticosteroids. *J Exp Med* **193**: 585–593.

Strickland, P., Morriss, R., Wearden, A., and Deakin, B. (1998). A comparison of salivary cortisol in chronic fatigue syndrome, community depression and healthy controls. *J Affect Disord* **47**: 191–194.

Subramaniam, N., Cairns, W., and Okret, S. (1997). Studies on the mechanism of glucocorticoid-mediated repression from a negative glucocorticoid response element from the bovine prolactin gene. *DNA Cell Biol* **16**: 153–163.

Takahasi, K.I., Fukushima, K., Sasano, H., Sasaki, I., Matsuno, S., Krozowski, Z.S., *et al.* (1999). Type II 11beta-hydroxysteroid dehydrogenase expression in human colonic epithelial cells of inflammatory bowel disease. *Dig Dis Sci* **44**: 2516–2522.

Tanimura, S.M. and Watts, A.G. (2001). Corticosterone modulation of ACTH secretogue gene expression in the paraventricular nucleus. *Peptides* **22**: 775–783.

Tonelli, L., Webster, J.I., Rapp, K.L., and Sternberg, E. (2001). Neuroendocrine responses regulating susceptibility and resistance to autoimmune/inflammatory disease in inbred rat strains. *Immunol Rev* **184**: 203–211.

Tsigos, C. (1999). Isolated glucocorticoid deficiency and ACTH receptor mutation. *Arch Med Res* **30**: 475–480.

Tsigos, C., Tsiotra, P., Garibaldi, L.R., Stavridis, J.C., Chrousos, G.P., and Raptis, S.A. (2000). Mutation of the ACTH receptor gene in a new family with isolated glucocorticoid deficiency. *Mol Genet Metab* **71**: 646–650.

van Denderen, J.C., Boersma, J.W., Zeinstra, P., Hollander, A.P., and van Neerbos, B.R. (1992). Physiological effects of exhaustive physical exercise in primary fibromyalgia syndrome (PFS): is PFS a disorder of neuroendocrine reactivity? *Scand J Rheumatol* **21**: 35–37.

van Haarst, A.D., Oitzl, M.S., and de Kloet, E.R. (1997). Facilitation of feedback inhibition through blockade of glucocorticoid receptors in the hippo-campus. *Neurochem Res* **22**: 1323–1328.

Vedhara, K., Cox, N.K.M., Wilcock, G.K., Perks, P., Hunt, M., Anderson, S., *et al.* (1999). Chronic stress in elderly carers of dementia patients and antibody response to influenza vaccination. *Lancet* **353**: 627–631.

Vottero, A., Kino, T., Combe, H., Lecomte, P., and Chrousos, G.P. (2002). A novel, *C*-terminal dominant negative mutation of the GR causes familial gluco-corticoid resistance through abnormal interactions with p160 steroid receptor coactivators. *J Clin Endocrinol Metab* **87**: 2658–2667.

Weaver, I.C., La Plante, P., Weaver, S., Parent, A., Sharma, S., Diorio, J., *et al.* (2001). Early environmental regulation of hippocampal glucocorticoid receptor gene expression: characterization of intracellular mediators and potential genomic target sites. *Mol Cell Endocrinol* **185**: 205–218.

Webster, E.L., Torpy, D.J., Elenkov, I.J., and Chrousos, G.P. (1998). Corticotropin-releasing hormone and inflammation. *Ann N Y Acad Sci* **840**: 21–32.

Webster, E.L., Barrientos, R.M., Contoreggi, C., Isaac, M.G., Ligier, S., Gabry, K.E., *et al.* (2002). Corticotropin releasing hormone (CRH) antagonist attenuates adjuvant induced arthritis: role of CRH in peripheral inflammation. *J Rheumatol* **29**: 1252–1261.

Webster, J.C., Jewell, C.M., Bodwells, J.E., Munck, A., Sar, M., and Cidlowski, J.A. (1997). Mouse glucocorticoid receptor phosphorylation status influences multiple functions of the receptor protein. *J Biol Chem* **272**: 9287–9293.

Webster, J.C., Oakley, R.H., Jewell, C.M., and Cidlowski, J.A. (2001). Pro-inflammatory cytokines regulate human glucocorticoid receptor gene expression and lead to the accumulation of the dominant negative β iso-form: a mechanism for the generation of glucocorticoid resistance. *Proc Natl Acad Sci USA* **98**: 6865–6870.

Webster, J.I. and Carlstedt-Duke, J. (2002). Involvement of multidrug resistance proteins (MDR) in the modulation of glucocorticoid response. *J Steroid Biochem Mol Biol* **82**: 277–288.

Webster, J.I., Tonelli, L., and Sternberg, E.M. (2002). Neuroendocrine regulation of immunity. *Annu Rev Immunol* **20**: 125–163.

Wei, T. and Lightman, S.L. (1997). The neuroendocrine axis in patients with multiple sclerosis. *Brain* **120**: 1067–1076.

Wick, G., Sgonc, R., and Lechner, O. (1998). Neuroendocrine-immune disturb-ances in animal models with spontaneous autoimmune diseases. *Ann N Y Acad Sci* **840**: 591–598.

Wilder, R.L., Calandra, G.B., Garvin, A.J., Wright, K.D., and Hansen, C.T. (1982). Strain and sex variation in the susceptibility to streptococcal cell wall-induced polyarthritis in the rat. *Arthritis Rheum* **25**: 1064–1072.

Wilder, R.L., Griffiths, M.M., Cannon, G.W., Caspi, R., Gulko, P.S., and Remmers, E.F. (2001). Genetic factors involved in central nervous system/immune interactions. *Adv Exp Med Biol* **493**: 59–67.

Wu, S.-M., Stratakis, C.A., Chan, C.H.Y., Hallermeier, K.M., Bourdony, C.J., Rennert, O.M., *et al.* (1998). Genetic heterogeneity of adrenocorticotropin (ACTH) resistance syndromes: identification of a novel mutation of the ACTH receptor gene in hereditary glucocorticoid deficiency. *Mol Genet Metab* **64**: 256–265.

Young, A.H., Sharpe, M., Clements, A., Dowling, B., Hawton, K.E., and Cowen, P.J. (1998). Basal activity of the hypothalamic-pituitary-adrenal axis in patients with the chronic fatigue syndrome (neurasthenia). *Biol Psychiat* **43**: 236–237.

8 Immunological properties of the peripheral nervous system

Ralf Gold, Bernd C. Kieseier, and Hans-Peter Hartung

Introduction

The peripheral nervous system (PNS) is a target for heterogeneous immune attacks mediated by different components of the systemic immune compartment. T cells, B cells, and macrophages can interact with endogenous, partially immune-competent glial cells and contribute to local inflammation. In this scenario, adaptive and innate immunity are functionally connected allowing for intensive interactions between hematogenic cells and glial elements of the PNS.

This chapter will cover the interaction of the immune system with the cellular and extracellular components in the PNS, immune functions of local glial cells such as Schwann cells and endoneurial macrophages, and their final outcome resulting in tissue inflammation or repair processes.

The animal model experimental autoimmune neuritis (EAN) allows direct monitoring of these immune responses *in vivo*. In EAN contributions to regulate autoimmunity in the PNS are made by adhesion molecules and by cytokines that orchestrate cellular interactions or even elimination of invading cells. Interestingly, several conventional and novel immunotherapeutic approaches allow a better understanding of immune regulation and its failure in the PNS. Finally this may help to develop improved, more specific immunotherapies.

The local immune circuit

The PNS has traditionally been considered as 'immunologically privileged', yet not as strictly as the central nervous system (CNS). This view has undergone revision within recent years. Some in the mid-1980s it was shown that indeed immune surveillance is operative in such tissues (Wekerle *et al.*, 1986*a*). Even vulnerable privileged sites like the nervous system are constantly patrolled by activated T lymphocytes. The PNS is separated from the external environment by the blood–nerve barrier (BNB), which does restrict access of immune cells and soluble mediators to a certain degree; however, this restriction is not complete, neither anatomically nor functionally. The BNB is practically absent at nerve roots, in dorsal root ganglia, and nerve terminals. Immune surveillance, as found in most organs, is present in the PNS as well: activated T and B lymphocytes can cross the BNB irrespective of their antigen specificity, and antigen-presenting cells, such as macrophages, are abundant in peripheral nerve tissue. Schwann cells also can function as antigen-presenting cells *in vitro* (Wekerle *et al.*, 1986*b*).

Triggering of autoreactive T- and B-cell responses: molecular mimicry and other immunological assaults

The mechanisms underlying breakdown of tolerance and thus generation of autoreactive T-cell and B-cell responses are clear in experimental models. There the autoimmune cascade is deliberately and artificially set off. In both acute and chronic immune neuropathies in humans the conditions allowing emergence of peripheral nerve-directed autoreactivity remain obscure.

If one of the regulatory mechanisms fails, a specific immune response is mounted against self antigens. This leads to expansion of autoreactive effector T cells, generation of autoantibodies through T-cell help, and may give rise to tissue damage. Autoaggressive responses may initiate autoimmune disease. The autoimmune response may persist because the immune system is not able to remove the autoantigen from the body, in contrast to foreign antigens; even worse, new hitherto hidden autoantigens can be released to amplify the immune response and broaden its epitope specificity, a process termed *epitope spreading* (Lehmann *et al.*, 1992).

It is conceivable that myelin-reactive T lymphocytes are contained in the immune repertoire of healthy individuals. Under normal conditions they are inactive or silenced by various modes of peripheral tolerance. Only recently has it been realized that many myelin proteins such as P0 are also expressed in thymic tissue, thus contributing to the development of immune tolerance (Visan *et al.*, 2004). Tolerance may break down when the individual is confronted by an infective organism that happens to share epitopes with endogenous peripheral myelin proteins such as P0 or P2. Such mimicry has been hypothesized to underlie Guillain–Barré syndrome (GBS) associated with cytomegalovirus infection (Adelman and Linington, 1992). Given the degeneracy of epitope recognition by T lymphocytes this notion may be considered. Another possibility is antigen non-specific T-cell activation mediated by cytokines (Benoist and Mathis, 1998).

This hypothesis may be viewed as a revival of the time-honored concept of bystander demyelination. Evidence to support a variation on this theme is available. The possibility of nerve injury mediated by activated, non-neural-specific T cells was studied by systemic transfer of ovalbumin-specific T cells, followed by intraneural injection of ovalbumin (Harvey *et al.*, 1995; Pollard *et al.*, 1995). Rapid endoneurial infiltration of T cells and macrophages occurred on the side injected with ovalbumin and was associated with a marked increase in BNB permeability. In the casein-injected control nerve only degeneration and macrophage infiltration was observed, which declined after 3 days. Histological and clinical features in this model were similar to those observed in P2-induced EAN. When given in combination with antimyelin antibodies primary demyelination or axonal degeneration was demonstrable by electrophysiological studies, thus replicating typical features of GBS.

Molecular mimicry based on structural similarities between micro-organisms and peripheral myelin may be more important for the generation of autoreactive B-cell responses. There is a large body of evidence indicating that infection with certain strains of the Gram-negative enteropathogen *Campylobacter jejuni* elicits antibody responses directed to gangliosides and related glycolipids on the myelin membrane and axolemma since carbohydrate sequences of these glycoconjugates are also contained in the lipopolysaccharide fraction of the micro-organism (Yuki, 1997; Yuki *et al.*, 1999). Based on these molecular similarities a model of human axonal GBS has been established that uses inoculation with a bovine brain ganglioside mixture or isolated GM1 (Yuki *et al.*, 2001).

Experimental autoimmune neuritis—a model to study immune regulation *in vivo* and to dissect induction and effector phases of the disease

Experimental autoimmune neuritis (EAN) is an animal model for human GBS, an acute demyelinating inflammatory disease of the peripheral nervous system (PNS), mediated by autoantigen-specific T cells (reviewed in Hartung *et al.* (1998)). EAN can be actively induced in Lewis rats by immunization with bovine P2 protein (Kadlubowski and Hughes, 1979) or recombinant human P2 protein (Weishaupt *et al.*, 1995), with a peptide (amino acids 53–78) spanning the neuritogenic epitope (Olee *et al.*, 1989),

or by adoptive transfer of neuritogenic T cells (AT-EAN) (Linington *et al.*, 1984). Further autoantigens that have been identified in EAN models in rats and mice are P0 (Linington *et al.*, 1992), peripheral myelin protein-22 (PMP22) (Gabriel *et al.*, 1998), and myelin-associated glycoprotein (MAG) (Weerth *et al.*, 1999); in rabbits galactocerebroside has been identified (Saida *et al.*, 1978). Since EAN replicates many clinical, electrophysiological and immunological aspects of GBS it has been widely used as a model to investigate disease mechanisms (see review in Maurer and Gold (2002)). Only EAN models in mice are still of limited reliability and value.

The immune response in EAN can be divided into an induction and an effector phase (Fig. 8.1). Adhesion molecules (AMs) are critically involved into these different phases. In the induction phase the injected autoantigen is presented to 'naïve' T cells by professional antigen-presenting cells (APC) such as macrophages or dendritic cells resulting in T-cell activation. Two

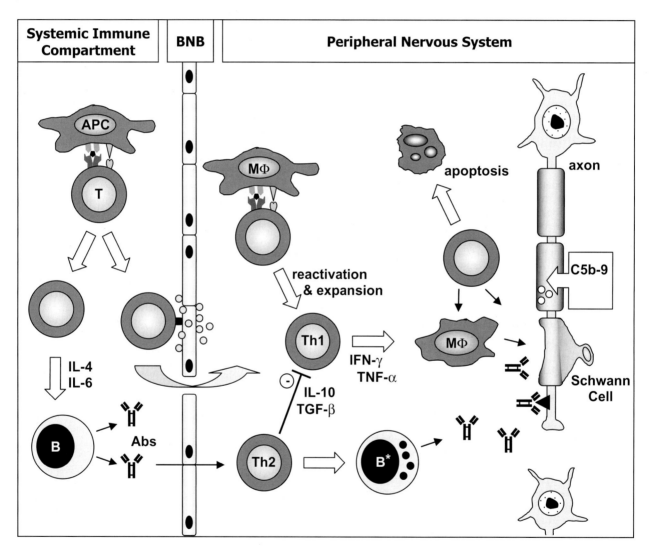

Fig. 8.1 Basic principles of cellular and humoral immune reponses within the peripheral nervous system (PNS). Autoreactive T cells (T) recognize a specific autoantigen presented by major histocompatibility complex Class II molecules and the simultaneous delivery of co-stimulatory signals on the cell surface of antigen-presenting cells (APCs), such as macrophages (MΦ), in the systemic immune compartment. An infection might trigger this event inducing molecular mimicry. These activated T lymphocytes can cross the blood–nerve barrier (BNB) in order to enter the PNS, a processs mediated in part by chemokines, cellular adhesion molecules, and matrix metalloproteinases (MMPs). Within the PNS, T cells activate macrophages that enhance phagocytic activity, production of cytokines, and the relases of toxic mediators, such as nitric oxide, MMPs, and pro-inflammatory cytokines, such as tumor necrosis factor-alpha (TNF-α) or interferon-gamma (IFN-γ). Autoantibodies (Abs), crossing the BNB or locally produced by B lymphocytes (B; Plasma cells, B*), contribute to the process of demyelination and axonal damage. Abs can mediate demyelination by antibody-dependent cellular cytotoxicity, can potentially block epitopes functionally relevant for nerve conduction, and can activate the complement system by the classical pathway yielding pro-inflammatory mediators and the lytic C5b-9 terminal complex. Termination of the inflammatory response is mediated, in part, by macrophages through the induction of T-cell apoptosis and the release of anti-inflammatory cytokines, such as interleukin-10 (IL-10) and transforming growth factor-beta (TGF-β).

external signals are crucially required for an effective T-cell activation by antigen presentation: the antigen-specific signal provided by the immunogenic peptide and presented in the context of major histocompatibility complex (MHC) molecules on APC, and the antigen-independent signal called co-stimulation and mediated by AMs of the integrin family such as αLβ2 (LFA-1, CD11a/CD18), α4β1 (VLA-4, CD49d/CD29), or αvβ3 (CD51/ CD61) and AMs of the immunoglobulin superfamily such as ICAM-1 (CD54), VCAM-1 (CD106), CD2, CD58, and, of special functional relevance, CTLA-4 (CD152), B7-1 (CD80) and B7-2 (CD86), ICOS, and ICOSL expressed on T cells or APC.

It is of note that the meticulous interaction of these co-stimulatory molecules is critical for maintenance of immune regulation. In the non-obese diabetic mouse (NOD), the co-stimulatory B7-1 and B7-2 molecules on immune cells have been shown to play distinct roles. Elimination of B7-2 expression by breeding NOD mice onto the B7-2-deficient background prevents diabetes, but leads to the development of a spontaneous autoimmune peripheral polyneuropathy (SAPP) (Salomon et al., 2001). Morphological analysis revealed significant demyelination, with a mononuclear cellular infiltrate, composed of dendritic cells, CD4+ T cells, and CD 8+ T cells.

Entry of inflammatory cells: the role of cell adhesion molecules, chemokines, and matrix metalloproteinases

The first important step in the pathogenesis of EAN is the presentation of autoantigen in the induction phase. This results in the physiological activation of disease-inducing T cells. Cellular adhesion molecules (CAMs) are essential for effective antigen presentation *in vitro* in rodents and humans. *In vivo*, inhibition of some of these co-accessory molecules such as CD2 (Jung et al., 1996), ICAM-1 (Archelos et al., 1993) or LFA-1 (Archelos et al., 1994) by monoclonal antibodies (mAbs) prevents adequate T-cell activation.

The specific function of individual CAMs was first elucidated by blocking their action with specific monoclonal antibodies in various animal models. Later the generation of knockout animals for the corresponding gene of a particular CAM became instrumental (see review in Archelos et al. (1999)). The mechanism of subsequent transendothelial migration across the BNB is a multistep process occurring in an ordered sequence : In the first step, CAMs are expressed on leukocytes and vascular endothelium, resulting in a slowing and attachment of the circulating immune cells along the vessel wall ('tethering' and 'rolling'). Since the flowing blood quickly dislodges cells that touch the vessel wall, adhesion molecules must act as

mechanical anchors in addition to their function as tissue-specific recognition molecules.

Archelos and colleagues extended their studies and recently confirmed the role of L-selectin in transendothelial migration in EAN (Archelos et al., 1997). Subsequently also VLA-4 and its ligand VCAM-1 were investigated (Enders et al., 1998). Blockade of VLA-4 (α4β1) by mAb was effective in EAN (Fig. 8.2). Similar to the situation in multiple sclerosis, this integrin seems to be the most important AM in transendothelial migration of T cells in rodent EAN and hence the most promising target candidate for therapeutic intervention in GBS. Surprisingly VLA-4 and VCAM-1 blockade are equally effective in enhancing T-cell apoptosis in the inflammatory lesion (Leussink et al., 2002). In addition to their binding function, mAb against VLA-4 also seem to be involved in blocking cellular signaling and thus abrogating survival of inflammatory T cells.

In a second step, chemokines come into play providing signals to direct leukocyte migration into the extravascular space. Since lymphocytes must be positioned correctly to interact with other cells, the pattern and anatomical distribution of chemokines within the target tissue as well as the types of chemokine receptors expressed on the cell surface become critically important in orchestrating the ongoing immune responses (Campbell et al., 1998; Moser and Loetscher, 2001).

Studies on the expression pattern of the chemokines interferon-gamma-inducible protein (IP)-10, monocyte chemoattractant protein (MCP)-1, macrophage inflammatory protein (MIP)-1α, MIP-1β, and regulated upon activation normal T-cell-expressed and secreted (RANTES) in sciatic nerves from animals with myelin-induced experimental autoimmune neuritis speak for a timely ordered sequence of expression (Kieseier et al., 2000): The mRNAs for MIP-1α and MIP-1β were found to be up-regulated with peak values at day 13 post-immunization (p.i.), preceding maximum disease severity. In contrast, mRNAs for MCP-1, RANTES, and IP-10 exhibited peak levels coincident with peak of the disease at day 15 p.i. Immunohistochemistry for IP-10 protein revealed immunoreactivity associated with perineurial endothelial cells. RANTES protein was localized immunohistologically to invading T lymphocytes.

Similar to EAN a differential pattern of chemotactic signals was defined in inflammatory disorders of the human PNS. Peak expression levels prior to or coincident with maximum clinical disease activity involved different chemokines such as CXCL10 (IP-10), CCL2 (MCP-1), CCL3 (MIP-1α), and CCL5 (RANTES) (Kieseier et al., 2002). Corresponding chemokine receptors were detected in the inflamed PNS, with CCR-1 and CCR-5 primarily expressed by endoneurial macrophages and CCR-2, CCR-4, and CXCR-3 by invading T lymphocytes (Fig. 8.3). Quantitative analysis revealed that CXCR-3 is highest in infiltrating T cells compared with the

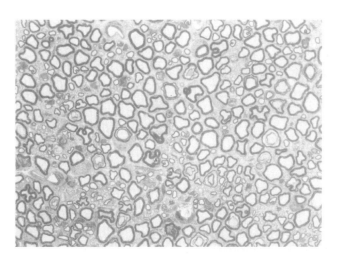 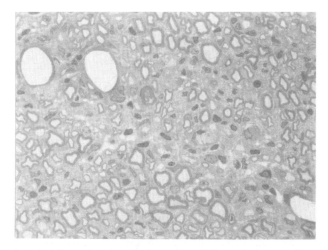

Fig. 8.2 VLA-4 therapy of active experimental autoimmune neuritis. Note the abundant perivascular inflammation, demyelination, and axonal damage in the control group (right side) which was treated with isotype control antibody only. In contrast, only rare demyelination can be seen in the treatment group (left side). Semithin sections stained with toluidine blue.

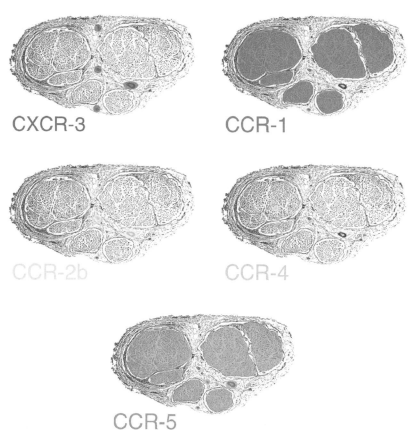

CXCR-3   CCR-1

CCR-2b   CCR-4

CCR-5

Fig. 8.3 Chemokine receptor expression. Consistent chemokine receptor expression patterns can be detected in inflammatory demyelinating neuropathies by immunohistochemistry: CCR-1 and CCR-5 are primarily expressed by endoneurial macrophages, whereas CCR-2, CCR-4, and CXCR-3 can be localized to invading T lymphocytes, suggesting that the latter might play a specific role in chemokine-mediated lymphocyte traffic into the inflamed peripheral nervous tissue.

other receptors. Its ligand CXCL10 mirrors the distribution of the cognate receptor within the inflamed PNS, and delineates endothelial cells as the primary cellular source of CXCL10, thus pointing to a pathogenic role for specific chemokine receptors and IP-10 in the generation of inflammatory demyelinating neuropathies (Kieseier *et al.*, 2002).

In a third step, matrix metalloproteinases (MMPs) are secreted by leukocytes in order to disrupt the BNB, thus facilitating transmigration of cells and of plasma-derived macromolecules into the parenchyma of the PNS. Up-regulation and expression of MMP-9 (92 kDa gelatinase) and MMP-7 (matrilysin), but not of other MMPs, were found by immunocytochemistry, reverse transcription polymerase chain reaction, and zymo-

graphy in the endoneurium and epineurium of the inflamed peripheral nerve (Leppert *et al.*, 1999; Kieseier *et al.*, 1999) (Fig. 8.4). Also, utilization of a comparable MMP pattern underlined pathophysiological similarities between EAN and GBS (Kieseier *et al.*, 1999). The selective expression of certain MMPs in inflammatory autoimmune disorders of the PNS and their varied cellular localizations suggest that these enzymes may play a crucial, but multifactorial, role in the process leading to disruption of the BNB. MMPs may therefore serve as potential targets for newer therapies that make use of specific inhibitors capable of preventing activation of MMPs. Such an approach has already been shown to have a beneficial effect on the disease course of EAN (Redford *et al.*, 1997).

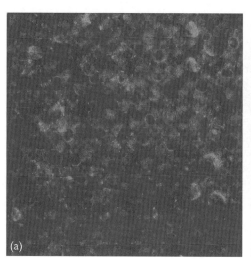
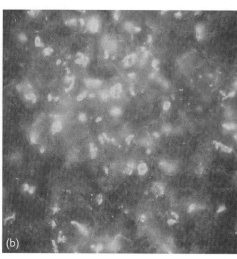

Fig. 8.4 Expression of matrix metalloproteinases (MMPs) in the inflamed nerve. Metalloproteinases mediate tissue invasion of inflammatory cells into the peripheral nervous system. Proteolytic activity of gelatinases. such as MMP-2 and MMP-9, can be visualized by *in situ* zymography in the sciatic nerve of animals with experimental autoimmune neuritis. In control animals only background fluorescence is observable (a), whereas in animals with maximum clinical disease severity strong proteolytic activity can be found within the inflamed nerve (b). (See also Plate 1 of the colour plate section at the center of this book.)

Amplification and termination of the local immune response: the role of cytokines

Concomitant with cellular infiltration, a broad range of cytokines is induced in EAN nerves (Gillen *et al.*, 1998; Kiefer *et al.*, 2001). Cytokines are mainly expressed by T cells and macrophages, but also to some extent by Schwann cells (see below). At disease onset, T cells and a subpopulation of macrophages express interferon (IFN)-γ, the prototype of a pro-inflammatory cytokine (Schmidt *et al.*, 1992). The key role of IFN-γ in disease initiation is underscored by antibody neutralization experiments, leading to attenuation of clinical EAN (Hartung *et al.*, 1990). IFN-γ is inducible by interleukin (IL)-18, a key mediator of innate immunity. In EAN, infiltrating macrophages strongly express IL-18. It is of note that patients with GBS may show increased IL-18 serum levels during the acute phase of their disease (Jander and Stoll, 2001). Thus IL-18 probably contributes to the amplification of the initial inflammatory response.

IFN-γ, moreover, activates macrophages to release tumor necrosis factor (TNF)-α to provide the appropriate local milieu for myelin damage(Stoll *et al.*, 1993). In further support of a detrimental role of TNF-α in EAN, experimental neutralization of TNF-α ameliorated demyelination (Stoll *et al.*, 1993). Interestingly, in GBS patients, circulating TNF-α correlated with electrophysiological signs of demyelination (Sharief *et al.*, 1997). Injection of TNF-α into nerves may cause inflammation, demyelination by inducing death of Schwann cells (Weishaupt *et al.*, 2001), and damage to endothelial cells (Said and Hontebeyrie Joskowicz, 1992), although this mechanism remained a matter of debate (Uncini *et al.*, 1999).

Yet it has to be considered that TNF-α is part of a complex cytokine network and may have a pivotal role in EAN. TNF-α also diminishes inflammation in nerves by inducing T-cell apoptosis. Apoptosis of T cells is an important mechanism for termination of immune responses (see below). Accordingly, neutralization of TNF-α by antibodies led to a prolonged persistence of T cells in EAN nerves (Weishaupt *et al.*, 2000). At present, it appears that in EAN neutralization of TNF-α-mediated myelin damage outweighs the ameliorating effects through T-cell removal.

In addition to IL-18, IL-12 is a key cytokine of the innate immune system (Trinchieri, 1995). The IL-12 family of cytokine proteins are released from macrophages and dendritic cells in response to pathogens, and bind to receptors on target cells, activating a variety of immune functions. Most of the available data in EAN have focused on IL-12. IL-12 exerts pro-inflammatory actions as a p35/40 heterodimer, but is immunosuppressive in the form of its IL-12 p40 homodimers. IL-12-mRNA+ cells have been described in EAN by *in situ* hybridization at onset of overt disease (Zhu *et al.*, 1997). Functionally, IL-12 injected into healthy peripheral nerve provoked inflammation and caused marked demyelination (Pelidou *et al.*, 1999). Thus it is conceivable that macrophage-derived IL-12 might promote inflammation at onset of EAN, while IL-12 p40 homodimers may have immunosuppressive effects during recovery. The recent discovery of IL-23 as another family member acting upstream of IL-12 (Cua *et al.*, 2003) showed that the perceived central role for IL-12 in autoimmune inflammation, specifically in the brain, has been misinterpreted and that IL-23, and not IL-12, is the critical upstream factor regulating this response. Recent evidence suggests that IL-23, expressed in the early inflammatory phase of the disease, might also be relevant in amplifying the ongoing immune response in the inflamed PNS (Kieseier *et al.*, in preparation).

Effector mechanisms of myelin destruction: macrophage-mediated mechanisms, antimyelin antibodies, and complement

Despite the crucial role of T-cell infiltration in EAN, their mere presence is not sufficient to induce clinical disease. Recruitment of macrophages is a crucial secondary step. The essential pathogenic role of macrophages in EAN was highlighted by depletion experiments. Macrophage depletion by intraperitoneal injections of silica quartz (Hartung *et al.*, 1988*b*) or, more selectively, by dichlormethylene diphosphonate-containing liposomes (Jung *et al.*, 1993), prevented all clinical, electrophysiological, and histological signs of EAN. There are two ways in which macrophages can destroy nerve tissue: by diffuse release of toxic factors or, more specifically, by adhering to and attacking the myelin sheath.

The functional significance of toxic macrophage factors in disease progression has been elucidated by pharmacological blocking experiments. Arachidonic acid metabolites, possibly synergizing with activated complement, could function as chemoattractants and secretagogues for inflammatory cells or could enhance vascular permeability and breach the BNB (Hartung *et al.*, 1988*b*). Reactive oxygen species such as superoxide anion, hydrogen peroxide, and hydroxyl radicals could inflict peroxidation injury on myelin, but may also act by generating chemotactic signals and by exerting cytotoxic effects on endothelial cells (Konat and Wiggins, 1985). Macrophage-derived neutral proteases and phospholipases induce myelin damage *in vitro*. Accordingly, microinjection of a proteinase into rat sciatic nerve produced inflammatory demyelination and treatment of EAN rats with proteinase inhibitors delayed development of clinical disease (Schabet *et al.*, 1991).

The hallmark of actively induced EAN and of typical human GBS cases is segmental demyelination that cannot be explained by diffuse release of toxic mediators. As a basic morphological observation macrophages adhere to nerve fibers at an early stage of disease development and often normally appearing nerve fibers are attacked (Griffin *et al.*, 1990). In contrast, after axotomy or nerve crush macrophages selectively infiltrate nerve fibers undergoing Wallerian degeneration, but they spare intact fibers (Stoll *et al.*, 1989). In EAN, macrophages strip off myelin lamellae from the axons, resulting in demyelination. The mechanisms by which initial T-cell infiltration leads to macrophage adherence on the surface of individual myelin sheaths are largely unknown. Possibly inflammatory mediators such as chemokines are crucially involved.

Humoral autoantibodies to myelin components can play a role in the pathogenesis of EAN and human autoimmune neuropathies. These antibodies may block nerve excitation or neuromuscular transmission, may enhance T-cell-mediated demyelination by complement-mediated lysis and ADCC effector mechanisms, and may also augment local T-cell activation in analogy to findings in myasthenia gravis (Schalke *et al.*, 1985). Polyvalent antibodies to various components of the PNS have been detected in hyperimmune serum of rabbits and guinea pigs with EAN. However, demyelination can only be triggered by these autoantibodies with prior disruption of the BNB. For this purpose, the AT-EAN model can be used in co-transfer studies to examine the putative demyelinating activity of sera from patients with GBS or chronic inflammatory polyneuropathy (Harvey *et al.*, 1995; Hadden *et al.*, 2001). Following an intravenous injection of a subneuritogenic cell dose, breakdown of the BNB is observed (Hadden *et al.*, 2002). Subsequent intravenous injection of purified IgG fractions from GBS/EAN then allows for examination of demyelinating activity by electrophysiology and/or histology.

In EAN increased antibody titers against peripheral myelin components could be measured in the bloodstream (Zhu *et al.*, 1994; Koehler *et al.*, 1996). They can gain access to nerves by T-cell-mediated disruption of the BNB (Spies *et al.*, 1995). Accordingly, a rapid increase in the passage of immunoglobulin into spinal roots, together with endoneurial infiltration of T lymphocytes and polymorphonuclear leukocytes, was demonstrated in AT-EAN. Accumulation of immunoglobulin was maximal during the worsening of neurological deficit, and declined rapidly before the onset of neurological recovery (Hadden *et al.*, 2002). In support of a decisive role of complement in the pathogenesis, decomplementation of animals with cobra venom factor partly suppressed EAN (Vriesendorp *et al.*, 1995; Feasby *et al.*, 1987). Moreover, in myelin-induced EAN, macrophages were concentrated in areas of strong terminal complement complex (TCC) accumulation on myelin sheaths and Schwann cells (Stoll *et al.*, 1991).

Functionally, TCC deposition on the surface of myelin sheaths may promote an influx of calcium, which is considered an important initial step in myelin breakdown and cytotoxicity in general. Additionally, macrophages in culture respond to TCC by liberating chemotactically active and pro-inflammatory eisosanoids which have been found to contribute to the pathogenesis of EAN (Hartung *et al.*, 1988*a,b*). Alternatively, TCC formation in myelin membranes may cause activation of myelin-associated neutral proteinases with subsequent hydrolysis of myelin proteins. It is conceivable that TCC-targeted myelin is selectively attacked by macrophages. In support of this notion, Hafer-Macko *et al.* (1996) showed TCC deposits on the outer surface of myelin sheaths in nerve specimens from demyelinating GBS, while in axonal GBS TCC was deposited axonally at paranodes. In both settings, macrophages adhered to nerve fibers at the location of TCC deposits. Schwann cells appear to escape TCC attacks, as shown *in vitro* by induction of cell-cycle activation, proliferation, and rescue from apoptotic cell death (Hila *et al.*, 2001). It was concluded from these *in vitro* studies that sublytic C5b-9 detected on Schwann cells *in vivo* during inflammatory neuropathies may even facilitate survival of Schwann cells to ensure remyelination (see below).

Local immune activation—the role of Schwann cells in cellular and humoral autoimmunity

The contribution of Schwann cells (Fig. 8.5) to the initiation and termination of an immune response in the PNS is still a matter of debate. In principle it has been shown that they possess all immune molecules of the trimolecular complex as a basic prerequisite to interact with invading T cells. Schwann cells *in vitro* constitutively express MHC Class I molecules at low levels but no significant numbers of MHC Class II molecules. Upregulation of MHC Class I or expression of MHC Class II can be induced by stimulation with IFN-γ or upon co-culture with activated T cells (Armati *et al.*, 1990). Interestingly, TNF-α synergizes with IFN-γ and further increases MHC expression which also has functional importance (Gold *et al.*, 1995). Moreover adhesion molecules such as ICAM-1 (CD54), which are constitutively expressed on cultured Schwann cells are up-regulated by these cytokines and may exert co-stimulatory functions (Fig. 8.6).

Thus pre-treated, Schwann cells have been shown to process exogenous P2 protein or its neuritogenic peptide for antigen presentation (Gold *et al.*, 1995). Under certain conditions they can even present endogenous myelin proteins like myelin basic protein (MBP) to autoaggressive lymphocytes in a MHC Class II-restricted manner (Wekerle *et al.*, 1986*b*). Although the relevance of MHC Class II expression on Schwann cells has been questioned in EAN (Schmidt *et al.*, 1990) and CIDP (Kiefer *et al.*, 2000) (see below), there is evidence that Schwann cells are capable of this immune

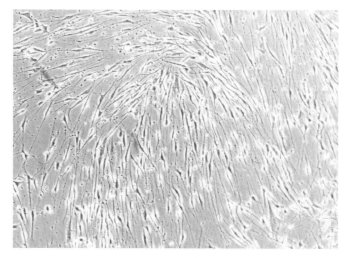

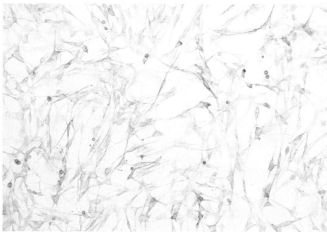

Fig. 8.5 Schwann cell culture. Neonatal rat Schwann cells after Thy 1.1-mediated immunopurification. They display a typical spindle shape and show cytoplasmic labelling with anti-S100 (below). High purity is mandatory to exclude experimental bias by contaminating fibroblasts.

function *in vivo* (Pollard *et al.*, 1987) and also express other co-stimulatory molecules in the inflamed nerve (Murata and Dalakas, 2000). A possible explanation for this discrepancy between the *in vitro* and *in vivo* situation

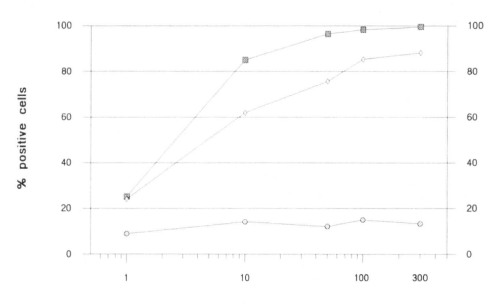

Fig. 8.6 Up-regulation of adhesion molecules (ICAMs) in Schwann cell cultures. Schwann cell cultures were treated with graded doses of TNF-α (circles), IFN-γ (diamonds), or both cytokines (squares) for 3 days. ICAM expression was monitored by fluorescence activated cell sorting (FACS) analysis.

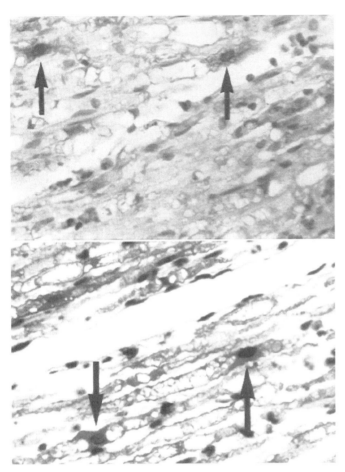

Fig. 8.7 Schwann cell apoptosis in experimental autoimmune neuritis. Schwann cells are detected by anti-S100 immunocytochemistry with morphological signs of apoptosis (arrows in upper figure). In double-labelling studies with the TUNEL technique apoptotic Schwann cells exhibit black nuclei (arrows in lower figure). (See also Plate 2 of the colour plate section.)

Schwann cells produce IL-1, a potent cytokine which promotes T-cell activation and proliferation (Skundric *et al.*, 2001), and also IL-6 which may bias the local cytokine milieu to a T helper 2 (Th2) type of reaction (Bolin *et al.*, 1995). Furthermore, Constable *et al.* (1994) reported that Schwann cells can be induced *in vitro* to secrete prostaglandin E_2 and thromboxane A_2. These immunomodulators may inhibit or stimulate T cells, depending on their level of production. Schwann cells are also endowed with a cytokine-inducible nitric oxide synthase (iNOS) which is rapidly up-regulated after simultaneous treatment with IFN-γ and TNF-α (Gold *et al.*, 1996). mRNA was detected within 12 h, and nitrite secretion as a measure of NO production was detectable after 24 h. Secretion of NO by Schwann cells exerts a strong suppressive effect on T-cell activation in a co-culture model (Gold *et al.*, 1996). Thus, Schwann cell-derived reactive oxygen intermediates have the potency to limit inflammatory demyelination, unless T cells are rescued by exogenous IL-2 (see below). Another mediator of steroid hormones, lipocortin-1 (annexin-1) may also contribute to the down-regulation of inflammatory reactions. Importantly, lipocortin-1 expression in sciatic nerve is also increased during recovery from EAN and may contribute to termination of the inflammatory reaction (Gold *et al.*, 1999).

Schwann cells are endowed on their membrane with a number of regulatory complement proteins such as CR1 (CD35), decay accelerating factor

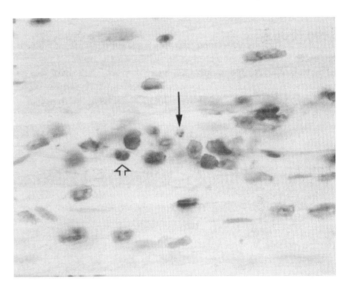

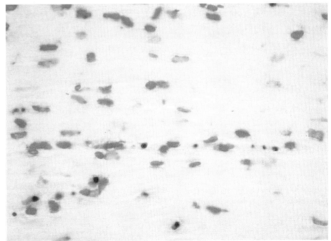

Fig. 8.8 T-cell apoptosis in experimental autoimmune neuritis. Top: T cells are detected by anti-T-cell immunocytochemistry with morphological apoptosis (open arrow) or apoptotic fragments (arrow). Bottom: double labelling for T cells and apoptotic nuclei by TUNEL stain.

may be provided by the findings of Tontsch and Rott (1993) and Neumann *et al.* (1995) who have demonstrated that viable, electrically active neurons indeed exert a regulatory function on glial cells.

It is of note that Schwann cells are also the source of a number of pro-inflammatory, co-stimulatory cytokines such as IL-1 and TNF-α (Skundric *et al.*, 2001). Given the autocrine and paracrine functions of these molecules, both feedback actions on Schwann cells and modulation of the pericellular immune circuitry are conceivable.

Schwann cells also express molecules that can terminate T-cell inflammation by induction of apoptosis (see below) and down-regulate immune functions. Fas and its ligand are central molecules of a family of death factors that regulate T-cell survival in the immune system. Recent findings from two groups show that Schwann cells do not express Fas (CD95) or Fas ligand (FasL) constitutively. However, pro-inflammatory T helper 1 (Th1) cytokines can up-regulate FasL or Fas on the surface of Schwann cells within 48 h (Wohlleben *et al.*, 2000; Bonetti *et al.*, 2003). Thus several potential scenarios are conceivable. First, cross-linking of Fas molecules on invading T cells by membrane-bound or secreted FasL could eliminate the autoaggressive immune effectors. This could explain T-cell apoptosis observed during the natural disease course of EAN (see below). Second, expression of Fas on Schwann cell membranes could render them susceptible to T-cell attack. Apoptotic elimination of Schwann cells is observed during EAN (Fig. 8.7) (Weishaupt *et al.*, 2001) and may further augment demyelination in the PNS. Local secretion of TNF-α is probably involved in regulation of apoptotic Schwann cell death.

CD55, membrane cofactor protein CD46, and CD59 (Koski *et al.*, 1996; Vedeler *et al.*, 1994). This ensemble of proteins serves to attenuate the pro-inflammatory and demyelinating properties of activated complement. On the other hand, while macrophages constitute the major source of complement at inflammatory foci, Schwann cells can also be induced, e.g. by IFN-α, TNF-α and IL-1β to generate the central complement component C3 (Dashiell *et al.*, 1997).

T-cell apoptosis in EAN—a physiological defense mechanism to terminate inflammation

The termination of ongoing PNS inflammation can be induced by continuous down-regulation of the vicious circle of the amplification–effector pathways. One such mode is silencing of macrophages, another is apoptosis of autoimmune T cells which occurs during the natural disease course of EAN (Fig. 8.8) (Zettl *et al.*, 1996). Although the rate of cellular apoptosis is much higher in EAE (Gold *et al.*, 1997), it is still a powerful mechanism for limiting damage in the inflamed nerve. The decisive natural mediator of T-cell apoptosis during neuritis has as yet not been identified. Possibly several of the above-mentioned effector pathway mechanisms such as secretion of NO, TNF-α < or lipocortins may act in concert to mediate T-cell death in the inflamed PNS.

Glucocorticosteroids are amongst the most efficient anti-inflammatory drugs which can eradicate infiltrating T cells through augmenting apoptosis. Based on the use of high-dose glucocorticosteroids in human disease, steroid 'pulse therapy' (10 mg/kg body weight) in rat EAN led to a four- to five-fold increase of T-cell apoptosis in the inflamed sciatic nerve (Zettl *et al.*, 1995). Antigen-specific therapy is of similar efficacy, but is as yet limited to experimental systems (Weishaupt *et al.*, 1997).

Summary and perspectives

In conclusion, great progress has been made in achieving a better understanding of the pathogenesis of inflammatory neuropathies. This is based on histological studies on human tissue and also on experimental models. As a result, newly developed drugs and compounds provided by the pharmaceutical industry have been successfully explored in experimental models, and will now enter the stage of controlled clinical trials. It is strongly hoped that in the future investigator-initiated trials will also receive governmental or international funding to test existing drugs, in particular in combination with already available effective treatments. In addition, more studies on neuritis models in genetically modified mice are needed.

References

Adelman, M. and Linington, C. (1992). Molecular mimicry and the autoimmune response to the peripheral nerve myelin PO glycoprotein. *Neurochem Res* 17: 887–891.

Archelos, J.J., Maurer, M., Jung, S., Toyka, K.V., and Hartung, H.P. (1993). Suppression of experimental allergic neuritis by an antibody to the intracellular adhesion molecule ICAM-1. *Brain* 116: 1043–1058.

Archelos, J.J., Maurer, M., Jung, S., *et al.* (1994). Inhibition of experimental autoimmune neuritis by an antibody to the lymphocyte function-associated antigen-1. *Lab Invest* 70: 667–675.

Archelos, J.J., Fortwängler, T., and Hartung, H.P. (1997). Attenuation of experimental autoimmune neuritis in the Lewis rat by treatment with an antibody to L-selectin. *Neurosc Lett* 235: 9–12.

Archelos, J.J., Previtali, S.C., and Hartung, H.P. (1999). The role of integrins in immune-mediated diseases of the nervous system. *Trends Neurosci* 22: 30–38.

Armati, P.J., Pollard, J.D., and Gatenby, P. (1990). Rat and human Schwann cells *in vitro* can synthesize and express MHC molecules. *Muscle Nerve* 13: 106–116.

Benoist, C. and Mathis, D. (1998). The pathogen connection. *Nature* 394: 227–228.

Bolin, L.M., Verity, N., Silver, J.E., Shooter, E.M., and Abrams, J.S. (1995). Interleukin-6 production by Schwann cells and induction in sciatic nerve injury. *J Neurochem* 64: 850–858.

Bonetti, B., Valdo, P., Ossi, G., *et al.* (2003). T-cell cytotoxicity of human Schwann cells: TNFalpha promotes fasL-mediated apoptosis and IFN gamma perforin-mediated lysis. *Glia* 43: 141–148.

Campbell, J.J., Hedrick, J., Zlotnik, A., Siani, M.A., Thompson, D.A., and Butcher, E.C. (1998). Chemokines and the arrest of lymphocytes rolling under flow conditions. *Science* 279: 381–384.

Constable, A.L., Armati, P.J., Toyka, K.V., and Hartung, H.P. (1994). Production of prostanoids by Lewis rat Schwann cells in vitro. *Brain Res* 635 : 75–80.

Cua, D.J., Sherlock, J., Chen, Y., *et al.* (2003). Interleukin-23 rather than interleukin-12 is the critical cytokine for autoimmune inflammation of the brain. *Nature* 421: 744–748.

Dashiell, S.M., Vanguri, P., and Koski, C. (1997). Inflammatory cytokines mediate dibutyryl cyclin AMP-induced C3 expression in glial cells. *Glia* 20: 308–321.

Enders, U., Lobb, R., Pepinsky, R.B., Hartung, H.-P., Toyka, K.V., and Gold, R. (1998). The role of the very late antigen-4 (VLA-4) and its counterligand vascular cell adhesion molecule-1 (VCAM-1) in the pathogenesis of experimental autoimmune neuritis (EAN) of the Lewis rat. *Brain* 121: 1257–1266.

Feasby, T.E., Gilbert, J.J., Hahn, A.F., and Neilson, M. (1987). Complement depletion suppresses Lewis rat experimental allergic neuritis. *Brain Res* 419: 97–103.

Gabriel, C.M., Hughes, R.A.C., Moore, S.E., Smith, K.J., and Walsh, F.S. (1998). Induction of experimental autoimmune neuritis with peripheral myelin protein-22. *Brain* 121: 1895–1902.

Gillen, C., Jander, S., and Stoll, G. (1998). Sequential expression of mRNA for proinflammatory cytokines and interleukin-10 in the rat peripheral nervous system: comparison between immune-mediated demyelination and Wallerian degeneration. *J Neurosci Res* 51: 489–496.

Gold, R., Toyka, K.V., and Hartung, H.P. (1995). Synergistic effect of IFN-gamma and TNF-alpha on expression of immune molecules and antigen presentation by Schwann cells. *Cell Immunol* 165: 65–70.

Gold, R., Zielasek, J., Kiefer, R., Toyka, K.V., and Hartung, H.P. (1996). Secretion of nitrite by Schwann cells and its effect on T-cell activation in vitro. *Cell Immunol* 168: 69–77.

Gold, R., Hartung, H.P., and Lassmann, H. (1997). T-cell apoptosis in autoimmune diseases: termination of inflammation in the nervous system and other sites with specialized immune-defense mechanisms. *Trends Neurosci* 20: 399–404.

Gold, R., Oehlschlaeger, M., Pepinsky, R.B., Sommer, C., Hartung, H.P., and Toyka, K.V. (1999). Increased lipocortin-1 expression in the sciatic nerve of Lewis rats with experimental autoimmune neuritis. *Acta Neuropathologica* 98: 583–589.

Griffin, J.W., Stoll, G., Li, C.Y., Tyor, W., and Cornblath, D.R. (1990). Macrophage responses in inflammatory demyelinating neuropathies. *Ann Neurol* 27(Suppl.): S64–S68.

Hadden, R.D.M., Gregson, N.A., Gold, R., Willison, H.J., and Hughes, R.A.C. (2001). Guillain-Barre syndrome serum and anti-Campylobacter antibody do not exacerbate experimental autoimmune neuritis. *J Neuroimmunol* 119: 306–316.

Hadden, R.D.M., Gregson, N.A., Gold, R., Smith, K.J., and Hughes, R.A.C. (2002). Accumulation of immunoglobulin across the 'blood-nerve barrier' in spinal roots in adoptive transfer experimental autoimmune neuritis. *Neuropathol Appl Neurobiol* 28: 489–497.

Hafer-Macko, C., Hsieh, S.T., Li, C.Y., *et al.* (1996). Acute motor axonal neuropathy: an antibody-mediated attack on axolemma. *Ann Neurol* 40: 635–644.

Hartung, H.P., Heininger, K., Schäfer, B., Fierz, W., and Toyka, K.V. (1988a). Immune mechanisms in inflammatory polyneuropathy. *Ann N Y Acad Sci* 540: 122–161.

Hartung, H.P., Schäfer, B., Heininger, K., Stoll, G., and Toyka, K.V. (1988b). The role of macrophages and eicosanoids in the pathogenesis of experimental allergic neuritis. Serial clinical, electrophysiological, biochemical and morphological observations. *Brain* 111: 1039–1059.

Hartung, H.P., Schäfer, B., Van der Meide, P.H., Fierz, W., Heininger, K., and Toyka, K.V. (1990). The role of interferon-gamma in the pathogenesis of experimental autoimmune disease of the peripheral nervous system. *Ann Neurol* 27: 247–257.

Hartung, H.-P., Toyka, K.V., and Griffin, J.W. (1998). Guillain–Barre syndrome and chronic inflammatory demyelinating polyneuropathy. In: *Clinical neuroimmunology* (ed. J. Antel, G. Birnbaum, and H.-P. Hartung), pp. 294–306. Blackwell Science, Oxford.

Harvey, G.K., Gold, R., Toyka, K.V., and Hartung, H.P. (1995). Nonneural-specific T lymphocytes can orchestrate inflammatory peripheral neuropathy. *Brain* 118: 1263–1272.

Hila, S., Soane, L., and Koski, C.L. (2001). Sublytic C5b-9-stimulated Schwann cell survival through PI 3-kinase-mediated phosphorylation of BAD. *Glia* 36: 58–67.

Jander, S. and Stoll, G. (2001). Interleukin-18 is induced in acute inflammatory demyelinating polyneuropathy. *J Neuroimmunol* 114: 253–258.

Jung, S., Huitinga, I., Schmidt, B., *et al.* (1993). Selective elimination of macrophages by dichlormethylene diphosphonate-containing liposomes suppresses experimental autoimmune neuritis. *J Neurol Sci* 119: 195–202.

Jung, S., Toyka, K., and Hartung, H.P. (1996). T cell directed immunotherapy of inflammatory demyelination in the peripheral nervous system—potent suppression of the effector phase of experimental autoimmune neuritis by anti-CD2 antibodies. *Brain* 119: 1079–1090.

Kadlubowski, M. and Hughes, R.A.C. (1979). Identification of the neuritogen for experimental allergic neuritis. *Nature* 277: 140–141.

Kiefer, R., Dangond, F., Mueller, M., Toyka, K.V., Hafler, D.A., and Hartung, H.P. (2000). Enhanced B7 costimulatory molecule expression in inflammatory human sural nerve biopsies. *J Neurol Neurosurg Psychiatryiat* 69: 362–368.

Kiefer, R., Kieseier, B.C., Stoll, G., and Hartung, H.P. (2001). The role of macrophages in immune-mediated damage to the peripheral nervous system. *Progr Neurobiol* 64: 109–127.

Kieseier, B.C., Seifert, T., Giovannoni, G., and Hartung, H.P. (1999). Matrix metalloproteinases in inflammatory demyelination—targets for treatment. *Neurology* 53: 20–25.

Kieseier, B.C., Krivacic, K., Jung, S., *et al.* (2000). Sequential expression of chemokines in experimental autoimmune neuritis. *J Neuroimmunol* 110: 121–129.

Kieseier, B.C., Tani, M., Mahad, D., *et al.* (2002). Chemokines and chemokine receptors in inflammatory demyelinating neuropathies: a central role for IP-10. *Brain* 125: 823–834.

Koehler, N.K., Martin, R., and Wietholter, H. (1996). The antibody repertoire in experimental allergic neuritis: evidence for PMP-22 as a novel neuritogen. *J Neuroimmunol* 71: 179–189.

Konat, G.W. and Wiggins, R.C. (1985). Effect of reactive oxygen species on myelin membrane proteins. *J Neurochem* 45: 1113–1118.

Koski, C.L., Estep, A.E., Sawant-Mane, S., Shin, M.L., Highbarger, L., and Hansch, G.M. (1996). Complement regulatory molecules on human myelin and glial cells: differential expression affects the deposition of activated complement proteins. *J Neurochem* 66: 303–12.

Lehmann, P.V., Forsthuber, T., Miller, A., and Sercarz, E.E. (1992). Spreading of T-cell autoimmunity to cryptic determinants of an autoantigen. *Nature* 358: 155–157.

Leppert, D., Hughes, P., Huber, S., *et al.* (1999). Matrix metalloproteinase up-regulation in chronic inflammatory demyelinating polyneuropathy and nonsystemic vasculitic neuropathy. *Neurology* 53: 62–70.

Leussink, V.I., Zettl, U.K., Jander, S., *et al.* (2002). Blockade of signaling via the very late antigen (VLA-4) and its counterligand vascular cell adhesion molecule-1 (VCAM-1) causes increased T cell apoptosis in experimental autoimmune neuritis. *Acta Neuropathol* 103: 131–136.

Linington, C., Izumo, S., Suzuki, M., Uyemura, K., Meyermann, R., and Wekerle, H. (1984). A permanent rat T cell line that mediates experimental allergic neuritis in the Lewis rat *in vivo*. *J Immunol* 133: 1946–1950.

Linington, C., Lassmann, H., Ozawa, K., Kosin, S., and Mongan, L. (1992). Cell adhesion molecules of the immunoglobulin supergene family as tissue-specific autoantigens: induction of experimental allergic neuritis (EAN) by P0 protein-specific T cell lines. *Eur J Immunol* 22: 1813–1817.

Maurer, M. and Gold, R. (2002). Animal models of immune-mediated neuropathies. *Curr Opin Neurol* 15: 617–622.

Moser, B. and Loetscher, P. (2001). Lymphocyte traffic control by chemokines. *Nat Immunol* 2: 123–128.

Murata, K. and Dalakas, M.C. (2000). Expression of the co-stimulatory molecule BB-1, the ligands CTLA-4 and CD28 and their mRNAs in chronic inflammatory demyelinating polyneuropathy. *Brain* 123: 1660–1666.

Neumann, H., Cavalie, A., Jenne, D.E., and Wekerle, H. (1995). Induction of MHC class I genes in neurons [see comments]. *Science* 269: 549–552.

Olee, T., Weise, M., Powers, J., and Brostoff, S. (1989). A T cell epitope for experimental allergic neuritis is an amphipathic alpha-helical structure. *J Neuroimmunol* 21: 235–240.

Pelidou, S.H., Deretzi, G., Zou, L.P., Quiding, C., and Zhu, J. (1999). Inflammation and severe demyelination in the peripheral nervous system induced by the intraneural injection of recombinant mouse interleukin-12. *Scand J Immunol* 50: 39–44.

Pollard, J.D., Baverstock, H., and McLeod, J.G. (1987). Class II antigen expression and inflammatory cells in the Guillain–Barre syndrome. *Ann Neurol* 21: 337–341.

Pollard, J.D., Westland, K.W., Harvey, G.K., *et al.* (1995). Activated T cells of non-neural specificity open the blood-nerve barrier to circulating antibody. *Ann Neurol* 37: 467–475.

Redford, E.J., Smith, K.J., Gregson, N.A., *et al.* (1997). A combined inhibitor of matrix metalloproteinase activity and tumour necrosis factor-α processing attenuates experimental autoimmune neuritis. *Brain* 120: 1895–1905.

Said, G. and Hontebeyrie Joskowicz, M. (1992). Nerve lesions induced by macrophage activation. *Res Immunol* 143: 589–599.

Saida, K., Saida, T., Brown, M.J., Silberberg, D.H., and Asbury, A.K. (1978). Antiserum-mediated demyelination *in vivo*: a sequential study using intraneural injection of experimental allergic neuritis serum. *Lab Invest* 39: 449–462.

Salomon, B., Rhee, L., Bour-Jordan, H., *et al.* (2001). Development of spontaneous autoimmune peripheral polyneuropathy in B7–2-deficient NOD mice. *J Exp Med* 194: 677–684.

Schabet, M., Whitaker, J.N., Schott, K., *et al.* (1991). The use of protease inhibitors in experimental allergic neuritis. *J Neuroimmunol* 31: 265–272.

Schalke, B.C., Klinkert, W.E., Wekerle, H., and Dwyer, D.S. (1985). Enhanced activation of a T cell line specific for acetylcholine receptor (AChR) by using anti-AChR monoclonal antibodies plus receptors. *J Immunol* 134: 3643–3648.

Schmidt, B., Stoll, G., Hartung, H.P., Heininger, K., Schäfer, B., Toyka, K.V. (1990). Macrophages but not Schwann cells express Ia antigen in experimental autoimmune neuritis. *Ann Neurol* 28: 70–77.

Schmidt, B., Stoll, G., van der Meide, P., Jung, S., and Hartung, H.P. (1992). Transient cellular expression of gamma-interferon in myelin- induced and T-cell line-mediated experimental autoimmune neuritis. *Brain* 115: 1633–1646.

Sharief, M.K., Ingram, D.A., and Swash, M. (1997). Circulating tumor necrosis factor-alpha correlates with electrodiagnostic abnormalities in Guillain–Barre syndrome. *Ann Neurol* 42: 68–73.

Skundric, D.S., Lisak, R.P., Rouhi, M., Kieseier, B.C., Jung, S., and Hartung, H.P. (2001). Schwann cell-specific regulation of IL-1 and IL-1Rα during EAN: possible relevance for immune regulation at paranodal regions. *J Neuroimmunol* 116: 74–82.

Spies, J.M., Pollard, J.D., Bonner, J.G., Westland, K.W., and McLeod, J.G. (1995). Synergy between antibody and P2-reactive T cells in experimental allergic neuritis. *J Neuroimmunol* 57: 77–84.

Stoll, G., Griffin, J.W., Li, C.Y., and Trapp, B.D. (1989). Wallerian degeneration in the peripheral nervous system: participation of both Schwann cells and macrophages in myelin degradation. *J Neurocytol* 18: 671–683.

Stoll, G., Schmidt, B., Jander, S., Toyka, K.V., and Hartung, H.P. (1991). Presence of the terminal complement complex (C5b-9) precedes myelin degradation in immune-mediated demyelination of the rat peripheral nervous system. *Ann Neurol* 30: 147–155.

Stoll, G., Jung, S., Jander, S., van der Meide, P., and Hartung, H.P. (1993). Tumor necrosis factor-alpha in immune-mediated demyelination and Wallerian degeneration of the rat peripheral nervous system. *J Neuroimmunol* **45**: 175–182.

Tontsch, U. and Rott, O. (1993). Cortical neurons selectively inhibit MHC class II induction in astrocytes but not in microglial cells. *Int Immunol* **5**: 249–254.

Trinchieri, G. (1995). Interleukin-12: a proinflammatory cytokine with immunoregulatory functions that bridge innate resistance and antigen-specific adaptive immunity. *Annu Rev Immunol* **13**: 251–276.

Uncini, A., Di Muzio, A., Di Guglielmo, G., *et al.* (1999). Effect of rhTNF-alpha injection into rat sciatic nerve. *J Neuroimmunol* **94**: 88–94.

Vedeler, C., Ulvestad, E., Bjorge, L., *et al.* (1994). The expression of CD59 in normal human nervous tissue. *Immunology* **82**: 542–547.

Visan, L., Visan, I.A., Weishaupt, A., *et al.* (2004). Tolerance induction by intrathymic expression of P0. *J Immunol* **172**: 1364–1370.

Vriesendorp, F.J., Flynn, R.E., Pappolla, M.A., and Koski, C.L. (1995). Complement depletion affects demyelination and inflammation in experimental allergic neuritis. *J Neuroimmunol* **58**: 157–165.

Weerth, S., Berger, T., Lassmann, H., and Linington, C. (1999). Encephalitogenic and neuritogenic T cell responses to the myelin- associated glycoprotein (MAG) in the Lewis rat. *J Neuroimmunol* **95**: 157–164.

Weishaupt, A., Giegerich, G., Jung, S., *et al.* (1995). T cell antigenic and neuritogenic activity of recombinant human peripheral myelin P2 protein. *J Neuroimmunol* **63**: 149–156.

Weishaupt, A., Gold, R., Gaupp, S., Giegerich, G., Hartung, H.P., and Toyka, K.V. (1997). Antigen therapy eliminates T cell inflammation by apoptosis: effective treatment of experimental autoimmune neuritis with recombinant myelin protein P2. *Proc Natl Acad Sci USA* **94**: 1338–1343.

Weishaupt, A., Gold, R., Hartung, T., *et al.* (2000). Role of TNF-α in high-dose antigen therapy in experimental autoimmune neuritis: inhibition of TNF-α by neutralizing antibodies reduces T-cell apoptosis and prevents liver necrosis. *J Neuropathol Exp Neurol* **59**: 368–376.

Weishaupt, A., Bruck, W., Hartung, T., Toyka, K.V., and Gold, R. (2001). Schwann cell apoptosis in experimental autoimmune neuritis of the Lewis rat and the functional role of tumor necrosis factor-alpha. *Neurosci Lett* **306**: 77–80.

Wekerle, H., Linington, C., Lassmann, H., and Meyermann, R. (1986*a*). Cellular immune reactivity within the CNS. *Trends Neurosci* **9**: 271–277.

Wekerle, H., Schwab, M., Linington, C., and Meyermann, R. (1986*b*). Antigen presentation in the peripheral nervous system: Schwann cells present endogenous myelin autoantigens to lymphocytes. *Eur J Immunol* **16**: 1551–1557.

Wohlleben, G., Ibrahim, S.M., Schmidt, J., Toyka, K.V., Hartung, H.P., and Gold, R. (2000). Regulation of Fas and FasL expression on rat Schwann cells. *Glia* **30**: 373–381.

Yuki, N. (1997). Molecular mimicry between gangliosides and lipopolysaccharides of *Campylobacter jejuni* isolated from patients with Guillain–Barre syndrome and Miller Fisher syndrome. *J Infect Dis* **176**: S150–S153.

Yuki, N., Ho, T.W., Tagawa, Y., *et al.* (1999). Autoantibodies to GM1b and GalNAc-GD1a: relationship to *Campylobacter jejuni* infection and acute motor axonal neuropathy in China. *J Neurol Sci* **164**: 134–138.

Yuki, N., Yamada, M., Koga, M., *et al.* (2001). Animal model of axonal Guillain–Barre syndrome induced by sensitization with GM1 ganglioside. *Ann Neurol* **49**: 712–720.

Zettl, U.K., Gold, R., Toyka, K.V., and Hartung, H.P. (1995). Intravenous glucocorticosteroid treatment augments apoptosis of inflammatory T cells in experimental autoimmune neuritis (EAN) of the Lewis rat. *J Neuropathol Exp Neurol* **54**: 540–547.

Zettl, U.K., Gold, R., Toyka, K.V., and Hartung, H.P. (1996). In situ demonstration of T cell activation and elimination in the peripheral nervous system during experimental autoimmune neuritis in the Lewis rat. *Acta Neuropathol* **91**: 360–367.

Zhu, J., Link, H., Weerth, S., Linington, C., Mix, E., and Qiao, J. (1994). The B cell repertoire in experimental allergic neuritis involves multiple myelin proteins and GM1. *J Neurol Sci* **125**: 132–137.

Zhu, J., Bai, X.F., Mix, E., and Link, H. (1997). Cytokine dichotomy in peripheral nervous system influences the outcome of experimental allergic neuritis: dynamics of mRNA expression for IL-1β, IL-6, IL-10, IL-12, TNF-α, TNF-β, and cytolysin. *Clin Immunol Immunopathol* **84**: 85–94.

9 Genetics of immune-mediated neurological diseases

David Brassat, Stephen L. Hauser, and Jorge R. Oksenberg

Introduction

Immune-mediated neurological impairment is a downstream outcome of a rather extensive and coordinated series of events that include peripheral lymphocyte activation, disruption of the blood–brain barrier, cellular infiltration into the brain parenchyma, local inflammation, and tissue injury. Cytokines, adhesion molecules, growth factors, antibodies, and other molecules (including free radicals, proteases, vasoactive amines, and excitatory neurotransmitters) induce and regulate numerous critical cell functions that perpetuate inflammation, leading to tissue injury, neurodegeneration, and neurological deficits (Diaz-Villoslada and Oksenberg, 1998). The nature and intensity of this response, as well as the physiological ability to restore homeostasis, are to a large extend conditioned by the unique amino acid sequences that define allelic variants on each of the participating molecules. Therefore, genes in their germline configuration play a primary role in determining who is at risk for developing such disorders, how the disease progresses, and how someone responds to therapy.

Narrowing the search and identifying candidate genes

Many clinical neuroinflammatory disorders are associated with an autoimmune reaction. There are approximately 30 autoimmune diseases, affecting 3–5% of the population. The central and peripheral nervous systems can be affected by either an organ-specific immunological reaction (multiple sclerosis, myasthenia gravis, idiopathic inflammatory myopathies, autoimmune peripheral neuropathies) or by a multisystem reaction such as in the systemic rheumatic diseases. The pathogenesis of autoimmune diseases is complex and multifactorial with a genetic component that is not strictly Mendelian and involves the interaction, either programmed or stochastic, of two or more genes, as well as a number of post-genomic DNA changes (see Box 9.1). These include genes that rearrange from their position in the germline to encode a vast variety of T-cell receptors and immunoglobulins, somatic mutations, post-transcriptional regulatory mechanisms, and incorporation of retroviral sequences. In addition, it is likely that interactions with infectious, nutritional, climatic, and/or other environmental influences affect genetic susceptibility considerably. This complex array of factors results in disregulation of the immune response, loss of self-tolerance, and the development of abnormal (i.e. autoimmune) inflammatory pathogenic responses against structural components of the peripheral (PNS) and/or central (CNS) nervous systems.

Although genetic elements in autoimmune/neuroinflammatory diseases are clearly present, the lack of an obvious and homogeneous mode of transmission has prevented the application of classical genetic epidemiological techniques for their identification and characterization. Statistical methods to identify *disease loci* have been available since the 1950s and have been applied successfully, for example, to discover the mutation in the M2 domain of the epsilon subunit of the acetylcholine receptor causing autosomal dominant congenital myasthenia gravis (Ohno *et al.*, 1995). How-

---

Box 9.1 Model of genetic contributions in immune-mediated neurologic diseases

- Multiple genes of moderate and cumulative effect dictate susceptibility and influence disease course.
- No major gene/locus with the exception of the *major histocompatibility complex*.
- Post-genomic (transcriptional) mechanisms.
- Unidentified non-heritable (environmental) factors.
- Unknown genetic parameters and mode of inheritance.
- Complex gene–gene and gene–environment interactions.
- Genetic heterogeneity may result in clinical isoforms.

Disease genes

- Genes with rare alleles but strong effects and penetrance (deletions, expansions, translocations, etc.).

Susceptibility genes

- Genes with common or rare alleles with weak but cumulative effects and penetrance (i.e. polymorphisms).

---

ever, only recently have newer techniques emerged for their application to the problem of detecting *susceptibility loci*. On 15 February 2001, the International Human Genome Sequencing Consortium and the private company Celera simultaneously reported the completion of the first draft of the human genome sequence with the declared goal of producing a finished sequence by early 2003. This historic scientific milestone provided a direct way to connect a chromosomal region with its DNA sequence and gene content, and dramatically changed our ability to examine genetic variation as it relates to human disease.

An early gain of the Human Genome Project was the development of detailed maps of highly polymorphic markers (i.e. microsatellites) for all chromosomes facilitating comprehensive (all-genome) screenings. Some authors proposed then that a reasonable approach for gene discovery in complex disorders involves first determining the chromosomal region of the genomic effect by linkage analysis. The establishment of genetic linkage requires the collection of family pedigrees with more than one affected member in order to track, with the help of the markers, the inheritance of discrete chromosomal segments that deviate from independent segregation and co-segregate with the disease (Fig. 9.1). The theoretical foundation and methodologies are currently available to examine this type of family data in a variety of ways based upon the structure of pedigrees in a given study (Haines and Pericak-Vance, 1998). For example, family collections may consist of extended multigenerational pedigrees with more than one affected individual or affected sib pairs, alone or with parents and other affected

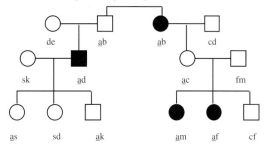

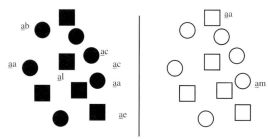

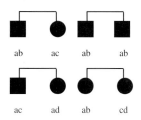

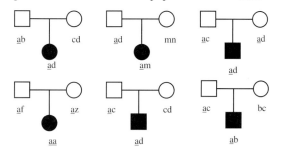

Fig. 9.1 Methods of genetic analysis.

sibs. The frequency and penetrance of the susceptibility allele may determine the optimal strategy for sample ascertainment. Once these regions in linkage with the trait have been identified and confirmed, a narrow and well-defined list of candidate genes can be compiled for analysis, even in the absence of a unifying model of pathogenesis. The potential of linkage mapping for gene identification in complex diseases was highlighted in a study of type 2 diabetes. The investigators followed original linkage data that implicated the distal long arm of chromosome 2 and identified a disease-associated intronic polymorphism in calpain-10, a ubiquitously expressed member of the calpain-like family of cysteine proteases (Horikawa *et al.*, 2000). The identification in 1996 of a locus linked to Crohn's disease on chromosome 16 resulted in the recent identification of a frameshift mutation in *NOD2*, a member of the Apaf-1/Ced-4 superfamily of apoptosis regulators, associated with disease susceptibility (Hugot *et al.*, 2001; Ogura *et al.*, 2001).

It has been argued, however, that because of the low relative risk conferred by any gene variant, incomplete penetrance, and the relative high frequency of the variant in the population at large, the linkage approach may require an unrealistically large number of samples for analysis in order to locate a (complex) disease gene (Risch, 2000). Alternatively, association studies of well-selected candidate genes may be more powerful for the detection of susceptibility alleles. Allelic association refers to a significantly increased or decreased frequency of a marker allele in individuals carrying a disease trait, and represents deviation from the random occurrence of the allele with respect to disease phenotype. Candidate genes are defined as

genes that are logical possibilities to play a role in a disease; for immune-mediated diseases, candidate genes might encode cytokines, immune receptors, and proteins involved in pathogen clearance. However, multiple polymorphisms within each candidate locus must be tested in adequately powered datasets to ensure that any true effect is identified. Recently, attention has focused on the goal to catalogue the entire DNA sequence variation in the human genome. Specifically, a genome-wide SNP (single nucleotide polymorphism) map has grown from an initial version with 4000 SNPs in 1998 (Wang *et al.*, 1998) to a map with more than 6 million SNPs by early 2004 (see www.ncbi.nlm.nih.gov/SNP/). SNPs (Fig. 9.2) are the most frequent form of genetic variation, comprising on average 1 per 1000 or 2000 bases with a total of over 10 million in the human genome. SNPs are thought to represent old and stable mutations, evenly distributed throughout the entire genome; such characteristics make them good markers for genetic studies, and their application does not require access to collections of multicase families. Although most SNPs are likely to be neutral with no phenotypic consequences, some may contribute to disease susceptibility and/or resistance, and may identify the 'causative' sequence difference. However, most genetic determinants of disease will not be included even in a sample of several hundred thousand SNPs, and, therefore, allelic associations with nearby SNPs are the key for gene identification through linkage disequilibrium (LD) mapping. LD refers to the presence of alleles at neighbouring loci segregating together more frequently than would be expected.

SNPs

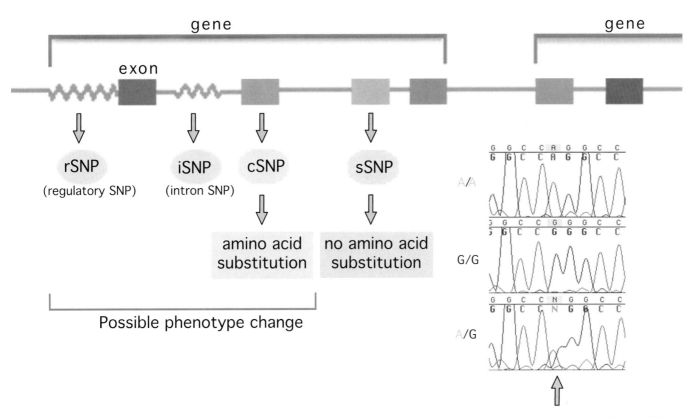

Fig. 9.2 Single-nucleotide polymorphisms (SNPs) associated with a phenotype can be used to pinpoint the responsible mutation. With an estimated 10 million SNPs in the human genome, genome-wide scans of all potential SNPs are impractical. It is possible, however, to group SNPs in co-inherited blocks, therefore reducing the number of SNPs required to map disease gene loci. Linkage disequilibrium (LD) mapping refers to the process of inferring the segregation of multiple SNPs covering discrete chromosomal segments by analysing a single SNP representative of the haplotype. It is of interest to note that LD patterns are not consistent across the genome or within specific regions across different populations.

Crude theoretical modelling of human population history suggested that variants which have a high population frequency are likely to be responsible for complex traits; the *common disease–common variant* hypothesis. Other observers argue that these common variants are too old to be responsible for complex diseases affecting non-African populations; the *common disease–rare variant* hypothesis. In either case, association studies using SNPs (frequent in the population or rare) may provide critical information for the final positional cloning of disease-associated genes. In all likelihood, the use of phenotypic (clinical and paraclinical), epidemiological, and demographic variables will assume increasing importance as stratifying elements, so that the question of genotype–phenotype correlation in neurological disease can be addressed.

Although numerous methods have been described that can increase genotyping throughput from hundreds of genotypes per day to thousands or even millions, it is a daunting task indeed to examine the whole genome, or even large chromosomal segments, in sufficient detail to ensure that no potentially relevant genetic variant is missed. For a direct genome screen, testing more than a million functionally relevant polymorphisms in exons and regulatory region in thousands of individuals might have to be undertaken. A powerful recent discovery is the finding that long-range disequilibrium exists in the human genome. The maintenance of these LD blocks with their limited number of haplotypes is most likely due to the non-uniform distribution of recombination, which tends to occur at 'hot spots' demarcating one block from the next. In simple terms, these blocks

can be considered the basic unit of inheritance. Therefore, rather than considering each individual chromosome as carrying a unique combination of SNPs, human chromosomes may be viewed as mosaics comprising blocks of SNP alleles with common patterns. Recent studies defined the long-range extent of correlations among SNPs and identified the existence of 'haplotype blocks' as a general feature of the genomic landscape (Martin *et al.*, 2000; Daly *et al.*, 2001; Jeffreys *et al.*, 2001; Gabriel *et al.*, 2002). On average, significant SNPs associations are seen at distances in the range of 60–100, with only two to four common patterns of variation (i.e. haplotypes) (Daly *et al.*, 2001; Reich *et al.*, 2001; Rioux *et al.*, 2001). Furthermore, between the genomic blocks there are short intervals where recombination is apparently most active in creating assortments of these patterns. Therefore, rather than each individual chromosome carrying a unique combination of SNP alleles, each chromosome is a simple mosaic of long common patterns of SNP alleles. The immediate implication of these observations is that it may be possible to use only a small fraction of the total genetic variation to serve as an adequate test for the remainder (Fig. 9.3). It is expected that there will be approximately 100 000 disequilibrium blocks. Assuming that three SNPs are required to interrogate fully the diversity associated with each haplotype, the whole genome could be screened using just 300 000 SNPs (~3% of all SNPs). Interestingly, at short distances African- and European-derived populations may show the same allelic combinations, at least for some chromosomal segments, but the extend of LD is markedly shorter in African chromosomes (less than 5 kilobases (kb)

SNPs

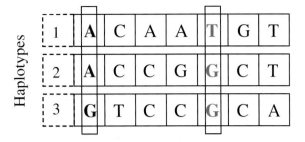

Fig. 9.3 About 10 million SNPs exist in human populations where the rarer SNP allele has a frequency of at least 1%. Alleles of SNPs that are close together tend to be inherited together. A set of associated SNP alleles in a region of a chromosome is called a 'haplotype'. Most chromosome regions have only a few common haplotypes (each with a frequency of at least 5%), which account for most of the variation from person to person in a population. A chromosome region may contain many SNPs, but only a few 'tag' SNPs can provide most of the information on the pattern of genetic variation in the region. In the figure, three haplotypes are shown. The two bold SNPs are sufficient to identify (tag) each of the three haplotyes. For example, if a chromosome has alleles A and T at these two tag SNPs, then it has the first haplotype. The HapMap Project (http://www.hapmap.org/) will identify 200 000 to 1 million tag SNPs, which describe the common patterns of genetic variation in humans. It will include the chromosome regions with sets of strongly associated SNPs, the haplotypes in those regions, and the SNPs that tag them. It will also note the chromosome regions where associations among SNPs are weak.

for some blocks in Yorubans for example) than in Caucasians or Asians (Reich *et al.*, 2001). Hence, although northern European chromosomes can be useful for mapping traits, this approach clearly provides diminishing returns for fine mapping studies, as the resolution and amount of new information will be limited. Populations with smaller LD blocks may allow fine mapping and the identification of the specific nucleotide substitutions associated with the phenotypic trait (Rioux *et al.*, 2001; Oksenberg *et al.*, 2004).

Genomics in immune-mediated neurological diseases

Diseases of the CNS with or without PNS involvement

Multiple sclerosis

Evidence of disease risk heritability in multiple sclerosis (MS) in the form of familial recurrence has long been known (Sadovnick *et al.*, 1996, 2000; Robertson *et al.*, 1996). The degree of familial aggregation can be determined by estimating the ratio of the prevalence in siblings versus the population prevalence of the disease (λs). For MS, λs is between 20 (0.02/0.001) and 40 (0.04/0.001) (Risch, 1992). Half-siblings (Sadovnick *et al.*, 1996) and adoption (Ebers *et al.*, 1995) studies confirm that genetic, and not environmental, factors are responsible for the familial clustering of cases. Concordant sibs tend to share age of symptom onset rather than year of

onset, and second- and third-degree relatives of MS patients are also at an increased risk. Concordance for early and late clinical features has been observed as well, suggesting that in addition to susceptibility, genes influence disease severity or other aspects of the clinical phenotype (Brassat *et al.*, 1999; Barcellos *et al.*, 2002; Kantarci *et al.*, 2002). In addition, twin studies from different populations consistently indicate pairwise concordance (20–40% in identical twin pairs compared with 2–5% in like-sex fraternal twin pairs) providing additional evidence for a genetic aetiology to MS (Sadovnick *et al.*, 1993; Mumford *et al.*, 1994). However, neither the recurrence rate nor the twin concordance supports the presence of a Mendelian trait. A simple model of inheritance for all MS is indeed unlikely and cannot account for the non-linear decrease in disease risk in families with increasing genetic distance from the proband. Modelling of the available data predicts that the MS-prone genotype results from multiple independent or interacting polymorphic genes, each exerting a small or at most a moderate effect to the overall risk.

High incidence rates are found in Scandinavia, Iceland, and the British Isles (about 1 in 1000) and the countries inhabited by their descendants. Relatively high incidence is also found among Sardinians, Parsis, and Palestinians (Rosati, 2001). MS is uncommon in Japan (2 per 100 000) and other Asian nations, in sub-Saharan Africa, the Indian subcontinent, and in the native populations of Oceania and the Americas. According to some observers, this characteristic geographical distribution implicates in the aetiology of MS a pathogen that is not ubiquitously distributed. However, this prevalence pattern can also be explained, at least in part, by the geographical clustering of northern Europeans and their descendants with susceptible genetic profiles. The high occurrence of MS in populations of northern European origin irrespective of geographical location and the observation of resistant ethnic groups residing in high-risk regions, as for example Gypsies in Bulgaria or Japanese in the United States, suggest that the differential risk observed in different population groups results primarily from genetic susceptibility or resistance (Rosati, 2001).

An important conceptual development in the understanding of MS genetics has been the recognition of locus heterogeneity, meaning that different genes can cause identical or similar forms of the disease. In a recent analysis of 184 multicase MS families, linkage and association to the HLA-DR locus, and a strong association with the specific DR2 haplotype (DRB1*1501, DQB1*0602) was confirmed (Barcellos *et al.*, 2002). Remarkably, all the linkage information and evidence for association derived from the families in which DR2 was present in at least one nuclear member (Table 9.1). No genetic effect of the HLA locus could be discerned in the DR2-negative family set. In fact, the results excluded linkage for at least 20 cM around HLA-DRB1 in the DR2-negative families. In addition, no evidence of association or excess transmission of other DRB1 or DQB1 alleles was detected. These data provide strong evidence that heterogeneity at the HLA locus exists in MS.

Another example of HLA locus heterogeneity in MS is provided by studies in Japanese patients. In this group, one form of MS is apparently characterized by disseminated CNS involvement and is associated with the HLA-DR2 haplotype whereas more restricted forms of disease in which optic nerve and or spinal cord involvement predominate and lesions are more severe and necrotizing, are not associated with HLA-DR2 (Kira *et al.*, 1996). Locus heterogeneity may not be present in all populations, however, underscoring the complex genetic nature of this disease (Ligers *et al.*, 2001). The strength of the association between primary progressive MS (PPMS) and HLA-DR2 is also uncertain. A number of small studies failed to show

Table 9.1 Locus heterogeneity in multiple sclerosis

| | Max LOD score (linkage) | | PDT (association) |
	Autosomal dominant	Autosomal recessive	P value
All families	3.80	2.91	0.0002
DR2-positive families	4.62	3.95	0.0002
DR2-negative families	−0.03	−0.04	0.87

PDT: pedigree disequilibrium test

any association between PPMS and DR2, although a larger study from Northern Ireland appeared to show the association (McDonnell and Hawkins, 1998). The implications of heterogeneity are considerable because they may reflect fundamentally distinct immunopathogenic mechanisms in different affected individuals. The pharmacogenomic consequences of HLA locus heterogeneity in MS are also important and could potentially explain individual differences in treatment response to glatiramer acetate, a molecular mimic of a region of myelin basic protein that is immunodominant in HLA-DR2-positive individuals (Fusco et al., 2001).

Genetic studies in MS in the previous decade were influenced by three large multistage whole-genome screens performed in multiple-affected families ascertained in the USA, UK, and Canada (Ebers et al., 1996; Multiple Sclerosis Genetics Group, 1996; Sawcer et al., 1996). A fourth study concentrated on a genetically isolated region of Finland but was based on a small number of families (Kuokkanen et al., 1997). Follow-up screenings in confirmatory and additional datasets have been completed as well. The studies all together identified about 60 genomic regions with a potential involvement in disease susceptibility, consistent with the long-held view that MS is a polygenic disorder. However, total or even predominant replication between the different screens was not present. This is in part due to the strategy of reporting all 'hits' suggestive of linkage, recognizing that false positives will be generated along with the true positives. It is also possible that the study design in each case underestimated the confounding influence of disease heterogeneity and the limitations of parametric methods of statistical analysis. It should be noted, however, that because each study used a somewhat overlapping but different set of genetic markers and different clinical inclusion criteria, the direct comparison of results is not straightforward. Nevertheless, a detailed analysis of the composite published data identified overlapping regions of interest, including 1p36–p33, 2p23–p21, 3p14–p13, 3q22–q24, 4q31–qter, 5p14–p12, 5q12–q13, 6p21–22, 6q22–27, 6q22–27, 7q21–q22, 17q22, 18p11, 19q12–13 (Oksenberg et al., 2001). In addition, meta-analysis of the raw and published data from the four original genomic scans singled out discrete overlapping MS susceptibility regions at chromosomes 5, 6, 16, 17, 19, and 22 (Wise et al., 1999; GAMES and the Transatlantic Multiple Sclerosis Genetics Cooperative, 2001; Games, 2003). In summary, evidence for linkage exceeding the threshold for genome-wide statistical significance is seen in the MHC region on chromosome 6p21. Additional regions were identified, but the overall data provide support primarily for chromosomes 19q13 and 17q21, making these the best-supported non-MHC regions of linkage. Consensus is emerging to consider them bonafide MS loci and designate the HLA region at 6p21.3, 19q13, and 17q21 as MS loci 1, 2, and 3 respectively. Although further work is necessary to better define the complete roster of MS loci, these studies represent real progress in mapping the full set of MS-associated genes.

MS1, chromosome 6p21.3, the major histocompatibility complex (MHC)

The HLA-DR2 haplotype (DRB1*1501, DQB1*0602) within the MHC is the strongest genetic effect identified in MS, and has consistently demonstrated both linkage and association in family and case–control studies. Using family data, the proportion of the total λ_s explained by the HLA-DR locus can be estimated (Multiple Sclerosis Genetics Group, 1998). At the upper end, under a multiplicative genetic model and assuming a λ_s of 15, the HLA-DR association can explain as much as 60% of the genetic aetiology of MS. At the lower end, under an additive model and assuming a λ_s of 40, it could explain as little as 17%. However, fine mapping studies have not settled whether the effect is explained by the *HLA-DRB1* gene itself, by another closely spaced gene within the Class II HLA region such as *HLA-DQB1*, or by some other nearby gene in close disequilibrium. Analysis has been made more complex by extensive LD across the 6p21 region and by the presence of more than 240 genes within this superlocus, many of which have roles in immune function and are thus plausible MS candidates. Results suggesting that loci of interest exist within the Class III (de Jong et al., 2002; Palacio et al., 2002) and/or telomeric to the Class I region (Shinar et al., 1998; Fogdell-Hahn et al., 2000; Marrosu et al., 2001; Rubio et al., 2002) have been reported as well. A dose effect of HLA-DR2 haplotypes on MS susceptibility has also been demonstrated; two copies of the

susceptibility haplotype increases disease risk (Barcellos et al., 2003). Furthermore this genotype modifies disease expression, as there was a paucity of benign MS and an increase of severe MS in individuals homozygous for DR2. These effects were unexpected because if the HLA-DRβ molecules confer susceptibility by presenting an encephalitogenic peptide, then a dominant effect would be expected. For example, in experimental allergic encephalomyelitis a single copy of a disease-associated MHC haplotype, when present in the context of an appropriate genetic background, is generally sufficient for the induction of susceptibility. One model to explain the dose effect of MHC genes on MS susceptibility and progression predicts that more than one gene within the HLA Class II region contributes to disease susceptibility; this might involve a dominantly acting susceptibility gene present on DR2 haplotypes plus the absence of a protective gene required for the maintenance of peripheral tolerance present on non-DR2 haplotypes.

MS2, chromosome 19q13

Genomic screens have shown support for linkage to this region and a meta-analysis (Wise et al., 1999) of all four pivotal genomic screens published results confimed 19q13 as a significant disease locus. Additional evidence for this region came from allelic association and from follow-up studies (Barcellos et al., 1997; Pericak-Vance et al., 2001; Haines et al., 2002; Schmidt et al., 2002). Overall, the effect of the 19q13 locus is likely to be moderate, with an estimated locus-specific $\lambda_s = 1.5$, thus accounting for 4–6% of the overall genetic component in MS. On chromosome 19q13 the minimal critical region spans about 70–80 cM. This region contains 380 genes including many attractive disease candidates. The well-documented involvement of apolipoprotein E (apoE) in neurological disease, for example, makes this gene an interesting candidate for MS studies. The apoE protein has long been associated with regeneration of axons and myelin after lesions of central and peripheral nervous tissue, and its isoforms have been shown to have differential effects on neuronal growth. Several studies excluded APOE as a susceptibility factor in MS, but have reported an association between the APOE-4 allele and more severe disease (Evangelou et al., 1999; Oliveri et al., 1999; Chapman et al., 2001; Fazekas et al., 2001). Another study reported some evidence for a protective effect of the APOE-2 allele, observing that the time to reach secondary progression for patients whose initial disease type was relapsing-remitting was significantly longer for APOE-2/3 genotypes compared with APOE-3/3 and -3/4 genotypes (Ballerini et al., 2000). In a multicase US familial dataset, the proportion of APOE-4 carriers was significantly higher in the severe disease group than the non-severe group (Schmidt et al., 2002). On the other hand, the proportion of APOE-2 carriers was significantly higher in the mild disease group than the non-mild group. Some biological support for the APOE-4 association with disease progression was suggested by an MRI investigation, which revealed more extensive tissue destruction or less efficient repair in MS APOE-4 carriers (Fazekas et al., 2000). Additional suggestive candidate genes in the 19q13 extended region include *TGFB1*, immunoglobulin-like transcripts (ILT genes), killer cell inhibitory receptors (KIR genes), the leukocyte-associated inhibitory receptors (*LAIR1* and *-2*), the Fc receptor, IL-11, the heavy chain of the MHC class I-like Fc receptor, and *APOC4*.

MS3, chromosome 17q21–23

The chromosomal segment 17q21 was highlighted first in the genome scan performed in MS pedigrees collected in the UK (Sawcer et al., 1996), and confirmed in Finnish families (Kuokkanen et al., 1997). On chromosome 17q21 the minimal critical region spans between 36 and 46 cM, and includes 331 genes. Further support for chromosome 17q21 was detected in follow-up studies of both populations (Chataway et al., 1998; Saarela et al., 2002; Sawcer et al., 2002), association screening in several European and migrant European populations (http://www.gene.cimr.cam.ac.uk/Msgenetics/GAMES), and as yet unpublished data in Canadian sib pairs. In a recently published analysis of 22 multicase Finnish families, the putative MS locus in chromosme 17q was mapped to a region of less than 4cM covering ~2.5 Mb at 17q22–23 (Saarela et al., 2002). Biologically relevant genes such as *MPO*, *ICAM2*, and *PECAM1* map in the immedaite vicinity. No evidence of linkage to this region was detected in French or American MS families (Fontaine *et al.*, 1999; Haines *et al.*, 2002).

Susceptibility genes versus modifiers

Clinical symptoms in MS are extremely variable. The course may be relapsing–remitting or progressive, severe or mild, and involve the neuraxis in a widespread fashion or predominantly affect spinal cord and optic nerve. Very little is known about the underlying cause of disease variability in MS. Earlier studies have reported intrafamilial concordance for disease course, disease severity, and age of onset (Barcellos *et al.*, 2002, 2003; Brassat *et al.*, 1999; Kantarci *et al.*, 2002). The clinical course and severity of MS may also differ between ethnic groups. Conceivably, this phenotypic aggregation is due to genetic sharing. In the MS disease model experimental allergic (or autoimmune) encephalomyelitis (EAE), it appears that MHC genes primarily influence penetrance, whereas other loci modulate specific

phenotypes such as topographic location of lesions in brain or spinal cord, demyelination, and severity of inflammation (Butterfield *et al.*, 2000). It is likely that a similar interplay of genetic factors operates in human disease. To assess the state of genotype–phenotype research in MS we have identified from the literature a set of gene polymorphisms that have been significantly associated with phenotypic endpoints (Table 9.2). The list omits many reports and probably include a few type 1 errors due to small sample sizes. In addition, series are retrospective, some phenotypic endpoints are questionable or not validated, and the confounding effects of drug treatment and/or stratification have not been generally considered. Finally, the assessment of modifier effects has often been piggybacked upon candidate gene susceptibility studies, further limiting their informativeness. Parenthetically, it may also be difficult to discriminate whether phenotypic diversity reflects aetiological heterogeneity, a modifying role of a specific gene, or some combination of the two.

Table 9.2 Examples of gene variants that have been associated with the multiple sclerosis phenotype

Gene/locus	Chromosomal location	Associated phenotype
GSTM1	1p13.3	Severe disability
IL1RA/IL1B	2q14.2	High protein expression and favourable prognosis
CCR5	3p21–24	Age of onset was approximately 3 years later in patients carrying the deletion
		Progression to disability was delayed in homozygotes and heterozygotes for the deletion
		Lower risk of recurrent disease activity
		Trend to reduced frequency in primary progressive MS (PPMS)
		Trend to smaller lesion burden
SPP1 (OPN)	4q21-q25	Patients with the wild-type 1284A genotype are less likely to have mild disease course and were at increased risk for a secondary-progressive clinical type
		Patients with the 9583 G/G genotype showed later disease onset
		No association with disease severity
IL4	5q31.1	Late onset. Late onset in homozygotes
HLA	6p21.3	HLA haplotypes have been reported to be associated with an earlier age of disease onset, gender dimorphism, severe, relapsing–remitting, and mild MS courses
		HLA haplotypes have been reported to have no influence on disease course
		No DRB1 association in some Asian populations who have a restricted disease, termed neuromyelitis optica, in which optic nerve and/or spinal cord involvement predominates
		A high prevalence of DR2 was observed in patients with acute unilateral optic neuritis. Its presence was associated with increased odds for developing definite MS. The association was most apparent among patients with signal abnormalities on the baseline brain MRI
		A number of small studies failed to show any association between PPMS and DR2, although a larger study from Northern Ireland appeared to show the association. Others suggested an association between PPMS and the HLA-DR4 haplotype although a *post hoc* analysis is consistent with an effect decreasing the risk for RRMS in HLA-DR4+ individuals, rather than increasing the risk for PPMS
CD24	6q21	50% of CD24 V/V patients with expanded disability status scale 6.0 reached the milestone in 5 years, whereas the CD24 A/V whereas the CD24 A/V and CD24 A/A patients did so in 16 and 13 years, respectively
ESR1	6q21.5	The P allele-positive patients had a significantly higher progression of disability and a worse ranked MS severity score. The study also suggests an interaction between the ESR1 genotype and DR2 in women with MS
		The study suggests an interaction between the ESR1 genotype and DR2 in women with MS
CD59	10q24.1	Gender dimorphism
CNTF	11q12	Patients with the CNTF –/– genotype had significantly earlier onset (17 versus 27 years) with predominant motor symptoms
		No correlation with age of onset, course, or severity
CRYAB	11q22.3–23.1	Non-inflammatory, neurodegenerative phenotype characterized by rapid PPMS course
MEFV	16p13.3	Rapid progression to disability in non-Ashkenazi Jewish patients
APOE	19q13.2	Increased severity, rate of progression, or disease brain activity
		No effect
		Decreased severity and progression to chronic progressive disease
TGFB1	19q13	Decreased severity defined as an Expanded Disability Status Scale (EDSS) score of <3 after 10 years of symptoms

Animal models

EAE can be induced in a variety of animal species, including non-human primates, by immunization with myelin proteins or their peptide derivatives, as well as by adoptive transfer of CD4+ activated cells specific for myelin components. A second, virally induced, animal model for MS uses the Theiler's murine virus from the picorna family to induce brain inflammation and injury of the myelin sheath. When studied in genetically susceptible animals, immunization induces brain inflammation accompanied by varied signs of neurological disease, ataxia, and paralysis, first in the tail and hindlimbs, then progressing to forelimb paralysis and eventual death. EAE and MS share common clinical, histological, immunological, and genetic features; hence EAE is widely considered to be a relevant model for the human disease. Genetic studies in EAE have been very informative in defining the complex interplay of multiple genes that can result in brain inflammation and demyelination. These studies have also been useful in validating EAE as an MS disease model. The best characterized EAE susceptibility gene resides within the MHC on murine chromosome 17 (Encinas et al., 1996). Induction and full clinical manifestations of EAE are strongly influenced by inherited polymorphisms of MHC Class II region genes; certain MHC haplotypes are more permissive for EAE whereas others are more resistant. The concept of susceptibility versus resistance in EAE is relative rather than absolute, as evidence demonstrates that modifications of the experimental protocol will induce detectable disease in strains previously considered resistant.

The use of classic genetics and whole-genome screening has identified several additional genetic regions that participate in conferring EAE susceptibility, including loci on chromosomes 3, 6, 7, 15, 17 (MHC in the mouse), 17 (distal to MHC) and X. Other regions, including segments on chromosomes 1 to 5, 7 to 12, and 14 to 18, have been implicated as containing disease-modifying genes. These studies provide compelling evidence for the hypothesis that susceptibility to autoimmune demyelination is in part genetically determined. A multiple-locus model is applicable; each locus may contribute to a specific stage of EAE pathology, although some loci are probably involved in several steps of the autoimmune process (Butterfield et al., 2000). However, no locus seems to be an absolute requirement for the susceptible phenotype; i.e. a susceptible EAE phenotype can be achieved in different crosses by different combinations of genotypes. As the actual roster of genes that contribute to EAE are identified, such genes will represent strong 'candidates' for testing in human disease.

Systemic lupus erythematosus (SLE)

SLE is a chronic multisystem autoimmune disease that affects primarily women of childbearing age (F:M ratio 9:1) and has a prevalence rate of 1 in 2500. Neuropsychiatric involvement (NP-SLE) is frequent. In some studies NP symptoms occur in about 50% of patients and carry a poor prognosis (Ainiala et al. 2001). The SLE λs is estimated to be over 20, indicating a strong genetic component. Concordance in identical twins is about 24%, compared with 2% in dizygotic twins (Deapen et al., 1992). SLE is more prevalent (3:1), more severe, and manifests at younger age in African-Americans than in European-Americans. Most people with homozygous deficiencies of early complement components (C1q, C2, C4) have SLE or a similar disease, suggesting that these genes are predisposing factors. A defective or deleted C4AQO allele is a common genetic marker associated with SLE in many ethnic groups (40–50% in patients compared with 15% in healthy controls).

Seven genome screens have been performed on various collections of multicase SLE pedigrees. Over 60 regions of interest were reported; seven of these meet or exceed the established threshold for significant linkage (LOD > 3.3 or P < 0.00005) (Table 9.3) (Kelly et al., 2002). Although the MHC locus at 6p21 has been consistently linked to SLE, it is noteworthy that the association appears to be weaker than in other autoimmune disorders. A modest association was found with HLA-DRB1*1501 and DRB1*0301 in Caucasians. Despite positive linkage, association results in other racial groups are conflicting. Dense microsatellite mapping in the HLA region in a collection of 334 families confirmed the role of HLA Class II DR2, DR3,

Table 9.3 Chromosomal segments linked to susceptibility to systemic lupus erythematosus

Locus	Max. LOD	Ethnicity
1q22–23	4.03	All
1q41–42	3.30	All
2q37	4.24	Icelandic/Swedish
4p16	3.62	European-American
6p21–p11	4.19	All
16q13	3.85	All
17p13	3.64	European-American

and DR8 haplotypes in conferring susceptibility, but only in Caucasian patients (Graham et al., 2002). Another region of interest discovered through linkage analysis is 1q22–23, harbouring the gene coding for the Fcγ receptor (Moser et al., 1998). This receptor is expressed on mononuclear phagocytic cells and is responsible for binding the Fc portion of the immune complex containing IgG. This gene was implicated in both association and linkage studies, particularly in African-American patients. Nath and colleagues reported significant linkage to chromosome 4p16 in a subset of Caucasian families with at least one patient showing either neurological or psychiatric symptoms (Nath et al., 2002). Rood and colleagues observed an association between IL-10 promoter polymorphisms and neuropsychiatric manifestations of SLE (Rood et al., 1999).

Sjögren's syndrome

Sjögren's syndrome (SS), or exocrinopathy, is a chronic, slowing progressive disease, characterized by exocrine gland dysfunction resulting from an immunological attack against the salivary and lacrimal glands. Primary SS defines an autoimmune component restricted to the exocrine glands, while secondary SS is accompanied by other autoimmune disorders, often involving connective tissues. The prevalence of primary SS is approximately 0.5 to 1%, with a 9:1 F:M ratio. Central nervous system involvement occurs in approximately 20% of patients with SS. The clinical presentation can mimic primary progressive MS (de Seze et al., 2001), although occurrence of SS in definite cases of primary progressive MS (PPMS) has been reported. The peripheral nervous system is involved in as many as 25% of cases. Results from association studies done in different ethnic backgrounds have shown a consistent effect of HLA Class II genes on SS susceptibility. For example, the frequency of HLA-DR3 was found significantly elevated in a primary SS British cohort (Foster et al., 1993). In a study of 45 French patients with primary SS, the highest relative risk was associated with the DRB1*15–DRB1*0301 heterozygous genotype, suggesting complex interactions between cis and trans genetic elements in the MHC (Jean et al., 1998). Other studies implicate the HLA-DQA1*0501 allele, regardless of the ethnic origin of the patient.

Non-obese diabetic (NOD) mice exhibit overlapping autoimmune endocrinopathy and exocrinopathy. More than 19 chromosomal intervals (Idd regions) have been identified as contributors to the diabetogenic phenotype. Using congenic crossing to non-susceptible C57BL/6 mice, Brayer and colleagues identified regions in chromosomes 1 (Idd5) and 3 (Idd3) that interact to influence susceptibility and resistance to the development of autoimmune exocrinopathy (Brayer et al., 2000). The mapping of (Idd5) and (Idd3) was recently confirmed by 2 independent groups (Cha et al., 2002; Boulard et al., 2002).

Sarcoidosis

Sarcoidosis is a chronic multisystem granulomatous disorder characterized by the accumulation of T helper 1 (Th1) type CD4+ T lymphocytes and mononuclear phagocytes in the affected organ. Sarcoidosis is a relatively common disease with a prevalence range of 1–60 per 100 000. In an unrestricted post-mortem Swedish study, the prevalence of sarcoidosis lesions was found to be over 640 per 100 000. The clinical expression in sarcoidosis is highly heterogeneous. Neurological clinical symptoms occur in approximately 5% of the patients, but reach as high as 25% in autopsy-based studies. The seventh cranial nerve is most frequently affected, but all components of the nervous system can be involved. Other clinical manifestations of neurosarcoidosis include vestibular dysfunction, isolated optic neuritis, and intracraneal mass lesion. Psychiatric disturbances have been described and seizures can occur. Genetic involvement in sarcoidosis is suggested by familial clustering and the frequent occurrence in some ethnic populations (African-Americans for example) compared with others (Caucasian-Americans), irrespective of geographical location. However, sarcoidosis has been described in all races, and although in the USA most patients are Black (10:1 to 17:1 ratio), in Europe the disease affects mostly Whites. Familial aggregation appears to be more prominent in populations of African descent (McGrath et al., 2000; Rybicki et al., 2001).

Genes for HLA-DRB1*13, TNF-α, immunoglobulin (GM and KM), complement receptor 1, angiotensin converting enzyme, TGF-α, TGF-β, vitamin D receptor, TAP, IL-1, IL-10, IL-18, CFTR, MIF, CCR2, and RANTES have all been implicated in case–control studies but require confirmation (Amoli et al., 2002; Pandey and Frederick, 2002; Takada et al., 2002; Zorzetto et al., 2002). Hydrophobic amino acids at position 11 (Pocket 6) in the *HLA-DRB1* gene may have a protective effect (Foley et al., 2001), whereas HLA-DQB1*0601 and HLA-DR3 were associated with cardiac sarcoidosis and the acute Lofgren's syndrome presentation respectively (Naruse et al., 2000).

Behçet's disease (BD)

Behçet's disease is a multisystem disorder with mucocutaneous (recurrent oral and genital ulcerations), ocular, arthritic, vascular, and central nervous system involvement. The disease has a worldwide distribution with a broad range of incidence: 0.5–1 per 250 000 in Europe and North America, 1 per 10 000 in Japan, and over 20 per 1500 in Turkey and the Middle and Far East. Neurological symptoms are rare, but overall are more common in northern Europeans. The most common manifestations include benign intracranial hypertension, pyramidal involvement, and psychiatric disturbances. Familial aggregation has been sporadically reported (Nishiura et al.; 1996; Gul et al., 2000). Susceptibility is strongly associated across ethnicities with the Class I HLA-B*5101/B*5103 alleles (Gul, 2001). Studies in HLA-B51 transgenic mice showed an excessive function of peripheral blood neutrophils with an increased superoxide release (Takeno et al., 1995). A linkage-based study performed in 28 Turkish multicase families found a region of interest 17 cM telomeric to HLA-B (Gul et al., 2001). Other genes reported to influence susceptibility include endothelial nitric oxide synthase, *IL6*, and *ICAM1* (Boiardi et al., 2001; Salvarani et al., 2002).

Diseases of the PNS

Guillain–Barré syndrome (GBS)

GBS represents a heterogeneous but related group of inflammatory disorders of the peripheral nervous system: acute inflammatory demyelinating polyneuropathy (AIDP), acute motor sensory axonal neuropathy (AMSAN), acute motor axonal neuropathy (AMAN), and the Miller–Fisher syndrome. All share acute onset and significant involvement of lymphocytes and antibodies in their pathogenesis (Hartung et al., 2002). Small case-controls studies suggest weak associations between GBS preceded by *Campylobacter* infection and specific alleles at the HLA Class II, TNF-α2, TCR, and IgGRII loci (Rees et al., 1995; Ma et al., 1998a,b; van der Pol et al., 2000). Additional data suggesting an important role for genetic factors affecting susceptibility and pathogenesis in autoimmune peripheral nerve disease came from a linkage study performed in the laboratory model experimental autoimmune neuritis (EAN). Eleven loci showed evidence of linkage in a rat F2 population that segregated with high levels of anti-PNM IgG (Dahlman et al., 2001). The colocalization of EAN loci with reported susceptibility loci for experimental arthritis and/or encephalomyelitis was observed. A potentially informative spontaneous model of autoimmune peripheral polyneuropathy was reported in B7-2-deficient NOD mice (Salomon et al., 2001).

Diseases of the nerve–muscle junction

Myasthenia Gravis (MG)

MG is an antibody-mediated autoimmune disease of the neuromuscular junction characterized by muscle weakness and fatigability. MG is a heterogeneous disease; subsets of patients can be cluster based on age at onset, gender, thymic anomalies, and antibody profiles. Familial aggregation of cases has been described but is uncommon. No twin studies are available in the literature. Early evidence implicating MHC genes came from genetic studies in murine laboratory models (Christadoss et al., 1981, 1982). In humans the HLA-DR3 haplotype was consistently found associated with disease in Caucasian patients (Zelano et al., 1999). In Japanese, infantile MG is perhaps associated with HLA-DR9, but any HLA association with adult MG remains unclear (Suzuki et al. 2001).

Interestingly, HLA-DR3 and HLA-DR7 appear to have opposing effects on the MG phenotype. Patients with thymus hyperplasia were associated with DR3 but not DR7. Conversely, in patients without hyperplasia but with high expression of antititin antibodies, an association with DR7 but not with DR3 was detected (Giraud et al., 2001). A possible association with the Class I allele HLA-B8, independent of HLA-DR3, was reported for early onset MG in a British cohort (Janer et al., 1999). The authors proposed that the region of maximal susceptibility extends from HSP70 (in Class III) past HLA-B and HLA-C at least 600 kb telomeric into the Class I region. Experimental MG in HLA-DQ transgenic animals showed that polymorphism at the HLA-DQ locus affects incidence and severity, at least in this laboratory model of the disease (Raju et al., 1998).

Because of the rarity of familial MG, whole genome linkage scans in humans have not been performed to date. The *IL1A* gene was associated with early onset but not with susceptibility in an Italian case–control study that included 421 patients and 995 controls (Sciacca et al., 2002). A series of studies from the Karolinska Institute by Lefvert, Sanjeevi and colleagues suggest associations with polymorphisms in *CTLA4*, *IL10*, *IL1B*, *TNF*, and *ADRB2* (β2-adrenergic receptor) genes, but exclude the *TAP* genes, *IL4*, and *IL6*.

Diseases of the muscle

Autoimmune inflammatory myopathies (AIMs)

AIMs (polymyositis, dermatomyositis, and related disorders) are a heterogeneous group of rare disorders affecting skeletal muscle. The presence of specific autoantibodies and autoreactive T cells in the affected muscle as well as up-regulation of cell surface activation molecules, MHC Class I, cytokines, chemokines, and metalloproteinases provides strong evidence for underlying autoimmune pathogenic mechanisms (Nagaraju, 2001). A role for genetic factors in conferring susceptibility is suggested by familial aggregation of cases (Shamim and Miller, 2000; Shamim et al., 2000). No twin studies are available in the literature. The HLA region is the strongest and most consistent effect identified in AIMs. In Caucasians patients of northern European descent, but not in mesoamericans, predisposition to inflammatory myopathy has been associated with the Class II HLA-DRB1*0301-DQA1*0501 haplotype (Arnett et al., 1996; Reed et al., 1998; Shamim et al., 2002). The association appears more significant in patients with high titres of myositis-specific autoantibodies, particularly anti-Jo-1. Genome scans have not been performed to date, but non-HLA genetic effects on risk (*IL1RN*, *TNFA*, *IL1A*, *IL1B*, *PRNP*, *APOE*, and *GM* allotypes) were reported and require confirmation.

Other neurological diseases with a neuroinflammatory component

Alzheimer's disease (AD)

The brain pathology of AD is well characterized: neurons of the cerebral cortex and hypocampus showing neurofibrillary tangles together with deposition of amyloid within senile plaques and cerebral blood vessels. The identification of susceptibility genes, most notably *APOE* on chromosome

19 (Corder *et al.*, 1993), has provided the foundation for rapid progress in understanding the mechanisms underlying neuronal death in this disease. Following the suggestion that apolipoprotein E has important immuno-modulatory functions, at least *in vitro*, the role of inflammation in AD was re-examined, and there is now compelling evidence that inflammatory processes play a role in the progression and pathology of neurodegenerative disorders. For example, the local up-regulation of inflammatory cytokines (IL-1, IL-6, TNF-α, NF-κB), acute phase proteins, activation of the complement cascade, and accumulation of microglia in damaged regions of AD is well documented. Interestingly, apoe-3 but not apoe-4 blocked the activation of microglia by the secreted derivative of β-amyloid precursor protein (Barger and Harmon, 1997). In addition, some studies suggest that anti-inflammatory drugs decrease the incidence and progression of AD. On the other hand, a protective role for the immune response is also conceivable (Wyss-Coray *et al.*, 2002). Genetic associations between polymorphisms in immune-related genes (*HLAA*, *TNFA*, *IL1*, *IL6*, and *SERPINA3* (α1-antichymotrypsin)) and AD susceptibility and/or progression have been reported, but require confirmation (Du *et al.*, 2000; Grimaldi *et al.*, 2000; Nicoll *et al.*, 2000; Alvarez *et al.*, 2002; Combarros *et al.*, 2002; Licastro *et al.*, 2000; Pola *et al.*, 2002; Zareparsi *et al.*, 2002).

Genetic susceptibility to neuro-AIDS and neuro-HTLV1 disease

Clinical disease of the nervous system accounts for a significant degree of morbidity in AIDS. HIV can cause a broad spectrum of neurological diseases due to secondary opportunistic infections, neoplasms, and drug toxicity. A primary link between HIV infection and neurological disease is suspected in HIV-related dementia (in up to 20% of the seropositive patients), and HIV-related peripheral neuropathies. Neurological problems may be inflammatory, demyelinating, or degenerative in nature. Several genes, including *CCR5*, *CCR2*, *CX3CR1*, *CCL5* (*RANTES*), *CXCL12* (*SDF1*), *IL10*, the *KIR* genes, and the p53 tumor suppressor gene as well as MHC-encoded genes have been described as host factors that may influence the pathogenesis and course of HIV disease. The role of genetic factors in HIV neuropathogenesis is unclear.

HIV-infected individuals heterozygous for CCR5-delta32 appear to be relatively protected against the development of HIV encephalopathy, and carriers of the monocyte chemoattractant protein-1 (MCP-1) 2578G allele have a 50% reduction in the risk of acquiring HIV. However, once HIV-1 infection is established, MCP-1-2578G carriers have a more rapid disease progression and a 4.5-fold increased risk of HIV-associated dementia (Gonzalez *et al.*, 2002). Similarly, APOE-4 carriers have more frequent HIV-related dementia and peripheral neuropathy (Corder *et al.*, 1998). Finally, the TNFA-308A allele was also implicated in susceptibility to HIV dementia (Quasney *et al.* 2001).

It is estimated that worldwide 10 to 20 million people are infected with the HTLV-1 virus. HTLV-1 is endemic in southwestern Japan and Okinawa. The development of clinical disease is rare (~95% HTLV-1 seropositive individuals remain unsymptomatic carriers). A progressive spastic or ataxic myelopathy develops in 2–3% of HTLV-1 seropositives, and it is likely to be associated with direct nervous system infection. HTLV-1-specific CD8+ T cells producing interferon-gamma (IFN-γ) and TNF-α can be detected in peripheral blood and in spinal cord lesions. Susceptibility and/or resistance associated with HLA Class I alleles remains controversial (Usuku *et al.*, 1988, 1990; Nishimura *et al.*, 1991; Shohat *et al.*, 1996; Seki *et al.*, 1999; Jeffery *et al.*, 2000; Vine *et al.*, 2002).

Adrenoleukodystrophy (ALD)

ALD is a peroxysomal genetic disorder characterized by progressive demyelination within the CNS, adrenal insufficiency, and accumulation of very-long-chain fatty acids. It is an X-linked Mendelian trait, due to a mutation in an ATP-binding cassette transporter gene (Mosser *et al.*, 1993). The clinical presentation is heterogeneous with a cerebral demyelinating form that affects mainly boys aged between 5 and 12 years (60% of ALD cases), or an adult form, which involves primarily the spinal cord (40%). This clinical heterogeneity can been observed even in the same kindred. Interestingly,

discordant phenotypes have been reported in three pairs of monozygotic twins, indicating that environmental or epigenetic factors are prominent in the clinical expression (Di Rocco *et al.*, 2001). An inflammatory reaction and demyelination that differ from the one observed in MS is characteristic of the ALD CNS pathology. The macrophages and T lymphocytes are localized more deeply into the brain lesions compared with a more peripheral localization in MS, suggesting that inflammation appears in reaction to a primary demyelinating process. Macrophages accumulate early in recent demyelinating lesions even in the absence of perivascular infiltration. Finally, the pattern of cytokine expression shows a prominent Th1 profile, with predominant TNF-α expression. Based on these findings, immuno-modulatory or suppressive drugs have been used (cyclophosphamide, IFN-β), although with very limited success. A bone marrow transplantation trial, performed in childhood-onset cerebral X-linked ALD, showed a long-term positive effect on neurological symptoms (Shapiro *et al.*, 2000).

Narcolepsy

Narcolepsy is a disorder affecting the ability to sustain wakefulness voluntarily and REM sleep regulation. It is characterized by excessive daytime sleepiness, cataplexy, sleep paralysis, and hypnagogic hallucination. Narcolepsy affects about 1 in 4000 people in the USA and appears to have a genetic basis. Although there is a high rate of discordance in identical twins, first-degree relatives of narcoleptic patients have about a 1% incidence, much higher than in the general population. The observation that all patients with cataplexy are carriers for HLA-DQB*0602 suggested the involvement of autoimmune mechanisms in disease pathogenesis. The study of different ethnic groups indicate that complex HLA-DR/DQ interactions underlie susceptibility in narcolepsy and that additional susceptibility loci are most likely involved (Rogers *et al.*, 1997; Mignot and Thorsby, 2001; Lin *et al.*, 2001; Mignot *et al.*, 2001). A mutation in the orexin (hypocretin) receptor 2 gene has been associated with canine narcolepsy (Lin *et al.*, 1999), and orexin-knockout mice exhibit a behavioural and physiological phenotype that mimics human narcolepsy (Chemelli *et al.*, 1999; Hara *et al.*, 2001).

Chronic focal encephalitis (CFE)

It is not uncommon to find evidence of active brain inflammation in patients with epilepsy. In a series of patients with medically refractory temporal lobe epilepsy who went to seizure surgery, approximately 5% had perivascular lymphocytic cuffing and varying degrees of neuronal degeneration on pathology (Laxer, 1991). While the temporal lobe epilepsy patients with inflammatory changes represent only a small percentage of patients going to seizure surgery, they represent a significant percentage (approximately 25%) of the patients for whom surgery fails to control their epilepsy. However, generally regarded as a secondary phenomenon of the diseased brain, the detailed study of these inflammatory responses in epilepsy has been generally neglected.

CFE is a rare and severe form of childhood epilepsy characterized by epilepsia partialis continua, atrophy, scarring, loss of cortical neurons, and chronic inflammation (Rasmussen *et al.*, 1958; Rasmussen, 1978). Unlike other epilepsies, CFE involves only one cerebral hemisphere and currently available antiepileptic drugs fail to halt its progression (Chinchilla *et al.*, 1994). A primary role for pathogenic antibodies in the aetiology of CFE has been debated for the last few years, since the initial report by Rogers and colleagues describing seizure activity in rabbits that developed high titres of antibodies after immunization with the *N*-terminal extracellular domain of glutamate receptor (GluR) subunit 3 (Rogers *et al.*, 1994). Of greater interest, neuropathological examinations in the immunized rabbits revealed lesions similar to those of CFE in humans: microglial nodules, and meningeal and perivascular lymphocytic infiltrates in the cerebral cortex. These findings led to the identification of circulating antibodies against GluR3 in CFE patients (Rogers *et al.*, 1994). More recently, the occurrence of GluR3 autoantibodies was extended to non-CFE epilepsy patients with severe, early onset disease and intractable seizures (Mantegazza *et al.*, 2002). In the original CFE series, GluR immunoreactivity correlated well with clinical findings and disease activity. Using epitope mapping and whole-cell patch-clamp recording techniques on fetal mouse cortical neurons in culture, it was shown that both CFE and rabbit antisera contain antibodies directed to two epitopes in the extracellular domain of the GluR3 subunit, and activate a non-NMDA GluR current in a subset of kainic acid-responsive neurons (Twyman et al., 1995). The finding that GluR3 antisera activates GluRs, suggest that the antibodies contribute directly to seizure development through GluR excitation and neuronal excitotoxicity. On the basis of these findings, it was proposed that antibody removal might be a useful adjunctive therapy in CFE, particularly for treatment of patients with acute deterioration such as status epilepticus. Partial success achieved by plasma exchange (PE) procedures supported the hypothesis that humoral factors may play a role in maintaining progression of the disease (Andrews et al., 1990, 1996; Antozzi et al., 1998). However, despite some degree of clinical improvement observed in a number of CFE cases treated with PE, anatomically partial, functionally complete hemispherectomy continues to be the chosen procedure for controlling seizures and stabilizing the patient's condition (Vining et al., 1993; Lilly, 2000). Pathological examination of resected cortical tissue typically shows profuse inflammation, mainly characterized by T-cell infiltrates. Molecular analysis of such specimens reveals the presence of clonally expanded T and B lymphocytes, suggesting an active immune reaction against discrete epitopes from neural antigens (Li et al., 1997; Baranzini et al., 1999). Furthermore, CFE specimens show a dramatic increase in the expression of several inflammation-related genes (i.e. IL1B, IGVH genes, and IL2RG among others) and a striking down-regulation of several GluRs, in particular mGluR4 (Baranzini et al. 2002).

There are no reports of HLA association with CFE that will support the autoimmune hypothesis for this disease. Evidence for a locus in the HLA region predisposing to idiopathic generalized epilepsy in the families of patients with juvenile myoclonic epilepsy has been obtained in independent groups of kindreds. However, other studies failed to show evidence of linkage to 6p21, suggesting that genetic heterogeneity exists within the most common epilepsy phenotype (Delgado-Escueta et al., 1994; Liu et al., 1995; Whitehouse et al., 1993).

Common genetic background for different autoimmune diseases

Autoimmune disorders share several characteristics including gender dimorphism, increasing prevalence throughout adult life with peak incidence between the ages of 20 and 40 years, a tendency for remission during pregnancy with transient deterioration or increased incidence of onset in the post-partum period, polygenic inheritance, specific associations with particular HLA alleles, and evidence that an environmental exposure of some type is involved. Familial clustering of multiple autoimmune diseases and the presence of autoantibodies generally associated with other autoimmune conditions have also been reported. A recent study found an increased prevalence of MS and SLE in the relatives of patients with juvenile rheumatoid arthritis (Prahalad et al., 2002). Similar data were obtained for relatives of patients with MS (Broadley et al., 2000; Heinzlef et al., 2002), idiopathic inflammatory myopathy (Ginn et al., 1998), and SLE (Corporaal et al., 2002). Although the significance of these findings is unclear, they suggest that common genetic susceptibility factors for autoimmunity may exist.

A meta-analysis of linkage results from 23 human and experimental immune-mediated diseases, including MS and EAE, detected overlapping of susceptibility loci, further supporting the hypothesis that the pathophysiology of clinically distinct autoimmune disorders may be controlled, at least in part, by a common set of genes (Becker et al., 1998). In a different meta-analysis based on non-parametric ranking methods applied to four MS genome scans and across 11 additional autoimmune disorders (insulin-dependent diabetes mellitus, rheumatoid arthritis (RA), inflammatory bowel disease (IBD), psoriasis), only the MHC region appears to be shared,

although minor contributions from chromosomes 6q, 11p, 16, and 17 were also detected (Wise et al., 1999). In a recent genome scan of RA, several linked regions were identified that had been previously implicated in studies of MS, SLE, or IBD (Jawaheer et al., 2001). Finally, a recently published study using cDNA array methodology revealed similar transcriptional profiles among four autoimmune disorders (Maas et al., 2002).

HLA and immune-mediated neurological diseases

As described above, the genetic contribution of the major histocompatibility complex (MHC) to susceptibility and pathogenesis of autoimmune diseases of the central and peripheral nervous system has been consistently established in numerous linkage and association studies (Table 9.4). The human MHC (the human leukocyte antigen (HLA) system) consists of linked gene clusters located at 6p21.3, spanning almost 4 million base pairs (Fig. 9.4). HLA molecules are cell surface glycoproteins whose primary role in an immune response is to display and present short antigenic peptide fragments to peptide/MHC-specific T cells. Many of the HLA Class I and II genes are highly polymorphic, resulting in the generation of enormously diverse numbers of different genotypic combinations or haplotypes. The polymorphic residues that define an HLA allele are constrained to exons 2 and 3 for Class I and exon 2 for Class II, and are clustered in the antigen-peptide-binding groove of the molecule, suggesting that polymorphism developed in response to evolutionary pressures. At the population level, this heterogeneity would ensure, for example, that even if a proportion of individuals succumbed to a new pathogen because of their inability to mount an efficacious immune response, others bearing distinct MHC molecules would be resistant. Although there is substantial variation in allele and haplotype frequencies among different populations, most populations studied to date show a relatively even distribution of allele frequencies at most HLA loci, suggesting balancing selection. Balancing selection is expected to lower the frequency of homozygotes and maintain multiple alleles in a population at appreciable frequencies due to heterozygote advantage and other selective forces. MHC heterozygosity advantage has been associated with long-term survival in HIV-infected individuals (Carrington et al., 1999; Penn et al., 2002). There are exceptions, nevertheless, suggestive of directional selection. Extreme skewed allele distributions were observed in some population groups, such as the very high frequency of HLA-A*2402 in Papua New Guinea Highlanders (Bugawan et al. 1999). Overall, however, mammalian susceptibility or resistance to infectious diseases has rarely been unambiguously linked to specific HLA haplotypes (Hill et al., 1992; Kaslow et al., 1996). As an alternative hypothesis to explain the extreme HLA polymorphism, recent data links the MHC polymorphism to the diversification of the cytotoxic T-lymphocyte repertoire by allowing the intrathymic generation of precursor pools from which high-avidity effector cells can be selected (Messaoudi et al., 2002). In either case, the ability to respond to an antigen, whether foreign or self, and the nature of that response, is to a large extent determined by the unique amino acid sequences of HLA alleles, an observation that powered the rationale for focusing on genetic associations between HLA genotypes and susceptibility

Table 9.4 Immune-mediated disorders and HLA relative risk

Disease	HLA haplotype/allele	Relative risk of carriers
Multiple sclerosis	DR2	4.1
Systemic lupus erythematosus	DR3	5.8
Myasthenia gravis	DR3	2
Narcolepsy	DQ6	>38
Sjögren's syndrome	DR3	9.7
Behçet's disease	B51	8.2

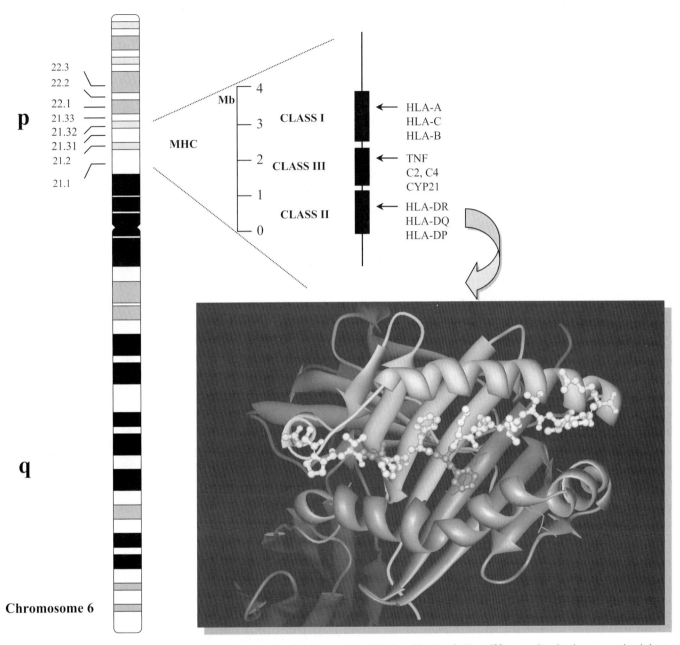

Fig. 9.4 The full sequence of the MHC region (6p21–23) was completed and reported in 1999. From 224 identified loci, 128 are predicted to be expressed and about 40% to have immune-response functions. The diagram shows the relative positions of Class I and II loci involved in antigen presentation. Other genes mapped in the MHC region include complement proteins, genes for the 21-hydroxylase, tumour necrosis factor, and heat-shock proteins, collectively known as Class III. The graphic representation of the crystal structure is a top view of HLA-DRA*0101, -DRB*1501 in complex with a putative MS autoantigen, the myelin basic protein peptide 85–99.

to autoimmune diseases, including those affecting the central and peripheral nervous systems (Begovich and Oksenberg, 2000).

The mechanisms underlying the genetic associations of HLA alleles with autoimmune diseases are not yet fully understood. One possibility is that DR2 molecules play a role in the selection of high-avidity autoreactive T cells within the embryonic thymic microenvironment. In MS, for example, the T-cell response against the 85–99 peptide of MBP is immunodominant in DRB1*1501-positive individuals (Pette *et al.*, 1990). Specific activation of these T cells occurs in the circulation of MS patients (Allegretta *et al.*, 1990) and in MS lesions T-cell receptors bearing antigen recognition CDR3 motifs likely to recognize this peptide are present (Oksenberg *et al.*, 1993). Structural data reveals a DRB-1501 structure different from other DRB molecules in that aromatic residues in the antigenic

peptide are preferred in the large hydrophobic P4 pocket of the peptide-binding domain (Smith *et al.* 1998). In the case of MBP, this pocket is primarily occupied by the aromatic side chain Phe92, acting as an important primary anchor and accounting for the high-affinity binding of the MBP peptide to the HLA-DRA0101/DRB1501 heterodimer. The polymorphic position DRB 71 (Ala in DRB1501) appears to be important in creating the necessary space for Phe side chain of MBP. In addition, it was found that two peptide side chains of the p85–99 MBP immunodominant peptide, Val89 and Phe92, are the primary anchors and account for the high-affinity binding of the MBP peptide to HLA-DRA0101/DRB1501 (Smith *et al.*, 1998; Gauthier *et al.*, 1998). The analysis also revealed that only two primary T-cell receptor contact residues of MBP p85–99 had to be conserved to properly stimulate antigen-specific clones. In addition, the crystal structure determination of a DRB5*0101–EBV peptide complex revealed a marked structural equivalence to the DRB1*1501–MBP peptide complex at the surface presented for TCR recognition (Lang *et al.*, 2002). The data suggest that microbial peptides with only limited sequence identity with a self-peptide could well activate autoreactive T cells.

Pharmacogenomics in immune-mediated neurological diseases

The field of pharmacogenomics focuses on genetic polymorphisms and how they translate into inherited differences in response to drug treatment. Several genomic variants in drug receptors, metabolizing enzymes, transporters, and targets have been linked to interindividual differences in efficacy and toxicity of medications (Roden and George, 2002). In neuroimmunological diseases, the pharmacogenomic literature is relatively sparse, but several laboratories are trying to address the question of genetic heterogeneity and the response to therapy by analysis of the correlation between different genotypes and clinical response to immunotherapeutic modalities. In recently published studies for example, an effect of the HLA-DR2 haplotype was observed in MS patients treated with Copaxone but not with IFN-β (Fusco *et al.*, 2001; Villoslada *et al.*, 2002). The type 1 interferons, which include about 14 cytokines (13 isotypes of IFN-α, one IFN-β), all share the same receptor, IFNAR, for binding. The two subunits of the receptor, IFNAR1 and IFNAR2, are coded by two different genes located close to each other on chromosome 21q22.1. A pharmacogenomic analysis of eight SNPs in the interferon receptor genes failed to show significant evidence of genotypic influences in the response to IFN-β in MS (Sriram *et al.* 2003).

Conclusion

The development of pathological inflammation or autoimmunity in genetically susceptible individuals involves at least two factors: (1) the loss of immune homeostasis, normally maintained through inhibitory signalling pathways, induction of anergy or apoptosis, and anti-idiotypic networks, and (2) the engagement and activation of lymphocytes by adjuvant signals including, conceivably, recurrent exposures to exogenous pathogens. New gene expression networks that incorporate multiple cell–cell and cell–matrix interactions are established and maintain the progression of neuroinflammatory and neurodegenerative processes. With the aid of high-capacity technologies, multidisciplinary and multianalytical approaches will decipher complete rosters of disease loci, and define useful and unifying conceptual models of neuronal pathogenesis. These studies need to be linked to the development of novel mathematical formulations, designed to identify modest genetic effects, interactions between multiple genes, and interactions between genetic, clinical, and environmental factors. Their characterization will help to define basic aetiologies, improve risk assessment, and influence therapeutics for degenerative, infectious, epileptic, and autoimmune neurological diseases.

Acknowledgements

The authors are supported by the National Multiple Sclerosis Society (US), the National Institute of Health, and the Nancy Davis and Sandler Foundations. David Brassat is a post-doctoral Fellow supported by the Association pour le Developpement de la Recherche et de l'Enseignement en Neurologie (ADREN).

References

Ainiala, H., Loukkola, J., Peltola, J., Korpela, M., and Hietaharju, A. (2001). The prevalence of neuropsychiatric syndromes in systemic lupus erythematosus. *Neurology* 57: 496–500.

Allegretta, M., Nicklas, J.A., Sriram, S., and Albertini, R.J. (1990). T cells responsive to myelin basic protein in patients with multiple sclerosis. *Science* 247: 718–721.

Alvarez, V., Mata, I.F., Gonzalez, P., Lahoz, C.H., Martinez, C., Pena, J., et al. (2002). Association between the TNFalpha-308 A/G polymorphism and the onset-age of Alzheimer disease. *Am J Med Genet* 114: 574–577.

Amoli, M.M., Donn, R.P., Thomson, W., Hajeer, A.H., Garcia-Porrua, C., Lueiro, M., et al. (2002). Macrophage migration inhibitory factor gene polymorphism is associated with sarcoidosis in biopsy proven erythema nodosum. *J Rheumatol* 29: 1671–1673.

Andrews, J.M., Thompson, J.A., Pyser, T.J., Walker, M.L., and Hammond, M.E. (1990). Chronic encephalitis, epilepsy, and cerebrovascular immune complex deposits. *Ann Neurol* 28: 88–90.

Andrews, P.I., Dichter, M.A., Berkovic, S.F., Newton, M.R., and McNamara, J.O. (1996). Plamapheresis in Rasmussen's encephalitis. *Neurology* 46: 242–246.

Antozzi, C., Granata, T., Aurisano, N., Zardini, G., Confalonieri, P., Airaghi, G., et al. (1998). Long-term selective IgG immuno-adsorption improves Rasmussen's encephalitis. *Neurology* 51: 302–305.

Arnett, F.C., Targoff, I.N., Mimori, T., Goldstein, R., Warner, N.B., and Reveille, J.D. (1996). Interrelationship of major histocompatibility complex class II alleles and autoantibodies in four ethnic groups with various forms of myositis. *Arthritis Rheum* 39: 1507–1518.

Ballerini, C., Campani, D., Rombola, G., Gran, B., Nacmias, B., Pia Amato, M., et al. (2000). Association of apolipoprotein E polymorphism to clinical heterogeneity of multiple sclerosis. *Neurosci Lett* 296: 174–176.

Baranzini, S.E., Jeong, M.C., Butunoi, C., Murray, R.S., Bernard, C.C., and Oksenberg, J.R. (1999). B cell repertoire diversity and clonal expansion in multiple sclerosis brain lesions. *J Immunol* 163: 5133–5144.

Baranzini, S.E., Laxer, K., Bollen, A., and Oksenberg, J.R. (2002). Gene expression analysis reveals altered brain transcription of glutamate receptors and inflammatory genes in a patient with chronic focal (Rasmussen's) encephalitis. *J Neuroimmunol* 128: 9–15.

Barcellos, L.F., Thomson, G., Carrington, M., Schafer, J., Begovich, A.B., Lin, P., et al. (1997). Chromosome 19 single-locus and multilocus haplotype associations with multiple sclerosis. *J Am Med Assoc* 15: 1256–1271.

Barcellos, L.F., Oksenberg, J.R., Green, A.J., Bucher, P., Rimmler, J.B., Schmidt, S., et al. (2002). Genetic basis for clinical expression in multiple sclerosis. *Brain* 125: 150–158.

Barcellos, L.F., Oksenberg, J.R., Begovich, A.B., Martin, E.R., Schmidt, S., Vittinghoff, E., et al. (2003). HLA-DR2 dose effect on susceptibility to multiple sclerosis and influence on disease course. *Am J Hum Genet* 72: 710–716.

Barger, S.W. and Harmon, A.D. (1997). Microglial activation by Alzheimer amyloid precursor protein and modulation by apolipoprotein E. *Nature* 388: 878–881.

Becker, K.G., Simon, R.M., Bailey-Wilson, J.E., Freidlin, B., Biddison, W., McFarland, H.F., et al. (1998). Clustering of non-major histocompatibility complex susceptibility candidate loci in human autoimmune diseases. *Proc Natl Acad Sci USA* 95: 9979–9984.

Begovich, A.B. and Oksenberg, J.R. (2000). Variation in genes regulating the immune system and relationship to disease. In: *Genetic Polymorphisms and Susceptibility to Disease* (ed. M.S. Miller and M. Cronin), pp. 139–74. Taylor and Francis, Philadelphia.

Boiardi, L., Salvarani, C., Casali, B., Olivieri, I., Ciancio, G., Cantini, F., et al. (2001). Intercellular adhesion molecule-1 gene polymorphisms in Behcet's disease. *J Rheumatol* 28: 1283–1287.

Boulard, O., Fluteau, G., Eloy, L., Damotte, D., Bedossa, P., and Garchon, H.J. (2002). Genetic analysis of autoimmune sialadenitis in nonobese diabetic mice: a major susceptibility region on chromosome 1. *J Immunol* 168: 4192–4201.

Brassat, D., Azais-Vuillemin, C., Yaouanq, J., Semana, G., Reboul, J., Cournu, I., et al. (1999). Familial factors influence disability in MS multiplex families. French Multiple Sclerosis Genetics Group. *Neurology* 52: 1632–1636.

Brayer, J., Lowry, J., Cha, S., Robinson, C.P., Yamachika, S., Peck, A.B., et al. (2000). Alleles from chromosomes 1 and 3 of NOD mice combine to influence Sjogren's syndrome-like autoimmune exocrinopathy. *J Rheumatol* 27: 1896–1904.

Broadley, S.A., Deans, J., Sawcer, S.J., Clayton, D., and Compston, D.A. (2000). Autoimmune disease in first-degree relatives of patients with multiple sclerosis. A UK survey. *Brain* **123**: 1102–1111.

Bugawan, T.L., Mack, S.J., Stoneking, M., Saha, M., Beck, H.P., and Erlich, H.A. (1999). HLA class I allele distributions in six Pacific/Asian populations: evidence of selection at the HLA-A locus. *Tissue Antigens* **53**: 311–319.

Butterfield, R.J., Blankenhorn, E.P., Roper, R.J., Zachary, J.F., Doerge, R.W., and Teuscher, C. (2000). Identification of genetic loci controlling the characteristics and severity of brain and spinal cord lesions in experimental allergic encephalomyelitis. *Am J Pathol* **157**: 637–645.

Carrington, M., Nelson, G.W., Martin, M.P., Kissner, T., Vlahov, D., Goedert, J.J., *et al.* (1999). HLA and HIV-1: heterozygote advantage and B*35-Cw*04 disadvantage. *Science* **283**: 1748–1752.

Cha, S., Nagashima, H., Brown, V.B., Peck, A.B., and Humphreys-Beher, M.G. (2002). Two NOD Idd-associated intervals contribute synergistically to the development of autoimmune exocrinopathy (Sjogren's syndrome) on a healthy murine background. *Arthritis Rheum* **46**: 1390–1398.

Chapman, J., Vinokurov, S., Achiron, A., Karussis, D.M., Mitosek-Szewczyk, K., Birnbaum, M., *et al.* (2001). APOE genotype is a major predictor of long-term progression of disability in MS. *Neurology* **56**: 312–316.

Chataway, J., Feakes, R., Coraddu, F., Gray, J., Deans, J., Fraser, M., *et al.* (1998). The genetics of multiple sclerosis: principles, background and update results of the UK systematic genome screen. *Brain* **121**: 1869–1887.

Chemelli, R.M., Willie, J.T., Sinton, C.M., Elmquist, J.K., Scammell, T., Lee, C., *et al.* (1999). Narcolepsy in orexin knockout mice: molecular genetics of sleep regulation. *Cell* **98**: 437–451.

Chinchilla, D., Dulac, O., Robaim, O., Plouin, P., Ponsot, G., Pinel, J.F., *et al.* (1994). Reappraisal of Rasmussen's syndrome with special emphasis on treatment with high doses of steroids. *J Neurol Neurosurg Psychiatry* **57**: 1325–1333.

Christadoss, P., Krco, C.J., Lennon, V.A., and David, C.S. (1981). Genetic control of experimental autoimmune myasthenia gravis in mice. II. Lymphocyte proliferative response to acetylcholine receptor is dependent on Lyt-1+23- cells. *J Immunol* **126**: 1646–1647.

Christadoss, P., Lennon, V.A., Krco, C.J., and David, C.S. (1982). Genetic control of experimental myasthenia gravis in mice. III. Ia molecules mediate cellular immune responsiveness to AChR. *J Immunol* **128**: 1141–1144.

Combarros, O., Sanchez-Guerra, M., Infante, J., Llorca, J., and Berciano, J. (2002). Gene dose-dependent association of interleukin-1A [-889] allele 2 polymorphism with Alzheimer's disease. *J Neurol* **249**: 1242–1245.

Corder, E.H., Saunders, A.M., Strittmatter, W.J., Schmechel, D.E., Gaskell, P.C., Small, G.W., *et al.* (1993). Gene dose of apolipoprotein E type 4 allele and the risk of Alzheimer's disease in late onset families. *Science* **261**: 921–923.

Corder, E.H., Robertson, K., Lannfelt, L., Bogdanovic, N., Eggertsen, G., Wilkins, J., *et al.*(1998). HIV-infected subjects with the E4 allele for APOE have excess dementia and peripheral neuropathy. *Nat Med* **4**: 1182–1184.

Corporaal, S., Bijl, M., and Kallenberg, C.G. (2002). Familial occurrence of autoimmune diseases and autoantibodies in a Caucasian population of patients with systemic lupus erythematosus. *Clin Rheumatol* **21**: 108–113.

Dahlman, I., Wallstrom, E., Jiao, H., Luthman, H., Olsson, T., and Weissert, R. (2001). Polygenic control of autoimmune peripheral nerve inflammation in rat. *J Neuroimmunol* **119**: 166–174.

Daly, M.J., Rioux, J.D., Schaffner, S.F., Hudson, T.J., and Lander, E.S. (2001). High-resolution haplotype structure in the human genome. *Nat Genet* **29**: 229–232.

de Jong, B.A., Huizinga, T.W., Zanelli, E., Giphart, M.J., Bollen, E.L., Uitdehaag, B.M., *et al.* (2002). Evidence for additional genetic risk indicators of relapse-onset MS within the HLA region. *Neurology* **59**: 549–555.

de Seze, J., Devos, D., Castelnovo, G., Labauge, P., Dubucquoi, S., Stojkovic, T., *et al.* (2001). The prevalence of Sjogren syndrome in patients with primary progressive multiple sclerosis. *Neurology* **57**: 1359–1363.

Deapen, D., Escalante, A., Weinrib, L., Horwitz, D., Bachman, B., Roy-Burman, P., *et al.* (1992). A revised estimate of twin concordance in systemic lupus erythematosus. *Arthritis Rheum* **35**: 311–318.

Delgado-Escueta, A.V., Serratosa, J.M., Liu, A., Weissbecker, K., Medina, M.T., Gee, M., *et al.* (1994). Progress in mapping human epilepsy genes. *Epilepsia* **35**: S29–S40.

Di Rocco, M., Doria-Lamba, L., and Caruso, U. (2001). Monozygotic twins with X-linked adrenoleukodystrophy and different phenotypes. *Ann Neurol* **50**: 424.

Diaz-Villoslada, P. and Oksenberg, J.R. (1998). Chronic inflammatory diseases of the nervous system. *Curr Opin Neurol* **11**: 235–240.

Du, Y., Dodel, R.C., Eastwood, B.J., Bales, K.R., Gao, F., Lohmuller, F., Muller, U., *et al.* (2000). Association of an interleukin 1 alpha polymorphism with Alzheimer's disease. *Neurology* **55**: 480–483.

Ebers, G.C., Sadovnick, A.D., and Risch, N.J. (1995). A genetic basis for familial aggregation in multiple sclerosis. Canadian Collaborative Study Group. *Nature* **377**: 150–151.

Ebers, G.C., Kukay, K., Bulman, D.E., Sadovnick, A.D., Rice, G., Anderson, C., *et al.* (1996). A full genome search in multiple sclerosis. *Nat Genet* **13**: 472–476.

Encinas, J.A., Weiner, H.L., and Kuchroo, V.K. (1996). Inheritance of susceptibility to experimental autoimmune encephalomyelitis. *J. Neurosci Res* **45**: 655–669.

Evangelou, N., Jackson, M., Beeson, D., and Palace, J. (1999). Association of the APOE epsilon4 allele with disease activity in multiple sclerosis. *J Neurol Neurosurg Psychiatryiat* **67**: 203–205.

Fazekas, F., Strasser-Fuchs, S., Schmidt, H., Enzinger, C., Ropele, S., Lechner, A., *et al.* (2000). Apolipoprotein E genotype related differences in brain lesions of multiple sclerosis. *J Neurol Neurosurg Psychiatryiat* **69**: 25–28.

Fazekas, F., Strasser-Fuchs, S., Kollegger, H., Berger, T., Kristoferitsch, W., Schmidt, H., *et al.* (2001). Apolipoprotein E epsilon 4 is associated with rapid progression of multiple sclerosis. *Neurology* **57**: 853–857.

Fogdell-Hahn, A., Ligers, A., Gronning, M., Hillert, J., and Olerup, O. (2000). Multiple sclerosis: a modifying influence of HLA class I genes in an HLA class II associated autoimmune disease. *Tissue Antigens* **55**: 140–148.

Foley, P.J., McGrath, D.S., Puscinska, E., Petrek, M., Kolek, V., Drabek, J., *et al.* (2001). Human leukocyte antigen-DRB1 position 11 residues are a common protective marker for sarcoidosis. *Am J Respir Cell Mol Biol* **25**: 272–277.

Fontaine, B., Cournu, I., Arnaud, I., Babron, M.C., Eichenbaum-Voline, S., Oksenberg, J.R., *et al.* (1999). Chromosome 17q22-q24 and multiple sclerosis genetic susceptibility. American-French Multiple Sclerosis Genetic Group. *Genes Immun* **1**: 149–150.

Foster, H., Stephenson, A., Walker, D., Cavanagh, G., Kelly, C., and Griffiths, I. (1993). Linkage studies of HLA and primary Sjogren's syndrome in multicase families. *Arthritis Rheum* **36**: 473–484.

Fusco, C., Andreone, V., Coppola, G., Luongo, V., Guerini, F., Pace, E., *et al.* (2001). HLA-DRB1*1501 and response to copolymer-1 therapy in relapsing- remitting multiple sclerosis. *Neurology* **57**: 1976–1979.

Gabriel, S.B., Schaffner, S.F., Nguyen, H., Moore, J.M., Roy, J., Blumenstiel, B., *et al.* (2002). The structure of haplotype blocks in the human genome. *Science* **296**: 2225–2229.

GAMES and the Transatlantic Multiple Sclerosis Genetics Cooperative (2003). A meta-analysis of whole genome linkage screens in multiple sclerosis. *J. Neuroimmunol* **143**: 39–46.

Gauthier, L., Smith, K.J., Pyrdol, J., Kalandadze, A., Strominger, J.L., Wiley, D.C., *et al.* (1998). Expression and crystallization of the complex of HLA-DR2 (DRA, DRB1*1501) and an immunodominant peptide of human myelin basic protein. *Proc Natl Acad Sci USA* **95**: 11828–11833.

Ginn, L.R., Lin, J.P., Plotz, P.H., Bale, S.J., Wilder, R.L., Mbauya, A., *et al.* (1998). Familial autoimmunity in pedigrees of idiopathic inflammatory myopathy patients suggests common genetic risk factors for many autoimmune diseases. *Arthritis Rheum* **41**: 400–405.

Giraud, M., Beaurain, G., Yamamoto, A.M., Eymard, B., Tranchant, C., Gajdos, P., *et al.* (2001). Linkage of HLA to myasthenia gravis and genetic heterogeneity depending on anti-titin antibodies. *Neurology* **57**: 1555–1560.

Gonzalez, E., Rovin, B.H., Sen, L., Cooke, G., Dhanda, R., Mummidi, S., *et al.* (2002). From the cover: HIV-1 infection and AIDS dementia are influenced by a mutant MCP-1 allele linked to increased monocyte infiltration of tissues and MCP-1 levels. *Proc Natl Acad Sci USA* **99**: 13795–13800.

Graham, R.R., Ortmann, W.A., Langefeld, C.D., Jawaheer, D., Selby, S.A., Rodine, P.R., *et al.* (2002). Visualizing human leukocyte antigen class II risk haplotypes in human systemic lupus erythematosus. *Am J Hum Genet* **71**: 543–553.

Grimaldi, L.M., Casadei, V.M., Ferri, C., Veglia, F., Licastro, F., Annoni, G., *et al.* (2000). Association of early-ons*et alz*heimer's disease with an interleukin-1 alpha gene polymorphism. *Ann Neurol* **47**: 361–365.

Gul, A. (2001). Behcet's disease: an update on the pathogenesis. *Clin Exp Rheumatol* **19**: S6–S12.

Gul, A., Inanc, M., Ocal, L., Aral, O., and Konice, M. (2000). Familial aggregation of Behcet's disease in Turkey. *Ann Rheum Dis* **59**: 622–625.

Gul, A., Hajeer, A.H., Worthington, J., Ollier, W.E., and Silman, A.J. (2001). Linkage mapping of a novel susceptibility locus for Behcet's disease to chromosome 6p22–23. *Arthritis Rheum* **44**: 2693–2696.

Haines, J.L. and Pericak-Vance, M.A. (1998). *Approaches to Gene Mapping in Complex Human Diseases*. Wiley-Liss, New York.

Haines, J.L., Bradford, Y., Garcia, M.E., Reed, A.D., Neumeister, E., Pericak-Vance, M.A., *et al.* (2002). Multiple susceptibility loci for multiple sclerosis. *Hum Mol Genet* **11**: 2251–2256.

Hara, J., Beuckmann, C.T., Nambu, T., Willie, J.T., Chemelli, R.M., Sinton, C.M., *et al.* (2001). Genetic ablation of orexin neurons in mice results in narcolepsy, hypophagia, and obesity. *Neuron* **30**: 345–354.

Hartung, H.P., Willison, H.J., and Kieseier, B.C. (2002). Acute immunoinflammatory neuropathy: update on Guillain–Barre syndrome. *Curr Opin Neurol* **15**: 571–577.

Heinzlef, O., Weill, B., Johanet, C., Sazdovitch, V., Caillat-Zucman, S., Tournier-Lasserve, E., *et al.* (2002). Anticardiolipin antibodies in patients with multiple sclerosis do not represent a subgroup of patients according to clinical, familial, and biological characteristics. *J Neurol Neurosurg Psychiatryiat* **72**: 647–649.

Hill, A.V., Elvin, J., Willis, A.C., Aidoo, M., Allsopp, C.E., Gotch, F.M., *et al.* (1992). Molecular analysis of the association of HLA-B53 and resistance to severe malaria. *Nature* **360**: 434–439.

Horikawa, Y., Oda, N., Cox, N.J., Li, X., Orho-Melander, M., Hara, M., *et al.* (2000). Genetic variation in the gene encoding calpain-10 is associated with type 2 diabetes mellitus. *Nat Genet* **26**: 163–175.

Hugot, J.P., Chamaillard, M., Zouali, H., Lesage, S., Cezard, J.P., Belaiche, J., *et al.* (2001). Association of NOD2 leucine-rich repeat variants with susceptibility to Crohn's disease. *Nature* **411**: 599–603.

Janer, M., Cowland, A., Picard, J., Campbell, D., Pontarotti, P., Newsom-Davis, J., *et al.* (1999). A susceptibility region for myasthenia gravis extending into the HLA-class I sector telomeric to HLA-C. *Hum Immunol* **60**: 909–917.

Jawaheer, D., Seldin, M.F., Amos, C.I., Chen, W.V., Shigeta, R., Monteiro, J., *et al.* (2001). A genomewide screen in multiplex rheumatoid arthritis families suggests genetic overlap with other autoimmune diseases. *Am J Hum Genet* **68**: 927–936.

Jean, S., Quelvennec, E., Alizadeh, M., Guggenbuhl, P., Birebent, B., Perdriger, A., *et al.* (1998). DRB1*15 and DRB1*03 extended haplotype interaction in primary Sjogren's syndrome genetic susceptibility. *Clin Exp Rheumatol* **16**: 725–728.

Jeffery, K.J., Siddiqui, A.A., Bunce, M., Lloyd, A.L., Vine, A.M., Witkover, A.D., *et al.* (2000). The influence of HLA class I alleles and heterozygosity on the outcome of human T cell lymphotropic virus type I infection. *J Immunol* **165**: 7278–7284.

Jeffreys, A.J., Kauppi, L., and Neumann, R. (2001). Intensely punctate meiotic recombination in the class II region of the major histocompatibility complex. *Nat Genet* **29**: 217–222.

Kantarci, O.H., de Andrade, M., and Weinshenker, B.G. (2002). Identifying disease modifying genes in multiple sclerosis. *J Neuroimmunol* **123**: 144–159.

Kaslow, R.A., Carrington, M., Apple, R., Park, L., Munoz, A., Saah, A.J., *et al.* (1996). Influence of combinations of human major histocompatibility complex genes on the course of HIV-infection. *Nat Genet* **2**: 405–411.

Kelly, J.A., Moser, K.L., and Harley, J.B. (2002). The genetics of systemic lupus erythematosus: putting the pieces together. *Genes Immun* **3**(Suppl. 1): S71–S85.

Kira, J., Kanai, T., Nishimura, Y., Yamasaki, K., Matsushita, S., Kawano, Y., *et al.* (1996). Western versus Asian types of multiple sclerosis: immunogenetically and clinically distinct disorders. *Ann Neurol* **40**: 569–574.

Kuokkanen, S., Gschwend, M., Rioux, J.D., Daly, M.J., Terwilliger, J.D., Tienari, P.J., *et al.* (1997). Genomewide scan of multiple sclerosis in Finnish multiplex families. *Am J Hum Genet* **61**: 1379–1387.

Lang, H.L., Jacobsen, H., Ikemizu, S., Andersson, C., Harlos, K., Madsen, L., *et al.* (2002). A functional and structural basis for TCR cross-reactivity in multiple sclerosis. *Nature Immunol* **3**: 940–943.

Laxer, K.D. (1991). Temporal lobe epilepsy with inflammatory pathologic changes. In: *Chronic Focal Encephalitis* (ed. F. Anderman) pp. 135–140. Butterworth Press, Montreal.

Li, Y., Uccelli, A., Laxer, K.D., Jeong, M.C., Vinters, H.V., Tourtellotte, W.W., *et al.* (1997). Local-clonal expansion of infiltrating T lymphocytes in chronic encephalitis of Rasmussen. *J Immunol* **158**: 1428–1437.

Licastro, F., Pedrini, S., Ferri, C., Casadei, V., Govoni, M., Pession, A., *et al.* (2000). Gene polymorphism affecting alpha1-antichymotrypsin and interleukin-1 plasma levels increases Alzheimer's disease risk. *Ann Neurol* **48**: 388–391.

Ligers, A., Dyment, D.A., Willer, C.J., Sadovnick, A.D., Ebers, G., Risch, N., *et al.* (2001). Evidence of linkage with HLA-DR in DRB1*15-negative families with multiple sclerosis. *Am J Hum Genet* **69**: 900–903.

Lilly, D.J. (2000). Functional hemispherectomy: radical treatment for Rasmussen's encephalitis. *J Neurosci Nurs* **32**: 89–92.

Lin, L., Faraco, J., Li, R., Kadotani, H., Rogers, W., Lin, X., *et al.* (1999). The sleep disorder canine narcolepsy is caused by a mutation in the hypocretin (orexin) receptor 2 gene. *Cell* **98**: 365–376.

Lin, L., Hungs, M., and Mignot, E. (2001). Narcolepsy and the HLA region. *J Neuroimmunol* **117**: 9–20.

Liu, A.W., Delgado-Escueta, A.V., Serratosa, J.M., Alonso, M.E., Medina, M.T., Gee, M.N., *et al.* (1995). Juvenile myoclonic epilepsy locus in chromosome 6p21.2–p11: linkage to convulsions and electroencephalography trait. *Am J Hum Genet* **57**: 368–381.

Ma, J.J., Nishimura, M., Mine, H., Kuroki, S., Nukina, M., Ohta, M., *et al.* (1998*a*). Genetic contribution of the tumor necrosis factor region in Guillain–Barre syndrome. *Ann Neurol* **44**: 815–818.

Ma, J.J., Nishimura, M., Mine, H., Kuroki, S., Nukina, M., Ohta, M., *et al.* (1998*b*). HLA and T-cell receptor gene polymorphisms in Guillain-Barre syndrome. *Neurology* **51**: 379–384.

Maas, K., Chan, S., Parker, J., Slater, A., Moore, J., Olsen, N., *et al.* (2002). Cutting edge: molecular portrait of human autoimmune disease. *J Immunol* **169**: 5–9.

Mantegazza, R., Bernasconi, P., Baggi, F., Spreafico, R., Ragona, F., Antozzi, C., *et al.* (2002). Antibodies against GluR3 peptides are not specific for Rasmussen's encephalitis but are also present in epilepsy patients with severe, early onset disease and intractable seizures. *J Neuroimmunol* **131**: 179–185.

Marrosu, M.G., Murru, R., Murru, M.R., Costa, G., Zavattari, P., Whalen, M., *et al.* (2001). Dissection of the HLA association with multiple sclerosis in the founder isolated population of Sardinia. *Hum Mol Genet* **10**: 2907–2916.

Martin, E.R., Gilbert, J.R., Lai, E.H., Riley, J., Rogala, A.R., Slotterbeck, B.D., *et al.* (2000). Analysis of association at single nucleotide polymorphisms in the APOE region. *Genomics* **63**: 7–12.

McDonnell, G.V. and Hawkins, S.A. (1998). Clinical study of primary progressive multiple sclerosis in Northern Ireland, UK. *J Neurol Neurosurg Psychiatryiat* **64**: 451–454.

McGrath, D.S., Daniil, Z., Foley, P., du Bois, J.L., Lympany, P.A., Cullinan, P., *et al.* (2000). Epidemiology of familial sarcoidosis in the UK. *Thorax* **55**: 751–754.

Messaoudi, I., Patino, J.A., Dyall, R., LeMaoult, J., and Nikolich-Zugich, J. (2002). Direct link between MHC polymorphism, T cell avidity, and diversity in immune defense. *Science* **298**: 1797–1800.

Mignot, E. and Thorsby, E. (2001). Narcolepsy and the HLA system. *N Engl J Med* **344**: 692.

Mignot, E., Lin, L., Rogers, W., Honda, Y., Qiu, X., Lin, X., *et al.* (2001). Complex HLA-DR and -DQ interactions confer risk of narcolepsy-cataplexy in three ethnic groups. *Am J Hum Genet* **68**: 686–699.

Moser, K.L., Neas, B.R., Salmon, J.E., Yu, H., Gray-McGuire, C., Asundi, N., *et al.* (1998). Genome scan of human systemic lupus erythematosus: evidence for linkage on chromosome 1q in African-American pedigrees. *Proc Natl Acad Sci USA* **95**: 14869–14874.

Mosser, J., Douar, A.M., Sarde, C.O., Kioschis, P., Feil, R., Moser, H., *et al.* (1993). Putative X-linked adrenoleukodystrophy gene shares unexpected homology with ABC transporters. *Nature* **361**: 726–730.

Multiple Sclerosis Genetics Group (1996). A complete genomic screen for multiple sclerosis underscores a role for the major histocompatibility complex. *Nat Genet* **13**: 469–471.

Multiple Sclerosis Genetics Group (1998). Linkage of the MHC to familial multiple sclerosis suggests genetic heterogeneity. *Hum Molec Genet* 7: 1229–1234.

Mumford, C.J., Wood, N.W., Kellar-Wood, H., Thorpe, J.W., Miller, D.H., Compston, D.A. *et al.* (1994). The British Isles survey of multiple sclerosis in twins. *Neurology* 44: 11–15.

Nagaraju, K. (2001). Update on immunopathogenesis in inflammatory myopathies. *Curr Opin Rheumatol* 13: 461–468.

Naruse, T.K., Matsuzawa, Y., Ota, M., Katsuyama, Y., Matsumori, A., Hara, M., *et al.* (2000). HLA-DQB1*0601 is primarily associated with the susceptibility to cardiac sarcoidosis. *Tissue Antigens* 56: 52–57.

Nath, S.K., Kelly, J.A., Reid, J., Lam, T., Gray-McGuire, C., Namjou, B., *et al.* (2002). SLEB3 in systemic lupus erythematosus (SLE) is strongly related to SLE families ascertained through neuropsychiatric manifestations. *Hum Genet* 111: 54–58.

Nicoll, J.A., Mrak, R.E., Graham, D.I., Stewart, J., Wilcock, G., MacGowan, S., *et al.* (2000). Association of interleukin-1 gene polymorphisms with Alzheimer's disease. *Ann Neurol* 47: 365–368.

Nishimura, Y., Okubo, R., Minato, S., Itoyama, Y., Goto, I., Mori, M., *et al.* (1991). A possible association between HLA and HTLV-I-associated myelopathy (HAM) in Japanese. *Tissue Antigens* 37: 230–231.

Nishiura, K., Kotake, S., Ichiishi, A., and Matsuda, H. (1996). Familial occurrence of Behcet's disease. *Japan J Ophthalmol* 40: 255–259.

Ogura, Y., Bonen, D.K., Inohara, N., Nicolae, D.L., Chen, F.F., Ramos, R., *et al.* (2001). A frameshift mutation in NOD2 associated with susceptibility to Crohn's disease. *Nature* 411: 603–606.

Ohno, K., Hutchinson, D.O., Milone, M., Brengman, J.M., Bouzat, C., Sine, S.M., *et al.* (1995). Congenital myasthenic syndrome caused by prolonged acetylcholine receptor channel openings due to a mutation in the M2 domain of the epsilon subunit. *Proc Natl Acad Sci USA* 92: 758–762.

Oksenberg, J.R., Panzara, M.A., Begovich, A.B., Mitchell, D., Erlich, H.A., Murray, R.S., *et al.* (1993). Selection for T-cell receptor Vb-Db-Jb gene rearrangements with specificity for a myelin basic protein peptide in brain lesions of multiple sclerosis. *Nature* 362: 68–70.

Oksenberg, J.R., Baranzini, S.E., Barcellos, L.F., and Hauser, S.L. (2001). Multiple sclerosis: genomic rewards. *J Neuroimmunol* 113: 171–184.

Oksenberg J.R., Barcellos, L.F., Cree, B.A.C., Baranzin, S.E., Bugawan, T.L., Khan, O., *et al.* (2004). Mapping multiple sclerosis susceptibility to the HLA-DR locus in African Americans. *Am J Hum Genet* 74: 160–167.

Oliveri, R.L., Cittadella, R., Sibilia, G., Manna, I., Valentino, P., Gambardella, A., *et al.* (1999). APOE and risk of cognitive impairment in multiple sclerosis. *Acta Neurol Scand* 100: 290–295.

Palacio, L.G., Rivera, D., Builes, J.J., Jimenez, M.E., Salgar, M., Anaya, J.M., *et al.* (2002). Multiple sclerosis in the tropics: genetic association to STR's loci spanning the HLA and TNF. *Mult Scler* 8: 249–255.

Pandey, J.P. and Frederick, M. (2002). TNF-alpha, IL1-beta, and immunoglobulin (GM and KM) gene polymorphisms in sarcoidosis. *Hum Immunol* 63: 485–491.

Penn, D.J., Damjanovich, K., and Potts, W.K. (2002). MHC heterozygosity confers a selective advantage against multiple- strain infections. *Proc Natl Acad Sci USA* 99: 11260–11264.

Pericak-Vance, M.A., Rimmler, J.B., Martin, E.R., Haines, J.L., Garcia, M.E., Oksenberg, J.R., *et al.* (2001). Linkage and association analysis of chromosome 19q13 in multiple sclerosis. *Neurogenetics* 3: 195–201.

Pette, M., Fujita, K., Kitze, B., Whitaker, J.N., Kappos, A., and Wekerle, H. (1990). Myelin basic protein specific T cell lines from MS patients and healthy individuals. *Neurology* 40: 1770–1776.

Pola, R., Flex, A., Gaetani, E., Lago, A.D., Gerardino, L., Pola, P., *et al.* (2002). The -74 G/C polymorphism of the interleukin-6 gene promoter is associated with Alzheimer's disease in an Italian population. *Neuroreport* 13: 1645–1647.

Prahalad, S., Shear, E.S., Thompson, S.D., Giannini, E.H., and Glass, D.N. (2002). Increased prevalence of familial autoimmunity in simplex and multiplex families with juvenile rheumatoid arthritis. *Arthritis Rheum* 46: 1851–1856.

Quasney, M.W., Zhang, Q., Sargent, S., Mynatt, M., Glass, J., and McArthur, J. (2001). Increased frequency of the tumor necrosis factor-alpha-308 A allele in adults with human immunodeficiency virus dementia. *Ann Neurol* 50: 157–162.

Raju, R., Zhan, W.Z., Karachunski, P., Conti-Fine, B., Sieck, G.C., and David, C. (1998). Polymorphism at the HLA-DQ locus determines susceptibility to experimental autoimmune myasthenia gravis. *J Immunol* 160: 4169–4174.

Rasmussen, T. (1978). Further observations on the syndrome of chronic encephalitis and epilepsy. *Appl. Neurophysiol.* 41: 1–12.

Rasmussen, T., Olszewski, J., and Lloyd-Smith, D. (1958). Focal seizures due to chronic localized encephalitis. *Neurology* 8: 435–455.

Reed, A.M., Pachman, L.M., Hayford, J., and Ober, C. (1998). Immunogenetic studies in families of children with juvenile dermatomyositis. *J Rheumatol* 25: 1000–1002.

Rees, J.H., Vaughan, R.W., Kondeatis, E., and Hughes, R.A. (1995). HLA-class II alleles in Guillain–Barre syndrome and Miller Fisher syndrome and their association with preceding Campylobacter jejuni infection. *J Neuroimmunol* 62: 53–57.

Reich, D.E., Cargill, M., Bolk, S., Ireland, J., Sabeti, P.C., Richter, D.J., *et al.* (2001). Linkage disequilibrium in the human genome. *Nature* 411: 199–204.

Rioux, J.D., Daly, M.J., Silverberg, M.S., Lindblad, K., Steinhart, H., Cohen, Z., *et al.* (2001). Genetic variation in the 5q31 cytokine gene cluster confers susceptibility to Crohn disease. *Nat Genet* 29: 223–228.

Risch, N. (1992). Corrections to linkage strategies for genetically complex traits. III. The effect of marker polymorphism on analysis of affected relative pairs. *Am J Hum Genet* 51: 673–675.

Risch, N. (2000). Searching for genetic determinants in the new millennium. *Nature* 405: 847–856.

Robertson, N.P., Fraser, M., Deans, J., Clayton, D., Walker, N., and Compston, D.A.S. (1996). Age-adjusted recurrence risks for relatives of patients with multiple sclerosis. *Brain* 119: 449–455.

Roden, D.M. and George, A.L. Jr (2002). The genetic basis of variability in drug responses. *Nat Rev Drug Discov* 1: 37–44.

Rogers, A.E., Meehan, J., Guilleminaul, C., Grumet, F.C., and Mignot, E. (1997). HLA DR15 (DR2) and DQB1*0602 typing studies in 188 narcoleptic patients with cataplexy. *Neurology* 48: 1550–1556.

Rogers, S.W., Andrews, P.I., Gahring, L.C., Whisenand, T., Cauley, K., Crain, B., *et al.* (1994). Autoantibodies to glutamate receptor GluR3 in Rasmussen's encephalitis. *Science* 265: 648–651.

Rood, M.J., Keijsers, V., van der Linden, M.W., Tong, T.Q., Borggreve, S.E., Verweij, C.L., *et al.* (1999). Neuropsychiatric systemic lupus erythematosus is associated with imbalance in interleukin 10 promoter haplotypes. *Ann Rheum Dis* 58: 85–89.

Rosati, G. (2001). The prevalence of multiple sclerosis in the world: an update. *Neurol Sci,* 22: 117–39.

Rubio, J.P., Bahlo, M., Butzkueven, H., van Der Mei, I.A., Sale, M.M., Dickinson, J.L., *et al.* (2002). Genetic dissection of the human leukocyte antigen region by use of haplotypes of Tasmanians with multiple sclerosis. *Am J Hum Genet* 70: 1125–1137.

Rybicki, B.A., Kirkey, K.L., Major, M., Maliarik, M.J., Popovich, J. Jr, Chase, G.A., *et al.* (2001). Familial risk ratio of sarcoidosis in African-American sibs and parents. *Am J Epidemiol* 153: 188–193.

Saarela, J., Schoenberg Fejzo, M., Chen, D., Finnila, S., Parkkonen, M., Kuokkanen, S., *et al.* (2002). Fine mapping of a multiple sclerosis locus to 2.5 Mb on chromosome 17q22–q24. *Hum Mol Genet* 11: 2257–2267.

Sadovnick, A.D., Armstrong, H., Rice, G.P.A., Bulman, D., Hashimoto, L., Paty, D.W., *et al.* (1993). A population-based study of multiple sclerosis in twins: update. *Ann Neurol* 33: 281–285.

Sadovnick, A.D., Ebers, G.C., Dyment, D.A., and Risch, N.J. (1996). Evidence for genetic basis of multiple sclerosis. *Lancet* 347: 1728–1730.

Sadovnick, A.D., Yee, I.M., and Ebers, G.C. (2000). Factors influencing sib risks for multiple sclerosis. *Clin Genet* 58: 431–435.

Salomon, B., Rhee, L., Bour-Jordan, H., Hsin, H., Montag, A., Soliven, B., *et al.* (2001). Development of spontaneous autoimmune peripheral polyneuropathy in B7-2- deficient NOD mice. *J Exp Med* 194: 677–684.

Salvarani, C., Boiardi, L., Casali, B., Olivieri, I., Ciancio, G., Cantini, F., *et al.* (2002). Endothelial nitric oxide synthase gene polymorphisms in Behcet's disease. *J Rheumatol* 29: 535–540.

Sawcer, S., Jones, H.B., Feakes, R., Gray, J., Smaldon, N., Chataway, J., *et al.* (1996). A genome screen in multiple sclerosis reveals susceptibility loci on chromosome 6p21 and 17q22. *Nat Genet* 13: 464–468.

Sawcer, S., Maranian, M., Setakis, E., Curwen, V., Akesson, E., Hensiek, A., et al. (2002). A whole genome screen for linkage disequilibrium in multiple sclerosis confirms disease associations with regions previously linked to susceptibility. Brain 125: 1337–1347.

Schmidt, S., Barcellos, L.F., DeSombre, K., Rimmler, J.B., Lincoln, R.R., Bucher, P., et al. (2002). Association of polymorphisms in the apolipoprotein E region with susceptibility to and progression of multiple sclerosis. Am J Hum Genet 70: 708–717.

Sciacca, F.L., Ferri, C., Veglia, F., Andreetta, F., Mantegazza, R., Cornelio, F., et al. (2002). IL-1 genes in myasthenia gravis: IL-1A -889 polymorphism associated with sex and age of disease onset. J Neuroimmunol 122: 94–99.

Seki, N., Yamaguchi, K., Yamada, A., Kamizono, S., Sugita, S., Taguchi, C., et al. (1999). Polymorphism of the 5'-flanking region of the tumor necrosis factor (TNF)-alpha gene and susceptibility to human T-cell lymphotropic virus type I (HTLV-I) uveitis. J Infect Dis 180: 880–883.

Shamim, E.A. and Miller, F.W. (2000). Familial autoimmunity and the idiopathic inflammatory myopathies. Curr Rheumatol Rep 2: 201–211.

Shamim, E.A., Rider, L.G., and Miller, F.W. (2000). Update on the genetics of the idiopathic inflammatory myopathies. Curr Opin Rheumatol 12: 482–491.

Shamim, E.A., Rider, L.G., Pandey, J.P., O'Hanlon, T.P., Jara, L.J., Samayoa, E.A., et al. (2002). Differences in idiopathic inflammatory myopathy phenotypes and genotypes between Mesoamerican Mestizos and North American Caucasians: ethnogeographic influences in the genetics and clinical expression of myositis. Arthritis Rheum 46: 1885–1893.

Shapiro, E., Krivit, W., Lockman, L., Jambaque, I., Peters, C., Cowan, M., et al. (2000). Long-term effect of bone-marrow transplantation for childhood-onset cerebral X-linked adrenoleukodystrophy. Lancet 356: 713–718.

Shinar, Y., Pras, E., Siev-Ner, I., Gamus, D., Brautbar, C., Israel, S., et al. (1998). Analysis of allelic association between D6S461 marker and multiple sclerosis in Ashkenazi and Iraqi Jewish patients. J Mol Neurosci 11: 265–269.

Shohat, B., Achiron, A., Narinski, R., Kochba, I., Sidi, Y., Sonada, S., et al. (1996). Possible HLA association with susceptibility to HTLV-1 tropical spastic paraparesis in Israel in Iranian Jews as compared to HTLV 1-associated myelopathy in Japan. Tissue Antigens 48: 136–138.

Smith, K.J., Pyrdol, J., Gauthier, L., Wiley, D.C., and Wucherpfennig, K.W. (1998). Crystal structure of HLA-DR2 (DRA*0101, DRB1*1501) complexed with a peptide from human myelin basic protein. J Exp Med 188: 1511–1520.

Sriram, U., Barcellos, L.F., Villoslada, P., Rio, J., Baranzini, S.E., Caillier, S., et al. (2003). Pharmacogenomic analysis of interferon receptor polymorphisms in multiple sclerosis. Genes Immun 4: 147–152.

Suzuki, S., Kuwana, M., Yasuoka, H., Tanaka, K., Fukuuchi, Y., and Kawakami, Y. (2001). Heterogeneous immunogenetic background in Japanese adults with myasthenia gravis. J Neurol Sci 189: 59–64.

Takada, T., Suzuki, E., Morohashi, K., and Gejyo, F. (2002). Association of single nucleotide polymorphisms in the IL-18 gene with sarcoidosis in a Japanese population. Tissue Antigens 60: 36–42.

Takeno, M., Kariyone, A., Yamashita, N., Takiguchi, M., Mizushima, Y., Kaneoka, H., et al. (1995). Excessive function of peripheral blood neutrophils from patients with Behcet's disease and from HLA-B51 transgenic mice. Arthritis Rheum 38: 426–433.

The Transatlantic Multiple Sclerosis Cooperative (2001). A meta-analysis of genomic screens in multiple sclerosis. Mult Scler 7: 3–11.

Twyman, R.E., Gahring, L.C., Spiess, J., and Rogers, S.W. (1995). Glutamate receptor antibodies activate a subset of receptors and reveal an agonist binding site. Neuron 14: 755–762.

Usuku, K., Sonoda, S., Osame, M., Yashiki, S., Takahashi, K., Matsumoto, M., et al. (1988). HLA haplotype-linked high immune responsiveness against HTLV-I in HTLV-I-associated myelopathy: comparison with adult T-cell leukemia/lymphoma. Ann Neurol 23: S143–S150.

Usuku, K., Nishizawa, M., Matsuki, K., Tokunaga, K., Takahashi, K., Eiraku, N., et al. (1990). Association of a particular amino acid sequence of the HLA-DR beta 1 chain with HTLV-I-associated myelopathy. Eur J Immunol 20: 1603–1606.

van der Pol, W.L., van den Berg, L.H., Scheepers, R.H., van der Bom, J.G., van Doorn, P.A., van Koningsveld, R., et al. (2000). IgG receptor IIa alleles determine susceptibility and severity of Guillain–Barre syndrome. Neurology 54: 1661–1665.

Villoslada, P., Barcellos, L., Rio, J., Begovich, A., Tintore, M., Sastre-Garriga, J., et al. (2002). The HLA locus and multiple sclerosis in Spain. Role in disease susceptibility, clinical course and response to interferon-beta. J Neuroimmunol 130: 194–201.

Vine, A.M., Witkover, A.D., Lloyd, A.L., Jeffery, K.J., Siddiqui, A., Marshall, S.E., et al. (2002). Polygenic control of human T lymphotropic virus type I (HTLV-I) provirus load and the risk of HTLV-I-associated myelopathy/tropical spastic paraparesis. J Infect Dis 186: 932–939.

Vining, E.P.G., Freeman, J.M., Brandt, J., Carson, B.S., and Uematsu, S. (1993). Progressive unilateral encephalopathy of childhood (Rasmussen's syndrome): a reappraisal. Epilepsia 34: 639–650.

Wang, D.G., Fan, J.B., Siao, C.J., Berno, A., Young, P., Sapolsky, R., et al. (1998). Large-scale identification, mapping, and genotyping of single- nucleotide polymorphisms in the human genome. Science 280: 1077–1082.

Whitehouse, W.P., Rees, M., Curtis, D., Sundqvist, A., Parker, K., Chung, E., et al. (1993). Linkage analysis of idiopathic generalized epilepsy (IGE) and marker loci on chromosome 6p in families of patients with juvenile myoclonic epilepsy: no evidence for an epilepsy locus in the HLA region. Am J Hum Genet 53: 652–662.

Wise, L.H., Lanchbury, J.S., and Lewis, C.M. (1999). Meta-analysis of genome searches. Ann Hum Genet 63: 263–272.

Wyss-Coray, T., Yan, F., Lin, A.H., Lambris, J.D., Alexander, J.J., Quigg, R.J., et al. (2002). Prominent neurodegeneration and increased plaque formation in complement-inhibited Alzheimer's mice. Proc Natl Acad Sci USA 99: 10837–10842.

Zareparsi, S., James, D.M., Kaye, J.A., Bird, T.D., Schellenberg, G.D., and Payami, H. (2002). HLA-A2 homozygosity but not heterozygosity is associated with Alzheimer disease. Neurology 58: 973–975.

Zelano, G., Settesoldi, D., Lino, M.M., Batocchi, A., Evoli, A., and Tonali, P.A. (1999). Thymic disorders and myasthenia gravis: genetic aspects. Ann Med 31(Suppl. 2): 46–51.

Zorzetto, M., Bombieri, C., Ferrarotti, I., Medaglia, S., Agostini, C., Tinelli, C., et al. (2002). Complement receptor 1 gene polymorphisms in sarcoidosis. Am J Respir Cell Mol Biol 27: 17–23.

10 Principles of immune–virus interactions in the nervous system

Pierre J. Talbot, Hélène Jacomy, and Edith Gruslin

Autoimmunity and viruses

Autoimmunity

The immune system must be able to defend the host from pathogens by triggering a response to non-self (foreign) antigens, while avoiding a response to its own (self) antigens. During the development of B cells, this tolerance is achieved by several mechanisms such as clonal deletion, anergy, maturation stop, and receptor editing (for a review see Tsubata and Honjo (2000)). Different mechanisms are involved in the induction of T-cell tolerance: peripheral tolerance, ignorance, regulatory cells, and clonal deletion. T-cell tolerance is induced in the thymus by clonal deletion of T cells in which the receptor (TCR) strongly recognizes complexes composed of self-peptide and the major histocompatibility complex (MHC) molecule (Kappler et al., 1987; Kretz-Rommel and Rubin, 2000). Some potentially autoreactive T cells escape this negative selection and proceed to the periphery. This is possible because of positive selection, either due to cells having a low affinity or avidity for a self-peptide linked to an MHC on the surface of a thymic antigen presenting cell (APC) (Datta, 2000), or, if cells are low in number, or it may simply be that the autoantigen is not expressed in the thymus (Benoist and Mathis, 1998). These T cells are benign as long as they are at rest. To be activated, the autoreactive cell must receive both a specific signal, a TCR linked to a self antigen–MHC complex, and a non-specific signal, from professional APC co-stimulation (Steinman, 1991; Barnaba, 1996). Once activated, the autoreactive T cell can induce either direct damage, by cytotoxic action or cytokine release, or indirect damage, by T-cell dependent pathogenic antibody production (Nauclér et al., 1996). However, natural killer (NK) T cells may protect the mouse from an autoimmune response (Gombert et al., 1996; Sharif et al., 2001; Singh et al., 2001). Once an autoimmune response is induced, damage may result, leading to autoimmune disease.

Autoimmune diseases affect 3 to 5% of the general population (Jacobson et al., 1997). These are triggered by a particular population of autoreactive T or B cells specific to a given antigen. They can be organ-specific or systemic, depending on whether the target antigen is expressed in only one organ or widely in the host (Marrack et al., 2001). Specific organ autoimmune disease, such as type 1 diabetes or multiple sclerosis (MS), is characterized by chronic inflammation, tissue destruction, and loss of function of the target organ (Shi et al, 2001). In spite of the association of some genes, such as MHC genes, with different autoimmune diseases (Merriman and Todd, 1995), the precise etiology of this kind of pathology remains unknown. Why are autoreactive cells, observed at physiological levels in normal subjects (Carnaud and Bach, 1993), activated at a specific moment leading to pathology for only some individuals? It is often suggested that triggering of the disease process requires an environmental factor, such as an infection, to activate an autoreactive population that was already present in a genetically predisposed individual (Aichele et al., 1996; Barnaba, 1996; Gianani and Sarvetnick, 1996). The following section describes different mechanisms that have been proposed to explain the activation of such a population following a viral infection. These mechanisms imply an immune response more harmful to the host than the original pathogen (Benoist and Mathis, 1998).

Bystander effects

In this scenario, autoreactive T cells are not specifically activated by a self antigen but by cytokines liberated at the inflammation site. The virus plays an adjuvant role in inducing inflammatory cytokine production to increase host protection, resulting in development of an autoimmune disease (Fairweather et al., 2001).

Thus, the host immune response would lead to specific T-cell activation following a viral infection. An activated T cell can bind to the vascular cell adhesion molecule (VCAM-1) on the endothelium by a very late antigen (VLA-4), and next bind to the endothelial wall (Fabbri et al., 1999). The T cell then penetrates the endothelial wall by extravasation and finds itself in the infected organ. Once at the site, the activated T cell secretes pro-inflammatory cytokines such as interferon-gamma (IFN-γ) and tumor necrosis factor-alpha (TNF-α), which play different roles (Boehm et al., 1997). These are in particular responsible for an increase in expression of adhesion molecules at the surface of the epithelial cell (Botazzo et al., 1983). In addition, IFN-γ induces chemokine secretion (as CCL2, also named MCP-1 (monocyte chemoattractant protein), RANTES, MIP (macrophage inflammatory protein)-1α and 1β) that is chemoattractant for monocytes and lymphocytes (Boehm et al, 1997). The increased presence of adhesion molecules combined with chemokine secretion results in a non-specific recruitment of inflammatory cells. In this way, a pool of T cells is conducted to the inflamed organ. Recruited T cells may then proliferate in response to cytokines, without any consideration for antigen specificity (Unutmaz et al., 1994; Tough et al., 1996). Memory T cells stimulated by pro-inflammatory cytokines even demonstrate an effector function. Thus, a cellular response is triggered with no stimulation from the TCR.

Nevertheless, the biological relevance of non-specific activation in autoimmunity is controversial. Some studies indicate that most of the CD8+ and CD4+ T cells found at the site of pathology are antigen-specific (Murali-Krishna et al., 1998; Haring et al., 2001). There is a lack of consensus concerning the non-specific activation of effector T cells suggested by some (Ehl et al., 1997; Murali-Krishna et al., 1998) and contested by others (Ke et al., 1998). Moreover, non-specific stimulation can have different effects depending on its duration and whether the cells are naïve or memory cells (Di Rosa and Barnaba, 1998).

If inflammation alone does not lead to a non-specific activation sufficient to induce an autoimmune disease it could, however, allow an autoreactive immune lymphocytic population a means to penetrate the target organ. Indeed, it is possible that autoreactive cells specific to a self antigen expressed in the target organ may be found amongst cells recruited to the inflamed site. In addition, an increase in cytokine production can contribute to division of activated T cells (Wucherpfennig, 2001). Thus, a reaction specifically directed towards a self antigen could be triggered (Barnaba, 1996).

Several factors contribute to the release of self and non-self antigens following inflammation due to a viral infection. Viral cytopathic effects, pro-inflammatory cytokine and chemokine recruitment and activation of non-specific T cells and monocytes at the inflammation site as well as the direct action of some cytokines cause cell death and tissue destruction, thus increasing antigen release (Barnaba, 1996; Horwitz and Sarvetnick, 1999). This increased presence of antigen promotes antigenic presentation.

In addition, there are several reasons why pro-inflammatory cytokines are responsible for an improvement in the efficiency of antigen presentation. They induce an increase in the expression of cell surface molecules, both co-stimulation (Panoutsakopoulou and Cantor, 2001) and MHC (Botazzo *et al.*, 1983) molecules. Furthermore, inflammatory response leads to complete maturation of dendritic cells that migrate towards secondary lymphoid organs to stimulate naïve T cells (Banchereau and

Steinman, 1998). In this context, the antigen-presenting cell (APC) will not only present viral antigen more efficiently, but also present self antigen released by damaged cells from the inflamed tissue.

To sum up, viral infection may induce an autoimmune response by causing inflammation at the infection site (see Fig. 10.1). Pro-inflammatory cytokines lead to non-specific immune cell recruitment and allow for T-cell activation. Autoreactive T cells specific to the self antigen present in the target organ may be found amongst the recruited cells. Moreover, tissue destruction causes release of self antigens. Autoreactive T cells present at

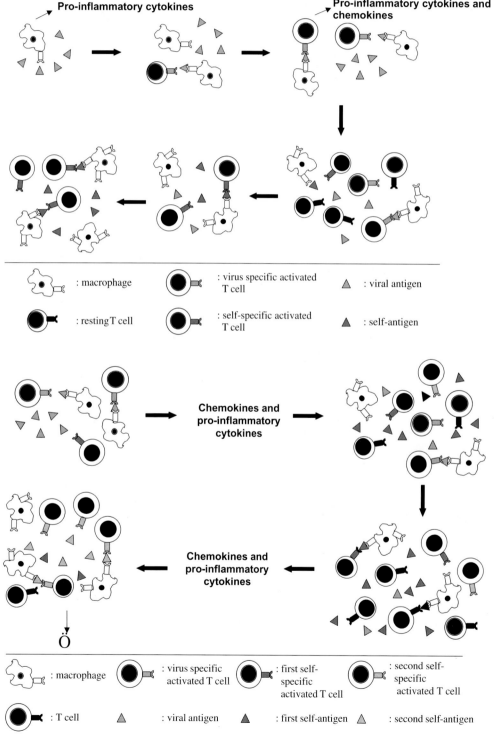

Fig. 10.1 Consequences of inflammation caused by a viral infection on induction of an autoimmune response. Phagocytosis of viral antigens by macrophages leads to release of pro-inflammatory cytokines and T-cell recruitment at the infection site. A T cell specific for viral antigen recognizes antigen presented by an antigen-presenting cell (APC), which leads to release of cytokines and chemokines in correlation with antigenic presentation efficiency. Death of the infected cell and tissue damage caused by inflammation allow release of self antigens. Amongst the population of recruited T cells found at the site can be a self-reactive subpopulation. The self-reactive T cell to which the self antigen is presented by an APC is activated and then divides. An autoimmune response is now engaged.

Fig. 10.2 Role of epitope (determinant) spreading in antoimmnne response following viral infection. In an inflammatory context, cell death and tissue damage lead to release of self antigens. The T cell recruited under these conditions and that is specific for a self antigen can then be activated. This T cell divides and a first autoimmune response takes place. Inflammation is maintained and tissue damage continues, thus exposing a second self antigen. A specific T cell recognizes this second self antigen and an autoimmune response is now directed against this antigen. A succession of autoimmune reactions is triggered in this inflammatory context.

the inflammation site may then respond via their TCR to a self antigen presented efficiently by APC in the context of an inflammation.

Epitope spreading

A second mechanism which may explain how a viral infection can lead to a chronic autoimmune disease is epitope spreading. Inflammation caused by an infection induces release of pro-inflammatory cytokines. These cytokines increase production of cellular (Frosch *et al.*, 1993; Opdenakker and Van Damme, 1994) and extracellular (Paroli *et al.*, 2000) proteases, which expose and degrade cryptic epitopes, thus facilitating their presentation by MHC (Kozwloski *et al.*, 1992; Sherman *et al.*, 1992; Accapezzato *et al.*, 1998). The immune response to the triggering antigen is then directed towards those antigens newly exposed at the inflammation site. Protease inhibitors can block the development of experimental allergic encephalomyelitis (EAE) (Brosnan *et al.*, 1980). Epitope spreading is the phenomenon by which autoreactive T cells are activated *de novo* by self antigen released following tissue damage caused by inflammation (Vanderlugt *et al.*, 2000) (see Fig. 10.2).

Epitope spreading has been demonstrated in the murine model of EAE (Lehmann *et al.*, 1992). Lehmann and his collaborators showed that the immunodominant epitope associated with induction of EAE was different from epitopes responsible for the immune response during the chronic stage of disease. Moreover, T cells from mice in which EAE was induced by myelin basic protein (MBP) showed a proliferative response to proteolipid protein (PLP) (Perry *et al.*, 1991; Cross *et al.*, 1993). Epitope spreading was found in an insulin-dependent murine model of diabetes (Kaufman *et al.*, 1993). Non-obese diabetic (NOD) mice were used by Lehmann's team in an experiment demonstrating that the immune response was initially directed towards glutamate decarboxylase, an antigen found in pancreatic islets, then toward others pancreatic beta cell antigens (Kaufman *et al.*, 1993). In addition, epitope spreading is supported by studies conducted with a murine model of demyelination induced by Theiler's murine encephalomyelitis virus (TMEV). The immune response induced by TMEV infection is first directed towards the virus, then towards epitopes from PLP and myelin oligodendrocyte glycoprotein (MOG) (Miller *et al.*, 1997).

The epitope spreading cascade follows a constant and predictable order (Tuohy *et al.*, 1998; Vanderlugt *et al.*, 2000). This order is determined by frequency and avidity of the T cells involved (Vanderlugt *et al.*, 2000; Tian *et al.*, 2001). Regression of the primary response could be explained by various mechanisms: clonal exhaustion and deletion at the periphery, T-cell anergy, or T-cell suppression by other cell populations (Tuohy *et al.*, 1999). In other respects, involvement of epitope spreading in pathogenicity has been demonstrated by tolerance studies in which the autoimmune response cascade was blocked. Thus, tolerance induction with TMEV epitopes before infection prevented disease induction (Karpus *et al.*, 1995), whereas induction of tolerance for different epitopes involved in the EAE epitope spreading cascade inhibited disease progression (McRae *et al.*, 1995; Yu *et al.*, 1996).

There is no more consensus concerning the theory of epitope (determinant) spreading as an explanation of the link between viral infections and autoimmune disease than for any other proposed theory. A longitudinal study conducted on the murine model of EAE induced by different peptides did not demonstrate epitope spreading, but rather a response remaining centered on the epitope used to induce the pathology (Takacs and Altmann, 1998). Furthermore, a study of rats before, during, and after EAE showed a natural heterogeneous response against MBP, which restricted itself to a dominant epitope during disease to become once again heterogeneous following remission (Mor and Cohen, 1993).

In short, the epitope spreading theory requires that the response directed against the antigen at the triggering of the disease attenuates itself to make way for new reactions directed against self antigens determined by a constant hierarchy. This phenomenon would contribute to the relapsing–remitting episodes and chronicity of autoimmune diseases.

Molecular mimicry

A third mechanism that has been proposed to link viral infections and autoimmune diseases is molecular mimicry. Molecular mimicry is based on the activation of autoreactive T cells following cross-recognition by TCR of a pathogen and a self epitope (Oldstone, 1987; Miller *et al.*, 2001) (see summary in Fig. 10.3). This recognition of different epitopes by the same TCR is possible because of the flexibility and degeneration of TCRs.

Nanda *et al.* (1995) have demonstrated that the TCR is flexible and can link different peptides presented by the same MHC molecule. Moreover, an analysis by substitution from a peptide antigen has shown that a peptide having only one amino acid in common with the starting peptide can be recognized by a TCR (Evavold *et al.*, 1995). Studies undertaken with combinatory peptide libraries demonstrate a still greater flexibility of TCR, concluding that T cells can recognize thousands of different peptides (Hemmer *et al.*, 1997, 2000). Transgenic mice expressing only one peptide associated with MHC Class II allowed positive selection of CD4+ T cells expressing different TCR (Ignatowicz *et al.*, 1996; Tourne *et al.*, 1997). These two approaches, that is to say one T cell recognizing several peptides and one MHC–peptide complex allowing the selection of different T cells, appear to demonstrate the degeneration of TCR recognition.

Homologies found between virus sequences and normal constituent host cells are well characterized (Lane and Hoeffler, 1980; Clarke *et al.*, 1983; Fujinami *et al.*, 1983; Haynes *et al.*; 1983; Talbot, 1997; Talbot *et al.*, 2001). Induction by a viral peptide of either antibodies having a double recognition or lymphoid cells proliferating upon autoantigen stimulation were demonstrated using rabbits immunized with a peptide of the polymerase from hepatitis B virus sharing a sequence of six consecutive amino acids with MBP (Fujinami and Oldstone, 1985). It was subsequently shown that sequence identity is not necessary for molecular mimicry: one TCR can recognize several peptides having a similar conformation (Wucherpfennig and Strominger, 1995).

Thus, T-cell receptors are flexible (Nanda *et al.*, 1995) and the same TCR can recognize peptides from different origins but having similar structure (Wucherpfennig and Strominger, 1995). Can an antigen from an infectious agent having a structure similar to a self antigen activate autoreactive cells resting in the periphery? Studies of transgenic mice expressing lymphocytic

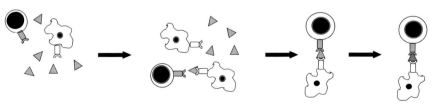

Fig. 10.3 Molecular mimicry in autoimmunity. During a viral infection, the T-cell receptor (TCR) recognizes a foreign antigen and the T cell is activated. Then, the latter can migrate to a target organ, where the TCR recognizes a self antigen. An autoimmune response follows.

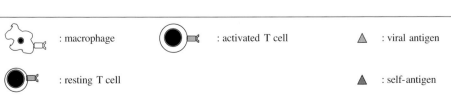

choriomeningitis virus (LCMV) glycoprotein or nucleoprotein on pancreatic beta cells demonstrated a strong cytotoxic response against viral antigen following LCMV infection (Ohashi *et al.*, 1991; Oldstone *et al.*, 1991). It is thus fair to say that viral antigen (considered in this case as a self antigen) in the periphery does not induce tolerance at the time of a subsequent infection. These experiments indicate an absence of tolerance or ignorance and open the door to the molecular mimicry principle, although they do not demonstrate the relevance of the mechanism in reality, where mimicry is never that exact (Albert and Inman, 1999).

Different experimental models suggest the presence of molecular mimicry following infection. *Salmonella typhimurium* infection involves a CD8+ T-cell response against an immunodominant epitope (GroEL); these CD8+ lymphocytes also recognize a peptide from a self protein (hsp60) (Lo *et al.*, 2000). In another model, transgenic mice expressing lymphocytic choriomeningitis virus (LCMV) glycoprotein or nucleoprotein on oligodendrocytes develop a CNS disease after a peripheral infection by LCMV (Evans *et al.*, 1996). Infection by a modified TMEV encoding a PLP peptide induced a demyelinating disease in mice (Olson *et al.*, 2001). Moreover, mouse infection by another modified TMEV coding for a *Haemophilus influenzae* peptide sharing six of 13 amino acids with a PLP immunodominant peptide induces a demyelinating disease (Olson *et al.*, 2001). Molecular mimicry is supported by another model: herpes simplex virus (HSV) induces herpes simplex keratitis (HSK). In this case, there is T-cell cross-reactivity between virus protein UL6 and a cornea antigen as well as an IgG2a derivate peptide (Avery *et al.*, 1995). Mice susceptible to HSK become resistant to it if they are tolerized by G2a peptide before infection (Avery *et al.*, 1995). Further, infection by an HSV mutant not expressing the epitope shared by cornea self antigen and IgG2a does not induce any autoimmune disease (Zhao *et al.*, 1998).

In humans, molecular mimicry is suggested in different neurological inflammatory diseases:

(1) in MS pathology by the presence of T cells recognizing both MBP and coronavirus (Talbot *et al.*, 1996, 2001);

(2) in Guillain–Barré syndrome by the high prevalence of *Campylobacter jejuni* infection preceding the appearance of disease (Rees *et al.*, 1995), coupled with a sharing of the epitopes of the micro-organism with gangliosides expressed in human peripheral nerves and the presence of autoantibodies against these gangliosides (Sheikh *et al.*, 1998);

(3) in patients affected by human T lymphotropic virus (HTLV-1), which is associated with myelopathy/tropical spastic paraparesis (HAM/TSP), a disease similar to MS, by the presence of antibodies recognizing both HTLV-1 and neurons (Levin *et al.*, 2002).

In addition, approximately 10% of arthritis observed in patients infected by *Borrelia burgdorferi,* causing Lyme disease, is resistant to antibiotic therapy (Benoist and Mathis, 2001). Persistence of arthritis in spite of the absence of spirochete DNA suggests an autoimmune disease similar to the association established between MHC and resistance to antibiotic therapy (Benoist and Mathis, 2001). The cross-reaction involved here occurs between bacterial outer surface protein A (OspA) and lymphocyte function-associated antigen 1 (LFA-1) (Gross *et al.*, 1998) and has been demonstrated at the clonal level (Trollmo *et al.*, 2001)

Once again, this theory is controversial. In Lyme disease, on the one hand, only 10% of anti-OspA clones also proliferate against LFA-1a. The absence of a murine model mitigates against establishing with certainty that molecular mimicry is not an epiphenomenon (Benoist and Mathis, 2001). In addition, molecular mimicry induced by HSV between virus UL6 peptide and a cornea antigen as an IgG2a peptide in the HSK model is also put in question by some observations. Deshande *et al.* (2001) did not succeed in demonstrating specific response to HSV UL6 peptide following infection of mice with HSV. Moreover, T cells recognizing peptide UL6 from mice immunized with this peptide fail to recognize either peptide G2a or HSK-infected cells (Deshande *et al.*, 2001). On the other hand, transgenic mice expressing only one TCR specific to ovalbumin developed HSK following HSV-1 infection, even if their TCR is monoclonal and does not show any detectable response against HSV-1 antigen (Deshande *et al.*, 2001).

In brief, molecular mimicry supports the idea that TCR can recognize both viral antigen and self antigen. During a viral infection, the T lymphocyte recognizes a viral peptide and is activated. Then, the T lymphocyte migrates to a target organ, where it cross-reacts with a self antigen. At this point, an autoimmune response is initiated.

Superantigen

Superantigens (SAg) are proteins, originating primarily from bacteria or a virus, that link MHC II of an APC to the Vβ domain of a TCR outside the antigen groove (Nakagawa and Harrison, 1996; Torres and Johnson, 1998)

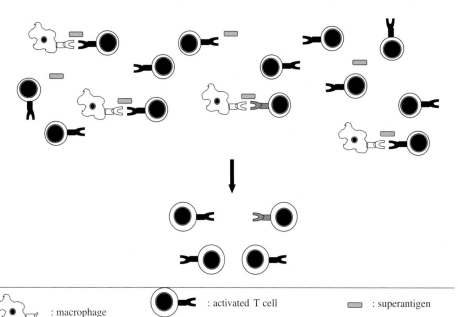

Fig. 10.4 Polyclonal activation of T cells by a superantigen (SAg). A SAg links MHC II and the Vβ domain of the T-cell receptor. Several T cells are activated this way, of which a fraction can be specific to a self antigen.

: macrophage   : activated T cell   : superantigen

: resting T cell   : self-specific activated T cell

(see Fig. 10.4). This contact between lateral areas of the TCR and MHC activates T cells with no regard for peptide–MHC specificity (Hodstev *et al.*, 1998). An important proportion (5 to 20%) of the T-cell population can be activated by this mechanism (Li *et al.*, 1999) and a part of this pool of activated T cells can be specific to a self antigen (Wucherpfennig, 2001).

In the PL/J mouse EAE, Vβ8 T cells are important for triggering disease (Acha-Orbea *et al.*, 1988). In mice immunized with an MBP peptide or having received T cells specific to MBP, injection of an SAg activating Vβ T cells (staphylococcal enterotoxin B, SEB) induces the following: (1) disease exacerbation in mice already affected, (2) relapses in remitting mice, or (3) appearance of symptoms in mice that had no clinical disease (Brocke *et al.*, 1993; Schiffenbauer *et al.*, 1993). Moreover, arthritis in mice immunized with collagen is exacerbated or triggered by SAg from *Mycoplasma arthritidis* (Cole and Griffiths, 1993). Therefore, SAg can lead to expansion of the autoreactive population and to clinical signs of disease (Schiffenbauer *et al.*, 1998).

SAg has been implicated in the autoimmune response in humans. For example, in rheumatoid arthritis patients, the Vβ14 T-cell frequency found in synovial fluid of the joints is higher than that found in peripheral blood (Paliard *et al.*, 1991). Moreover, SAg can activate synoviocytes to express different pro-inflammatory cytokines and chemokines (Mourad *et al.*, 1992; Mehindate *et al.*, 1994). Activation of T cells by SAg presented by synovial cells is also possible (Origuchi *et al.*, 1995). The implication of SAg in type 1 diabetes was suggested by the results of a study demonstrating a selective expansion of the Vβ7 T-cell population infiltrating the pancreas of diabetic patients (Conrad *et al.*, 1994). Moreover, the proportion of Vβ7 T cells in mononucleated cells of peripheral blood was found to be higher in patients than in controls; this proportion is also higher in recently diagnosed patients than in those with long-established chronic diabetes (Luppi *et al.*, 2000). In addition, an endogenous retrovirus coding for a SAg inducing Vβ7 T-cell proliferation has been isolated and found in diabetic patients, but not in controls (Conrad *et al.*, 1997). Overall, these studies suggest that SAg can be associated with autoimmune diseases.

Evidence of an association between SAg and autoimmune disease in humans is more circumstantial (Schiffenbauer *et al.*, 1998). Of the three mechanisms described above, the role of SAg in autoimmune diseases has not been consistently observed in different studies. For example, results of work by Conrad *et al.* (1994) implied that SAg is coded by an endogenous retrovirus in type 1 diabetes. Whereas another research team was unable to detect the DNA of this retrovirus in any subject, either diabetic or controls (Muir *et al.*, 1999), and other laboratories refer to the ubiquity of the sequence of the retrovirus involved, in both diabetics and in controls (Badenhoop *et al.*, 1999; Jaeckel *et al.*, 1999), or at least to a highly homologous sequence (Kim *et al.*, 1999). The results of these studies seriously challenge the plausibility of an association between SAg and an autoimmune pathology in humans.

Finally, SAg could activate several lymphocytes having a certain Vβ. Autoreactive cells can be found amongst the activated T-cell pool. Thus, SAg may play a role in autoimmune reaction and be involved in relapses and exacerbations of disease (Wucherpfennig, 2001). Although some studies undertaken with animal models and a few observations on humans are consistent with this theory, it remains controversial. The final proof to end this controversy has not yet been achieved.

Conclusions on autoimmunity and viruses

Different theories explaining the link between infections and autoimmune diseases have been presented in this section. Autoreactive T cells may be activated (1) indirectly in an inflammatory context, (2) through epitope (determinant) spreading, (3) as a result of a cross-reactivity of TCR between self and non-self antigen or (4) through a superantigen. None of these theories is accepted unequivocally as the explanation for the etiology of autoimmune pathology. Nevertheless, it is important to bear in mind that these mechanisms are not mutually exclusive. It is possible that they are involved in different steps of the autoimmune pathway (Wucherpfennig, 2001).

Viruses in the central nervous system (CNS)

Virus and microglial cell activation

Microglial cells seem to act as APC in the CNS in the course of local immune responses (for a review see Aloisi (2001) and Cross and Woodroofe (2001)). These cells can be transformed from a resting state to an activated state in certain pathophysiological conditions. This activation is characterized by morphological and immunophenotypical changes (Gehrmann *et al.*, 1995; Nakajima and Kohsoka, 1998; Streit *et al.*, 1999). Microglial cells are one of the principal elements of initiation of defense mechanisms against toxic agents in the CNS. However, activated microglial cells can also be responsible for damage to surrounding cells, following pro-inflammatory cytokine secretion. Neurotoxicity of microglial cells is suspected in several experimental and natural encephalopathies.

Microglial cells can be the targets of some viruses or they can be recruited by different pro-inflammatory signals produced following infections. Some viruses are neurotropic for glial cells, meaning that they can infect these cells in the nervous system, including microglial cells residing in the CNS. Viruses can also infect monocytes, which can become macrophage/microglial cells of the CNS. This infection can be acute or chronic and can lead to a persistence of the virus in the cells. Microglial cells are the main target of human or simian immunodeficiency virus (HIV or SIV) in the brain, an infection that leads to the development of dementia associated with neuro-AIDS (Xiong *et al.*, 2000; Smits *et al.*, 2000; Lawrence and Major, 2002; Williams and Hickey, 2002). Nevertheless, the mechanisms underlying neurological deterioration associated with HIV remain unclear. There is no formal proof indicating that activated microglial cells really lead to the development of neurodegenerative lesions, such as those found in Alzheimer's disease, HIV-related dementia, or multiple sclerosis (MS). The role of microglial cells as targets or potentializators of these pathologies remains to be determined.

Positive effects of immune factors release by microglial cells: lessons from studies with murine coronavirus

Some strains of the murine coronavirus 'mouse hepatitis virus' (MHV) are neurotropic and neuroinvasive and can cause neurological disorders in rodents in a biphasic fashion, from acute encephalitis to chronic and recurring demyelination (Haring and Perlman, 2001). The antiviral effect of CD8+ T cells seems to be related to direct lysis of infected cells. However, CD8+ and CD4+ T cells can also have an indirect impact through cytokine secretion (Biron, 1994). Several findings indicate that cytokines contribute to virus clearance as well as protection from MHV. During CNS infection by MHV-JHM, there is a notable increase of mRNA encoding interleukin(IL)-1 (α and β), IL-4, IL-6, IL-10, TNF-α, and IFN-γ at the point at which the virus is cleared, which coincides in time with infiltration of mononucleated cells (Pearce *et al.*, 1994; Parra *et al.*, 1997). Release of IL-6, TNF-α, and iNOS is also seen in the CNS during acute MHV-JHM infection (Sun *et al.*, 1995; Stohlman *et al.*, 1995*b,c*; Lane *et al.*, 1997) while IL-1β, IL-6, TNF-α, and iNOS are found in the CNS of chronically infected mice (Sun *et al.*, 1995). Moreover, MHV-JHM infection of endothelial cells and astrocytes induces IL-6 production (Joseph *et al.*, 1993). IL-6 has been described as essential to myelomonocyte recruitment and glial cell activation (Penkowa *et al.*, 1999, 2000).

IFN-γ seems to be involved in resistance to MHV infection (in some mouse strains or as a function of age) by a mechanism linked to macrophages (Lucchiari and Pereira, 1989, 1990). It has been demonstrated that neutralization of IFN-γ secretion induced by MHV-JHM infection causes a major increase in pathology and precipitates death of the mice (Smith *et al.*, 1991). IFN-γ seems to be essential for optimal activation and migration of macrophages or microglial cells in the white matter of the spinal cord, but does not seem to facilitate lymphocyte entry into the CNS (Pewe and Perlman, 2002). It is now well known that oligodendrocytes proliferate in response to CNS lesions in demyelinating disease. Studies have shown that there are factors in demyelinating lesions that aid in the proliferation and differentiation of the progenitors of glial cells in oligodendrocytes, in order to repair myelin (Prayoonwiwat and Rodriguez, 1993). In the same way, grafting of microglial cells after spinal cord damage can promote the development of neuritis (Rabchevsky and Streit, 1997). *In vitro*, activated microglial cells can secrete neurotrophic factors such as brain-derived neurotrophic factor (BDNF) or nerve growth factor (NGF) (Heese *et al.*, 1997; Nakajima *et al.*, 2002). It has also been shown, *in vitro*, that activated microglial cells interact with astrocytes and can increase local release of IL-6, which could increase astrocyte reaction and neuroprotection (Eskes *et al*, 2002). Taken together these findings are evidence of a positive role of microglial cells and the release of some factors in the remyelination process.

Negative effects of immune factors release by microglial cells

Production of inflammatory molecules may have a cytotoxic effect on the surrounding cells in the CNS. Indeed, oligodendrocytes are susceptible to exposure to TNF-α or IL-1 (Oldstone, 1991). The activation of macrophages and microglial cells by inflammatory mediators, such as basic fibroblast growth factor (bFGF) or NGF, increases the expression and activity of cathepsin S (a cysteine lysosomal protease) on macrophage/microglial cells (Liuzzo *et al.*, 1999). *In vitro*, cathepsin S is able to degrade MBP as β-amyloid peptide, which explains the attainment of a fragile balance between the recruitment of macrophages/microglial cells by inflammatory signals and the start of tissue damage. However, cathepsin S activity can be beneficial and necessary for the elimination of the remains of myelin.

A recent study demonstrated that coadministration of pro-inflammatory mediators (IFN-γ, TNF-α) in cerebrospinal fluid affects mature oligodendrocytes and activates microglial cells, which is then accompanied by astrocyte activation and the proliferation of oligodendrocyte precursors (Kong *et al.*, 2002). This demonstrates a toxic effect of molecules secreted by glial cells on the mature oligodendrocytes of the CNS at the same time as their ability to stimulate oligodendrocyte precursors in the adult brain.

Activated microglial cells are suspected of playing a pathogenic role in immune-mediated neurodegenerative disease. Thus, microglial cell activation by IFN-γ induces a marked reduction in neuron survival. Transgenic mice in which IFN-γ expression is under the transcriptional control of the MBP gene reveal hypomyelination and reactive gliosis (macrophages/microglial cells), indicating that IFN-γ is a key element in immune-mediated demyelination (Corbin *et al.*, 1996). *In vitro* studies support the hypothesis that microglial cells are at the source of release of neurocytotoxic free radicals, such as NO, which would explain the additional mechanisms of immune-mediated CNS damage. Moreover, NO production decreases NGF released by astrocytes (Xiong *et al.*, 1999).

Recently, the development of transgenic mice has contributed a great deal to an understanding of the role of some cytokines. IL-12 is a cytokine produced by microglial cells that can regulate cellular immunity locally in the CNS. In transgenic mice having astrocytes that produce IL-12, immunization induces an immune CNS pathology, infiltration of T cells (CD4+ and CD8+) and macrophages/microglial cells, and the expression of cytokines (IFN-γ and TNF), chemokines (IP-10 and RANTES), MHC Class II molecules, and NO synthase-2 (Lassman *et al.*, 2001). This indicates that the cytokine environment in tissue can dramatically influence intrinsic immune response and associated pathology. In the same way, transgenic mice producing IL-3 chronically develop motor difficulties at the demyelination and remyelination phases associated with proliferation, recruitment, and activation of macrophages/microglial cells (Chiang *et al.*, 1996).

In conclusion, neurotrophic and neurotoxic roles have been attributed to microglial cells in neurodenegerative diseases. These cells may increase neurodegeneration associated with the presence of a virus in releasing neurotoxic and/or pro- or anti-inflammatory molecules. On the other hand, they may support regeneration by releasing growth factors or isolating and eliminating infected (or damaged) neurons as well as myelin fragments. A better understanding of parameters governing the fragile balance between the negative and the positive effects of microglial cell activation remains essential to our knowledge of the pathogenesis of several neurodegenerative diseases, whether or not infectious agents are involved.

Human coronavirus, strain OC43 (HCoV-OC43), a newly recognized CNS pathogen

The coronaviruses are suspected of being among a number of viruses infecting the CNS. Coronaviruses are a family of respiratory and enteric viruses infecting animals and humans. Human coronaviruses (HCoV) have been implicated in the etiology of multiple sclerosis (MS), an autoimmune disease. Several studies have demonstrated, with the help of different techniques, the preponderance of HCoV in the brains of MS patients relative to the normal brain (Murray *et al.*, 1992; Stewart *et al.*, 1992; Arbour *et al.*, 2000). Moreover, coronaviruses can activate T cells reactive for myelin in MS patients (Talbot *et al.*, 1996, 2001; Boucher *et al.*, 2001). However, the link between the presence of the virus and the disease remains uncertain. Coronavirus could contribute to MS by an indirect mechanism, namely by the activation of glial cells and by the release of pro-inflammatory cytokines that could contribute to myelin destruction. The HCoV-OC43 strain can infect primary cultures of microglial cells, enriched to 90% from adult human brains (Bonavia *et al.*, 1997). These adult microglial cells do not produce infectious virus, unlike fetal microglial cells which are susceptible to a productive infection (Bonavia *et al.*, 1997). In addition, HCoV-OC43 can also infect macrophages from peripheral blood (Collins, 1998; Miletti *et al.*, 2004). Other studies on established cell lines demonstrate that CHME-5 cells (immortalized fetal microglial cells) are susceptible to acute infection but do not act as a reservoir for HCoV-OC43 (Arbour *et al.*, 1999a). This same cell line is resistant to an infection by the HCoV-229E strain (Arbour *et al.*, 1999b). CHME-5 cell infection with HCoV-OC43 induces modulation of metalloproteinases MMP-2 and MMP-9 and release of nitric oxide by the iNOS gene (Edwards *et al.*, 2000). However, cell infection by HCoV-OC43 does not induce release of IL-6, TNF-α, or MCP-1. Release of pro-inflammatory molecules following viral infection could influence CNS degeneration. Indeed, MMP-9 contributes to myelin degradation and supports the passage of leukocytes through the blood–brain-barrier (BBB) (Goetzl *et al.*, 1996; Chandler *et al.*, 1997). MMP-2 can cleave to and activate MMP-9 (Fridman *et al.*, 1995). In addition, MMPs can influence cytokine release, which itself increases NO release (Ogura and Esumi, 1996). It has been shown that iNOS is increased in the brain of MS patients (Bagasra *et al.*, 1995). Thus, viral infection may cause damage in inducing release of pro-inflammatory molecules from infected cells. These mediators may have an effect on other cell types and induce a chain-reaction release of molecules which are toxic to the brain and may result in lesions. It is reasonable to suppose that once the coronavirus is in the CNS, its neurotoxic potential can be responsible for direct lesions of target cells and/or indirect lesions in inducing an inflammatory response (Edwards *et al.*, 2000) or an autoimmune response by molecular mimicry (Talbot *et al.*, 1996, 2001).

In mice, intracerebral inoculation of HCoV-OC43 induces a spongiform encephalopathy, associated with a strong inflammatory reaction. *In vivo*, the favorite target of the virus is the neuron, acute infection by HCoV-OC43 causing neural degeneration (Jacomy and Talbot, 2003), while the virus can infect astrocytes and microglial cells *in vitro* (Jacomy and Talbot, 2001). Pathology induced by the virus is not orchestrated by the immune system, but the inflammatory reaction plays an important role in elimination of the virus and animal survival. A strong signal of activated microglial cells appears when the virus is already widely distributed throughout the CNS and remains after the complete clearance of the virus. There are no data on cytokine production or inflammation mediators at this time. However, a strong immunoreactivity against the Mac2 protein (also named galectin-3, a marker of activated microglial cells) is detectable at the inflammation peak (Jacomy and Talbot, 2003), whereas mRNA appears from the first days of the infection.

Murine coronavirus (MHV)

Most of the studies on murine coronaviruses (MHV) were conducted using strains JHM and A59 in mice and rats (Wege, 1995). MHV-infected mice develop a chronic encephalomyelitis, which is in large part mediated by the immune system (Dalziel *et al.*, 1986; Fleming *et al.*, 1986; Kristensson *et al.*

1986; Wang et al., 1990; Sun and Perlman, 1995). Myelin destruction and the infiltration of inflamed cells looks like that seen in MS patients. Thus, infection of rodents by MHV represents one of the experimental models for the study of mechanisms involved in the immune demyelination process.

Once in the CNS, the target cells for virus are astrocytes, microglial cells, oligodendrocytes, and neurons (Dalziel et al., 1986; Fleming et al., 1986; Massa et al., 1986; Perlman and Ries, 1987; Kyuwa and Stohlman, 1990; Pearce et al., 1994; Stohlman et al., 1995a). Coronavirus infection persists in CNS white matter, particularly in astrocytes and microglial cells (Perlman and Ries, 1987; Sun et al., 1995). The virus has been detected in several forms: RNA (Fleming et al., 1994; Adami et al., 1995), proteins (Kyuwa and Stohlman, 1990), and infectious particles (Knobler et al., 1982). Thus, it seems that the immune system is unable to completely eliminate the virus from the CNS.

Immune response in the CNS following coronavirus infection

Acute infection

Acute infection of the CNS causes a local inflammatory response, during which different cell populations are recruited: macrophages, NK, CD4+ and CD8+ T cells and B cells (Williamson et al., 1991).

Initially, several chemokines are transcribed in the CNS following MHV infection: macrophage inflammatory protein (MIP)-1β, CCL2 and 3, RANTES, MIP-2, and CXCL10 (also named IP-10) (Lane et al., 1998). These chemokines allow the recruitment of mononucleated cells into the CNS (Marten et al., 2001a). Firstly, NK cells and macrophages infiltrate the CNS (Marten et al., 2001a). Then, CD4+ and CD8+ lymphocytes enter the infection site, where they seem to be of major importance in clearing the virus (Williamson and Stohlman, 1990). In fact, SCID and nude mice, which do not have functional T cells, are unable to clear the virus (Marten et al., 2001a). Furthermore, mice depleted in CD4+ or CD8+ before infection clear the virus more slowly (Williamson and Stohlman, 1990). In addition, an important proportion of the T cells, up to 50% of CD8+ and approximately 30% of CD4+, found in the CNS are virus-specific (Bergmann et al., 1999; Haring et al., 2001). CD8+ cells play an antiviral role in two ways: (1) they carry out cytolysis with perforin, which controls viral replication in astrocytes and microglial cells (Lin et al., 1997), and (2) they secrete IFN-γ, which contributes to elimination of virus from oligodendrocytes (Parra et al., 1999). Although IFN-γ secretion by CD4+ T cells can contribute to control of viral replication in oligodendrocytes (Marten et al., 2001a), their role seems to be more that of support to antiviral response from CD8+ (Stohlman et al., 1998). Thus, cytokine secretion by CD4+ T cells can increase CD8+ T-cell expansion, while secreted chemokines can help cytotoxic T-cell and macrophage infiltration into the CNS (Marten et al., 2001a). Finally, antibodies produced by B cells are particularly known for their role in protection against neural infection (Buchmeier et al., 1984) and prevention of virus reactivation (Lin et al., 1999), but a study conducted with mature B-cell-deficient mice concluded that B cells are important actors in clearance of primary infection of the CNS (Matthews et al., 2001).

Persistent infection

When the immune system does not eliminate MHV completely, infection can persist in mice, mostly in astrocytes and microglial cells (Perlman and Ries, 1987; Sun and Perlman, 1995). During persistent infection, NK cells and macrophages are eliminated from the CNS (Marten et al., 2001a). CD8+ T cells present in the CNS at that time have lost their cytolytic activity, although they are still able to secrete IFN-γ and CD69, an activation marker, is expressed on their surface (Bergmann et al., 1999). Survival or recruitment of CD8+ and CD4+ T cells appears to depend on persistence of the virus (Marten et al., 2000b). It should be noted that B cells impede re-emergence of the virus and allow persistence of MHV in the CNS (Lin et al., 1999).

Demyelination

Infection of the CNS by MHV-A59 and MHV-JHM is responsible for myelin destruction (Pappenheimer, 1958; Lampert et al., 1973; Herndon

et al., 1975; Lavi et al., 1984). Several mechanisms have been proposed to explain this virus-induced demyelination. The death of oligodendrocytes following the cytopathic effect of MHV infection was first proposed to explain myelin destruction (Lampert et al., 1973; Powell and Lampert, 1975).

However, it is clear that the immune system is involved in this process, as indicated by studies conducted with immunosuppressed mice infected with MHV-JHM. Indeed, SCID (Houtman et al., 1995), RAG-1–/– (Wu and Perlman, 1999), and irradiated immunocompetent mice (Wang et al., 1990) have shown no demyelination following infection by murine coronavirus. The adoptive transfer of splenocytes from mice immunized with MHV to immunosuppressed mice resulted in demyelination (Wang et al., 1990; Houtman et al., 1995; Wu and Perlman, 1999). Demyelination has also been observed following transfer of splenocytes depleted in CD4+ or CD8+ lymphocytes, but not after transfer of splenocytes depleted of CD4+ and CD8+ T cells (Wu et al., 2000). In addition, demyelination following MHV infection was observed in nude mice, with B cells but without functional T cells (Houtman and Fleming, 1996b). All these studies suggest a role for the immune system in demyelination. But how is the immune system involved in this pathologic process?

First, the immune response could be directly involved. In this hypothesis, viral infection causes a defense reaction that eliminates infected cells (Houtman and Fleming, 1996a). Thus, infected oligodendrocytes may become the target for cytotoxic mechanisms. Nevertheless, neither Fas expression nor perforin expression, both involved in cytolytic mechanisms, nor IFN-γ are associated with demyelination (Parra et al., 2000; Lin et al., 1997 ; Parra et al., 1999). A direct role for cytotoxic T cells in demyelination is not yet supported by clear observations (Marten et al., 2001b).

Second, the immune response could play an indirect role in establishing demyelination. For example, cytokines or toxic products released by macrophages/microglial cells responding to a viral infection can damage surrounding oligodendrocytes (Houtman and Fleming, 1996a). Microglial cells can be recruited from monocytes circulating through the intact blood–brain barrier and rapidly differentiate in resident microglial cells (Lawson et al., 1992). Microglial cells are activated by different signals associated with lesions or disease and can become phagocytic cells that produce their own cytotoxic molecules (Smith, 2001; Cheepsunthorn et al., 2001; Bohatschek et al., 2001). Moreover, activated microglial cells express several receptors involved in attaching and ingesting myelin fragments (Smith, 2001). In addition, following MHV infection, CD4+ T cells contribute to demyelination and inflammation by producing RANTES, a chemokine that recruits macrophages to the CNS (Lane et al., 2000). Macrophage recruitment is correlated in time with myelin destruction (Wu and Perlman, 1999). Loss of the chemokine CCR5 receptor is associated with diminution of the severity of demyelination (Glass et al., 2001), whereas CCR2 loss impedes leukocyte activation and precipitates death in animals (Chen et al., 2001). Microglial cells are the main immune cells of the CNS and play a critical role in the defense of the organism against infectious agents. However, their activation may also be responsible for damage to the CNS.

Third, MHV infection can initiate an autoimmune response directed against one or many CNS antigens (Stohlman and Hinton, 2001). Myelin-specific T cells have been detected in rats following MHV infection (Watanabe et al., 1983). Adoptive transfer of these cells causes CNS inflammation and clinical symptoms (Watanabe et al., 1983). In mice, the frequency of cells that are autoreactive without antigenic stimulation increases following MHV infection (Kyuwa et al., 1991). However, the presence of self-reactive cells specific to a CNS antigen remains to be demonstrated (Marten et al., 2001). Nevertheless, we have recently obtained evidence for activation of MBP-reactive T cells following MHV-A59 infection of C57BL/6 mice, without any reactivity to control antigens, ovalbumin, or lung lysates (Gruslin et al., 2004).

In conclusion, MHV is neurotropic and neuroinvasive. The CNS-directed immune response leads to elimination of the virus from the CNS, even though sterile immunity is not achieved and the virus can persist. Several mechanisms have been proposed to explain demyelination induced by viral infection. Even if the viral cytopathic effect on oligodendrocytes is one hypothesis that has been formulated, involvement of the immune system has also been clearly demonstrated. The immune response could lead to demyelination either directly, indirectly, by activating an autoimmune response, or by a combination of one or more of these mechanisms.

References

Accapezzato, D., Nisini, R., Paroli, M., Bruno, G., Bonino, F., Houghton, M., *et al.* (1998). Generation of an MHC class II-restricted T cell epitope by extracellular processing of hepatitis delta antigen. *J Immunol* 160: 5262–5266.

Acha-Orbea, H., Mitchell, D.J., Timmermann, L., Wraith, D.C., Tausch, G.S., Waldor, M.K., *et al.* (1988). Limited heterogeneity of T cell receptors from lymphocytes mediating autoimmune encephalomyelitis allows specific immune intervention. *Cell* 54: 263–273.

Adami, C., Pooley, J., Glomb, J., Stecker, E., Fazal, F., Fleming, J.O., *et al.* (1995). Evolution of mouse hepatitis virus (MHV) during chronic infection: quasi-species nature of the persisting MHV RNA. *Virology* 209: 337–346.

Aichele, P., Bachmann, M.F., Hengartner, H., and Zinkernagel, R.M. (1996). Immunopathology of organ specific autoimmunity as a consequence of virus infection. *Immunol Rev* 152: 21–45.

Albert, L.J. and Inman, R.D. (1999). Molecular mimicry and autoimmunity. *N Engl J Med* 341: 2068–2074.

Aloisi, F. (2001). Immune function of microglia. *Glia* 36: 165–179.

Arbour, N., Côté, G., Lachance, C., Tardieu, M., Cashman, N.R., and Talbot, P.J. (1999a). Acute and persistent infection of human neural cell lines by human coronavirus OC43. *J Virol* 73: 3338–3350.

Arbour, N., Ekandé, S., Côté, G., Lachance, C., Chagnon, F., Tardieu, M., *et al.* (1999b). Persistent infection of human oligodendrocytic and neuroglial cell lines by human coronavirus 229E. *J Virol* 74: 3326–3337.

Arbour, N., Day, R., Newcombe, J., and Talbot, P.J. (2000). Neuroinvasion by human respiratory coronaviruses and association with multiple sclerosis. *J Virol* 74: 8913–8921.

Avery, A.C., Zhao, Z.S., Rodriguez, A., Bikoff, E.K., Soheilian, M., Foster, C.S., *et al.* (1995). Resistance to herpes stromal keratitis conferred by an IgG2a-derived peptide. *Nature* 376: 431–434.

Badenhoop, K., Donner, H., Neumann, J., Herwig, J., Kurth, R., Usadel, K.H., *et al.* (1999). IDDM patients neither show humoral reactivities against endogenous retroviral envelope protein nor do they differ in retroviral mRNA expression from healthy relatives or normal individuals. *Diabetes* 48: 215–218.

Bagasra, O., Michaels, F.H., Zheng, Y.M., Bobroski, L.E., Spitsin, S.V., Fu, Z.F., *et al.* (1995). Activation of the inducible form of nitric oxide synthase in the brains of patients with multiple sclerosis. *Proc Natl Acad Sci USA* 92: 12041–12045.

Bancherau, J. and Steinman, R.M. (1998). Dendritic cells and the control of immunity. *Nature* 392: 245–252.

Barnaba, V. (1996). Viruses, hidden self-epitopes and autoimmunity. *Immunol Rev* 152: 47–66.

Benoist, C. and Mathis, D. (1998). The pathogen connection. *Nature* 394: 227–228.

Benoist, C. and Mathis, D. (2001). Autoimmunity provoked by infection: how good is the case for epitope mimicry? *Nat Immunol* 2: 797–801.

Bergmann, C.C., Altman, J.D., Hinton, D., and Stohlman, S.A. (1999). Inverted immunodominance and impaired cytolytic function of CD8+ T cells during viral persistence in the central nervous system. *J Immunol* 163: 3379–3387.

Biron, C.A. (1994). Cytokines in the generation of immune responses to, and resolution of, virus infection. *Curr Opin Immunol* 6: 530–538.

Boehm, U., Klamp, T., Groot, M., and Howard, J.C. (1997). Cellular responses to interferon-gamma. *Ann Rev Immunol* 15: 749–795.

Bohatschek, M., Kloss, C.U., Kalla, R., and Raivich, G. (2001). *In vitro* model of microglial deramification: ramified microglia transform into amoeboid phagocytes following addition of brain cell membranes to microglia-astrocyte cocultures. *J Neurosci Res* 64: 508–522.

Bonavia, A., Arbour, N., Wee Yong, V., and Talbot, P.J. (1997). Infection of primary cultures of human neural cells by human coronavirus 229E and OC43. *J Virol* 71: 800–806.

Bottazzo, G.E., Pujol-Borell, B.R., Hanafusa, T., and Feldmann, M. (1983). Role of aberrant HLA-DR expression and antigen presentation in induction of endocrine autoimmunity. *Lancet* 2: 1115–1119.

Boucher, A., Denis, F., Duquette, P., and Talbot, P.J. (2001). Generation from multiple sclerosis patients of long-term T-cell clones that are activated by both human coronavirus and myelin antigens. *Adv Exp Med Biol* 494: 355–362.

Boucher, A., Tremblay, M., Arbour, N., Edwards, J., Day, R., Newcombe, J., *et al.* (2001b). The role of neuroinvasive human coronaviruses in autoimmune processes associated with multiple sclerosis. In: *Genes and Viruses in Multiple Sclerosis* (ed. O.R. Hommes, H. Wekerle, and M. Clanet), pp. 209–220. Elsevier, Amsterdam.

Brocke, S., Gaur, A., Piercy, C., Gautam, A., Gijbels, K., Fathman, C.G., *et al.* (1993). Induction of relapsing paralysis in experimental autoimmune encephalomyelitis by bacterial superantigen. *Nature* 365: 642–644.

Brosnan, C.F., Cammer, W., Norton, W.T., and Bloom, B.R. (1980). Proteinase inhibitors suppress the development of experimental allergic encephalomyelitis. *Nature* 285: 235–337.

Buchmeier, M.J., Lewicki, H.A., Talbot, P.J., and Knobler, R.L. (1984). Murine hepatitis virus-4 (strain JHM)-induced neurologic disease is modulated *in vivo* by monoclonal antibody. *Virology* 132: 261–270.

Carnaud, C. and Bach, J.F. (1993). Cellular basis of T-cell autoreactivity in autoimmune diseases. *Immunol Res* 12: 131–148.

Chandler, S., Miller, K.M., Clements, J., Lury, J., Corkill, D., Anthony, D.C., *et al.* (1997). Matrix metalloproteinases, tumor necrosis factor and multiple sclerosis: an overview. *J Neuroimmunol* 72: 155–161.

Cheepsunthorn, P., Radov, L., Menzies, S., Reid, J., and Connor, J.R. (2001). Characterization of a novel brain-derived microglial cell line isolated from neonatal rat brain. *Glia* 35: 53–62.

Chen, B.P., Kuziel, W.A., and Lane, T.E. (2001). Lack of CCR2 results in increased mortality and impaired leukocyte activation and trafficking following infection of the central nervous system with a neurotropic coronavirus. *J Immunol* 167: 4585–4592.

Chiang, C.S., Powell, H.C., Gold, L.H., Samimi, A., and Campbell, I.L. (1996). Macrophage/microglial-mediated primary demyelination and motor disease induced by the central nervous system production of interleukin-3 in transgenic mice. *J Clin Invest* 97: 1512–1524.

Clarke, M.F., Gelmann, E.P., and Reitz, M.S. Jr (1983). Homology of human T-cell leukemia virus envelope gene with class I HLA gene. *Nature* 305: 60–62.

Cole, B.C. and Griffiths, M.M. (1993). Triggering and exacerbation of autoimmune arthritis by the *Mycoplasma arthritidis* superantigen MAM. *Arthritis Rheum* 36: 994–1002.

Collins, A.R. (1998). Human macrophages are susceptible to coronavirus OC43. *Adv Exp Med Biol* 440: 635–639.

Conrad, B., Weidmann, E., Trucco, G., Rudert, W.A., Behboo, R., Ricordi, C., *et al.* (1994). Evidence for superantigen involvement in insulin-dependent diabetes mellitus aetiology. *Nature* 371: 351–355.

Conrad, B., Weissmahr, R.N., Boni, J., Arcari, R., Schupbach, J., and Mach, B. (1997). A human endogenous retroviral superantigen as candidate autoimmune gene in type I diabetes. *Cell* 90: 303–313.

Corbin, J.G., Kelly, D., Rath, E.M., Baerwald, K.D., Suzuki, K., and Popko, B. (1996). Targeted CNS expression of interferon-gamma in transgenic mice leads to hypomyelination, reactive gliosis, and abnormal cerebellar development. *Mol Cell Neurosci* 7: 354–370.

Cross, A.H., Tuohy, V.K., and Raine, C.S. (1993). Development of reactivity to new myelin antigens during chronic relapsing autoimmune demyelination. *Cell Immunol* 146: 261–269.

Cross, A.K. and Woodroofe, M.N. (2001). Immunoregulation of microglial functional properties. *Microsc Res Tech* 54: 10–17.

Dalziel, R.G., Lampert, P.W., Talbot, P.J., and Buchmeier, M.J. (1986). Site-specific alteration of murine hepatitis virus type 4 peplomer glycoprotein E2 results in reduced neurovirulence. *J Virol* 59: 463–471.

Datta, S.K. (2000). Positive selection for autoimmunity. *Nat Med* 6: 259–261.

Desforges, M., Miletti, T., Gagnon, M., and Talbot, P.J. Human monocytic cells: possible vector of human coronavirus into the central nervous system (in preparation).

Deshande, S.P., Lee, S., Zheng, M., Song, B., Knipe, D., Kapp, J.A., et al. (2001). Herpes simplex virus-induced keratitis: evaluation of the role of molecular mimicry in lesion pathogenesis. *J Virol* 75: 3077–3088.

Di Rosa, F. and Barnaba, V. (1998). Persisting viruses and chronic inflammation: understanding their relation to autoimmunity. *Immunol Rev* 164: 17–27.

Edwards, J.A., Denis, F., and Talbot, P.J. (2000). Activation of glial cells by human coronavirus OC43 infection. *J Neuroimmunol* 108: 73–81.

Ehl, S., Hombach, J., Aichele, P., Hengartner, H., and Zinkernagel, R.M. (1997). Bystander activation of cytotoxic T cells: studies on the mechanism and evaluation of *in vivo* significance in a transgenic mouse model. *J Exp Med* 185: 1241–1251.

Eskes, C., Honegger, P., Juillerat-Jeanneret, L., and Monnet-Tschudi, F. (2002). Microglial reaction induced by noncytotoxic methylmercury treatment leads to neuroprotection via interactions with astrocytes and IL-6 release. *Glia* 37: 43–52.

Evans, C.F., Horwitz, M.S., Hobbs, M.V., and Oldstone, M.B. (1996). Viral infection of transgenic mice expressing a viral protein in oligodendrocytes leads to chronic central nervous system autoimmune disease. *J Exp Med* 184: 2371–2384.

Evavold, B.D., Sloan-Lancaster, J., Wilson, K.J., Rothbard, J.B., and Allen, P.M. (1995). Specific T cell recognition of minimally homologous peptides: evidence for multiple endogenous ligands. *Immunity* 2: 655–663.

Fabbri, M., Bianchi, E., Fumagalli, L., and Pardi, R. (1999). Regulation of lymphocyte traffic by adhesion molecules. *Inflamm Res* 48: 239–246.

Fairweather, D., Kaya, Z., Shellam, G.R., Lawson, C.M., and Rose, N.R. (2001). From infection to autoimmunity. *J Autoimmun* 16: 175–186.

Fleming, J.O., Trousdale, M.D., el Zaatari, F.A., Stohlman, S.A., and Weiner, L.P. (1986). Pathogenicity of antigenic variants of murine coronavirus JHM selected with monoclonal antibodies. *J Virol* 58: 869–875.

Fleming, J.O., Houtman, J.J., Alaca, H., Hinze, H.C., McKenzie, D., Aiken, J., et al. (1994). Persistence of viral RNA in the central nervous system of mice inoculated with MHV-4. In: *Coronaviruses* (ed. H. Laude and J.F. Vautherot), pp. 327–332. Plenum Press, New York.

Fridman, R., Toth, M., Pena, D., and Mobashery, S. (1995). Activation of pro-gelatinase B (MMP-9) by gelatinase A (MMP-2). *Cancer Res* 55: 2548–2555.

Frosch, S., Bonifas, U., Eck, H.P., Bockstette, M., Droege, W., Rude, E., et al. (1993). The efficient bovine insulin presentation capacity of bone marrow-derived macrophages activated by granulocyte-macrophage colony-stimulating factor correlates with a high level of intracellular reducing thiols. *Eur J Immunol* 23: 1430–1434.

Fujinami, R.S. and Oldstone, M.B.A. (1985). Amino acid homology between the encephalitogenic site of myelin basic protein and virus: mechanism for autoimmunity. *Science* 230: 1043–1045.

Fujinami, R.S., Oldstone, M.B., Wroblewska, Z., Frankel, M.E., and Koprowski, H. (1983). Molecular mimicry in virus infection: crossreaction of measles virus phosphoprotein or of herpes simplex virus protein with human intermediate filaments. *Proc Natl Acad Sci USA* 80: 2346–2350.

Gehrmann, J., Matsumoto, Y., and Kreutzberg, G.W. (1995). Microglia: intrinsic immuneffector cell of the brain. *Brain Res Rev* 20: 269–287.

Gianani, R. and Sarvetnick, N. (1996). Viruses, cytokines, antigen, and autoimmunity. *Proc Natl Acad Sci USA* 93: 2257–2259.

Glass, W.G., Liu, M.T., Kuziel, W.A., and Lane, T.E. (2001). Reduced macrophage infiltration and demyelination in mice lacking the chemokine receptor CCR5 following infection with a neurotropic coronavirus. *Virology* 288: 8–17.

Goetzl, E.J., Banda, M.J., and Leppert, D. (1996). Matrix metalloproteinases in immunity. *J Immunol* 156: 1–4.

Gombert, J.M., Herbelin, A., Tancrede-Bohin, E., Dy, M., Carnaud, C., and Bach, J.F. (1996). Early quantitative and functional deficiency of NK1(+)-like thymocytes in the NOD mouse. *Eur J Immuno,* 26: 2989–2998.

Gross, D.M., Forsthuber, T., Tary-Lehmann, M., Etling, C., Ito, K., Nagy, Z.A. et al. (1998). Identification of LFA-1 as a candidate autoantigen in treatment-resistant Lyme arthritis. *Science* 281: 703–706.

Gruslin, E.G., Moisan, S., St Pierre, Y., Desforges, M., and Talbot, P.J. (in press). Transcriptome profile within the mouse central nervous system and activation of myelin-reactive T cells following murine coronavirus infection. *J Neuroimmunol.*

Haring, J. and Perlman, S. (2001). Mouse hepatitis virus. *Curr Opin Microbio,* 4: 462–466.

Haring, J.S., Pewe, L.L., and Perlman, S. (2001). High-magnitude, virus-specific CD4 T-cell response in the central nervous system of coronavirus-infected mice. *J Virol* 75: 3043–3047.

Haynes, B.F., Robert-Guroff, M., Metzgar, R.S., Franchini, G., Kalyanaraman, V.S., Palker, T.J., et al. (1983). Monoclonal antibody against human T cell leukemia virus p19 defines a human thymic epithelial antigen acquired during ontogeny. *J Exp Med* 157: 907–920.

Heese, K., Fiebich, B.L., Bauer, J., and Otten, U. (1997). Nerve growth factor (NGF) expression in rat microglia is induced by adenosine A2a-receptors. *Neurosci Lett* 231: 83–86.

Hemmer, B., Fleckenstein, B.T., Vergelli, M., Jung, G., McFarland, H., Martin, R., et al. (1997). Identification of high potency microbial and self ligands for a human autoreactive class II-restricted T cell clones. *J Exp Med* 185: 1651–1659.

Hemmer, B., Jacobsen, M., and Sommer, N. (2000). Degeneracy in T-cell antigen recognition—implications for the pathogenesis of autoimmune diseases. *J Neuroimmunol* 107: 148–153.

Herndon, R.M., Griffin, D.E., McCormick, U., and Weiner, L.P. (1975). Mouse hepatitis virus-induced recurrent demyelination. A preliminary report. *Arch Neurol* 32: 32–35.

Hodstev, A.S., Choi, Y., Spanopoulou, E., and Posnett, D.N. (1998). Mycoplasma superantigen is a CDR3-dependent ligand for the T cell antigen receptor. *J Exp Med* 187: 319–327.

Horwitz, M.S. and Sarvetnick, N. (1999). Viruses, host responses, and autoimmunity. *Immunol Re,* 169: 241–253.

Houtman, J.J. and Fleming, J.O. (1996a). Pathogenesis of mouse hepatitis virus-induced demyelination. *J Neurovirol* 2: 361–376.

Houtman, J.J. and Fleming, J.O. (1996b). Dissociation of demyelination and viral clearance in congenitally immunodeficient mice infected with murine coronavirus JHM. *J Neurovirol* 2: 101–110.

Houtman, J.J., Hinze, H.C., and Fleming, J.O. (1995). Demyelination induced by murine coronavirus JHM infection of congenitally immunodeficient mice. *Adv Exp Med Biol* 380: 159–163.

Ignatowicz, L., Kappler, J., and Marrack, P. (1996). The repertoire of T cells shaped by a single MHC/peptide ligand. *Cell* 84: 521–529.

Jacobson, D.L., Gange, S.J., Rose, N.R., and Graham, N.M. (1997). Epidemiology and estimated population burden of selected autoimmune diseases in the United States. *Clin Immunol Immunopathol* 84: 223–243.

Jacomy, H. and Talbot, P.J. (2001) Susceptibility of murine CNS to OC43 infection. *Adv Exp Med Biol* 494: 101–107.

Jacomy, H. and Talbot, P.J. (2003). Vacuolating encephalopathy in mice infected by human coronavirus OC43. *Virology* 315: 20–33.

Jaeckel, E., Heringlake, S., Berger, D., Brabant, G., Hunsmann, G., and Manns, M.P. (1999). No evidence for association between IDDMK(1,2)22, a novel isolated retrovirus, and IDDM. *Diabetes* 48: 209–214.

Joseph, J., Grun, J.L., Lublin, F.D., and Knobler, R.L. (1993). Interleukin-6 induction *in vitro* in mouse brain endothelial cells and astrocytes by exposure to mouse hepatitis virus (MHV-4, JHM). *J Neuroimmunol* 42: 47–52.

Kappler, J.W., Roehm, N., and Marrack, P. (1987). T cell tolerance by clonal elimination in the thymus. *Cell* 49: 273–280.

Karpus, W.J., Pope, J.G., Peterson, J.D., Dal Canto, M.C., Miller, S.D. (1995). Inhibition of Theiler's virus-mediated demyelination by peripheral immune tolerance induction. *J Immunol* 155: 947–957.

Kaufman, D.L., Clare-Salzler, M., Ian, J., Forsthuber, T., Ting, G.S., Robinson, P., et al. (1993). Spontaneous loss of T-cell tolerance to glutamic acid decarboxylase in murine insulin-dependent diabetes. *Nature* 366: 69–72.

Ke, Y., Ma, H., and Kapp, J.A. (1998). Antigen is required for the activation of effector activities, whereas interleukin 2 is required for the maintenance of memory in ovalbumin-specific, CD8+ cytotoxic T lymphocytes. *J Exp Med* 187: 49–57.

Kim, A., Jun, H.S., Wong, L., Stephure, D., Pacaud, D., Trussell, R.A., et al. (1999). Human endogenous retrovirus with a high genomic sequence homology with IDDMK(1,2)22 is not specific for Type 1 (insulin-dependent) diabetic patients but ubiquitous. *Diabetologia* 42: 413–418.

Knobler, R.L., Lampert, P.W., and Oldstone, M.B.A. (1982). Virus persistence and recurring demyelination produced by a temperature-sensitive mutant of MHV-4. *Nature* 298: 279–298.

Kong, G.Y., Kristensson, K., and Bentivoglio, M. (2002). Reaction of mouse brain oligodendrocytes and their precursors, astrocytes and microglia, to pro-inflammatory mediators circulating in the cerebrospinal fluid. *Glia* **37**: 191–205.

Kozwloski, S., Corr, M., Takeshita, T., Boyd, L.F., Pendleton, C.D., Germain, R.N., *et al.* (1992). Serum angiotensin-1 converting enzyme activity processes a human immunodeficiency virus 1 gp160 peptide for presentation by major histocompatibility complex class 1 molecules. *J Exp Med* **175**: 1417–1422.

Kretz-Rommel, A. and Rubin, R.L. (2000). Disruption of positive selection of thymocytes causes autoimmunity. *Nat Med* **6**: 298–305.

Kristensson, K., Holmes, K.V., Duchala, C.S., Zeller, N.K., Lazzarini, R.A., and Dubois-Dalcq, M. (1986). Increased levels of myelin basic protein transcripts in virus-induced demyelination. *Nature* **322**: 544–547.

Kyuwa, S. and Stohlman, S.A. (1990). Pathogenesis of a neurotropic murine coronavirus, strain JHM in the central nervous system of mice. *Semin Virol* **1**: 273–280.

Kyuwa, S., Yamaguchi, K., Toyoda, Y., and Fujiwara, K. (1991). Induction of self-reactive T cells after murine coronavirus infection. *J Virol* **65**: 1789–1795.

Lampert, P.W., Sims, J.K., and Kniazeff, A.J. (1973). Mechanism of demyelination in JHM virus encephalomyelitis. *Acta Neuropathol* **24**: 76–85.

Lane, D.P. and Hoeffler, W.K. (1980). SV40 large T shares an antigenic determinant with a cellular protein of molecular weight 68,000. *Nature* **288**: 167–170.

Lane, T.E. and Buchmeier, M.J. (1997). Murine coronavirus infection: a paradigm for virus-induced demyelinating disease. *Trends Microbiol* **5**: 9–14.

Lane, T.E., Paoletti, A.D., and Buchmeier, M.J. (1997). Disassociation between the *in vitro* and *in vivo* effects of nitric oxide on a neurotropic murine coronavirus. *J Virol* **71**: 2202–2210.

Lane, T.E., Asensio, V.C., Yu, N., Paoletti, A.D., Campbell, I.L., and Buchmeier, M.J. (1998). Dynamic regulation of alpha- and beta-chemokine expression in the central nervous system during mouse hepatitis virus-induced demyelinating disease. *J Immunol* **160**: 970–978.

Lane, T.E., Liu, M.T., Chen, B.P., Asensio, V.C., Samawi, R.M., Paoletti, A.D., *et al.* (2000). A central role for CD4⁺ T cells and RANTES in virus-induced central nervous system inflammation and demyelination. *J Virol* **74**: 1415–1424.

Lassmann, H., Bruck, W., and Lucchinetti, C. (2001). Heterogeneity of multiple sclerosis pathogenesis: implications for diagnosis and therapy. *Trends Mol Med* **7**: 115–121.

Lavi, E., Gilden, D.H., Wroblewska, Z., Rorke, L.B., and Weiss, R. (1984). Experimental demyelination produced by the A59 strain of mouse hepatitis virus. *Neurology* **34**: 597–603.

Lawrence, D.M. and Major, E.O. (2002). HIV-1 and the brain: connections between HIV-1-associated dementia, neuropathology and neuroimmunology. *Microbes Infect* **4**: 301–308.

Lawson, L.J., Perry, V.H., and Gordon, S. (1992). Turnover of resident microglia in the normal adult mouse brain. *Neuroscience* **48**: 405–415.

Lehmann, P.V., Forsthuber, T., Miller, A., and Sercarz, E.E. (1992). Spreading of T-cell autoimmunity to cryptic determinants of an autoantigen. *Nature* **358**: 155–157.

Levin, M.C., Lee, S.M., Kalume, F., Morcos, Y., Dohan, F.C Jr, Hasty, K.A., *et al.* (2002). Autoimmunity due to molecular mimicry as a cause of neurological disease. *Nat Med* **8**: 509–513.

Li, H., Llera, A., Malchiodi, E.L., and Mariuzza, R.A. (1999). The structural basis of T cell activation by superantigens. *Annu Rev Immunol* **17**: 435–466.

Lin, M.T., Hinton, D.R., Marten, N.W., Bergmann, C.C., and Stohlman, S.A. (1999). Antibody prevents virus reactivation within the central nervous system. *J Immunol* **162**: 7358–7368.

Lin, M.Y., Stohlman, S.A., and Hinton, D.R. (1997). Mouse hepatitis virus is cleared from the central nervous system of mice lacking perforin-mediated cytolysis. *J Virol* **71**: 383–391.

Liuzzo, J.P., Petanceska, S.S., and Devi, L.A. (1999). Neurotrophic factors regulate cathepsin S in macrophages and microglia: Aarole in the degradation of myelin basic protein and amyloid beta peptide. *Mol Med* **5**: 334–343.

Lo, W.F., Woods, A.S., DeCloux, A., Cotter, R.J., Metcalf, E.S., and Soloski, M.J. (2000). Molecular mimicry mediated by MHC class Ib molecules after infection with Gram-negative pathogens. *Nat Med* **6**: 215–218.

Lucchiari, M.A. and Pereira, C.A. (1989). A major role of macrophage activation by interferon-gamma during mouse hepatitis virus type 3 infection. I. Genetically dependent resistance. *Immunobiology* **180**: 12–22.

Lucchiari, M.A. and Pereira, C.A. (1990). A major role of macrophage activation by interferon-gamma during mouse hepatitis virus type 3 infection. II. Age-dependent resistance. *Immunobiology* **181**: 31–39.

Luppi, P., Zanone, M.M., Hyoty, H., Rudert, W.A., Haluszczak, C., Alexander, A.M., *et al.* (2000). Restricted TCR V beta gene expression and enterovirus infection in type I diabetes: a pilot study. *Diabetologia* **43**: 1484–1497.

Marrack, P., Kappler, J., and Kotzin, B. (2001). Autoimmune disease: why and where it occurs. *Nat Med* **7**: 899–905.

Marten, N.W., Stohlman, S.A., and Bergmann, C.C. (2000). Role of viral persistence in retaining CD8(+) T cells within the central nervous system. *J Virol* **74**: 7903–7910.

Marten, N.W., Stohlman, S.A., and Bergmann, C.C. (2001*a*). MHV infection of the CNS: mechanisms of immune-mediated control. *Viral Immunol* **14**: 1–18.

Marten, N.W., Hohman, R., Stohlman, S.A., Atkinson, R.D., Hinton, D.R., and Bergmann, C.B. (2001*b*). Acute CNS infection is insufficient to mediate chronic T cell retention. *Adv Exp Med Biol* **494**: 349–354.

Massa, P.T., Wege, H., and ter Meulen, V. (1986). Analysis of murine hepatitis virus (JHM strain) tropism toward Lewis rat glial cells *in vitro*. Type I astrocytes and brain macrophages (microglia) as primary glial cell targets. *Lab Invest* **55**: 318–327.

Matthews, A.E., Weiss, S.R., Shlomchik, M.J., Hannum, L.G., Gombold, J.L., and Paterson, Y. (2001). Antibody is required for clearance of infectious murine hepatitis virus A59 from the central nervous system, but not the liver. *J Immunol* **167**: 5254–5263.

McRae, B.L., Vanderlugt, C.L., Dal Canto, M.C., and Miller, S.D. (1995). Functional evidence for epitope spreading in the relapsing pathology of experimental autoimmune encephalomyelitis». *J Exp Med* **182**: 75–85.

Mehindate, K., Al-Daccak, R., Scall, T.J., and Mourad, W. (1994). Induction of chemokine gene expression by major histocompatibility complex class II ligands in human fibroblast-like synoviocytes. Different regulation by interleukin-4 and dexamethasone. *J Biol Chem* **269**: 32063–32069.

Merriman, T.R. and Todd, J.A. (1995). Genetics of autoimmune disease. *Curr Opin Immunol* **7**: 786–792.

Miller, S.D., Vanderlugt, C.L., Begolka, W.S., Pao, W., Yauch, R.L., Neville, K.L., *et al.* (1997). Persistent infection with Theiler's virus leads to CNS autoimmunity via epitope spreading. *Nat Med* **3**: 1133–1136.

Miller, S.D., Olson, J.K., and Croxford, J.L. (2001). Multiple pathways to induction of virus-induced autoimmune demyelination: lessons from Theiler's virus infection. *J Autoimm* **16**: 219–227.

Mor, F. and Cohen, I.R. (1993). Shifts in the epitopes of myelin basic protein recognized by Lewis rat T cells before, during and after the induction of experimental autoimmune encephalomyelitis. *J Clin Invest* **92**: 2199–2206.

Mourad, W., Mehindate, K., Schall, T.J., and McColl, S.R. (1992). Engagement of major histocompatibility complex class II molecules by superantigens induces inflammatory cytokine gene expression in human rheumatoid fibroblast-like synoviocytes. *J Exp Med* **175**: 613–616.

Muir, A., Ruan, Q.G., Marron, M.P., and She, J.X. (1999). The IDDMK(1,2)22 retrovirus is not detectable in either mRNA or genomic DNA from patients with type 1 diabetes. *Diabetes* **48**: 219–222.

Murali-Krishna, K., Altman, J.D., and Suresh, M. (1998). Counting antigen-specific CD8 T cells: a reevaluation of bystander activation during viral infection. *Immunity* **8**: 177–187.

Murray, R.S., Brown, B., Brian, D., and Cabirac, G.F. (1992). Detection of coronavirus RNA and antigen in multiple sclerosis brain. *Ann Neurol* **31**: 525–553.

Nakagawa, K. and Harrison, L.C. (1996). The potential roles of endogenous retroviruses in autoimmunity. *Immunol Rev* **152**: 193–236.

Nakajima, K. and Kohsaka, S. (1998). Functional roles of microglia in the central nervous system. *Hum Cell* **11**: 141–155.

Nakajima, K., Tohyama, Y., Kohsaka, S., and Kurihara, T. (2002). Ceramide activates microglia to enhance the production/secretion of brain-derived neurotrophic factor (BDNF) without induction of deleterious factors *in vitro*. *J Neurochem* **80**: 697–705.

Nanda, N.K., Arzoo, K.K., Getsen, H.M., Sette, A., and Sercarz, E.E. (1995). Recognition of multiple peptide cores by a single T cell receptor. *J Exp Med* **182**: 531–539.

Nauclér, C.S., Larsson, S., and Möller, E. (1996). A novel mechanism for virus-induced autoimmunity in humans. *Immunol Rev* **152**: 175–192.

Ogura, T. and Esumi, H. (1996). Nitric oxide synthase expression in human neuroblastoma cell line induced by cytokines. *Neuroreport* **7**: 853–856.

Ohashi, P.S., Oehen, S., Buerki, K., Pircher, H., Ohashi, C.T., Odermatt, B., *et al.* (1991). Ablation of 'tolerance' and induction of diabetes by virus infection in viral antigen transgenic mice. *Cell* **65**: 301–317.

Oldstone, M.B. (1987). Molecular mimicry and autoimmune disease. *Cell* **50**: 819–820.

Oldstone, M.B. (1991). Molecular anatomy of viral persistence. *J Virol* **65**: 6381–6386.

Oldstone, M.B., Nerenberg, M., Southern, P., Preice, J., and Lewicki, H. (1991). Virus infection triggers insulin-dependent diabetes mellitus in a transgenic model: role of anti-self (virus) immune response. *Cell* **65**: 319–331.

Olson, J.K., Croxford, J.L., Calenoff, M.A., Dal Canto, M.C., and Miller, S.D. (2001). A virus-induced molecular mimicry model of multiple sclerosis. *J Clin Invest* **108**: 311–318.

Opdenakker, G. and Van Damme, J. (1994). Cytokine-regulated proteases in autoimmune diseases. *Immunol Today* **15**: 103–107.

Origuchi, T., Eguchi, K., Kawabe, Y., Mizokami, A., Ida, H., and Nagataki, S. (1995). Synovial cells are potent antigen-presenting cells for super-antigen, staphylococcal enterotoxin B (SEB). *Clin Exp Immunol* **99**: 345–351.

Paliard, X., West, S.G., Lafferty, J.A., Clements, J.R., Kappler, J.W., Marrack, P., *et al.* (1991). Evidence for the effects of a superantigen in rheumatoid arthritis. *Science* **253**: 325–329.

Panoutsakopoulou, V. and Cantor, H. (2001). On the relationship between viral infection and autoimmunity. *J Autoimmun* **16**: 341–345.

Pappenheimner, A.M. (1958). Pathology of infection with the JHM virus. *J Natl Cancer Inst* **20**: 879–901.

Paroli, M., Schiaffella, E., Di Rosa, F., and Barnaba, V. (2000). Persisting viruses and autoimmunity. *J Neuroimmunol* **107**: 201–204.

Parra, B., Hinton, D.R., Lin, M.T., Cua, D.J., and Stohlman, S.A. (1997). Kinetics of cytokine mRNA expression in the central nervous system following lethal and nonlethal coronavirus-induced acute encephalomyelitis. *Virology* **233**: 260–270.

Parra, B., Hinton, D.R., Marten, N.W., Bergmann, C.C., Lin, M.T., Yang, C.S., *et al.* (1999). IFN-gamma is required for viral clearance from central nervous system oligodendroglia. *J Immunol* **162**: 1641–1647.

Parra, B., Lin, M.T., Stohlman, S.A., Bergmann, C.C., Atkinson, R., and Hinton, D.R. (2000). Contributions of Fas–Fas ligand interactions to the pathogenesis of mouse hepatitis virus in the central nervous system. *J Virol* **74**: 2447–2450.

Pearce, B.D., Hobbs, M.V., McGraw, T.S., and Buchmeier, M.J. (1994). Cytokine induction during T-cell-mediated clearance of mouse hepatitis virus from neurons *in vivo*. *J Virol* **68**: 5483–5495.

Penkowa, M., Moos, T., Carrasco, J., Hadberg, H., Molinero, A., Bluethmann, H., *et al.* (1999). Strongly compromised inflammatory response to brain injury in interleukin-6-deficient mice. *Glia* **25**: 343–357.

Penkowa, M., Giralt, M., Carrasco, J., Hadberg, H., and Hidalgo, J. (2000). Impaired inflammatory response and increased oxidative stress and neuro-degeneration after brain injury in interleukin-6-deficient mice. *Glia* **32**: 271–285.

Perlman, S. and Ries, D. (1987) The astrocyte is a target cell in mice persistently infected with mouse hepatitis virus, strain JHM. *Microb Pathogen* **3**: 309–314.

Perry, L.L., Barzaga-Gilbert, E., and Trotter, J.L. (1991). T cell sensitization to proteolipid protein in myelin basic protein-induced relapsing experimental allergic encephalomyelitis. *J Neuroimmunol* **33**: 7–15.

Pewe, L. and Perlman, S. (2002). Cutting edge: CD8 T cell-mediated demyelination is IFN-gamma dependent in mice infected with a neurotropic coronavirus. *J Immunol* **168**:1547–1551.

Powell, H.C. and Lampert, P.W. (1975). Oligodendrocytes and their myelin-plasma membrane connections in JHM mouse hepatitis virus encephalomyelitis. *Lab Investig* **33**: 440–445.

Prayoonwiwat, N. and Rodriguez, M. (1993). The potential for oligodendrocyte proliferation during demyelinating disease. *J Neuropathol Exp Neurol* **52**: 55–63.

Rabchevsky, A.G. and Streit, W.J. (1997). Grafting of cultured microglial cells into the lesioned spinal cord of adult rats enhances neurite outgrowth. *J Neurosci Res* **47**: 34–48.

Rees, J.H., Soudain, S.E., Gregson, N.A., and Hughes, R.A.C. (1995). *Campylobacter jejuni* infection and Guillain–Barré syndrome. *N Engl J Med* **333**: 1374–1379.

Schiffenbauer, J., Johnson, H.M., Butfiloski, E.J., Wegrzyn, L., and Soos, J.M. (1993). Staphyloccocal enterotoxins can reactivate experimental allergic encephalomyelitis. *Proc Natl Acad Sci USA* **90**: 8543–8546.

Schiffenbauer, J., Soos, J., and Johnson, H. (1998). The possible roles of bacterial superantigens in the pathogenesis of autoimmune disorders. *Immunol Today* **19**: 117–120.

Sharif, S., Arreaza, G.A., Zucker, P., Mi, Q.S., Sondhi, J., Naidenko, O.V., *et al.* (2001). Activation of natural killer T cells by alpha-galactosylceramide treatment prevents the onset and recurrence of autoimmune Type 1 diabetes. *Nat Med* **7**: 1057–1062.

Sheikh, K.A., Ho, T.W., Nachamkin, I., Li, C.Y., Cornblath, D.R., Asbury, A.K., *et al.* (1998). Molecular mimicry in Guillain–Barre syndrome. *Ann N Y Acad Sci* **845**: 307–321.

Sherman, L.A., Burke, T.A., and Biggs, J.A. (1992). Extracellular processing of peptide antigens that bind class 1 major histocompatibility molecules. *J Exp Med* **175**: 1221–1226.

Shi, F.D., Ljunggren, H.G., and Sarvetnick, N. (2001). Innate immunity and autoimmunity: from self-protection to self-destruction. *Trends Immunol* **22**: 97–101.

Singh, A.K., Wilson, M.T., Hong, S., Olivares-Villagomez, D., Du, C., Stanic, A.K., *et al.* (2001). Natural killer T cell activation protects mice against experimental autoimmune encephalomyelitis. *J Exp Med* **194**: 1801–1811.

Smith, A.L., Barthold, S.W., de Souza, M.S., and Bottomly, K. (1991). The role of gamma interferon in infection of susceptible mice with murine coronavirus, MHV-JHM. *Arch Virol* **121**: 89–100.

Smith, M.E. (2001). Phagocytic properties of microglia in vitro: implications for a role in multiple sclerosis and EAE. *Microsc Res Tech* **54**: 81–94.

Smits, H.A., Boven, L.A., Pereira, C.F., Verhoef, J., and Nottet, H.S. (2000). Role of macrophage activation in the pathogenesis of Alzheimer's disease and human immunodeficiency virus type 1-associated dementia. *Eur J Clin Invest* **30**: 526–535.

Steinman, R.M. (1991). The dendritic cell system and its role in immunogenicity. *Ann Rev Immunol* **9**: 271–296.

Steiman, L (1996). Multiple sclerosis: a coordinated immunological attack against myelin in the central nervous system. *Cell*, **85**, 299–302.

Stewart, J.N., Mounir, S., and Talbot, P.J. (1992). Human coronavirus gene expression in the brains of multiple sclerosis patients. *Virology* **191**: 502–505.

Stohlman, S.A. and Hinton, D.R. (2001). Viral induced demyelination. *Brain Pathol* **11**: 92–106.

Stohlman, S.A., Bergmann, C.C., van der Veen, R.C., and Hinton, D.R. (1995*a*). Mouse hepatitis virus-specific cytotoxic T lymphocytes protect from lethal infection without eliminating virus from the central nervous system. *J Virol* **69**: 684–694.

Stohlman, S.A., Hinton, D.R., Cua, D., *et al.* (1995*b*). Tumor necrosis factor expression during mouse hepatitis virus-induced demyelinating encephalomyelitis. *J Virol* **69**: 5898–5903.

Stohlman, S.A., Yao, Q., Bergmann, C.C., Tahara, S.M., Kyuwa, S., and Hinton, D.R. (1995*c*). Transcription and translation of proinflammatory cytokines following JHMV infection. *Adv Exp Med Biol* **380**: 173–178.

Stohlman, S.A., Bergmann, C.C., Lin, M.T., Cua, D.J., and Hinton, D.R. (1998). CTL effector function within the central nervous system requires CD4+ T cells. *J Immunol* **160**: 2896–2904.

Streit, W.J., Walter, S.A., and Pennell, N.A. (1999). Reactive microgliosis. *Prog Neurobiol* **57**: 563–581.

Sun, N., Grzybicki, D., Castro, R.F., Murphy, S., and Perlman, S. (1995). Activation of astrocytes in the spinal cord of mice chronically infected with a neurotropic coronavirus. *Virology* **213**: 482–493.

Sun, N. and Perlman, S. (1995). Spread of a neurotropic coronavirus to spinal cord white matter via neurons and astrocytes. *J Virol* **69**: 633–641.

Takacs, K. and Altmann, D.M. (1998). The case against epitope spread in experimental allergic encephalomyelitis. *Immunol Rev* **164**: 101–110.

Talbot, P.J. (1997). Virus-induced autoimmunity in multiple sclerosis: the coronavirus paradigm. *Adv Clin Neurosci* **7**: 215–233.

Talbot, P.J., Paquette, J.-S., Ciurli, C., Antel, J.P., and Ouellet, F. (1996). Myelin basic protein and human coronavirus 229E cross-reactive T cells in multiple sclerosis. *Ann Neurol* **39**: 233–240.

Talbot, P.J., Arnold, D., and Antel, J. (2001) Virus-induced autoimmune reactions in the nervous system. *Curr Topics Microbiol Immunol* **253**: 247–271.

Tian, J., Gregory, S., Adorini, L., and Kaufman, D.L. (2001). The frequency of high avidity T cells determines the hierarchy of determinant spreading. *J Immunol* **166**: 7144–7150.

Torres, B.A. and Johnson, H.M. (1998). Modulation of disease by superantigens. *Curr Opin Immunol* **10**: 465–470.

Tough, D.F., Borrow, P., and Sprent, J. (1996). Induction of bystander T cell proliferation by viruses and type 1 interferon *in vivo*. *Science* **272**: 1947–1950.

Tourne, S., Miyazaki, T., Oxenius, A., Klein, L., Fehr, T., Kyewski, B., *et al.* (1997). Selection of a broad repertoire of CD4+ T cells in H-2Ma0/0 mice. *Immunity* **7**: 187–195.

Trollmo, C., Meyer, A.L., Steere, A.C., Hafler, D.A., and Huber, B.T. (2001). Molecular mimicry in Lyme arthritis demonstrated at the single cell level: LFA-1a$_L$ is a partial agonist for outer surface protein A-reactive T cells. *J Immunol* **166**: 5286–5291.

Tsubata, T. and Honjo, T. (2000). B cell tolerance and autoimmunity. *Rev Immunogenet* **2**: 18–25.

Tuohy, V.K., Yu, M., Yin, L., Kawczak, J.A., Johnson, J.M., Mathisen, P.M. *et al.* (1998). The epitope spreading cascade during progression of experimental autoimmune encephalomyelitis and multiple sclerosis. *Immunol Rev* **164**: 93–100.

Tuohy, V.K., Yu, M., Yin, L., Kawczak, J.A., and Kinkel, P.R. (1999). Regression and spreading of self-recognition during the development of autoimmune demyelinating disease. *J Autoimmun* **13**: 11–20.

Unutmaz, D., Pileri, P., and Abrignani, S. (1994). Antigen-independent activation of naive and memory resting T cells by a cytokine combination. *J Exp Med* **180**: 1159–1164.

Vanderlugt, C.L., Neville, K.L., Nikcevich, K.M., Eagar, T.N., Bluestone, J.A., and Miller, S.D. (2000). Pathologic role and temporal appearance of newly emerging autoepitopes in relapsing experimental autoimmune encephalomyelitis. *J Immunol* **164**: 670–678.

Wang, F.I., Stohlman, S.A., and Fleming, J.O. (1990). Demyelination induced by murine hepatitis virus JHM strain (MHV-4) is immunologically mediated. *J Neuroimmunol* **30**: 31–41.

Watanabe, R., Wege, H., and ter Meulen, V. (1983). Adoptive transfer of EAE-like lesions from rats with coronavirus-induced demyelinating encephalomyelitis. *Nature* **305**: 150–153.

Wege, H. (1995). Immunopathological aspects of coronavirus infections. *Springer Semin Immunopathol* **17**: 133–148.

Williams, K.C. and Hickey, W.F. (2002). Central nervous system damage, monocytes and macrophages, and neurological disorders in AIDS. *Ann Rev Neurosci* **25**: 537–562.

Williamson, J.S.P. and Stohlman, S. (1990). Effective clearance of mouse hepatitis virus from the CNS requires both CD4+ and CD8+ T cells. *J Virol* **64**: 4590–4592.

Williamson, J., Sykes, S.P.K., and Stohlman, S. (1991). Characterization of brain infiltrating mononuclear cells during infection with mouse hepatitis virus strain JHM. *J Neuroimmunol* **32**: 199–207.

Wu, G.F. and Perlman, S. (1999). Macrophage infiltration, but not apoptosis, is correlated with immune-mediated demyelination following murine infection with a neurotropic coronavirus. *J Virol* **73**: 8771–8780.

Wu, G.F., Dandekar, A.A., Pewe, L., and Perlman, S. (2000). CD4 and CD8 T cells have redundant but not identical roles in virus-induced demyelination. *J Immunol* **165**: 2278–2286.

Wucherpfennig, K.W. (2001). Mechanisms for the induction of autoimmunity by infectious agents. *J Clin Invest* **108**: 1097–1104.

Wucherpfennig, K.W. and Strominger, J.L. (1995). Molecular mimicry in T cell-mediated autoimmunity: viral peptides activate human T cell clones specific for myelin basic protein. *Cell* **80**: 695–705.

Xiong, H., Yamada, K., Jourdi, H., Kawamura, M., Takei, N., Han, D., *et al.* (1999). Regulation of nerve growth factor release by nitric oxide through cyclic GMP pathway in cortical glial cells. *Mol Pharmacol* **56**: 339–347.

Xiong, H., Zeng, Y.C., Lewis, T., Zheng, J., Persidsky, Y., and Gendelman, H.E. (2000). HIV-1 infected mononuclear phagocyte secretory products affect neuronal physiology leading to cellular demise: relevance for HIV-1-associated dementia. *J Neurovirol* **6**(Suppl. 1):S14–S23.

Yu, M., Johnson, J.M., and Tuohy, V.K. (1996). A predictable sequential determinant spreading cascade invariably accompanies progression of experimental autoimmune encephalomyelitis: a basis for peptide-specific therapy after onset of clinical disease. *J Exp Med* **183**: 1777–1788.

Zhao, Z.S., Granucci, F., Yeh, L., Schaffer, P.A., and Cantor, H. (1998). Molecular mimicry by herpes simplex virus-type 1: autoimmune disease after viral infection *Science* **279**: 1344–1347.

11 Immunity to bacterial infections

Uwe Koedel and H. Walter Pfister

Bacterial infections involving the central nervous system (CNS) are often life-threatening. Even if treated adequately, the prognosis for bacterial infections of the CNS remains serious. The case fatality rate reaches more than 30% depending on the causative agent and the site of infection. Many survivors, up to one-third, develop long-term sequelae including neurologic deficits and neuropsychologic impairment (Mathisen and Johnson, 1997; Koedel et al., 2002). The intent of this chapter is to provide an overview of the current state of knowledge on the following questions: (1) How is the CNS protected against bacterial infections? (2) How do bacteria gain access to the CNS? (3) How does the host organism react to bacterial infections within the CNS compartment? Are there any differences in the immune response between the CNS and non-CNS tissues? Are there any differences in the immune response between different compartments within the CNS? What are the consequences of the host imune response to bacterial infections within the CNS?

Anatomical barriers: protection against infection

The CNS is well defended against bacterial infection. The brain and the spine are covered by three connective tissue membranes called meninges (Fig. 11.1). The pia mater is the membrane closest to the brain and the spinal cord, the arachnoid is the middle membrane, and the dura mater is

the outermost membrane. Together, these membranes constitute a protective barrier against bacterial invasion from the external environment.

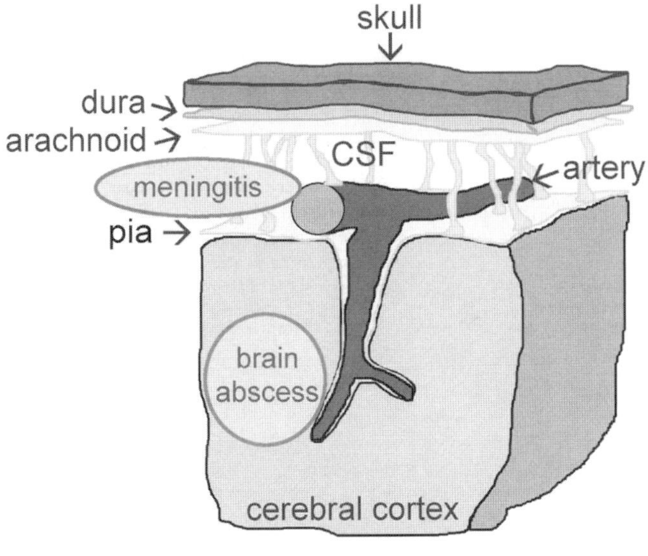

Invasion of the brain by blood-borne bacteria (from the internal environment) is restricted by two physiological barriers which separate the bloodstream from the CNS: the blood–brain barrier and the blood–cerebrospinal fluid (CSF) barrier (Fig. 11.2). The blood–brain barrier, interposed between the circulatory system and the CNS, is formed by microvascular endothelial cells (Huber et al., 2001). These cells differ from their peripheral counterparts in three important aspects: (1) they have tight junctions with extremely high electrical resistance, (2) they have sparse

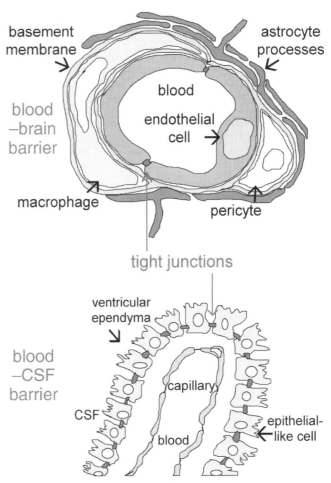

Fig. 11.1 Diagram of the brain, its coverings, and spaces involved in infections of the central nervous system (CNS). Bacterial infections of the CNS can be divided into two broad categories—those which involve primarily the meninges (meningitis) and those which are confined primarily to the parenchyma (e.g. brain abscess). CSF = cerebrospinal fluid.

Fig. 11.2 Schematic diagram of the blood–brain barrier and blood–cerebrospinal fluid (CSF) barrier. Both cerebromicrovascular endothelial cells and choroidal epithelial-like cells form tight junctions restricting the non-specific transport of ions, proteins, cells, and pathogens into the CNS microenvironment.

pinocytic activity, and (3) they have specific carrier and transport systems. In combinations, these features restrict the non-specific transport of ions, proteins, cells, and pathogens into the CNS microenviroment (Gloor *et al.*, 2001).

The blood–CSF barrier is located at the choroid plexuses and the arachnoid membrane situated between the dura and the CSF (Strazielle and Ghersi-Egea, 2000). The choroid plexuses, with their relatively large vascular surface area, are the major interface between the blood and the CSF. The plexuses contain fenestrated (permeable) capillaries and venules. The external covering of the plexuses is the site of the barrier between blood and CSF and is composed of epithelial-like cells. An occluding band of tight junctions close to the CSF side of these cells restricts transport via the paracellular pathway, although the junctions are slightly more permeable than those of the blood–brain barrier.

Possible routes of infection

In order to invade the CNS, the pathogen must cross the physiological barriers between the CNS and the environment. Bacteria can penetrate into the CNS from the environment if there is a break in the continuity of the protective layers (skull, spinal column, meninges). Such a discontinuity may be due to congenital defects (encephalocele, meningomyelocele) or may be caused by trauma or surgical procedures. Bacteria can also spread to the CNS from infected adjacent air sinuses, the middle ear, and the mastoids. They can reach the CNS either directly through the bone, especially in areas where the bone plate is thin, or along veins or nerves.

Bacteria can also be conveyed to the CNS from distant sites of infection by the bloodstream. In this case, the pathogen must cross a monolayer either of endothelial cells (blood–brain barrier) or epithelial cells (blood–CSF barrier) expressing tight junctions. How can a pathogen cope with this task? The pathogen can employ three strategies including (1) paracellular passage by disruption of the tight junctions or endothelial/epithelial injury, (2) transcellular transport by active or passive transcytosis, and (3) traversal of the barriers using leukocytes as 'Trojan horses' (Fig. 11.3) (Nassif *et al.*, 2002). Only a limited number of pathogens are capable of crossing the blood–brain/CSF barrier and invading the CNS. This suggests that bacteria presenting brain tropism have specific attributes. For example, although

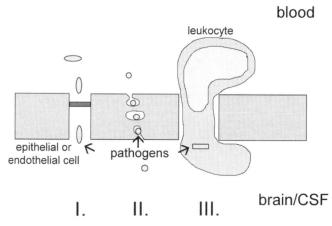

Fig. 11.3 Mechanisms of bacterial transmigration across the blood–brain/CSF barrier. The pathogen can employ three strategies including (I) paracellular passage by disruption of the tight junctions or endothelial/epithelial injury, (II) transcellular transport by active or passive transcytosis, and (III) traversal of the barriers using leukocytes as 'Trojan horses'.

quite different genetically and physiologically, major meningeal pathogens have intriguing similarities. *Streptococcus pneumoniae*, *Neisseria meningitidis*, and *Haemophilus influenzae* are capable of asymptomatic carriage in the nasopharynx, but can also cause devastating disease. They share certain structural features such as phosphorylcholine moieties, IgA proteases, and polysaccharide capsules, as well as certain physiological features such as phase variations, DNA transformation, and autolysis (for review see Tzeng and Stephens (2000), McCullers and Tuomanen (2001), and Marrs *et al.* (2001)). Thus, consideration of the pathogenesis of one of these bacteria, e.g. *S. pneumoniae*, as in this chapter (Fig. 11.4), may yield insight into the pathogenesis of the others.

The preferred route by which *S. pneumoniae* transits across the blood–brain barrier is thought to be through endothelial cells rather than between them (Ring *et al.*, 1998). Invasion requires prior adhesion of the pathogen to the endothelial cell surface. Simple attachment occurs to

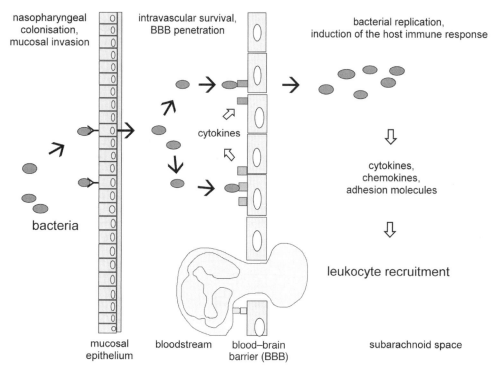

Fig. 11.4 Pathogenic steps leading to the initiation of bacterial meningitis. Effective invasion of the central nervous system involves multiple interactions between the pathogen and the host that sequentially result in mucosal colonization, invasion into, and survival within the intravascular space, and traversal of the blood–brain barrier. Replication and autolysis of bacteria in the subarachnoid space leads to the release of bacterial components into the cerebrospinal fluid that, in turn, are known stimuli for the release of pro-inflammatory host factors.

several glycoconjugates (Cundell and Tuomanen, 1994). Pneumococcal invasion and transmigration is promoted by activation of endothelial cells which increases the amount of surface-expressed platelet-activating factor (PAF) receptor that in turn binds phosphorylcholine of the pneumococcal cell wall (Cundell et al., 1995). The PAF receptor is known to be rapidly internalized after interaction with its natural ligand. Accordingly, the pneumococcus seems to invade the endothelial cell in a vacuole together with the PAF receptor. Within the endothelial cell, the pathogen undergoes different fates including death within the vacuole and transmigration through the cell. Only transparent pneumococci appear to possess the ability to transcytose through endothelial monolayers in a significant proportion (Ring et al., 1998). The morphological phenotypes, termed opaque and transparent because of their appearance when viewed with oblique transmitted light on transparent agar surfaces, are the result of a process termed phase variation. Phenotype variations are associated with differences in the expression of a variety of surface determinants that contribute to the ability of the pathogen to interact with the host (Overweg et al., 2000). In S. pneumoniae, the transparent variants produce increased amounts of the cell wall components teichoic acid and cholin binding protein (Cbp) A, whereas the opaque variant is associated with larger amounts of capsular polysaccharide and the cell wall component pneumococcal suface protein (Psp) A (Kim and Weiser, 1998). As a result of the expression patterns of the phenotypic variants, transparent variants are more suited than opaque for colonization and invasion while opaque variants survive better than transparent once in the bloodstream. Thus, phase variation is an important mechanism that allows the meningeal pathogen to adapt to the dramatic changes in the host environment (bloodstream, endothelial surface, intra- and intercellular space) on its way into the CNS.

Syndromes of CNS infections: terminology and major causative agents

The infecting bacteria cause an inflammatory reaction in the area invaded. Depending on the location of the infection, bacterial infections of the CNS can be divided into two broad categories—those which involve primarily the meninges and those which are confined primarily to the parenchyma. The term '(lepto)meningitis' generally refers to infection of the arachnoid membrane, the pia mater, and the CSF within the subarachnoid space (Fig. 11.1) (Townsend and Scheld, 1998; Rajnik and Ottolini, 2000). Meningitis is the most common bacterial infection involving the CNS. Extension of the inflammatory process into the underlying brain leads to a meningoencephalitis. The term 'encephalitis' means a diffuse parenchymal inflammation of the brain. In contrast to encephalitis, a brain abscess is a circumscribed region of infection within the brain parenchyma. The abscess is initially characterized by a focal area of inflammation and edema (early cerebritis stage). Expansion of cerebritis and the development of a central necrotic focus are seen in the late cerebritis stage. The necrotic center cavitates and becomes filled with pus, and a vascular zone of brain tissue with macrophages, mononuclear cells, and reactive astrocytes surrounds the cavity. Later, collagen (derived from vascular

cells) laid down in this reactive zone forms a thick capsule that walls off the infection (Flaris and Hickey, 1992).

The causative agents of bacterial mening(oencephal)itis vary with host age and with the route of infection. The most common organisms of acute bacterial meningitis in children and adults are S. pneumoniae and N. meningitidis. H. influenzae is infrequent now in young children thanks to vaccination. In newborns, the most common organisms are beta hemolytic streptococcus group B and Escherichia coli, less often Staphylococcus aureus and Listeria monocytogenes. In the elderly, S. pneumoniae (over 50% of cases) is the predominant cause of acute bacterial meningitis; Gram-negative bacteria and L. monocytogenes reappear (Schuchat et al., 1997). The prototypic infectious agent for chronic mening(oencephal)itis is Mycobacterium tuberculosis. Chronic meningitis is an inflammation of the meninges lasting more than 4 weeks. This form of meningitis is fairly rare in developed countries.

Brain abscesses are frequently polymicrobial, and the most etiologic agents in clinical series have been microaerophilic streptococci (Streptococcus viridans) and anaerobic bacteria (Gortvai et al., 1987). Additional microorganisms such as S. aureus and facultative anaerobic Gram-negative bacteria (e.g. Enterobacteriaceae) may also be involved, depending on the underlying source (e.g. infected air sinuses or middle ear, bacterial endocarditis) (Mathisen and Johnson, 1997).

Combined, bacterial infection of the CNS can be categorically divided into infections of the meninges and the parenchyma. Meningeal infections are primarily caused by different pathogens from parenchymal infections. Are there also differences in the immune reactivity between these two CNS compartments?

What do we know about the immune system within the CNS?

The immune system of vertebrates has been conceptionally divided into two parts: innate and acquired immunity (Table 11.1) (Parkin and Cohen, 2001). Acquired immunity is mediated by two classes of specialized cells, T and B lymphocytes. Since each lymphocyte displays a single kind of structurally unique receptor, the repertoire of antigen receptors in the entire lymphocyte population is very large and diverse. The size and diversity of this receptor repertoire increase the probability that an individual lymphocyte will encounter an antigen that binds to its receptor, thus triggering activation and proliferation. This process, termed clonal expansion, is absolutely necessary for the establishment of an efficient immune response. However, acquired immunity has two major limitations. First, antigen receptors are unable to determine the source of the antigen for which they are specific (they are unable to discriminate between self versus non-self). Second, initiation of acquired immunity takes typically 4–7 days to occur, which allows more than enough time for most pathogens to damage the host (Medzhitov and Janeway, 2000). In contrast, the effector mechanisms of innate immunity are activated immediately after infection and rapidly combat replicating microbial invaders. The major players of innate immunity are phagocytes such as macrophages,

Table 11.1 Major differences between innate and acquired immunity

Innate immune system	Acquired immune system
Immediate maximal response	Lag time (3–4 days) between exposure and maximal response
No immmunologic memory	Immunologic memory
Not antigen specific	Antigen specific
Receptors:	Receptors
Germline encoded	Generated somatically
In almost all multicellular organisms	Only in vertebrates
Recognition of conserved molecular patterns	Recognition of details of molecular structure
(Relatively) perfect self/non-self discrimination	Imperfect self/non-self discrimination
Only hundreds of different receptors	Over 100 000 000 000 different receptors

neutrophils, and dendritic cells (DC). The main functions of these cells were thought for a long time to be phagocytosis of pathogens in a non-specific manner, digestion of pathogens, and presentation of pathogen-derived antigens to T cells. However, recent identification of the Toll-like receptor (TLR) family has made clear that innate immunity has considerable specificity. Innate immunity can recognize conserved pathogen-associated molecular patterns (PAMP) through pattern recognition receptors (PRRs), such as TLRs. Recognition of pathogens then triggers cytokine production and upregulation of co-stimulatory molecules on phagocytes (especially DCs), leading to T helper (Th) cell differentiation (Akira *et al.*, 2001; Akira and Hemmi, 2003). Thus, innate immunity is closely linked to acquired immunity.

The CNS poses an interesting challenge for the immune system. The CNS, unlike many other tissues, has a limited capacity for self-repair; mature neurons lack the ability to regenerate, and neural stem cells, although they exist even in the adult brain, have a limited ability to generate new functional neurons in response to injury (Bjorklund and Lindvall, 2000*a,b*). For this reason, the CNS requires a particular degree of protection, for example against microbial infection. However, the weapons used by the immune system to defend the organism against pathogens can be deleterious to the function and survival of CNS neurons. Indeed, in a variety of mouse models of CNS pathology, neurodegeneration is more readily initiated or exacerbated in immunocompetent mice than in mice lacking competent immune systems (Carson and Sutcliffe, 1999). Thus, the immune reactivity within the CNS must be limited to the essential minimum in order to avoid unwanted side-effects ('bystander' killing of healthy CNS neurons). Nevertheless, it must be sufficient to identify and remove potentially dangerous structures (such as microbes) (Wekerle, 2002). What do we know about the immune reactivity within the brain parenchyma?

Today it is clear that the intact CNS tissue constitutes a milieu unfavorable for immune responses. For example, in contrast to other tissue macrophages, microglia do not express major histocompatibility complex (MHC) Class I or II antigens in their quiescent state (Carson, 2002). Without MHC proteins expressed on cell membranes, there is no presentation of antigenic peptides to T lymphocytes. Perhaps of even more importance, DCs, the most potent antigen-presenting cells (APC) in the body, are absent from the normal brain parenchyma (Pashenkov and Link, 2002). DCs are specialized for the transport of antigen to lymph nodes and for activation of antigen-inexperienced naive T lymphocytes. In addition, normal physiologically active neurons have a general suppressive potential that prevents (and limits) the development of inflammatory/immune responses (Neumann, 2001). For instance, microglia are kept in a quiescent state in the intact CNS tissue by local interactions between the CD200 receptor, expressed by neurons, and its ligand, expressed on microglial cells. Moreover, MHC Class II inducibility of microglia and astrocytes (non-professional CNS APCs) by the pro-inflammatory interferon-γ was suppressed by electrically active neurons (e.g. via indirect electrical coupling due to changes in ion concentrations)(Wekerle, 2002). However, the absence of immune responsiveness applies only to the normal CNS tissue. During the course of various pathological processes, genes are activated changing the immunologically silent CNS tissue into a milieu allowing inflammation and enabling antigen-specific immune responses (Neumann, 2001). Thus, the immune reactivity within the brain parenchyma seems to be inducible, becoming available on temporary demand.

What do we know about the immune reactivity within the CSF compartments (the leptomeninges, the choroid plexus, and the CSF)? In contrast to microglia, macrophages in the leptomeninges and the choroid plexus have a more up-regulated, active phenotype than brain microglial cells. They constitutively express MHC antigens (Matyszak, 1998). Moreover, DCs are normally present in all non-neural structures that are in direct contact with the CSF, namely the leptomeninges and the choroid plexus (Pashenkov *et al.*, 2003). In addition, PRRs, essential triggers for an immediate (innate) immune response, are widely expressed within the CSF compartment, but are virtually absent within the brain parenchyma. For instance, TLR2- and TLR4-expressing cells are present along the leptomeninges and choroid plexus under normal conditions, but are nearly

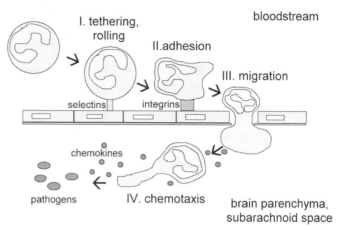

Fig. 11.5 Leukocyte–endothelial adhesion cascade. Leukocytes in the main bloodstream tether, roll (I), adhere (II), emigrate (III), and chemotax (IV) towards the site of infection.

undetectable in parenchymal structures (Laflamme and Rivest, 2001; Laflamme *et al.*, 2001). Thus, in contrast to the brain parenchyma, immune reactivity within the CSF compartment seems to be constitutive and similar to that in peripheral organs, like the skin.

What is the impact of the marked differences in immune reactivity between these CNS compartments on acute inflammatory reactions to bacterial stimuli?

Acute inflammatory reactions to bacterial antigens within the CNS

A central feature of the acute inflammatory reaction is the recruitment of neutrophils to a site of infection to eradicate the pathogens. Neutrophil migration from the vasculature occurs as a multistep process, dictated by the sequential activation of cell adhesion molecules (CAM) on both neutrophils and endothelial cells (for mored detailled information see also Wagner and Roth, 2000 and Krieglstein and Granger, 2001). The adhesion cascade can be divided into three sequential steps of rolling, firm adhesion, and emigration (Fig. 11.5).

Neutrophil rolling on endothelial cells is mediated by the selectin family of adhesion molecules. The selectins are lectin-like molecules that are expressed on leukocytes (L-selectin), endothelial cells (E-selectin), and platelets (P-selectin). L-selectin is constitutively expressed on neutrophils, with the highest expression level found on neutrophils newly released from the bone marrow. During very early stages of infection, the release of granulocyte- and granulocyte-macrophage colony stimulating factors (G-CSF and GM-CSF) stimulate division of myeloid precursors in the bone marrow, releasing millions of the cells into the circulation and causing characteristic neutrophil leukocytosis. P-selectin is stored in specific granules that are present in platelets and endothelial cells from where it can be rapidly mobilized to the cell surface after stimulation. The second endothelial selectin, E-selectin, is not stored in pre-formed granules but requires gene transcription for expression. Thus, peak cell surface expression of E-selectin needs several hours to occur after exposure to appropriate stimuli. Cytokines, bacterial products, and oxidants are known to promote the expression of P- and E-selectin in endothelial cells. The major ligands for all selectins are cell surface glycans that possess a specific sialyl-Lewis X-type structure; L-selectin may also serve as a ligand for P- and E-selectin (Krieglstein and Granger, 2001).

Firm adhesion of neutrophils to the endothelium is mediated by integrins. Because integrins on neutrophils do not bind well unless they are activated, a triggering step is required for integrin activation. The triggering signal is postulated to be either a receptor-mediated event to inflam-

Table 11.2 Adhesion molecules involved in neutrophil–endothelial cell adhesion

	Adhesion molecule	Localization	Ligand	Function
Selectin family	L-selectin	Neutrophil	P-/E-selectin, GlyCAM, CD14 etc.	Rolling
	P-selectin	Endothelial cell, platelets	L-selectin, PSGL-1 etc.	Rolling
	E-selectin	Endothelial cell	L-selectin, ESL-1 etc.	Rolling
Integrin family	CD11a/CD18 (LFA-1)	Neutrophil	ICAM-1, ICAM-2	Adherence, migration
	CD11b/CD18 (MAC-1)	Neutrophil, monocyte	ICAM-1, iC3b, Fb	Adherence, migration
	CD11c/CD18	Neutrophil, monocyte	iC3b, Fb?	Adherence, migration
Immunoglobulin supergene family	ICAM-1	Endothelial cell, monocyte	CD11a/CD18, CD11b/CD18	Adherence, migration
	ICAM-2	Endothelial cell	CD11a/CD18	Adherence, migration
	VCAM-1	Endothelial cell	CD49d/CD29	Adherence, migration
	PECAM-1	Endothelial cell, leukocytes, platelets	PECAM-1	Adherence, migration

CAM, cell adhesion molecule; GlyCAM, glycosylation dependent CAM; PSGL-1, P-selectin glycoprotein ligand 1; ESL-1, E-selectin ligand-1; LFA, lymphocyte function-associated antigen; MAC, macrophage antigen; ICAM, intercellular CAM; Fb, fibronectin; iC3B, complement 3b fragment; VCAM, vascular endothelial CAM; PECAM, platelet endothelial CAM.

matory factors (such as IL-1β, IL-8, bacterial cell wall products) or an event propagated from signals from activated selectins (Williams and Solomkin, 1999; Sedgwick *et al.*, 2000; Alon and Feigelson, 2002). Integrins are a group of heterodimeric transmembrane glycoproteins that are composed of non-covalently linked α and β subunits which together form an extra-cellular ligand binding site. At present, eight different β subunits that associate with one of 16 α subunits are known (Wagner and Roth, 2000). Neutrophil binding is primarily mediated by two integrins that consist of β2 (CD18) subunits (Table 11.2). These are the macrophage antigen-1 (MAC-1; CD11b/CD18) and lymphocyte-asssociated function antigen-1 (LFA-1; CD11a/CD18). MAC-1 has emerged as the more critical β2-containing integrin in most models of neutrophil-dependent inflammation, such as pneumococcal meningitis. Pre-formed MAC-1 is stored within neutrophil granules where it can be rapidly (within minutes) mobilized to the cell surface after exposure to inflammatory stimuli such as LPS or TNF-α. Inflammatory stimuli also can induce transcription and translation of MAC-1, thus prolonging integrin involvement during inflammation (Wagner and Roth, 2000). The ligand specificity of integrins is largely determined by the α subunits and falls into two groups: a variety of extracellular matrix proteins and cell surface molecules of the immuno-globulin (Ig) supergene family. The Ig superfamily include a broad range of molecules such as intercellular adhesion molecule (ICAM)-1 and -2, vascular cell adhesion molecule (VCAM)-1, or platelet-endothelial cell adhesion molecule (PECAM)-1. The most important complementary endothelial ligand for MAC-1 appears to be ICAM-1 which exhibits low constitutive presentation on the cell surface of the resting endothelium, but is markedly induced by exposure of the endothelium to inflammatory stimuli. VCAM-1-dependent adhesion represents an alternate pathway of neutrophil–endothelial interaction. VCAM-1 can be profoundly up-regulated on the endothelial cell surface after cytokine challenge. It binds selectively to β1 integrins like VLA-4 (α4β1) which has recently been identified on the cell surface of activated neutrophils.

Although the mechanisms of neutrophil extravasation are not fully understood, it is clear that PECAM-1 is critical for the passage of neutrophils between endothelial cells. Found on neutrophils, platelets, and endothelial cells, PECAM-1 can serve as its own ligand and form homodimers with molecules on opposing cells. PECAM-1 is concentrated at intercellular junctions of endothelial cells and, thus, may act as a homing receptor to locate the transendothelial portal of the migrating neutrophils (Wagner and Roth, 2000).

The directed emigration of neutrophils from the vasculature to the site of infection requires sequential interactions with different chemokines present in different anatomical locations. Chemokines are small molecules that are structurally and functionally related to form a family of proteins subdivided into four distinct subfamilies according to the number and spacing of the conserved *N*-terminal cysteines (Gerard and Rollins, 2001; Proudfoot, 2002). The CC or β chemokines, and the CXC or α chemokines, are the largest groups and contain four conserved cysteines. In the CC family the first two cysteines are adjacent, while in the CXC family they are separated by one amino acid. An important subclass of CXC chemokines is characterized by the presence of the glutamic acid–leucine–arginine (ELR) motif preceding the first conserved cysteine. The ELR CXC chemokines are potent neutrophil chemoattractants, whereas CXC chemokines without the ELR motif are inactive toward neutrophils (Table 11.3). The best-studied ELR CXC chemokine is human IL-8. However, at least six additional human ELR CXC chemokines have been described including growth-related oncogene (GRO)-α, GRO-β, and GRO-γ, endothelial cell-derived neutrophil-activating peptide-78 (ENA-78), granulocyte chemotactic protein-2 (GCP-2), and neutrophil-activating peptide-2 (NAP-2) (Rollins, 1997; Luster, 1998). Two human receptors for the ELR CXC chemokines have been identified, CXCR1 and CXCR2. Whereas CXCR1 is selective for IL-8, human CXCR2 is activated by all seven ELR CXC chemokines. Humans and rodents have genes for similar but non-identical sets of ELR CXC chemokines. In mice, no ortholog of human IL-8 has been discovered so

Table 11.3 Neutrophil chemoattractants and their receptors

ELR CXC chemokine	Species	Receptor
IL-8, GCP-2	Human	CXCR1
IL-8, GRO-α, -β, -γ, ENA78, NAP-2	Human	CXCR2
MIP-2, KC, LIX	Mouse	CXCR2
Other chemoattractants: PAF, LTB4, C5a, bacterial peptides		

IL, interleukin; GCP, granulocyte chemotactic protein; GRO, growth-related oncogene; ENA, endothelial cell-derived neutrophil-activating peptide; NAP, neutrophil-activating peptide; MIP, macrophage inflammatory protein; KC, keratinocyte-derived cytokine; LIX, LPS-induced CXC chemokine; PAF, platelet activating factor; LTB, leukotriene B; C5, complement factor 5.

far. Moreover, mice seem to lack a functional homolog of CXCR1. However, mouse neutrophils express a receptor homologous to human CXCR2 that mediates neutrophil chemotaxis in response to murine ELR CXC chemokines KC, macrophage inflammatory protein (MIP)-2, and LPS-induced CXC chemokine (LIX) (Rovai et al., 1998). KC and MIP-2 are related to the three human GRO chemokines, whereas LIX is equally closely related to both ENA-78 and GCP-2. Besides CXCR receptors, neutrophils have at least four additional receptors that can mediate directed migration of neutrophils into and through tissue. Unique receptors exist for PAF, complement protein (e.g. C5a), arachidonic acid metabolites (e.g. LTB4), and bacterial peptides (e.g. fMLP). In contrast to ELR CXC chemokines, these molecules attract neutrophils and monocytes with equal potency (Rollins, 1997; Wagner and Roth, 2000).

What do we know about acute inflammatory responses to bacterial stimuli, such as E. coli LPS or bacille Calmette–Guérin (BCG)? When LPS or heat-killed BCG (given at a small dose of 10^4 organisms) were inoculated in the skin, extensive neutrophil recruitment occurred within a few hours. Intratracheal or intraperitoneal inoculation of LPS or BCG yields similar results. Within the CNS, the meninges and choroid plexuses respond to both LPS and BCG in a manner reminiscent of a peripheral inflammatory response. In contrast, direct intracerebral inoculation of E. coli LPS causes only minimal recruitment of neutrophils and delayed monocyte entry (Andersson et al., 1992; Montero-Menei et al., 1994, 1996). Neutrophils were also scarce when a small dose of BCG (10^4 organisms) was inoculated intracerebrally. However, when the dose of heat-killed BCG was increased to 10^5 organisms, an immune response that was comparable to that in peripheral tissues became detectable (Matyszak and Perry, 1995, 1996). Therefore, the brain parenchyma seems to be more resistant to acute inflammatory reactions, but with large doses of pathogens this resistance is overridden and the normal inflammatory response, characterized by rapid and extensive neutrophil recruitment, is restored (Matyszak, 1998). This atypical kinetic of neutrophil recruitment to the brain parenchyma may be the result of deficient or delayed expression of adhesion molecules and/or chemotactic factors.

A wealth of recent information indicates that the expression of CAMs on the brain endothelium follows a similar pattern to that found in peripheral organs. In detail, ICAM-1 is expressed on only a small number of parenchymal microvessels, whereas VCAM-1 expression is virtually absent in normal brain tissue (Washington et al., 1994; Brosnan et al., 1995). Studies using cultured human and murine cerebromicrovascular endothelial cells have supported these findings (Wong and Dorovini-Zis, 1995; Barkalow et al., 1996; Vastag et al., 1999). Stimulation of isolated brain endothelial cells with pro-inflammatory cytokines induces ICAM-1 and VCAM-1 expression in a similar way as for non-brain endothelial cells (like those derived from umbilical veins) (Stins et al., 1997). Likewise, following intracerebral injection of the pro-inflammagen LPS, ICAM-1 and VCAM-1 are readily up-regulated on brain endothelium in a time course comparable with that demonstrated on non-CNS endothelium (Bell and Perry, 1995). The endothelial selectins E-selectin and P-selectin cannot be detected in normal CNS (Gotsch et al., 1994; Carvalho-Tavares et al., 2000). Like ICAM-1 and VCAM-1, a significant increase in brain expression of both selectins is induced by pro-inflammatory cytokines and LPS with a maximum expression at the cell surface 3–4 h after stimulation. Thus, the time course of brain selectin expression resembles that in peripheral organs, but both are clearly more weakly expressed in the brain parenchyma than in any other tissue (Gotsch et al., 1994; Carvalho-Tavares et al., 2000). The chief difference, however, is that the brain tissue lacks constitutive P-selectin expression, and thus is devoid of the rapid pathway of P-selectin-mediated neutrophil adhesion. This pathway is characterized by the rapid translocation of P-selectin from intracellular storage granules to the cell surface after stimulation (e.g. with histamine) (Carvalho-Tavares et al., 2000). The lack of stored P-selectin may lead to delayed leukocyte–neutrophil interactions, but may not explain the higher threshold for initiating an immune response within the brain parenchyma.

Apart from adhesion molecules, the regulated expression of chemokines is a critical determinant in regulating the leukocyte recruitment cascade (Johnston and Butcher, 2002). There has been a recent explosion of research

into chemokines. The list of chemokines that have been identified to be present in brain tissues and cells include MCP-1 (monocyte chemoattractant protein-1), MIP-1α and -1β, RANTES (regulated on activation, normal T-cell expressed and secreted), IL-8, GRO-β (in rodents: MIP-2 and KC), IP-10 (interferon-γ-inducible protein-10), SDF-1α (stromal cell-derived factor-1), and fractalkine. Of these, only SDF-1β and fractalkine have been shown to be constitutively expressed in the brain (Mennicken et al., 1999; Bajetto et al., 2001). Up-regulation of selective cytokines has been described in numerous neuroimmunological, neurodegenerative, and neuroinfectious diseases (Anthony et al., 2002; Biber et al., 2002; Ransohoff, 2002). For example, in an experimental brain abscess model in which live S. aureus (encapsulated in agarose beads) were implanted in rodent brains, early and sustained expression of KC became detectable in the brain which correlated with the appearance of neutrophils in the abscess (Kielian and Hickey, 2000). In addition, two CC chemokines, MCP-1 and IP-10, were induced within 24 h of staphylococcal implantation and preceded the influx of macrophages and lymphocytes into the brain. However, there was no significant up-regulation in the expression of MIP-2, RANTES, or fractalkine expression (Kielian and Hickey, 2000). In a mouse model of cortical injury plus topical LPS application, a rapid and transient induction of diverse chemokines, namely KC, MCP-1, MIP-1α and -1β, and IP-10 was oberseved, whereas RANTES was induced more slowly and in a more sustained fashion than the other chemokines (Hausmann et al., 1998). To test the biological effects of chemokines in the CNS environment studies in which recombinant chemokines were injected directly into the brain parenchyma have been conducted. Intrahippocampal injections of MCP-1, RANTES, and IP-10 were found to be chemotactic for monocytes, whereas IL-8 and MIP-2 provoked a dramatic recruitment of neutrophils into the brain parenchyma (Bell et al., 1996). Similarly, transgenic mice expressing murine MCP-1 or KC (under the control of the myelin basic protein promotor) showed specific leukocyte recruitment (monocytes for MCP-1 and neutrophils for KC) without additional stimuli (Fuentes et al., 1995; Tani et al., 1996). Thus, it is now clear that appropriate chemoattractants alone are sufficient to induce leukocyte entry into the CNS. However, it is possible that stromal cells in the brain parenchyma do not synthesize sufficient quantities of appropriate chemokines in response to inflammatory stimuli, and that this contributes to the partial resistance of the brain parenchyma to acute inflammation. This hypothesis is supported by recent work showing (1) that the brain parenchyma in adult rodents is more resistant to acute inflammation than that of either juvenile or old rodents, and (2) that this age-related susceptibility to inflammation seems to be due to age-related changes in the brain expression of chemokines and cytokines (Anthony et al., 1998; Terao et al., 2002). Although the exact mechanisms underlying the (possibly) inadequate release of cytokines and chemokines in response to inflammatory/ infectious stimuli is still unclear, it is conceivable that this phenomenon may be caused by the (relative) lack and/or age-related changes in the expression of PRRs within the brain parenchyma. What do we know about the PRRs within the CNS?

Pattern recognition receptors in the CNS: a brief overview

Recognition of microbial non-self plays a crucial role in the host defense. The recognition strategy is based on the detection of constitutive and conserved molecular patterns that are essential products of microbial metabolism. These structures are called pathogen-associated molecular patterns (PAMP). PAMPs have three common features (Medzhitov, 2001; Medzhitov and Janeway, 2002):

1. PAMPs are produced only by microbes (and not by host cells). Thus, recognition of PAMPs by the innate immune system allows the distinction between self and non-self.

2. PAMPs are usually invariant structures shared by entire classes of pathogens. This allows limited classes of germline receptors to detect the presence of virtually any bacterial infection.

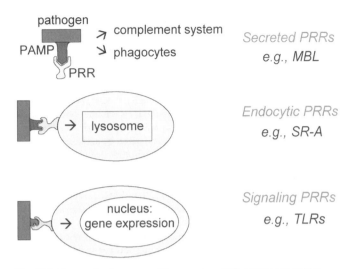

Fig. 11.6 Classes of pattern recognition receptors: PRR, pattern recognition receptor; PAMP, pathogen-associated molecular pattern; MBL, mannose-binding lectin; SR-A, (macrophage) class A scavenger receptor; TLR, Toll-like receptor.

3. PAMPs are usually essential for survival or pathogenicity of microorganisms. Mutations or loss of PAMPs are, therefore, either lethal for the microorganisms or they greatly attenuate their adaptive fitness.

Several structurally and functionally distinct classes of PRRs have evolved to recognize PAMPs and to induce various host defense pathways. Structurally, PRRs belong to several protein families. Calcium-dependent lectin domains, scavenger-receptor protein domains, and leucine-rich repeat domains are often involved in pattern recognition. Functionally, PRRs can be divided into three classes: secreted, endocytic, and signaling PRRs (Fig. 11.6).

Secreted PRRs bind to microbial cells and flag them for recognition by the complement system and phagocytes. The best-characterized receptor of this class is mannan-binding lectin (MBL), a member of the collectin family of proteins (Fraser et al., 1998; Kawasaki, 1999; Fujita, 2002). The collectins, in turn, belong to the calcium-dependent (C-type) lectin superfamily characterized by the presence of the C-type carbohydrate recognition domain (CRD). In addition to MBL, lung surfactant protein (SP)-A and -D, bovine conglutinin, collectin-43 (CL-43), CL-L1 (liver), and CL-P1 (placenta) belong to this protein family (Gadjeva et al., 2001; Lu et al., 2002). MBL is synthesized predominantly in the liver and is secreted into the blood circulation. The serum concentrations of MBL are highly variable in healthy populations and this is genetically controlled by polymorphism/mutations in both the promotor and coding regions of the MBL gene. As an acute phase protein, the expression of MBL can be further up-regulated during infection/inflammation. Apart from the liver, low expression of MBL has also been found in kidney, spleen, muscle, testis, intestine, and the brain (Wagner et al., 2003). MBL can bind to an array of carbohydrate structures on the surface of Gram-negative and Gram-positive bacteria and yeast, as well as some viruses and parasites. On binding to its target, MBL activates the complement system via MBL-associated serine protease (MASP)-1 and MASP-2, of which the latter cleaves complement protein 4 (C4) and C2 to generate a C3 convertase independent of antigen–antibody complexes (Petersen et al., 2000). The expression of MASPs in the CNS or by primary brain cells has not yet been reported. The recent discovery of MASP mRNA in a human glioma cell line may be a first, albeit weak, hint at a possible involvement of the MBL pathway in the detection and defense of bacterial infections of the CNS. Further studies are needed to verify whether this is the case. The need for such studies is underlined by reports demonstrating that:

(1) MBL enhances complement activation and opsonophagocytosis/killing of major CNS pathogens (especially *N. meningitidis*) *in vitro* (Jack et al., 1998, 2001b; Neth et al., 2002);

(2) variant MBL alleles and MBL deficiencies seem to be associated with an increased risk for invasive meningococcal and pneumococcal disease (*N. meningitidis* and *S. pneumoniae* are the most important CNS pathogens)(Bax et al., 1999; Roy et al., 2002); and

(3) apart from complement activation, MBL appears to act as an important regulator of inflammatory pathways and, as such, may also affect the severity of bacterial CNS disease (Jack et al., 2001a; Takahashi et al., 2002).

Endocytic pattern recognition receptors occur on the surface of phagocytes. On recognizing PAMPs on a microbial cell, these receptors mediate the uptake and delivery of the pathogen into the lysosomes where it is destroyed. Pathogen-derived proteins can then be processed, and the resulting peptide can be presented by MHC molecules on the surface of the phagocyte. Class A scavenger receptors (SR-A) are endocytic PRRs (Yamada et al., 1998; Gough and Gordon, 2000; Husemann et al., 2002; Peiser et al., 2002b). The classical SR-A is a trimeric integral membrane glycoprotein which exists in two forms, type I and II, generated by alternative splicing of a single gene product, with the larger type I receptor differing from the type II receptor in having a 110-amino-acid SR cysteine-rich (SRCR) domain at the C-terminus of the protein. Both SR-AI and SR-AII have been shown to have nearly identical ligand-binding properties which have been shown to be mediated through the collagenous domain. The exact functional significance of the SRCR domain found in SR-AI remains to be clarified. The first suggestion that SR-A may play a role in innate immunity came from studies examining the binding of microbial surface components LPS of Gram-negative bacteria and lipoteichoic acid (LTA) of Gram-positive bacteria to the receptor. Hampton et al. (1991) were the first to demonstrate that lipid IV_A forms of bacterial endotoxin bind to SR-A and that other SR ligands can reduce the clearance of LPS from the circulation. Subsequently, Dunne et al. (1994) demonstrated that SR-A also recognizes LTA of a number of Gram-positive bacteria including *Streptococcus pyogenes*, *S. aureus*, and *L. monocytogenes* (Dunne et al., 1994). The range of pathogens to which SR-A is known to bind has been expanded by other studies, and includes *N. meningitidis* and *M. tuberculosis* (Zimmerli et al., 1996; Peiser et al., 2002a). SR-AI and SR-AII are constitutively present on mononuclear phagocytes, e.g. Kupffer cells, dendritic cells, and peritoneal and alveolar macrophages. In the normal adult brain, SR-As are expressed by perivascular macrophages surrounding arterioles and by macrophages within the meninges and the choroid plexuses, but not by resident microglia. In neonate brains, however, SR-As were also detectable, albeit at low amounts, on several microglial populations suggesting a developmental regulation of brain SR-A expression. Moreover, SR-A expression by microglia can be up-regulated by intracerebral administration of pro-inflammatory stimuli such as LPS or IL-1 (Yamada et al., 1998; Husemann et al., 2002). The functional role of these receptors in bacterial brain infections remains to be clarified. It can be speculated that SR-As play an essential role in the clearance of bacteria from the CNS, especially from the CSF compartment, as was reported for peripheral infections. For example, mice deficient in both SR-AI and SR-AII were more susceptible to intraperitoneal infection with *S. aureus* (which is also frequently found in brain abscesses) (Thomas et al., 2000). SR-AI/II-deficient mice displayed an impaired ability to clear bacteria from the site of infection despite of normal killing of *S. aureus* by neutrophils, and die as a result of disseminated infection (Thomas et al., 2000). In addition, SR-AI/II-deficient mice also showed an increased susceptibility to lethal, intravenous infection with *L. monocytogenes* (a major causative agent of bacterial meningoencephalitis), presumably due to an impaired capability to phagocytose and kill *L. monocytogenes* (Ishiguro et al., 2001).

Signaling receptors recognize PAMPs and activate signal transduction pathways that induce the expression of a variety of immune response genes, including pro-inflammatory cytokines. The recently identified receptors of the Toll family appear to have a major role in the initiation of acute immune and inflammatory responses (Akira et al., 2001; Medzhitov, 2001; Janeway and Medzhitov, 2002; Takeda et al., 2003). Toll receptors are type I transmembrane proteins that are evolutionarily conserved between insects

Table 11.4 Toll-like receptors and their ligands (with special emphasis on molecular patterns of CNS pathogens)

TLR family	Ligands
TLR1	Triacyl lipopeptides (*Mycobacteria* species)
	Soluble factors (*Neisseria meningitidis*)
TLR2	Peptidoglycan (*Streptococcus pneumoniae, Staphylococcus aureus, Listeria monocytogenes?*)
	Lipoteichoic acid (*Streptococcus pneumoniae, Staphylococcus aureus*)
	Lipoarabinomannan (*Mycobacteria* species)
	Porins (*Neisseria* species)
	Atypical LPS (e.g. *Leptospira interrogans*)
	HSP70 (host)
TLR4	LPS (Gram-negative bacteria; e.g. *Escherichia coli, Neisseria meningitidis*)
	HSP60 (*Chlamydia* pneumoniae)
	HSP60, HSP70 (host)
	Type III repeat extra domain A of fibronectin (host)
	Fibrinogen (host)
	Oligosacccharides of hyaluronic acid (host)
	Polysaccharide fragments of heparan sulfate (host)
TLR5	Flagellin (e.g. *Escherichia coli*)
TLR6	Diacyl lipopeptides (e.g. *Mycoplasma* species)
TLR9	CpG DNA (bacteria)

and humans. Toll was first identified as an essential molecule for embryonic patterning in *Drosophila* and was subsequently shown to be a key regulator in antifungal immunity (Lemaitre *et al.*, 1996). A homologous family of Toll receptors, the so-called TLRs, exist in mammals. Based on the similarity in the intracellular domain (the Toll-IL-1R or TIR domain), TLRs are related to IL-1 receptors (IL-1Rs). However, the extracellular portions of both receptors are structurally unrelated: IL-1Rs possess an IgG-like domain whereas TLRs bear leucine-rich repeats (LRR) in their extracellular domain. Although the actual mechanism of ligand recognition is still not known, available work provide evidence for a direct interaction between the LRR domain of TLRs and specific PAMPs (Medzhitov, 2001; Takeda *et al.*, 2003). To date, 10 TLRs (TLR1–10) have been reported in human and mouse, respectively (Akira and Hemmi, 2003). Each TLR recognizes specific components of pathogens (Table 11.4) (Takeda and Akira, 2003).

TLR2 is involved in the recognition of components of a variety of pathogens. These include lipoproteins from a variety of pathogens, peptidoglycan and lipoteichoic acid from Gram-positive bacteria, lipoarabinomannan from mycobacteria, and a phenol-soluble modulin from *Staphylococcus epidermidis*. In addition, TLR2 recognizes atypical LPS from *Leptospira interrrogans* or *Porphyromonas gingivalis*. The mechanism by which TLR2 recognizes such a broad spectrum of microbial components is—at least in part—explained by the cooperation of TLR2 with TLR1 and TLR6. Thus, the introduction of a dominant negative form of TLR6 in macrophages inhibited TNF-α production in response to peptidoglycan, but not to bacterial lipopeptides, both of which are recognized by TLR2 (Ozinsky *et al.*, 2000). Analyses of TLR6- and TLR1-deficient mice further revealed their importance for the discrimination of structural differences between lipopeptides. Thus, macrophages from TLR6-deficient mice did not respond to diacyl lipopeptides whereas macrophages from TLR2-deficient mice showed an impaired immune response to triacyl peptides. Thus, TLR1 and TLR6 functionally associate with TLR2 and participate in the discrimination of lipopeptides. In addition to PAMPs, TLR2 also appears to interact with endogenous molecules, liberated during inflammation and/or necrotic cell death (Li *et al.*, 2001; Vabulas *et al.*, 2001).

TLR4 functions as a signal transducing receptor for LPS. The recognition of LPS by TLR4 is complex and requires several accessory molecules. LPS first binds to serum LPS-binding protein (LBP) which functions by transferring LPS to a glycophosphoinositol-anchored cell surface molecule CD14. An additional critical component of the LPS receptor is the small protein MD-2 which lacks a transmembrane domain and is expressed on the cell surface in association with TLR4. Although the exact mechanism of LPS recognition by TLR4 remains to be clarified, several lines of evidence indicate that TLR4 might, in fact, interact with LPS directly. The interaction, however, is clearly aided by CD14 and MD-2. In addition to LPS, TLR4 is implicated in the recognition of several other ligands, including lipoteichoic acid, heat shock proteins (HSP60, HSP70, HSPGp96), fibronectin 7EDA domain, and oligosaccharides of hyaluronan (Takeuchi *et al.*, 1999; Okamura *et al.*, 2001; Termeer *et al.*, 2002; Vabulas *et al.*, 2002a,b). Thus, TLR4 also seems to be involved in the recognition of several endogenous ligands involved in the inflammatory process.

TLR5 is involved in the recognition of flagellin from Gram-positive and Gram-negative bacteria. Flagellated bacteria, but not non-flagellated bacteria, activate TLR5. For example, expression of *L. monocytogenes* flagellin in non-flagellated *E. coli* conferred ability to activate TLR5 whereas deletion of the flagellin gene from *Salmonella typhimurium* abrogated TLR5-stimulating activity (Akira *et al.*, 2001).

Perhaps the most enigmatic example of pattern recognition is the recognition of unmethylated CpG motifs in bacterial DNA by TLR9. In vertebrates, the frequency of CpG motifs is severely suppressed and the cytosine residues of the CpG motif are highly methylated which leads to complete abrogation of immunostimulatory activity. Because bacteria lack cytosine methylation and their DNA contains more CpG motifs than that of vertebrates, CpG motifs might signal the presence of microbial infection. The essential role of TLR9 in the recognition of bacterial DNA was shown using TLR9-deficient mice (Hemmi *et al.*, 2000). Another fascinating aspect of CpG DNA recognition is that the optimal response of mouse versus human cells requires slightly different CpG DNA ligands. It was shown that a CpG motif (GACGT) that optimally stimulates mouse cells is also a more potent activator of transfected mouse TLR9 compared with human TLR9. The

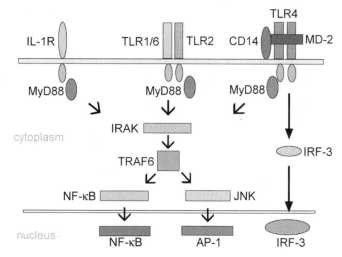

Fig. 11.7 Toll signaling pathway. The interleukin-1 receptor (IL-1R) family and Toll-like receptor (TLR) family members share several signaling components, including the adaptor MyD88, the protein kinase IRAK (IL-1R-associated kinase) and TRAF6 (TNF receptor-associated factor 6). TRAF6 can activate NF-κB and JNK (c-Jun N-terminal kinase) that, in turn, can result in NF-κB- and AP-1-dependent gene transcription. In case of TLR4, additional signaling pathways have been reported, for example LPS-induced activation of IRF-3 (IFN regulatory factor-3). TLR2 recognizes a broad range of structurally unrelated ligands in combination with several other TLRs, including TLR1 and TLR6. Recognition of its ligand LPS (lipopolysaccharide) by TLR4 is aided by two accessory proteins: CD14 and MD-2.

opposite was observed when a CpG motif (GTCGTT) with optimal immuno-stimulatory activity for human cells was used (Bauer *et al.*, 2001). This finding indicates that TLR9 itself can discriminate between two immuno-stimulatory CpG motifs, and therefore can supposedly recognize CpG motifs directly. No bacterial ligands have yet been identified for other members of the TLR family (e.g. TLR3, TLR7, or TLR10).

Activation of signal transduction pathways by TLRs leads to the induction of various genes that encode proteins involved in the host defense, including inflammatory cytokines, chemokines, MHC, and co-stimulatory molecules. Mammalian TLRs also induce a variety of effector molecules such as inducible nitric oxide synthase (iNOS) and antimicrobial peptides which can directly kill microbial pathogens. Because TLRs share sequence similarity with IL-Rs in their intracellular domain, it is not surprising that downstream events are mediated by common components (Fig. 11.7). Upon binding of ligand to TLR or IL-1R, the first intracellular event is the recruitment of MyD88 to the receptor complex. MyD88 then links the receptor complex to IL-1R-associated protein kinase (IRAK). IRAK is autophosphorylated following activation, subsequently dissociates from the complex and associates with TNF receptor-associated factor 6 (TRAF6). The next steps in the pathway downstream of TLR/IL-1R are the TRAF6-dependent activations of the IkB kinase (IKK) complex and the mitogen-activated protein kinase (MAPK) kinase TAK-1 (transforming growth factor-β-activated kinase 1) which, in turn, activates the Rel family transcription factor NF-κB (nuclear factor-κB) as well as the c-Jun-*N*-terminal kinase (JNK) and the p38 MAPK (Akira *et al.*, 2001; Girardin *et al.*, 2002). This signaling cascade seems to be shared by all members of the Toll and IL-1R families. Analysis of MyD88-deficient macrophages, however, showed several unexpected features of the signaling downstream of TLR4 (and TLR3). For example, LPS could induce NF-κB, JNK, and p38 in MyD88-deficient cells, although this activation is delayed compared with wild-type macrophages and insufficient for the induction of cytokine gene expression (Kawai *et al.*, 1999). In addition, DCs from MyD88-deficient, but not from TLR4-deficient, mice showed normal functional maturation in response to LPS (Kaisho *et al.*, 2001). Moreover, LPS stimulation of MyD88-deficient macrophages led to the induction of several interferon (IFN)-inducible genes, such as IP-10 (Kawai *et al.*, 2001). Expression of these genes is TLR4-dependent, and probably occurs through the activation of IFN regulatory factor-3 (IRF-3). IRF-3 confers the induction of IFN-β and subsequent activation of STAT1 (signal transducer and activator of transscription 1) which, in turn, leads to the expression of IFN-inducible genes (Toshchakov *et al.*, 2002). Thus, IRF-3 plays an important role in MyD88-independent TLR4 signaling. Recently, a novel protein containing a TIR domain and designated TIR domain-containing adaptor protein (TIRAP)/MyD88-adaptor-like (Mal) was identified (Horng *et al.*, 2001; Fitzgerald *et al.*, 2001). Initial *in vitro* studies suggested that TIRAP/Mal is a possible adaptor involved in LPS-induced, MyD88-independent signaling. However, generation of TIRAP/Mal-deficient mice revealed that this molecule functions as an adaptor in the MyD88-dependent signaling pathway via TLR2 and TLR4, and may provide specificity in the downstream signaling of individual TLRs (Horng *et al.*, 2002). Thus other, as yet unidentified, TIR domain-containing molecules may be responsible for MyD88-independent signaling.

While the expression of TLRs in blood cells and peripheral tissues has been extensively studied over the past few years (Hornung *et al.*, 2002; Zarember and Godowski, 2002), little information has been published on TLR expression within the CNS.

In murine CNS, expression of TLR4 and TLR2 has been recently documented (Laflamme and Rivest, 2001; Laflamme *et al.*, 2001; 2003). A low to moderate TLR4 mRNA hybridization signal was found in the lepto-meninges, choroid plexus, and in circumventricular organs in normal CNS. Scattered small cells also displayed a convincing TLR4 mRNA hybridization signal within the brain parenchyma (Laflamme and Rivest, 2001). Lehnardt *et al.* (2002) have shown that microglia are the only CNS glial cells that express high levels of TLR4, whereas astrocytes and oligodendrocytes express none. A quite similar regional expression pattern has been described for TLR2 with the exception that there was no positive hybridization signal across the brain parenchyma of healthy mice (Laflamme *et al.*,

2001). During endotoxemia (induced by intraperitoneal challenge with *E. coli* LPS), a robust and transient transcriptional activation of the gene encoding TLR2 in the murine brain was detectable, whereas the gene encoding TLR4 was down-regulated in the cerebral tissue of LPS-challenged mice (Laflamme and Rivest, 2001; Laflamme *et al.*, 2001). In contrast to LPS, peptidoglycan and lipoteichoic acid, known ligands for TLR2, failed to modulate TLR2 mRNA transcription in the murine brain (Laflamme *et al.*, 2001).

More recently, expression of TLRs in the human CNS has been documented (Bsibsi *et al.*, 2002). The major finding of this study was that human adult microglia express a wide range of TLR family members, including TLR1 through TLR8, at least *in vitro*. Expression of TLR2, TLR3, and to some extent also TLR1 and TLR4 was also found in human astrocytes and oligodendrocytes. Since murine astrocytes and oligodendrocytes appear not to be able to express TLR4 (Lehnardt *et al.*, 2002), human glial cells do not necessarily display the same TLR profile as rodent glial cells. In addition, immunohistochemical examination of brain and spinal cord sections from patients with multiple sclerosis (MS) and from control donors revealed high expression of both TLR4 and TLR3 in all active MS lesions, especially in perivascular areas at the borders and in the center of lesions, while in healthy white matter or normal-appearing white matter in MS patients TLR expression was barely detectable (Bsibsi *et al.*, 2002). All in all, these studies provided evidence for broad and regulated expression of several different TLRs in human and rodent CNS. These findings warrant investigations on the role of TLRs in controlling immune and neuro-degenerative processes in the CNS. Up to now, only two studies focusing on the functional role of TLR2 in acute brain inflammation have been published (Echchannaoui *et al.*, 2002; Koedel *et al.*, 2003).

After intracerebral inoculation with a small dose of *S. pneumoniae* (10³ organims), TLR2-deficient mice showed an earlier time of death than wild-type mice (Echchannaoui *et al.*, 2002). With ceftriaxone treatment, none of the wild-type but about one-third of the TLR2-deficient mice died. In addition, TLR2-deficient mice showed higher CNS bacterial titers, higher TNF-α activity in the CSF, and more pronounced blood–brain barrier breaching than wild-type mice (Echchannaoui *et al.*, 2002). When mice were challenged intracisternally with 10⁵ colony forming units of *S. pneumoniae* (the 'classic' model of meningitis (Koedel and Pfister, 1999)), TLR2-deficient mice also showed an increase in disease severity (Koedel *et al.*, 2003). The aggravation of the clinical course was associated with higher bacterial titers in the CNS and in the blood in TLR2-deficient mice, while the expression of meningitis-relevant inflammatory mediators such as IL-1β, TNF-α, IL-16, MIP2, and iNOS (Koedel *et al.*, 2002) was quite similar in both TLR2-deficient and wild-type mice. Together, these studies showed that TLR2 plays a significant role in a murine model of experimental pneumococcal meningitis. Nonetheless, a robust immune response was established in TLR2-deficient mice upon infection, pointing at TLR2-independent cellular recognition of *S. pneumoniae* (cell wall) products. Additional cell culture experiments in which HEK293 cells transfected with single TLRs were exposed to ceftriaxone-killed pneumococci implicated TLR4 as another potential candidate for sensing pneumococcal infection (Koedel *et al.*, 2003; Malley *et al.*, 2003). However, its role *in vivo* remains to be analysed, and further pattern recognition receptors remain to be implicated in recognition of pneumococcal infection of the host organism. Further studies are also warranted to investigate the role of TLRs in the recognition of other bacterial CNS infections, for example *L. monocytogenes* meningoencephalitis, tuberculous meningitis, or brain abscesses due to *S. aureus*.

The host immune response: a protective or autodestructive host reaction?

Once microbial pathogens reach the CNS, they are likely to survive because host defenses in the CNS appear to be largely ineffective in killing them. What are the reasons for this regional immunodeficiency?

Table 11.5 Host defense mechanisms against major CNS pathogens: central role of neutrophils

Pathogen	Host defense
Streptococcus pneumoniae	Complement-mediated opsonophagocytosis, dominant role of the classical complement pathway
Neisseria meningitidis	Direct complement-mediated bacteriolysis. Complement-mediated opsonophagocytosis, all three pathways of complement activation involved
Streptococcus agalactiae	Complement- and antibody-mediated opsonophagocytosis
Escherichia coli	Opsonophagocytosis, bacterial killing mediated by oxidants and proteolytic enzymes
Staphylococcus aureus	Complement-mediated opsonophagocytosis, dominant role of the alternative pathway
Listeria monocytogenes and Mycobacterium tuberculosis	Bacterial killing by neutrophils during the early phase of infection. Immunoregulatory role of neutrophils

Neutrophils are the host immune cells that are the first to migrate into tissue in response to invading microbes. One of their principal roles in immune responses is thought to be phagocytosis and killing of bacteria via generation of oxidants and release of lytic enzymes and antimicrobial peptides. Numerous studies using in vitro assays and/or animal models of systemic infection have highlighted the extraordinary role of neutrophils in the host defense against infection by extracellular pathogens. Recent work has shown that neutrophils also play a protective role against infection by intracellular pathogens. For example, when mice were rendered neutropenic (either by treatment with antineutrophil antibodies or with cyclophosphamide), they had significantly higher bacterial burdens than non-neutropenic controls, irrespective whether they were infected systemically with the extracellular pathogens S. pneumoniae and S. aureus or with the intracellular pathogens L. monocytogenes or M. tuberculosis (Verdrengh and Tarkowski, 1997; Lopez et al., 2000; Pedrosa et al., 2000; Wang et al., 2002). Although the definite mechanisms underlying the bactericidal effects of neutrophils against extra- and intracellular pathogens are far from clear, several aspects of their bactericidal activities have been elucidated by in vitro and in vivo studies (Table 11.5). It seems clear that complement-mediated neutrophil phagocytosis is the dominant host defense mechanism against systemic infection with S. pneumoniae (AlonsoDeVelasco et al., 1995). The classical pathway appears to be the decisive pathway for activation of the complement system during innate immunity to S. pneumoniae (Brown et al., 2002). The host defense against systemic N. meningitidis infection seems to be provided by both direct complement-mediated bacteriolysis and complement- and antibody-induced neutrophil phagocytosis (Tzeng and Stephens, 2000). All three pathways (the classical, the MBL/lectin, and the alternative pathway)(Walport, 2001a,b) may contribute to the deposition of the principal complement opsonins C3b and iC3b onto N. meningitidis (Fijen et al., 2000). Bound complement protein C1q (component of the classical pathway) appears to act synergistically with IgG to increase the association of extracellular Streptococcus agalactiae and neutrophils, thereby facilitating opsonophagocytosis mediated by C3b and IgG (Butko et al., 1999; Spellerberg, 2000). Intracellular destruction of S. agalactiae by neutrophils may depend mainly on the production of oxidants (Cheng et al., 2001). In addition to oxidants, proteolytic enzymes (namely elastase) and antimicrobial peptides seem to contribute to bacterial killing of E. coli by neutrophils (Belaaouaj et al., 2000; Porro et al., 2001). In contrast to E. coli, S. aureus appears to be broadly protected against antimicrobial peptides (Peschel et al., 2001). The major host defense mechanism against this extracellular pathogen may be complement-mediated opsonophagocytosis by neutrophils, whereby the alternative pathway seems to be the major pathway for complement activation (Lowy, 1998; Peschel and Collins, 2001). As mentioned above, neutrophils have also been demonstrated to be key cells in the early resistance of mice

to infections with intracellular pathogens, such as L. monocytogenes or M. tuberculosis (Rogers and Unanue, 1993; Conlan and North, 1994; Sugawara et al., 2001; Portnoy et al., 2002; van Crevel et al., 2002). Apart from direct killing of intracellular pathogens (e.g. by the release of antimicrobial peptides), neutrophils may also exert important immunoregulatory functions. They may release cytokines, chemokines, lytic enzymes, and antimicrobial peptides, thus triggering and/or supporting the activation of macrophages and the recruitment of activated lymphocytes (Lopez et al., 2000; Pedrosa et al., 2000). All in all, neutrophils and neutrophil-dependent mechanisms are thought to play a vital role in the host defense against pathogens that are known to be the major causes of CNS infections.

Although virtually absent in the normal CNS, neutrophil invasion into the CNS occurs with bacterial multiplication and/or the presence of bacterial components. However, neutrophils do not succeed in phagocytosing and killing microbes in the CNS. The reasons for this functional deficit has been clarified only in part. One is the virtual absence of major components of the complement pathways within the CNS (Gasque et al., 2000) The concentrations of the other major bacterial opsonin, immunoglobulin, are also low in normal CNS. Although complement and immunoglobulin concentrations appear to increase in the presence of bacterial CNS infection, they likewise remain below concentrations optimal for opsonic activity (Smith et al., 1977; Simberkoff et al., 1980; Stahel et al., 1997a,b). Thus, the CNS can be conceptualized as a compartment of partial immunodeficiency facilitating (nearly) unrestrained proliferation of microbes which, if untreated, can overwhelm the host until death. The dramatic difference in the efficiency of the host defense against micobes between the CNS and the periphery can be illustrated by comparing the prognosis of two invasive pneumococcal diseases, pneumococcal meningitis and pneumococcal pneumonia. The intracisternal inoculation of 10^4 colony forming units of S. pneumoniae type 3 in C57BL/6 mice resulted in the death of all infected mice whereas only one-quarter of the mice died after intratracheal application of an identical dose of this pneumococcal strain (Gerber et al., 2001; Rijneveld et al., 2001). Similar data have also been reported for humans. Thus, in the pre-antibiotic era, pneumococcal meningitis was a lethal disease (Toomey and Roach, 1939). In contrast, 75% of patients survived pneumococcal pneumonia (Heffron, 1979).

As mentioned above, elevated numbers of neutrophils within the CNS are a hallmark of bacterial CNS infections. It is well known that besides their physiologic functions in the clearance of invading microorganisms (that they do not fulfill sufficiently within the CNS), activated neutrophils have a remarkable potential to cause tissue damage. This is attributable to their capability of releasing a complex assortment of potentially tissue-destructive agents including reactive oxidants and proteolytic enzymes (Bellingan, 2000; Nussler et al., 1999). Over the past years, different experimental strategies including disruption of genes encoding for CXCRs or CAMs and treatment with antibodies designed to prevent leukocyte–endothelial interactions or to deplete neutrophils have been used to assess the role of neutrophils in bacterial infection-associated brain damage. First, Tuomanen et al. (1989) demonstrated that treatment with anti-CD18 antibodies dramatically reduced inflammation, tissue damage, and mortality in experimental pneumococcal meningitis. Similar results were also obtained in an experimental model of H. influenzae meningitis (Saez-Llorens et al., 1991) as well as in experimental pneumococcal meningitis by using different antileukocyte–endothelial interaction strategies including application of anti-ICAM1-antibodies (Weber et al., 1995) or fucoidin, a selectin blocker (Granert et al., 1998). In contrast to bacterial meningitis, antineutrophil strategies exerted no effect, or even unfavorable effects, in experimental models of S. aureus brain infection. Thus, the extent of tissue necrosis and the regional increase of blood–brain barrier permeability were not reduced by neutrophil depletion in a rodent model of staphylococcal cerebritis (Lo et al., 1998). In a murine staphylococcal brain abscess model, neutrophil-depleted mice and mice deficient in CXCR2, the sole receptor for the neutrophil chemoattractants MIP2 and KC, consistently demonstrated even more severe brain abscesses (Kielian et al., 2001). Similarly, treatment with antineutrophil antibodies enhanced lesion formation in the brain of mice infected with L. monocytogenes (Lopez et al., 2000). In the latter studies, the antineutrophil strategy also resulted in an, albeit minor, increase in the bacterial burden within the CNS, whereas this approach did not affect the multiplication of *S. pneumoniae* within the CSF. All in all, these data suggest that neutrophils (and the acute immune response) can exert both protective and harmful effects in bacterial CNS infections. Their pathogenic role seems to be dependent upon the causative agent and the site of infection. However, further studies are warranted to get a more precise picture of their function in bacterial CNS infections.

Conclusion and future tasks

Bacterial infections involving the CNS are often life-threatening. Although it is well known that bacterial infections of the CNS result in an exaggerated and sustained inflammatory response, the mechanisms of immune activation to major CNS pathogens are largely unknown. Recognition of bacterial infections appears to be dependent on specific PRRs. The expression patterns of most PRRs (e.g. TLRs, MBL, SR-As) in the normal and inflamed CNS are still insufficiently characterized. Moreover, the functional role of PRRs in the CNS is nearly completely unknown. In addition, the microbicidal mechanisms present in the normal CNS and induced by infection have to be investigated. For example, are antimicrobial peptides produced by brain cells? If yes, do they also have other immune functions beside bacterial killing? Finally, the definite role of neutrophils and CNS macrophages in both the host defense against microbes and the induction of brain damage has to be more precisely characterized. These investigations would provide the basis for adjuvant treatment strategies of bacterial brain infections which are absolutely necessary to improve their bad prognosis.

References

Akira, S. and Hemmi, H. (2003). Recognition of pathogen-associated molecular patterns by TLR family. *Immunol Lett* **85**: 85.

Akira, S., Takeda, K., and Kaisho, T. (2001). Toll-like receptors: critical proteins linking innate and acquired immunity. *Nat Immunol* **2**: 675.

Alon, R. and Feigelson, S. (2002). From rolling to arrest on blood vessels: leukocyte tap dancing on endothelial integrin ligands and chemokines at sub-second contacts. *Semin Immunol* **14**: 93.

AlonsoDeVelasco, E., Verheul, A.F., Verhoef, J., and Snippe, H. (1995). *Streptococcus pneumoniae*: virulence factors, pathogenesis, and vaccines. *Microbiol Rev* **59**: 591.

Andersson, P.B., Perry, V.H., and Gordon, S. (1992). The acute inflammatory response to lipopolysaccharide in CNS parenchyma differs from that in other body tissues. *Neuroscience* **48**: 169.

Anthony, D.C., Blond, D., Dempster, R., and Perry, V.H. (2002). Chemokine targets in acute brain injury and disease. *Prog Brain Res* **132**: 507.

Anthony, D., Dempster, R., Fearn, S., Clements, J., Wells, G., Perry, V.H., *et al.* (1998). CXC chemokines generate age-related increases in neutrophil-mediated brain inflammation and blood-brain barrier breakdown. *Curr Biol* **8**: 923.

Bajetto, A., Bonavia, R., Barbero, S., Florio, T., and Schettini, G. (2001). Chemokines and their receptors in the central nervous system. *Front Neuroendocrinol* **22**: 147.

Barkalow, F.J., Goodman, M.J., and Mayadas, T.N. (1996). Cultured murine cerebral microvascular endothelial cells contain von Willebrand factor-positive Weibel-Palade bodies and support rapid cytokine-induced neutrophil adhesion. *Microcirculation* **3**: 19.

Bauer, S., Kirschning, C.J., Hacker, H., Redecke, V., Hausmann, S., Akira, S., *et al.* (2001). Human TLR9 confers responsiveness to bacterial DNA via species-specific CpG motif recognition. *Proc Natl Acad Sci USA* **98**: 9237.

Bax, W.A., Cluysenaer, O.J., Bartelink, A.K., Aerts, P.C., Ezekowitz, R.A., and Van Dijk, H. (1999). Association of familial deficiency of mannose-binding lectin and meningococcal disease. *Lancet* **354**: 1094.

Belaaouaj, A., Kim, K.S., and Shapiro, S.D. (2000). Degradation of outer membrane protein A in *Escherichia coli* killing by neutrophil elastase. *Science* **289**: 1185.

Bell, M.D. and Perry, V.H. (1995). Adhesion molecule expression on murine cerebral endothelium following the injection of a proinflammagen or during acute neuronal degeneration. *J Neurocytol* **24**: 695.

Bell, M.D., Taub, D.D., and Perry, V.H. (1996). Overriding the brain's intrinsic resistance to leukocyte recruitment with intraparenchymal injections of recombinant chemokines. *Neuroscience* **74**: 283.

Bellingan, G. (2000). Leukocytes: friend or foe. *Intensive Care Med* **26**(Suppl. 1): S111.

Biber, K., Zuurman, M.W., Dijkstra, I.M., and Boddeke, H.W. (2002). Chemokines in the brain: neuroimmunology and beyond. *Curr Opin Pharmacol* **2**: 63.

Bjorklund, A. and Lindvall, O. (2000a). Cell replacement therapies for central nervous system disorders. *Nat Neurosci* **3**: 537.

Bjorklund, A. and Lindvall, O. (2000b). Self-repair in the brain. *Nature* **405**: 892.

Brosnan, C.F., Cannella, B., Battistini, L., and Raine, C.S. (1995). Cytokine localization in multiple sclerosis lesions: correlation with adhesion molecule expression and reactive nitrogen species. *Neurology* **45**: S16.

Brown, J.S., Hussell, T., Gilliland, S.M., Holden, D.W., Paton, J.C., Ehrenstein, M.R., *et al.* (2002). The classical pathway is the dominant complement pathway required for innate immunity to *Streptococcus pneumoniae* infection in mice. *Proc Natl Acad Sci USA* **99**: 16969.

Bsibsi, M., Ravid, R., Gveric, D., and van Noort, J.M. (2002). Broad expression of Toll-like receptors in the human central nervous system. *J Neuropathol Exp Neurol* **61**: 1013.

Butko, P., Nicholson-Weller, A., and Wessels, M.R. (1999). Role of complement component C1q in the IgG-independent opsonophagocytosis of group B streptococcus. *J Immunol* **163**: 2761.

Carson, M.J. (2002). Microglia as liaisons between the immune and central nervous systems: functional implications for multiple sclerosis. *Glia* **40**: 218.

Carson, M.J. and Sutcliffe, J.G. (1999). Balancing function vs. self defense: the CNS as an active regulator of immune responses. *J Neurosci Res* **55**: 1.

Carvalho-Tavares, J., Hickey, M.J., Hutchison, J., Michaud, J., Sutcliffe, I.T., and Kubes, P. (2000). A role for platelets and endothelial selectins in tumor necrosis factor-alpha-induced leukocyte recruitment in the brain microvasculature. *Circ Res* **87**: 1141.

Cheng, Q., Carlson, B., Pillai, S., Eby, R., Edwards, L., Olmsted, S.B., *et al.* (2001). Antibody against surface-bound C5a peptidase is opsonic and initiates macrophage killing of group B streptococci. *Infect Immun* **69**: 2302.

Conlan, J.W. and North, R.J. (1994). Neutrophils are essential for early anti-Listeria defense in the liver, but not in the spleen or peritoneal cavity, as revealed by a granulocyte-depleting monoclonal antibody. *J Exp Med* **179**: 259.

Cundell, D.R. and Tuomanen, E.I. (1994). Receptor specificity of adherence of *Streptococcus pneumoniae* to human type-II pneumocytes and vascular endothelial cells in vitro. *Microb Pathog* **17**: 361.

Cundell, D.R., Gerard, N.P., Gerard, C., Idanpaan-Heikkila, I., and Tuomanen, E.I. (1995). *Streptococcus pneumoniae* anchor to activated human cells by the receptor for platelet-activating factor. *Nature* **377**: 435.

Dunne, D.W., Resnick, D., Greenberg, J., Krieger, M., and Joiner, K.A. (1994). The type I macrophage scavenger receptor binds to Gram-positive bacteria and recognizes lipoteichoic acid. *Proc Natl Acad Sci USA* **91**: 1863.

Echchannaoui, H., Frei, K., Schnell, C., Leib, S.L., Zimmerli, W., and Landmann, R. (2002). Toll-like receptor 2-deficient mice are highly susceptible to *Streptococcus pneumoniae* meningitis because of reduced bacterial clearing and enhanced inflammation. *J Infect Dis* **186**: 798.

Fijen, C.A., Bredius, R.G., Kuijper, E.J., Out, T.A., De Haas, M., De Wit, A.P., *et al.* (2000). The role of Fcgamma receptor polymorphisms and C3 in the immune defence against *Neisseria meningitidis* in complement-deficient individuals. *Clin Exp Immunol* **120**: 338.

Fitzgerald, K.A., Palsson-McDermott, E.M., Bowie, A.G., Jefferies, C.A., Mansell, A.S., Brady, G., *et al.* (2001). Mal (MyD88-adapter-like) is required for Toll-like receptor-4 signal transduction. *Nature* **413**: 78.

Flaris, N.A. and Hickey, W.F. (1992). Development and characterization of an experimental model of brain abscess in the rat. *Am J Pathol* **141**: 1299.

Fraser, I.P., Koziel, H., and Ezekowitz, R.A. (1998). The serum mannose-binding protein and the macrophage mannose receptor are pattern recognition molecules that link innate and adaptive immunity. *Semin Immunol* **10**: 363.

Fuentes, M.E., Durham, S.K., Swerdel, M.R., Lewin, A.C., Barton, D.S., Megill, J.R., et al. (1995). Controlled recruitment of monocytes and macrophages to specific organs through transgenic expression of monocyte chemoattractant protein-1. J Immunol 155: 5769.

Fujita, T. (2002). Evolution of the lectin-complement pathway and its role in innate immunity. Nat Rev Immunol 2: 346.

Gadjeva, M., Thiel, S., and Jensenius, J.C. (2001). The mannan-binding-lectin pathway of the innate immune response. Curr Opin Immunol 13: 74.

Gasque, P., Dean, Y.D., McGreal, E.P., VanBeek, J., and Morgan, B.P. (2000). Complement components of the innate immune system in health and disease in the CNS. Immunopharmacology 49: 171.

Gerard, C. and Rollins, B.J. (2001). Chemokines and disease. Nat Immunol 2: 108.

Gerber, J., Raivich, G., Wellmer, A., Noeske, C., Kunst, T., Werner, A., et al. (2001). A mouse model of Streptococcus pneumoniae meningitis mimicking several features of human disease. Acta Neuropathol 101: 499.

Girardin, S.E., Sansonetti, P.J., and Philpott, D.J. (2002). Intracellular vs extracellular recognition of pathogens–common concepts in mammals and flies. Trends Microbiol 10: 193.

Gloor, S.M., Wachtel, M., Bolliger, M.F., Ishihara, H., Landmann, R., and Frei, K. (2001). Molecular and cellular permeability control at the blood-brain barrier. Brain Res Brain Res Rev 36: 258.

Gortvai, P., De Louvois, J., and Hurley, R. (1987). The bacteriology and chemotherapy of acute pyogenic brain abscess. Br J Neurosurg 1: 189.

Gotsch, U., Jager, U., Dominis, M., and Vestweber, D. (1994). Expression of P-selectin on endothelial cells is upregulated by LPS and TNF-alpha in vivo. Cell Adhes Commun 2: 7.

Gough, P.J. and Gordon, S. (2000). The role of scavenger receptors in the innate immune system. Microbes Infect 2: 305.

Granert, C., Raud, J., and Lindquist, L. (1998). The polysaccharide fucoidin inhibits the antibiotic-induced inflammatory cascade in experimental pneumococcal meningitis. Clin Diagn Lab Immunol 5: 322.

Hampton, R.Y., Golenbock, D.T., Penman, M., Krieger, M., and Raetz, C.R. (1991). Recognition and plasma clearance of endotoxin by scavenger receptors. Nature 352: 342.

Hausmann, E.H., Berman, N.E., Wang, Y.Y., Meara, J.B., Wood, G.W., and Klein, R.M. (1998). Selective chemokine mRNA expression following brain injury. Brain Res 788: 49.

Heffron, R. (1979). Pneumonia with Special Reference to Pneumococcus Lobar Pneumonia. Harvard University Press, Cambridge, MA.

Hemmi, H., Takeuchi, O., Kawai, T., Kaisho, T., Sato, S., Sanjo, H., et al. (2000). A Toll-like receptor recognizes bacterial DNA. Nature 408: 740.

Horng, T., Barton, G.M., and Medzhitov, R. (2001). TIRAP: an adapter molecule in the Toll signaling pathway. Nat Immunol 2: 835.

Horng, T., Barton, G.M., Flavell, R.A., and Medzhitov, R. (2002). The adaptor molecule TIRAP provides signalling specificity for Toll-like receptors. Nature 420: 329.

Hornung, V., Rothenfusser, S., Britsch, S., Krug, A., Jahrsdorfer, B., Giese, T., et al. (2002). Quantitative expression of toll-like receptor 1–10 mRNA in cellular subsets of human peripheral blood mononuclear cells and sensitivity to CpG oligodeoxynucleotides. J Immunol 168: 4531.

Huber, J.D., Egleton, R.D., and Davis, T.P. (2001). Molecular physiology and pathophysiology of tight junctions in the blood-brain barrier. Trends Neurosci 24: 719.

Husemann, J., Loike, J.D., Anankov, R., Febbraio, M., and Silverstein, S.C. (2002). Scavenger receptors in neurobiology and neuropathology: their role on microglia and other cells of the nervous system. Glia 40: 195.

Ishiguro, T., Naito, M., Yamamoto, T., Hasegawa, G., Gejyo, F., Mitsuyama, M., et al. (2001). Role of macrophage scavenger receptors in response to Listeria monocytogenes infection in mice. Am J Pathol 158: 179.

Jack, D.L., Dodds, A.W., Anwar, N., Ison, C.A., Law, A., Frosch, M., et al. (1998). Activation of complement by mannose-binding lectin on isogenic mutants of Neisseria meningitidis serogroup B. J Immunol 160: 1346.

Jack, D.L., Read, R.C., Tenner, A.J., Frosch, M., Turner, M.W., and Klein, N.J. (2001a). Mannose-binding lectin regulates the inflammatory response of human professional phagocytes to Neisseria meningitidis serogroup B. J Infect Dis 184: 1152.

Jack, D.L., Jarvis, G.A., Booth, C.L., Turner, M.W., and Klein, N.J. (2001b). Mannose-binding lectin accelerates complement activation and increases serum killing of Neisseria meningitidis serogroup C. J Infect Dis 184: 836.

Janeway, C.A.J. and Medzhitov, R. (2002). Innate immune recognition. Annu Rev Immunol 20: 197.

Johnston, B. and Butcher, E.C. (2002). Chemokines in rapid leukocyte adhesion triggering and migration. Semin Immunol 14: 83.

Kaisho, T., Takeuchi, O., Kawai, T., Hoshino, K., and Akira, S. (2001). Endotoxin-induced maturation of Myd88-deficient dendritic cells. J Immunol 166: 5688.

Kawai, T., Adachi, O., Ogawa, T., Takeda, K., and Akira, S. (1999). Unresponsiveness of MyD88-deficient mice to endotoxin. Immunity 11: 115.

Kawai, T., Takeuchi, O., Fujita, T., Inoue, J., Muhlradt, P.F., Sato, S., et al. (2001). Lipopolysaccharide stimulates the MyD88-independent pathway and results in activation of IFN-regulatory factor 3 and the expression of a subset of lipopolysaccharide-inducible genes. J Immunol 167: 5887.

Kawasaki, T. (1999). Structure and biology of mannan-binding protein, MBP, an important component of innate immunity. Biochim Biophys Acta 1473: 186.

Kielian, T. and Hickey, W.F. (2000). Proinflammatory cytokine, chemokine, and cellular adhesion molecule expression during the acute phase of experimental brain abscess development. Am J Pathol 157: 647.

Kielian, T., Barry, B., and Hickey, W.F. (2001). CXC chemokine receptor-2 ligands are required for neutrophil-mediated host defense in experimental brain abscesses. J Immunol 166: 4634.

Kim, J.O. and Weiser, J.N. (1998). Association of intrastrain phase variation in quantity of capsular polysaccharide and teichoic acid with the virulence of Streptococcus pneumoniae. J Infect Dis 177: 368.

Koedel, U. and Pfister, H.-W. (1999). Models of experimental bacterial meningitis: role and limitations. Infect Dis Clin North Am 13: 549.

Koedel, U., Scheld, W.M., and Pfister, H.W. (2002). Pathogenesis and pathophysiology of pneumococcal meningitis. Lancet Infect Dis 2: 721.

Koedel, U., Angele, B., Rupprecht, T., Wagner, H., Roggenkamp, A., Pfister, H.W., et al. (2003). Toll-like receptor 2 participates in mediation of immune response in experimental pneumococcal meningitis. J Immunol 170: 438.

Krieglstein, C.F. and Granger, D.N. (2001). Adhesion molecules and their role in vascular disease. Am J Hypertens 14: 44S.

Laflamme, N. and Rivest, S. (2001). Toll-like receptor 4: the missing link of the cerebral innate immune response triggered by circulating Gram-negative bacterial cell wall components. FASEB J 15: 155.

Laflamme, N., Soucy, G., and Rivest, S. (2001). Circulating cell wall components derived from Gram-negative, not Gram-positive, bacteria cause a profound induction of the gene-encoding Toll-like receptor 2 in the CNS. J Neurochem 79: 648.

Laflamme, N., Echchannaoui, H., Landmann, R., and Rivest, S. (2003). Cooperation between toll-like receptor 2 and 4 in the brain of mice challenged with cell wall components derived from Gram-negative and Gram-positive bacteria. Eur J Immunol 33: 1127.

Lehnardt, S., Lachance, C., Patrizi, S., Lefebvre, S., Follett, P.L., Jensen, F.E., et al. (2002). The Toll-like receptor TLR4 is necessary for lipopolysaccharide-induced oligodendrocyte injury in the CNS. J Neurosci 22: 2478.

Lemaitre, B., Nicolas, E., Michaut, L., Reichhart, J.M., and Hoffmann, J.A. (1996). The dorsoventral regulatory gene cassette spatzle/Toll/cactus controls the potent antifungal response in Drosophila adults. Cell 86: 973.

Li, M., Carpio, D.F., Zheng, Y., Bruzzo, P., Singh, V., Ouaaz, F., et al. (2001). An essential role of the nf-kappab/toll-like receptor pathway in induction of inflammatory and tissue-repair gene expression by necrotic cells. J Immunol 166: 7128.

Lo, W.D., Chen, R., Boue, D.R., and Stokes, B.T. (1998). Effect of neutrophil depletion in acute cerebritis. Brain Res 802: 175.

Lopez, S., Marco, A.J., Prats, N., and Czuprynski, C.J. (2000). Critical role of neutrophils in eliminating Listeria monocytogenes from the central nervous system during experimental murine listeriosis. Infect Immun 68: 4789.

Lowy, F.D. (1998). Staphylococcus aureus infections. N Engl J Med 339: 520.

Lu, J., Teh, C., Kishore, U., and Reid, K.B. (2002). Collectins and ficolins: sugar pattern recognition molecules of the mammalian innate immune system. Biochim Biophys Acta 1572: 387.

Luster, A.D. (1998). Chemokines—chemotactic cytokines that mediate inflammation. N Engl J Med 338: 436.

Malley, R., Henneke, P., Morse, S.C., Cieslewicz, M.J., Lipsitch, M., Thompson, C.M., et al. (2003). Recognition of pneumolysin by Toll-like receptor 4 confers resistance to pneumococcal infection. Proc Natl Acad Sci USA 100: 1966.

Marrs, C.F., Krasan, G.P., McCrea, K.W., Clemans, D.L., and Gilsdorf, J.R. (2001). Haemophilus influenzae—human specific bacteria. Front Biosci 6: E41.

Mathisen, G.E. and Johnson, J.P. (1997). Brain abscess. Clin Infect Dis 25: 763.

Matyszak, M.K. (1998). Inflammation in the CNS: balance between immunological privilege and immune responses. Prog Neurobiol 56: 19.

Matyszak, M.K. and Perry, V.H. (1995). Demyelination in the central nervous system following a delayed-type hypersensitivity response to bacillus Calmette–Guerin. Neuroscience 64: 967.

Matyszak, M.K. and Perry, V.H. (1996). A comparison of leucocyte responses to heat-killed bacillus Calmette–Guerin in different CNS compartments. Neuropathol Appl Neurobiol 22: 44.

McCullers, J.A. and Tuomanen, E.I. (2001). Molecular pathogenesis of pneumococcal pneumonia. Front Biosci 6: D877.

Medzhitov, R. (2001). Toll-like receptors and innate immunity. Nat Rev Immunol 1: 135.

Medzhitov, R. and Janeway, C.J. (2000). Innate immunity. N Engl J Med 343: 338.

Medzhitov, R. and Janeway, C.A.J. (2002). Decoding the patterns of self and non-self by the innate immune system. Science 296: 298.

Mennicken, F., Maki, R., De Souza, E.B., and Quirion, R. (1999). Chemokines and chemokine receptors in the CNS: a possible role in neuroinflammation and patterning. Trends Pharmacol Sci 20: 73.

Montero-Menei, C.N., Sindji, L., Pouplard-Barthelaix, A., Jehan, F., Denechaud, L., and Darcy, F. (1994). Lipopolysaccharide intracerebral administration induces minimal inflammatory reaction in rat brain. Brain Res 653: 101.

Montero-Menei, C.N., Sindji, L., Garcion, E., Mege, M., Couez, D., Gamelin, E., et al. (1996). Early events of the inflammatory reaction induced in rat brain by lipopolysaccharide intracerebral injection: relative contribution of peripheral monocytes and activated microglia. Brain Res 724: 55.

Nassif, X., Bourdoulous, S., Eugene, E., and Couraud, P.O. (2002). How do extracellular pathogens cross the blood-brain barrier? Trends Microbiol 10: 227.

Neth, O., Jack, D.L., Johnson, M., Klein, N.J., and Turner, M.W. (2002). Enhancement of complement activation and opsonophagocytosis by complexes of mannose-binding lectin with mannose-binding lectin-associated serine protease after binding to Staphylococcus aureus. J Immunol 169: 4430.

Neumann, H. (2001). Control of glial immune function by neurons. Glia 36: 191.

Nussler, A.K., Wittel, U.A., Nussler, N.C., and Beger, H.G. (1999). Leukocytes, the Janus cells in inflammatory disease. Langenbecks Arch Surg 384: 222.

Okamura, Y., Watari, M., Jerud, E.S., Young, D.W., Ishizaka, S.T., Rose, J., et al. (2001). The extra domain A of fibronectin activates Toll-like receptor 4. J Biol Chem 276: 10229.

Overweg, K., Pericone, C.D., Verhoef, G.G., Weiser, J.N., Meiring, H.D., De Jong, A.P., et al. (2000). Differential protein expression in phenotypic variants of Streptococcus pneumoniae. Infect Immun 68: 4604.

Ozinsky, A., Underhill, D.M., Fontenot, J.D., Hajjar, A.M., Smith, K.D., Wilson, C.B., et al. (2000). The repertoire for pattern recognition of pathogens by the innate immune system is defined by cooperation between toll-like receptors. Proc Natl Acad Sci USA 97: 13766.

Parkin, J. and Cohen, B. (2001). An overview of the immune system. Lancet 357: 1777.

Pashenkov, M. and Link, H. (2002). Dendritic cells and immune responses in the central nervous system. Trends Immunol 23: 69.

Pashenkov, M., Teleshova, N., and Link, H. (2003). Inflammation in the central nervous system: the role for dendritic cells. Brain Pathol 13: 23.

Pedrosa, J., Saunders, B.M., Appelberg, R., Orme, I.M., Silva, M.T., and Cooper, A.M. (2000). Neutrophils play a protective nonphagocytic role in systemic Mycobacterium tuberculosis infection of mice. Infect Immun 68: 577.

Peiser, L., De Winther, M.P., Makepeace, K., Hollinshead, M., Coull, P., Plested, J., et al. (2002a). The class A macrophage scavenger receptor is a major pattern recognition receptor for Neisseria meningitidis which is independent of lipopolysaccharide and not required for secretory responses. Infect Immun 70: 5346.

Peiser, L., Mukhopadhyay, S., and Gordon, S. (2002b). Scavenger receptors in innate immunity. Curr Opin Immunol 14: 123.

Peschel, A. and Collins, L.V. (2001). Staphylococcal resistance to antimicrobial peptides of mammalian and bacterial origin. Peptides 22: 1651.

Peschel, A., Jack, R.W., Otto, M., Collins, L.V., Staubitz, P., Nicholson, G., et al. (2001). Staphylococcus aureus resistance to human defensins and evasion of neutrophil killing via the novel virulence factor MprF is based on modification of membrane lipids with L-lysine. J Exp Med 193: 1067.

Petersen, S.V., Thiel, S., Jensen, L., Vorup-Jensen, T., Koch, C., and Jensenius, J.C. (2000). Control of the classical and the MBL pathway of complement activation. Mol Immunol 37: 803.

Porro, G.A., Lee, J.H., de Azavedo, J., Crandall, I., Whitehead, T., Tullis, E., et al. (2001). Direct and indirect bacterial killing functions of neutrophil defensins in lung explants. Am J Physiol Lung Cell Mol Physiol 281: L1240.

Portnoy, D.A., Auerbuch, V., and Glomski, I.J. (2002). The cell biology of Listeria monocytogenes infection: the intersection of bacterial pathogenesis and cell-mediated immunity. J Cell Biol 158: 409.

Proudfoot, A.E. (2002). Chemokine receptors: multifaceted therapeutic targets. Nature Rev Immunol 2: 106.

Rajnik, M. and Ottolini, M.G. (2000). Serious infections of the central nervous system: encephalitis, meningitis, and brain abscess. Adolesc Med 11: 401.

Ransohoff, R.M. (2002). The chemokine system in neuroinflammation: an update. J Infect Dis 186(Suppl. 2): S152.

Rijneveld, A.W., Florquin, S., Branger, J., Speelman, P., van Deventer, S.J., and Van der Poll, T. (2001). TNF-alpha compensates for the impaired host defense of IL-1 type I receptor-deficient mice during pneumococcal pneumonia. J Immunol 167: 5240.

Ring, A., Weiser, J.N., and Tuomanen, E.I. (1998). Pneumococcal trafficking across the blood-brain barrier. Molecular analysis of a novel bidirectional pathway. J Clin Invest 102: 347.

Rogers, H.W. and Unanue, E.R. (1993). Neutrophils are involved in acute, non-specific resistance to Listeria monocytogenes in mice. Infect Immun 61: 5090.

Rollins, B.J. (1997). Chemokines. Blood 90: 909.

Rovai, L.E., Herschman, H.R., and Smith, J.B. (1998). The murine neutrophil-chemoattractant chemokines LIX, KC, and MIP-2 have distinct induction kinetics, tissue distributions, and tissue-specific sensitivities to glucocorticoid regulation in endotoxemia. J Leukoc Biol 64: 494.

Roy, S., Knox, K., Segal, S., Griffiths, D., Moore, C.E., Welsh, K.I., et al. (2002). MBL genotype and risk of invasive pneumococcal disease: a case-control study. Lancet 359: 1569.

Saez-Llorens, X., Jafari, H.S., Severien, C., Parras, F., Olsen, K.D., Hansen, E.J., et al. (1991). Enhanced attenuation of meningeal inflammation and brain edema by concomitant administration of anti-CD18 monoclonal antibodies and dexamethasone in experimental Haemophilus meningitis. J Clin Invest 88: 2003.

Schuchat, A., Robinson, K., Wenger, J.D., Harrison, L.H., Farley, M., Reingold, A.L., et al. (1997). Bacterial meningitis in the United States in 1995. Active Surveillance Team. N Engl J Med 337: 970.

Sedgwick, J.D., Riminton, D.S., Cyster, J.G., and Korner, H. (2000). Tumor necrosis factor: a master regulator of leukocyte movement. Immunol Today 21: 110.

Simberkoff, M.S., Moldover, N.H., and Rahal, J.J. (1980). Absence of detectable bactericidal and opsonic activities in normal and infected human cerebrospinal fluids. J Lab Clin Med 95: 362.

Smith, H., Bannister, B., and O'Shea, M.J. (1977). Cerebrospinal fluid immunoglobulins in meningitis. Lancet 2: 591.

Spellerberg, B. (2000). Pathogenesis of neonatal Streptococcus agalactiae infections. Microbes Infect 2: 1733.

Stahel, P.F., Frei, K., Eugster, H.P., Fontana, A., Hummel, K.M., Wetsel, R.A., et al. (1997a). TNF-alpha-mediated expression of the receptor for anaphylatoxin C5a on neurons in experimental Listeria meningoencephalitis. J Immunol 159: 861.

Stahel, P.F., Frei, K., Fontana, A., Eugster, H.P., Ault, B.H., and Barnum, S.R. (1997b). Evidence for intrathecal synthesis of alternative pathway complement activation proteins in experimental meningitis. Am J Pathol 151: 897.

Stins, M.F., Gilles, F., and Kim, K.S. (1997). Selective expression of adhesion molecules on human brain microvascular endothelial cells. J Neuroimmunol 76: 81.

Strazielle, N. and Ghersi-Egea, J.F. (2000). Choroid plexus in the central nervous system: biology and physiopathology. J Neuropathol Exp Neurol 59: 561.

Sugawara, I., Mizuno, S., Yamada, H., Matsumoto, M., and Akira, S. (2001). Disruption of nuclear factor-interleukin-6, a transcription factor, results in severe mycobacterial infection. *Am J Pathol* **158**: 361.

Takahashi, K., Gordon, J., Liu, H., Sastry, K.N., Epstein, J.E., Motwani, M., *et al.* (2002). Lack of mannose-binding lectin-A enhances survival in a mouse model of acute septic peritonitis. *Microbes Infect* **4**: 773.

Takeda, K. and Akira, S. (2003). Toll receptors and pathogen resistance. *Cell Microbiol* **5**: 143.

Takeda, K., Kaisho, T., and Akira, S. (2003). Toll-like receptors. *Annu Rev Immunol* **21**: 335.

Takeuchi, O., Hoshino, K., Kawai, T., Sanjo, H., Takada, H., Ogawa, T., *et al.* (1999). Differential roles of TLR2 and TLR4 in recognition of Gram-negative and Gram-positive bacterial cell wall components. *Immunity* **11**: 443.

Tani, M., Fuentes, M.E., Peterson, J.W., Trapp, B.D., Durham, S.K., Loy, J.K., *et al.* (1996). Neutrophil infiltration, glial reaction, and neurological disease in transgenic mice expressing the chemokine N51/KC in oligodendrocytes. *J Clin Invest* **98**: 529.

Terao, A., Apte-Deshpande, A., Dousman, L., Morairty, S., Eynon, B.P., Kilduff, T.S., *et al.* (2002). Immune response gene expression increases in the aging murine hippocampus. *J Neuroimmunol* **132**: 99.

Termeer, C., Benedix, F., Sleeman, J., Fieber, C., Voith, U., Ahrens, T., *et al.* (2002). Oligosaccharides of hyaluronan activate dendritic cells via toll-like receptor 4. *J Exp Med* **195**: 99.

Thomas, C.A., Li, Y., Kodama, T., Suzuki, H., Silverstein, S.C., and El Khoury, J. (2000). Protection from lethal gram-positive infection by macrophage scavenger receptor-dependent phagocytosis. *J Exp Med* **191**: 147.

Toomey, J.A. and Roach, F. (1939). Pneumococcus meningitis. *Ohio Sate Med J* **35**: 841.

Toshchakov, V., Jones, B.W., Perera, P.Y., Thomas, K., Cody, M.J., Zhang, S., *et al.* (2002). TLR4, but not TLR2, mediates IFN-beta-induced STAT1alpha/beta-dependent gene expression in macrophages. *Nat Immunol* **3**: 392.

Townsend, G.C. and Scheld, W.M. (1998). Infections of the central nervous system. *Adv Intern Med* **43**: 403.

Tuomanen, E.I., Saukkonen, K., Sande, S., Cioffe, C., and Wright, S.D. (1989). Reduction of inflammation, tissue damage, and mortality in bacterial meningitis in rabbits treated with monoclonal antibodies against adhesion-promoting receptors of leukocytes. *J Exp Med* **170**: 959.

Tzeng, Y.L. and Stephens, D.S. (2000). Epidemiology and pathogenesis of *Neisseria meningitidis*. *Microbes Infect* **2**: 687.

Vabulas, R.M., Ahmad-Nejad, P., Da Costa, C., Miethke, T., Kirschning, C.J., Hacker, H., *et al.* (2001). Endocytosed HSP60s use toll-like receptor 2 (TLR2). and TLR4 to activate the toll/interleukin-1 receptor signaling pathway in innate immune cells. *J Biol Chem* **276**: 31332.

Vabulas, R.M., Ahmad-Nejad, P., Ghose, S., Kirschning, C.J., Issels, R.D., and Wagner, H. (2002*a*). HSP70 as endogenous stimulus of the Toll/interleukin-1 receptor signal pathway. *J Biol Chem* **277**: 15107.

Vabulas, R.M., Braedel, S., Hilf, N., Singh-Jasuja, H., Herter, S., Ahmad-Nejad, P., *et al.* (2002*b*). The endoplasmic reticulum-resident heat shock protein Gp96 activates dendritic cells via the Toll-like receptor 2/4 pathway. *J Biol Chem* **277**: 20847.

van Crevel, R., Ottenhoff, T.H., and van der Meer, J.W. (2002). Innate immunity to *Mycobacterium tuberculosis*. *Clin Microbiol Rev* **15**: 94.

Vastag, M., Skopal, J., Voko, Z., Csonka, E., and Nagy, Z. (1999). Expression of membrane-bound and soluble cell adhesion molecules by human brain microvessel endothelial cells. *Microvasc Res* **57**: 52.

Verdrengh, M. and Tarkowski, A. (1997). Role of neutrophils in experimental septicemia and septic arthritis induced by *Staphylococcus aureus*. *Infect Immun* **65**: 2517.

Wagner, J.G. and Roth, R.A. (2000). Neutrophil migration mechanisms, with an emphasis on the pulmonary vasculature. *Pharmacol Rev* **52**: 349.

Wagner, S., Lynch, N.J., Walter, W., Schwaeble, W.J., and Loos, M. (2003). Differential expression of the murine mannose-binding lectins a and C in lymphoid and nonlymphoid organs and tissues. *J Immunol* **170**: 1462.

Walport, M.J. (2001*a*). Complement. First of two parts. *N Engl J Med* **344**: 1058.

Walport, M.J. (2001*b*). Complement. Second of two parts. *N Engl J Med* **344**: 1140.

Wang, E., Simard, M., Ouellet, N., Bergeron, Y., Beauchamp, D., and Bergeron, M.G. (2002). Pathogenesis of pneumococcal pneumonia in cyclo-phosphamide-induced leukopenia in mice. *Infect Immun* **70**: 4226.

Washington, R., Burton, J., Todd, R.F., Newman, W., Dragovic, L., and Dore-Duffy, P. (1994). Expression of immunologically relevant endothelial cell activation antigens on isolated central nervous system microvessels from patients with multiple sclerosis. *Ann Neurol* **35**: 89.

Weber, .J.R, Angstwurm, K., Bürger, W., Einhäupl, K.M., and Dirnagl, U. (1995). Anti ICAM-1 (CD 54). monoclonal antibody reduces inflammatory changes in experimental bacterial meningitis. *J Neuroimmunol* **63**: 63.

Wekerle, H. (2002). Immune protection of the brain—efficient and delicate. *J Infect Dis* **186**(Suppl. 2): S140.

Williams, M.A. and Solomkin, J.S. (1999). Integrin-mediated signaling in human neutrophil functioning. *J Leukoc Biol* **65**: 725.

Wong, D. and Dorovini-Zis, K. (1995). Expression of vascular cell adhesion molecule-1 (VCAM-1). by human brain microvessel endothelial cells in primary culture. *Microvasc Res* **49**: 325.

Yamada, Y., Doi, T., Hamakubo, T., and Kodama, T. (1998). Scavenger receptor family proteins: roles for atherosclerosis, host defence and disorders of the central nervous system. *Cell Mol Life Sci* **54**: 628.

Zarember, K.A. and Godowski, P.J. (2002). Tissue expression of human Toll-like receptors and differential regulation of Toll-like receptor mRNAs in leukocytes in response to microbes, their products, and cytokines. *J Immunol* **168**: 554.

Zimmerli, S., Edwards, S., and Ernst, J.D. (1996). Selective receptor blockade during phagocytosis does not alter the survival and growth of *Mycobacterium tuberculosis* in human macrophages. *Am J Respir Cell Mol Biol* **15**: 760.

12 Animal models of neurologic disease

Iain L. Campbell and Trevor Owens

Introduction

Neuroimmunological disorders exemplified by multiple sclerosis (MS) and Guillain–Barré syndrome (GBS) are heterogeneous, with evidence supporting a compound etiopathogenesis involving interactions between the environment (for example, microbes and chemicals) and the genotype. The culmination of this interaction is a host response targeted to the nervous system that involves elements of both the immune system and the local milieu. Post mortem and biopsy analysis of diseased tissue has defined the cellular and molecular components of this response which is characterized by the presence of activated and non-activated immune cells (i.e. T cells, macrophages, and granulocytes) in lesion areas, by prominent gliosis, and in advancing disease damage to and loss of oligodendrocytes or Schwann cells and ultimately the neurons they ensheath. When activated or responding to perturbation in their immediate environment each of these different cell types has the potential to produce an array of soluble effectors (for example, chemokines, cytokines, growth factors, complement factors, and proteases) that often form interacting functional networks that serve a number of important functions involved in further coordinating the host response and in the repair of tissue injury. These host-derived factors are also extremely potent modifiers of both cellular structure and function, which besides their beneficial actions may also possess considerable pathogenic potential. Typically, neuroimmune disorders such as MS evolve over a considerable time so that the information provided by post mortem and biopsy analysis is largely descriptive, limited to late-stage disease, and reflects the complex combination of causative and compensatory processes. This of course makes it very difficult to identify pathogenic mechanisms and prove that a given cellular response or molecular alteration is crucially involved in a direct cause and effect relationship. It is also obvious that many features of neuroimmunological diseases are difficult if not impossible to replicate and study using simple *in vitro* systems such as cell culture. An experimental approach that offers a solution to these issues is the application of animal model systems that more closely replicate in one or more major aspects the diseased human nervous system.

Animal models have proven to be a relevant and informative experimental approach for the study of neuroimmune processes. Animal models replicate the complex, dynamic, and interactive milieu of the nervous and immune systems and facilitate analysis of the consequences of the encounter and interaction of these organ systems. They are amenable to manipulation at many different levels and are therefore ideally suited for hypothesis testing and defining the role of basic cellular processes and molecular mechanisms in disease. Further, not only do animal models aid in the identification of pivotal targets for therapeutic intervention, but they also provide a vehicle for the pre-clinical testing and validation of potential therapeutic strategies.

In the field of neuroimmunology there is a broad diversity of animal models available for study and the choice of which to use ultimately rests with the specific question or process being addressed. In general, and for the purposes of further discussion in this chapter, animal models can be grouped into one of two categories (see Fig. 12.1). The first of these are the induced models of inflammatory or autoimmune diseases of the CNS. The most widely studied examples in this category of animal models that will be discussed here include experimental autoimmune encephalomyelitis (EAE; modeling human MS) and experimental autoimmune neuritis (EAN; modeling human GBS). These classical models of nervous system autoimmune disease are established by active immunization of (most commonly) rodents, with a neural-specific autoantigen. Autoreactive T cells induced in these models may also be further propagated *in vitro* and re-introduced into normal hosts to achieve adoptive transfer of disease. The second and more recent category relies on the ability to manipulate the mouse genome to generate genetically engineered animal models of human nervous system disease. Genetically engineered animals fall into two distinct types which in simple terms are represented by mutant mice with gene expression either added ('transgenic') or lost ('knockout'). Transgenic technology involves the use of tissue-specific promoter sequences to direct the expression of ectopic genes to specific tissues while knockout technology employs homologous recombination and insertion of a targeting vector to inactivate or disrupt an endogenous gene. Not surprisingly, through the power of this technology, the neuroimmunology field over the last decade has witnessed an unprecedented explosion in the availability of new animal models for study.

This chapter will describe these different categories of animal models in more detail highlighting their relevance to neuroimmunological disease and utility for understanding basic pathogenic mechanisms. Like all paradigms both the inducible and the genetically manipulated animal models each have their advantages and drawbacks that will also be further highlighted.

Experimental autoimmune diseases

Demyelinating diseases of the central or peripheral nervous systems can be induced in animals by immunization with myelin antigens. The pathology of ensuing disease thus reflects the autoimmune response against myelin antigens. This is also assumed to be the case in clinical neurological diseases such as MS or GBS, although the etiology of these diseases remains unknown.

Experimental autoimmune encephalomyelitis (EAE)

Encephalomyelitis occurs in response to immunization with central nervous system (CNS) myelin, or when the CNS is infected with virus. EAE (the acronym also covers experimental allergic encephalomyelitis) describes inflammatory disease induced by immunization with myelin antigens (Martin *et al.*, 1992, Owens and Sriram, 1995). EAE can probably be induced in any animal. Routes to induction and the spectrum of pathologies vary between species, strains, and antigens. Unifying features are immunization with myelin antigens in adjuvant and inflammatory infiltration to the CNS. Immunization induces a T-lymphocyte response to myelin antigens. T cells and other leukocytes enter the CNS by extravasation across the blood–brain barrier endothelia and basal laminae. Within the CNS, T cells are reactivated by recognition of antigen presented by local and infiltrating antigen-presenting cells. Activated T cells initiate an inflamma-

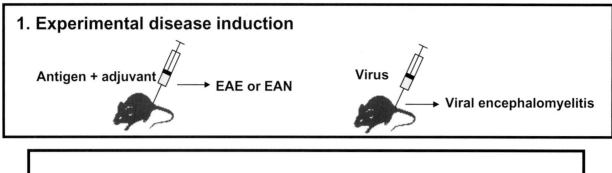

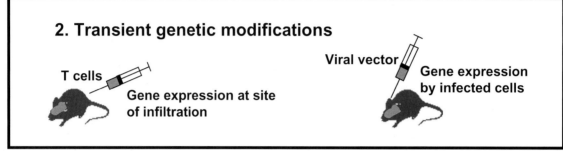

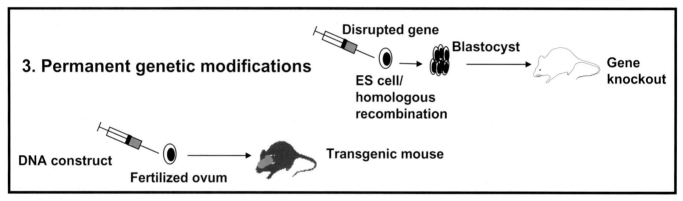

Fig. 12.1 Animal models for neurologic disease. Three categories of animal models are shown, as described in the text. (1) Experimental models of disease involve immunization of mice with neural antigens, usually those from myelin, or infection with neurotropic viruses that provoke an immune response against neural tissue. (2) Gene delivery to the nervous system can be mediated by cells with tropism for the nervous system, such as myelin-specific T cells, or neurotropic or nervous system-targeted viruses. Both T cells and viruses can be engineered to express genes of choice in the targeted tissue. (3) Permanent genetic modification can be achieved through transgenesis, by which genes with nervous-tissue-specific promoters are introduced to fertilized embryos, or knockouts, by which genes are disrupted throughout the whole animal, by targeted introduction of genetic elements to specific sites in the genome by homologous recombination. Approaches (1) and (2) may be applied separately or together, in combination with transgenic and knockout animals (3).

tory response in the CNS that includes production of cytokines and chemokines, activation of co-infiltrating leukocytes and resident glia, cellular cytotoxicity, and elaboration of inflammatory and cytotoxic mediators that converge to myelin damage. In many models of EAE, animals remit from symptoms, and in some models subsequently relapse. Chronic disease can be directly induced or may occur after relapse.

EAE can be transferred from immunized animals to naïve recipients. CD4+ T cells, that recognize antigenic peptides in association with Class II major histocompatibility complex (MHC) molecules, are essential for transfer of disease. Neither B cells nor immunoglobulin can transfer EAE. Two recent reports showed that CD8+ T cells can transfer EAE (Huseby et al., 2001; Sun et al., 2001), these await wider confirmation. Perivascular infiltrates of MHC Class II-restricted CD4+ T cells and macrophages, associated with demyelinating lesions, are a prominent feature of EAE in most mouse models. Inflammation occurs predominantly in the spinal cord. Antimyelin antibodies have been shown to enhance demyelination in EAE (Linington et al., 1993; Genain et al., 1995, 1996), although neither B cells nor antibodies are necessary for disease (Lyons et al., 2002; Oliver et al., 2003). Axonal damage also occurs in EAE, and has been attributed to glutamate-mediated cytotoxicity (Smith et al., 2000; Pitt et al., 2000), although cellular cytotoxicity may also contribute (Neumann et al., 2002).

Encephalitogens

With few exceptions (such as the astrocyte protein S100β), the antigens used to induce EAE are myelin proteins or peptides of these proteins. The disease that is induced by S100β does not involve demyelination (Kojima et al., 1994). The myelin proteins most commonly used to induce EAE are myelin basic protein (MBP), proteolipid protein (PLP), and myelin oligodendrocyte glycoprotein (MOG) (Martin et al., 1992). Other myelin proteins that have been shown to be encephalitogenic include myelin-associated oligodendrocytic basic protein (MOBP) (Maatta et al., 1998; Holz et al., 2000; Kaye et al., 2000) and myelin-associated glycoprotein (MAG) (Weerth et al., 1999; Morris-Downes et al., 2002). Instances of myelin antigens that did not induce EAE, e.g. CNPase, may reflect strain- or species-specific tolerance (Birnbaum et al., 1996; Morris-Downes et al., 2002), as has been shown for PLP and MBP (Huseby and Goverman, 2000; Klein et al., 2000).

Pathology

The strain and species of animal often dictate the choice of antigen and immunization protocol, and together this leads to a heterogeneity of disease outcomes. The two most commonly described mouse EAE systems in the recent literature are MBP-induced EAE in SJL/J mice, which is a relapsing–

Table 12.1 Selected examples of differing pathologies and progressions of EAE

Encephalitogen	Mouse/rat strain	Characteristics of EAE
MBP	SJL/J	Relapsing/remitting, demyelinating (Owens and Sriram, 1995)
	Lewis rat	Non-relapsing, no demyelination (Linington et al., 1993)
	C3H	CD8+ T-cell-mediated (Huseby et al., 2001)
MOG	C57Bl/6, 129/J	Chronic/relapsing, demyelinating (Slavin et al., 1998)
	A.SW	Rapidly progressing, neutrophilia (Tsunoda et al., 2000)
PLP	SJL/J or (SWR × SJL/J)F$_1$	Relapsing/remitting, demyelinating (Sobel et al., 1990; Tuohy et al., 1989)
S100β	Rat	No demyelination (Kojima et al., 1994)

remitting disease, and MOG-induced disease in C57Bl/6 mice, a disease that shows a chronic/relapsing progression. The pathology of both is dominated by T cells and macrophages with focal demyelination centering on perivascular infiltrates. Rodent MOG-induced EAE in C57Bl/6 mice is independent of either B cells or immunoglobulin (Oliver et al., 2003). By contrast, non-demyelinating CNS inflammation in Lewis rat was converted to a demyelinating disease by co-administration of anti-MOG antibodies (Linington et al., 1993). In ASW mice, immunization with MOG induces a form of EAE that includes a diffuse antibody and complement-mediated demyelinating pathology, CNS neutrophilia, and reduced rather than elevated levels of the cytokine interferon-gamma (IFN-γ) (Tsunoda et al., 2000). Interestingly, disseminated neutrophilia and demyelination are also seen in the CNS of either IFN-γ- or IFN-γ-receptor-deficient SJL/J or C57Bl/6 mice with EAE (Tran et al., 2000b). A chronic demyelinating disease that shows little T-cell dependence in its progressive phase can be induced in mice that over-express either IFN-γ or tumor necrosis factor (TNF) in the CNS (Taupin et al., 1997; Renno et al., 1998). These examples are selected to illustrate that EAE is not a monolithic disease, despite points in common between all models (see Table 12.1).

Experimental autoimmune neuritis (EAN)

Peripheral nerve inflammation and demyelination is induced by immunization of animals (usually rodents) with peripheral myelin proteins such as P0 or P2 (Gold et al., 2000; Zou et al., 2000). Peripheral nerve inflammation ensues from induction of an antimyelin T-cell response. The target tissue includes both spinal cord roots and axons, but the roots are favored, as in GBS, the human disease which is modeled by this immunization (Hartung et al., 1998; Gold et al., 2000). Resident endoneurial macrophages subserve an equivalent role to microglia, acting as antigen-presenting cells in tandem with infiltrating macrophages, and probably contributing to the segmental demyelination that is a hallmark of pathology in EAN and GBS (Kiefer et al., 2001).

Adjuvants

Both EAE and EAN depend on the induction of aggressive T-cell responses against self antigens. Breaking of self-tolerance is achieved through use of adjuvants, most commonly complete Freund's adjuvant (CFA), which includes *Mycobacterium tuberculosis* organisms, and pertussis toxin, from *Bordetella pertussis*. Adjuvants work through mimicking the co-stimulation-inducing effects of pathogenic infections, so that the immune system becomes 'fooled' into responding to antigens to which it should not. This somewhat teleological understanding is at the root of studies of the innate immune response, and there is both a strong belief and much evidence for infection as a primary trigger for autoimmune disease. Demyelination can also be induced by viral infection, and the immune processes that underlie this are reasonably assumed to model those that occur in neuroautoimmune diseases such as MS.

Viral encephalomyelitis

Experimental models of virally induced demyelination have particular appeal in that adjuvants are avoided (see below) and physiologically relevant processes of autoimmune induction may be assumed to operate.

Virally induced models of encephalomyelitis (see Chapter 10) complement EAE as systems for studying CNS inflammatory demyelinating disease. These include the picornavirus Theiler's murine encephalomyelitis virus (TMEV) (Drescher et al., 1997), JHM coronavirus (Talbot et al., 2001), and mouse hepatitis virus (MHV) (Buchmeier and Lane, 1999). TMEV is injected intracerebrally to induce a persisting infection whose pathology includes demyelination and immune infiltration. Virally infected glial cells direct a CD4+ and CD8+ T-cell infiltrate. A CD4+ T-cell response is not always required for continued antiviral CD8+ T-cell co-infiltration and demyelinating pathology, as shown by disease induction in MHC Class II-deficient mice (Njenga et al., 1996). Although TMEV-induced demyelination can occur in absence of MHC Class I (and therefore of CD8+ T cells), clinical symptoms of axonal dysfunction were greatly reduced in mice that lacked MHC Class I and CD8+ T cells (Rivera-Quinones et al., 1998). As virus-specific T-cell responses progress, myelin-specific T-cell responses are initiated (Katz-Levy et al., 1999, 2000). This phenomenon of epitope spreading illustrates the link between infection and autoimmunity (discussed in Chapter 2). Importantly for our discussion, there is considerable overlap between the immune events in antiviral and autoimmune responses in the CNS.

Immune events in the induction of demyelinating pathology

The events that follow from immunization of an animal to establishment and progression of inflammatory neurological disease are generalizable between diseases, both clinical and experimental. Many of them represent attractive targets for therapeutic or experimental intervention. The cellular and molecular events described below are part of a common pathway that is broadly applicable to experimental, viral, and clinical inflammatory diseases of the central and peripheral nervous systems.

Antigen presentation and co-stimulation

The induction of an immune response requires antigen presentation and co-stimulation (see Chapters 2 and 5). The CD4+ T cells that are critical for disease are activated by recognition of antigenic peptides associated with Class II MHC molecules on antigen-presenting cells. Primary T-cell activation is critically dependent on, and secondary responses are enhanced by, co-stimulatory signals delivered through T-cell surface molecules such as CD28, by ligation of co-stimulatory ligands such as CD80/B7.1 and CD86/B7.2 (Chambers and Allison 1999). This is also true for adjuvant-primed immunizations such as those that induce EAE and EAN (Chang et al., 1999; Kiefer et al., 2000), although may be less critical for the induction of antiviral responses to TMEV (Johnson et al., 1999). Furthermore, the secondary responses within nervous tissue that are essential for the induction of actual inflammation are optimized by co-stimulation to a significant extent.

Entry of immune cells to the nervous system

The process of immune cell entry to a tissue involves interactions between chemokines and their receptors, adhesion molecules and their receptors, and proteases and their substrates (Owens et al., 1998; Miller, 1999). All of these are influenced, if not directed by cytokines, and in experimental disease are ultimately directed by the activated T lymphocytes that initiate immune cell entry in the first place. In the CNS, an adhesion molecule and chemokine-directed interaction with endothelial cells promotes adhesion of leukocytes to and transmigration across vascular endothelium into the perivascular space. Events in perivascular space may include interaction with perivascular macrophages, and matrix metalloproteinase-mediated migration across the basement membrane, part of a complex barrier that is includes astrocyte cell processes and also receives contributions from microglia (Yong et al., 1998; Prat et al., 2001). Both blood–brain barrier-associated glial cells and endothelial cells are themselves sources of chemokines and express adhesion ligands (Engelhardt et al., 1994; Prat et al., 2001). It has been suggested that population migration depends on preceding (pre-clinical) interactions between individual cytokine-secreting T cells and blood–brain barrier-associated glial cells, and that the cytokine TNF plays a critical role in these initial interactions (Murphy et al., 2002). Matrix metalloproteinase (MMP) enzymes are implicated in the migration process, and may be thought to play a particular role in migration into and through the CNS parenchyma, although this remains to be verified (Yong et al., 2001). The related ADAM (a disintegrin and metalloproteinase) enzymes may also contribute to this process. Access of the immune system to the peripheral nervous system is not constrained by a blood–brain barrier, but nevertheless involves a similar hierarchy of events as for immune cell entry to other tissues. Thus, EAN can be blocked by antibodies against adhesion molecules, as well as by co-stimulation blockade or deficiency in ligands (Archelos et al., 1994, 1997; Enders et al., 1998; Previtali et al., 1998; Kiefer et al., 2001).

Antigen presentation in the nervous system

Another general principle that applys to antigen- and virus-induced experimental demyelinating diseases is that recognition of antigen within the CNS is required for induction of pathology. Candidate antigen-presenting cells include macrophages which have co-infiltrated with T cells, and CNS-resident microglia (Hickey and Kimura, 1988; Becher et al., 2001). Dendritic cells may infiltrate, and whether they are among the antigen-presenting cells resident in the CNS that can induce primary T-cell responses is unresolved (De Vos et al., 2002; Dittel et al., 1999; Serafini et al., 2000). The phenomenon of epitope spreading suggests recruitment of naïve T cells to inflammatory responses (Miller et al., 1995), which argues either for primary inductive antigen presentation in the CNS, or antigen traffic to peripheral lymph nodes.

Effector functions

Antigen presentation in the CNS leads to induction of effector function. Effector functions include cytokine secretion, cellular cytotoxicity, induction of inflammatory mediators such as reactive nitrogen and oxygen species, and antibody plus complement-mediated tissue damage. The primary effector function of T cells that infiltrate the CNS is cytokine production. The myelin-specific CD4+ T cells that induce EAE are of the T helper 1 (Th1)-cytokine-secreting type (Martin et al., 1992). Th1 cytokines are associated with inflammation and include IFN-γ and TNF (Janeway et al., 1999). Th1 CD4+ T cells are specialized for entry to tissues by virtue of expression of selected adhesion ligands and chemokine receptors (Baron et al., 1993; Borges et al., 1997). The alternative Th2 cytokine profile is associated with anti-inflammatory responses and neutralizing antibodies. Th2 cytokines include interleukins (IL)-4, 5 and 10 (Chapter 2). In the absence of regulatory T cells, Th2 cells may also induce EAE (Lafaille et al., 1997). The pro-inflammatory cytokines IFN-γ and TNF induce expression of MHC and adhesion molecules, and of chemokines, and in this way they promote inflammation. They are both also implicated in activation of glial cells and macrophages in the CNS. IFN-γ itself induces TNF production by a variety of cell types. Many other cytokines are implicated in EAE, including IL-1β and IL-6.

Other inflammatory mediators include nitric oxide, produced by the IFN-γ-inducible enzyme inducible nitric oxide synthase (iNOS, or NOS2). NO can combine with superoxide (O_2–) to generate the highly oxidative peroxynitrite (ONOO–) moiety. These reactive oxygen and nitrogen species are part of the armamentarium of macrophages and granulocytes in antiparasite responses and have been proposed to both mediate cytotoxicity and regulate inflammation in the CNS (Cross et al., 1997; Willenborg et al., 1999b).

Glia

Glial cells that normally reside in the CNS are activated in EAE and contribute to the inflammatory milieu. Microglia are CD45+ cells, of the same bone marrow-derived lineage as macrophages. They are phagocytic and express MHC Class II and co-stimulator ligands. Microglia have been implicated as antigen-presenting cells for T-cell responses in the CNS (Smith et al., 1992). It has been suggested that they may mediate demyelination (Sriram and Rodriguez, 1997). Both microglia and astrocytes are sources of cytokines and chemokines in the CNS (Merrill and Benveniste, 1996; Asensio and Campbell, 1999). The proximity of both cell types to the blood–brain barrier makes them ideal candidates for control of leukocyte entry (Miller, 1999; Prat et al., 2001).

Cytotoxicity

Direct cellular cytotoxicity can be mediated by cytotoxic CD8+ T cells, acting via targeted release of perforin and granzyme enzymes. CD8+ T cells are rare in most models of EAE but oligodendrocytes and neurons are both induced to express MHC Class I in the inflamed CNS and so a role for CD8+ T cells is certainly possible (Neumann et al., 2002). There is evidence for MHC-independent killing of oligodendrocytes by CD4+ T cells, so-called bystander killing (Ruijs et al., 1993; Vergelli et al., 1997). Cytotoxicity may also be mediated by macrophages, microglia, and neutrophils, through antibody-directed cellular cytotoxicity (Janeway et al., 1999).

B cells and antibodies

Even though B-cell-deficient mice are fully susceptible to EAE, there may be a role for antibody and complement in demyelination in some models of EAE. The example of demyelination in Lewis rats (Kojima et al., 1994) has been cited above. Pertinent here is that mice in which the complement inhibitor sCrry was over-expressed in the CNS were resistant to EAE (Davoust et al., 1999).

Protection and repair in EAE

T cells, macrophages, and antimyelin antibodies have been shown to mediate neuroprotective or regenerative roles in the CNS (David et al., 1990; Rodriguez et al., 1996; Huang et al., 1999; Kerschensteiner et al., 1999; Yoles et al., 2001). This can reflect production of neurotrophins, clearance of debris to facilitate repair, or other mechanisms. For instance, NOS2-deficient mice develop very severe EAE compared with controls, arguing that NO is protective in EAE (Fenyk-Melody et al., 1998; Sahrbacher et al., 1998). Similarly, IFN-γ-deficient mice develop a lethal, non-remitting form of EAE, so this cytokine, although pro-inflammatory, may also exert regulatory functions (Ferber et al., 1996; Krakowski and Owens, 1996; Willenborg et al., 1996). Proliferative responses of IFN-γ-deficient T cells are exacerbated and this may reflect lack of an IFN-γ-inducible NO-mediated regulatory circuit (Willenborg et al., 1999a; Tran et al., 2000b). It has been suggested that remission from EAE correlates to production of Th2 cytokines and/or to the anti-inflammatory cytokine transforming growth factor (TGF)-β (Kennedy et al., 1992; Khoury et al., 1992; Antel and Owens, 1999). However, this has not achieved consensus.

These experimental animal models represent a mainstay of research into inflammatory neurologic disease. They have identified fundamental principles, that immune responses induced in lymphoid tissue have access to nervous tissue, that cytokine-directed processes of chemoattraction and adhesion are critical for immune cell entry to nervous tissue, and that antigen presentation within the target tissue is critical for elaboration of pathologic and repair processes. These models remain 'gold standards'. Nevertheless, the need for either adjuvants or viral infection introduces complexity that can make interpretation difficult, and there are limitations to what can be achieved through use of systemically administered reagents such as blocking antibodies in dissecting the mechanism. For these reasons, the experimental animal models of neurologic disease are complemented by genetic models. Generally, these have targeted genes that were first identified from the experimental models.

Genetically engineered animal models

Over the past 15–20 years, advances in the fields of molecular biology, molecular genetics, cellular biology, and embryology have laid the foundations for two great advances in experimental biology. They are (1) the tools for the targeted introduction and expression and stable germline transmission of ectopic genes in the mouse, and (2) the identification and cloning of a vast number of mammalian genes critical in the functioning of the immune and nervous systems in normal and disease states. Most simply put, through genetic manipulation of the mouse genome it became possible to determine in the intact immune or nervous system and organism, the cause and effect relationships between a suspected pathogenic gene and the development of disease. There are a number of methods for introducing genes into animals. However, as we mentioned above, the most widely embraced techniques for generating gene manipulations in mice involve producing either transgenic (gain of function) or knockout (loss of function) mutations (for detailed reviews see Capecchi (1994), Murphy and Carter (1993) and Pinkert (1994)). In either case, once made, the stable mutant lines generated provide an unrestricted source of animals identical for the introduced genetic and molecular alteration, thus permitting systematic analysis of the molecular, cellular, and clinical phenotypes.

Transgenic mice

Approach

In order to generate transgenic mice a fusion gene (i.e. a transgene) construct is microinjected directly into the pro-nucleus of fertilized mouse ova, which are then implanted in the oviduct of pseudopregnant recipient mice. Progeny are screened using complementary probes to elements of the transgene construct that are not normally present in the host genome, usually by Southern blotting or by polymerase chain reaction (PCR) analysis.

Crucial to the creation of transgenic mice is the design and construction of the transgene. The objective of this approach is a functional gene that will undergo the necessary transcriptional, post-transcriptional, and translational processing to yield the proper bioactive gene product. In its simplest form, the transgene construct is chimeric, and consists of an upstream transcriptional control unit (the promoter) joined to the coding sequence (the expressed gene; this requires the availability of either the complete genomic sequence or a full length cDNA for the gene of interest) and a downstream regulatory sequence (the polyadenylation signal) to facilitate correct processing of the primary RNA transcript.

The choice of which promoter construct to use is a critical decision that depends largely on the experimental objective and the nature of the protein to be expressed. Generally, promoters can be classified into two categories depending on whether transcriptional control is or is not restricted to a specific tissue. In experimental neuroimmunology tissue-specific promoters for the targeting of transgene expression to either the CNS or immune cells such as T lymphocytes, have been widely embraced. This is understandable when the underlying objectives for engineering new models of neuroimmune disease are considered. Thus, transgene constructs have been designed either around recapitulating putative effector

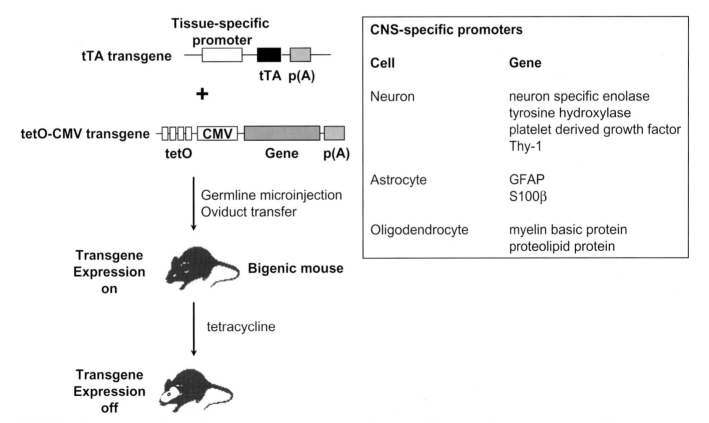

CNS-specific promoters	
Cell	**Gene**
Neuron	neuron specific enolase tyrosine hydroxylase platelet derived growth factor Thy-1
Astrocyte	GFAP S100β
Oligodendrocyte	myelin basic protein proteolipid protein

Fig. 12.2 Development of tetracycline-inducible transgenic mice. A transgene construct is made in which the tetracycline transcriptional activator, tTA, is cloned downstream of a tissue-specific promoter together with a polyadenylation p(A) signal sequence. A second transgene is constructed in which the gene of interest to be expressed is cloned downstream of the tetO–CMV minimal promoter. Equimolar combinations of these two transgene constructs are then microinjected into fertilized ova which are then implanted into the oviduct of pseudopregnant mice. In bigenic mice, administration of tetracycline (in this example tetracycline will bind to tTA and switch off transcriptional activity of the CMV promoter) can be used to control transgene expression.

mechanisms associated with localized immune processes in the CNS or to challenge the immune system's mechanisms of tolerance towards CNS autoantigens. A variety of promoter constructs are available that permit the transcriptional targeting of transgenes to specific cells of the CNS or the immune system (see Fig. 12.2). CNS examples include neuron-specific enolase (Forss-Petter et al., 1990), myelin basic protein for oligodendrocytes (Gow et al., 1992), and glial fibrillary acidic protein for astrocytes (Mucke et al., 1991), while those that target immune cells include the Eμ enhancer for lymphocytes for B cells (Harris et al., 1988), proximal Lck for T cells (Wildin et al., 1991), and the scavenger receptor A for macrophages (Horvai et al., 1995). It should be noted that at present a promoter for microglial-specific transgene targeting is not available.

Once transgenic progeny are obtained it is important to verify the level of transgene expression and its anatomical distribution. The spatial pattern of transgene expression is related to the characteristics of the promoter employed, while the chromosomal site of integration plays an important role in determining the level of expression (Murphy and Carter, 1993; Pinkert, 1994). Depending on the regulatory properties of the promoter and the nature of the transgene-encoded protein, this product itself may also contribute to both the pattern and levels of expression. The absolute level of expression often varies from one transgenic line to another, reflecting effects of sequences surrounding the integration sites. Although measurement at the protein level is the most compelling evidence for a functional transgene, expression is commonly measured at the RNA level in cases where protein levels are below the detectable limits.

Considerations

The greatest advantage of the transgenic approach is that it uniquely permits the targeted delivery of a single gene product to a specific tissue compartment and thus allows the study of the function of that gene in a non-invasive and anatomically relevant fashion. However, there are also potential disadvantages and pitfalls associated with this technology of which we will consider the more important here. From the outset, the choice of which promoter (and therefore cell) to target with transgene expression is not a trivial one. First, targeting a cell that does not normally produce the gene of interest may yield interesting results. However, these may be artifactual and bear little relevance to the role of that gene in a disease process. Second, such a strategy could actually result in artifactual toxic effects of transgene expression in certain sensitive cells. One such cell in the CNS is the oligodendrocyte. Transgenic experiments designed to develop new models for CNS autoimmunity in which expression of MHC Class I were targeted to oligodendrocytes using the MBP promoter produced mice with motor disease. However, this turned out to be due to direct toxic effects of the transgene expression on developing oligodendrocytes and was not associated with any immune process in the white matter (Turnley et al., 1991).

The tissue specificity and temporal expression of the introduced gene is determined largely by the nature of the promoter used in the transgene and by the site in the genome into which the transgene becomes integrated. Although many gene promoters show tissue-restricted expression, this is not always absolute. For example, the GFAP promoter used to target the expression of transgenes to the astrocyte in the CNS can also be active in enteric glia of the gut (Bush et al., 1998). Promoter 'leakiness' resulting from positional effects at the chromosomal site of integration can also occur. In view of these considerations it is always important to establish the tissue specificity for the expression of transgenes. The process of chromosomal insertion of the transgene is a largely random one giving rise to the potential for the disruption of endogenous gene function either directly via the integration of the foreign DNA within critical regulatory or coding regions or through positional effects leading to altered transcriptional activity of the endogenous gene. In order to rule out the possibility of such an insertional mutation, it is important to develop and study independent transgenic lines for a given transgene to establish that any phenotype observed is reproducible and transgene dose-dependent. The issue of transgene dose is also worth considering, since production of transgene-encoded

molecules at supraphysiologic levels may also result in actions and phenotypes that are not normally encountered during disease processes. Comparison of the expression levels of the transgene product with those found during experimentally induced disease can therefore further validate the relevance of a transgenic model.

A final drawback to the conventional transgenic approach is that transgene expression cannot be controlled in a temporal fashion. This can result in the expression of the transgene occurring throughout the life of the animal, increasing the potential for developmental effects and compensatory processes. A good example here is the cytokine IFN-γ. IFN-γ is not produced normally in the CNS, but rather by activated T cells and natural killer (NK) cells entering the CNS in response to stimuli such as infection or during an autoimmune episode. Transgenic mice developed with IFN-γ under the control of the MBP (Corbin et al., 1996) or GFAP (LaFerla et al., 2000) promoters die soon after birth with minimal immune involvement. However, some lines of such transgenic mice had a severe abnormality in cerebellar development with hypomyelination and disturbed granule neuron proliferation and patterning. Others showed vascular occlusions that were not further characterized (Renno et al., 1998). These findings therefore highlighted toxic effects of IFN-γ that were particularly pronounced in the developing brain and limited the intended utility of these transgenic mice for studying the contribution of IFN-γ to immune-mediated demyelination in the adult CNS. The solution to this problem would be to employ strategies that permit tight temporal control of transgene expression. Such methodologies allowing the conditional control of transgene expression are discussed further below.

Gene knockout mice

Approach

Compared with transgenic mice, gene disruption by homologous recombination represents a technically more challenging and, time wise, more lengthy approach to manipulation of the mouse genome. In spite of this, because of its ability to allow precise targeting and mutation of specific genes in the animal, the application of this technique has grown rapidly. The generic vector (see Fig. 12.2) used in this strategy typically consists of a homologous cloned genomic DNA into which is inserted coding sequences for two antibiotic resistance marker genes that permit selection of positive embryonal stem (ES) cells. The first marker, commonly the neo^r gene, is inserted within an exon of the targeting homologous genomic DNA while the second marker, typically the herpes simplex thymidine kinase (HSV-tk) gene, is placed downstream immediately adjacent to the region of homology with the targeted chromosomal gene. Following introduction of the vector into ES cells by transfection or electroporation, successful homologous recombination between the vector and the targeted gene will result in disruption of the chromosomal gene and insertion of the neo^r and exclusion of the HSV-tk gene. However, more commonly, the targeting vector will insert at random sites in the genome of the ES cells thus necessitating selection and enrichment of the desired mutant cells. Initially, the ES cells are exposed to gancyclovir which kills those cells bearing the negative selectable marker thymidine kinase. A second round of selection is then performed, treating the surviving ES cells with neomycin that selects for cells in which the cloned gene with the neo^r, replaced the targeted sequence in the chromosome. This process results in a pure population of ES cells that carry a targeted mutation in one chromosome.

The ES cells, which are typically derived from the 129/J strain, are then microinjected into blastocyst stage embryos, derived from a black mouse, often of the C57BL/6 background. After oviduct implantation into pseudopregnant surrogate mothers offspring can be sorted according to coat color. Chimeric pups, with a mixture of brown and black shading, contain cells from both mouse strains whereas black pups are considered to be negative for the ES cells. Chimeric males are then further interbred with C57BL/6 females. Offspring with evidence of ES lineage, i.e. brown coats, are then screened by Southern blot hybridization for evidence of the targeted mutation. Males and females carrying the mutation are then interbred producing mice that are homozygous for the targeted gene resulting in a complete disruption of the functional gene.

Considerations

There are a number of important caveats that must be considered in interpreting the effects of gene mutations in whole animal studies (Steinman, 1997). Like promoter-driven transgene expression, the conventional 'gene knockout' approach described above is also non-conditional in that temporal and spatial control of the mutation is not possible. Thus, the loss of gene function mutation is present throughout the life of the animal and in every cell of the organism. Consequently, the effects of the targeted mutation might be widespread, involving peripheral organs as well as the CNS making, it very difficult to discern primary from secondary or compensatory changes. If the gene happens to be irreplaceable, disruption may be lethal at an embryonic or post-natal stage (e.g. as occurs with targeted disruption of the gp130 subunit gene of the IL-6 receptor cytokine superfamily (Yoshida et al., 1996)) making further analysis of neuroimmune processes impossible. Even in the circumstance that a gene knockout produces apparently healthy, viable mice, peripheral tissues may still have structural or functional changes that could significantly influence subsequent immune and CNS disease processes. A good case in point here is the TNF superfamily of cytokines and receptors. Mice that lack TNF, LT-α, LT-β or the corresponding receptors for these ligands show to varying extents a variety of abnormalities associated with defective lymphoid organogenesis resulting in the absence of lymph nodes (LN) or Peyer's patches (PP) and altered splenic or lymph node architecture (Kassiotis and Kollias, 2001). This of course is a major complication that needs to be considered when these mice are used to study the role of these immune effector genes in neuroimmune disease processes such as EAE. Fortunately, more recent technical advances (see following discussion), should address these concerns by making it possible to control the time and the site of such gene knockouts.

An additional concern that warrants consideration here is the one of mouse background strain. The influence of the genetic background of the mouse can have far-reaching consequences that could contribute in a negative or positive fashion to the mutant phenotype (Jabs et al., 2002). In particular, when it comes to the study of immune responses the impact of factors such as the MHC haplotype can vary tremendously between different strains of mice. As noted above, ES cells derived from the 129/J genetic background are most commonly used for targeting mutations. Importantly, mice wild type for these backgrounds have a propensity for agenesis of the corpus callosum which does not occur in many other backgrounds such as C57BL/6 (Muller et al., 1994). This spontaneous developmental abnormality is also expressed to a variable degree in hybrid offspring and clearly has the potential to influence disease processes in the brain. Controlling for influences of genetic background strain is a major challenge in the study of knockout models. Depending on the nature of the processes under study it might be appropriate to maintain mice on the 129/J background, but in many cases this may not be the case, when the only solution is extensive backcrossing to derive mice congenic for the desired inbred genetic background. However, even through backcrossing, flanking genes that are tightly linked to the site of the targeted mutation will lead to the creation of individually variable congenic segments that possibly could influence the phenotype independent of the targeted gene mutation. The use of directly targeted, disease-susceptible mouse strains represents a solution to this problem, facilitated by the availability of ES cells derived from other inbred strains of mice (e.g. C57BL/6 (Korner et al., 1997)).

Knock-ins

The same principles that allow targeting of a disrupting element to a gene locus by homologous recombination also allow complete replacement of the gene by a modified version. Site-specific integration of transgenes has the advantage that the substituted gene remains under control of the same regulatory elements as the one it replaced, so that levels and kinetics of expression are unaffected. By targeting transgenes to specific sites, all trans-

genic founders will have the same copy number. Inclusion of promoter elements in the targeted transgene allows copy number and gross regulation to be equivalent between mice, while gene-specific promoter may vary with transgene design (Bronson et al., 1996; Mak et al., 2001).

One recent application of this approach was the substitution of the TNF gene by a mutated uncleavable allele that lacked the recognition sequence for the TACE enzyme that cleaves TNF to generate a soluble cytokine. The mice therefore selectively lacked soluble TNF and only generated a membrane-bound form (Ruuls et al., 2001). This revealed distinct roles for membrane-bound versus soluble TNF. Membrane TNF plays a greater role in the organization of lymphoid tissue whereas soluble TNF was shown to be critical for the induction of EAE.

Conditional transgenic and knockout models

As is apparent from the above discussion, the inability to control temporally the expression of a transgene or a targeted gene knockout represents a major drawback with the pioneer generation of these technologies. This frontier, however, has been propelled forward by the advent of technologies that permit the fine control of genetic manipulations in time and space. The ability to switch gene expression 'on' or 'off' in a tissue-specific fashion at defined times offers the potential for unparalleled opportunities for elucidating gene function in normal and disease states (for more extensive reviews see Ryding et al. (2001) and Yamamoto et al. (2001)).

Regulatable promoters have been designed that permit precise temporal control over transgene expression. These fall into two broad categories, the eukaryotic-based and prokaryotic-based inducible systems. Examples of eukaryotic-based regulatable promoter systems include metallothionein, interferon, and hormone-dependent promoters. However, due to the pleiotropic effects and/or toxicity of the switch or inducer, the use of these systems has been largely restricted to cell culture. These limitations of the eukaryotic-based systems led to the investigation of regulatable systems that exploit the unique transcriptional controls of prokaryotic operons. The best defined and most widely used of these to direct inducible transgene expression is based on the Escherichia coli tet operon.

The tet operon controls the expression of the tetracycline resistance gene in E. coli. Expression of this gene is repressed by the tetracycline repressor (tetR), which binds to the tetracycline operator sequence (tetO) and thereby silences transcription. Repression is removed in the presence of tetracycline which binds avidly to the tetR, thus preventing tetR from binding to tetO. Pioneering studies by Gossen and Bujard (1992) that exploited this system led to the development of the tetracycline transactivator (tTA) regulatable system which permitted transgene expression to be controlled in a simple on/off fashion by tetracycline (Fig. 12.2). In the tTA regulatable system, tetR is converted into a transcriptional activator (tTA) by combining it with the activation domains of the herpes simplex virus VP16 protein. The tTA binds to a series of tandemly arranged tetO sequences that are fused with a cytomegalovirus (CMV) minimal promoter resulting in transcriptional activation. In the presence of tetracycline (which binds to tTA), tTA is incapacitated and cannot bind to the tetO–CMV minimal promoter DNA, blocking transcriptional activity.

Adapting this regulatable system to mice requires that the animals are bigenic with respect to the tTA and the tetO–CMV transgenes. This is commonly achieved by the generation of two independent transgenic lines: one carrying the transgene of interest under the control of the tetO–CMV and the other in which a tissue-specific promoter is used to drive expression of the tTA to a particular tissue or cell. Interbreeding of the two lines will result in a proportion of progeny with both transgenes. Since the minimal promoter itself confers no tissue specificity, control of transgene expression is determined by the site of expression of tTA. An alternative to this time-consuming and laborious approach is to microinject equimolar mixtures of these two transgenes directly into the germline (Ray et al., 1997). Since both transgenes are likely to be co-integrated into the same chromosomal site, a number of the progeny founders will be bigenic. A further advantage of this is that the expression of both transgenes is coordinately controlled within the same cell. Irrespective of the method used to produce the bigenic mice, silencing of the transgene expression is attained by the oral administration (in food or drinking water) of tetracycline or more commonly its less toxic analog doxycycline, which has a higher tTA binding affinity. Significant reductions in transgene expression can occur within 2 days of doxycycline treatment and this repression is reversible, with full re-induction by 7 days after removal of doxycycline (Tremblay *et al.*, 1998).

Several groups have successfully applied this approach to express transgenes in the CNS (Yamamoto *et al.*, 2001), although, none have involved neuroimmune studies. A drawback with this initial tTA regulatable system concerns the use of doxycycline in order to keep transgene expression silent. The consequences of long-term or developmental exposure to this inducer are not known. Recent studies indicate that doxycycline can inhibit microglial activation and suppress CNS inflammation (Yrjanheikki *et al.*, 1998). Therefore the tTA regulatable system is not suitable for many experimental situations. More recent modifications have been introduced to get around this problem. Reverse tTA (rtTA) is a mutagenized form of tTA that requires tetracycline to bind to tetO to activate transgene expression (Gossen *et al.*, 1995). In the basal state transcriptional activity of the mini-

mal promoter is silent, but can be activated by administration of doxycycline. Unfortunately, problems with this system have precluded its widespread use in the CNS. These include increased background or leaky expression from the minimal promoter and the requirement for much higher levels of doxycycline to drive rtTA induction of transgene expression. To address these problems the variant rtTA2s–M2 was recently generated (Urlinger *et al.*, 2000). This has virtually no background activity, greatly enhanced doxycycline sensitivity, and increased stability. While to date, use of the rtTA2s–M2 system has not been reported in mice, in principle its considerable enhancements should make it the favored approach for temporal control of transgene expression in the CNS.

The advent of the tet regulatable system offers a potentially ideal approach for turning transgenes on and off. A second system that has co-evolved is the Cre/loxP recombination system that makes it possible to control the site of a gene ablation (Fig. 12.3). Cre recombinase is a site-specific recombinase that catalyses intra-and intermolecular recombination between loxP sites. In this procedure, the cloned gene to be disrupted is flanked by loxP recognition sequences and introduced by homologous recombination in ES cells. Transgenic mice bearing the loxP modified gene

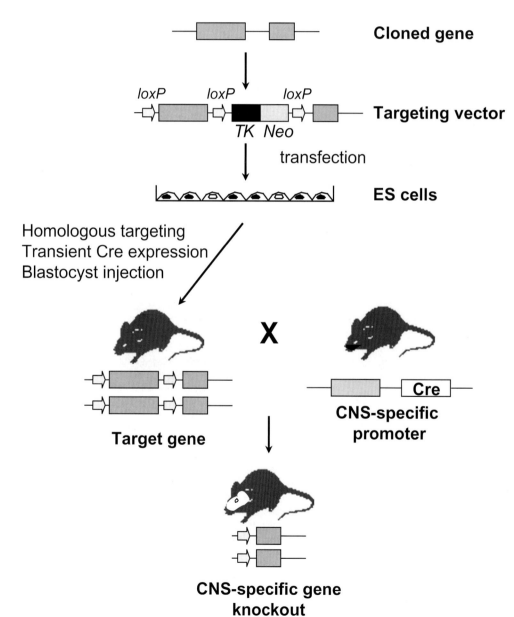

Fig. 12.3 CNS-restricted gene ablation by Cre recombinase. A targeting vector is created from the cloned endogenous gene in which a coding region and an adjacent cassette with the *TK* and *Neo* genes are flanked by loxP sites. The targeting vector is then introduced into embryonic stem (ES) cells by transfection. After homologous recombination and selection with neomycin, the genetically modified ES cells are transiently transfected with Cre recombinase resulting in removal of the antibiotic cassette from the recombined gene. Further gancyclovir treatment selects for positive cell clones that are screened by Southern analysis for the recombined gene flanked by the loxP sequences. ES cells containing the floxed gene are introduced into blastocyst stage pre-implantation embryos (derived from black mice) and transferred to the oviduct of pseudopregnant recipients. To achieve tissue-specific gene disruption, mutant mice with the loxP gene are bred with transgenic mice expressing Cre recombinase under the control of the CNS-specific promoter. The loxP flanked target gene will only be 'knocked out' in the specific tissues, expressing the Cre recombinase—in the case of the example shown here this would be the CNS.

can be bred to homozygosity and then crossed with transgenic mice expressing the Cre recombinase gene constitutively under the control of a cell-type-specific promoter. In bigenic mice, cell-specific gene inactivation will then occur as a result of excision of the 'floxed' gene by the Cre recombinase. The activity and tissue specificity of the Cre transgenics can be effectively monitored using reporter lines carrying a reporter gene such as LacZ, whose expression requires excision of loxP-flanked stop sequences. Although a variety of CNS- and leukocyte-specific promoter Cre recombinase transgenic mice are available that have been used successfully for the tissue- or cell-specific ablation of many different genes, this system has yet to be applied in the study of gene function in experimental neuroimmunology.

Since the expression of Cre recombinase in the transgenic mice is under the transcriptional control of a cell-type-specific promoter, the timing for the inactivation of the floxed target gene is characteristic of the promoter type used. Therefore, to have temporal control over Cre-mediated recombination several strategies, including the use of the tet-inducible system, have been employed to drive inducible Cre recombinase. Mostly this system has been used to achieve inducible gene knockouts. This strategy permits the inactivation of a gene in the adult mouse and therefore overcomes the problem of lethality in the case of an essential developmental gene or developmental compensation due to redundancy. Many cases of the application of inducible gene knockouts to study gene function in neurobiology and immunology can now be found in the literature (Yamamoto et al., 2001). However, the application of inducible gene knockouts to address basic problems in neuroimmunology at this time still awaits realization.

Gene delivery to the central nervous system

Insertion or deletion of genes in the genome is a powerful manipulation. However, disease-relevant genetic manipulation often calls for transient or reversable effects, and in particular may call for alterations of gene expression in adult animals. Conditional promoters make this possible, but construction of each animal is laborious and, using current technology, fraught with difficulties that often lead to failure. These considerations promote interest in methods for de novo gene expression in the nervous system of otherwise normal animals.

Viral vectors for gene delivery

Viruses represent organisms that are naturally selected for gene delivery to mammalian cells. The neurotropism of certain viruses makes them ideal candidates for gene delivery to the central nervous system. The ideal virus for gene delivery would retain the ability to infect cells (e.g. retain infectivity and tropism) while losing the ability to replicate within the cell. Under normal circumstances the nervous system is dominated by non-dividing cells, so viral vectors for gene delivery to neural cells should not require a dividing cell as host. Those that do would tend to target inflammatory cells (which may have other advantages). Whether a virus integrates into the host genome or remains epigenetically associated influences the stability of expression. Those that integrate may exert undesired effects on the host genome, beyond those of the exogene that they deliver. Finally, most viruses are both pathogenic and immunogenic, and a balance must be struck between deletion of those capabilities that renders them biologically inactive, versus retention of sufficient capability to infect and deliver the gene of interest.

Neurotropic viruses that have been used as vectors in the nervous system include herpes simplex virus-1 (HSV-1). Viruses that infect non-dividing cells, with a broad tropism, include adenoviruses, adenoassociated virus (AAV), and lentiviruses. For a current review on this topic see Hsich et al. (2002).

Herpesvirus is neurotropic and can be introduced to the CNS via direct inoculation or via intrathecal or intraventricular injection. Replication-defective HSV-1-encoded IFN-γ was introduced to the CNS of mice with EAE, where it abrogated disease (Furlan et al., 2001), consistent with results from direct injection of IFN-γ in one other study (Voorthuis et al., 1990) but in apparent contradiction to findings from direct injection of IFN-γ to unmanipulated spinal cord (Simmons and Willenborg 1990). Similar vectors have been used for CNS-directed cytokine gene delivery in rhesus monkeys (Poliani et al., 2001).

Adenovirus is a DNA virus with a broad tropism. One of the major clinical issues confronting use of adenovirus as a therapeutic is the possibility that immune response against viral antigens would compromise the recipient through induction of chronic inflammation (Thomas et al., 2000). This is overcome by use of 'gutless' high-capacity vectors (Thomas et al., 2000). These are helper-dependent, which increases the technical complexity of their growth and purification. However, such adenoviruses have been shown to survive in the CNS for as long as 90 days, in contrast to weeks at most for first-generation viruses (Zou et al., 2002). Gutless adenoviruses can, indeed must, accommodate very large amounts (over 30 kilobases) of foreign DNA. This allows introduction of genomic promoter and flanking regulatory regions as well as the intron-containing genomic gene sequence. As such, they have many potential advantages despite the difficulty of handling such large amounts of DNA. For experimental purposes, the first-generation vectors have allowed transient expression of cytokines and chemokines in the CNS of adult animals, with useful results. Adenoviral vectors have been used to introduce suicide genes such as p53 to gliomas in rodent models, and to introduce chemokines to murine CNS (Bell et al., 1996; Gilbert et al., 2001; Li et al., 1997). Adenovirus-encoded MIP-2 induced neutrophilia (Bell et al., 1996), and IL-10 delivered by adenovirus vector was protective (Croxford et al., 1998, 2001).

Lentiviruses derived from human immunodeficiency virus-1 (HIV-1) infect non-dividing cells and have the potential advantages of long-term transgene expression, integration into the host chromosome (unlike adenovirus), and absence of induction of an inflammatory immune response. Lentiviruses have been used for delivery of GDNF or fluorescent protein constructs to rat brain, by intrastriatal injection. Both studies showed that lentivirus vectors were neurotropic (Georgievska et al., 2002, Lai and Brady, 2002). Rabies-G pseudotyping of lentiviral vectors enabled their retrograde transport to the nervous system following peripheral administration (Mazarakis et al., 2001).

Routes of administration

Viruses can be administered for expression in the CNS by three routes. They can be administered distally from the CNS, to access the CNS via natural targeting. This is a possibility for herpesviruses, that can access the CNS via retrograde transport along axons. The advantage of this route is that physiologically appropriate sites are infected. However, due to the need to use non-replicating and otherwise-modified viruses as vectors, this may not always be an optimal route for infection, and target specificity imposes limits to the range of expression that can be achieved. Viral vectors can also be administered by intrathecal or intraventricular injection to the subdural space, for access to the CNS via ependymal routes. This has been used for both adenovirus and for HSV-1 vectors (Martino et al., 2001). It has the advantage of not inducing damage to tissue, especially when intrathecal injections are used, and ensuring delivery to the CNS, but may not result in dependable entry of virus to CNS parenchyma. Finally, viral vectors can be directly injected into the CNS by intracerebral injection. The advantage of this lies in precision of location, but accompaning tissue damage inevitably induces inflammation.

Gene delivery by infiltrating T cells

For gene delivery one can also exploit the fact that lymphocytes and myeloid cells have the capacity to infiltrate the CNS. T lymphocytes that were transfected with IL-10 or with PDGF-α (a survival factor for oligodendrocytes) were used to alleviate EAE (Mathisen et al., 1997, 1999; Mathisen and Tuohy, 2000). This may be viewed as an experimental manipulation that parallels the natural ability of T cells to exert protective effects in the CNS (Kerschensteiner *et al.*, 1999; Schwartz *et al.*, 1999; Schwartz and Moalem, 2001). An analogous approach was used to deliver IL-12 p40 to the CNS to alleviate EAE (Costa *et al.*, 2001). In this case the T cells were engineered to produce a molecule (IL-12 p40) that functions as an antagonist of IFN-γ-mediated inflammation.

Genes targeted in transgenic/knock-out models and findings

Cytokines/chemokines

Given the central role of cytokines and chemokines in directing immune responses in the CNS, it is not surprising that they should be among the most commonly targeted genes in genetic dissection of disease mechanisms. Recent reviews have covered the findings from such studies in detail (Owens *et al.*, 2001; Wang *et al.*, 2002a). An overview of the major findings is provided in Table 12.2.

Over-expression of cytokines considered to be pro-inflammatory has in all cases resulted in either spontaneous disease or exacerbation of inducible inflammatory conditions. In general, the spontaneous diseases induced by individual cytokines are specific in that they reflect the unique functions of these molecules. For example, astrocyte expression of IL-3 (Chiang *et al.*, 1996), a cytokine that acts primarily on macrophages, promotes the accumulation of highly activated macrophage/microglia in the white matter resulting in demyelinating disease. On the other hand, similarly targeted expression of the Th1 cytokine gene IL-12 (Pagenstecher *et al.*, 2000) results in a prominent active T-cell meningoencephalitis. Over-expression of chemokines has resulted in, as expected, movement of leukocytes either towards or into the CNS, with consequences dependent on the chemokine in question. However, and in contrast with cytokines, for many pro-inflammatory chemokines, e.g. CCL2 (MCP-1) (Fuentes *et al.*, 1995) or

CXCL10 (Boztug *et al.*, 2002), this migration of leucocytes into the CNS was not associated with the activation of these cells and the development of spontaneous disease.

Knockout experiments have targeted a number key genes involved in cytokine actions including the cytokine, its receptor, and downstream components of the signal transduction pathway. Generally, these have generated findings that are consistent with the effects of antibodies or other antagonists of the targeted molecule. One notable exception has been the cytokine IFN-γ, abrogation of which resulted in mice that had increased susceptibility to EAE (Ferber *et al.*, 1996; Krakowski and Owens, 1996; Willenborg *et al.*, 1996; Owens *et al.*, 2001). At first glance this appears at odds with the perception of IFN-γ as a pro-inflammatory mediator, although it is consistent with the fact that blocking antibodies exacerbated EAE (Billiau *et al.*, 1988; Duong *et al.*, 1992). Although the susceptibility of IFN-γ-deficient mice seemed unexpected, this actually reflects an incomplete understanding of the normal physiological role of this cytokine. IFN-γ is not only pro-inflammatory but has been described to have antiproliferative and immune-regulatory effects. One can speculate that effects of IFN-γ are themselves influenced by the state of the systems into which it is introduced. Thus, *de novo* introduction of IFN-γ to otherwise uninflamed nervous tissue induced or promoted inflammation (Simmons and Willenborg, 1990; Sethna and Lampson, 1991), whereas up-regulation or abrogation in the context of ongoing inflammation has revealed regulatory effects (Billiau *et al.*, 1988; Voorthuis *et al.*, 1990; Furlan *et al.*, 2001). It is important to consider which of these modalities is to be modeled when designing genetic manipulations. In a clinical context, the inflammatory status of patients who are intended recipients of IFN-γ therapy would need to be carefully defined.

Other unexpected findings from knockouts may have more to do with lack of correspondence to MS than to the effects of the knockout *per se*. Thus, mice that are deficient in TNF are, as one might expect, refractory to induction of EAE, although disease is induced with a delay. That delay reflects initial dependence on TNF for induction of critical chemokine sig-

Table 12.2 Major neuroimmunological findings in mice with transgenic production or knockout of different cytokines and chemokines or their receptors

Cytokine/chemokine	Effects of ectopic expression in CNS	Effects of knockout
IFN-α	Neurodegeneration. T-cell inflammation	Not done (Akwa *et al.*, 1998)
IFN-γ	Neurodegeneration. Demyelination	Increased susceptibility to EAE (Corbin *et al.*, 1996; Renno *et al.*, 1998; LaFerla *et al.*, 2000; Krakowski and Owens, 1996)
TNFα	Demyelination. Neurodegeneration. Mixed leukocyte infiltrates. Macrophage/microglial activation	Delayed onset of EAE (Probert *et al.*, 1995; Renno *et al.*, 1995; Stalder *et al.*, 1998; Korner *et al.*, 1997)
IL-3	Demyelination. Macrophage infiltration and activation	Not known (Chiang *et al.*, 1996)
IL-6	Neurodegeneration. Intrinsic inflammation	Resistant to EAE (Campbell *et al.*, 1993; Eugster *et al.*, 1998)
IL-4	No effect	Exacerbated EAE (Falcone et al., 1998, Poliani et al., 2001)
IL-10	Alleviated EAE	Exacerbated EAE (Nagelkerken *et al.*, 1997; Samoilova *et al.*, 1998)
IL-12	Meningoencephalitis	Pagenstecher *et al.* (2000)
IL-12p40		Resistant to EAE (Segal *et al.*, 1998)
IL-12p35		Susceptible to EAE (Becher *et al.*, 2002)
CCL2/ MCP-1	No clinical symptoms. Perivascular leukocytes	Resistant to EAE (Fuentes *et al.*, 1995; Huang *et al.*, 2001; Karpus *et al.*, 1995)
CCL-3	Not done	Susceptible to EAE (Tran *et al.*, 2000a)
CCL21	Dysmyelination. Inflammation/ CNS neutrophilia	Chen *et al.* (2002)
CXCL1/KC/GRO-α	CNS neutrophilia	Not done (Tani *et al.*, 1996)
CXCL10	No symptoms. CNS neutrophilia	Boztug *et al.* (2002)
CCR-5	Not done	Susceptible to EAE (Tran *et al.*, 2000a). Resistant to MHV encephalomyelitis (Lane *et al.*, 2000)
CCR1	Not done	Mildly resistant to EAE (Rottman *et al.*, 2000)
CCR2	Not done	Resistant to EAE (Fife *et al.*, 2000; Izikson *et al.* 2000). Increased mortality with decreased T-cell influx in MHV encephalomyelitis (Chen *et al.*, 2001)

nals that direct T-cell entry to the CNS (Murphy *et al.*, 2002). However, targeting of TNF in MS resulted in worsening of disease in many cases (Arnason, 1999), and indeed may have induced demyelinating disease in some recipients of therapy for rheumatoid arthritis (Sicotte and Voskuhl, 2001). Reasons for this discrepancy remain unclear, but may include differential TNF receptor signaling and the fact that the sTNFR drugs used did not penetrate the blood–brain barrier, unlike their ready access to the arthritic joint (Feldmann and Maini, 2001).

Co-stimulator ligands and receptors are also logical targets for genetic intervention. Knockout of either CD80 or CD86 has reduced susceptibility to EAE, and mice that lack both co-stimulator ligands are entirely unsusceptible to disease (Chang *et al.*, 1999). Unexpectedly, knockout or blockade of the ICOS ligand, that is implicated in co-stimulation of memory T-cell responses, enhanced susceptibility to EAE, which identifies a regulatory role for this ligand that had not been appreciated (Jabs *et al.*, 2001).

Transgenic over-expression of co-stimulator ligands in the CNS has not been directly attempted, partly due to lack of a microglial-specific promoter. However, one study describes the serendipitous finding that a transgene targeted to T cells was also ectopically expressed in microglia of the CNS and macrophages of the peripheral NS (Zehntner *et al.*, 2003)). These mice show a spontaneous demyelinating disease with onset in adult animals, that is dominated by CD8+ T cells.

Targeting receptor and signal transduction molecules

Transgenic expression of cytokine or chemokine receptors has not been described. Knockouts of receptors have been informative. Mice deficient in the receptor for IFN-γ are by and large similar in their EAE susceptibility to mice that lack IFN-γ. Other cytokine– or chemokine–receptor interactions are not so monogamous as those of IFN-γ. TNF acts through either of two receptors and knockout of these has dramatically different effects. Lack of TNFRI generates mice with reduced responsiveness to EAE, whereas susceptibility is enhanced by TNFRII deficiency (Eugster *et al.*, 1999). Similarly, many chemokines act through multiple receptors (Ransohoff *et al.*, 1996; Asensio and Campbell, 1999) so that knockouts of either receptors or chemokines have not necessarily recapitulated results expected from blockade of the primary ligand. Mice deficient in MIP-1α are susceptible to EAE, although anti-MIP-1α Mabs blocked disease (Karpus *et al.*, 1995; Tran *et al.*, 2000a). Similarly, CCR5-deficient mice are susceptible, but CCR2- or MCP-1-deficient mice are resistant (Tran *et al.*, 2000a; Fife *et al.*, 2000; Izikson *et al.*, 2000; Huang *et al.*, 2001). The logic that cytokine or chemokine action is as much regulated through receptor expression and action as at the level of production is compelling. Tissue-specific and conditional expression of receptors is likely to prove informative in the future.

A complementary approach to receptor knockout has been to target key signaling molecules that are coupled to receptor activation. Specific STAT (signal transducers and activators of transcription) molecules are critical for signaling through receptors for a variety of cytokines (Aaronson and Horvath, 2002). Mice that are null for STAT4 (which is critical for IL-12-mediated differentiation of CD4+ T cells into a Th1 phenotype) are resistant to induction of EAE (Chitnis *et al.*, 2001). In contrast, mice that lack STAT6 (which is involved in the IL-4-mediated differentiation of Th2 cells) develop more severe EAE (Chitnis *et al.*, 2001). These findings confirm the essential contribution of these STAT molecules to IL-12 and IL-4 function and further highlight the pivotal role of regulatory CD4 T cells in modulating EAE. The NF-κB family of transcription factors are highly activated at sites of inflammation and participate in receptor signaling mediated by a number of cytokines including TNF and IL-1. Mice lacking NF-κB1 are quite resistant to the development of EAE and show a profound impairment in CD4+ T-cell differentiation (Hilliard *et al.*, 1999). The dramatic results obtained by knockout of these different signal transduction molecules suggest they might serve as key targets for therapeutic intervention in neuroimmune disorders. Against this backdrop, however, it should be noted that knockout of STAT-1 (which mediates type I and type II IFN

receptor signaling) revealed unexpected and novel signaling pathways in an IFN-α transgenic mouse, so that the neurodegenerative/inflammatory phenotype induced by the transgene was actually exacerbated in mice lacking the signaling intermediate (Wang *et al.*, 2002b).

Antigen receptors

The myelin antigen specificity of EAE and evidence for restricted TCR Vβ usage and skewed CDR3 spectratypes in MS lesions make a compelling case that antigen-specific T cells are critical to induction of MS. As a logical test of this, transgenic mice have been generated that express TCRs which are specific for known encephalitogenic epitopes of myelin proteins. These use endogenous TCR promoters and are constructed by crossing individual transgenics expressing the relevant TCR-α and TCR-β genes. The majority of T cells in these animals express the potentially encephalitogenic specificity. Interestingly, such TCR transgenic mice have shown either low or no spontaneous incidence of encephalomyelitis (Goverman, 1999). Incidences of disease that arose independent of experimental manipulation have reflected either environmental stimuli or removal of endogenous regulatory elements (Goverman *et al.*, 1993; Lafaille *et al.*, 1997). The latter occurs in RAG-deficient transgenics (Lafaille *et al.*, 1997; Van de Keere and Tonegawa, 1998). Backcrossing such mice to RAG-deficient mice, which cannot recombine TCR or immunoglobulin genes and so lack T and B cells, ensures that the myelin-specific TCR becomes the animal's only specificity.

Another approach to the question of TCR specificity and induction of autoimmune inflammatory disease in the nervous system involves 'humanizing' mice. This approach involves expression of human MHC Class II molecules in mice (Taneja and David, 1999). These mice can then be crossed with transgenics that express TCRs which recognize antigenic peptides presented by the human MHC. In some cases further transgenes that encode human CD4, CD8, or co-stimulator molecules have been crossed in, to optimize interaction between T cells and human MHC-expressing antigen-presenting cells in the multitransgenic mouse (Altmann *et al.*, 1995; Madsen *et al.*, 1999). In one specific instance, mice were created that express the HLA-DRB5*0101/DRB1*1501 (HLA-DR2) haplotype which is associated with susceptibility to MS. These mice were crossed to transgenic mice that express human α/β TCRs with specificity for myelin basic protein peptides presented by HLA-DRB1*1501, and human CD4 (Madsen *et al.*, 1999). Only a small percentage of these transgenics developed spontaneous autoimmune disease, despite the fact that T cells could recognize and be activated by myelin peptide. When backcrossed to RAG-deficient mice, the incidence of spontaneous disease increased. The TCR in question crossreactively recognizes a peptide from Epstein–Barr virus, presented by a distinct MHC Class II haplotype (DRB5*0101) that is tightly linked to DRB1*1501 (Lang *et al.*, 2002). Such cross-reactivity is of interest as a potential inducing stimulus for MS. In a separate study, adoptive transfer of HLA-DR2-restricted PLP-specific mouse T cells into a mouse that expressed HLA-DRB1*1502 induced encephalitis (Kawamura *et al.*, 2000).

The complementary approach has been to generate immunoglobulin transgenics, using IgH/IgL transgenes that confer specificity for myelin. A knock-in transgenic mouse expressing anti-MOG antibodies showed no spontaneous autoimmunity, but developed exacerbated EAE when immunized, even with myelin antigens other than MOG (Litzenburger *et al.*, 1998). Interestingly, B cells in these mice underwent receptor editing, replacing kappa light chains with lambda (Litzenburger *et al.*, 2000). This phenomenon of light-chain editing potentially alters the antigen specificity of B cells during their development and is assumed to reflect censoring of autoimmune specificities. Editing of the MOG-specific Igκ light chain also occurred in MOG-deficient mice, suggesting that a cross-reactive determinant directed B-cell development.

Complement

Complement activation is linked to several effector processes in EAE and MS (see above). A number of complement pathway genes have been manipulated in transgenic and knockout models in an effort to pinpoint their function in EAE. Astrocyte-targeted production of a soluble broad-spectrum physiological complement inhibitor in transgenic mice attenuates EAE (Davoust *et al.*, 1999). Rats deficient for C6 cannot form the membrane attack complex, and despite comparable T-cell responses and CNS inflammation are resistant to EAE with markedly reduced demyelination and axonal damage (Tran *et al.*, 2002c; Mead *et al.*, 2002). In all these findings suggest an important role for complement activation in myelin injury and cytotoxicity towards oligodendrocytes and neurons. Other studies, however, have been less conclusive. In particular, mice null for C3, a key component of complement activation, were found to either have decreased (Nataf *et al.*, 2000) or no change (Calida *et al.*, 2001) in their EAE severity. Finally, a recent study in knockout mice that lacked the receptor for the potent complement anaphylatoxin C5a demonstrates that these animals are fully susceptible to EAE indicating that C5a is not involved (Reiman *et al.*, 2002).

Concluding remarks

The application of molecular biology to engineer novel animal models has greatly expanded our ability to study aspects of neurological disease. Emerging technologies of tissue-specific and conditional gene expression and ablation will soon allow us to model the dynamics of disease, not just the mechanics. Nevertheless, it remains the case that each model represents only one facet of clinical disease, or as has been suggested, each animal model reflects an individual patient. One must not lose sight of the fundamental issues underlying study of complex and elegant genetic models. Thus, choice of antigen, adjuvants, and background genetics remain critical determinants of the outcome of experimental systems. Design, creation, and interpretation of these animal models require an almost holistic understanding of immunology, neurobiology, and molecular biology, as well as animal and clinical science. Study of these animal models is therefore an exercise in integrative multidisciplinary research, which is justified by the intellectual payback and the advances in our understanding of neurological disease.

References

Aaronson, D.S. and Horvath, C.M. (2002). A road map for those who know JAK-STAT. *Science* 296: 1653–1655.

Akwa, Y., Hassett, D.E., Eloranta, M.L., *et al.* (1998). Transgenic expression of IFN-α in the central nervous system of mice protects against lethal neurotropic viral infection but induces inflammation and neurodegeneration. *J Immunol* 161: 5016–5026.

Altmann, D.M., Douek, D.C., Frater, A.J., Hetherington, C.M., Inoko, H., and Elliott, J.I. (1995). The T cell response of HLA-DR transgenic mice to human myelin basic protein and other antigens in the presence and absence of human CD4. *J Exp Med* 181: 867–875.

Antel, J.P. and Owens, T. (1999). Immune regulation and CNS autoimmune disease. *J Neuroimmunol* 100: 181–189.

Archelos, J.J., Maurer, M., Jung, S., *et al.* (1994). Inhibition of experimental autoimmune neuritis by an antibody to the lymphocyte function-associated antigen-1. *Lab Invest* 70: 667–675.

Archelos, J.J., Fortwangler, T., and Hartung, H..P (1997). Attenuation of experimental autoimmune neuritis in the Lewis rat by treatment with an antibody to L-selectin. *Neurosci Lett* 235: 9–12.

Arnason, B. (1999). TNF neutralization in MS: results of a randomized, placebo-controlled multicenter study. *Neurology* 53: 457–465.

Asensio, V.C. and Campbell, I.L. (1999). Chemokines in the CNS: plurifunctional mediators in diverse states. *Trends Neurosci* 22: 504–512.

Baron, J.L., Madri, J.A., Ruddle, N.H., Hashim, G., and Janeway, J.C.A. (1993). Surface expression of a4 integrin by CD4 T cells is required for their entry into brain parenchyma. *J Exp Med* 177: 57–68.

Becher, B., Durell, B.G., Miga, A.V., Hickey, W.F., and Noelle, R.J. (2001). The clinical course of experimental autoimmune encephalomyelitis and inflammation is controlled by the expression of CD40 within the central nervous system. *J Exp Med* 193: 967–974.

Becher, B., Durell, B.G., and Noelle, R.J. (2002). Experimental autoimmune encephalitis and inflammation in the absence of interleukin-12. *J Clin Invest* 110: 493–497.

Bell, M.D., Taub, D.D., Kunkel, S.J., *et al.* (1996). Recombinant human adenovirus with rat MIP-2 gene insertion causes prolonged PMN recruitment to the murine brain. *Eur J Neurosci* 8: 1803–1811.

Billiau, A., Heremans, H., Vandekerckhove, F., Dijkmans, R., Sobis, H., Meulepas, E., *et al.* (1988). Enhancement of experimental allergic encephalomyelitis in mice by antibodies against IFN-gamma. *J Immunol* 140: 1506–1510.

Birnbaum, G., Kotilinek, L., Schlievert, P., Clark, H.N., Trotter, J., Horvath, E., *et al.* (1996). Heat shock proteins and experimental autoimmune encephalomyelitis (EAE): I. Immunization with a peptide of the myelin protein 2′,3′ cyclic nucleotide 3′ phosphodiesterase that is cross-reactive with a heat shock protein alters the course of EAE. *J Neurosci Res* 44: 381–396.

Borges, E., Tietz, W., Steegmaier, M., Moll, T., Hallmann, R., Hamann, A., *et al.* (1997). P-selectin glycoprotein ligand-1 (PSGL-1) on T helper 1 but not on T helper 2 cells binds to P-selectin and supports migration into inflamed skin. *J Exp Med* 185: 573–578.

Boztug, K., Carson, M.J., Pham-Mitchell, N., Asensio, V.C., DeMartino, J.A., and Campbell, I.L. (2002). Leukocyte infiltration, but not neurodegeneration, in the CNS of transgenic mice with astrocyte production of the CXC chemokine ligand 10. *J Immunol* 169: 467–473.

Bronson, S.K., Plaehn, E.G., Kluckman, K.D., Hagaman, J.R., Maeda, N., and Smithies, O. (1996). Single-copy transgenic mice with chosen-site integration. *Proc Natl Acad Sci USA* 93: 9067–9072.

Buchmeier, M.J. and Lane, T.J. (1999). Viral-induced neurodegenerative disease. *Curr Opin Microbiol* 2: 398–402.

Bush, T.G., Savidge, T.C., Freeman, T.C., Cox, H.J., Campbell, E.A., Mucke, L., *et al.* (1998). Fulminant jejunoileitis following ablation of enteric glia in adult transgenic mice. *Cell* 93: 189–201.

Calida, D.M., Constantinescu, C., Purev, E., Zhang, G.X., Ventura, E.S., Lavi, E., *et al.* (2001). Cutting edge: C3, a key component of complement activation, is not required for the development of myelin oligodendrocyte glycoprotein peptide-induced experimental autoimmune encephalomyelitis in mice. *J Immunol* 166: 723–726.

Campbell, I.L., Abraham, C.R., Masliah, E., Kemper, P., Inglis, J.D., Oldstone, M.B.A., *et al.* (1993). Neurologic disease induced in transgenic mice by the cerebral overexpression of interleukin 6. *Proc Natl Acad Sci USA* 90: 10061–10065.

Capecchi, M. (1994). Targeted gene replacement. *Sci Am* 270: 52–59.

Chambers, C.A. and Allison, J.P. (1999). Costimulatory regulation of T cell function. *Curr Opin Cell Biol* 11: 203–210.

Chang, T.T., Jabs, C., Sobel, R.A., Kuchroo, V.K., and Sharpe, A.H. (1999). Studies in B7-deficient mice reveal a critical role for B7 costimulation in both induction and effector phases of experimental autoimmune encephalomyelitis. *J Exp Med* 190: 733–740.

Chen, B.P., Kuziel, W.A., and Lane, T.E. (2001). Lack of CCR2 results in increased mortality and impaired leukocyte activation and trafficking following infection of the central neurous system with a neurotropic coronavirus. *J Immunol* 167: 4585–4592.

Chen, S.-C., Leach, M.W., Chen, Y., Cai, X.-Y., Sullivan, L., Wiekowski, M., *et al.* (2002). Central nervous system inflammation and neurological disease in transgenic mice expressing the CC chemokine CCL21 in oligodendrocytes. *J Immunol* 168: 1009–1017.

Chiang, C.S., Powell, H.C., Gold, L.H., Samimi, A., and Campbell, I.L. (1996). Macrophage/microglial-mediated primary demyelination and motor disease induced by the central nervous system production of interleukin-3 in transgenic mice. *J Clin Invest* 97: 1512–1524.

Chitnis, T., Najafian, N., Benou, C., Salama, A.D., Grusby, M.J., Sayegh, M.H., *et al.* (2001). Effects of targeted disruption of STAT4 and STAT6 on the induction of experimental autoimmune encephalomyelitis. *J Clin Invest* 108: 739–747.

Corbin, J.G., Kelly, D., Rath, E.M., Baerwald, K.D., Suzuki, K., and Popko, B. (1996). Targeted CNS expression of interferon-γ in transgenic mice leads to hypomyelination, reactive gliosis, and abnormal cerebellar development. *Mol Cell Neurosci* 7: 354–370.

Costa, G.L., Sandora, M.R., Nakajima, A., Nguyen, E.V., Taylor-Edwards, C., Slavin, A.V., *et al.* (2001). Adoptive immunotherapy of experimental autoimmune encephalomyelitis vis T cell delivery of the IL-12 p40 subunit[1]. *J Immunol* 167: 2379–2387.

Cross, A.H., Manning, P.T., Stern, M.K., and Misko, T.P. (1997). Evidence for the production of peroxynitrite in inflammatory CNS demyelination. *J Neuroimmunol* 80: 121–130.

Croxford, J.L., Triantaphyllopoulos, K., Podhajcer, O.L., Feldmann, M., Baker, D., and Chernajovsky, Y. (1998). Cytokine gene therapy in experimental allergic encephalomyelitis by injection of plasmid DNA-cationic liposome complex into the central nervous system. *J Immunol* 160: 5181–5187.

Croxford, J.L., Feldmann, M., Chernajovsky, Y., and Baker, D. (2001). Different therapeutic outcomes in experimental allergic encephalomyelitis dependent upon the mode of delivery of IL-10: a comparison of the effects of protein, adenoviral or retroviral IL-10 delivery into the central nervous system. *J Immunol* 166: 4124–4130.

David, S., Bouchard, C., Tsatas, O., and Giftochristos, N. (1990). Macrophages can modify the nonpermissive nature of the adult mammalian central nervous system. *Neuron* 5: 463–469.

Davoust, N., Nataf, S., Reiman, R., Holers, M.V., Campbell, I.L., and Barnum, S.R. (1999). Central nervous system-targeted expression of the complement inhibitor sCRRY prevents experimental allergic encephalomyelitis. *J Immunol* 163: 6551–6556.

De Vos, A.F., Van Meurs, M., Brok, H.P., Boven, L.A., Hintzen, R.Q., Van Der Valk, P., *et al.* (2002). Transfer of central nervous system autoantigens and presentation in secondary lymphoid organs. *J Immunol* 169: 5415–5423.

Dittel, B.N., Visintin, I., Merchant, R.M., and Janeway, C.A. Jr (1999). Presentation of the self antigen myelin basic protein by dendritic cells leads to experimental autoimmune encephalomyelitis. *J Immunol* 163: 32–39.

Drescher, K.M., Pease, L.R., and Rodriguez, M. (1997). Antiviral immune responses modulate the nature of central nervous system (CNS) disease in a murine model of multiple sclerosis. *Immunol Rev* 159: 177–193.

Duong, T.T., St Louis, J., Gilbert, J.J., Finkelman, F.D., and Strejan, G.H. (1992). Effect of anti-interferon-gamma and anti-interleukin-2 monoclonal antibody treatment on the development of actively and passively induced experimental allergic encephalomyelitis in the SJL/J mouse. *J Neuroimmunol* 36: 105–115.

Enders, U., Lobb, R., Pepinsky, R.B., Hartung, H.P., Toyka, K.V., and Gold, R. (1998). The role of the very late antigen-4 and its counterligand vascular cell adhesion molecule-1 in the pathogenesis of experimental autoimmune neuritis of the Lewis rat. *Brain* 121: 1257–1266.

Engelhardt, B., Conley, F.K., and Butcher, E.C. (1994). Cell adhesion molecules on vessels during inflammation in the mouse central nervous system. *J Neuroimmunol* 51: 199–208.

Eugster, H.P., Frei, K., Kopf, M., Lassmann, H., and Fontana, A. (1998). IL-6-deficient mice resist myelin oligodendrocyte glycoprotein-induced autoimmune encephalomyelitis. *Eur J Immunol* 28: 2178–2187.

Eugster, H.-P., Frei, K., Bachmann, R., Bluethmann, H., Lassmann, H., and Fontana, A. (1999). Severity of symptoms and demyelination in MOG-induced EAE depends on TNFR1. *Eur J Immunol* 29: 626–632.

Falcone, M., Rajan, A.J., Bloom, B.R., and Brosnan, C.F. (1998). A critical role for IL-4 in regulating disease severity in experimental allergic encephalomyelitis as demonstrated in IL-4-deficient C57BL/6 mice and BALB/c mice. *J Immunol* 160: 4822–4830.

Feldmann, M. and Maini, R.N. (2001). Anti-TNF alpha therapy of rheumatoid arthritis: what have we learned? *Annu Rev Immunol* 19: 163–196.

Fenyk-Melody, J.E., Garrison, A.E., Brunnert, S.R., Weidner, J.R., Shen, F., Shelton, B.A., *et al.* (1998). Experimental autoimmune encephalomyelitis is exacerbated in mice lacking the *NOS2* gene. *J Immunol* 1998: 2940–2946.

Ferber, I.A., Brocke, S., Taylor-Edwards, C., Ridgway, W., Dinisco, C., Steinman, L., *et al.* (1996). Mice with a disrupted IFN-γ gene are susceptible to the induction of experimental autoimmune encephalomyelitis (EAE). *J Immunol* 156: 5–7.

Fife, B.T., Huffnagle, G.B., Kuziel, W.A., and Karpus, W.J. (2000). CC chemokine receptor 2 is critical for induction of experimental autoimmune encephalomyelitis. *J Exp Med* 192: 899–905.

Forss-Petter, S., Danielson, P.E., Catsicus, S., Battenberg, E., Price, J., Nerenberg, M., *et al.* (1990). Transgenic mice expressing beta-galactosidase in mature neurons under neuron-specific enolase promoter control. *Neuron* 5: 187–197.

Fuentes, M.E., Durham, S.K., Swerdel, M.R., Lewin, A.C., Barton, D.S., Megill, J.R., *et al.* (1995). Controlled recruitment of monocytes and macrophages to specific organs through transgenic expression of monocyte chemoattractant protein-1. *J Immunol* 155: 5769–5776.

Furlan, R., Brambilla, E., Ruffini, F., Poloano, P.L., Bergami, A., Marconi, P.C., *et al.* (2001). Intrathecal delivery of IFN-γ protects C57BL/6 mice from chronic-progressive experimental autoimmune encephalomyelitis by increasing apoptosis of central nervous system-infiltrating lymphocytes. *J Immunol* 167: 1821–1829.

Genain, C.P., Nguyen, M.H., Letvin, N.L., Pearl, R., Davis, R.L., Adelman, M., *et al.* (1995). Antibody facilitation of multiple sclerosis-like lesions in a non-human primate. *J Clin Invest* 96: 2966–2974.

Genain, C.P., Abel, K., Belmar, N., Villinger, F., Rosenberg, D.P., Linington, C., *et al.* (1996). Late complications of immune deviation therapy in a nonhuman primate. *Science* 274: 2054–2057.

Georgievska, B., Kirik, D., Rosenblad, C., Lundberg, C., and Bjorklund, A. (2002). Neuroprotection in the rat Parkinson model by intrastriatal GDNF gene transfer using a lentiviral vector. *Neuroreport* 13: 75–82.

Gilbert, R., Nalbantoglu, J., Howell, J.M., Davies, L., Flectcher, S., Amalfitano, A, *et al.* (2001). Dystrophin expression in muscle following gene transfer with a fully deleted ('gutted') adenovirus is markedly improved by trans-acting adenoviral gene products. *Hum Gene Ther* 12: 1741–1755.

Gold, R., Hartung, H.P., and Toyka, K.V. (2000). Animal models for auto-immune demyelinating disorders of the nervous system. *Mol Med Today* 6: 88–91.

Gossen, M. and Bujard, H. (1992). Tight control of gene expression in mammalian cells by tetracycline-responsive promoters. *Proc Natl Acad Sci USA* 89: 5547–5551.

Gossen, M., Freundlieb, S., Bender, G., Muller, G., Hillen, W., and Bujard, H. (1995). Transcriptional activation by tetracyclines in mammalian cells. *Science* 268: 1766–1769.

Goverman, .J (1999). Tolerance and autoimmunity in TCR transgenic mice specific for myelin basic protein. *Immunol Rev* 169: 147–159.

Goverman, J., Woods, A., Larson, L., Weiner, L.P., Hood, L., and Zaller, D.M. (1993). Transgenic mice that express a myelin basic protein-specific T cell receptor develop spontaneous autoimmunity. *Cell* 72: 551–560.

Gow, A., Friedrich, J.V.L., and Lazzarini, R.A. (1992). Myelin basic protein gene contains separate enhancers for oligodendrocyte and Schwann cell expression. *J Cell Biol* 119: 605–616.

Harris, A.W., Pinkert, C.A., Crawford, M., Landgdon, W.Y., Brinster, R.L., and Adams, J.M. (1988). The Emu-myc transgenic mouse. A model for high-incidence spontaneous lymphoma and leukemia of early B cells. *J Exp Med* 167: 353–371.

Hartung, H.P., van der Meche, F.G., and Pollard, J.D. (1998). Guillain–Barre syndrome, CIDP and other chronic immune-mediated neuropathies. *Curr Opin Neurol* 11: 497–513.

Hickey, W.F. and Kimura, H. (1988). Perivascular microglial cells of the CNS are bone marrow-derived and present antigen *in vivo*. *Science* 239: 290–292.

Hilliard, B., Samoilova, E.B., Liu, T.-S.T., Rostami, A., and Chen, Y. (1999). Experimental autoimmune encephalomyelitis in NK-κB-deficient mice: roles of NF-κB in the activation and differentiation of autoreactive T cells. *J Immunol* 163: 2937–2943.

Holz, A., Bielekova, B., Martin, R., and Oldstone, M.B. (2000). Myelin-associated oligodendrocytic basic protein: identification of an encephalitogenic epitope and association with multiple sclerosis. *J Immunol* 164: 1103–1109.

Horvai, A., Palinski, W., Wu, H., Moulton, K.S., Kalla, K., and Glass, C.K. (1995). Scavenger receptor A gene regulatory elements target gene expression to macrophages and foam cells of atherosclerotic lesions. *Proc Natl Acad Sci USA* 92: 5391–5395.

Hsich, G., Sena-Esteves, M., and Breakefield, X.O. (2002). Critical issues in gene therapy for neurologic disease. *Hum Gene Ther* 13: 579–604.

Huang, D.R., Wang, J., Kivisakk, P., Rollins, B.J., and Ransohoff, R.M. (2001). Absence of monocyte chemoattractant protein 1 in mice leads to decreased local macrophage recruitment and antigen-specific T helper cell type 1 immune response in experimental autoimmune encephalomyelitis. *J Exp Med* 193: 713–726.

Huang, D.W., McKerracher, L., Braun, P.E., and David, S. (1999). A therapeutic vaccine approach to stimulate axon regeneration in the adult mammalian spinal cord. *Neuron* **24**: 639–647.

Huseby, E.S. and Goverman, J. (2000). Tolerating the nervous system: a delicate balance. *J Exp Med* **191**: 757–760.

Huseby, E.S., Liggitt, D., Brabb, T., Schnabel, B., Ohlen, C., and Goverman, J. (2001). A pathogenic role for myelin-specific CD8(+) T cells in a model for multiple sclerosis. *J. Exp Med* **194**: 669–676.

Izikson, L., Klein, R.S., Charo, I.F., Weiner, H.L., and Luster, A.D. (2000). Resistance to experimental autoimmune encephalomyelitis in mice lacking the CC chemokine receptor (CCR)2. *J Exp Med* **192**: 1075–1080.

Jabs, C., McAdam, A.J., Greenfield, E.A., Freeman, G.J., Sharpe, A.H., and Kuchroo, V.K. (2001). The role of ICOS costimulatory pathway in the induction and regulation of EAE 9abstract0. *J Neuroimmunol* **118**: 77.

Jabs, C., Greve, B., Chang, T.T., Sobel, R.A., Sharpe, A.H., and Kuchroo, V.K. (2002). Genetic background determines the requirement for B7 costimulation in induction of autoimmunity. *Eur J Immunol* **32**: 2687–2697.

Janeway, C., Travers, P., Walport, M., and Capra, J. (1999) *Immunobiology: The Immune System in Health and Disease*. Garland, New York.

Johnson, A.J., Njenga, M.K., Hansen, M.J., Kuhns, S.T., Chen, L., Rodriguez, M., et al. (1999). Prevalent class I-restricted T-cell response to the Theiler's virus epitope Db:VP2121–130 in the absence of endogenous CD4 help, tumor necrosis factor alpha, gamma interferon, perforin, or costimulation through CD28. *J Virol* **73**: 3702–3708.

Karpus, W.J., Lukacs, N.W., McRae, B.L., Strieter, R.M., Kunkel, S.L., and Miller, S.D. (1995). An important role for the chemokine macrophage inflammatory protein-1α in the pathogenesis of the T cell-mediated autoimmune disease, experimental autoimmune encephalomyelitis. *J Immunol* **155**: 5003–5010.

Kassiotis, G. and Kollias, G. (2001). TNF and receptors in organ-specific autoimmune disease: multi-layered functioning mirrored in animal models. *J Clin Invest* **107**: 1507–1508.

Katz-Levy, Y., Neville, K.L., Girvin, A.M., Vanderlugt, C.L., Pope, J.G., Tan, L.J., et al. (1999). Endogenous presentation of self myelin epitopes by CNS-resident APCs in Theiler's virus-infected mice. *J Clin Invest* **104**: 599–610.

Katz-Levy, Y., Neville, K.L., Padilla, J., Rahbe, S., Begolka, W.S., Girvin, A.M., et al. (2000). Temporal development of autoreactive Th1 responses and endogenous presentation of self myelin epitopes by central nervous system-resident APCs in Theiler's virus-infected mice. *J Immunol* **165**: 5304–5314.

Kawamura, K., Yamamura, T., Yokoyama, K., Chui, D.H., Fukui, Y., Sasazuki, T., et al. (2000). Hla-DR2-restricted responses to proteolipid protein 95–116 peptide cause autoimmune encephalitis in transgenic mice. *J Clin Invest* **105**: 977–984.

Kaye, J.F., Kerlero de Rosbo, N., Mendel, I., Flechter, S., Hoffman, M., Yust, I., et al. (2000). The central nervous system-specific myelin oligodendrocytic basic protein (MOBP) is encephalitogenic and a potential target antigen in multiple sclerosis (MS). *J Neuroimmunol* **102**: 189–198.

Kennedy, M.K., Torrance, D.S., Picha, K.S., and Mohler, K.M. (1992). Analysis of cytokine mRNA expression in the central nervous system of mice with experimental autoimmune encephalomyelitis reveals that IL-10 mRNA expression correlates with recovery. *J Immunol* **149**: 2496–2505.

Kerschensteiner, M., Gallmeier, E., Behrens, L., Leal, V.V., Misgeld, T., Klinkert, W.E., et al. (1999). Activated human T cells, B cells, and monocytes produce brain-derived neurotrophic factor in vitro and in inflammatory brain lesions: a neuroprotective role of inflammation? *J Exp Med* **189**: 865–870.

Khoury, S.J., Hancock, W.W., and Weiner, H.L. (1992). Oral tolerance to myelin basic protein and natural recovery from experimental autoimmune encephalomyelitis are associated with downregulation of inflammatory cytokines and differential upregulation of transforming growth factor beta, interleukin 4, and prostaglandin E expression in the brain. *J Exp Med* **176**: 1355–1364.

Kiefer, R., Dangond, F., Mueller, M., Toyka, K.V., Hafler, D.A., and Hartung, H.P. (2000). Enhanced B7 costimulatory molecule expression in inflammatory human sural nerve biopsies. *J Neurol Neurosurg Psychiatryiat* **69**: 362–368.

Kiefer, R., Kieseier, B.C., Stoll, G., and Hartung, H.P. (2001). The role of macrophages in immune-mediated damage to the peripheral nervous system. *Prog Neurobiol* **64**: 109–127.

Klein, L., Klugmann, M., Nave, K.A., and Kyewski, B. (2000). Shaping of the autoreactive T-cell repertoire by a splice variant of self protein expressed in thymic epithelial cells [see comments]. *Nat Med* **6**: 56–61.

Kojima, K., Berger, T., Lassmann, H., Hinze-Selch, D., Zhang, Y., Gehrmann, J., et al. (1994). Experimental autoimmune panencephalitis and uveoretinitis transferred to the Lewis rat by T lymphocytes specific for the S100 beta molecule, a calcium binding protein of astroglia. *J Exp Med* **180**: 817–829.

Korner, H., Riminton, D.S., Strickland, D.H., Lemckert, F.A., Pollard, J.D., and Sedgwick, J.D. (1997). Critical points of tumor necrosis factor action in central nervous system autoimmune inflammation defined by gene targeting. *J Exp Med* **186**: 1585–1590.

Krakowski, M. and Owens, T. (1996). Interferon-gamma confers resistance to experimental allergic encephalomyelitis. *Eur J Immunol* **26**: 1641–1646.

Lafaille, J.J., Keere, F.V., Hsu, A.L., Baron, J.L., Haas, W., Raine, C.S., et al. (1997). Myelin basic protein-specific T helper 2 (Th2) cells cause experimental autoimmune encephalomyelitis in immunodeficient hosts rather than protect them from the disease. *J Exp Med* **186**: 307–312.

LaFerla, F.M., Sugarman, M.C., Lane, T.E., and Leissring, M.A. (2000). Regional hypomyelination and dysplasia in transgenic mice with astrocyte-targeted expression of interferon-γ. *J Mol Neurosci* **15**: 45–59.

Lai, Z. and Brady, R.O. (2002). Gene transfer into the central nervous system in vivo using a recombinant lentivirus vector. *J Neurosci Res* **67**: 363–371.

Lane, T.E., Liu, M.T.C., Chen, B.P.C., et al. (2000). A central role for CD4+ T-cells and RANTES in virus-induced central nervous system inflammation and demyelination. *J Virol* **74**: 1415–1424.

Lang, H.L., Jacobsen, H., Ikemizu, S., Andersson, C., Harlos, K., Madsen, L., et al. (2002). A functional and structural basis for TCR cross-reactivity in multiple sclerosis. *Nat Immunol* **3**: 940–943.

Li, H., Lochmuller, H., Yong, V.W., Karpati, G., and Nalbantoglu, J. (1997). Adenovirus-mediated wild-type p53 gene transfer and overexpression induces apoptosis of human glioma cells independent of endogenous p53 status. *J Neuropathol Exp Neurol* **56**: 872–878.

Linington, C., Berger, T., Perry, L., Weerth, S., Hinze-Selch, D., Zhang, Y., et al. (1993). T cells specific for the myelin oligodendrocyte glycoprotein mediate an unusual autoimmune inflammatory response in the central nervous system. *Eur J Immunol* **23**: 1364–1372.

Litzenburger, T., Fassler, R., Bauer, J., Lassmann, H., Linington, C., Wekerle, H., et al. (1998). B lymphocytes producing demyelinating autoantibodies: development and function in gene-targeted transgenic mice. *J Exp Med* **188**: 169–180.

Litzenburger, T., Bluthmann, H., Morales, P., Pham-Dinh, D., Dautigny, A., Wekerle, H., et al. (2000). Development of myelin oligodendrocyte glycoprotein autoreactive transgenic B lymphocytes: receptor editing in vivo after encounter of a self-antigen distinct from myelin oligodendrocyte glycoprotein. *J Immunol* **165**: 5360–5366.

Lyons, J.A., Ramsbottom, M.J., and Cross, A.H. (2002). Critical role of antigen-specific antibody in experimental autoimmune encephalomyelitis induced by recombinant myelin oligodendrocyte glycoprotein. *Eur J Immunol* **32**: 1905–1913.

Maatta, J.A., Kaldman, M.S., Sakoda, S., Salmi, A.A., and Hinkkanen, A.E. (1998). Encephalitogenicity of myelin-associated oligodendrocytic basic protein and 2',3'-cyclic nucleotide 3'-phosphodiesterase for BALB/c and SJL mice. *Immunology* **95**: 383–388.

Madsen, L.S., Andersson, E.C., Jansson, L., Krogsgaard, M., Andersen, C.B., Engberg, J., et al. (1999). A humanized model for multiple sclerosis using HLA-DR2 and a human T- cell receptor. *Nat Genet* **23**: 343–347.

Mak, T.W., Penninger, J.M., and Ohashi, P.S. (2001). Knockout mice: a paradigm shift in modern immunology. *Nat Rev Immunol* **1**: 11–19.

Martin, R., McFarland, H.F., and McFarlin, D.E. (1992). Immunological aspects of demyelinating diseases. *Annu Rev Immunol* **10**: 153–187.

Martino, G., Furlan, R., Comi, G., and Adorini, L. (2001). The ependymal route to the CNS: an emerging gene-therapy approach for MS. *Trends Immunol* **22**: 483–490.

Mathisen, P.M. and Tuohy, V.K. (2000). Gene therapy in experimental autoimmune encephalomyelitis. *J Clin Immunol* **20**: 327–333.

Mathisen, P.M., Yu, M., Johnson, J.M., Drazba, J.A., and Tuohy, V.K. (1997). Treatment of experimental autoimmune encephalomyelitis with genetically modified memory T cells. *J Exp Med* **186**: 159–164.

Mathisen, P.M., Yu, M., Yin, L., *et al.* (1999). Th2 T cells expressing transgene PDGF-A serve as vectors for gene therapy in autoimmune demyelinating disease. *J Autoimmun* 13: 31–38.

Mazarakis, N.D., Azzouz, M., Rohll, J.B., Ellard, F.M., Wilkes, F.J., Olsen, A.L., *et al.* (2001). Rabies virus glycoprotein pseudotyping of lentiviral vectors enables retrograde axonal transport and access to the nervous system after peripheral delivery. *Hum Mol Genet* 10: 2109–2121.

Mead, R.J., Singhrao, S.K., Neal, J.W., Lassmann, H., and Morgan, B.P. (2002). The membrane attack complex of complement causes severe demyelination associated with acute axonal injury. *J Immunol* 168: 458–465.

Merrill, J.E. and Benveniste, E.N. (1996). Cytokines in inflammatory brain lesions: helpful and harmful. *Trends Neurosci* 19: 331–338.

Miller, D.W. (1999). Immunobiology of the blood-brain barrier. *J Neurovirol* 5: 570–578.

Miller, S.D., McRae, B.L., Vanderlugt, C.L., Nikcevich, K.M., Pope, J.G., Pope, L., *et al.* (1995). Evolution of the T-cell repertoire during the course of experimental immune-mediated demyelinating diseases. *Immunol Rev* 144: 225–244.

Morris-Downes, M.M., McCormack, K., Baker, D., Sivaprasad, D., Natkunarajah, J., and Amor, S. (2002). Encephalitogenic and immunogenic potential of myelin-associated glycoprotein (MAG), oligodendrocyte-specific glycoprotein (OSP) and 2′,3′-cyclic nucleotide 3′-phosphodiesterase (CNPase) in ABH and SJL mice. *J Neuroimmunol* 122: 20–33.

Mucke, L., Oldstone, M.B.A., Morris, J.C., and Nerenberg, M.I. (1991). Rapid activation of astrocyte-specific expression of GFAP-lacZ transgene by focal injury. *New Biol* 3: 465–474.

Muller, U., Cristina, N., Li, Z.-W., Wolfer, D.P., Lipp, H.-P., Rulicke, T., *et al.* (1994). Behavioral and anatomical deficits in mice homozygous for a modified β-amyloid precursor protein gene. *Cell* 79: 755–765.

Murphy, C.A., Hoek, R.M., Wiekowski, M.T., Lira, S.A., and Sedgwick, J.D. (2002). Interactions between hemopoietically derived TNF and central nervous system-resident glial chemokines underlie initiation of autoimmune inflammation in the brain. *J Immunol* 169: 7054–7062.

Murphy, D. and Carter, D.A. (eds) (1993). *Transgenesis Techniques: Principles and Protocols.* Humana Press, Totowa, NJ.

Nagelkerken, L., Blauw, B., and Tielemans, M. (1997). IL-4 abrogates the inhibitory effect of IL-10 on the development of experimental allergic encephalomyelitis in SJL mice. *Int Immunol* 9: 1243–1251. (Published erratum in *Int Immunol* 9: 1773.)

Nataf, S., Carroll, S.L., Wetsel, R.A., Szalai, A.J., and Barnum, S.R. (2000). Attenuation of experimental autoimmune demyelination in complement-deficient mice. *J Immunol* 165: 5867–5873.

Neumann, H., Medana, I.M., Bauer, J., and Lassmann, H. (2002). Cytotoxic T lymphocytes in autoimmune and degenerative CNS diseases. *Trends Neurosci* 25: 313–319.

Njenga, M.K., Pavelko, K.D., Baisch, J., Lin, X., David, C., Leibowitz, J., *et al.* (1996). Theiler's virus persistence and demyelination in major histocompatibility complex class II-deficient mice. *J Virol* 70: 1729–1737.

Oliver, A.R., Lyon, G.M. and Ruddle, N.H. (2003). Rat and human myelin oligodendrocyte glycoproteins induce experimental autoimmune encephalomyelitis by different mechanisms in C57BL/6 mice. *J Immunol* 171: 462–468.

Owens, T. and Sriram, S. (1995). The immunology of multiple sclerosis and its animal model, experimental allergic encephalomyelitis. *Neurol Clin* 13: 51–73.

Owens, T., Tran, E., Hassan-Zahraee, M., and Krakowski, M. (1998). Immune cell entry to the CNS–a focus for immunoregulation of EAE. *Res Immunol* 149: 781–9 (discussion 844–6, 55–60).

Owens, T., Wekerle, H., and Antel, J. (2001). Genetic models for CNS inflammation. *Nat Med* 7: 161–166.

Owens, T., Murphy, T., and Minton, K. (2002). VIth International Congress of Neuroimmunology. Edinburgh, Scotland, September 3–7, 2001. *J Neuroimmunol* 124: 4–8.

Pagenstecher, A., Lassmann, S., Carson, M.J., Kincaid, C.L., Stalder, A.K., and Campbell, I.L. (2000). Astrocyte-targeted expression of IL-12 induces active cellular immune responses in the central nervous system and modulates experimental allergic encephalomyelitis. *J Immunol* 164: 4481–4492.

Pinkert, C.A. (ed.) (1994). *Transgenic Animal Technology.*, Academic Press, San Diego, CA.

Pitt, D., Werner, P., and Raine, C.S. (2000). Glutamate excitotoxicity in a model of multiple sclerosis. *Nat Med* 6: 67–70.

Poliani, P.L., Brok, H., Furlan, R., Ruffini, F., Bergami, A., Desina, G., *et al.* (2001). Delivery to the central nervous system of a nonreplicative herpes simplex type 1 vector engineered with the interleukin 4 gene protects rhesus monkeys from hyperacute autoimmune encephalomyelitis. *Hum Gene Ther* 12: 905–920.

Prat, A., Biernacki, K., Wosik, K., and Antel, J.P. (2001). Glial cell influence on the human blood-brain barrier. *Glia* 36: 145–155.

Previtali, S.C., Archelos, J.J., and Hartung, H.P. (1998). Expression of integrins in experimental autoimmune neuritis and Guillain–Barre syndrome. *Ann Neurol* 44: 611–621.

Probert, L., Akassoglou, K., Pasparakis, M., Kontogeorgos, G., and Kollias, G. (1995). Spontaneous inflammatory demyelinating disease in transgenic mice showing central nervous system-specific expression of tumor necrosis factor α. *Proc Natl Acad Sci USA* 92: 11294–11298.

Ransohoff, R.M., Glabinski, A., and Tani, M. (1996). Chemokines in immune-mediated inflammation of the central nervous system. *Cytokine Growth Factor Rev* 7: 35–46.

Ray, P., Tang, W., Wang, P., Homer, R., Kuhn III, C., Flavell, R.A., *et al.* (1997). Regulated overexpression of interleukin 11 in the lung. *J Clin Invest* 100: 2501–2511.

Reiman, R., Gerard, C., Campbell, I.L., and Barnum, S.R. (2002). Disruption of the C5a receptor gene fails to protect against experimental allergic encephalomyelitis. *Eur J Immunol* 32: 1157–1163.

Renno, T., Krakowski, M., Piccirillo, C., Lin, J.-Y., and Owens, T. (1995). TNF-α expression by resident microglia and infiltrating leukocytes in the central nervous system of mice with experimental allergic encephalomyelitis. *J Immunol* 154: 944–953.

Renno, T., Taupin, V., Bourbonniere, L., Verge, G., Tran, E., De Simone, R., *et al.* (1998). Interferon-γ in progression to chronic demyelination and neurological deficit following acute EAE. *Mol Cell Neurosci* 12: 376–389.

Rivera-Quinones, C., McGavern, D., Schmelzer, J.D., Hunter, S.F., Low, P.A., and Rodriguez, M. (1998). Absence of neurological deficits following extensive demyelination in a class I-deficient murine model of multiple sclerosis. *Nat Med* 4: 187–193.

Rodriguez, M., Miller, D.J., and Lennon, V.A. (1996). Immunoglobulins reactive with myelin basic protein promote CNS remyelination. *Neurology* 46: 538–545.

Rottman, J.B., Slavin, A.J., Silva, R., Weiner, H.L., Gerard, C.G., and Hancock, W.W. (2000). Leukocyte recruitment during onset of experimental allergic encephalomyelitis is CCR1 dependent. *Eur J Immunol* 30: 2372–2377.

Ruijs, T.C., Louste, K., Brown, E.A., and Antel, J.P. (1993). Lysis of human glial cells by major histocompatibility complex- unrestricted CD4+ cytotoxic lymphocytes. *J Neuroimmunol* 42: 105–111.

Ruuls, S.R., Hoek, R.M., Ngo, V.N., McNeil, T., Lucian, L.A., Janatpour, M.J., *et al.* (2001). Membrane-bound TNF supports secondary lymphoid organ structure but is subservient to secreted TNF in driving autoimmune inflammation. *Immunity* 15: 533–543.

Ryding, A.D.S., Sharp, M.G.F., and Mullins, J.J. (2001). Conditional transgenic technologies. *J Endocrinol* 171: 1–14.

Sahrbacher, U.C., Lechner, F., Eugster, H.P., Frei, K., Lassmann, H., and Fontana, A. (1998). Mice with an inactivation of the inducible nitric oxide synthase gene are susceptible to experimental autoimmune encephalomyelitis. *Eur J Immunol* 28: 1332–1338.

Samoilova, E.B., Horton, J.L., and Chen, Y. (1998). Acceleration of experimental autoimmune encephalomyelitis in interleukin-10-deficient mice: roles of interleukin-10 in disease progression and recovery. *Cell Immunol* 188: 118–124.

Schwartz, M. and Moalem, G. (2001). Beneficial immune activity after CNS injury: prospects for vaccination. *J Neuroimmunol* 113: 185–192.

Schwartz, M., Moalem, G., Leibowitz-Amit, R., and Cohen, I.R. (1999). Innate and adaptive immune responses can be beneficial for CNS repair. *Trends Neurosci* 22: 295–299.

Segal, B.M., Dwyer, B.K., and Shevach, E.M. (1998). An interleukin (IL)-10/IL-12 immunoregulatory circuit controls susceptibility to autoimmune disease. *J Exp Med* 187: 537–546.

Serafini, B., Columba-Cabezas, S., Di Rosa, F., and Aloisi, F. (2000). Intracerebral recruitment and maturation of dendritic cells in the onset and progression of experimental autoimmune encephalomyelitis. *Am J Pathol* **157**: 1991–2002.

Sethna, M.P. and Lampson, L.A. (1991). Immune modulation within the brain: recruitment of inflammatory cells and increased major histocompatibility antigen expression following intracerebral injection of interferon-γ. *J Neuroimmunol* **34**: 121–132.

Sicotte, N.L. and Voskuhl, R.R. (2001). Onset of multiple sclerosis associated with anti-TNF therapy. *Neurology* **57**: 1885–1888.

Simmons, R.D. and Willenborg, D.O. (1990). Direct injection of cytokines into the spinal cord causes autoimmune encephalomyelitis-like inflammation. *J Neurol Sci* **100**: 37–42.

Slavin, A., Ewing, C., Liu, J., Ichikawa, M., Slavin, J., and Bernard, C.C. (1998). Induction of a multiple sclerosis-like disease in mice with an immunodominant epitope of myelin oligodendrocyte glycoprotein. *Autoimmunity* **28**: 109–120.

Smith, T., Groom, A., Zhu, B., and Turski, L. (2000). Autoimmune encephalomyelitis ameliorated by AMPA antagonists. *Nat Med* **6**: 62–66.

Smith, T.W., DeGirolami, U., and Hickey, W.F. (1992). Neuropathology of immunosuppression. *Brain Pathol* **2**: 183–194.

Sobel, R.A., Tuohy, V.K., Lu, Z.J., Laursen, R.A., and Lees, M.B. (1990). Acute experimental allergic encephalomyelitis in SJL/J mice induced by a synthetic peptide of myelin proteolipid protein. *J Neuropathol Exp Neurol* **49**: 468–479.

Sriram, S. and Rodriguez, M. (1997). Indictment of the microglia as the villain in multiple sclerosis. *Neurology* **48**: 464–470.

Stalder, A.K., Carson, M.J., Pagenstecher, A., Asensio, V.C., Kincaid, C., Benedict, M., *et al.* (1998). Late-onset chronic inflammatory encephalopathy in immune-competent and severe combined immune-deficient (SCID) mice with astrocyte-targeted expression of tumor necrosis factor. *Am J Pathol* **153**: 767–783.

Steinman, L. (1997). Some misconceptions about understanding autoimmunity through experiments with knockouts. *J Exp Med* **185**: 2039–2041.

Sun, D., Whitaker, J.N., Huang, Z., Liu, D., Coleclough, C., Wekerle, H., *et al.* (2001). Myelin antigen-specific CD8+ T cells are encephalitogenic and produce severe disease in C57BL/6 mice. *J Immunol* **166**: 7579–7587.

Talbot, P.J., Arnold, D., and Antel, J.P. (2001). Virus-induced autoimmune reactions in the CNS. *Curr Top Microbiol Immunol* **253**: 247–271.

Taneja, V. and David, C.S. (1999). HLA class II transgenic mice as models of human diseases. *Immunol Rev* **169**: 67–79.

Tani, M., Fuentes, M.E., Peterson, J.W., Trapp, B.D., Durham, S.K., Loy, J.K., *et al.* (1996). Neutrophil infiltration, glial reaction, and neurological disease in transgenic mice expressing the chemokine N51/KC in oligodendrocytes. *J Clin Invest* **98**: 529–539.

Taupin, V., Renno, T., Bourbonniere, L., Peterson, A.C., Rodriguez, M., and Owens, T. (1997). Increased severity of experimental autoimmune encephalomyelitis, chronic macrophage/microglial reactivity, demyelination in transgenic mice producing tumor necrosis factor-α in the central nervous system. *Eur J Immunol* **27**: 905–913.

Thomas, C.E., Schiedner, G., Kochanek, S., Castro, M.G., and Lowenstein, P.R. (2000). Peripheral infection with adenovirus causes unexpected long-term brain inflammation in animals injected intracranially with first-generation, but not with high-capacity, adenovirus vectors: toward realistic long-term neurological gene therapy for chronic diseases. *Proc Natl Acad Sci USA* **97**: 7482–7487.

Tran, E.H., Kuziel, W.A., and Owens, T. (2000a). Induction of experimental autoimmune encephalomyelitis in C57BL/6 mice deficient in either the chemokine macrophage inflammatory protein-1α or its CCR5 receptor. *Eur J Immunol* **30**: 1410–1415.

Tran, E.H., Prince, E.N., and Owens, T. (2000b). IFN-gamma shapes immune invasion of the central nervous system via regulation of chemokines. *J Immunol* **164**: 2759–2768.

Tran, G.T., Hodgkinson, S.J., Carter, N., Killingsworth, M., Spicer, S.T., and Hall, B.M. (2002c). Attenuation of experimental allergic encephalomyelitis in complement component 6-deficient rats associated with reduced complement C9 deposition, P-selectin expression, and cellular infiltrate in spinal cords. *J Immunol* **168**: 4293–4300.

Tremblay, P., Meiner, Z., Gaou, M., Heinrich, C., Petromilli, C., Lisse, T., *et al.* (1998). Doxycycline control of prion protein transgene expression modulates prion disease in mice. *Proc Natl Acad Sci USA* **95**: 12580–12585.

Tsunoda, I., Kuang, L.Q., Theil, D.J., and Fujinami, R.S. (2000). Antibody association with a novel model for primary progressive multiple sclerosis: induction of relapsing-remitting and progressive forms of EAE in H2s mouse strains. *Brain Pathol* **10**: 402–418.

Tuohy, V.K., Lu, Z., Sobel, R.A., Laursen, R.A., and Lees, M.B. (1989). Identification of an encephalitogenic determinant of myelin proteolipid protein for SJL mice. *J Immunol* **142**: 1523–1527.

Turnley, A.M., Morahan, G., Okano, H., Bernard, O., Mikoshiba, K., Allison, J., *et al.* (1991). Dysmyelination in transgenic mice resulting from expression of class I histocompatibility molecules in oligodendrocytes. *Nature* **353**: 566–569.

Urlinger, S., Baron, U., Thellmann, M., Hasan, M.T., Bujard, H., and Hillen, W. (2000). Exploring the sequence space for tetracycline-dependent transcriptional activators: novel mutations yield expanded range and sensitivity. *Proc Natl Acad Sci USA* **97**: 7963–7968.

Van de Keere, F. and Tonegawa, S. (1998). CD4(+) T cells prevent spontaneous experimental autoimmune encephalomyelitis in anti-myelin basic protein T cell receptor transgenic mice. *J Exp Med* **188**: 1875–1882.

Vergelli, M., Hemmer, B., Muraro, P.A., Tranquill, L., Biddison, W.E., Sarin, A., *et al.* (1997). Human autoreactive CD4+ T cell clones use perforin- or Fas/Fas ligand- mediated pathways for target cell lysis. *J Immunol* **158**: 2756–2761.

Voorthuis, J.A., Uitdehaag, B.M., De Groot, C.J., Goede, P.H., van der Meide, P.H., and Dijkstra, C.D. (1990). Suppression of experimental allergic encephalomyelitis by intraventricular administration of interferon-gamma in Lewis rats. *Clin Exp Immunol* **81**: 183–188.

Wang, J., Asensio, V.C., and Campbell, I.L. (2002a). Cytokines and chemokines as mediators of protection and injury in the central nervous system assessed in transgenic mice. *Curr Top Microbiol Immunol* **265**: 23–48.

Wang, J., Schreiber, R.D., and Campbell, I.L. (2002b). STAT1 deficiency unexpectedly and markedly exacerbates the pathophysiological actions of IFN-α in the central nervous system. *Proc Natl Acad Sci USA* **99**: 16209–16214.

Weerth, S., Berger, T., Lassmann, H., and Linington, C. (1999). Encephalitogenic and neuritogenic T cell responses to the myelin- associated glycoprotein (MAG) in the Lewis rat. *J Neuroimmunol* **95**: 157–164.

Wildin, R.S., Garvin, A.M., Pawar, S., Lewis, D.B., Abraham, K.M., Forbush, K.A. *et al.* (1991). Developmental regulation of lck gene expression in T-lymphocytes. *J Exp Med* **173**: 383–393.

Willenborg, D.O., Fordham, S., Bernard, C.A., Cowden, W.B., and Ramshaw, I.A. (1996). IFN-γ plays a critical down-regulatory role in the induction and effector phase of myelin oligodendrocyte glycoprotein-induced autoimmune encephalomyelitis. *J Immunol* **157**: 3223–3227.

Willenborg, D.O., Fordham, S.A., Staykova, M.A., Ramshaw, I.A., and Cowden, W.B. (1999a). IFN-γ is critical to the control of murine autoimmune encephalomyelitis and regulates both in the periphery and in the target tissue: a possible role for nitric oxide. *J Immunol* **163**: 5278–5286.

Willenborg, D.O., Staykova, M.A., and Cowden, W.B. (1999b). Our shifting understanding of the role of nitric oxide in autoimmune encephalomyelitis: a review. *J Neuroimmunol* **100**: 21–35.

Yamamoto, A., Hen, R., and Dauer, W.T. (2001). The ons and offs of inducible transgenic technology: a review. *Neurobiol Dis* **8**: 923–932.

Yoles, E., Hauben, E., Palgi, O., Agranov, E., Gothilf, A., Cohen, A., *et al.* (2001). Protective autoimmunity is a physiological response to CNS trauma. *J Neurosci* **21**: 3740–3748.

Yong, V.W., Krekowski, C.A., Forsyth, P.A., Bell, R., and Edwards, D.R. (1998). Matrix metalloproteinases and diseases of the CNS. *Trends Neurosci* **21**: 75–80.

Yong, V.W., Power, C., Forsyth, P., and Edwards, D.R. (2001). Metalloproteinases in biology and pathology of the nervous system. *Nat Rev Neurosci* **2**: 502–511.

Yoshida, K., Taga, T., Saito, M., Suematsu, S., Kumanogoh, A., Tanaka, T., *et al.* (1996). Targeted disruption of gp 130, a common signal transducer for the interleukin 6 family of cytokines, leads to myocardial and hematological disorders. *Proc Natl Acad Sci USA* **93**: 407–411.

Yrjanheikki, J., Keinanen, R., Pellikka, M., Hokfelt, T., and Koistinaho, J. (1998). Tetracyclines inhibit microglial activation and are neuroprotective in global brain ischemia. *Proc Natl Acad Sci USA* **95**: 15769–15774.

Zehntner, S.P., Briseboise, M., Tran, E., Owens, T., and Fournier, S. (2003). Constitutive expression of a costimulatory ligand on antigen-presenting cells in the nervous system drives demyelinating disease. *Faseb J* **17**: 1910–1912.

Zou, L., Yotnda, P., Zhao, T., Yuan, X., Long, Y., Zhou, H., *et al.* (2002). Reduced inflammatory reactions to the inoculation of helper-dependent adenoviral vectors in traumatically injured rat brain. *J Cereb Blood Flow Metab* **22**: 959–970.

Zou, L.P., Ljunggren, H.G., Levi, M., Nennesmo, I., Wahren, B., Mix, E., *et al.* (2000). P0 protein peptide 180–199 together with pertussis toxin induces experimental autoimmune neuritis in resistant C57BL/6 mice. *J Neurosci Res* **62**: 717–721.

13 Acute disseminated encephalomyelitis

Alex Tselis and Robert P. Lisak

Introduction

Acute disseminated encephalomyelitis (ADEM) is a generally monophasic inflammatory disease of the white matter of the central nervous system (CNS) (Cohen and Lisak, 1987; Johnson and Griffin, 1987; Lisak, 1994; Tselis and Lisak, 1995). The relation of ADEM to multiple sclerosis (MS), another inflammatory disease of the CNS white matter, is an important issue and is discussed later in the chapter.

It has long been noted that following recovery from a viral infection, a few patients develop an acute or subacute neurologic disease. The original virus probably does not cause this neurologic disease because (1) no virus has been *consistently* isolated from the brains of fatal cases or from cerebrospinal fluid (CSF) samples of non-fatal cases; (2) the pathology of ADEM in fatal cases is different from that of an acute viral encephalitis; and (3) the same clinical and pathologic disease occurs consequent to other circumstances that do not involve infection, such as vaccination with non-viable organisms.

Post-infectious encephalomyelitis was first reported in 1790. It occurred in a 23-year-old woman who had lower extremity weakness and urinary retention about a week after a measles rash, and who had a similar syndrome 10 years earlier after a bout of smallpox (Croft, 1969; Johnson and Griffin, 1987). The prototypical post-infectious encephalomyelitis follows measles. This once was the most common precipitant of ADEM because of the high incidence of measles in the population. No virus could be isolated from, or detected by immunostaining in, the brains of patients with 'measles encephalomyelitis' (Gendelman et al., 1984), as the measles-associated ADEM was called in the literature. (In the older literature, the nomenclature was confusing, in that a febrile encephalopathy associated with or following a particular viral illness was labeled with that illness, thus measles encephalomyelitis, varicella encephalomyelitis, rubella encephalomyelitis, and so forth, so that a direct viral infection of the brain and a post-infectious encephalomyelitis were given the same name.)

It soon became apparent that a clinically and pathologically similar illness occasionally followed vaccination with killed or attenuated microorganisms, usually (but not necessarily) viruses (Fenichel, 1982). In particular, post-vaccination encephalomyelitis frequently followed smallpox (Spillane and Wells, 1964) and rabies vaccination (which was first noted by Pasteur himself) (Applebaum et al., 1953). The post-rabies vaccination encephalomyelitis is also known in the older literature as a *neuroparalytic accident*, a term that broadly encompassed any neurologic complication of rabies vaccination, including acute inflammatory demyelinating polyneuropathy. Indeed neuroparalytic accidents secondary to immunization with vaccine containing nervous system tissue are, in retrospect, the first instances of experimental allergic encephalomyelitis. The pathology in the cases involving the CNS is indistinguishable from that of other forms of ADEM (Shirali and Otani, 1959).

Eventually it became clear that ADEM can arise 'spontaneously' or can follow a bacterial (Reik et al., 1985), mycoplasmal (Decaux et al., 1980; Fisher et al., 1983; Fernandez et al., 1993), or viral infection (Miller et al., 1956); a vaccination (Spillane and Wells, 1964; Schlenska, 1977); an insect

sting (Means et al., 1973); administration of a medication Russell, 1937; Fisher and Gilmour, 1939; Marsh, 1952; Cohen et al., 1985) or tetanus antitoxin (Williams and Chafee, 1961); or other illness (Cohen and Lisak, 1987; Johnson and Griffin, 1987; Lisak, 1994; Tselis and Lisak, 1995). The disease can also occur after disseminated tuberculosis (Kopp et al., 1978) and possibly neurobrucellosis (Shakir et al., 1987). Other cases have been self-induced, following injections of animal tissues, particularly lamb brain and porcine hypophysis, given as some sort of 'health tonics' and 'natural therapies' (Sotelo et al., 1984; Goebel et al., 1986). All of these different types of encephalomyelitis share common clinical and pathologic features (Seitelberger, 1967), and hence are all considered by most as ADEM. In rare instances, there may be concomitant demyelination in both the central and peripheral nervous systems, a combination of ADEM and Guillain–Barré syndrome, either simultaneously (Kinoshita et al., 1996) or in rapid succession (Nadkarni and Lisak, 1993). A patient who was vaccinated against hepatitis A during a subacute diarrheal illness later shown to be due to *Campylobacter jejuni*, developed both ADEM and a severe motor axonal polyneuropathy consistent with axonal Guillain–Barré syndrome (Huber et al., 1999). His brain MRI showed multiple lesions in the basal ganglia and in the left cerebral peduncle. Electromyography showed acute denervation changes and he was found to have a high titer (>50 000 units (normal levels are <800 units)) of anti-GM1 IgG antibodies, as well as high titers of complement-fixing antibody to *C. jejuni*, which subsequently decreased in the convalescent phase.

Recently, a form of 'brain inflammation' was reported that may be an iatrogenic ADEM. This was associated with a trial of a therapeutic vaccine, AN-1792, intended to treat Alzheimer's disease, by inducing antibodies (and possibly also cell-mediated immunity) to a aggregates of a fragment of beta-amyloid (Aβ), Aβ42. Aggregates of Aβ42 form a major constituent of the amyloid plaques in Alzheimer's disease (Birmingham and Frantz, 2002). The vaccine consisted of aggregates of synthetic Aβ42 fragment of amyloid precursor protein (APP), with a plant-derived adjuvant molecule (QS-21). In this trial, meningoencephalitis occurred in 18/298 (6%) of patients randomized to the vaccine, and in none of the 74 randomized to placebo (Orgogozo et al., 2003). Most patients developed the illness after two injections of the vaccine. Most patients had headache, lethargy, and confusion; in addition, some had superimposed seizures, focal weakness, and ataxia. Imaging studies showed variable abnormalities, including variable combinations of white matter abnormalities, meningeal enhancement, and cortical lesions. Almost all patients had a moderate mononuclear pleocytosis, and only one had oligoclonal bands on a follow-up cerebrospinal fluid (CSF) examination. No anti-Aβ42 antibodies were seen in baseline CSF examination in the small number of patients in which this was tested. On follow-up examination, anti-Aβ42 IgG antibodies were found in 6/8 and IgM antibodies in 4/8. Some patients were treated with variable regimens of corticosteroids, and seemed to benefit (Orgogozo et al., 2003). There appeared to be no relation between anti Aβ42 titers and severity of illness. It is known from animal studies that injection of Aβ with adjuvant into mice can induce experimental allergic encephalomyelitis (EAE), an animal model of ADEM (see below) (Furlan et al., 2003). However, the adjuvant used in the animal model consisted of complete Freund's adjuvant as well as intravenous pertussis toxin, both of which strongly enhance the antigeniticity of the vaccine, and often give rise to autoimmune reactions. In one autopsied case of the disease, there was good evidence of clearance of amyloid plaques without much difference in the other pathological features of Alzheimer's disease such as neurofibrillary tangles and neuropil threads. There was also demyelination and macrophage infiltration, and a CD4+ T-cell meningoencephalitis, typical of inflammatory demyelination (Nicoll et al., 2003).

Post-infectious or post-vaccination white matter inflammation can be highly focal clinically and even pathologically, and affect only the optic nerve, the spinal cord, or the cerebellum. Such allied syndromes with focal monophasic inflammatory demyelination (optic neuritis, transverse myelitis, and cerebellar ataxia) appear to have triggers similar to those of ADEM. Thus optic neuritis may follow a vaccination (Kazarian and Gager, 1978) and acute transverse myelitis may follow simultaneous immunization with diphtheria, tetanus, and polio (Whittle and Roberton, 1977) or infection with varicella (McCarthy and Amer, 1978) or Mycoplasma pneumoniae (Yoshizawa, et al., 1982). Neuromyelitis optica may also follow varicella (Chusid, et al. 1982). Bilateral optic neuritis, followed a week later by transverse myelitis, can occur after rubella vaccination (Kline et al., 1982). Optic neuritis has also been associated with Lyme disease, but whether this is due to direct infection by Borrelia burgdorferi or is a form of post-infectious white matter inflammation is not clear (Schecter, 1986; Jacobson et al., 1991). Bilateral optic neuritis has occurred after vaccination with the trivalent measles, mumps, and rubella vaccine (Kazarian and Gager, 1978). Indeed, any vaccination can be followed by dysfunction at any level of the nervous system (Miller and Stanton, 1954).

Patients can also develop acute hemorrhagic leukoencephalitis (AHLE), a severe form of ADEM (Hurst, 1947; Byers, 1975). AHLE is characterized by a more fulminant clinical course, with hemorrhagic necrosis of the white matter and a high fatality rate. The relation of all these conditions to the quintessential inflammatory demyelinating CNS disease of humans, MS, is unclear.

An acute febrile encephalopathy reportedly coincides with or follows systemic infections, viral and possibly also bacterial. The histopathology is not that of an encephalomyelitis. We discuss this in more detail later.

Virus-induced demyelination

The notion of virally induced demyelination involves certain philosophical subtleties. The mere detection of a virus in a tissue does not establish that the virus is pathogenetically involved in disease of that tissue, especially with the development of extremely sensitive methods of detecting viral genomes. In many cases, especially with viruses which are known to be present in a latent (or reactivated) state (particularly herpesviruses), detection of the virus merely establishes its presence, possibly as an 'innocent bystander', and does not at all imply an etiological role for the virus in the disease.

The detection of Epstein–Barr virus (EBV) DNA in the CSF has been reported in four patients with post-infectious neurological complications, one with ADEM and one each with Guillain–Barré syndrome, polyradiculitis, and transverse myelitis (Weinberg et al., 2002). These patients had pleocytosis and a low quantity ('load') of EBV in the CSF. This would be compatible with EBV being carried along as a 'passenger' in B lymphocytes, which are known to be latently infected with EBV. These patients were compared with 10 patients with EBV encephalitis and 14 immunosuppressed (12 AIDS and two post-transplant) patients with primary CNS lymphoma (which is an EBV-driven neoplasm). In both of these other groups, the viral load in the CSF was far higher than that in the post-infectious patients, and they had comparable (EBV encephalitis) or less (primary CNS lymphoma) pleocytosis than the post-infectious patients. The high viral load in diseases known to be directly caused by EBV and low viral load in diseases which are not thought so to be caused suggests that detection of virus in demyelinat-

ing lesions must be viewed with circumspection, especially when such viruses are known to be present in a latent form.

This point is further illustrated in a study of 15 patients with AHLE, all of whom died within 4 weeks of onset (An et al., 2002). The brains of these patients were compared with the brains of 10 controls who had died in road accidents. Histopathological examination showed a typical hemorrhagic inflammatory demyelination in all cases. Herpes simplex virus (HSV) was found in four cases, varicella zoster virus (VZV) in two and human herpes virus-6 (HHV6) in one. No cases showed cytomegalovirus (CMV) or EBV. When tested, viral DNA and antigens were found only in cells in the inflammatory region, particularly macrophages and endothelial and other vascular cells, but not in glia or neurons, as would occur with direct viral infection of the CNS. Among the controls, HSV, but no other virus, was found in two. This shows that detection of virus in the brain, with new very sensitive techniques, does not necessarily imply a pathogenetic role for the virus.

Occasionally, direct viral infections of the brain and spinal cord can cause demyelination with relative axonal and neuronal sparing. It is rare for these infections to be confused with ADEM. An example may be EBV infection, which is also an associated trigger of ADEM (Bray et al., 1992; Paskavitz et al., 1995). In several patients, an acute EBV infection with neurologic manifestations was followed by either a progressive or a relapsing and remitting white matter disease (Bray et al., 1992). Whether this was a purely demyelinating disease is unknown. Acute infection with human immunodeficiency virus (HIV) is very rarely associated with an ADEM-like syndrome (Jones et al., 1988; Gray et al., 1991; von Giesen et al., 1994), with pathologically confirmed demyelination and relative axonal sparing in the lesions, but this is uncommon enough that any causal relation is unclear. Human T-lymphotropic virus (HTLV) type 1-associated myelopathy (tropical spastic paraparesis) is documented to have direct demyelinating effects (Robertson and Cruikshank, 1972; Vernant et al., 1987; Osame et al., 1987). It is unknown how these arise, although it is known that HTLV-1 infects CD8+ T lymphocytes, which become activated and proliferate. However, these cells are directed against HTLV-1 antigens and not myelin. The virus does not infect oligodendrocytes, so that direct viral lysis of myelin-producing cells does not occur. HTLV-1 does infect primary cultures of human microglia, activating them and inducing cytokine production, which may be directly toxic to myelin (McKendall, 1994). Despite the activation of immune cells in HTLV-1 disease, the main clinical outcome of this is a mild immune deficiency, although adult T-cell leukemia/lymphoma and tropical spastic paraparesis are the usual associated diseases, occurring in about 5% of all patients with HTLV-1 infections (McKendall, 1994). HIV leukoencephalopathy, commonly seen with advanced HIV disease, is characterized by an apparent deficit of myelin (myelin pallor) of unclear nature (Kliehues et al., 1985). This has been cited as a possible example of demyelination (Budka, 1989), but further studies showed that the intensity of immunostaining for myelin basic protein (MBP) from affected areas was normal, no lipid-laden macrophages were detected, and neither active demyelination nor demyelinating axons were seen, which suggests that no classic inflammatory demyelination takes place (Power et al., 1993). Instead the pathogenesis appears to have some relationship to alterations in the blood–brain barrier (Power et al., 1993), but the nature of this relationship is still not completely clear. These blood–brain barrier alterations are inferred from the presence of serum proteins in the brain parenchyma, localized to neurons and glia, in which they are usually absent. This is different from the alterations seen in the blood–rain barrier seen with ADEM and MS, in which there is a more specific inflammatory reaction surrounding small cerebral venules in the deep white matter, with an associated perivenular demyelination in which both cellular and humoral factors have access to the brain parenchyma. More recently, an unprecedented phenomenon has been described in HIV patients whose immune systems reconstitute when the patients take highly active antiretroviral therapy (HAART). This suppresses viral replication and allows a rebound in the number of CD4 cells. In a small proportion of such patients, new inflammatory lesions occur at sites of residual antigen (or low-level replicating pathogen), such as CMV retinitis (DeSimone et al.,

2000). This so-called immune reconstitution syndrome has been invoked to explain inflammatory damage to the white matter in seven cases of diffuse neurological deterioration occurring in patients with advanced HIV disease treated with HAART, in whom CD4 counts increased and diagnostic investigation revealed no other cause of white matter disease (Langford et al., 2002). MRI of the brain showed either multifocal white matter hyperintensities on T_2 imaging, or more diffuse lesions, which tended to be more prominent in the centrum semiovale, corpus callosum, and optic radiations, and less likely in the frontal poles. Gross pathology shows white matter atrophy and, occasionally, cavitation in severe cases. Microscopically, both demyelination and axonal damage are seen in the context of an intense perivascular infiltration with HIV-infected monocytes and astrogliosis. The pathology did not, however, mimic that of ADEM or MS, with perivenular demyelination and relative axonal sparing (Langford et al., 2002).

Subacute sclerosing panencephalitis, a chronic progressive measles virus infection of the brain in young persons, is characterized in part by inflammatory demyelination (Swoveland and Johnson, 1989). Similarly, progressive rubella panencephalitis, a chronic progressive rubella virus disease of the brain, is also characterized by prominent white matter involvement (Townsend et al., 1975). The white matter involvement proceeds beyond demyelination, with axonal fragmentation present as well (Townsend et al., 1976). Neither of these clinically resembles ADEM, however. Progressive multifocal leukoencephalopathy, a papovavirus infection of the brain lytic for oligodendrocytes (and transforming for astrocytes), is seen in patients with advanced immunodeficiency secondary to acquired immunodeficiency syndrome (AIDS), cancer chemotherapy, or immunosuppression after transplantation, and rarely without obvious associations. The characteristic lesions consist of demyelination with little or no accompanying inflammation (Major et al., 1992). Demyelination occurs rarely in varicella-zoster virus (VZV) encephalitis in AIDS patients (Ryder et al., 1986; Amlie-Lefond et al., 1995). Clinically, this is a slowly progressive disease characterized by prominent cognitive difficulties, especially memory loss, and multifocal motor deficits (Amlie-Lefond et al., 1995). The lesions in AIDS-associated VZV encephalitis cover a broad pathologic spectrum, including a leukoencephalitis in which a vasculopathy gives rise to both necrosis and demyelination, often in the same lesion (Ryder et al., 1986; Gray et al., 1994). Additionally, demyelination is probably due to direct infection of oligodendrocytes by VZV, since some of the demyelinated areas are ringed with oligodendrocytes containing viral inclusions (Amlie-Lefond et al., 1995; Gray et al., 1994). Other cells, including macrophages, endothelial cells, and occasionally neurons, are also infected (Gray et al., 1994). Finally, it was recently proposed that demyelination can be caused directly by infection of the brain by human herpesvirus-6 (HHV-6) in immunosuppressed transplant recipients and AIDS patients (Knox and Carrigan, 1995). HHV-6 was recently added to the list of possible etiologic agents in MS (Challoner et al., 1995).

A number of viruses can cause demyelination in animal models (Weller, 1991; Fazakerley and Buchmeier, 1992). These include Theiler's virus (an enterovirus) (Lipton, 1975), herpesvirus (Kastrukoff et al., 1987), and coronavirus (Dal Canto and Rabinowitz, 1982; Lavi and Weiss, 1989). Other model viral demyelinating syndromes include those include those due to Chandipura and vesicular stomatitis viruses (both rhabdoviruses), canine distemper virus, Venezuelan equine encephalomyelitis virus, and Semliki Forest virus (Dal Canto and Rabinowitz, 1982). Almost all of these are enveloped viruses. A prominent virally induced inflammatory demyelinating disease in nature is the retroviral infection visna, which infects both lungs and brain in sheep (Georgsson, 1994).

ADEM can follow a frank viral encephalitis (Koenig et al., 1979), just as it can follow any other viral disease. A patient with biopsy-proved herpes simplex encephalitis who presented with headache, fever, memory loss, and a pleocytosis of 150/mm³ was treated with adenine arabinoside, and improved almost back to baseline status. After 2 weeks of therapy, his neurologic exam showed only a minimal aphasia, and his CSF pleocytosis had decreased by half. A month later, his condition began to deteriorate, and he did not respond to a second course of adenine arabinoside. A repeat

biopsy showed inflammatory demyelination, typical of ADEM. In two patients with rabies, extensive demyelination was found at autopsy, along with the perivenular inflammatory infiltrates typical of ADEM (Toro et al., 1977; Nelson and Berry, 1993). The pathogenesis of this finding was unclear, but may well have been due to concurrent rabies encephalitis and ADEM. One of the two patients received a partial (Nelson and Berry, 1993) and one had completed (Toro et al., 1977) a full course of rabies vaccination when the fatal illness began. In one patient, demyelination was seen in the frontal lobes and in the cervical and thoracic regions of the spinal cord as well as the cervical nerve roots (Nelson and Berry, 1993). In addition, a widespread rabies encephalitis with characteristic viral inclusions (Negri bodies and lyssa bodies) was noted and confirmed by inoculation into suckling mice (Nelson and Berry, 1993). It is possible also that in these cases the vaccine triggered the ADEM.

With the possible exception of acute EBV infection, directly involving the CNS and which, as noted already, can be a trigger for ADEM, few viral demyelinating diseases are likely to be confused with ADEM.

Epidemiology

Epidemiologic studies of ADEM are complicated by the by the fact that this is an uncommon disease. The figures for ADEM vary considerably according to the precipitating disease. ADEM occurs after measles (1:1000), vaccinia (given as an inoculation against smallpox) (Spillane and Wells, 1964) (1:63 to 1:300 000), varicella (about 1:10 000), and rubella cases (1:20 000) (Miller et al., 1956). It has also occurred after mumps and rarely, scarlet fever, a bacterial infection (Miller et al., 1956).

The disease has an interesting age distribution: ADEM and the restricted syndromes do not appear to occur in very young children (less than about 2 or 3 years old). There are rare apparent exceptions. This rarity of ADEM in young children presumably has to do with the immature state of the myelin, although differences in the immune system may also be involved. However, an acute toxic encephalopathy can be seen in very young children under circumstances typically associated with ADEM, and is characterized by a rapidly progressive disease with prominent drowsiness and coma, as well as seizures (McNair Scott, 1967). The histopathology is bland, without the white matter perivenular infiltrates typical of ADEM. The incidence of this toxic encephalopathy is uncertain (McNair Scott, 1967). We discuss this entity in more detail later.

A very rough estimate of the incidence of ADEM can be obtained from a study of all encephalitis patients admitted to the London Hospital (Kennard and Swash, 1981) over a 15-year period, between 1963 and 1978. Encephalitis was defined as an acute, rapidly progressive illness with diffuse or multifocal inflammatory involvement of the nervous system with other causes excluded. Three subgroups were defined: (1) one group in which a virus was definitely linked to the encephalitis, (2) one group in which no causal or antecedent virus could be implicated in the encephalitis, and (3) one group in which the viral illness had occurred in the month before the onset of the neurologic illness, and was separated from it by a period of normal health. Of 60 patients who fulfilled the criteria for encephalitis, at least one-third were thought to have post-infectious encephalomyelitis, by virtue of the fact that they had had an antecedent viral illness that had completely resolved in the month before the onset of the neurologic illness (Kennard and Swash, 1981). It should be noted that it is possible that some cases of post-infectious encephalomyelitis may have been missed, because in some viral exanthems the associated ADEM can overlap the systematic viral disease (Lisak, 1994; Johnson and Griffin, 1987). While there is likely to be some referral bias in this series, and therefore some imprecision in the estimate of the proportion, the above-cited figures provide a rough estimate (probably low) of the proportion of ADEM among all encephalitis patients.

ADEM can occur after immunization with vaccines to prevent measles, diphtheria/tetanus, rubella, and pertussis (Fenichel, 1982). Given the very large number of vaccinations performed against these diseases, the incidence of ADEM is rare enough to suggest coincidence rather than causality

(Fenichel, 1982). On the other hand, after vaccination with rabies vaccine containing neural antigens, the incidence of ADEM is between 1:7000 and 1:50 000 and yet a casual connection is not doubted (Hemachudha *et al.*, 1987a). In a series of 61 patients in Thailand with neurologic complications that occurred after they received Semple-type rabies vaccine, 36 had 'major' complications: 12 had encephalitis, seven had myelitis, 13 had meningitis, and four had GBS (Hemachudha *et al.*, 1987a). All were treated with dexamethasone and all recovered completely. The other 25 patients had 'minor' complications consisting of headache, backache, fever, and no pleocytosis. It has been estimated in Thailand that between 1 in 400 and 1 in 220 recipients of Semple virus rabies vaccine develop ADEM (Hemachudha *et al.*, 1987a). Other vaccines reported to have ADEM as sequelae include influenza (Warren, 1956; Woods and Ellison, 1964; Rosenberg, 1970; Yahr and Lobo-Antunes, 1972; Cherington, 1977; Gross *et al.*, 1978; Saito *et al.*, 1980), hepatitis B (Trevisani *et al.*, 1993; Kaplanski *et al.*, 1995), and Japanese B encephalitis (Ohtaki *et al.*, 1992; 1995). The period between influenza vaccination and the onset of the encephalitis could be exceedingly short—only a few hours, in two patients (Warren, 1956; Gross *et al.*, 1978). Both patients were confused, with one having right-sided weakness and hemisensory loss and the other having incontinence and marked pleocytosis (Warren, 1956; Gross *et al.*, 1978). One of the patients (Warren, 1956) had strong local reactions to previous influenza vaccinations. In the other patient (Gross *et al.*, 1978), skin testing to chicken protein elicited a strong reaction, 35 mm in diameter, within 10 minutes. Hepatitis B vaccination in one patient was followed 21 days later by an illness characterized by headache, backache, flaccid paraplegia, lower extremity areflexia, and urinary retention, which was attributed to transverse myelitis (Trevisani *et al.*, 1993). This illness largely resolved in 2 weeks, except for some residual bladder dysfunction. All of these vaccines are of enveloped viruses. We are unaware of any well-documented reports of ADEM following polio vaccination, for example, and the main neurologic complication of this is a clinical poliomyelitis resulting from the reversion of an attenuated strain to a virulent strain. The only post-vaccination report was of a case of myelitis after multiple vaccinations with diphtheria, tetanus, and polio vaccine, which is hardly convincing evidence of an autoimmune poliovirus vaccine-induced myelitis. One case of a patient with myelitis and decreased visual acuity in the left eye following oral polio vaccine was reported, with abnormal signal in the spinal cord, but the isolation of poliovirus from the CSF makes it difficult to ascribe the illness to a parainfectious mechanism of disease rather than a direct infection of the cord (Ozawa *et al.*, 2000).

More recently, eight patients with ADEM following vaccination with hepatitis B vaccine were reported from France. All developed symptoms of demyelination, five of them multifocal, within 4 days to 10 weeks of vaccination. Two of the patients had possible symptoms of demyelination in the past, but no definite history of demyelinating disease. The disease was remitting and relapsing in seven of the patients, and monophasic in one. All patients had abnormal MRIs, with persistent MRI activity in four of five patients (Tourbah *et al.*, 1999). Although there is molecular mimicry between the hepatitis B polymerase and myelin basic protein, the vaccine only contains hepatitis B surface antigen. While interesting, such a case series provides no real evidence of causality, because of the recall bias inherent in this type of report. This report occasioned much controversy in France, and other subsequent cases were reported, but calculations of the expected number of new MS cases (1–3/100 000 per year) showed that the disease incidence in the vaccinees (0.65/100 000 per year) was actually less than would have been expected, so that the risk of MS following vaccination is unlikely to be increased (Monteyne and Andre, 2000). Furthermore, a population-based study of the incidence of MS in hepatitis B vaccine recipients in British Columbia showed no link between hepatitis B vaccination and MS (Sadovnick and Scheifele, 2000).

ADEM can also occur after administration of a medication (Russell, 1937; Fisher and Gilmour, 1939; Marsh, 1952; Cohen *et al.*, 1985), but such reports are rare enough that a causal link is unlikely. Furthermore, the apparent post-medication ADEM may have been due to the original illness for which the medication was given.

There are additional reasons why we cannot quantify the incidence of ADEM accurately. For measles, previously a common antecedent, the above-quoted incidence of ADEM may be an underestimate, as patients may have a subclinical form of the disease; indeed, a high proportion of measles patients have minor neurologic and behavioral abnormalities, electroencephalographic (EEG) abnormalities, and CSF pleocytosis (Hanninen *et al.*, 1980). Other systemic infections, such as EBV disease (Gautier-Smith, 1965), varicella (Griffith *et al.*, 1970), and mumps, can cause a mild viral encephalitis that can be confused with ADEM clinically, and so its incidence can be overestimated if the illness due to the viral encephalitis is ascribed to ADEM, or underestimated if the illness due to ADEM is ascribed to a viral encephalitis. Indeed, many viral exanthems can be associated with CSF (Ojala, 1947) and EEG abnormalities (Gibbs *et al.*, 1959) without any obvious brain pathology. Other systemic infections such as legionellosis, *B. burgdorferi* infection, and *Mycoplasma* infection can also cause encephalopathies that may be erroneously ascribed to ADEM.

The epidemiology of the clinically and pathologically restricted forms of ADEM mentioned previously, such as optic neuritis, acute cerebellar ataxia, and transverse myelitis, is also not totally understood. These interesting forms of ADEM are discussed in more detail later. Over the years 1951 to 1985, 92 children with a diagnosis of optic neuritis were referred to the Hospital for Sick Children, Great Ormond Street, a major referral center. After exclusion of patients with clear causes of optic neuropathy (leukemia, syphilis, diabetes, hypertension, vitamin deficiency, etc.), there were 39 patients (Kriss *et al.*, 1988). A population-based study of optic neuritis in Olmstead County, Minnesota, was performed using the unique comprehensive Mayo Clinic records-linkage system, and 156 patients who had optic neuritis between 1935 and 1991 were identified (Rodriguez *et al.*, 1995). Patients were included if (1) there was rapid visual loss with no evidence for any other local or systemic disease, (2) there were clinical signs of optic neuritis, and (3) if the diagnosis was made by a Mayo Clinic ophthalmologist. The incidence rate was found to be 5.5/100 000 per year, based on 156 patients 'captured' in the years 1935 to 1991, and the prevalence was 115/100 000 (prevalence date 1 December 1991). The incidence and prevalence were age- and sex-adjusted to the 1951 US White population. In neither of these studies were there any details about previous infections or other illnesses or vaccinations. In another study of optic neuritis in childhood, 21 patients with optic neuritis (defined as sudden reduction of visual acuity, sudden visual field defects, and an afferent papillary defect) were seen in the University Children's Hospital in Helsinki from 1970 to 1985 (Riikonen *et al.*, 1988). Of these, five were diagnosed with other diseases, nine were diagnosed with optic neuritis associated with MS (either because of previous history or subsequent events), and seven were believed to have idiopathic optic neuritis. Of the patients who went on to develop MS, five of the nine had common respiratory infections or vaccinations 3 days to 1 month before the onset of the optic neuritis.

A report from a tertiary medical care center reviewed 40 patients who presented with acute childhood ataxia during a 10-year period (Gieron-Korthals *et al.*, 1995). All presented to the emergency room and were subsequently admitted. The most common established etiology was post-infectious acute cerebellar ataxia, which was diagnosed in 14 (35%) of the patients. The next most common causes were drug ingestion (32.5%) and GBS (12.5%). Post-infectious cerebellar ataxia (cerebellitis) usually is associated with VZV infections, generally following chickenpox in children (Miller *et al.*, 1956), but it can follow other viral infections as EBV mononucleosis (Bergen and Grossman, 1975; Cleary *et al.*, 1980). Its incidence is uncertain, although it is clear that it is high on the list of differential diagnoses for acute cerebellar ataxia in children.

In a population-based study of acute transverse myelitis carried out in Israel, the average annual incidence rate was 1.34/million per year, based on 62 cases presenting between 1955 and 1975 (Berman *et al.*, 1981). Patients with other known neurologic disease or injury were excluded. It was found that 23 (37%) of the patients had a preceding infection. Lipton and Teasdall (1973) looked at the records of patients seen at Johns Hopkins Hospital from 1929 to 1967 who had an acute transverse myelopathy as above and for whom follow-up data at 5 years or later or at autopsy could be obtained. Thirty-four such patients were found. Twelve (35%) of these patients had a preceding viral-like illness. Another retrospective study of acute transverse myelitis, using similar criteria, 'captured' 32 cases from five neurologic departments in Denmark over a period of 12 years (Christensen et al., 1990). A history of preceding viral infection was obtained in 12 (37.5%) patients.

Clinical presentation and outcome

ADEM has a broad clinical spectrum of presentation. It can range from a subclinical episode, detected by the appearance of multifocal white matter abnormalities on brain magnetic resonance images (MRIs) made for other reasons, to a fulminant, rapidly progressive disease with seizures and coma, leading to death. It is likely that ADEM and AHLE have a similar but not identical underlying pathogenesis (Russell, 1955), as both occur under the same circumstances, with ADEM evolving to AHLE in some patients (Dangood et al., 1991). This hypothesis is also supported by work done on the animal models experimental allergic encephalomyelitis (EAE) and hyperacute EAE by Levine (1974) (see below).

The neurologic symptoms usually begin 1 to 3 weeks after the time of infection, although in exanthems, especially measles, the illness tends to begin sooner, 2 to 7 days after the rash occurs. The onset tends to be abrupt, which may be a point of differentiation (Johnson et al., 1984) from the slightly more gradual onset of a viral encephalitis that ADEM most closely resembles. Rarely, the illness is concurrent with or even precedes the rash. The symptoms consist of headache, fever, nausea, vomiting, confusion, delirium, obtundation, and coma, and evolve over several days. Often superimposed on this global dysfunction are focal abnormalities, including hemiparesis, hemisensory loss, ataxia, visual loss, and paraparesis (Miller et al., 1956). The latter three may be clinical expressions of a coexistent cerebellar ataxia, optic neuritis, or transverse myelitis, respectively. Seizures, myoclonus, and memory loss have also been reported. Occasionally, there may be dystonia, chorea, athetosis, and rigidity with lesions in the basal ganglia (Donovan and Lenn, 1989). MRIs of the two patients described by Donovan and Lenn (1989) showed abnormal signal in the putamens bilaterally and the globus pallidus, and extending through the cerebral peduncles to the substantia nigra; interestingly, the lesions were bilaterally symmetric. There is often gradual recovery, which can be surprisingly complete. However, patients with seizures and coma tend to have a less positive outcome (Miller et al., 1956). The case mortality rate historically was 10 to 20% (Miller et al., 1956). However, recent series suggest a more benign outcome. In a series of 84 pediatric ADEM patients, there were no deaths and 89% had either complete or minimally abnormal signs on examination (Tenembaum et al., 2002). There was no clear relationship between the initial appearance of the brain MRI and ultimate outcome. In another series of 35 pediatric ADEM patients, no patients died, and 57% had a complete recovery. In those with residual deficits, roughly equal proportions had motor, visual, and cognitive/behavioral impairment (Dale et al., 2000). It should be clear that the differentiation of ADEM or AHLE from other encephalitides and occasionally from toxic–metabolic encephalopathies can be very difficult.

Of the 62 patients with acute transverse myelitis evaluated by the previously cited Israeli study (Berman et al., 1981), more than one-third had a good recovery while one-third had only a 'fair' recovery. The time to maximum improvement was 4 weeks to 3 months. In the study by Lipton and Teasdall (1973), most of the patients (85%) had a thoracic sensory level. Half of the patients had CSF pleocytosis on presentation, and one-third had an increased CSF protein concentration. Most of the early deaths (five patients) occurred in the days before respiratory support methods were available, and were due to respiratory failure and pneumonia—all occurred before 1950. Of the patients who survived, roughly two-thirds had a good or fair outcome and became ambulatory. Lipton and Teasdall (1973) classified the outcomes as follows: (1) good outcome—normal gait, normal mic-

turition or minimal urgency, and no or minimally abnormal neurologic signs; (2) fair outcome—functional and ambulatory but with an abnormal gait, urinary urgency, and persistent signs of spinal cord dysfunction; and (3) poor outcome—chair bound or bedridden, incontinent, and severe sensory deficits. Recovery can take many months, but most of the patients who were able to walk did so within 3 to 6 months. Patients who retained deep tendon reflexes and posterior column function were more likely to recover than were those who did not. Only three patients were treated with steroids (doses not reported), and so the efficacy of this therapy could not be evaluated. In the Danish study (Christensen et al., 1990), of the 29 surviving patients who were followed for an average of 12 years, roughly one-third of each had a good, fair, or poor outcome. Patients with back pain and signs of spinal shock were particularly likely to have a poor outcome. It is interesting to note that only one patient (3%) of the 29 in this study eventually developed MS. Another study (Ropper and Poskanzer, 1978) evaluated 52 patients with acute transverse myelitis at the Massachusetts General Hospital. The investigators noted typically four types of initial symptoms of the disease: (1) bilateral lower extremity paresthesias, (2) bilateral lower extremity weakness, (3) back pain, and (4) urinary retention, the latter being uncommon. Three distinct tempos of disease were discerned: (1) smoothly progressive over 2 weeks, (2) progressive in a slow or stuttering manner over 10 days to 4 weeks, and (3) explosive in onset. Patients with type 1 or 2 disease tended to have a fair to good outcome (as classified by Lipton and Teasdall (1973)), whereas patients with an explosive onset, especially those with back pain (which may reflect the degree of swelling), had a poor outcome, with only one of 11 patients becoming ambulatory again. MS developed in seven (13%) of the 52 patients, but the mode of onset and tempo could not be used to predict which patients these would be. The degree of pleocytosis and increase in CSF protein concentration were also not predictive of outcome.

The question of the risk of development of MS after ADEM or one of the isolated demyelinating lesions is an important one, and is discussed in more detail below. It should be noted, however, that in the older studies, especially of myelitis, optic neuritis, and brainstem syndromes, MRI of the brain was not done, and thus only crude predictions of the risk of development of MS could be made.

Pathology

The neuropathology of ADEM is that of a perivenular inflammatory myelinopathy. In ADEM, the brain is often grossly swollen, with macroscopic engorgement of veins in the white matter. Microscopically, there is perivascular edema with mononuclear infiltration, mostly with lymphocytes and macrophages (Fig. 13.1). Plasma cells and granulocytes are rarely seen. There is proliferation of endothelial cells. The hallmark pathology is that of demyelination, with relative axonal sparing.(Figs 13.2 and 13.3) This demyelination occurs around small veins. The pathology is uniform and appears to be independent of the particular inciting agent (Hart and Earle, 1975). This appearance is similar to that of EAE in animals (Hart and Earle, 1975). EAE is a disease induced in animals by administration of neural tissue (and certain antigens) with adjuvant, as well as by passive administration of activated sensitized T cells and T-cell lines or clones (Rivers and Schwentker, 1935; Levine, 1974). Rabies post-vaccinal encephalomyelitis, which used to occur after the inoculation of attenuated (Pasteur and Fermi vaccines) or inactivated (Semple vaccine) rabies virus grown in neural tissue, is an example of EAE in humans (Shiraki and Otani, 1959). The Semple vaccine was replaced by the duck embryo rabies vaccine in the late 1950s, but this was also associated with neuroparalytic accidents, including transverse myelitis, although less commonly than with the earlier vaccines (Label and Batts, 1982). The newer human diploid cell strain vaccine (HDCV), free of neural tissue, is not associated with rabies post-vaccinal encephalomyelitis, although one case of a GBS-like syndrome after the administration of HDCV has been reported (Bernard et al., 1982). EAE reportedly occurred in a laboratory worker as a result of a laboratory accident in which a

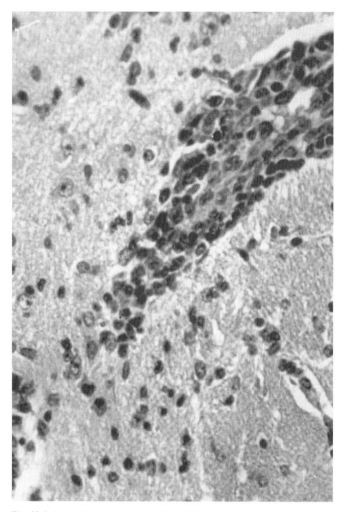

Fig. 13.1 Acute disseminated encephalomyelitis. Perivascular edema with mononuclear infiltration, mostly with lymphocytes and macrophages, is seen.

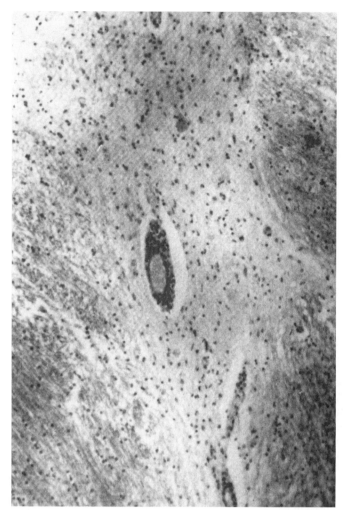

Fig. 13.2 Experimental autoimmune encephalomyelitis. Demyelination is seen surrounding a small vein. Intact myelin can be seen at the three corners of the photomicrograph.

mixture of complete Freund's adjuvant and guinea pig CNS tissue was inoculated via a broken test tube. Twenty-five days later, headache, fever, and a partial lateral rectus palsy developed, and there was a mild pleocytosis with a raised CSF protein concentration. The patient was treated with corticosteroids and the illness resolved completely. Conversion from protein purified derivative (PPD) negative to PPD positive showed that the amount of Freund's adjuvant was enough to induce a delayed hypersensitivity cell-mediated immune reaction (Drachman *et al.*, 1974).

In AHLE the pathology is a continuation of that seen in ADEM. Macroscopically, the brain is swollen and distended; punctate hemorrhages and ring-like hemorrhagic lesions are seen grossly. Microscopically, there is fibrinoid necrosis and infiltration of the vessels with neutrophils and occasional eosinophils. There is exudation of serum proteins. Red blood cells and granulocytes are distributed around the vessels. Ring hemorrhages associated with venous thrombosis are seen. The pathology does not involve gray matter. The picture is identical to that of hyperacute EAE in animals (Levine, 1974; Hart and Earle, 1975) (Fig. 13.4). Adams and Kubik (1952) and Russell (1955) pointed out the continuum between AHLE and ADEM, and Levine (1974) demonstrated the continuum between EAE and hyperacute EAE.

Pathogenesis

This is most likely a T-cell-mediated autoimmune disease directed against a myelin/oligodendrocytes antigen, probably MBP (Paterson, 1960; Lisak and

Zweiman, 1977). The evidence for this is indirect. First, there is a strong similarity between ADEM and EAE, and between AHLE and hyperacute EAE, which are known to be T-cell mediated, since the disease may be transferred to naive recipient animals by lymphocytes but not by serum (Paterson, 1960). Second, *in vitro* studies of blood and CSF lymphocytes from ADEM patients demonstrate increased T-cell reactivity to MBP (Paterson, 1960; Lisak and Zweiman, 1977). Similar results have been reported for transverse myelopathy (Abramsky and Teitekbaum, 1977). However, MBP need not be the only relevant antigen. Proteolipid protein (PLP) and myelin-oligodendrocyte glycoprotein (MOG) would be other possibilities since they also induce EAE. However, no studies have been done to test T-cell reactivity to MBP, PLP, and MOG in the same ADEM patients. It may be pertinent to note that localized models of EAE, corresponding possibly to some of the focal demyelinating syndromes (e.g. optic neuritis and myelitis) have been studied (Levine, 1974). In these, EAE is induced in an animal after mechanical injury to focal areas of the brain. The resulting inflammatory demyelinating lesions localize at the site of the previous mechanical injury (Levine, 1974), and this may be a useful model of the focal forms of ADEM.

The reason for the cell-mediated immune reaction directed against myelin is not known. Several possibilities are as follows.

One possible pathogenetic mechanism is that of 'molecular mimicry', in which certain peptide, carbohydrate, or lipid epitopes on an infecting virus

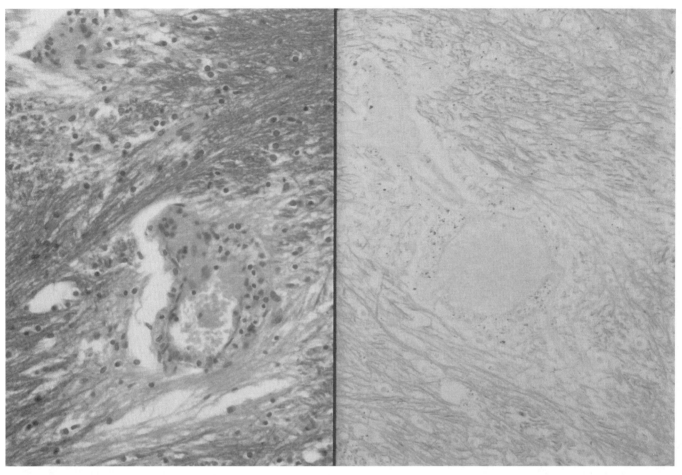

Fig. 13.3 Acute disseminated encephalomyelitis in a human patient. Left figure shows myelin staining absent immediately around a small venule (H&E stain.) The right figure shows relative preservation of axons surrounding a venule in adjacent section, although there is some rarefaction immediately around the venule, possibly due to edema (Bielschowsky stain.) (See also Plate 3 of the colour plate section at the center of this book.)

or other antigen are similar to epitopes on myelin (Lisak *et al.*, 1968; Jahnke *et al.*, 1985; Fujinami and Oldstone, 1985). Other examples of molecular mimicry of possible pathogenic significance include the cross-reactivity between *C. jejuni* and GQ$_{1b}$ ganglioside in the Fisher–Miller variant of GBS (Jacobs *et al.*, 1995); *C. jejuni* and GM$_1$ ganglioside in the acute motor axonal neuropathy variant of GBS (Oomes *et al.*, 1995; Rees *et al.*, 1995); and some Gram-negative bacteria and the α subunit of the acetylcholine receptor (AChR), and herpes simplex virus and the AChR α subunit, in myasthenia gravis (Stefansson *et al.*, 1985; Schwimmbeck *et al.*, 1989). If cross-reactive T cells are exposed to this antigen, they will expand clonally. Activated cross-reactive T cells can cross the blood–brain barrier. They may then be retained in the CNS, where they could open up the blood–brain barrier and recruit other lymphocytes and macrophages, leading to inflammation and demyelination.

Another possible mechanism is that of viruses or other antigens non-specifically activating T cells. Such activated T cells can cross the blood–brain barrier. If a non-specific activated T cell does not find any recognizable epitopes, it will migrate out of the CNS leaving no real trace of its passage. On the other hand, if the non-specifically activated T cell happens to be one that recognizes an epitope on myelin, it will expand clonally and trigger the inflammatory reaction, as described already. Some microbial antigens act as 'superantigens', which can activate broad classes of CD4+ T cells by binding simultaneously to the major histocompatibility complex (MHC) Class II molecule of an antigen-presenting cell and to the Vβ region of the T-cell receptor (TCR). Such a superantigen can therefore activate a very large fraction (up to 1 in 50) of the CD4+ T cells in the body. Some of

these could be myelin-reactive, and will find themselves in the brain, with the consequences discussed above (Burns *et al.*,1992). Such a mechanism has been postulated to occur in a post-streptococcal ADEM case, in which myelin-reactive T-cell clones were generated from the patient's peripheral blood mononuclear cells. These cells displayed cross-reactivity with *Streptococcus pyogenes* antigens and expressed mRNA patterns with a T2-bias, stimulating, at least in part, a humoral immune response. This is reminiscent of the anti-MOG antibody model of EAE discussed above, although the antibody specificity of the humoral immune reaction is not known (Jorens *et al.*, 2000).

A third possible pathogenic mechanism is that of inhibition of suppressor T cells. Some viral infections suppress certain types of CD4+ suppressor T cells. If any of these are myelin-specific suppressor cells, the removal of their influence by a virus (or some other means) may result in the spontaneous activation of myelin-specific CD4+ T cells, and thence to CNS inflammation and demyelination as described already.

Another less likely possibility includes the direct infection of the oligodendrocytes or astrocytes, leading to an immune reaction. Unlike progressive multifocal leukoencephalopathy or subacute sclerosing panencephalitis, infection of these cells has never been demonstrated in ADEM. Finally, it is possible (though never demonstrated) that endothelial cells are infected, impairing the blood–brain barrier and allowing cells or myelinotoxic factors into the brain, resulting in demyelinating lesions. However, this would not explain how killed microbial products in vaccines could induce ADEM or AHLE, although such vaccines may be compatible with a mechanism requiring systemic cytokine-induced alteration of endothelial cells.

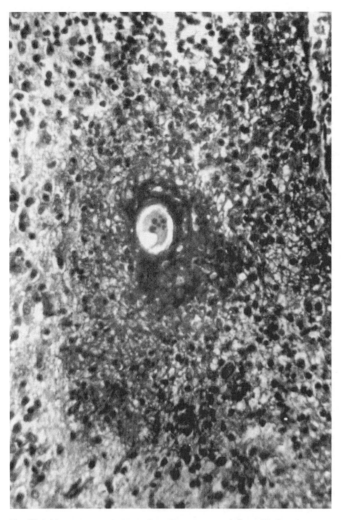

Fig. 13.4 Hyperacute experimental autoimmune encephalomyelitis in a rat. A ring hemorrhage associated with venous thrombosis is seen surrounding the venule at the center of the photomicrograph. Red blood cells and granulocytes are distributed around the vessel. (Courtesy of Dr Seymour Levine.)

A final possibility is that viral infection of certain cells in the brain induces the expression of MHC Class II molecules, which along with viral antigen are necessary for the presentation of viral antigens to helper-inducer T lymphocytes. Some brain cells, such as astrocytes and microglia, can be induced to express MHC Class II molecules and act as antigen-presenting cells. It is known that exposure of astrocytes to measles virus or the JHM strain of mouse coronavirus can induce MHC Class II molecules. If such glial cells, primed to do so by a previous measles infection, present myelin antigens to T lymphocytes that would otherwise not be stimulated or activated, the stage would be set for an indirect virus-induced demyelination (ter Meulen, 1989).

It is certainly possible that different mechanisms could be involved with different types of triggers and in different patients. The possibilities mentioned above are certainly not mutually exclusive.

Some clues to the pathogenesis can be obtained from studies of post-measles ADEM and post-rabies vaccination encephalomyelitis. In one study of measles patients in Peru (Johnson et al., 1984), the proliferative responses of blood lymphocytes to MBP from patients with post-measles ADEM were compared with those from patients with uncomplicated measles or with other neurologic diseases, and normal control subjects. The ADEM lymphocytes showed statistically significantly higher reactivity to

MBP than those from the other patient groups. Such T-cell responses were also seen in individual patients with post-rabies vaccination ADEM, post-varicella cerebellar ataxia, and seizures and stupor occurring after rubella (Johnson et al., 1984). In no patient was there intrathecal synthesis of antimeasles antibody. In another study (Griffin et al., 1989), the concentration of soluble CD8 (a measure of immune activation of cytotoxic and/or suppressor T cells) was measured in CSF samples obtained from patients with post-measles ADEM and compared with those of control groups with CNS infections and peripheral neuropathy. There was again a statistically significant increase in the levels of soluble CD8 in the CSF from post-measles ADEM patients compared with those in the other groups. In another study, patients with ADEM after vaccination with Semple rabies vaccine were compared with vaccinated control subjects without neurologic disease and unvaccinated rabies patients (Hemachudha et al., 1987a). In this study, three (50%) of the six ADEM patients had lymphocytes showing proliferative responses to MBP. No lymphocytes from vaccinated control subjects had such responses. Lymphoproliferation was also seen in 40% (2/5) of unvaccinated rabies patients, however. The results of both these studies are consistent with ADEM being a cell-mediated immune disease. However, unlike in EAE, it has not been proved that the cell-mediated immunity in human ADEM is a cause rather than an effect.

Indeed, there may be a role for humoral immunity to play in ADEM. A study comparing patients who had major neurologic complications (mostly ADEM, and GBS in a few) after vaccination with Semple rabies vaccine with vaccinated control subjects (who did receive Semple rabies vaccine but who did not develop ADEM) found that the levels of serum and CSF antibodies to MBP were higher in the patients (both ADEM and GBS) than the control subjects (Hemachudha et al., 1987b). This is not unprecedented, as in some animal models of EAE, the superimposition of a humoral response (by injection of anti-MOG antibody) on a cell-mediated response enhances the severity and demyelination of the resulting EAE, and some animal species may have involvement of both T- and B-cell responses to EAE (Alvord et al., 1992). Furthermore, some cases of ADEM are triggered by bacterial organisms, such as group A β-hemolytic streptococcus (see below), which mainly incite a humoral immune response (Dale et al., 2001). Also, there has been at least one reasonably well-documented response to plasmapheresis in an ADEM patient, after failure of high-dose intravenous methylprednisolone (Shah et al., 2000). Finally, in a recently published study of the use of plasmapheresis in fulminant demyelinating diseases of the central nervous system (in which patients with MS, ADEM, myelopathy, and so forth were entered), there was some evidence of response of the disease to this modality (Weinshenker et al., 1999). Since plasmapheresis would be expected to affect humoral immune factors more than cell-mediated immunity, it suggests the involvement of more than cell-mediated immunity in the pathogenesis of ADEM. Finally, a systematic pathologic study of 396 demyelinating lesions in MS patients showed several subtypes of myelin damage, one of which was attributed to the direct effects of antibody and activated complement on myelin, in which IgG and complement deposition was located at the sites of maximal myelin damage (Lucchinetti et al., 2000). These antibody-dependent ('Pattern 2') lesions were stated to resemble those seen in the anti-MOG-mediated EAE model mentioned above.

All the viral infections and vaccines that have a proven or highly likely link to ADEM involve enveloped viruses. The implications of this observation are unclear. However, the literature reports myelitis, along with some brainstem signs, occurring in a patient about 2 or 3 weeks after an episode of acute hepatitis A (a member of the picornavirus family, which are not enveloped) (Tyler et al., 1986). Whether this myelitis occurred as a result of direct infection or post-infectious demyelination was not determinable from the case narrative. It is known that many picornaviruses are neurotropic. However, in many patients with ADEM following non-specific upper respiratory infections or gastroenteritis, a specific diagnosis of a virus is never made, and it is possible that adenoviruses and enteroviruses (neither of which are enveloped) may trigger ADEM. The 'classic' triggering viruses, such as measles, cause illnesses that have very characteristic clinical presentations and findings, and are thus easy to diagnose. Since illnesses caused by enteroviruses and adenoviruses are non-specific, there may be an ascertainment bias in favor of enveloped viruses. However, that said, there is still no well-documented case of a non-enveloped virus triggering ADEM.

Diagnosis

The diagnosis rests on a compatible clinical picture of an acute or subacute febrile neurologic illness, frequently with alterations in mental status, occurring following a non-specific viral (or other) illness or immunization, along with characteristic findings. Therefore, it is often difficult to diagnose. There is no definitive laboratory test for ADEM or AHLE, short of biopsy. Usually there are no systemic findings in ADEM, while in AHLE there may be an acute phase reaction, with a significantly increased erythrocyte sedimentation rate (ESR), increased C-reactive protein value, and proteinuria (Lisak, 1994). Acute transverse myelitis, optic neuritis, and cerebellar ataxia also have a fairly rapid onset, with characteristic findings on examination, and each has a list of other possible diagnoses to be ruled out, because the alternative diagnosis of spinal cord compression is a neurologic emergency and demands immediate definitive therapy. Other conditions that generally need to be considered include syphilis, acute viral infections, systemic collagen vascular disease, CNS vasculitis (occasionally), and (rarely) vitamin B_{12} deficiency, all of which can affect both the optic nerve and spinal cord simultaneously or sequentially. Devic's syndrome can be the presentation of ADEM.

Electroencephalography and evoked potentials

There are no specific changes on the EEG. The EEG usually shows non-specific generalized slowing, often with high voltage, and asymmetry (Ziegler, 1966), and appears to correlate with disease activity. In a series of 84 pediatric patients with ADEM, 51 had EEGs done during the acute illness (Tenembaum et al., 2002). Forty (78%) of these patients showed diffuse slowing, five (10%) had focal slowing, and one (2%) had focal temporal spikes. Interestingly, five patients had normal EEGs.

In a series of patients with acute transverse myelopathy (Ropper et al., 1982), evoked potential testing showed abnormal somatosensory evoked potentials from peroneal but not from median nerve stimulation, as one would expect from disease in the thoracic region of the cord, which is the most commonly involved level. Other modalities, such as visual evoked potentials and brainstem auditory evoked potentials, were normal in patients with acute transverse myelitis (Ropper et al., 1982). At the same time, 72% of MS patients had at least one abnormality in the battery of somatosensory, brainstem auditory, and visual evoked potentials (Ropper et al., 1982). Thus, an evoked potential battery frequently showed at least one abnormality in MS patients while there were few or no abnormalities (other than somatosensory evoked potentials) in patients with acute transverse myelitis (Ropper et al., 1982).

Cerebrospinal fluid

The CSF findings are often abnormal in ADEM and AHLE but non-specific. In ADEM, there is often a mild mononuclear pleocytosis, with a mild elevation in protein concentration, but the cell count and protein values are normal in approximately one-third of patients (Miller et al., 1956). In one well-studied series of 18 patients with post-measles ADEM, eight (44%) patients had elevated CSF protein levels (although most of these were <100 mg/dl) and 13 (72%) had a lymphocytic pleocytosis (although most of those had fewer than 100 cells/µl) (Johnson et al., 1984). There may be abnormalities of immunoglobulins and increased MBP (a non-specific indicator of damage to myelin) in a subset of patients, but in a measles ADEM study only one of 12 patients had an increased CSF IgG index (Johnson et al., 1984). In one study of adult patients with ADEM, 65% were reported to have CSF oligoclonal bands (Schwarz et al., 2001). In the group

who developed MS, 11/14 (80%) had CSF oligoclonal bands, while 15/26 (58%) in the pure ADEM did. These proportions were not statistically significantly different in the two groups. The proportion of ADEM patients with CSF oligoclonal bands was rather higher than would ordinarily be expected. The reasons for this are unknown, but may involve a high-risk population. Pediatric ADEM patients tend not to have oligoclonal bands in the CSF. In a study of 84 pediatric patients with ADEM, only 28% had CSF abnormalities, with either lymphocytic pleocytosis (<180 cells/µl) or increased protein (Tenembaum et al., 2002). No oligoclonal bands were seen in the CSF in 96% of patients, while in the 4% in which these were present, the patients had a preceding herpes simplex encephalitis. Increased myelin basic protein was found in only 11% of the patients. In a study of 31 pediatric ADEM patients in Australia, CSF was obtained in 29, with pleocytosis present in 18 patients, 90% of whom had 52 white blood cells (WBCs)/µl or less (Hynson et al., 2001). The highest cell count was 268 WBCs/µl. Most cells were lymphocytes. Only one patient (3%) had oligoclonal bands present in the CSF.

In AHLE, there is often a neutrophilic pleocytosis and erythrocytes in the CSF. The protein concentration is usually increased; in 25% of patients it is more than 200 mg/dl, with levels as high as 1000 mg/dl. In about 10% of reported patients with AHLE, the CSF is entirely normal (Byers, 1975). It should be noted that an illness of fever, encephalopathy, focal neurologic findings, pleocytosis, and red blood cells in the CSF is also compatible with acute herpes encephalitis.

In a series (Lipton and Teasdall, 1973) of 30 patients with acute transverse myelitis, 14 had a normal CSF cell count and protein level. Ten patients had an elevated CSF protein concentration and 15 had pleocytosis. Determinations of the CSF IgG concentration and IgG index in 16 patients showed elevations in six patients. Oligoclonal bands were found in one of 13 CSF samples tested for this abnormality. In another study (Ropper and Poskanzer, 1978) of 52 patients with transverse myelitis, 18 had pleocytosis of more than four cells, with six patients having between 200 and 300 white blood cells. All instances of pleocytosis resolved in 3 months. Furthermore, 18 of the patients had an increased CSF protein level (50 mg/dl), with the highest level being 203 mg/dl. The CSF IgG was more than 12% of the protein in six of the 12 patients in which this was tested during the acute illness.

In optic neuritis, pleocytosis is not uncommon, being present in eight of 21 patients with the isolated disease (Kriss et al. 1988) in the Great Ormond Street study. In that series, only five of the 21 patients had an isolated increased CSF protein level, without pleocytosis. In 11 of the 21 patients, the CSF was entirely normal. In another study from Finland of patients with optic neuritis, most were found to have mild pleocytosis at onset, as well as oligoclonal bands and an increased IgG index. However, the numbers from that study were a little difficult to interpret because the series had an admixture of MS patients (Riikonen et al., 1988). Of 25 Swedish patients with isolated optic neuritis, 15 (60%) had mononuclear pleocytosis, six (24%) had an increased protein level, six (24%) had oligoclonal bands, and four (16%) had an elevated relative IgG index. The pleocytosis was never very great, with a maximum of 30 cells in one patient, and consisted mostly of lymphocytes. In another series of 48 Finnish patients (Nikoskelainen et al., 1981) with optic neuritis, 24 (50%) had a WBC count of more than 5 cells/µl. In a more recent study (Rolak et al., 1996) of 457 optic neuritis patients, the CSF was examined in 83 patients. A pleocytosis of 6 cells/µl or higher was seen in 30 (36%) of the patients but the highest count was 27 cells/µl. Oligoclonal bands were seen in 38 (50%) of the 76 patients in whom this was tested. Increased IgG synthesis rates were noted in 10 (43%) of the 23 patients tested, and IgG indices were elevated in 10 (22%) of the 46 patients in whom this was tested. However, it is difficult to tell what biases might be present, because not all patients in this study had CSF testing.

Neuroimaging

Computed tomography (CT) scans of the brain may show hypodense white matter lesions, occasionally with mass effect, sometimes with enhancement (see Fig. 13.5). Often, the CT scans appear unremarkable in ADEM and

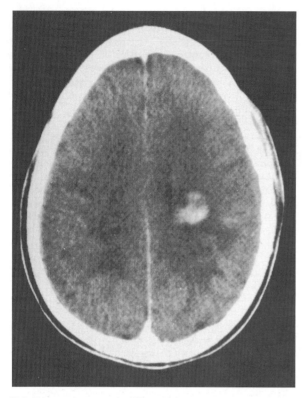

Fig. 13.5 Computed tomography (CT) scan of acute disseminated encephalomyelitis showing enhancing lesions in the deep white matter of the left hemisphere.

therefore are not very sensitive. In one series of 11 patients, four had normal-appearing brain CT scans, while seven had abnormalities that included cortical enhancing lesions, lucencies in the deep white matter and basal ganglia, and edema of the brainstem (Lukes and Norman, 1983). The initial brain CT scan often appeared normal, with abnormalities developing several days after the beginning of the clinical illness. The correlation between the CT abnormalities and clinical findings was limited (Lukes and Norman, 1983). One patient with autopsy-confirmed ADEM had a large area of hypodensity in the white matter with no mass effect and no enhancement (Loizou and Cole, 1982). In three patients with biopsy-proved AHLE, brain CT revealed white matter hypodensities and enhancement in only one lesion in one patient (Valentine *et al.*, 1982). The results were similar in an autopsied subject: an area of non-enhancing white matter hypodensity, with mass effect, corresponding to the findings of edema with petechial hemorrhages and congested vessels (Watson *et al.*, 1984). In a pathologically confirmed case of AHLE, confluent white matter lesions were noted asymmetrically in the subcortical white matter extending from the ependyma to the gray–white junction (Kuperan *et al.*, 2003). In one patient with a stuttering course of ADEM, the findings on serial brain CT paralleled the clinical state (Walker and Gawler, 1989). This was a 7-year-old girl who developed spastic weakness in the right leg after an upper respiratory tract infection. She was treated with low-dose prednisone. About 6 weeks later, this weakness had resolved and was replaced by right upper extremity weakness. She improved over the next 2 weeks, but then bulbar weakness developed with increased lower extremity tone. Dramatic improvement occurred with prednisone, and symptoms did not recur after the prednisone dose was tapered over the next few months. At the time of each new deficit, brain CT showed enlargements of the old and the emergence of new lesions. The CT abnormalities had completely disappeared by the time of the follow-up examination, when the clinical deficits had completely resolved. In another report of two patients with AHLE, serial brain CT again showed findings that paralleled the patient's state (Sucherowsky *et al.*, 1983).

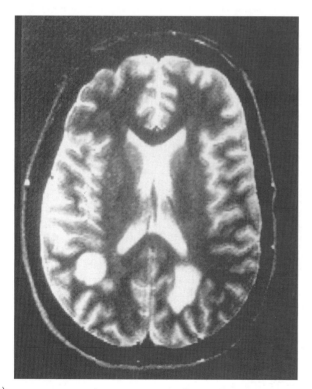

(a)

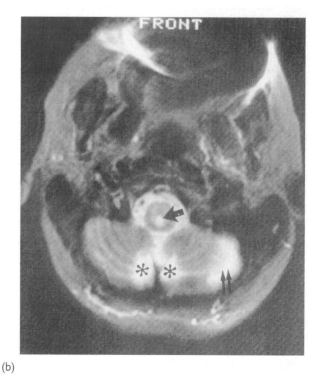

(b)

Fig. 13.6 (a) T_2-weighted MRI of the brain showing bilateral areas of increased intensity in white matter of the occipital lobe on the left and parietal lobe on the right. (b) Proton density-weighted image showing areas of abnormally increased signal in the brainstem (thick arrow), the cerebellar vermis bilaterally (asterisks), and left cerebellar hemisphere (double arrows).

MRI of the brain is a useful technique and shows multiple prominent white matter lesions, with increased signal on T_2-weighted images (Figs 13.6(a) and 13.7) and proton density-weighted images (Fig. 13.6(b)) and decreased signal on T_1-weighted images (Fig. 13.8), the latter often enhancing after administration of diethylenetriamine-pentaacetic acid gadolinium (see Fig. 13.8) (Atlas *et al.*, 1986; Epperson *et al.*, 1988; Caldemeyer

et al., 1991). The lesions as seen by MRI may vary in size, even in the same patient, and tend to be larger than the pathologic lesions, most likely due to surrounding edema (Fig. 13.9). Hyperintense lesions on T_2-weighted images (Fig. 13.10) and enhancing lesions on T_1-weighted images (Fig. 13.11) can be quite small and diffuse. In two children with ADEM,

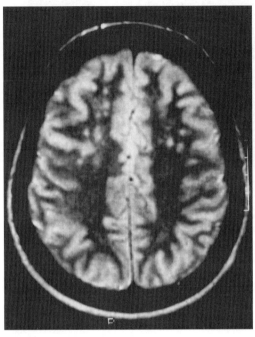

Fig. 13.7 Multiple small areas of abnormally increased signal in the white matter of the frontal lobe bilaterally, in a T_2-weighted image.

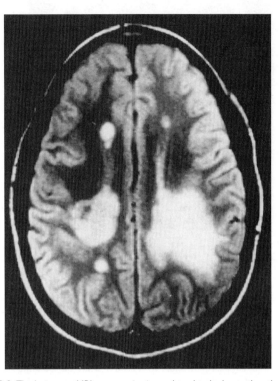

Fig. 13.9 The lesions on MRI may vary in size and tend to be larger than the pathologic lesions, most likely because of the surrounding edema as seen in the areas of increased signal on the proton-density weighted image. Note the penetration of the edema along the white matter tracts, especially in the left hemisphere.

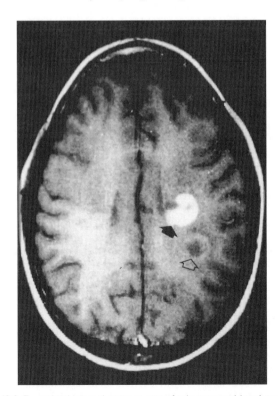

Fig. 13.8 T_1-weighted image showing an area of enhancement (closed arrow) and an area of decreased intensity (open arrow) in a patient with acute disseminated encephalomyelitis.

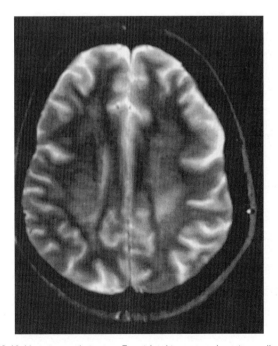

Fig. 13.10 Hyperintense lesions on T_2-weighted images can be quite small and diffuse (arrows).

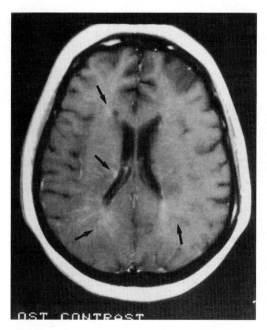

Fig. 13.11 Enhancing lesions on T_1-weighted images can be quite small and diffuse (arrows).

both T_1- and T_2-weighted MRIs of the brain showed multiple white matter abnormalities (Perdue *et al.*, 1985). These tended to resolve with clinical improvement. MRI often shows abnormal signal in the deep gray matter structures such as the thalamus and basal ganglia. In one study of 31 pediatric ADEM patients, 32% had an abnormal signal in the thalamus and 39% in the basal ganglia (Hynson *et al.*, 2001).

In acute transverse myelitis, the cord is often enlarged, sometimes with patchy areas of decreased signal on T_1-weighted images (Fig. 13.12) and increased signal on T_2-weighted images (Fig. 13.13), as well as diffuse or patchy areas of enhancement (Figs 13.14(a) and (b)) (Sanders *et al.*, 1990; Holtas *et al.*, 1993). Cord enlargement can occur in the absence of increased

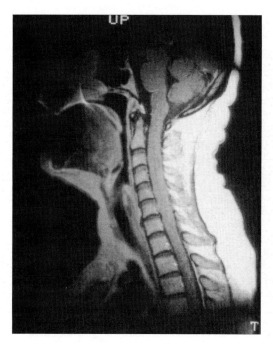

Fig. 13.12 In acute transverse myelitis, the cord is often enlarged, sometimes with patchy areas of decreased signal (arrows), as on this T_1-weighted image.

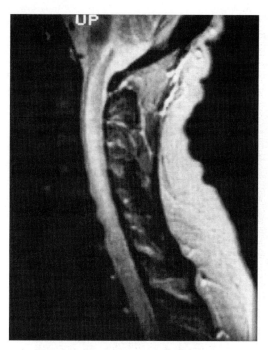

Fig. 13.13 In a patient with acute transverse myelitis, T_2-weighted MRIs may show patchy and diffuse areas of increased signal.

signal on T_2-weighted images (Merine *et al.*, 1987). In one series of seven patients with acute transverse myelopathy (Holtas *et al.*, 1993), the degree of cord enlargement, persistence of increased signal intensity, and poor outcome were correlated. Cord atrophy and persisting increased signal in the cord on late MRIs suggested that further recovery was unlikely (Holtas *et al.*, 1993). The difficulty with this last series, however, is that two of these patients had systemic lupus erythematosus, one had sarcoidosis, and one had giant cell arteritis. Therefore, what the results of that study mean for acute transverse myelitis and ADEM are unclear. The MRI findings of two patients with ADEM (including spinal cord involvement) following *Mycoplasma pneumoniae* infection were reported by Francis *et al.* (1988). These showed scattered multifocal lesions of the white matter during a work-up of acute neurologic symptoms that followed *M. pneumoniae*-associated upper respiratory tract illnesses (Francis *et al.*, 1988). In one of the patients, who was quadriplegic and ventilator dependent, MRI showed an atrophic cervical region of the cord late in the illness, as well as scattered lesions in the cerebral white matter.

In a review of 84 cases of ADEM in a pediatric population, Tenembaum *et al.* (2002) divided the brain MRI appearances into four groups: (1) small (<5 mm) lesions in 62%; (2) large confluent white matter lesions, some with 'tumor-like appearance' asymmetrically placed in 24%; (3) symmetric bithalamic involvement in 12% (small lesions in half of these patients, large lesions in the other half); and (4) acute hemorrhagic encephalomyelitis. An interesting observation was that the patients with symmetric bithalamic involvement did not have 'extrapyramidal' signs (such as rigidity or tremor or dystonia) but that those with asymmetric involvement of the thalamus or basal ganglia did, in four out of 12 (67%) cases (Fig. 13.15).

Therapy

There have been no clinical trials of any proposed therapies for this disease, and so there is no proven specific therapy. Symptomatic and supportive therapy is important, as many patients will recover meaningful function if they survive the acute illness. Clearly, reduction of a malignant fever, maintenance of vital functions (including intubation for respiratory or bulbar compromise) and fluid and electrolyte balance, nutrition, avoidance of decubiti and urinary tract infections, and treatment of seizures are import-

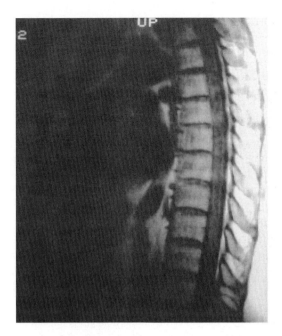

(a)

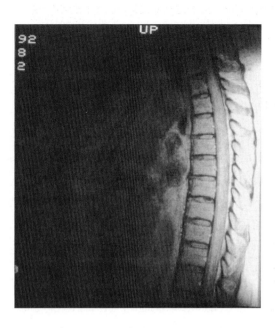

(b)

Fig. 13.14 Enhancement of the spinal cord in a patient with acute transverse myelitis on T_1-weighted images may be diffuse or patchy. (a) This pre-contrast T_1-weighted image of the thoracic region of the spinal cord in a patient with transverse myelitis shows areas of patchy diffuse decreased signal. (b) This post-contrast image of the same spinal cord shows diffuse enhancement. Note how the enhancement effaces the patchy abnormalities seen on the non-contrast image.

ant. Treatment of cerebral edema (by hyperventilation and the use of osmotic agents) is important if there is a threat of herniation of brain matter from one intracranial compartment to another, especially if vital brainstem centers are involved. Rehabilitation and physical therapy are important in the recovery phase.

Corticosteroids

The rationale for the use of corticosteroids is that they decrease edema, reduce inflammation, and restore the blood–brain barrier (thus reducing the diffusion of plasma proteins and migration of additional activated immune cells into the brain). Many neurologists treat patients with pulse doses of intravenous corticosteroids and then discharge them on a schedule to taper the oral prednisone doses (Lisak, 1994). Very good responses have been reported (Pasternak *et al.*, 1980), but these remain anecdotal. In a few patients improvement was seen during the administration of corticosteroids, with worsening occurring when the drugs were discontinued and improvement occurring when the drugs were reinstituted, which suggests strongly that corticosteroids do have a genuine effect (Ziegler, 1966). Patients with AHLE may also respond to corticosteroids (Byers, 1975). In a

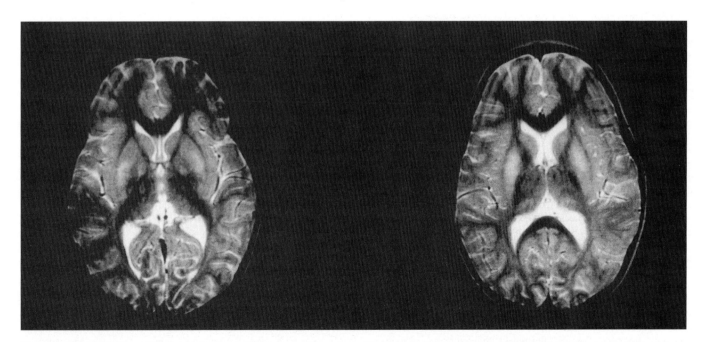

Fig. 13.15 MRI of ADEM in a child, showing increased signal in the caudate nucleus of the basal ganglia bilaterally. (Courtesy, Dr L Zhou, Department of Neurology, Wayne State University.)

series of 121 non-randomized pediatric patients with ADEM, 43 were treated with corticosteroids and the others were not. Of those treated with steroids, onset of improvement occurred in 5.46 days, while in the others, improvement began in 15.6 days. The time to maximal recovery was no different between the two groups (Rust *et al.*, 1997). The results are difficult to interpret, since patients were not randomized, and the authors state that the steroid-treated group tended to have more severe illness. However, it is important to be aware that no studies have been done formally to show efficacy.

Plasmapheresis

A few reports on the use of plasmapheresis for ADEM described dramatic recovery in some patients (Newton, 1981; Cotter *et al.*, 1983; Seales and Greer, 1991; Stricker *et al.*, 1992). However, some of these patients (Seales and Greer, 1991) were simultaneously treated with other immunosuppressive therapies, such as corticosteroids and cyclophosphamide. In two patients, there appeared to be improvement with plasmapheresis after there was no immediate response to high-dose corticosteroids (Kanter *et al.*, 1995). It is possible that the response ascribed to the plasmapheresis might have been a delayed response to the corticosteroids or spontaneous improvement. Furthermore, a series of six patients who had fulminant MS relapses, confirmed by biopsy, and who were unresponsive to high-dose intravenous methylprednisolone, improved dramatically after one or two courses of plasmapheresis (Rodriguez *et al.*, 1993). Again, the same caveat applies.

More recently, there has been some suggestive evidence for the beneficial role of plasmapheresis in the treatment of corticosteroid-unresponsive CNS demyelination. In the case of a pregnant woman with subacute multifocal neurological deficits, including a bilateral optic neuritis, right-sided weakness, mid-thoracic sensory level and urinary difficulty, occurring 2 weeks after a mild gastroenteritis, MRI of the brain showed multiple white matter lesions (Shah *et al.*, 2000). Intravenous methylprednisolone had no effect, and indeed the patient progressed to severe bilateral loss of vision (to hand motion only) and difficulty with ambulation. She was started on plasmapheresis, after giving birth to a healthy baby boy, and improved markedly, almost back to baseline, with visual acuity of 20/25 bilaterally (although there were significant visual field defects), after the second session (of a total of five sessions of 2.5 l exchanged each session). Five days after completing the plasmapheresis, her vision again deteriorated to hand motion in the right eye and 20/200 in the left. Another course of plasmapheresis was instituted (six exchanges), with improvement in vision. Again, there was deterioration of vision a week after the second course of pheresis was completed and again further pheresis resulted in improvement to near normal visual acuity. The patient was put on maintenance plasmapheresis, weekly for 4 weeks, every other week for four treatments, and every month for three treatments. Improvement in visual acuity was sustained. This case illustrates the potential benefit of plasmapheresis in ADEM, since the patient served as her own control.

Also, a recent trial of plasmapheresis was published in which 22 patients with severe acute inflammatory central demyelination were randomized to true or sham plasmapheresis after failing high-dose intravenous methylprednisolone (or equivalent corticosteroid) (Weinshenker *et al.*, 1999). The treatment consisted of seven exchanges every 2 days. Twelve of the patients had MS (group A) and the other 10 (group B) had various demyelinating diseases (transverse myelitis four, ADEM one, Marburg variant of MS one, neuromyelitis optica two, recurrent myelitis one, and focal cerebral demyelination one). Patients who had significantly improved clinically after the first (true or sham pheresis) treatment (phase 1) received no further treatment, while those who were no better were crossed over to the other arm (phase 2, sham or true pheresis, respectively). Regarding patients in phase 1 only, 5/11 on active pheresis improved while only 1/11 on sham pheresis did so, with a trend to statistical significance ($P = 0.0743$). If considered on the basis of all sessions of 2-week courses of pheresis, 8/19 (42.1%) improved on true pheresis versus 1/17 (5.9%) on sham pheresis, again a suggestive trend. The main difficulties with interpreting the results of this study are that multiple different demyelinating diseases, with differ-

ent pathogeneses, are being compared and it is not clear that what works for some of these entities works for others.

The rationale for plasmapheresis appears to be that it has efficacy in GBS, an acute or subacute demyelinating disease of the peripheral nervous system, and that a circulating factor may have some role in its pathogenesis (Guillain–Barré Syndrome Study Group, 1985; Stricker *et al.*, 1992). On the other hand, GBS and ADEM are different diseases. In GBS, humorally mediated mechanisms are likely to be at least as important as cell-mediated ones, and in some varieties of GBS more important, whereas ADEM is likely mostly cell mediated, although a humoral component may be important in some cases. Given some of the reported improvements, plasmapheresis is reasonable to try when more conventional therapy with corticosteroids fails, recognizing that improvement is not proof of efficacy.

Other modalities

Multiple other treatments have been tried at one time or another. A patient with progressive gait difficulty, fever, somnolence, and anorexia with onset a week after a non-specific viral syndrome was treated with intravenous immunoglobulin at a dose of 400 mg/kg for 5 days and showed clear clinical improvement within 24 h. MRI showed the typical white matter lesions (Kleiman and Brunquell, 1995). There was virtually complete resolution of his clinical deficits 6 days after the intravenous immunoglobulin was started. The MRI abnormalities also resolved 6 months later.

Another patient developed increasing headache and white matter abnormalities on MRI after a bout of viral meningitis. CSF analysis demonstrated pleocytosis and the EEG was abnormal. He had intermittent episodes of delirium and psychosis. The response to dexamethasone (Decadron) was remarkable, and the dose was tapered. Several weeks later, he had a relapse, which responded to methylprednisolone. Further relapses were accompanied by increasing MRI white matter abnormalities, and responded to corticosteroids. One episode consisted of a mass lesion, the biopsy of which revealed demyelination. He was then started on intravenous immunoglobulin, 400 mg/kg every month, and had no further episodes for the next 6 months (Hahn *et al.*, 1996). Other reports of the apparent efficacy of intravenous immunoglobulin have appeared (Pradhan *et al.*, 1999; Straussberg *et al.*, 2001), but most of these patients also received intravenous corticosteroids, and no controlled trials have been done.

A patient with apparent ADEM characterized by progressive spastic paraparesis, ataxia, and dysarthria over 5 months (Salazar *et al.*, 1981) had a mild-to-moderate pleocytosis with increased protein, MBP, and IgG values as well as five oligoclonal bands in the CSF. He was treated with high-dose prednisone, without response. He was then put on polyinosinic–polycytidylic acid–polylysine stabilized with carboxymethylcellulose (poly-ICLC) and the prednisone dose was tapered. His improvement was remarkable. Poly-ICLC is a potent interferon inducer and probably has immunomodulating effects, but the nature of these is unclear. Furthermore, the nature of this patient's illness is not completely clear, as the presentation was rather atypical.

In another report (Abramsky *et al.*, 1977), three patients with ADEM were treated with copolymer-1 (now called glatiramer acetate), which had previously been shown to prevent or improve EAE (Teitelbaum *et al.*, 1971), and all three had a complete recovery within 3 weeks, although this would not be totally unexpected without treatment, given the natural history of the disease.

Finally, hypothermia has been tried in a man with ADEM and refractory brain edema. The patient developed fever, confusion, and multifocal neurological deficits following an upper respiratory infection due to *M. pneumoniae*. MRI of the brain showed abnormal white matter. CSF exam showed a pleocytosis of 1429 WBCs/μl, and moderately increased CSF protein. The patient became progressively more comatose despite intravenous prednisolone and decompressive craniectomy. He was treated with hypothermia because of its possible anti-edema and anti-inflammatory effects. His vital signs became stabilized. Rewarming resulted in further deterioration, with stabilization on repeat cooling. Eventually, the patient could be rewarmed but had severe residual deficits (Takata *et al.*, 1999).

There is no way to fully evaluate these therapeutic modalities short of a controlled clinical trial.

Relationship of acute disseminated encephalomyelitis and restricted syndromes to multiple sclerosis

The isolated syndromes of acute optic neuritis, transverse myelitis, and acute cerebellar ataxia, which can occur in association with or following a viral illness or vaccination, and in which there is inflammatory white matter involvement, have an uncertain relation to ADEM (Lisak, 1994). Some of these syndromes are clearly manifestations of other autoimmune diseases, and some new associations have been described recently. In two patients, recurrent episodes of acute optic neuritis and transverse myelitis, responsive to corticosteroids, recurred for years. Their illnesses were believed to be consistent with MS, until high antinuclear antibody (ANA) titers developed in both and multiorgan disease in one, years after the onset of the neurological symptoms (Kira and Goto, 1994). However, a coincidence of two diseases was not ruled out and patients with MS may have elevated ANA titers (Dore-Duffy et al., 1982; Barned et al., 1995). Another patient with long-standing ulcerative colitis developed transverse myelitis. Work-up showed a lesion in the cervical region of the spinal cord and smaller lesions in the brain. She was thought to have MS until dermatomyositis and fibrosing alveolitis developed; the Jo-1 serum antibody titer was positive (Ray et al., 1994). The occurrence of more than one immunopathologic disorder in an individual patient is always a possibility. Indeed there is abundant evidence for such concordance in the literature (Seyfert et al., 1990).

The precise relation of the various forms of ADEM (including isolated demyelinative syndromes not otherwise linked with systemic autoimmune disease) to MS is unknown (Hartung and Grossman, 2001). It is clear that some patients with ADEM eventually develop MS, but the proportion is not known exactly. The data from older studies are conflicting. In a series of 27 (of 34) surviving patients with ADEM, acute transverse myelitis, and neuromyelitis optica, MS had not developed by follow-up, over an average of several years, although there were a few recurrences reproducing the original illness (Miller and Evans, 1953). In another study, roughly one-quarter of 29 patients with acute disseminated encephalomyelitis went on to develop MS (Thygesen, 1949). However, this study was done in Denmark, where the prevalence of MS is extremely high, and so it is difficult to generalize this result to other populations. A study of 86 Swedish patients with isolated optic neuritis showed that abnormal CSF, defined as the presence of pleocytosis or oligoclonal banding, was predictive of the development of MS (Sandberg-Wollheim et al., 1990). In that study, 64% of the patients with normal CSF were free of MS at 15 years of follow-up, as compared with 48% of the patients with abnormal CSF. Younger age at onset of optic neuritis and female gender also increased the risk of MS. The presence of HLA-DR2 also slightly increased the risk for developing MS. MRI data were not examined for their prognostic value in this study. In a more recent series of 40 adults with ADEM, also done in a high-risk area (Germany), 14 (35%) developed clinically definite MS after a mean period of 38 months (Schwarz et al., 2001). Risk factors for development of MS in this study were: younger age, absence of a prior, triggering infection, longer duration of symptoms before admission to hospital, and the presence of infratentorial lesions on MRI. In this study, the presence of oligoclonal bands in the CSF was not predictive of the subsequent development of MS. In another study of 121 pediatric ADEM patients, the risk of MS was highest in those with the illness occurring at age 12 years or more, those presenting with hemiparesis or a Devic's type syndrome, and those with an increased CSF IgG index (Rust et al., 1997).

Because optic neuritis is not rare, determining the relation of acute optic neuritis to subsequent MS takes on importance. In the Mayo Clinic study discussed previously (Rodriguez et al., 1995), the patients with isolated optic neuritis were analysed using life-table methods to find the risk for progression to MS. Of these patients, 39% had progressed to definite MS by 10 years of follow-up, 49% by 20 years, 54% by 30 years, and 60% by 40 years. Venous sheathing as seen on ophthalmoscopy and recurrent optic neuritis were risk factors for progression. Because CSF examinations were not done, the effect of the presence of oligoclonal bands on the risk of progression to MS could not be examined. Furthermore, brain MRI was not performed, and therefore the relative risk of progression to MS in those with abnormal appearing MRIs also could not be determined.

The results of the Optic Neuritis Treatment Trial are of interest and may have pathogenetic implications. This study examined how three regimens affecting visual function of a cohort of patients with acute optic neuritis (Optic Neuritis Study Group, 1992). The regimens were very high-dose intravenous methylprednisolone (1 g/day) followed by tapered doses of oral prednisone (beginning at 60 mg/day), a course of tapered doses of oral prednisone, and placebo designed to resemble the oral prednisone course. Patients were included if they showed signs of optic neuritis but had none of the systemic diseases associated with optic neuritis (such as syphilis or lupus erythematosus), although patients with MS were admitted to the study. The oral prednisone and placebo groups were double-blinded, but the intravenous methylprednisolone group had the fewest relapses, while the oral prednisone group had the most. In a post hoc analysis (Optic Neuritis Study Group, 1993), after patients with a diagnosis of MS at the time of randomization were excluded, the progression of the different groups to clinically definite MS was examined. The intravenous methylprednisolone group had the lowest rate of progression to MS. The entire cohort was stratified according to the lesion burden seen on cranial MRI, and those with the highest lesion burden had the greatest risk of progression to MS. When the intravenous methylprednisolone group was stratified according to the MRI lesion burden, the subgroup with the highest risk of progression had the most reduction in this risk. In the isolated optic neuritis subgroup, the MRI lesion burden was most predictive of progression to MS, with possibly a second independent contribution to the risk of progression from the presence of oligoclonal bands (Rolak et al., 1996).

It is possible that the apparent efficacy was only a reflection of the study design. It may reflect the ineffectiveness of the single-blind design (Silberberg, 1992) in masking who the intravenous methylprednisolone-treated patients were only from the study physicians. It is possible that placebo effects, which are known to be strong in MS, were sufficiently different in the intravenous methylprednisolone group to account for some of the effect (Silberberg, 1992). However, a real effect of the methylprednisolone on the evolution of the disease may also be occurring. A possible mechanism of such a long-term effect is as follows. In EAE, the range of epitopes on the MBP molecule recognized by T cells increases during the course of disease. Initially, only one or a very small number of epitopes is recognized by T cells. As an attack of the disease progresses, more and more epitopes on the MBP molecule are recognized. Also, the TCR gene usage to the myelin antigen broadens during the course of the disease, giving an increased number of distinct TCR molecules reacting to a specific epitope on MBP (and possible PLP and MOG). There is some evidence that similar dynamics take place in MS (Lehmann et al., 1992, 1993; Mor and Cohen, 1993; Cross et al., 1993; Sun et al., 1993). It is therefore possible that intravenous methylprednisolone had some effect in restricting the progressive broadening of the T-cell response (intra-antigen or interantigen determinant or epitope spreading), and therefore in inhibiting or delaying the subsequent waves of immune reactivity against other myelin antigens and epitopes, which would express clinically as attacks of MS (Lehmann et al., 1992, 1993). In EAE, clonotypic therapy started within the first 3 days can prevent or cure the disease (Lehmann et al., 1992). For optic neuritis in humans, all this is speculative, and if the phenomenon of delay of MS is real other effects of corticosteroids, such as effects on vascular endothelial cell activation (e.g. expression of intercellular adhesion molecules such as ICAM-1 and ICAM-2) need to be evaluated. A trial needs to be carried out to look specifically at the development of MS following treatment with intravenous methylprednisolone for isolated syndromes such as optic neuritis, brainstem events such as internuclear ophthalmoplegia, and myelitis (Silberberg, 1992). Unfortunately the trials of first attack of demyelinating disease likely to go on to develop MS (CHAMPS and ETOMS) did not include an arm with repeated doses of corticosteroid, to compare with low-dose interferon-β1a, in addition to the placebo arm.

In a study (Ford *et al.*, 1992) of partial acute transverse myelitis performed prospectively from 1985 to 1987 at the Montreal Neurological Institute, 15 patients with incomplete spinal cord involvement of at least one segment were evaluated and followed. Patients with identifiable causes were excluded, as were patients with complete quadriplegia or paraplegia or spinal shock. In this study, 12 patients (80%) progressed to clinically or laboratory-supported definite MS over an average follow-up time of 38.5 months. Of the patients with periventricular white matter abnormalities at onset, 93% were eventually diagnosed with definite MS.

In a study of patients with isolated brainstem or spinal cord demyelinating lesions (Miller *et al.*, 1989), evaluation included brain MRI as well as CSF examination, at onset. Of the 38 patients with a spinal cord syndrome (almost all of whom had an incomplete transverse myelopathy), 14 (42%) developed MS. The likelihood of progression to MS was strongest in those with disseminated involvement, as determined by MRI or clinical criteria or both (relative risk = 36), and with oligoclonal bands in the CSF (relative risk = 25). There appears to be a greater risk of progression to MS in patients with a partial transverse myelitis than in those with a complete transverse myelitis, in which all function below the involved spinal level is lost. Thus, an illness characterized by a fever, a depressed level of consciousness, and complete myelitis is unlikely to progress to MS (see below). This is especially likely to be true in patients with only a lesion in the spinal cord and none in the brain, as detected by MRI.

Another study (Morrisey *et al.*, 1993) examined the question of the relation of isolated demyelinative syndromes to the subsequent development of MS. This 5-year follow-up study examined what features (specifically, number of lesions on brain MRI, presence of CSF oligoclonal bands, and HLA haplotypes) present at the onset of an isolated optic nerve, brainstem, or spinal cord lesions were predictive of subsequent MS. The predictors, from strongest to weakest, were abnormal-appearing brain MRI, the presence of oligoclonal bands in the CSF, and the presence of the HLA-DR2 haplotype. There was a dose–response effect on the risk conferred by an abnormal MRI: of those with more than four lesions on MRI, 28 (85%) of 33 patients went on to develop clinically definite MS, whereas only one (17%) of six with a single lesion and only two (6%) of 32 with no lesions developed MS during the period of observation. In the three clinical groups, for patients with abnormal-appearing MRIs, those presenting with optic neuritis had the highest risk, and those with isolated spinal cord syndrome the lowest risk of developing MS. The overall risk ratio (RR) of an abnormal MRI versus a normal MRI was 38. The RR for the presence versus the absence of CSF oligoclonal bands was 5.2 and that for the presence versus the absence of HLA-DR2 was 3.2. While most study results suggest that MRI is the most useful predictor, there have been studies suggesting that oligoclonal bands may be at least as useful (Sandberg-Wollhheim *et al.*, 1990). The reason for this difference is unclear, but the magnetic field strength of the MRI apparatus used in the study by Sandberg-Wollhheim *et al.* (1990) was 0.3 T, while that used by Morrisey *et al.* (1993) was 0.5 T, which may account in part for the discrepancy, since the latter field strength would be somewhat more sensitive and reveal more lesions.

Some long-term data from the study of Brex *et al.* (2002) is of interest. In this study, 109 patients with isolated demyelinating lesions were evaluated by neurological and MRI examination at baseline, at 1 year (109 patients), at 5 years (89 patients), and at 10 years (81 patients). The initial and 5-year scans were done at 0.5 T, but the 10- and 14-year scans were done at 1.5 T. Some of the patients were further evaluated after 10 years, and 71 patients of the original cohort were followed for a mean of 14.1 years. At baseline, 21 patients had normal MRI scans, and only four (19%) of them developed clinically definite MS, over a median time of 7.5 years. Of 50 patients with an abnormal MRI at baseline, 44 (88%) developed clinical definite MS within a median time of 2 years. New lesions on subsequent MRIs were more common (98%) in patients destined to develop clinically definite MS

than those who did not (38%). The burden of disease on the MRI at baseline was predictive of the amount of disability at 14 years. This suggests that overall MRI abnormality (burden of lesions and presence of new lesions on follow-up scans) is predictive of the risk of developing MS, which corroborates the results of other studies quoted above, and the ultimate degree of disability.

Similar findings were observed in the 10-year follow-up study of 81 patients seen at Queen Square (O'Riordan *et al.*, 1998). Of the patients with an abnormal brain MRI at the onset of a clinically isolated demyelinating episode, 83% went on to develop MS, while only 11% of those with normal MRIs did. Of these latter patients, all had a benign form of the disease (relapsing–remitting with EDSS < 3). Of the patients with abnormal MRIs, a greater disease burden was predictive of greater severity of disease (EDSS) and type of disease (more often remitting relapsing with EDSS > 3 or secondary progressive rather than benign). The risk of progression to MS was found to be greater for optic neuritis (89%) and brainstem syndrome (91%) than myelopathy (67%).

A variant of optic neuritis is bilateral simultaneous optic neuritis. Since 1984, when a study at the Institute of Neurology at Queen Square was conducted (Parkin *et al.*, 1984), it has been thought that bilateral simultaneous optic neuritis led to MS only rarely in children and uncommonly in adults. In that study MS developed in only two of 11 adults with simultaneous bilateral optic neuritis, whereas it developed in eight of 20 with sequential optic neuritis. The children were followed for an average of 32 years while the adults were followed for an average of 37 years. A recent United Kingdom follow-up study of bilateral simultaneous optic neuritis analyzed 23 patients (Morrisey *et al.*, 1995). The entry criterion was acute (<14 days from onset to peak) or subacute (14–120 days from onset to peak) visual loss that occurred in both eyes simultaneously, defined as visual loss occurring in the two eyes within 2 weeks of each other. All patients had clinical assessments, brain MRI, HLA typing, and mitochondrial DNA analysis, and 50% had CSF electrophoresis. MS had developed in only five patients (22%) by the time of follow-up. MS had failed to develop in most patients (61%) after a mean follow-up of 50 months after the onset of bilateral simultaneous optic neuritis. These latter patients were found to have low rates of risk factors for the subsequent development of MS, such as multiple white matter abnormalities on brain MRI, HLA-DR15/DQw6 haplotype, and the presence of oligoclonal bands. Of interest is that four (17%) of the patients with bilateral simultaneous optic neuritis were found to have mitochondrial DNA point mutations indicating Leber's hereditary optic neuropathy. This study concluded that a lower proportion of patients with bilateral simultaneous optic neuritis than with acute unilateral optic neuritis proceed to develop MS. A significant proportion (about 20% of patients in the United Kingdom study) of patients with bilateral simultaneous optic neuritis have Leber's hereditary optic neuropathy.

As noted already, patients with complete transverse myelopathy do not seem to develop MS. In the Danish study discussed, of the 29 surviving patients who were followed for an average of 12 years (Christensen *et al.*, 1990), MS developed in only one (3%). In the Massachusetts General Hospital study (Ropper and Poskanzer, 1978), MS developed in seven (13%) of the 52 patients with acute transverse myelitis. On the other hand, in the Montreal Neurological Institute study (Ford *et al.*, 1992), 12 (80%) of 15 patients progressed to clinically or laboratory-supported definite MS over an average follow-up of 38.5 months. In the Queen Square study of patients with isolated brainstem or isolated spinal cord demyelinating lesions (Miller *et al.*, 1989), MS developed in 14 (42%) of 38 patients with transverse myelopathy. The reasons for the discrepancy among these studies are not completely clear, but may have to do with whether the study was prospective or retrospective, with whether the transverse myelopathy was complete (with total loss of neurological function below the affected level) or incomplete, and with different criteria for MS and follow-up times. Thus, some studies used both clinical and MRI criteria (Miller *et al.*, 1989; Ford *et al.*, 1992) for MS whereas others used only clinical criteria (Christensen *et al.*, 1990). Patients with complete transverse myelitis seem to be less likely to progress to MS.

It should be noted that the MRI appearances of both the brain (Kesselring *et al.*, 1990) and the spinal cord (Sze, 1992) can be very similar in ADEM and

MS. Furthermore, the multiple white matter abnormalities seen in the brain in normal ageing can superficially resemble those seen in multiple sclerosis. In a comparison of brain MRIs of 49 normal asymptomatic subjects with those of 50 MS patients, no areas of increased signal were noted in normal subjects aged less than 50 years, while multiple lesions were found in older normal subjects. Overall, MS patients had a larger number and size of lesions, which more frequently abutted the ventricles and were more frequently situated infratentorially than the normal healthy subjects (Fazekas *et al.*, 1988). For a positive MRI diagnosis of MS, the authors suggested that at least two of the following three criteria be satisfied: lesions have a size greater than 6 mm, abutting ventricular bodies, and infratentorial location, which had a sensitivity of 88% and a specificity of 100%. In a later study of 74 patients with clinically isolated syndromes, MRI characteristics predictive of MS were determined (Barkhof *et al.*, 1997). The criteria found to be most significant were: presence of juxtacortical lesions, gadolinium enhancement, periventricular lesions, and infratentorial lesions. The observed risk of development of clinically definite MS, with a median follow-up of 9 months, depended on the number of criteria satisfied: 16% with one criterion, 11% with two criteria, 54% with three, 75% with four, and 87% with five.

Recurrent and relapsing acute disseminated encephalomyelitis

A rare recurrent illness, which has been called multiphasic disseminated encephalomyelitis (MDEM), has been described for both ADEM (Alcock and Hoffman, 1962; Durston and Milnes, 1970; Poser *et al.*, 1978) and AHLE (Lamarche *et al.*, 1972), but more recent reports suggest that such recurrences are not so rare, particularly in children. In a series of 48 children with disseminated inflammatory CNS disease seen at the Great Ormond Street Hospital between 1985 and 1999, seven (15%) satisfied the criteria of MDEM, which is defined as a recurrence of the original ADEM illness immediately after full or partial resolution of the ADEM (Dale *et al.*, 2000). In another series of 84 children with ADEM seen at the National Pediatric Hospital in Buenos Aires, Argentina between 1988 and 2000, 10% had a biphasic course (Tenembaum *et al.*, 2002). In a series of 31 pediatric ADEM cases, definite relapses were reported to occur in four patients (Hynson *et al.*, 2001). Finally, in a large series reported in abstract form, 39 out of 121 patients developed recurrences of their ADEM (Rust *et al.*, 1997). In adults, MDEM remains apparently uncommon and was present in only one (2%)

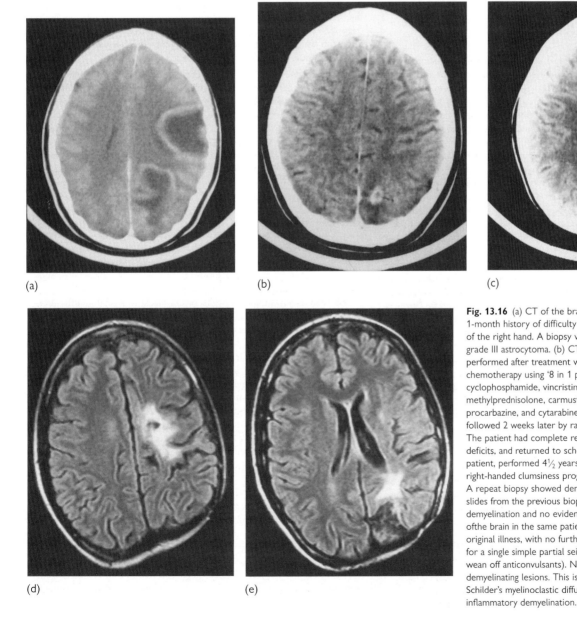

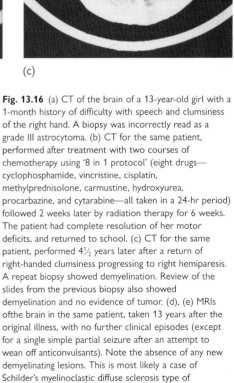

Fig. 13.16 (a) CT of the brain of a 13-year-old girl with a 1-month history of difficulty with speech and clumsiness of the right hand. A biopsy was incorrectly read as a grade III astrocytoma. (b) CT for the same patient, performed after treatment with two courses of chemotherapy using '8 in 1 protocol' (eight drugs—cyclophosphamide, vincristine, cisplatin, methylprednisolone, carmustine, hydroxyurea, procarbazine, and cytarabine—all taken in a 24-hr period) followed 2 weeks later by radiation therapy for 6 weeks. The patient had complete resolution of her motor deficits, and returned to school. (c) CT for the same patient, performed 4½ years later after a return of right-handed clumsiness progressing to right hemiparesis. A repeat biopsy showed demyelination. Review of the slides from the previous biopsy also showed demyelination and no evidence of tumor. (d), (e) MRIs of the brain in the same patient, taken 13 years after the original illness, with no further clinical episodes (except for a single simple partial seizure after an attempt to wean off anticonvulsants). Note the absence of any new demyelinating lesions. This is most likely a case of Schilder's myelinoclastic diffuse sclerosis type of inflammatory demyelination.

out of a consecutive series of 52 Taiwanese patients with the diagnosis of post-infectious encephalomyelitis (Hung *et al.*, 2001). In another series of 40 adults diagnosed with ADEM at the University of Heidelberg between 1988 and 1999, 14 had a second clinical episode (35%), but these were diagnosed as multiple sclerosis rather than MDEM. No details are provided about the recurrent illnesses, however. It is of interest that most patients in this series had oligoclonal bands in their spinal fluids (Schwarz *et al.*, 2001).

Recurrent acute transverse myelitis has also been reported (Lamarche *et al.*, 1972; Tippett *et al.*, 1991).

Some points of differentiation between recurrent ADEM and MS, which may resemble each other very closely, include the following: ADEM begins rather abruptly, evolving in an obvious way over several hours or possibly days, whereas an MS exacerbation/relapse tends to take longer, although this is not absolute. Also, episodes of ADEM tend to be febrile and cause prominent changes in mental status (delirium, confusion, disorientation), whereas MS relapses are afebrile and usually consist of focal neurological deficits. Finally, recurrences of ADEM usually mimic the first episode. Of course, patients with multiple recurrences of ADEM without delirium or changes in the level of consciousness may be difficult to distinguish from patients with clinically restricted MS.

Acute disseminated encephalomyelitis with mass lesions

An unusual variant of demyelinating disease, with large demyelinating lesions having a mass effect that can be confused with tumors, has been reported (Kepes, 1993; Peterson *et al.*, 1993). The diagnosis of tumor was made initially in several such patients on the basis of imaging and biopsy, and unnecessary therapy with high-dose radiation and chemotherapy was given, with rather poor results (Peterson *et al.*, 1993). In about 10% of patients in one study of a total of 31 such patients, the lesions recurred after 9 months to 12 years (Kepes, 1993) (Fig. 13.16). In seven of these patients the lesions were multifocal. Interestingly, three patients had systemic malignancies. In 11 patients, the symptoms resolved after treatment with corticosteroids. The disease tends to have a sudden onset, and followed an influenza vaccination in one patient. Since there was an abrupt onset, a good response to steroids, and unlikely recurrence, the disease resembled ADEM. It is not clear whether this is a distinct form of demyelinating disease, distinguished by having lesions with a mass effect, or whether it is a form of ADEM. Indeed, mass lesions mimicking neoplasms can also occur with AHLE. In two patients with well-documented AHLE, the entire clinical courses were 6 weeks and 3 months. Instead of an abrupt onset, the patients had a steadily progressive course, with cerebral CT scans showing multiple mass lesions that were diagnosed as tumors (Huang *et al.*, 1988). The correct diagnosis was made when tissue was obtained at surgery. The disease in some of these patients is reminiscent of an entity known as *myelinoclastic diffuse sclerosis* (the label given to a well-defined subset of patients previously given the vague diagnosis of Schilder's disease) (Poser, 1985; Afifi *et al.*, 1994). The diagnostic criteria for this entity are: (1) at least one large, discrete, bilateral, myelin-destroying, axon-sparing ('myelinoclastic') lesion in the centrum semiovale; (2) no other lesions demonstrable in the CNS (by clinical, paraclinical, or imaging methods); (3) normal peripheral nerve, adrenal, and peroxisomal (very long chain fatty acids) function; and (4) a histology typical of MS. Patients identified to have myelinoclastic diffuse sclerosis have had apparently dramatic responses to corticosteroid therapy and in one patient, to cyclophosphamide (Poser, 1985). A 40-year-old woman showed some response to pulsed methylprednisolone (Dresser *et al.*, 1991) (see Fig. 13.16 for a likely case of Schilder's myelinoclastic diffuse sclerosis.)

Post-streptococcal acute disseminated encephalomyelitis (PSADEM) and pediatric autoimmune neuropsychiatric disorders associated with streptococcal infections (PANDAS)

In the past few years it has become apparent that there may be an unusual form of post-infectious encephalomyelitis following streptococcal infec-

tions, particularly in children. The illness characteristically follows a febrile pharyngitis, with serology consistent with acute streptococcal infection, and presents with labile affect, particularly inappropriate laughter, along with rigidity, dystonia, and resting tremor, but no tics or chorea. Some patients have confusion, somnolence, rarely seizures and focal weakness. In half the patients, the movement disorder was a prominent manifestation (Dale *et al.*, 2001). In a report of 10 patients, mild leucocytosis and slightly increased ESR (mean 38 mm/hr) were noted, along with pleocytosis in 4/10 and increased CSF protein in 7/10. Only one patient had intrathecal synthesis of oligoclonal bands. The brain MRI showed high-intensity lesions on T_2-weighted images in the basal ganglia in eight of the 10 patients, as well as in some of the deep gray nuclei (thalamus, subthalamus), white matter of the hemispheres, and one in the spinal cord. The frequency of basal ganglia lesions was statistically significantly higher in the patient group (80%) than in a control group of non-post-streptococcal ADEM patients (4/22, 18%) (Dale *et al.*, 2001). The patients were found to have increased serum levels of antibasal ganglia antibodies, by immunosorbent assay, relative to controls with other post-streptococcal disease and controls with other inflammatory CNS diseases. The serum antibasal ganglia antibodies in one patient were found to bind to large striatal neurons by fluorescent immunostaining. Nine of the patients were treated with intravenous methylprednisolone and improved rapidly. Two patients had relapses, both triggered by pharyngitis, but recovered to baseline. Two patients (not the ones with relapses) had residual problems, one with obsessive–compulsive disorder and the other with hemidystonia (Dale *et al.*, 2001).

This presentation, in which labile affect and a movement disorder follow a streptococcal pharyngitis, is reminiscent of Sydenham's chorea (also called St Vitus' dance), which was first described by Sydenham in 1686, and is part of the rheumatic fever syndrome (Jummani and Okin, 2001). Rheumatic fever is a syndromic complex consisting of major (chorea, carditis, polyarthritis, erythema marginatum or subcutaneous nodules) and minor (fever, arthralgia, increased ESR or C-reactive protein, prolonged PR interval on the electrocardiogram) manifestations. The Jones criteria for the diagnosis of rheumatic fever include two major or one major and two minor manifestations, along with serological evidence of a preceding group A β-hemolytic streptococcal (GABHS) infection, such as raised anti-streptolysin O (ASO) or anti-DNAse B (ADB) antibody titers in the recent past. (Often the Sydenham's chorea occurs several months after the acute infection, and ASO or ADB titers may have decreased back to normal range when the chorea occurs.) Other conditions which can mimic Sydenham's chorea include Wilson's disease, lupus erythematosus, drug reactions, and metabolic and neurodegenerative diseases.

Sydenham's chorea typically begins several weeks to several months after a GABHS infection, usually a pharyngitis, and presents (often abruptly) with emotional lability, obsessive–compulsive symptoms, decreased attention span, and nightmares, restlessness, and facial grimacing followed by restlessness progressing to frank chorea, which can be quite diffuse and severe enough to interfere with walking (occasionally severe enough to confine the patient to a wheelchair), speech, dressing, and feeding (Swedo, 1994). Sydenham's chorea may recur during pregnancy and occur as a manifestation of lupus erythematosus. Antibodies to basal ganglia neurons are found in these patients and are cross-reactive with the M antigen of *Streptococcus* (Husby *et al.*, 1976). Half the patients have non-specific EEG abnormalities and early studies of brain imaging showed normal results, or non-specific abnormalities (Swedo *et al.*, 1993). More recently, brain MRIs done on Sydenham's chorea patients have shown abnormal signal in the striatum (Kienzle *et al.*, 1991; Giedd *et al.*, 1995). Another study showed abnormal signal in the basal ganglia with swelling in the acute phase of the disease and residual cystic changes on repeat imaging (Emery and Vieco, 1997). Basal ganglia lesions are not necessarily the only imaging abnormality seen, however. In a case of Sydenham's chorea, multiple areas of increased signal on T_2-weighted imaging were noted in the white matter, with sparing of the basal ganglia (Robertson and Smith, 2002). SPECT scans of the brain in early Sydenham's chorea show increased perfusion of the basal ganglia, and serial SPECT in a single case of Sydenham's chorea showed hyperperfusion of the basal ganglia in the acute, symptomatic stage of the disease (Barsottini *et al.*, 2002), with normal perfusion on resolution of the disease (Lee *et al.*, 1999).

The natural history of Sydenham's chorea is that of spontaneous, though sometimes slow, recovery, although patients with persistent (and possibly permanent) residua have been reported, both clinically (Church *et al.*, 2002) and on MRI (Emery and Vieco, 1997). Therapy for Sydenham's chorea is not standardized, but patients have been treated with pimozide, benzodiazepines, and haloperidol. There may be some evidence of efficacy of plasmapheresis, but the data are very limited. Prednisone is of uncertain efficacy (Swedo, 1994). Penicillin will need to be used to eradicate GABHS, if present, and patients should be continued on prophylactic penicillin to prevent further episodes of rheumatic fever, particularly to prevent any possible future episodes of rheumatic carditis.

More recently, a syndrome of obsessive–compulsive disorder, along with tics, has been noted to follow GABHS pharyngitis, by one to several months (Swedo *et al.*, 1998). Because of the relative prominence of psychiatric manifestations in this syndrome, unlike Sydenham's chorea, in which movement disorder predominates, it has been named pediatric autoimmune neuropsychiatric disorder associated with streptococcal infection (PANDAS). In a series of 50 cases, Swedo *et al.* (1998) noted that there was an acute onset of obsessive–compulsive disorder or a tic disorder (strongly resembling Tourette's syndrome) beginning after GABHS infection (usually pharyngitis), along with emotional lability, bedtime fears, oppositional behavior, separation anxiety, and hyperactivity, but no chorea. This syndrome occurred in children aged 2 to 12 years with a mean around 6.5 years. The cerebral localization of PANDAS is similar to that of Sydenham's chorea (Bottas and Richter, 2002). Unlike Sydenham's chorea, which is usually self-limited, PANDAS will often relapse after subsequent episodes of GABHS infection. Furthermore, while Sydenham's chorea is part of the acute rheumatic fever complex, with a high incidence of carditis (which may be severe or very mild and indeed subclinical) and arthritis, these are not seen in PANDAS. The therapy of PANDAS is not established, although there is preliminary evidence of the efficacy of plasmapheresis and intravenous immunoglobulin (IV Ig) over placebo in a trial of 30 children, who were being treated with serotonin re-uptake inhibitors for obsessive–compulsive disorder or clonidine or neuroleptics for tics (Perlmutter *et al.*, 1999). The subjects were randomized in a 1:1:1 ratio, and both clinically and statistically significant improvements, using standard neuropsychological rating scales for assessment, were noted in the treated groups compared with the placebo group, with only one child in each of the treatment groups not responding. The plasma exchange group improved first (within a week) while the IV Ig group took longer (more than 3 weeks). Of the 17 children seen in follow-up, three children were retreated with either pheresis or IV Ig, each having an exacerbation following GABHS pharyngitis. The others had sustained improvement.

The precise relationship between post-streptococcal ADEM, Sydenham's chorea, and PANDAS is not completely clear, although they seem to have inflammation of the basal ganglia as a common feature (Dale, 2003). Part of the difficulty in assessing the relationship is the lack of pathological data. Old reports suggest the presence of a mild inflammatory reaction in the basal ganglia and the cortex in Sydenham's chorea, which suggests a gray matter inflammation in the deep nuclei of the brain (Buchanan, 1941; Colony and Malamud, 1956). This would be consistent with the imaging data discussed above. However, white matter lesions have been seen in this disease. Also, gray matter involvement has been documented for PANDAS by imaging, but not by histopathologic data, and the clinical differences between PANDAS and Sydenham's chorea make it difficult to identify these as being the same disorder (Murphy *et al.*, 2000). It is interesting that in the post-streptococcal ADEM cases there was both gray and white matter involvement on MRI, and that some of the patients had behavioral abnormalities reminiscent of those seen in Sydenham's chorea and PANDAS, in which there is prominent involvement of the basal ganglia.

There is yet another possible twist to the post-streptococcal ADEM story. von Economo's encephalitis or encephalitis lethargica is a disease which broke out in a pandemic from about 1915 to about 1926 or so. It was thought to be an acute viral encephalitis, with a mortality rate of about 30%

of symptomatic cases. Survivors often had disabling psychiatric and movement disorders, as well described in Oliver Sacks' *Awakenings* (Sacks, 1999). Recently, it was suggested that von Economo's encephalitis was really a form of post-streptococcal ADEM (Dale *et al.* 2003). In a report of 20 cases of encephalitis which had clinical descriptions similar to those of von Economo's encephalitis, abnormal signal was noted in the deep gray structures of 40%, similar to that seen in the post-streptococcal ADEM patients. The patients had positive ASO titers and antibodies to basal ganglia antigens. These latter antigens were localized to neurons, as shown by immunohistochemistry. This is a fascinating speculation, which merits greater study. Although viral encephalitis is often an epidemic disease, post-infectious ADEM rarely is, unless the relevant strain of *Streptococcus* has a particularly strongly immunogenic antigen cross-reacting (in any of the senses discussed in the pathogenesis section above) with neuronal antigens in the basal ganglia.

Acute toxic encephalopathy

A small number of reports have described an acute post-viral illness that resembles ADEM in some respects but in which only cerebral edema is found at autopsy, with no inflammatory infiltrates (such as are found in ADEM) (Poser, 1985). Some patients, particularly following the use of aspirin in varicella and influenza B infections (Reye *et al.*, 1963; Griffith *et al.*, 1970) had concomitant liver failure, and this was recognized as a distinct post-viral syndrome—Reye's syndrome (Reye *et al.*, 1963; Davis, 1989). Other such syndromes have been seen without liver disease, and seem to occur in children younger than 2 or 3 years (Lyon *et al.*, 1961; McNair Scott, 1967), a population group in which ADEM is rare (Lyon *et al.*, 1961; Alvord, 1965; McNair Scott, 1967). However, many of these patients (Lyon *et al.*, 1961) had multiple confounding factors such as prolonged febrile seizures, aspiration pneumonia, and anoxic encephalopathy, and it is unclear whether a truly unique clinicopathologic entity of para-infectious non-inflammatory encephalopathy exists, other than Reye's syndrome. Most notorious of these toxic encephalopathies are those purported to occur after pertussis vaccination (Miller *et al.*, 1981). A review of the studies linking pertussis vaccination to toxic encephalopathies with residual neurologic damage showed that the evidence is at best inconclusive, with such cases being very rare (Wentz and Marcuse, 1991). However, there is a slight association of acute encephalopathy with pertussis vaccination, but this is non-specific: it occurs when febrile seizures occur, developmental delays begin, other diseases are common, or other confounders are present. In some of these patients, pathologic changes are noted in the cerebral microvasculature, and include perivascular edema and lymphocytic infiltrates, fibrinoid necrosis, endothelial proliferation, and neutrophilic and eosinophilic infiltrates in the vascular wall. This vasculopathy was believed to be out of proportion to demyelination, and has been asserted to be an independently existing disease entity. The pathogenesis of this is unclear, but the direct vascular damage suggests that it is mediated possibly by immune complexes (Alvord, 1965; Reik, 1980).

A possible example of such an immune complex-mediated encephalopathy, characterized by a post-diarrheal biphasic illness with fever, rash, seizures, very high ESR (150 mm/hr), positive ANA titer (1:320), and MRI showing more gray than white matter involvement, reportedly occurred in patients who had *C. jejuni* enteritis (Nasralla *et al.*, 1983). A brain biopsy specimen showed gliosis and a vasculopathy characterized by scattered lymphocytes and lipid-laden perivascular macrophages. The patient, who had baseline cerebral palsy, responded dramatically to high-dose intravenous methylprednisolone, with resolution of seizures and a return of the ESR and ANA to normal values. Another example is an acute transverse myelopathy that occurred after a febrile upper respiratory tract infection and progressed to a spastic quadriparesis and bilateral optic neuropathy (Renkawek *et al.*, 1985). The patient became dependent on a respirator and died 18 months later. Autopsy showed diffuse demyelination in the cerebral hemispheres with occasional perivascular and interstitial mononuclear infiltrates, and necrosis of the cervical and upper thoracic regions of the spinal cord. Scattered areas of vasculitis were seen and deposits of immunoglobulins and complement components were found in blood vessel walls. No viral inclusions were noted and the results of a previous work-up for collagen-vascular disease were negative. This appears to be an immune-complex-mediated encephalopathy with deposition of immune complexes (and complement) in the cerebral vasculature, leading to inflammatory demyelination.

An interesting form of acute encephalopathy is the so-called acute necrotizing encephalopathy of childhood, which has mostly been reported in the Far East (Mizuguchi, 1997). This occurs in young children, usually between the ages of 6 and 18 months, although one case was 11 years old. Usually, there is a viral prodrome, most often an upper respiratory illness, which is followed, in a few hours to a couple of days, by seizures in about half the cases and somnolence or delirium in a third, and intractable vomiting in the rest. The patients become comatose within a day or so, and become rigid, with abnormal pupils and decorticate or decerebrate posturing, suggestive of a central herniation syndrome. Laboratory studies show abnormal liver enzymes but no hypoglycemia or hyperammonemia, and increased urea nitrogen and C-reactive protein. Liver biopsy shows fatty change of a form different from that seen in Reye's syndrome. The mortality rate is about 30% over all. It is very high in younger patients, but is lower in children older than 4 years, those with normal liver enzyme levels, and those with minimal brainstem signs. The unifying finding that ties these otherwise non-specific cases together is that of bilaterally symmetric abnormal signal in the thalamus (by CT or MRI), seen in all cases, and abnormalities in the cerebral white matter, cerebellar nuclei, and upper brainstem tegmentum, each seen in about half the cases. The MRI lesions are of low and high intensity on T_1- and T_2-weighted images, respectively, initially, but eventually high-intensity areas appear in the T_1-weighted images, probably reflecting petechial hemorrhages in the tissue. Neuropathological findings in the gray matter include petechial hemorrhages around small vessels, edema, and necrosis of neurons and glial cells, but no perivascular inflammatory infiltrates. The white matter shows only perivascular edema, but no hemorrhages or inflammatory infiltrates (Mizuguchi, 1997). There has been one report of a relapsing case of acute necrotizing encephalopathy in a 4-year-old who had typical manifestations following an influenza A infection. He had severe sequelae (muteness, spastic quadriplegia, dementia) despite treatment with vidarabine, prednisone, IV Ig, phenytoin, and phenobarbital. A year later, he had an episode of high fever, somnolence, and increased rigidity, following an adenovirus infection. Treatment with high-dose intravenous methylprednisolone (400 mg/day) resulted in rapid improvement back to baseline. In the first episode, MRI of the brain showed thalamic, putaminal, and pontine lesions, with enhancement, which partly resolved during convalescence. In the second episode, lesions were noted in the cerebellum, as well as the pons. The latter were residual from the first episode, but the cerebellar lesions were new (Suwa *et al.*, 1999). The nature of this encephalopathy is unclear, and therapy is supportive, although it would not be unreasonable to try high-dose corticosteroids, plasmapheresis, or IV Ig in appropriate situations.

The clinical picture of acute toxic encephalopathy is by no means unique, and may be seen in any child with prolonged febrile seizures, hypoxia, and metabolic disturbance (Lyon *et al.*, 1961). Furthermore, the pathologic changes are often non-specific, and many of them are compatible with an agonal state (Lyon *et al.*, 1961). Some of the pathologic changes are variations of normal in the immature brain of a young child. Thus, small vessels in children are often more cellular than those in adults, giving rise to an incorrect impression of endothelial proliferation (Lyon *et al.*, 1961). The existence, therefore, of a separate, clinicopathologic entity of acute toxic encephalopathy is still controversial.

Future directions

Three major issues remain to be resolved: (1) the best therapy for acute disseminated encephalomyelitis, (2) the pathogenesis of the disease, and (3) the relation of a single demyelinative episode to the risk of subsequently developing MS and, as a corollary, what to do about such individuals. We

have only partial answers. The definitive answers will be difficult to obtain because this is an uncommon disease and in everyday practice is probably underdiagnosed. The first issue, that of the most efficacious therapy, requires a multicenter clinical trial that would need to be sustained for several years. There is a precedent, however, in the multicenter trials for herpes encephalitis, another relatively uncommon disease (Schlitt and Whitley, 1990). The pathogenesis of the disease can continue to be explored by investigating the animal model EAE. More direct and clinically relevant clues can be sought by obtaining immune cells from both blood and CSF of patients with the disease and examining the TCR gene usage and state of activation. Finally, the risk of subsequent development of MS after a single demyelinative episode can only be determined by further longitudinal follow-up, including MRI, of such patients.

References

Abramsky, O., Teitelbaum, D., and Arnon, R. (1977). Effect of a synthetic polypeptide (Cop-1) on patients with multiple sclerosis and acute disseminated encephalomyelitis. *J Neurol Sci* **31**: 433–438.

Adams, R. and Kubik, C. (1952). The morbid anatomy of the demyelinative diseases. *Am J Med* **12**: 510–546.

Afifi, A., Bell, W.E., Menezes, A.H., and Moore, S.A. (1994). Myelinoclastic diffuse sclerosis (Schilder's disease): report of a case and a review of the literature. *J Child Neurol* **9**: 398–403.

Alcock, N. and Hoffman, H. (1962). Recurrent encephalomyelitis in childhood. *Arch Dis Child* **37**: 40.

Alvord, E. Jr (1965). Pathogenesis of experimental allergic encephalomyelitis: introductory remarks. In: *Research in Demyelinating Diseases* (ed. L. Scheinberg, M. Kies, and E. Alvord Jr), pp. 245–255. New York Academy of Science, New York.

Alvord, E. Jr, Rose, L., and Richards, T. (1992). Chronic experimental allergic encephalomyelitis as a model of multiple sclerosis. In: *Myelin: Biology and Chemistry* (ed. R. Martenson), pp. 849–891. CRC Press, Boca Raton, FL.

Amlie-Lefond, C., Kleinschmidt-DeMasters, B.K., and Mahalingam, R., *et al.* (1995). The vasculopathy of varicella-zoster virus encephalitis. *Ann Neurol* **37**: 784–790.

An, S., Groves, M., Martinian, L., Kuo, L.T., *et al.* (2002). Detection of infectious agents in brain of patients with acute hemorrhagic leukoencephalitis. *J Neurovirol* **8**: 439–446.

Applebaum, E., Greenberg, M., and Nelson, J. (1953). Neurological complications following antirabies vaccination. *J Am Med Assoc* **151**: 188–191.

Atlas, S., Grossman, R.I., Goldberg, H.I., *et al.* (1986). MR diagnosis of acute disseminated encephalomyelitis. *J Comput Assist Tomogr* **10**: 798–801.

Barkhof, F., Filippi, M., Miller, D.H., *et al.* (1997). Comparison of MRI criteria at first presentation to predict conversion to clinically definite multiple sclerosis. *Brain* **120**: 2059–2069.

Barned, S., Goodman, A., and Mattson, D. (1995). Frequency of antinuclear antibodies in multiple sclerosis. *Neurology* **45**: 384–385.

Barsottini, O., Ferraz, H.B., Seviliano, M.M., *et al.* (2002). Brain SPECT imaging in Sydenham's chorea. *Brazil J Med Biol Res* **35**: 431–436.

Bergen, D. and Grossman, H. (1975). Acute cerebellar ataxia of childhood associated with infectious mononucleosis. *J Pediatr* **87**: 833–834.

Berman, M., Feldman, S., Alter, M., *et al.* (1981). Acute transverse myelitis: incidence and etiologic considerations. *Neurology* **31**: 966–971.

Bernard, K., Smith, P.W., Kader, F.J., *et al.* (1982). Neuroparalytic illness and human diploid cell rabies vaccine. *J Am Med Assoc* **248**: 3136–3138.

Birmingham, K. and Frantz, S. (2002). Set back to Alzheimer vaccine studies. *Nat Med* **8**: 199–200.

Bottas, A. and Richter, M. (2002). Pediatric autoimmune neuropsychiatric disorders associated with streptococcal infections (PANDAS). *Pediatr Infect Dis J* **21**: 67–71.

Bray, P., Culp, K.W., McFarlin, D.E., *et al.* (1992). Demyelinating disease after neurologically complicated primary Epstein–Barr virus infection. *Neurology* **42**: 278–282.

Brex, P., Ciccarelli, O., O'Riordan, J.I., *et al.* (2002). A longitudinal study of abnormalities on MRI and disability from multiple sclerosis. *N Engl J Med* **346**: 158–164.

Buchanan, D. (1941). Pathologic changes in chorea. *Am J Dis Child* **62**: 443–445.

Budka, H. (1989). Human immunodeficiency virus (HIV)-induced disease of the central nervous system: pathology and implications for pathogenesis. *Acta Neuropathol* **77**: 225–236.

Burns, J., Littlefield, K., Gill, J., Trottr, J.L. (1992). Bacterial toxin superantigens activate human T lymphocytes reactive with myelin antigens. *Ann Neurol* **32**: 352–357.

Byers, R. (1975). Acute hemorrhagic leukoencephalitis: report of 3 cases and a review of the literature. *Pediatrics* **56**: 727–735.

Caldemeyer, K., Harris, T.M., Smith, R.R., Edwards, M.K. (1991). Gadolinium enhancement in acute disseminated encephalomyelitis. *J Comput Assist Tomo* **15**: 673–675.

Challoner, P., Smith, K.T., Parker, J.D., *et al.* (1995). Plaque-associated expression of human herpesvirus 6 in multiple sclerosis. *Proc Natl Acad Sci USA* **92**: 7440–7444.

Cherington, C. (1977). Locked-in syndrome after 'swine flu' vaccination. *Arch Neurol* **34**: 258.

Christensen, P., Wermuth, L., Hinge, H.H., Bomers, K. (1990). Clinical course and long-term prognosis of acute transverse myelitis. *Acta Neurol Scand* **81**: 431–435.

Church, A., Cardoso, F., Dale, R.C., Lees, A.J., Thompson, E.J., Giovannoni, G. (2002). Anti-basal ganglia antibodies in acute and persistent Sydenham's chorea. *Neurology* **59**: 227–231.

Chusid, M., Williamson, S.J., Murphy, J.V., Ramey, L.S. (1979). Neuromyelitis optica (Devic disease) following varicella infection. *J Pediatr* **95**: 737–738.

Cleary, T., Henle, W., and Pickering, L. (1980). Acute cerebellar ataxia associated with Epstein–Barr virus infection. *J Am Med Assoc* **243**: 148–149.

Cohen, J. and Lisak, R. (1987). Acute disseminated encephalomyelitis. In: *Clinical Neuroimmunology* (ed. J. Aarli, W. Behan, and P. Behan), pp. 192–213. Blackwell Scientific, Oxford.

Cohen, M., Day, C., and Day, J. (1985). Acute disseminated encephalomyelitis as a complication of treatment with gold. *Br Med J* **290**: 1170–1180.

Colony, H. and Malamud, N. (1956). Sydenham's chorea. A clinicopathologic study. *Neurology* **6**: 672–676.

Cotter, F., Bainbridge, D., and Newland, A. (1983). Neurological deficit associated with *Mycobacterium pneumoniae* reversed by plasma exchange. *Br Med J* **286**: 22.

Croft, P. (1969). Parainfectious and postvaccinal encephalomyelitis. *Postgrad Med J* **45**: 392–400.

Cross, A., Tuohy, V., and Raine, C. (1993). Development of reactivity to new myelin antigens during chronic relapsing autoimmune demyelination. *Cell Immunol* **146**: 261–265.

Dal Canto, M. and Rabinowitz, S. (1982). Experimental models of virus-induced demyelination of the central nervous system. *Ann Neurol* **11**: 109–127.

Dale, R. (2003). Autoimmunity and the basal ganglia: new insights into old diseases. *Q J Med* **96**: 183–191.

Dale, R., de Sousa, Cl, Chong, W.K., Cox, T.C.S., Harding, B.N., Neville, B.G.R. (2000). Acute disseminated encephalomyelitis, multiphasic disseminated encephalomyelitis and multiple sclerosis in children. *Brain* **123**: 2407–2422.

Dale, R., Church, A.J., Cardoso, F, Goddard, E., Cox, T.C.S., Chong, WLK. (2001). Poststreptococcal acute disseminated encephalomyelitis with basal ganglia involvement and autoreactive antibasal ganglia antibodies. *Ann Neurol* **50**: 588–595.

Dale, R.C., Church, A.J., Surtees, R.A.H., Lees, A.J., Adcock, J.E., Harding, B., *et al.* (2003). Encephalitis lethargica syndrome: 20 new cases and evidence of basal ganglia autoimmunity. *Brain* **127**: 21–33.

Dangood, F., Lacomis, D., Schwartz, R.B., *et al.* (1991). Acute disseminated encephalomyelitis progressing to hemorrhagic encephalitis. *Neurology* **41**: 1697–1698.

Davis, L. (1989). Influenza virus and Reye's syndrome. In: *Clinical and Molecular Aspects of Neurotropic Virus Infection* (ed. D. Gilden and H. Lipton), pp. 173–202. Kluwer Academic: Norwell, MA.

Decaux, G., Szyper, M, Extors, M., *et al.* (1980). Central nervous system complications of *Mycoplasma pneumoniae*. *J Neurol Neurosurg Psychiatry* **43**: 883–887.

DeSimone, J., Pomerantz, R., and Babinchak, T. (2000). Inflammatory reactions in HIV-infected persons after initiation of highly active antiretroviral therapy. *Ann Intern Med* **133**: 447–454.

Donovan, M. and Lenn, N. (1989). Postinfectious encephalomyelitis with localized basal ganglia involvement. *Pediatr Neurol* **5**: 311–313.

Dore-Duffy, P., Donaldson, J.O., Rothman, B.L., Zurier, R.B. (1982). Antinuclear antibodies in multiple sclerosis. *Arch Neurol* **39**: 504–506.

Drachman, D., Paterson, P., and Bornstein, M. (1974). Experimental allergic encephalomyelitis in man: a laboratory accident. *Neurology* **24**: 364.

Dresser, L., Tourian, A., and Anthony, D. (1991). A case of myelinoclastic diffuse sclerosis in an adult. *Neurology* **41**: 316–318.

Durston, J. and Milnes, J. (1970). Relapsing encephalomyelitis. *Brain* **93**: 715–730.

Emery, E. and Vieco, P. (1997). Sydenham chorea: magnetic resonance imaging reveals permanent basal ganglia injury. *Neurology* **48**: 531–533.

Epperson, L., Whittaker, J., and Kapila, A. (1988). Cranial MRI in acute disseminated encephalomyelitis. *Neurology* **38**: 332–333.

Fazakerley, J. and Buchmeier, M. (1992). Virus-induced demyelination. In: *Myelin: Biology and Chemistry* (ed. R. Martenson), pp. 893–932. CRC Press, Boca Raton, FL.

Fazekas, F., Offenbacher, H., Fuchs, S., Schmidt, R., Niederkorn, K., Horner, S., Lechner, H. (1988). Criteria for an increased specificity of MRI interpretation in elderly subjects with suspected multiple sclerosis. *Neurology* **38**: 1822–1825.

Fenichel, G. (1982). Neurological complications of immunization. *Ann Neurol* **12**: 119–128.

Fernandez, C., Bortolussi, R., Gordon, K., *et al.* (1993). *Mycoplasma pneumoniae* infection associated with central nervous system complications. *J Child Neurol* **8**: 27–31.

Fisher, J. and Gilmour, J. (1939). Encephalomyelitis following administration of sulphanilamide. *Lancet* **2**: 301–305.

Fisher, R., Clark, A.W., Wolinsky, J.S., *et al.* (1983). Postinfectious leukoencephalitis complicating *Mycoplasma pneumoniae* infection. *Arch Neurol* **40**: 109–113.

Ford, B., Tampieri, D., and Francis, G. (1992). Long-term followup of acute transverse myelopathy. *Neurology* **42**: 250–252.

Francis, D., Brown, A., Miller, D.H., *et al.* (1988). MRI appearances of the CNS manifestations of *Mycoplasma pneumoniae*: a report of two cases. *J Neurol* **235**: 441–443.

Fujinami, R. and Oldstone, M. (1985). Amino acid homology between the encephalitogenic site of myelin basic protein and virus: mechanism for autoimmunity. *Science* **230**: 1043–1045.

Furlan, R., Brambilla, E., Sanvito, R., Roccatagliata, L., Olivieri, S., Bergami, A., Pluchino, S., *et al.* (2003). Vaccination with amyloid-beta peptide induces autoimmune encephalomyelitis in C57/BL6 mice. *Brain* **126**: 285–291.

Gautier-Smith, P. (1965). The neurological complications of glandular fever (infectious mononucleosis). *Brain* **88**: 323–334.

Gendelman, H., Wolinsky, J., and Johnson, R. (1984). Measles encephalomyelitis: lack of evidence of viral invasion of the central nervous system and quantitative study of the nature of demyelination. *Ann Neurol* **15**: 353–360.

Georgsson, G. (1994). Neuropathologic aspects of lentiviral infection. *Ann NY Acad Sci* **724**: 50–67.

Gibbs, F., Gibbs, E.L., Carpenter, P.R., Spies, H.W. (1959). Electroencephalographic abnormality in 'uncomplicated' childhood diseases. *J Am Med Assoc* **171**: 1050–1055.

Giedd, J., Rapoport, J., and Kruesi, M. (1995). Sydenham's chorea: magnetic resonance imaging of the basal ganglia. *Neurology* **45**: 2199–2202.

Gieron-Korthals, M., Westberry, K., and Emmanuel, P. (1995). Acute childhood ataxia: 10 year experience. *J Child Neurol* **9**: 381–384.

Goebel, H., Walther, G., and Meuth, M. (1986). Fresh cell therapy followed by fatal coma. *J Neurol* **233**: 242–247.

Gray, F., Chimelli, L., Mohr, M., *et al.* (1991). Fulminating multiple sclerosis-like leukoencephalopathy revealing human immunodeficiency virus infection. *Neurology* **41**: 105–109.

Gray, F., Belec, L., Lescs, M.C., *et al.* (1994). Varicella-zoster virus infection of the central nervous system in the acquired immune deficiency syndrome. *Brain* **117**: 987–999.

Griffin, D., Ward, B.J., Jauregui, E., *et al.* (1989). Immune activation in measles. *N Engl J Med* **320**: 1667–1672.

Griffith, J., Salam, M., and Adams, R. (1970). The nervous system diseases associated with varicella. A critical commentary with additional notes on the syndrome of acute encephalopathy and fatty hepatosis. *Acta Neurol Scand* **46**: 279–300.

Gross, W., Ravens, K., and Hansen, H. (1978). Meningoencephalitis syndrome following influenza vaccination. *J Neurol* **217**: 219–222.

Guillain–Barré Syndrome Study Group (1985). Plasmapheresis and acute Guillain–Barré syndrome. *Neurology* **35**: 1096–1104.

Hahn, J., Siegler, D., and Enzmann, D. (1996). Intravenous gamma-globulin therapy in recurrent acute disseminated encephalomyelitis. *Neurology* **46**: 1173–1174.

Hanninen, P., Arstila, P., Lang, H., *et al.* (1980). Involvement of the central nervous system in acute uncomplicated measles virus infection. *J Clin Microbiol* **11**: 610–613.

Hart, M. and Earle, K. (1975). Haemorrhagic and perivenous encephalitis: a clinical-pathological report of 38 cases. *J Neurol Neurosurg Psychiatry* **38**: 585–591.

Hartung, H. and Grossman, R. (2001). ADEM: distinct disease or part of the MS spectrum? *Neurology* **56**: 1257–1260.

Hemachudha, T., Phanuphak, P., Johnson, R.T., *et al.* (1987*a*). Neurologic complications of Semple-type rabies vaccine: clinical and immunological studies. *Neurology* **37**: 550–556.

Hemachudha, T., Griffin, D.E., Giffels, J.J., *et al.* (1987*b*). Myelin basic protein as an encephalitogen in encephalitis and polyneuritis following rabies vaccinations. *N Engl J Med* **316**: 369–374.

Holtas, S., Basibuyuk, N., and Fredriksson, K. (1993). MRI in acute transverse myelopathy. *Neuroradiology* **35**: 221–226.

Huang, C., Chu, N., Chen, T., Shaw, C. (1988). Acute hemorrhagic leukoencephalitis with a prolonged clinical course. *J Neurol Neurosurg Psychiatry* **51**: 870–874.

Huber, S., Kappos, L., Fuhr, P., Wetzel, S, Steck, A. (1999). Combined acute disseminated encephalomyelitis and acute motor axonal neuropathy after vaccination for hepatitis A and infection with *Campylobacter jejuni*. *J Neurol* **246**: 1204–1206.

Hung, K.-L., Liao, H.-T., and Tsai, M.-L. (2001). The spectrum of postinfectious encephalomyelitis. *Brain Dev* **23**: 42–45.

Hurst, E. (1947). Acute hemorrhagic leukoencephalitis: a previously undefined entity. *Med J Aust* **2**: 1.

Husby, G., Van de Rijn, I., Zabvriskie, J.B., Abdin, Z.H., Willaims, R.C. (1976). Antibodies reacting with cytoplasm of subthalamic and caudate nuclei neurons in chorea and acute rheumatic fever. *J Exp Med* **144**: 1094–1100.

Hynson, J., Kornberg, A., coleman, L., Shield, L., Harvey, A., Kean, M. (2001). Clinical and neuroradiologic features of acute disseminated encephalomyelitis in children. *Neurology* **56**: 1308–1312.

Jacobs, B., Endtz, H, van der Meche, F.G.A., *et al.* (1995). Serum anti-GQ1b IgG antibodies recognize surface epitopes on *Campylobacter jejuni* from patients with Miller–Fisher syndrome. *N Engl J Med* **37**: 260–264.

Jacobson, D., Marx, J., and Dlesk, A. (1991). Frequency and clinical significance of Lyme seropositivity in patients with isolated optic neuritis. *Neurology* **41**: 706–711.

Jahnke, U., Fischer, E., and Alvord, E. Jr (1985). Sequence homology between certain viral proteins and proteins related to encephalomyelitis and neuritis. *Science* **229**: 282–284.

Johnson, R. and Griffin, D. (1987). Postinfectious encephalomyelitis. In: *Infections of the Nervous System* (ed. P. Kennedy and R. Johnson), pp. 209–226. Butterworth, New York.

Johnson, R., Griffin, D.E., Hirsch, R.J., *et al.* (1984). Measles encephalomyelitis—clinical and immunological studies. *N Engl J Med* **310**: 137–141.

Jones, H., Ho, D., Forgacs, P., *et al.* (1988). Acute fulminating fatal leukoencephalopathy as the only manifestation of human immunodeficiency virus infection. *Ann Neurol* **23**: 519–522.

Jorens, P., VanderBorght, A., Ceulemans, B., Van Bever, H.P., Bossaert, L.L., Ieven, M., *et al.* (2000). Encephalomyelitis-associated antimyelin autoreactivity induced by streptococcal exotoxins. *Neurology* **54**: 1433–1441.

Jummani, R. and Okin, M. (2001). Sydenham chorea. *Arch Neurol* **58**: 311–313.

Kanter, D., Horensky, D., sperling, R.A., *et al.* (1995). Plasmapheresis in fulminant acute disseminated encephalomyelitis. *Neurology* **45**: 824–827.

Kaplanski, G., Retornaz, F., and Durand, J. (1995). Central nervous system demyelination after vaccination against hepatitis B and HLA haplotype. *J Neurol Neurosurg Psychiatry* **58**: 758–759.

Kastrukoff, L., Lau, A., and Kim, S. (1987). Multifocal CNS demyelination following peripheral inoculation with herpes simplex virus type 1. *Ann Neurol* **22**: 52–59.

Kazarian, E. and Gager, W. (1978). Optic neuritis complicating measles, mumps and rubella vaccination. *Am J Ophthalmol* **86**: 544–547.

Kennard, C. and Swash, M. (1981). Acute viral encephalitis. Its diagnosis and outcome. *Brain* **104**: 129–148.

Kepes, J. (1993). Large focal tumor-like demyelinating lesions of the brain: intermediate entity between multiple sclerosis and acute disseminated encephalomyelitis? A study of 31 patients. *Ann Neurol* **33**: 18–27.

Kesselring, J., Miller, D.H., Robb, S.A., *et al.* (1990). Acute disseminated encephalomyelitis. MRI findings and the distinction from multiple sclerosis. *Brain* **113**: 291–302.

Kienzle, G., Breger, R.K., Chun, R.W.M., Zupanc, M.L., Sackett, J.F. (1991). Sydenham chorea: MR manifestations in two cases. *Am J Neuroradiol* **12**: 73–76.

Kinoshita, A., Hayashi, M., Miyamoto, K., *et al.* (1996). Inflammation demyelination radiculitis in a patient with acute disseminated encephalomyelitis (ADEM). *J Neurol Neurosurg Psychiatry* **60**: 87–90.

Kira, J. and Goto, I. (1994). Recurrent opticomyelitis associated with anti-DNA antibody. *J Neurol Neurosurg Psychiatry* **57**: 1124–1125.

Kleiman, M. and Brunquell, P. (1995). Acute disseminated encephalomyelitis: response to intravenous immunoglobulin? *J Child Neurol* **10**: 481–483.

Kliehues, P., Lang, W., and Burger, P. (1985). Progressive diffuse leukoencephalopathy in patients with acquired immune deficiency syndrome (AIDS). *Acta Neuropathol* **68**: 333–339.

Kline, L., Margulies, S., and Oh, S. (1982). Optic neuritis and myelitis following rubella vaccination. *Arch Neurol* **39**: 443–444.

Knox, K. and Carrigan, D. (1995). Active human herpesvirus 6 (HHV-6) infection of the central nervous system in patients with AIDS. *J Acq Immun Def Synd* **9**: 69–73.

Koenig, H., Rabinowitz, S., Day, E., Miller, V.T. (1979). Post-infectious encephalomyelitis after successful treatment of herpes simplex encephalitis with adenine arabinoside. Ultrastructural observations. *N Engl J Med* **300**: 1089–1093.

Kopp, N., Groslambert, R., Pasquier, B., *et al.* (1978). Leucoencephalite aigue hemorrhagique au cours d'une tuberculose. *Rev Neurol (Paris)* **134**: 313–323.

Kriss, A., Francis, D.A., Cuender, F., *et al.* (1988). Recovery after optic neuritis in childhood. *J Neurol Neurosurg Psychiatry* **51**: 603–608.

Kuperan, S., Ostrow, P., Landi, M.K., Bakshi, R. (2003). Acute hemorrhagic leukoencephalitis vs ADEM: FLAIR MRI and neuropathology findings. *Neurology* **60**: 721–722.

Label, L. and Batts, D. (1982). Transverse myelitis caused by duck embryo rabies vaccine. *Arch Neurol* **39**: 426–430.

Lamarche, J., Behan, P.O., Segarra, J.M., Feldman, R.G. (1972). Recurrent acute necrotizing hemorrhagic encephalopathy. *Acta Neuropathol* **22**: 79–87.

Langford, T., Letendre, S., Marcotte, T., Ellis, R.J., McCutchan, J., Grant, I., *et al.* (2002). Severe demyelinating leukoencephalopathy in AIDS patients on antiretroviral therapy. *AIDS* **16**: 1019–1029.

Lavi, E. and Weiss, S. (1989). Coronaviruses. In: *Clinical and Molecular Aspects of Neurotropic Virus Infection* (ed. D. Gilden and H. Lipton), pp.101–139. Kluwer Academic, Norwell, MA.

Lee, P., Nam, H.S., Lee, K.Y., Lee, B.I., Lee, J.D. (1999). Serial brain SPECT images in a case of Sydenham chorea. *Arch Neurol* **56**: 237–240.

Lehmann, P., Forsthuber, Miller, A., Sercarz, E.E. (1992). Spreading of T-cell autoimmunity to cryptic determinants of an autoantigen. *Nature* **358**: 155–157.

Lehmann, P., Sercarz, E., Forsthuber, T., *et al.* (1993). Determinant spreading and the dynamics of the autoimmune T-cell repertoire. *Immunol Today* **14**: 203–208.

Levine, S. (1974). Hyperacute, neutrophilic and localized forms of experimental allergic encephalomyelitis: a review. *Acta Neuropathol* 28: 179–189.

Lipton, H. (1975). Theiler's virus infection in mice: an unusual biphasic disease process leading to demyelination. *Infect Immun* 11: 1147–1155.

Lipton, H. and Teasdall, R. (1973). Acute transverse myelopathy in adults. A follow-up study. *Arch Neurol* 28: 252–257.

Lisak, R. (1994). Immune-mediated parainfectious encephalomyelitis. In: *Handbook of Neurovirology* (ed. R. McKendall and W. Stroop), pp. 173–186. Marcel Dekker, New York.

Lisak, R. and Zweiman, B. (1977). *In vitro* cell-mediated immunity of cerebrospinal fluid lymphocytes to myelin basic protein in primary demyelinating diseases. *N Engl J Med* 297: 850–853.

Lisak, R., Heinze, R., Falk, G., Kies, M.W. (1968). Search for antiencephalitogen antibody in human demyelinative diseases. *Neurology* 18: 122–128.

Loizou, L. and Cole, G. (1982). Acute cerebral demyelination: clinical and pathological correlation with computed tomography. *J Neurol Neurosurg Psychiatry* 45: 725–728.

Lucchinetti, C., Bruck, W., Parisi, J., Scheithauer, B., Rodriguez, M. Lassmann, H. (2000). Heterogeneity of multiple sclerosis lesions: implications for the pathogenesis of demyelination. *Ann Neurol* 47: 707–717.

Lukes, S. and Norman, D. (1983). Computed tomography in acute disseminated encephalomyelitis. *Ann Neurol* 13: 567–572.

Lyon, G., Dodge, P., and Adams, R. (1961). The acute encephalopathies of obscure origin in infants and children. *Brain* 84: 680–708.

Major, E., Ameniya, K., Tornatore, C.S., *et al.* (1992). Pathogenesis and molecular biology of progressive multifocal leukoencephalopathy, the JC virus-induced demyelinating disease of the human brain. *Clin Microbiol Rev* 5: 49–73.

Marsh, K. (1952). Streptomycin-PAS hypersensitivity treated with ACTH. *Lancet* 2: 606–608.

McCarthy, J. and Amer, J. (1978). Postvaricella acute transverse myelitis: a case presentation and review of the literature. *Pediatrics* 62: 202–204.

McKendall, R. (1994). HTLV-1 diseases. In: *Handbook of Neurovirology* (ed. R. McKendall and W. Stroop), pp. 737–772. Dekker, New York.

McNair Scott, T. (1967). Postinfectious and vaccinal encephalitis. *Med Clin N Am* 51: 701–717.

Means, E., Barron, K., and Van Dyne, B. (1973). Nervous system lesions after sting by yellow jacket. *Neurology* 23: 881–890.

Merine, K., Wang, U., Kumar, A., *et al.* (1987). CT myelography and MR imaging of acute transverse myelitis. *J Comput Assist Tomo* 11: 606–608.

Miller, D., Ross, E.M., Alderslade, R., *et al.* (1981). Pertussis immunization and serious acute neurological illness in children. *Br Med J* 282: 1595–1599.

Miller, D., Ormerod, I., Rudge, P., *et al.* (1989). The early risk of multiple sclerosis following isolated acute syndromes of the brainstem and spinal cord. *Ann Neurol* 26: 635–639.

Miller, H. and Evans, M. (1953). Prognosis in acute disseminated encephalomyelitis: with a note on neuromyelitis optica. *Q J Med* 22: 347–379.

Miller, H. and Stanton, J. (1954). Neurological sequelae of prophylactic inoculation. *Q J Med* 23: 1–27.

Miller, H., Stanton, J., and Gibbons, J. (1956). Para-infectious encephalomyelitis and related syndromes. A critical review of the neurological complications of certain specific fevers. *Q J Med* 25: 427–505.

Mizuguchi, M. (1997). Acute necrotizing encephalopathy of childhood: a novel form of acute encephalopathy prevalent in Japan and Taiwan. *Brain Dev* 19: 81–92.

Monteyne, P. and Andre, F. (2000). Is there a causal link between hepatitis B vaccination and multiple sclerosis? *Vaccine* 18: 1994–2001.

Mor, F. and Cohen, I. (1993). Shifts in the epitopes of myelin basic protein recognized by Lewis rat T cells before, during and the induction of experimental allergic encephalomyelitis. *J Clin Invest* 92: 2199–2206.

Morrisey, S., Miller, D.H., Kendall, B.E., *et al.* (1993). The significance of brain magnetic resonance imaging abnormalities at presentation with clinically isolated syndromes suggestive of multiple sclerosis. A 5-year followup study. *Brain* 116: 135–146.

Morrisey, S., Borruat, F.X., Miller, D.H., *et al.* (1995). Bilateral simultaneous optic neuropathy in adults: clinical, imaging, serological, and genetic studies. *J Neurol Neurosurg Psychiatry* 58: 70–74.

Murphy, T., Goodman, W.K., Ayoub, E.M., Voeller, K.K. (2000). On defining Sydenham's chorea: where do we draw the line? *Biol Psych* 47: 851–857.

Nadkarni, K. and Lisak, R. (1993). Guillain–Barre syndrome (GBS) with bilateral optic neuritis and central white matter disease. *Neurology* 43: 842–843.

Nasralla, C., Pay, N., Goodpasture, H.C., *et al.* (1983). Postinfectious encephalopathy in a child following *Campylobacter jejuni* enteritis. *Am J Neuroradiol* 14: 444–448.

Nelson, D. and Berry, R. (1993). Fatal rabies associated with extensive demyelination. *Arch Neurol* 50: 317–322.

Newton, R. (1981). Plasma exchange in acute post-infectious demyelination. *Dev Med Child Neurol* 23: 538–543.

Nicoll, J.A.R., Wilkinson, D., Homes, C., Steart, P., Markham, H., and Weller, R.O. (2003). Neuropathology of human Alzheimer disease after immunization with amyloid-b peptide: a case report. *Nat Med* 9: 448–452.

Nikoskelainen, E., Frey, H., and Salmi, A. (1981). Prognosis of optic neuritis with special reference to cerebrospinal fluid immunoglobulins and measles virus antibodies. *Ann Neurol* 9: 545–550.

O'Riordan, J., Thompson, A.J., Kingsley, D.P.E., MacManus, D.G., Kendall, B.E., Rudge, P., McDonald, W.I., Miller, D.H. (1998). The prognostic value of brain MRI in clinically isolated syndromes of the CNS. A 10-year follow-up. *Brain* 121: 495–503.

Ohtaki, E., Murakami, Y., Komori, H., *et al.* (1992). Acute disseminated encephalomyelitis after Japanese B encephalitis vaccination. *Pediatr Neurol* 8: 137–139.

Ohtaki, E., Matsuishi, T., Hirano, Y., Maekawa, K. (1995). Acute disseminated encephalomyelitis after treatment with Japanese B encephalitis vaccine (Nakayama–Yoken and Beijing strains). *J Neurol Neurosurg Psychiatry* 59: 316–317.

Ojala, A. (1947). On changes in the cerebrospinal fluid during measles. *Ann Med Int Fenn* 36: 321–331.

Oomes, P., Jacobs, B.C., Hazenberg, M.P.H., *et al.* (1995). Anti-GM1 IgG antibodies and *Campylobacter* bacteria in Guillain–Barre syndrome: evidence of molecular mimicry. *Ann Neurol* 38: 170–175.

Optic Neuritis Study Group (1992). A randomized, controlled trial of corticosteroids in the treatment of optic neuritis. *N Engl J Med* 326: 581–588.

Optic Neuritis Study Group (1993). The effect of corticosteroids for acute optic neuritis on the subsequent development of multiple sclerosis. *N Engl J Med* 329: 1764–1769.

Orgogozo, J.M., Gilman, S., Dartigues, J.F., Laurent, B., Puel, M., Kirby, L.C., *et al.* (2003). Subacute meningoencephalitis in a subset of patients with AD after Ab42 immunization. *Neurology* 61: 46–54.

Osame, M., Matsumoto, M., Usuki, K., *et al.* (1987). Chronic progressive myelopathy with elevated antibodies to human lymphotropic virus type 1 and adult T-cell leukemia-like cells. *Ann Neurol* 21: 117–122.

Ozawa, H., Noma, S., Yoshida, Y., Sekine, H. Hashimoto, T. (2000). Acute disseminated encephalomyelitis associated with poliomyelitis vaccine. *Pediatr Neurol* 23: 177–179.

Parkin, P., Hierons, R., and McDonald, W. (1984). Bilateral optic neuritis. A long term followup. *Brain* 107: 951–964.

Paskavitz, J., Anderson, C.A., Filley, C.M. *et al.* (1995). Acute arcuate fiber demyelinating encephalopathy following Epstein–Barr virus infection. *Ann Neurol* 38: 127–131.

Pasternak, J., Devivo, C., and Prensky, A. (1980). Steroid-responsive encephalomyelitis in childhood. *Neurology* 30: 481–486.

Paterson, P. (1960). Transfer of allergic encephalomyelitis in rats by means of lymph node cells. *J Exp Med* 111: 119–136.

Perdue, Z., Bale, Jr, J.F., Dunn, V.K., Bell, W.E. (1985). Magnetic resonance imaging in childhood disseminated encephalomyelitis. *Pediatr Neurol* 1: 370–374.

Perlmutter, S., Leitmam, S., Garvey, M.A., Hamburger, S., Feldman, E., Leonard, H.L., Swedo, S.E. (1999). Therapeutic plasma exchange and intravenous immunoglobulin for obsessive-compulsive disorder and tic disorders in childhood. *Lancet* 354: 1153–1158.

Peterson, K., Rosenblum, M.K., Powers, J.M., *et al.* (1993). Effect of brain irradiation on demyelinating lesions. *Neurology* 43: 2105–2112.

Poser, C. (1985). Myelinoclastic diffuse sclerosis. In: *Demyelinating Diseases* (ed. J. Koetsier), pp. 419–428. Elsevier, Amsterdam.

Poser, C., Roman, G., and Emery, E. (1978). Recurrent disseminated vasculo-myelinopathy. *Arch Neurol* **36**: 166.

Power, C., Kong, P.A., Crawford, T., *et al.* (1993). Cerebral white matter changes in acquired immunodeficiency syndrome dementia: alterations of the blood-brain barrier. *Ann Neurol* **34**: 339–350.

Pradhan, S., Gupta, R.P., Shashank, S., Pandey, N. (1999). Intravenous immuno-globulin therapy in acute disseminated encephalomyelitis. *J Neurol Sci* **165**: 56–61.

Ray, D., Bridger, J., Hawnar, J., *et al.* (1994). Transverse myelitis as the presenta-tion of Jo-1 antibody syndrome (myositis and fibrosing alveolitis) in long-standing ulcerative colitis. *Br J Rheumatol* **32**: 1105–1108.

Rees, J., Gregson, N., and Hughes, R. (1995). Anti-ganglioside antibodies in Guillain-Barre syndrome and their relationship to *Campylobacter jejuni* infection. *Ann Neurol* **38**: 809–816.

Reik, L.J. (1980). Disseminated vasculomyelinopathy: an immune complex disease. *Ann Neurol* **7**: 291–296.

Reik, L.J., Smith, L., Khan, A., Nelson, W. (1985). Demyelinating encephalopathy in Lyme disease. *Neurology* **35**: 267–269.

Renkawek, K., Majkowska-Wierzbicka, J., and Krajewski, S. (1985). Necrotic changes of the spinal cord with immune-complex-mediated vasculitis in a case of allergic encephalomyelitis. *J Neurol* **232**: 368–373.

Reye, R., Morgan, G., and Baral, J. (1963). Encephalopathy and fatty infiltration of the viscera. *Lancet* **2**: 742–752.

Riikonen, R., Donner, M., and Erkkila, H. (1988). Optic neuritis in children and its relationship to multiple sclerosis: a clinical study of 21 children. *Dev Med Child Neurol* **30**: 349–359.

Rivers, T. and Schwentker, F. (1935). Encephalomyelitis accompanied by myelin destruction experimentally produced in monkeys. *J Exp Med* **61**: 689–702.

Robertson, W. and Smith, C. (2002). Sydenham's chorea in the age of MRI: a case report and review. *Pediatr Neurol* **27**: 65–67.

Robertson, W. and Cruikshank, E. (1972). Jamaican (tropical) neuropathy. In: *Pathology of the Nervous System* (ed. J. Minckler), pp. 2466–2476 McGraw-Hill, New York.

Rodriguez, M., Karnes, W.E., Bartleson, J.D., Pineda, A.A. (1993). Plasmapheresis in acute episodes of fulminant CNS inflammatory demyelination. *Neurology* **43**: 1100–1104.

Rodriguez, M., Siva, A., and Cross, S.E.A. (1995). Optic neuritis: a population-based study in Olmsted County, Minnesota. *Neurology* **45**: 1253–1258.

Rolak, L., Beck, R.W., Paty, D.W., *et al.* (1996). Cerebrospinal fluid in acute optic neuritis: experience of the optic neuritis treatment trial. *Neurology* **46**: 368–372.

Ropper, A. and Poskanzer, D. (1978). The prognosis of acute and subacute trau-matic myelopathy based on early signs and symptoms. *Ann Neurol* **4**: 51–59.

Ropper, A., Miett, T., and Chiappa, K. (1982). Absence of evoked potential abnormalities in acute transverse myelopathy. *Neurology* **32**: 80–82.

Rosenberg, G. (1970). Meningoencephalitis following an influenza vaccination. *N Engl J Med* **283**: 1209.

Russell, D. (1937). Changes in the central nervous system following arsphen-amine medication. *J Pathol Bacteriol* **45**: 357–366.

Russell, D. (1955). The nosological unity of acute hemorrhagic leucoencephalitis and acute disseminated encephalomyelitis. *Brain* **78**: 369–376.

Rust, R., Dodson, W., Prensky, A.L., Chun, R., Devivo, D., Dodge, P.R., *et al.* (1997). Classification and outcome of acute disseminated encephalomyelitis. *Ann Neurol* **42**: 491.

Ryder, J., Croen, K., Kleinschmidt-DeMasters, B.K., *et al.* (1986). Progressive encephalitis three months after resolution of cutaneous zoster in a patient with AIDS. *Ann Neurol* **19**: 182–188.

Sacks O. (1999). *Awakenings*. Vintage Books, New York.

Sadovnick, A. and Scheifele, D. (2000). School-based hepatitis B vaccination programme and adolescent multiple sclerosis. *Lancet* **355**: 549–550.

Saito, H., Endo, M., Takase, S., Itahara, K. (1980). Acute disseminated encephalo-myelitis after influenza vaccination. *Arch Neurol* **37**: 564–566.

Salazar, A., Engel, W., and Levy, H. (1981). PolyICLC in the treatment of post-infectious demyelinating encephalomyelitis. *Arch Neurol* **38**: 382–383.

Sandberg-Wollheim, M., *et al.* (1990). A long term prospective study of optic neuritis: evaluation of risk factors. *Ann Neurol* **27**: 386–393.

Sanders, K., Khandji, A., and Mohr, J. (1990). Gadolinium-MRI in acute trans-verse myelopathy. *Neurology* **40**: 1614–1616.

Schecter, S. (1986). Lyme disease with associated optic neuropathy. *Am J Med* **81**: 143–145.

Schlenska, G. (1977). Unusual neurological complications following tetanus toxoid administration. *J Neurol* **215**: 299–302.

Schlitt, M. and Whitley, R. (1990). Viral diseases: herpes simplex encephalitis. In: *Controlled Clinical Trials in Neurological Disease* (ed. R. Porter and B. Schoenberg), pp. 393–406. Kluwer Academic: Norwell, MA.

Schwarz, S., Mohr, A., Nauth, M., Wildermann, B., Storch-Hegenlocher, B. (2001). Acute disseminated encephalomyelitis. A follow-up study of 40 adult patients. *Neurology* **56**: 1313–1318.

Schwimmbeck, P. Dyrberg, T., Drachman, D.B., Oldstone, M.B.A. (1989). Molecular mimicry and myasthenia gravis: an autoantigenic site of the acetylcholine receptor a subunit that has biologic activity and reacts immunochemically with herpes simplex virus. *J Clin Invest* **84**: 1174–1180.

Seales, D. and Greer, M. (1991). Acute hemorrhagic leukoencephalopathy: a suc-cessful recovery. *Arch Neurol* **48**: 1086–1088.

Seitelberger, F. (1967). Autoimmunologic aspects of cerebral diseases. *Pathol Eur* **2**: 233–256.

Seyfert, S., Klapps, P., Meisel, C., *et al.* (1990). Multiple sclerosis and other autoimmune diseases. *Acta Neurol Scand* **81**: 37–42.

Shah, A., Tselis, A., and Mason, B. (2000). Acute disseminated encephalomyelitis in a pregnant woman successfully treated with plasmapheresis. *J Neurol Sci* **174**: 147–151.

Shakir, R., Al-Din, A., Araj, G.F., *et al.* (1987). Clinical categories of neurobrucell-osis. *Brain* **110**: 213–223.

Shiraki, H. and Otani, S. (1959). Clinical and pathological features of rabies post-vaccinal encephalomyelitis in man. Relationship to multiple sclerosis and to experimental 'allergic' encephalomyelitis in animals. In: *Allergic Encephalo-myelitis* (ed. M. Kies and E. Alvord), pp. 58–136. Charles C. Thomas, Springfield, IL.

Silberberg, D. (1992). Corticosteroids and optic neuritis. *N Engl J Med* **326**: 1808–1810.

Sotelo, J., Enriquez, R.G., Najera, R., Zermeno, F. (1984). Allergic encephalo-myelitis associated with holistic medicine (injection of porcine hypophysis). *Lancet* **2**: 702.

Spillane, J. and Wells, C. (1964). The neurology of Jennerian vaccination. A clin-ical account of the neurological complications which occurred during the smallpox epidemic in South Wales in 1962. *Brain* **87**: 1–44.

Stefansson, K., Dieperink, M.E., Richman, D.P., *et al.* (1985). Sharing of antigenic determinants between the nicotinic acetylcholine receptor and proteins in *Escherichia coli*, *Proteus vulgaris*, and *Klebsiella pneumoniae*: possible role in the pathogenesis of myasthenia gravis. *N Engl J Med* **312**: 221–225.

Straussberg, R., Schonfeld, T., Weitz, R., Karmazyn, B., Harel, L. (2001). Improve-ment of atypical acute disseminated encephalomyelitis with steroids and intravenous immunoglobulins. *Pediatr Neurol* **24**: 139–143.

Stricker, R., Miller, R., and Kiprov, D. (1992). Role of plasmapheresis in acute dis-seminated (postinfectious) encephalomyelitis. *J Clin Apheresis* **7**: 173–179.

Sucherowsky, O., Sweeney, V.P., Berry, K., Bratty, P.J.A. (1983). Acute hemor-rhagic leukoencephalopathy. A clinical, pathological, and radiological cor-relation. *Can J Neurol Sci* **10**: 63–67.

Sun, D., Le, J., Yang, S., *et al.* (1993). Major role of antigen-presenting cells in the response of rat encephalitogenic T cells to myelin basic proteins. *J Immunol* **151**: 111–118.

Suwa, K., Yamagata, T., Momoi, M.Y., Kawakami, A., Kikuchi, Y., Miyao, M., Hirokawa, H., Oikawa, T. (1999). Acute relapsing encephalopathy mimicking acute necrotizing encephalopathy in a 4-year-old boy. *Brain Dev* **21**: 554–558.

Swedo, S. (1994). Sydenham's chorea. A model for childhood autoimmune neuropsychiatric disease. *J Am Med Assoc* **272**: 1788–1791.

Swedo, S., Leonard, H.L., Schapiro, M.D., Casey, B.J., Mannheim, G.B., Lenane, M.C. Rettew, D.C. (1993). Sydenham's chorea: physical and psychological symptoms of St Vitus dance. *Pediatrics* **91**: 706–713.

Swedo, S., Leonard, H.L., Garvey, M. Mittleman, B., Allen, A.J., Perlmutter, S., Dow, S., Zamkoff, J., Dubbert, B.K., Lougee, L. (1998). Pediatric auto-immune neuropsychiatric disorders associated with streptococcal infections: clinical description of the first 50 cases. *Am J Psych* **155**: 264–271.

Swoveland, P. and Johnson, K. (1989). Subacute sclerosing panencephalitis and other paramyxovirus infections. In: *Viral Diseases* (ed. R. McKendall), pp. 412–437. Elsevier Science, Amsterdam.

Sze, G. (1992). MR imaging of the spinal cord: current status and future advances. *Am J Radiol* **159**: 149–159.

Takata, T., Hirakawa, M., Sakurai, M., Kanazawa, I. (1999). Fulminant form of acute disseminated encephalomyelitis: successful treatment with hypothermia. *J Neurol Sci* **165**: 94–97.

Teitelbaum, D., Meshorer, A., Hirshfeld, T., Arnon, R., Sela, M. (1971). Suppression of experimental allergic encephalomyelitis by a synthetic polypeptide. *Eur J Immunol* **1**: 242–248.

Tenembaum, S., Chamoles, N., and Fejerman, N. (2002). Acute disseminated encephalomyelitis. A long-term follow-up study of 84 pediatric patients. *Neurology* **59**: 1224–1231.

ter Meulen, V. (1989). Virus-induced cell-mediated autoimmunity. In: *Concepts in Viral Pathogenesis* (ed. A. Notkins and M. Oldstone), pp. 297–303. Springer, New York.

Thygesen, P. (1949). Prognosis in the initial stage of disseminated primary demyelinating disease of the central nervous system. *Arch Psych Neurol* **61**: 339–351.

Tippett, D., Fishman, P., and Panitch, H. (1991). Recurrent transverse myelitis. *Neurology* **41**: 703–706.

Toro, G., Vergara, I., and Roman, G. (1977). Neuroparalytic accidents of antirabies vaccination with suckling mouse brain vaccine. *Arch Neurol* **34**: 694–700.

Tourbah, A., Gout, O., Liblau, R., Lyon-Caen, O., Bougniot, C, Iba-Zizen, M.T., Cabanis, E.A. (1999). Encephalitis after hepatitis B vaccination: recurrent disseminated encephalitis or MS? *Neurology* **53**: 396–401.

Townsend, J., Baringer, J.R., Wolinsky, J.S. (1975). Progressive rubella panencephalitis. Late onset after congenital rubella. *N Engl J Med* **292**: 990–993.

Townsend, J., Wolinsky, J., and Baringer, J. (1976). The neuropathology of progressive rubella panencephalitis of late onset. *Brain* **99**: 81–90.

Trevisani, G., Gattinari, G.C., Caraceni, P., *et al.* (1993). Transverse myelitis following hepatitis B vaccination. *J Hepatol* **19**: 317–318.

Tselis, A. and Lisak, R. (1995). Acute disseminated encephalomyelitis and isolated central nervous system demyelinative syndromes. *Curr Opin Neurol* **8**: 227–229.

Tyler, K., Gross, R., and Cascino, G. (1986). Unusual viral causes of transverse myelitis: hepatitis A and cytomegalovirus. *Neurology* **36**: 855–858.

Valentine, A., Kendall, B., and Harding, B. (1982). Computed tomography in acute hemorrhagic leukoencephalitis. *Neuroradiology* **22**: 215–219.

Vernant, J., Maurs, L., Gessain, A., *et al.* (1987). Endemic tropical spastic paraparesis associated with human lymphotropic virus type 1: a clinical and seroepidemiological study of 25 cases. *Ann Neurol* **21**: 123–130.

von Giesen, H.-J., Arendt, G., Neuen-Jacob, E., *et al.* (1994). A pathologically distinct new form of HIV associated encephalopathy. *J Neurol Sci* **121**: 215–221.

Walker, R. and Gawler, J.)1989). Serial cerebral CT abnormalities in relapsing acute disseminated encephalomyelitis. *J Neurol Neurosurg Psychiatry* **52**: 1100–1102.

Warren, W. (1956). Encephalopathy due to influenza vaccine. *Arch Intern Med* **97**: 803–805.

Watson, R., Ballinger, W., and Quisling, R. (1984). Acute hemorrhagic leukoencephalitis: diagnosis by computed tomography. *Ann Neurol* **15**: 611–612.

Weinberg, A., Li, S., Palmer, M., Tyler, K.L. (2002). Quantitative CSF PCR in Epstein-Barr virus infections of the central nervous system. *Ann Neurol* **52**: 543–548.

Weinshenker, B., P'Brien, P.C., Petterson, T.M., Noseworthy, J.H., Luccinetti, C.F., Dodick, D.W., Pineda, A.A., Stevens, L.N., Rodriguez, M. (1999). A randomized trial of plasma exchange in acute central nervous system inflammatory demyelinating disease. *Ann Neurol* **46**: 878–886.

Weller, R. (1991). Animal models of demyelinating disease. *Curr Opin Neurol Neurosurg* **4**: 221–226.

Wentz, K. and Marcuse, E. (1991). Diphtheria–tetanus–pertussis vaccine and serious neurological illness: an updated review of the epidemiological evidence. *Pediatrics* **87**: 287–297.

Whittle, E. and Roberton, N. (1977). Transverse myelitis after diphtheria, tetanus, and polio immunization. *Br Med J* **2**: 1450.

Williams, H. and Chafee, F. (1961). Demyelinating encephalomyelitis in a case of tetanus treated with antitoxin. *N Engl J Med* **264**: 489–491.

Woods, C. and Ellison, G. (1964). Encephalopathy following influenza immunization. *J Pediatr* **65**: 745–748.

Yahr, M. and Lobo-Antunes, J. (1972). Relapsing encephalomyelitis following the use of influenza vaccine. *Arch Neurol* **27**: 182–183.

Yoshizawa, T., Tsukuda, A., Maki, Y., Kanazawa, I. (1982). Transverse myelitis associated with *Mycoplasma pneumoniae* infections. *Eur Neurol* **21**: 48–51.

Ziegler, D. (1966). Acute disseminated encephalomyelitis. Some therapeutic and diagnostic considerations. *Arch Neurol* **14**: 476–488.

14 Tissue pathology of multiple sclerosis

Don J. Mahad, Bruce D. Trapp, and Richard M. Ransohoff

Multiple sclerosis (MS)

General aspects

MS, an inflammatory demyelinating neurodegenerative disease of the CNS (Charcot, 1868; Waxman, 1998), is a common cause of disability in adults in North America and Europe (Sadovnick and Ebers, 1993). Over 1 million individuals are estimated to have MS, worldwide (Compston, 1990). The peak age of onset is in the third decade of life and the life expectancy is reduced by approximately 5 years (Compston *et al.*, 1998; Weinshenker, 1998). Eighty per cent of individuals with MS develop progressive neurological impairment either from the clinical onset of the disease (defined as primary progressive MS (PPMS), accountable for 15–20% of all MS patients (Thompson *et al.*, 2000)) or following a period of intermittent episodes of neurological dysfunction, which may be associated with a stepwise increase in residual neurological impairment (defined as secondary progressive MS (SPMS), accountable for 60–65% of all MS patients (Fig. 14.1) (Lublin and Reingold, 1996)). The clinical phase of the disease with intermittent episodes of neurological dysfunction (Schumacher, 1974) in the absence of continuous progression of neurological impairment, is defined as relapsing–remitting MS (RRMS, Fig. 14.1) (Weinshenker *et al.*, 1989). The remaining 20% of patients with MS do not progress and remain in the RRMS phase, with a proportion having a benign course (Mackay and Hirano, 1967; Compston *et al.*, 1998). Clinically 'silent' cases with neuropathological features of MS have been reported using autopsy tissue (Mackay and Hirano, 1967; Ghatak *et al.*, 1974; Morariu and Klutzow 1976; Heinsen *et al.*, 1995). However, the symptoms and signs of these cases may have been subtle and remained unnoticed. Although the aetiology of MS is unknown, genetic and environmental factors play a role in the pathogenesis. The genetic susceptibility is reported to be due to multiple genes with small effects rather than a single gene with a large effect (2001). Viral infections that prime the immune system during childhood are recognized as a predisposing environmental factor (Compston *et al.*, 1986; Kennedy and Steiner, 1994; Weinshenker, 1996).

Tissue pathology; historical context

Jean Martin Charcot's clinicopathological description, which followed Carswell's depiction of the MS lesion and Cruveilhier's association of pathological features with the clinical presentation, is considered as a milestone in the understanding of the pathogenesis of MS (McDonald, 1994; Trapp *et al.*, 1999c). Inflammation, demyelination, axonal loss, gliosis, and loss of oligodendrocytes are the cardinal neuropathological features of MS. There have been significant advances in the understanding of the mechanisms that lead to the pathological features and the relative contribution of these pathological features to the temporal evolution of MS lesions and to the natural history of MS. However, direct evidence supporting a pathogenic role for some of the mechanisms and relative contribution of pathological features to lesion evolution is limited, partly due to the lack of availability of effective therapeutic agents (Hohlfeld, 1997) and limited accessibility to CNS tissue during life.

We summarize and discuss the neuropathological features of MS, the underlying mechanisms of tissue damage, the changes in neuropathological features with temporal evolution of lesions, and the recent advances in the understanding of the clinicopathological correlation of MS as well as the heterogeneity of white matter and cortical MS lesions.

Inflammation in MS

Components of the inflammatory infiltrate in MS tissue

The cellular components of the inflammatory infiltrate in MS consist of T lymphocytes (cytotoxic (CD8), T helper (CD4) type 1 and type 2),

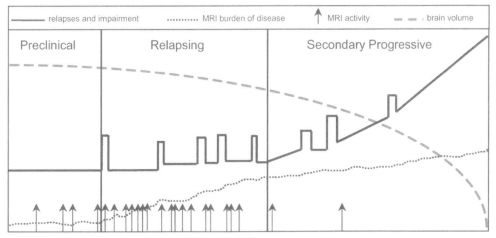

Fig. 14.1 The natural history of multiple sclerosis. During the pre-clinical stage of MS, both MRI activity (arrows), based on the presence of gadolinium-enhanced lesions or the appearance of new lesions on T_2-weighted images, and MRI burden of disease (dotted line), based on lesion load measurement on normalized T_2 images, indicate the presence of biological disease. During the relapsing remitting (RR) phase of MS, the MRI activity (arrows) is much greater than the relapse rate. The stepwise deterioration during the RR phase is associated with inflammatory activity and is due to inflammatory axonal transection. During the secondary progressive stage, brain atrophy indicating axonal loss and MRI disease burden continue to increase despite the reduction of MRI activity.

B lymphocytes, monocytes, macrophages, and activated microglia and are summarized below.

T cells

In MS, pathogenic roles have been implicated for CD4+ and CD8+ lymphocytes as well as γδ T-cells. Several studies suggest a pathogenic role for T helper 1 (Th1) lymphocytes in MS: CD4+ cells are present in all patterns of MS lesions (Lucchinetti et al., 2000) and MS is associated with the major histocompatibility (MHC) Class II haplotype; the intravenous administration of interferon-gamma (IFN-γ) (a Th1 cytokine), which activates macrophages and induces cytokines and chemokines, leads to worsening of MS (Panitch et al., 1987); the percentage of IFN-γ-producing T cells in peripheral blood mononuclear cells (PBMCs) from MS patients significantly correlates with MRI disease activity (Calabresi et al., 1998); elevated interleukin (IL)-12 and reduced IL-10 serum levels are associated with increased disease activity (Comabella et al., 1998; Boxel-Dezaire et al., 1999); Th1-related cytokines are expressed within MS lesions (Benveniste, 1992; Woodroofe, 1995); chemokine receptor expression patterns (CXCR3, CCR5) on inflammatory cells in MS lesions are consistent with the Th1 phenotype (Bonecchi et al., 1998; Sallusto et al., 1998); the increase in cerebrospinal fluid (CSF) interferon-γ inducible protein (IP-10)/CXCL10 and the decrease in CSF macrophage chemoattractant protein (MCP)-1/CCL2 levels in MS patients are indicative of IFN-γ-mediated processes (Sorensen et al., 1999; Franciotta et al., 2001; Mahad et al., 2002); the significant reduction in MRI-defined new lesion formation and peripheral lymphocyte counts following treatment with Campath-1H is associated with a decrease in Th1 cell differentiation while the increase in Th2 cell differentiation following Campath-1H is associated with the development of Grave's thyroid eye disease (a Th2/antibody-mediated disease) (Coles et al., 1999). However, many approaches directed at Th1 immunoregulation have resulted in disappointment (Hohlfeld, 1997), suggesting a pathogenic role for Th2 lymphocytes, cytotoxic T lymphocytes (CTLs) as well as monocytes, microglia, and macrophages (Lassmann et al., 1998, 2001).

Th2 cytokines (IL-4 and IL-10) are detectable in acute and chronic MS lesions (Benveniste, 1992). The expression of CCR3 on lymphocytes in tissue from cases with fulminant variants of MS, Devic's type neuromyelitis optica (NMO), and Marburg's type of acute MS suggests a pathogenic role for Th2 lymphocytes (Weinshenker 1995; Lucchinetti et al., 2002).

CD8+ cells are enriched in areas of active demyelination in MS tissue and are located in close proximity to demyelinating axons (Babbe et al., 2000; Neumann et al., 2002). A recent study, using single cells obtained through micromanipulation and polymerase chain reaction (PCR) reported a more prominent clonal expansion in CD8+ than CD4+ cell populations in active MS lesions (Babbe et al., 2000) and the number of CD8+ cells in MS lesions correlated better with the degree of axonal transection than CD4+ cells (Bitsch et al., 2000; Kuhlmann et al., 2002).

Studies that report the ratio of CD4 to CD8 T cells in MS tissue are not in agreement, most probably due to differential capacity of T cells to survive, undergo apoptosis (Pender and Rist, 2001), and proliferate as well as due to technical reasons (Booss et al., 1983; Hauser et al., 1986; Woodroofe et al., 1986; Hayashi et al., 1988; Sobel et al., 1988; Raine, 1994). The functional and molecular processes responsible for these observations are unclear (Neumann et al., 2002). Recent studies have identified CD8+ T cells predominantly within the parenchyma and CD4+ T cells predominantly in the perivascular cuffs (Babbe et al., 2000; Gay et al., 1997).

γδ T cells with cytotoxic properties act via the recognition of stress proteins such as heat shock protein (HSP) 60, 65, and αβ-crystalline and are capable of secreting large quantities of IFN-γ, independent of MHC expression (Gay et al., 1997). One to ten per cent of T cells in MS lesions have been shown to be γδ T cells, which are said to play a prominent role during the later stages of MS (Wucherpfennig et al., 1992).

B cells, antibody, and complement

Although the role of B cells in immune surveillance in the CNS is unknown, B cells and humoral mechanisms play a definitive role in inflammatory demyelination (Lucchinetti et al., 2002). The presence of oligoclonal bands (OCBs) in the CSF and MS lesions provides evidence for the existence of clonally expanded B cells producing immunglobulin (Ig) G (Lucchinetti et al., 2000; Hickey, 2001). Pathogenic roles for B cells are implicated during early and late stages of MS (Gay et al., 1997; Storch et al., 1998) and the presence of numerous B lymphocytes within NMO lesions is associated with a prominent complement activation and a severe clinical phenotype (Prineas and Graham, 1981; Lucchinetti et al., 2000, 2002).

Monocytes, macrophages, and microglia

The majority of the inflammatory infiltrate in MS lesions consists of phagocytic macrophages, which are derived from either monocytes or microglia (Bruck et al., 1995; Trebst et al., 2001). Macrophages are an essential mediator of in vivo demyelination (Brosnan et al., 1981; Huitinga et al., 1990). Whether the majority of the phagocytic macrophages in active MS lesions are derived from monocytes or microglia is unclear as the surface markers are indistinguishable once monocytes and microglia differentiate into phagocytic macrophages (Li et al., 1996; Trebst et al., 2001). Activated microglia have been observed in the periplaque white matter as well as in non-lesional/normal appearing white matter prior to the arrival of blood-derived inflammatory cells, attributing a pathogenic role for microglia at an early stage of lesion evolution (Woodroofe, 1986; Hayes et al., 1987). Activated microglia surround transected axons in the white matter and non-phosphorylated neurofilament-positive axons and neurites in the cortical lesions (Peterson et al., 2001; Trapp et al., 1998). Further, activated microglia express vascular cell adhesion molecule (VCAM)-1 and are closely opposed to oligodendrocytes, suggesting a pathogenic role in oligodendrocyte dysfunction (Peterson et al., 2001).

Immunopathogenesis

The immune-mediated pathogenesis of MS is based on several observations: the presence of inflammatory infiltrate which correlates with axonal transection and demyelination within MS lesions (Charcot 1868; Ferguson et al., 1997; Trapp et al., 1998; Bitsch et al., 2000; Trebst et al., 2001; Kuhlmann et al., 2002); the ability of CNS antigen-specific T cells to orchestrate inflammatory demyelination in animal models (experimental allergic encephalomyelitis, EAE) (Ransohoff et al., 1996); MS susceptibility genes linked to those involved in immune responses, in particular MHC Class II (The Transatlantic MS Genetics Cooperative, 2001); modulation of disease by anti-inflammatory agents (Rudick et al., 1999).

Several studies support a primary role for inflammation in the pathogenesis of MS, at least in a subset of MS patients: demyelination in the absence of inflammation is a rare observation in MS, with the exception of cortical MS lesions and cases treated with immunosuppressants (Woodroofe et al., 1986; Compston et al., 1998); biopsies of gadolinium-enhanced acute MS lesions show perivascular inflammation independent of associated demyelination (Compston et al., 1998); inflammatory infiltrate is present in tissue devoid of myelin, namely the retina in EAE (Kojima et al., 1994); successful active and passive transfer of EAE in genetically susceptible animals provides evidence for T-cell-mediated disease induction (Skundric et al., 1993; Tani and Ransohoff, 1994; Ransohoff et al., 1996).

The recruitment of inflammatory cells across the blood–brain barrier and migration within the brain parenchyma

The majority of the inflammatory infiltrate in MS is derived from the bone marrow and recruited across the blood–brain barrier (BBB) in a multistep process consisting of leukocyte deceleration, tethering, rolling, arrest, and diapedesis (Springer, 1994; Butcher and Picker, 1996). Several molecules are implicated in the recruitment of leukocytes into the CNS, namely integrins, cell adhesion molecules (CAM), chemokines, chemokine receptors, and matrix metalloproteases (MMPs) (Kieseier et al., 1999). ICAM (intercellular cell adhesion molecule)-1, ICAM-2, ICAM-3 and VCAM-1, two immunoglobulin superfamily CAMs, are implicated in CNS inflammation. Chemokines, chemoattractant cytokines, consist of over 40 members divided into four subfamilies based on their structure. CC and CXC subfamilies contain the majority of the chemokines (CCL1–28 and CXCL1–16) (Zlotnik and Yoshie, 2000). Chemokine receptors are G-protein coupled receptors, and to date we know of 10 CC receptors (CCR1–10) and six CXC receptors (CXCR1–6). The ligand–chemokine receptor interactions are complicated, as more than one chemokine can activate a given chemokine receptor and vice versa, within a subfamily (Zlotnik and Yoshie, 2000).

The expression of integrins and cell adhesion molecules in MS lesions

ICAM-1, ICAM-3, and VCAM-1 are expressed with differing temporal and spatial patterns within lesional and non-lesional white matter in MS as well as in other neuroinflammatory diseases (encephalitis, adrenoleukodystrophy, subacute sclerosing panencephalitis, tropical spastic paraparesis) and neurodegenerative diseases (amyotrophic lateral sclerosis, olivopontocerebellar degeneration, Parkinson's disease, and CNS infarcts) (Sobel et al., 1988; Cannella and Raine, 1995; Bo et al., 1996; Love and Barber, 2001; Peterson et al., 2002).

ICAM-1 expression, which is colocalized to the luminal surface of brain endothelial cells, is most prominent in MS lesions (81% of lesions (Bo et al., 1996)). Thirty-seven per cent of blood vessels in non-lesional MS white matter expressed ICAM-1 compared with 10% in control brains (Bo et al., 1996; Navratil et al., 1997). Within MS lesions, ICAM-1 expression is most prominent in acute lesions (Sobel et al., 1988), although Cannella and Raine (1995) reported, using a somewhat subjective scoring system, maximum staining in chronic silent lesions. The up-regulation of ICAM-2 was not detected in MS lesions. ICAM-3 is expressed mainly on lymphocytes and monocytes in perivascular cuffs and lesion edges (Bo et al., 1996). ICAM-3 expression on monocytes decreased during maturation into macrophages (Bo et al., 1996). LFA-1 (leukocyte function antigen), which binds to ICAMs, is expressed on activated microglia in MS lesions. The co-expression of LFA-1 and ICAM-3 on the majority of lymphocytes in MS lesions is consistent with the role of LFA-1/ICAM-3 interaction in lymphocyte recruitment. LFA-1 expression on microglia and ICAM-3 on lymphocytes suggests a role in lymphocyte–microglial interaction as part of antigen presentation in MS.

VCAM-1 expression was most prominent at the border of active MS lesions (Peterson et al., 2002). Based on morphology, VCAM-1+ cells were identified as lymphocytes and monocytes in the perivascular spaces, large lipid-filled macrophages in the cores and borders of active lesions, and activated microglia in association with oligodendrocyte somata in peri-

lesional white matter (Cannella and Raine, 1995; Peterson et al., 2002). VLA-4 (very late activation antigen), which binds to VCAM-1, was seen on perivascular lymphocytes and monocytes in chronic active MS lesions (Cannella and Raine, 1995). VCAM-1 and VLA-4 are also expressed in non-inflammatory CNS tissue, for example in ALS and olivopontocerebellar degeneration (OPCD), but the expression in control brain tissue was minimal. Consistent with a pathogenic role of VLA-4 in MS, intravenous administration of a humanized monoclonal antibody against human α4 integrin led to a significant reduction of new lesion formation, as defined by gadolinium-enhanced MRI (Tubridy et al., 1999; Miller et al., 2003).

The expression of chemokines and chemokine receptors in MS lesions

Several studies have reported the expression of chemokines and chemokine receptors in MS tissue, implicating a pathogenic role in the recruitment and retention of inflammatory infiltrate and providing insight into the evolution of lesions and monocyte differentiation in MS tissue.

Chemokines expressed in MS lesions

CCL2, CCL3, CCL4, CCL5, and CXCL10 are expressed in MS lesions and are summarized in Table 14.1.

MCP-1 (monocyte chemoattractant protein-1/CCL2), a potent monocyte chemoattractant in vivo, is expressed in MS lesions with much greater intensity of staining in acute lesions compared with sections of control brain tissue or normal appearing white matter (NAWM) (McManus et al., 1998; Simpson et al., 1998; van der Voorn et al., 1999). CCL2 also chemoattracts memory T lymphocytes, dendritic cells, natural killer (NK) cells, and microglia (Fuentes et al., 1995; Sozzani et al., 1995). Hypertrophic astrocytes are the main source of CCL2 in MS lesions and the intensity of CCL2 staining in the cytoplasm and processes of astrocytes was reduced as the lesions became chronic (McManus et al., 1998; van der Voorn et al., 1999; Nygardas et al., 2000).

MIP-1α/CCL3 and MIP-1β/CCL4, RANTES (regulated upon activation of normal T-cell expressed and secreted)/CCL5 are expressed within MS lesions and chemoattract CCR1-, CCR3-, and/or CCR5-bearing T cells and monocytes. In active MS lesions, CCL3 is expressed on microglia and macrophages (Simpson et al., 1998), whereas CCL5 is expressed on perivascular cells, blood vessel endothelial cells, and to a lesser extent on perivascular astrocytes (Hvas et al., 1997; Simpson et al., 1998; Woodroofe et al., 1999; Boven et al., 2000)

Immunoreactivity to CXCL10/IP-10, a potent lymphocyte chemoattractant, is observed on cell bodies and foot processes of reactive astrocytes in

Table 14.1 An overview of chemokines in MS tissue

Chemokine	Chemokines receptor(s) activated by the chemokine[a]	Expression in MS CNS tissue
CCL2	CCR2	Astrocytes and inflammatory cells express in active lesions (McManus et al., 1998; Simpson et al., 1998; van der Voorn et al., 1999a; Woodroofe et al., 1999)
CCL3	CCR1, CCR5	Microglia and macrophages express in active lesions (Simpson et al., 1998; Woodroofe et al., 1999; Boven et al., 2000)
CCL4	CCR1, CCR3, CCR5	Inflammatory cells and activated neuroglia express in active lesions (Simpson et al., 1998; Woodroofe et al., 1999; Boven et al., 2000)
CCL5	CCR1, CCR3, CCR5	Perivascular cells and astrocytes express in active lesions (Simpson et al., 1998; Boven et al., 2000).
CXCL10	CXCR3	Astrocytes express in active lesions (Balashov et al., 1999; Sorensen et al., 1999, 2002; Simpson et al., 2000b)

[a]Information from Zlotnik and Yoshie (2000).

CCL2/MCP-1, macrophage chemoattractant protein 1; CCL3/MIP-1α< macrophage inflammatory protein-1α; CCL4/MIP-1β< macrophage inflammatory protein-1β; CCL5/RANTES, regulated upon activation of normal T-cell expressed and secreted; CXCL10/IP-10, interferon-γ inducible protein-10.

active MS lesions and on the endothelium in non-lesional white matter (NLWM) (Sorensen *et al.*, 1999, 2002; Simpson *et al.*, 2000*b*). CXCL10 was not expressed in silent/inactive MS lesions or in control brain tissue (Balashov *et al.*, 1999; Simpson *et al.*, 2000*b*). Double staining for CXCL10 and CXCR3 showed a significant correlation between CXCL10+ cellular elements and CXCR3+ perivascular cells (Sorensen *et al.*, 2002). CXCL10 levels in the CSF from patients with MS correlated with the clinical disease activity and the CSF leukocyte count (Balashov *et al.*, 1999; Sorensen *et al.*, 1999, 2002; Mahad *et al.*, 2002).

Chemokine receptors expressed in MS lesions

Several chemokine receptors are expressed on the cellular inflammatory infiltrate in MS lesions (Table 14.1)

CCR1, a receptor for CCL3, CCL5, and CCL7, is expressed in newly arrived monocytes in early active MS lesions (Lucchinetti *et al.*, 1996; Trebst *et al.*, 2001). The majority (90%) of CSF monocytes expressed CCR1, independent of disease status (Kivisakk *et al.*, 2002; Trebst *et al.*, 2001). As the monocytes differentiate into macrophages *in vivo*, in accordance with lesion maturation from early active through late active to inactive stages (Lucchinetti *et al.*, 1996), CCR1 expression significantly decreased, consistent with the *in vitro* observations of activation-related down-regulation of CCR1 on monocytes (Trebst *et al.*, 2001).

CCR2, the receptor for CCL2, is expressed on microglia and macrophages in chronic active lesions and on perivascular mononuclear cells in both white matter lesions and unaffected cortex (Simpson *et al.*, 2000*a*).

CCR3, which is a receptor for CCL5, CCL7, and CCL8, is expressed at a low levels on macrophages in active MS lesions (Simpson *et al.*, 2000*a*) and on lymphocytes in NMO lesions (Lucchinetti *et al.*, 2002).

CCR5, a receptor for CCL3, CCL4, and CCL5, is expressed on perivascular lymphocytes, activated microglia, and macrophages in active MS lesions (Balashov *et al.*, 1999; Sorensen *et al.*, 1999; Simpson *et al.*, 2000*a*; Trebst *et al.*, 2001). CCR5 is likely to play a pathogenic role in MS, as patients with non-functional CCR5 due to a 32δ mutation had delayed age of onset of familial MS and a lower risk of recurrent clinical disease activity (Barcellos *et al.*, 2000; Sellebjerg *et al.*, 2000). However, 32δ mutation of the CCR5 gene was not protective against MS (Bennetts *et al.*, 1997). Approximately 80% of monocytes and 56% of T cells in the CSF expressed CCR5, independent of disease status (Kivisakk *et al.*, 2002; Trebst *et al.*, 2001) and CCR5 expression in MS lesions increases with lesion maturation predominantly due to CCR5 expression by activated microglia as they differentiate into phagocytic macrophages (Trebst *et al.*, 2001).

CCR8, expressed on activated microglia and phagocytic macrophages in MS tissue, is selectively expressed in the CNS (Trebst *et al.*, 2003).

CXCR3, the receptor for CXCL9 and CXCL10, is expressed by perivascular lymphocytes in active MS lesions and CXCR3+ T cells increase in number with lesion evolution (Balashov *et al.*, 1999; Sorensen *et al.*, 1999, 2002; Simpson *et al.*, 2000*b*).

Demyelination in MS

Inflammation may mediate demyelination in MS either directly or through interaction with oligodendrocytes as suggested by the correlation between the degree of inflammation and demyelinating activity (Bitsch *et al.*, 2000; Trebst *et al.*, 2001) and the presence of several patterns of myelin injury in MS: myelin stripping by lymphocytes and macrophages found between myelin sheaths; receptor-mediated phagocytosis of myelin suggested by coated pits on macrophages; vesicular disruption of myelin predominant in acute cases; dying-back oligodendrogliopathy leading to loss of myelin-associated glycoprotein (MAG), which is expressed in the most distal part of the oligodendrocytes (Trapp and Quarles, 1984; Trapp *et al.*, 1989).

These patterns of myelin injury highlight distinct mechanisms of demyelination: cell mediated; autoantibody, and complement mediated; cytokine and soluble molecule mediated; oligodendrocyte mediated.

Cell-mediated demyelination

Following antigen presentation, reactivated CD4+ T cells orchestrate the immune response in the CNS through secretion of cytokines, chemokines, and activation of macrophages, which produce proteolytic enzymes, cytokines, and free radicals (Selmaj *et al.*, 1991; Bo *et al.*, 1994). Cell-mediated demyelination occurs either as a direct result or through the secretion of pro-inflammatory cytokines. CD4+ T cells may directly destroy oligodendrocytes through interaction with Fas antigen. By analogy to the Theiler's murine encephalomyelitis virus (TMEV) model, CD8 cells may be directly cytotoxic to oligodendrocytes and neurons in MS (Rivera-Quinones *et al.*, 1998; Neumann *et al.*, 2002) and perforins secreted by CD8 and γδ T cells directly injure oligodendrocytes *in vitro* (Scolding *et al.*, 1990).

Antibody- and complement-mediated demyelination

Antibodies facilitate demyelination through antibody-dependent, cell-mediated cytoxicity (ADCC), Fc-receptor-mediated cytokine release by macrophages, NK cells, myelin opsonization, and complement activation. The presence of plasma cells, CSF oligoclonal bands and antibodies, and complement factors in MS lesions suggest a pathological role in demyelination in MS (Esiri, 1977). Antibodies against myelin oligodendrocyte protein (MOG), which is expressed on the outer surface of myelin sheaths and oligodendrocyte plasma membranes, is more prevalent in the serum from patients with active MS (Egg *et al.*, 2001).

Table 14.2 An overview of chemokine receptors in MS tissue

Chemokine receptors	Chemokines that activate the receptor[a]	Expression in MS tissue
CCR1	CCL3, 5, 7, 14, 15, 16, and 23	Newly infiltrating monocytes in active MS lesions (Trebst *et al.*, 2001)
CCR2	CCL2, 7, and 13	Macrophages in active MS lesions (Simpson *et al.*, 2000*a*)
CCR3	CCL5, 7, 8, 11, 13, 15, 24, and 26	Low levels of expression on macrophages in active MS lesions. In NMO, CCR3 is expressed on T-cells (Simpson *et al.*, 2000*a*; Lucchinetti *et al.*, 2002)
CCR5	CCL3, 4, and 5.	Perivascular lymphocytes, infiltrating monocytes and activated microglia and macrophages in active MS lesions (Balashov *et al.*, 1999; Sorensen *et al.*, 1999; Simpson *et al.*, 2000*a*; Trebst *et al.*, 2001)
CCR8	CCL1	Activated microglia and phagocytic macrophages in active lesions (Trebst *et al.*, 2003)
CXCR3	CXCL9, 10, and 11	Perivascular lymphocytes in active MS lesions (Balashov *et al.*, 1999; Sorensen *et al.*, 1999; Simpson *et al.*, 2000*b*)

[a]Information from Zlotnik and Yoshie (2000).

Cytokine- and other soluble-factor-mediated demyelination

The expression of IL-1α, IL-2, IL-6, IFN-γ, and tumour necrosis factor (TNF)-α have been reported in MS tissue (Hulshof *et al.*,; Woodroofe and Cuzner, 1993). The intravenous administration of IFN-γ, induced MS relapses (Panitch *et al.*, 1987). However, the neutralization of TNF increased MRI activity, indicating the complex role of cytokines in MS (van Oosten *et al.*, 1996). Cytokines may cause direct injury to myelin as well as damage the oligodendrocytes through induction of apoptosis via Fas, TNF-related apoptosis-inducing ligand (TRAIL) receptor 2, and TNF receptors p55 and p75. Fas and p75 have been detected on oligodendrocytes in or near MS lesions (Bonetti and Raine, 1997) and Bcl-2, which protects against apoptosis, is expressed in association with remyelination in MS lesions, suggesting a preservative role on oligodendrocytes (Kuhlmann *et al.*, 1999).

Oligodendrocyte-mediated demyelination

Loss of oligodendrocytes in chronic inactive MS lesions has been a consistent observation (Lucchinetti *et al.*, 1999; Lassmann *et al.*, 2001). A recent study, which described the fate of oligodendrocytes in early stages of MS and in actively demyelinating lesions, identified two major groups of oligodendrocyte pathology based on the presence (group I) or the absence (group II) of oligodendrocyte recruitment (Lucchinetti *et al.*, 1999). In group I and II, oligodendrocytes were invariably reduced during active stages of demyelination. Group I contained increased numbers of oligodendrocytes within inactive or remyelinating areas whereas in group II oligodendrocyte recruitment to inactive plaques was absent. Less extensive destruction of oligodendrocytes together with a greater role for antibody-mediated demyelination (MOG) may preserve oligodendrocyte precursors during active demyelination (as oligodendrocyte precursors do not express MOG) whereas extensive destruction in group II may also destroy oligodendrocyte precursors (Lucchinetti *et al.*, 1996)).

Direct injury to the oligodendrocytes may mediate demyelination in MS as suggested by differential loss of MAG in a subtype of MS lesions (Itoyama *et al.*, 1982; Gendelman *et al.*, 1985; Lucchinetti *et al.*, 2000). Differential loss of MAG, also reported in association with JC virus-infected oligodendrocytes in progressive multifocal leukoencephalopathy (PML) and in white matter ischaemia, is indicative of oligodendrocyte dysfunction (Itoyama *et al.*, 1982; Gendelman *et al.*, 1985; Aboul-Enein *et al.*, 2003). Oligodendrocytes express receptors for several cytokines (IL-2, IL-1a and b, IFN-γ, IL-6, TNF-α) (Merrill and Scolding, 1999) and may be injured by immune-mediated mechanisms, which may coincidently also damage compact myelin through myelin stripping, vesicular disruption, or antibody-mediated mechanisms. Oligodendrocytes also express death signals (Fas and p75) in MS lesions (Trapp *et al.*, 1999a) and demyelination due to extensive apoptosis has been recognized in a subset of MS lesions.

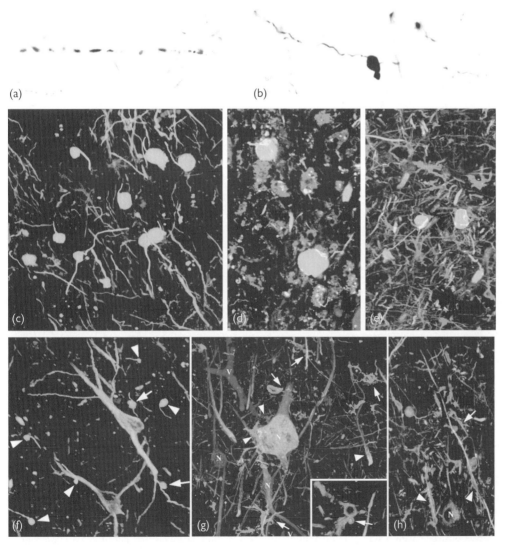

Fig. 14.2 Characteristics of axonal pathology in white matter MS lesions (a)–(e) and neuronal pathology in cortical MS lesions (f)–(h) with associated activated microglia and macrophages. (a, b). Discontinuous staining for non-phosphorylated neurofilaments (a) with constricted and dilated axons containing large swellings (b). (c) stacked confocal image showing terminal axonal ovoids with single or dual axonal connections. Macrophages (d in red) and microglia (e in red) surround and engulf terminal axonal swellings (c and d in green). In cortical lesions, neurofilament-positive ovoids representing terminal ends of neurites were abundant in cortical lesions (f). Activated microglia (g and h in red) extended processes to neurites and neurofilament positive (g and h in green) neurons in the cortex. (See also Plate 4 of the colour plate section at the center of this book.)

Axonal injury, degeneration, and loss

Axonal injury in MS

Several pathological characteristics of axonal injury in active and chronic active MS lesions have been reported using immunohistochemistry and confocal microscopy with computer-based three-dimensional reconstructs: the presence of amyloid precursor protein (APP) immunoreactive axons; increase in non-phosphorylated axonal neurofilaments; the presence of axonal ovoids indicative of axonal transection; change in axonal calibre (Figs 14.2(A–E)) (Trapp *et al.*, 1998).

APP is a neuronal protein transported by fast antegrade axonal transport, and can only be detected when the axoplasmic flow is compromised (Ferguson *et al.*, 1997). Two groups have reported APP immunoreactive axons in active and chronic active MS lesions and significantly correlated the number of APP immunoreactive axons with the density of macrophages in the lesions (Ferguson *et al.*, 1997; Bitsch *et al.*, 2000). APP immunoreactive axons were also present in remyelinating lesions (Bitsch *et al.*, 2000).

Phosphorylation of axons, which is facilitated by myelination, leads to an increase in neurofilament spacing and axonal calibre (Trapp 1998b). The presence of non-phosphorylated neurofilaments, in axons and axonal ovoids, is a sensitive marker of axonal pathology. As the formation of terminal axonal ovoids is a transient event, each terminal ovoid detected by a non-phosphorylated neurofilament or APP indicates a single recently transected axon. Terminal axonal ovoids were more abundant and larger in active lesions (11 236/mm^3) than in either the active rim (3138/mm^3) or the centre (875/mm^3) of chronic active lesions. NLWM (17/mm^3) and control white matter (1/mm^3) also had axonal ovoids, although the numbers were much less than in the lesions. The transected axons were demyelinated and the extent of axonal transection was independent of the disease duration of MS (2–27 years). In the centre of active lesions, macrophages surrounded the transected axons (Fig. 14.2(D)), whereas in the edge of active lesions the terminal ovoids but not the axons were surrounded by microglia (Fig. 14.2(E)). In addition to transection of axons, loss of axonal calibre and discontinuation of non-phosphorylated neurofilament staining in active lesions were also observed as features of axonal injury and degeneration (Fig. 14.2(A) and (B)).

Axonal loss in MS

Using autopsy tissue from MS cases with long-standing MS (disease duration from 12–39 years and mean EDSS of 7.5) and a triangulation method of quantitation, Bjartmar *et al.* (2000) reported 68% loss of axonal numbers and 60% loss of axonal density in chronic inactive spinal cord MS lesions. The extent of axonal loss correlated with neurological disability but not with disease duration or the degree of spinal cord atrophy, which was greater in the cervical than lumbar spine. The majority (seven out of 10) of the chronic lesions were atrophic (17–45% loss of volume) and others were hypertrophic in comparison with site-matched control tissue. The lack of correlation between axonal loss and volume loss of spinal cord lesions may be due to other factors, such as axonal atrophy, demyelination, inflammation-related oedema, and astrogliosis, which influence the volume of MS lesions. The proportion of white matter and grey matter areas were similar in MS and control cervical and lumbar spine cords, indicating that the loss of spinal cord volume in MS is due to a combination of both grey and white matter loss. This study also validated the biological implications of the *in vivo* studies of axonal loss and injury using magnetic resonance spectroscopy to detected levels of *N*-acetyl aspartate (NAA) (Bjartmar *et al.*, 2000). NAA, localized primarily in the neurons and neuronal processes, is produced in the mitochondria and transported to the cytoplasm. Although the function of NAA is unknown, reduction of NAA levels represents either reversible neuronal and axonal dysfunction or irreversible axonal and neuronal loss. NAA levels detected by high-performance liquid chromatography (HPLC) were reduced by 53–55% in whole spinal cord sections with inactive lesions compared with controls and reduction of NAA levels significantly correlated with the degree of axonal loss. Consistent with MRS

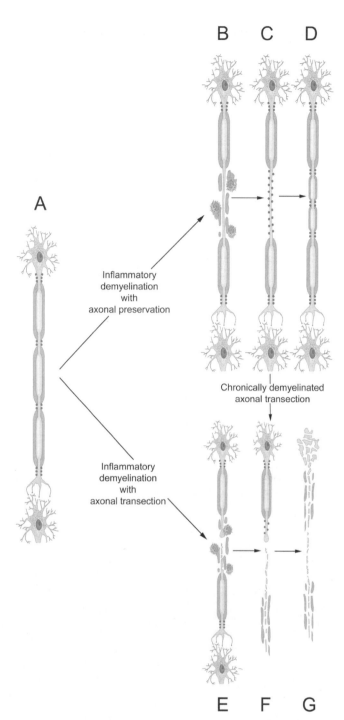

Fig. 14.3 The neuropathological features associated with neurological dysfunction in MS. (A) Normal myelinated axon with nodal sodium channel distribution. (B) Inflammation-mediated demyelination of axons without axonal transection. (C, D) Redistribution of sodium channels along the naked axon and remyelination lead to partial or complete resolution of symptoms. (E)–(G) Axonal transection and demyelination mediated by inflammation (E), which lead to degeneration of the distal axonal segment (F) and Wallerian degeneration (G). Chronically demyelinated (naked) axons (C) with redistributed sodium channels may undergo axonal transection and Wallerian degeneration (F and G).

findings, NAA levels were significantly reduced in demyelinated axons and myelinated axons in NLWM. Potentially reversible processes such as altered neuronal and axonal metabolism, demyelination, conduction block, and redistribution of axonal sodium channels may alter the NAA levels in demyelinated and myelinated axons. Further evidence for axonal loss as the cause of irreversible disability in MS is suggested by the studies of 'clinically silent' cases with neuropathological features of MS at autopsy, where axons were well preserved (Ghatak et al., 1974).

In active MS lesions, Bitsch et al. (2000) reported 35% loss of axons. Axonal loss, based on APP accumulation, in chronic active lesions was greater than in active lesions (Ferguson et al., 1997). The extent of axonal loss in NLWM would depend on whether or not the axons have been transected elsewhere due to a proximal or a distal lesion (Bjartmar et al., 2001; Trapp 1998b). A case study of MS with a 9 month disease duration and a brainstem lesion causing Ondine's curse, reported 22% loss of axons in the distal NLWM (cervical 6–7, without evidence of myelin degradation), consistent with Wallerian degeneration (Bjartmar et al., 2001).

Pathogenesis of axonal injury and axonal loss

Axonal damage or loss can be the result of several mechanisms: inflammatory axonal transection (inflammatory neurodegeneration); chronic demyelination related axonal transection and degeneration; Wallerian degeneration; ischaemia or pressure-related mechanical damage from surrounding oedema (Fig. 14.3) (Trapp et al., 1999b).

Inflammatory axonopathy

The correlation between the extent of axonal transection and the degree of inflammation (Ferguson et al., 1997; Trapp 1998b; Bitsch et al., 2000) suggests a causative role in MS, although direct evidence from clinical trials using anti-inflammatory agents is not yet available. In particular, CD8+ T lymphocytes, macrophages, and microglia have been implicated in inflammatory axonopathy (Bitsch et al., 2000; Kuhlmann et al., 2002). CD8 T lymphocytes may facilitate axonal damage through secretion of perforins resulting in pore formation on cell membranes and subsequent entry of ions (Murray et al., 1998). Further, nitric oxide, proteolytic enzymes, cytokines, and free radicals produced by macrophages in active and chronic active MS lesions may lead to axonopathy, particularly of demyelinated axons (Selmaj et al., 1991; Bo et al., 1994; Hohlfeld, 1997). Activated microglia surround axonal ovoids in the NLWM (probably due to Wallerian degeneration) and damaged neuritis (non-phosphorylated neurofilamnet+) in the grey matter lesions (Figs 14.2(E), (G), and (H)). Although microglia can mediate inflammation in neurodegenerative diseases (Gonzalez-Scarano and Baltuch, 1999), whether the association with ovoids and neuritis is deleterious or protective is unknown. Evidence for an immune response directed specifically against axons in the CNS is lacking.

Chronic demyelination related axonopathy

The presence of axonal ovoids (indicating recent transection) in chronically demyelinated axons in the centre of chronic active lesions (Trapp 1998b) and in inactive lesions suggests a pathogenic role for chronic demyelination in axonal damage (Ferguson et al., 1997; Bitsch et al., 2000). Signalling from myelin-forming cells is important for the viability of myelinated axons (Yin et al., 1998) and axonal signalling influences CNS myelination (Colello and Pott, 1997).

Myelin gene defects in humans provide insight into the dependency of axons on myelin. Pelizaeus–Merzbacher disease (PMD) is a human neurodegenerative disease due to proteolipidprotein (PLP) gene mutations, deletions, or duplications, which affects the CNS and causes spastic paraplegia, cerebellar ataxia, psychomotor developmental delay, and dystonia (Garbern et al., 1999; Inoue et al., 1999) The pathological processes in myelin gene defects are likely to be due to the gain of toxic functions rather than due to loss of physiological functions.

The chronically demyelinated axons are at risk of further damage due to exposure to cytokines and other pro-inflammatory agents (Fig. 14.3). Several studies have associated relapses, or recurrence of symptoms associated with previous relapses, with up-regulation of systemic cytokines. Although these inflammatory agents may not damage the demyelinated axons directly, they anatomically identify axons that are vulnerable (at risk)

and subsequently may cause irreversible disability through chronic demyelination-related axonopathy (Coles et al., 1999).

Axonal loss secondary to Wallerian degeneration

Wallerian degeneration, which follows axonal transection, entails the breakdown of the distal portion of the axon and the removal of the corresponding myelin sheath (Fig. 14.3). The disintegration of the axonal cytoskeleton is thought to be due the activation of proteases and the rise in intracellular calcium (Johnson et al., 1991). Once transected the axon may continue to conduct for up to a week (Compston et al., 1998). In the CNS, axonal loss due to Wallerian degeneration may occur within days with immediate functional consequences, while the loss of myelin may occur over months or years following the initial axonal transection (Griffin et al., 1992; Simon et al., 2000; Bjartmar et al., 2001). Axonal loss of 22% in NLWM, in the absence of loss of myelin, was reported distal to a brainstem lesion of approximately 9 months' duration since diagnosis (Bjartmar et al., 2001).

Temporal pattern of inflammation, axonal injury, and axonal loss and clinicopathological correlation

Inflammatory infiltrate in MS tissue is most prominent during the early stages of MS and decreases with increasing disease duration (Fig. 14.1) (Kuhlmann et al., 2002). The decrease is most striking for CD3+ T cells within lesions and CD8+ T cells in the periplaque white matter (Kuhlmann et al., 2002), whereas microglial activation remains steady in the periplaque white matter but tends to decrease within lesions with increasing disease duration (Kuhlmann et al., 2002). Inflammatory infiltrate in MS directly contributes to both reversible (relapse) (1993; Johnson et al., 1998), and irreversible disability (progression) through conduction block, demyelination, and acute axonal transection (Fig. 14.1) (Rudick et al., 1999). The recovery from relapse is partly due to the resolution of the inflammatory environment as well as remyelination (Trapp et al., 1999b) and the stepwise increase in irreversible disability, which follows a proportion of MS and NMO relapses, is consistent with inflammatory acute axonal transection (Lucchinetti et al., 2002) (Fig. 14.1). The lack of irreversible or progressing disability in early phases of RRMS when the rate of inflammatory axonal transection is greatest is due to the ability of the CNS to compensate for the loss of axons up to a threshold level, which may be due to redundant neuronal pathways and axonal sprouting. The onset of primary progressive MS, where the progression is not preceded by relapses despite MRI evidence of CNS inflammation, may be due to CNS inflammation in sites where symptomatology is silent or subtle.

The extent of inflammation during the early stages of MS determines the subsequent clinical course. The time taken to the onset of a defined EDSS in SPMS is dependent on the relapse rate during the first 2 years from diagnosis (Ebers, 2001). The disease continued to progress in SPMS patients treated with Campath-1H, despite the suppression of formation of new inflammatory lesions defined by gadolinium-enhanced MRI and relapses and the progression was dependent on the number of inflammatory lesions prior to commencement of Campath-1H (Coles et al., 1999).

Heterogeneity of white matter and cortical MS lesions

Subtypes of white matter MS lesions

The heterogeneity of clinical presentation and response to treatment may be due to the heterogeneity of neuropathology and disease-modifying and susceptibility gene effects (Ebers et al., 1996; Hohlfeld, 1997; Lucchinetti et al., 2000). Hence, one of the most important recent advances in the understanding of MS pathogenesis has been due to the recognition of subtypes of

MS lesions (white matter and cortical) and patterns of oligodendrocyte loss. Four patterns of white matter MS lesions have been described, based on the expression of myelin proteins in phagocytic macrophages, structure of the plaque, deposition of activated complement components, and the patterns of oligodendrocyte injury (Lassmann *et al.*, 2001; Lassmann, 2002). Lesions of patterns I and II are centred around venules and have sharply demarcated lesional edges resembling the pathology of EAE. The main difference between patterns II and III is the extensive deposition of activated complement at the site of active demyelination, present in pattern II. The number of oligodendrocytes was reduced in active lesions but increased in inactive regions with evidence of remyelination. Pattern III lesions are not centred around venules and have indistinct boarders. The complete loss of MAG with partially reduced myelin basic protein (MBP) and PLP in pattern III contrasts with the even loss of myelin proteins in other patterns. Pattern IV was only observed in a small number of patients, all with PPMS (Lucchinetti *et al.*, 2000). Features of pattern IV were similar to pattern I but additionally had extensive loss of oligodendrocytes in inactive plaque with sparse remyelination. The immunological and neurobiological mechanisms underlying these patterns of MS are yet to be characterized. The heterogeneity of lesional patterns between patients, but not within patients, is clinically relevant and the discovery of paraclinical, *in vivo*, markers to distinguish between these patterns is eagerly awaited. Such *in vivo* sub-classification of MS will enable improved selection of patients for clinical trials as well as identify a subset of MS patients who may require novel therapeutic strategies (Lassmann, 2002).

Subtypes of cortical MS lesions

Subtypes of cortical lesions have also been reported with potentially interesting pathogenic mechanisms (Peterson *et al.*, 2001). Type I lesions, accounting for 34% of cortical lesions, were termed leukocortical as the cortex and the adjacent white matter was involved. Type II lesions, confined to the cortex and containing a vessel at the centre, made up 16% of 112 cortical lesions. The remaining 50% of the lesions, type III, extended from the pial surface into cortical layers 3 or 4. Compared with white matter lesions, the numbers of CD68+ cells were decreased by six-fold and CD3+ cells decreased by 13-fold in the cortical lesions. Over 90% of CD68+ cells in the cortex were activated microglia. Cortical lesions contained significantly more transected neurites than non-lesional cortex and the number of neurites correlated with the demyelinating activity defined using MHC Class II expression within lesions. Lack of perivascular cuffs and more than a 10-fold decrease in the inflammatory infiltrate in cortical lesions may be due to several reasons: decreased or lack of expression of adhesion molecule and chemokines within cortical lesions; expression of molecules that may inhibit endothelial–leukocyte interaction in the cortex; decreased capacity of the cortical extracellular space to expand.

Acknowledgements

We would like to thank Dr Grahame Kidd, Dr Ansi Chang, and Dr John Peterson for help with illustrations.

References

Aboul-Enein, F., Rauschka, H., Kornek, B., *et al.* (2003). Preferential loss of myelin-associated glycoprotein reflects hypoxia- like white matter damage in stroke and inflammatory brain diseases. *J Neuropathol Exp Neurol* 1: 25–33.

Babbe, H., Roers, A., Waisman, A., *et al.* (2000). Clonal expansions of CD8(+) T cells dominate the T cell infiltrate in active multiple sclerosis lesions as shown by micromanipulation and single cell polymerase chain reaction. *J Exp Med* 3: 393–404.

Balashov, K.E., Rottman, J.B., Weiner, H.L., and Hancock, W.W. (1999). CCR5(+) and CXCR3(+) T cells are increased in multiple sclerosis and their ligands MIP-1alpha and IP-10 are expressed in demyelinating brain lesions. *Proc Natl Acad Sci USA* 12: 6873–6878.

Barcellos, L.F., Schito, A.M., Rimmler, J.B., *et al.* (2000). CC-chemokine receptor 5 polymorphism and age of onset in familial multiple sclerosis. Multiple Sclerosis Genetics Group. *Immunogenetics* 4–5: 281–288.

Bennetts, B.H., Teutsch, S.M., Buhler, M.M., Heard, R.N., and Stewart, G.J. (1997). The CCR5 deletion mutation fails to protect against multiple sclerosis. *Hum Immunol* 1: 52–59.

Benveniste, E.N. (1992). Inflammatory cytokines within the central nervous system: sources, function, and mechanism of action. *Am J Physiol* 1(1): C1–16.

Bitsch, A., Schuchardt, J., Bunkowski, S., Kuhlmann, T., and Bruck, W. (2000). Acute axonal injury in multiple sclerosis. Correlation with demyelination and inflammation. *Brain* 1174–1183.

Bjartmar, C., Kidd, G., Mork, S., Rudick, R., and Trapp, B.D. (2000). Neurological disability correlates with spinal cord axonal loss and reduced N-acetyl aspartate in chronic multiple sclerosis patients. *Ann Neurol* 6: 893–901.

Bjartmar, C., Kinkel, R.P., Kidd, G., Rudick, R.A., and Trapp, B.D. (2001). Axonal loss in normal-appearing white matter in a patient with acute MS. *Neurology* 7: 1248–1252.

Bo, L., Dawson, T.M., Wesselingh, S., *et al.* (1994). Induction of nitric oxide synthase in demyelinating regions of multiple sclerosis brains. *Ann Neurol* 5: 778–786.

Bo, L., Peterson, J.W., Mork, S., *et al.* (1996). Distribution of immunoglobulin superfamily members ICAM-1, -2, -3, and the beta 2 integrin LFA-1 in multiple sclerosis lesions. *J Neuropathol Exp Neurol* 10: 1060–1072.

Bonecchi, R., Bianchi, G., Bordignon, P.P., *et al.* (1998). Differential expression of chemokine receptors and chemotactic responsiveness of type 1 T helper cells (Th1s) and Th2s. *J Exp Med* 1: 129–134.

Bonetti, B. and Raine, C.S. (1997). Multiple sclerosis: oligodendrocytes display cell death-related molecules in situ but do not undergo apoptosis. *Ann Neurol* 1: 74–84.

Booss, J., Esiri, M.M., Tourtellotte, W.W., and Mason, D.Y. (1983). Immunohistological analysis of T lymphocyte subsets in the central nervous system in chronic progressive multiple sclerosis. *J Neurol Sci* 1–3: 219–232.

Boven, L.A., Montagne, L., Nottet, H.S., and De Groot, C.J. (2000). Macrophage inflammatory protein-1alpha (MIP-1alpha), MIP-1beta, and RANTES mRNA semiquantification and protein expression in active demyelinating multiple sclerosis (MS) lesions. *Clin Exp Immunol* 2: 257–263.

Boxel-Dezaire, A.H., Hoff, S.C., van Oosten, B.W., *et al.* (1999). Decreased interleukin-10 and increased interleukin-12p40 mRNA are associated with disease activity and characterize different disease stages in multiple sclerosis. *Ann Neurol* 6: 695–703.

Brosnan, C.F., Bornstein, M.B., and Bloom, B.R. (1981). The effects of macrophage depletion on the clinical and pathologic expression of experimental allergic encephalomyelitis. *J Immunol* 2: 614–620.

Bruck, W., Porada, P., Poser, S., *et al.* (1995). Monocyte/macrophage differentiation in early multiple sclerosis lesions. *Ann Neurol* 5: 788–796.

Butcher, E.C. and Picker, L.J. (1996). Lymphocyte homing and homeostasis. *Science* 272: 60–66.

Calabresi, P.A., Fields, N.S., Farnon, E.C., *et al.* (1998). ELI-spot of Th-1 cytokine secreting PBMC's in multiple sclerosis: correlation with MRI lesions. *J Neuroimmunol* 2: 212–219.

Cannella, B. and Raine, C.S. (1995). The adhesion molecule and cytokine profile of multiple sclerosis lesions. *Ann Neurol* 4: 424–435.

Charcot, M. (1868). Histologie de la sclerose en plaques. *Gaz Hop Civ Milit* 140: 554–558 and 141: 557–558.

Colello, R.J. and Pott, U. (1997). Signals that initiate myelination in the developing mammalian nervous system. *Mol Neurobiol* 1: 83–100.

Coles, A.J., Wing, M.G., Molyneux, P., *et al.* (1999). Monoclonal antibody treatment exposes three mechanisms underlying the clinical course of multiple sclerosis. *Ann Neurol* 3: 296–304.

Comabella, M., Balashov, K., Issazadeh, S., Smith, D., Weiner, H.L., and Khoury, S.J. (1998). Elevated interleukin-12 in progressive multiple sclerosis correlates with disease activity and is normalized by pulse cyclophosphamide therapy. *J Clin Invest* 4: 671–678.

Compston, A., Ebers, G.C., Lassmann, H., McFarland, H.F., Matthews, B., and Wekerle, H. (1998). In: *McAlpine's Multiple Sclerosis*.

Compston, D.A. (1990). The dissemination of multiple sclerosis. *J R Coll Phys Lond* 3: 207–218.

Compston, D.A., Vakarelis, B.N., Paul, E., McDonald, W.I., Batchelor, J.R., and Mims, C.A. (1986). Viral infection in patients with multiple sclerosis and HLA-DR matched controls. *Brain* 325–344.

Ebers, G.C. (2001). Natural history of multiple sclerosis. *J Neurol Neurosurg Psychiatry* ii16–ii19.

Ebers, G.C., Kukay, K., Bulman, D.E., et al. (1996). A full genome search in multiple sclerosis. *Nat Genet* 4: 472–476.

Egg, R., Reindl, M., Deisenhammer, F., Linington, C., and Berger, T. (2001). Anti-MOG and anti-MBP antibody subclasses in multiple sclerosis. *Mult Scler* 5: 285–289.

Esiri, M.M. (1977). Immunoglobulin-containing cells in multiple-sclerosis plaques. *Lancet* 2(8036): 478.

Ferguson, B., Matyszak, M.K., Esiri, M.M., and Perry, V.H. (1997). Axonal damage in acute multiple sclerosis lesions. *Brain* 393–399.

Franciotta, D., Martino, G., Zardini, E., et al. (2001). Serum and CSF levels of MCP-1 and IP-10 in multiple sclerosis patients with acute and stable disease and undergoing immunomodulatory therapies. *J Neuroimmunol* 1–2: 192–198.

Fuentes, M.E., Durham, S.K., Swerdel, M.R., et al. (1995). Controlled recruitment of monocytes and macrophages to specific organs through transgenic expression of monocyte chemoattractant protein-1. *J Immunol* 12: 5769–5776.

Garbern, J., Cambi, F., Shy, M., and Kamholz, J. (1999). The molecular pathogenesis of Pelizaeus–Merzbacher disease. *Arch Neurol* 10: 1210–1214.

Gay, F.W., Drye, T.J., Dick, G.W., and Esiri, M.M. (1997). The application of multifactorial cluster analysis in the staging of plaques in early multiple sclerosis. Identification and characterization of the primary demyelinating lesion. *Brain* 1461–1483.

Gendelman, H.E., Pezeshkpour, G.H., Pressman, N.J., et al. (1985). A quantitation of myelin-associated glycoprotein and myelin basic protein loss in different demyelinating diseases. *Ann Neurol* 3: 324–328.

Ghatak, N.R., Hirano, A., Lijtmaer, H., and Zimmerman, H.M. (1974). Asymptomatic demyelinated plaque in the spinal cord. *Arch Neurol* 6: 484–486.

Gonzalez-Scarano, F. and Baltuch, G. (1999). Microglia as mediators of inflammatory and degenerative diseases. *Annu Rev Neurosci* 219–240.

Griffin, J.W., George, R., Lobato, C., Tyor, W.R., Yan, L.C., and Glass, J.D. (1992). Macrophage responses and myelin clearance during Wallerian degeneration: relevance to immune-mediated demyelination. *J Neuroimmunol* 2–3: 153–165.

Hauser, S.L., Bhan, A.K., Gilles, F., Kemp, M., Kerr, C., and Weiner, H.L. (1986). Immunohistochemical analysis of the cellular infiltrate in multiple sclerosis lesions. *Ann Neurol* 6: 578–587.

Hayashi, T., Morimoto, C., Burks, J.S., Kerr, C., and Hauser, S.L. (1988). Dual-label immunocytochemistry of the active multiple sclerosis lesion: major histocompatibility complex and activation antigens. *Ann Neurol* 4: 523–531.

Hayes, G.M., Woodroofe, M.N., and Cuzner, M.L. (1987). Microglia are the major cell type expressing MHC class II in human white matter. *J Neurol Sci* 1: 25–37.

Heinsen, H., Lockemann, U., and Puschel, K. (1995). Unsuspected (clinically silent) multiple sclerosis. Quantitative investigations in one autoptic case. *Int J Legal Med* 5: 263–266.

Hickey, W.F. (2001). Basic principles of immunological surveillance of the normal central nervous system. *Glia* 2: 118–124.

Hohlfeld, R. (1997). Biotechnological agents for the immunotherapy of multiple sclerosis. Principles, problems and perspectives. *Brain* 865–916.

Huitinga, I., van Rooijen, N., De Groot, C.J., Uitdehaag, B.M., and Dijkstra, C.D. (1990). Suppression of experimental allergic encephalomyelitis in Lewis rats after elimination of macrophages. *J Exp Med* 4: 1025–1033.

Hulshof, S., Montagne, L., De Groot, C.J., and van d V Cellular localization and expression patterns of interleukin-10, interleukin-4, and their receptors in multiple sclerosis lesions.

Hvas, J., McLean, C., Justesen, J., et al. (1997). Perivascular T cells express the pro-inflammatory chemokine RANTES mRNA in multiple sclerosis lesions. *Scand J Immunol* 2: 195–203.

Inoue, K., Osaka, H., Imaizumi, K., et al. (1999). Proteolipid protein gene duplications causing Pelizaeus–Merzbacher disease: molecular mechanism and phenotypic manifestations. *Ann Neurol* 5: 624–632.

Itoyama, Y., Webster, H.D., Sternberger, N.H., et al. (1982). Distribution of papovavirus, myelin-associated glycoprotein, and myelin basic protein in progressive multifocal leukoencephalopathy lesions. *Ann Neurol* 4: 396–407.

Johnson, G.V., Greenwood, J.A., Costello, A.C., and Troncoso, J.C. (1991). The regulatory role of calmodulin in the proteolysis of individual neurofilament proteins by calpain. *Neurochem Res* 8: 869–873.

Johnson, K.P., Brooks, B.R., Cohen, J.A., et al. (1998). Extended use of glatiramer acetate (Copaxone) is well tolerated and maintains its clinical effect on multiple sclerosis relapse rate and degree of disability. Copolymer 1 Multiple Sclerosis Study Group. *Neurology* 3: 701–708.

Kennedy, P.G. and Steiner, I. (1994). On the possible viral aetiology of multiple sclerosis. *Q J Med* 9: 523–528.

Kieseier, B.C., Seifert, T., Giovannoni, G., and Hartung, H.P. (1999). Matrix metalloproteinases in inflammatory demyelination: targets for treatment. *Neurology* 1: 20–25.

Kivisakk, P., Trebst, C., Liu, Z., et al. (2002). T-cells in the cerebrospinal fluid express a similar repertoire of inflammatory chemokine receptors in the absence or presence of CNS inflammation: implications for CNS trafficking. *Clin Exp Immunol*

Kojima, K., Berger, T., Lassmann, H., et al. (1994). Experimental autoimmune panencephalitis and uveoretinitis transferred to the Lewis rat by T lymphocytes specific for the S100 beta molecule, a calcium binding protein of astroglia. *J Exp Med* 3: 817–829.

Kuhlmann, T., Lucchinetti, C., Zettl, U.K., Bitsch, A., Lassmann, H., and Bruck, W. (1999). Bcl-2-expressing oligodendrocytes in multiple sclerosis lesions. *Glia* 1: 34–39.

Kuhlmann, T., Lingfeld, G., Bitsch, A., Schuchardt, J., and Bruck, W. (2002). Acute axonal damage in multiple sclerosis is most extensive in early disease stages and decreases over time. *Brain* 125: 2202–2212.

Lassmann, H. (2002). Mechanisms of demyelination and tissue destruction in multiple sclerosis. *Clin Neurol Neurosurg* 3: 168–171.

Lassmann, H., Raine, C.S., Antel, J., and Prineas, J.W. (1998). Immunopathology of multiple sclerosis: report on an international meeting held at the Institute of Neurology of the University of Vienna. *J Neuroimmunol* 2: 213–217.

Lassmann, H., Bruck, W., and Lucchinetti, C. (2001). Heterogeneity of multiple sclerosis pathogenesis: implications for diagnosis and therapy. *Trends Mol Med* 3: 115–121.

Li, H., Cuzner, M.L., and Newcombe, J. (1996). Microglia-derived macrophages in early multiple sclerosis plaques. *Neuropathol Appl Neurobiol* 3: 207–215.

Love, S. and Barber, R. (2001). Expression of P-selectin and intercellular adhesion molecule-1 in human brain after focal infarction or cardiac arrest. *Neuropathol Appl Neurobiol* 6: 465–473.

Lublin, F.D. and Reingold, S.C. (1996). Defining the clinical course of multiple sclerosis: results of an international survey. National Multiple Sclerosis Society (USA) Advisory Committee on Clinical Trials of New Agents in Multiple Sclerosis. *Neurology* 4: 907–911.

Lucchinetti, C.F., Bruck, W., Rodriguez, M., and Lassmann, H. (1996). Distinct patterns of multiple sclerosis pathology indicates heterogeneity on pathogenesis. *Brain Pathol* 3: 259–274.

Lucchinetti, C., Bruck, W., Parisi, J., Scheithauer, B., Rodriguez, M., and Lassmann, H. (1999). A quantitative analysis of oligodendrocytes in multiple sclerosis lesions. A study of 113 cases. *Brain* 2279–2295.

Lucchinetti, C., Bruck, W., Parisi, J., Scheithauer, B., Rodriguez, M., and Lassmann, H. (2000). Heterogeneity of multiple sclerosis lesions: implications for the pathogenesis of demyelination. *Ann Neurol* 6: 707–717.

Lucchinetti, C.F., Mandler, R.N., McGavern, D., et al. (2002). A role for humoral mechanisms in the pathogenesis of Devic's neuromyelitis optica. *Brain* 1450–1461.

Mackay, R.P. and Hirano, A. (1967). Forms of benign multiple sclerosis. Report of two 'clinically silent' cases discovered at autopsy. *Arch Neurol* 6: 588–600.

Mahad, D.J., Howell, S.J., and Woodroofe, M.N. (2002). Expression of chemokines in the CSF and correlation with clinical disease activity in patients with multiple sclerosis. *J Neurol Neurosurg Psychiatry* 4: 498–502.

McDonald, W.I. (1994). Rachelle Fishman-Matthew Moore Lecture. The pathological and clinical dynamics of multiple sclerosis. *J Neuropathol Exp Neurol* 4: 338–343.

McManus, C., Berman, J.W., Brett, F.M., Staunton, H., Farrell, M., and Brosnan, C.F. (1998). MCP-1, MCP-2 and MCP-3 expression in multiple sclerosis lesions: an immunohistochemical and in situ hybridization study. *J Neuroimmunol* 1: 20–29.

Merrill, J.E. and Scolding, N.J. (1999). Mechanisms of damage to myelin and oligodendrocytes and their relevance to disease. *Neuropathol Appl Neurobiol* 6: 435–458.

Miller, D.H., Khan, O.A., Sheremata, W.A., *et al.* (2003). A controlled trial of natalizumab for relapsing multiple sclerosis. *N Engl J Med* 1: 15–23.

Morariu, M. and Klutzow, W.F. (1976). Subclinical multiple sclerosis. *J Neurol* 1: 71–76.

Murray, P.D., McGavern, D.B., Lin, X., *et al.* (1998). Perforin-dependent neurologic injury in a viral model of multiple sclerosis. *J Neurosci* 18: 7306–7314.

Navratil, E., Couvelard, A., Rey, A., Henin, D., and Scoazec, J.Y. (1997). Expression of cell adhesion molecules by microvascular endothelial cells in the cortical and subcortical regions of the normal human brain: an immunohistochemical analysis. *Neuropathol Appl Neurobiol* 1: 68–80.

Neumann, H., Medana, I.M., Bauer, J., and Lassmann, H. (2002). Cytotoxic T lymphocytes in autoimmune and degenerative CNS diseases. *Trends Neurosci* 6: 313–319.

Nygardas, P.T., Maatta, J.A., and Hinkkanen, A.E. (2000). Chemokine expression by central nervous system resident cells and infiltrating neutrophils during experimental autoimmune encephalomyelitis in the BALB/c mouse. *Eur J Immunol* 7: 1911–1918.

Panitch, H.S., Hirsch, R.L., Haley, A.S., and Johnson, K.P. (1987). Exacerbations of multiple sclerosis in patients treated with gamma interferon. *Lancet* 1(8538): 893–895.

Pender, M.P. and Rist, M.J. (2001). Apoptosis of inflammatory cells in immune control of the nervous system: role of glia. *Glia* 2: 137–144.

Peterson, J.W., Bo, L., Mork, S., Chang, A., and Trapp, B.D. (2001). Transected neurites, apoptotic neurons, and reduced inflammation in cortical multiple sclerosis lesions. *Ann Neurol* 50: 389–400.

Peterson, J.W., Bo, L., Mork, S., Chang, A., Ransohoff, R.M., and Trapp, B.D. (2002). VCAM-1-positive microglia target oligodendrocytes at the border of multiple sclerosis lesions. *J Neuropathol Exp Neurol* 6: 539–546.

Prineas, J.W. and Graham, J.S. (1981). Multiple sclerosis: capping of surface immunoglobulin G on macrophages engaged in myelin breakdown. *Ann Neurol* 10: 149–158.

Raine, C.S. (1994). The Dale E. McFarlin Memorial Lecture: the immunology of the multiple sclerosis lesion. *Ann Neurol* S61–S72.

Ransohoff, R.M., Glabinski, A., and Tani, M. (1996). Chemokines in immune-mediated inflammation of the central nervous system. *Cytokine Growth Factor Rev* 1: 35–46.

Rivera-Quinones, C., McGavern, D., Schmelzer, J.D., Hunter, S.F., Low, P.A., and Rodriguez, M. (1998). Absence of neurological deficits following extensive demyelination in a class I-deficient murine model of multiple sclerosis. *Nat Med* 2: 187–193.

Rudick, R.A., Cookfair, D.L., Simonian, N.A., *et al.* (1999). Cerebrospinal fluid abnormalities in a phase III trial of Avonex (IFNbeta-1a) for relapsing multiple sclerosis. The Multiple Sclerosis Collaborative Research Group. *J Neuroimmunol* 93(1–2): 8–14.

Sadovnick, A.D. and Ebers, G.C. (1993). Epidemiology of multiple sclerosis: a critical overview. *Can J Neurol Sci* 20: 17–29.

Sallusto, F., Lenig, D., Mackay, C.R., and Lanzavecchia, A. (1998). Flexible programs of chemokine receptor expression on human polarized T helper 1 and 2 lymphocytes. *J Exp Med* 187: 875–883.

Schumacher, G.A. (1974). Critique of experimental trials of therapy in multiple sclerosis. *Neurology* 24(11): 1010–1014.

Scolding, N.J., Jones, J., Compston, D.A., and Morgan, B.P. (1990). Oligodendrocyte susceptibility to injury by T-cell perforin. *Immunology* 70(1): 6–10.

Sellebjerg, F., Madsen, H.O., Jensen, C.V., Jensen, J., and Garred, P. (2000). CCR5 delta32, matrix metalloproteinase-9 and disease activity in multiple sclerosis. *J Neuroimmunol* 102(1): 98–106.

Selmaj, K., Raine, C.S., Cannella, B., and Brosnan, C.F. (1991). Identification of lymphotoxin and tumor necrosis factor in multiple sclerosis lesions. *J Clin Invest* 3: 949–954.

Simon, J.H., Kinkel, R.P., Jacobs, L., Bub, L., and Simonian, N. (2000). A Wallerian degeneration pattern in patients at risk for MS. *Neurology* 5: 1155–1160.

Simpson, J.E., Newcombe, J., Cuzner, M.L., and Woodroofe, M.N. (1998). Expression of monocyte chemoattractant protein-1 and other beta-chemokines by resident glia and inflammatory cells in multiple sclerosis lesions. *J Neuroimmunol* (2): 238–249.

Simpson, J., Rezaie, P., Newcombe, J., Cuzner, M.L., Male, D., and Woodroofe, M.N. (2000a). Expression of the beta-chemokine receptors CCR2, CCR3 and CCR5 in multiple sclerosis central nervous system tissue. *J Neuroimmunol* (1–2): 192–200.

Simpson, J.E., Newcombe, J., Cuzner, M.L., and Woodroofe, M.N. (2000b). Expression of the interferon-gamma-inducible chemokines IP-10 and Mig and their receptor, CXCR3, in multiple sclerosis lesions. *Neuropathol Appl Neurobiol* 2, 133–142.

Skundric, D.S., Kim, C., Tse, H.Y., and Raine, C.S. (1993). Homing of T cells to the central nervous system throughout the course of relapsing experimental autoimmune encephalomyelitis in Thy-1 congenic mice. *J Neuroimmunol* (1–2): 113–121.

Sobel, R.A., Hafler, D.A., Castro, E.E., Morimoto, C., and Weiner, H.L. (1988). The 2H4 (CD45R) antigen is selectively decreased in multiple sclerosis lesions. *J Immunol* (7): 2210–2214.

Sorensen, T.L., Tani, M., Jensen, J., *et al.* (1999). Expression of specific chemokines and chemokine receptors in the central nervous system of multiple sclerosis patients. *J Clin Invest* (6): 807–815.

Sorensen, T.L., Trebst, C., Kivisakk, P., *et al.* (2002). Multiple sclerosis: a study of CXCL10 and CXCR3 co-localization in the inflamed central nervous system. *J Neuroimmunol* (1–2): 59–68.

Sozzani, S., Sallusto, F., Luini, W., *et al.* (1995). Migration of dendritic cells in response to formyl peptides, C5a, and a distinct set of chemokines. *J Immunol* (7): 3292–3295.

Springer, T.A. (1994). Traffic signals for lymphocyte recirculation and leukocyte emigration: the multistep paradigm. *Cell* (2): 301–314.

Storch, M.K., Piddlesden, S., Haltia, M., Iivanainen, M., Morgan, P., and Lassmann, H. (1998). Multiple sclerosis: in situ evidence for antibody- and complement- mediated demyelination. *Ann Neurol* (4): 465–471.

Tani, M. and Ransohoff, R.M. (1994). Do chemokines mediate inflammatory cell invasion of the central nervous system parenchyma? *Brain Pathol* (2): 135–143.

The IFNB Multiple Sclerosis Study Group (1993). Interferon beta-1b is effective in relapsing-remitting multiple sclerosis. I. Clinical results of a multicenter, randomized, double- blind, placebo-controlled trial. *Neurology* (4): 655–661.

The Transatlantic Multiple Sclerosis Genetics Cooperative (2001). A meta-analysis of genomic screens in multiple sclerosis. *Mult Scler* (1): 3–11.

Thompson, A.J., Montalban, X., Barkhof, F., *et al.* (2000). Diagnostic criteria for primary progressive multiple sclerosis: a position paper. *Ann Neurol* (6): 831–835.

Trapp, B.D. and Quarles, R.H. (1984). Immunocytochemical localization of the myelin-associated glycoprotein. Fact or artifact? *J Neuroimmunol* (4): 231–249.

Trapp, B.D., Andrews, S.B., Cootauco, C., and Quarles, R. (1989). The myelin-associated glycoprotein is enriched in multivesicular bodies and periaxonal membranes of actively myelinating oligodendrocytes. *J Cell Biol* (5): 2417–2426.

Trapp, B.D., Peterson, J., Ransohoff, R.M., Rudick, R., Mork, S., and Bo, L. (1998). Axonal transection in the lesions of multiple sclerosis. *N Engl J Med* (5): 278–285.

Trapp, B.D., Bo, L., Mork, S., and Chang, A. (1999a). Pathogenesis of tissue injury in MS lesions. *J Neuroimmunol* (1): 49–56.

Trapp, B.D., Ransohoff, R., and Rudick, R. (1999b). Axonal pathology in multiple sclerosis: relationship to neurologic disability. *Curr Opin Neurol* (3): 295–302.

Trapp, B.D., Ransohoff, R.M., Fisher, E., and Rudick, R.A. (1999c). Neuro-degeneration in Multiple Sclerosis: Relationship to Neurological Disability. *The Neuroscientist* 48–57.

Trebst, C., Sorensen, T.L., Kivisakk, P., *et al.* (2001). CCR1+/CCR5+ mononuclear phagocytes accumulate in the central nervous system of patients with multiple sclerosis. *Am J Pathol* (5): 1701–1710.

Trebst, C., Staugaitis, S., Kivisakk, P., *et al.* (2003). CC chemokine receptor 8 (CCR8) in the central nervous system is associated with phagocytic macrophages. *Am J Pathol* (2): 427–438.

Tubridy, N., Behan, P.O., Capildeo, R., *et al.* (1999). The effect of anti-alpha4 integrin antibody on brain lesion activity in MS. The UK Antegren Study Group. *Neurology* (3): 466–472.

van Oosten, B.W., Barkhof, F., Truyen, L., *et al.* (1996). Increased MRI activity and immune activation in two multiple sclerosis patients treated with the monoclonal anti-tumor necrosis factor antibody cA2. *Neurology* (6): 1531–1534.

van der Voorn, P., Tekstra, J., Beelen, R.H., Tensen, C.P., van der Valk, P., and De Groot, C.J. (1999). Expression of MCP-1 by reactive astrocytes in demyelinating multiple sclerosis lesions. *Am J Pathol* (1): 45–51.

Waxman, S.G. (1998). Demyelinating diseases–new pathological insights, new therapeutic targets. *N Engl J Med* (5): 323–325.

Weinshenker, B.G. (1995). The natural history of multiple sclerosis. *Neurol Clin* (1): 119–146.

Weinshenker, B.G. (1996). Epidemiology of multiple sclerosis. *Neurol Clin* (2): 291–308.

Weinshenker, B.G. (1998). The natural history of multiple sclerosis: update 1998. *Semin Neurol* (3): 301–307.

Weinshenker, B.G., Bass, B., Rice, G.P., *et al.* (1989). The natural history of multiple sclerosis: a geographically based study. I. Clinical course and disability. *Brain* 133–146.

Woodroofe, M.N. (1995). Cytokine production in the central nervous system. *Neurology* (6, Suppl. 6): S6–S10.

Woodroofe, M.N. and Cuzner, M.L. (1993). Cytokine mRNA expression in inflammatory multiple sclerosis lesions: detection by non-radioactive in situ hybridization. *Cytokine* (6): 583–588.

Woodroofe, M.N., Bellamy, A.S., Feldmann, M., Davison, A.N., and Cuzner, M.L. (1986). Immunocytochemical characterisation of the immune reaction in the central nervous system in multiple sclerosis. Possible role for microglia in lesion growth. *J Neurol Sci* (2–3): 135–152.

Woodroofe, N., Cross, A.K., Harkness, K., and Simpson, J.E. (1999). The role of chemokines in the pathogenesis of multiple sclerosis. *Adv Exp Med Biol* 135–150.

Wucherpfennig, K.W., Newcombe, J., Li, H., Keddy, C., Cuzner, M.L., and Hafler, D.A. (1992). Gamma delta T-cell receptor repertoire in acute multiple sclerosis lesions. *Proc Natl Acad Sci USA* (10): 4588–4592.

Yin, X., Crawford, T.O., Griffin, J.W., *et al.* (1998). Myelin-associated glycoprotein is a myelin signal that modulates the caliber of myelinated axons. *J Neurosci* (6): 1953–1962.

Zlotnik, A. and Yoshie, O. (2000). Chemokines: a new classification system and their role in immunity. *Immunity* (2): 121–127.

15 The immunology of multiple sclerosis

Gary Birnbaum and Jack Antel

Introduction

This chapter is based on two hypotheses. The first is that multiple sclerosis (MS) is one disease, or at least a syndrome of similar diseases with similar etiologies. The second is that immunological factors play a key role in the pathogenesis of the disease. There is support for both of these hypotheses, but as this chapter will delineate, there are other possibilities.

A fundamental unknown regarding the pathogenesis of MS is the site of the abnormality that initiates the disease process. Do persons with MS have an altered central nervous system (CNS) such that there is a normal immunological response to this alteration, or is there a normal CNS in persons with MS and an alteration in that individual's immune system is responsible for triggering the disease? There are data in support of both hypotheses.

Initial concepts of MS

The clinical and pathologic features of multiple sclerosis (MS) were described in the mid-1800s and by the 1870s had been synthesized into a recognizable entity by Charcot and colleagues (Charcot, 1877). Vulpian had introduced the term 'sclerose en plaque disseminata' in 1867. Hammond (1871) referred to the entity as 'cerebro-spinal sclerosis' to distinguish it from a wide array of disorders resulting from trauma, infection, or unknown causes that contained the term 'sclerosis' referring to the scarring observed at different anatomic sites within the CNS. Charcot emphasized the loss of the myelin sheath with relative, but not absolute, preservation of axons. He referred to the observation by Reinfleisch in 1863 of inflammation around a vessel in the center of MS lesions. This can be viewed as the beginning of a continuing debate regarding the relative contributions of immune-mediated versus 'neurodegenerative' processes as a basis for the disease pathology (Hoeber, 1922). The presence of inflammation at the site of tissue destruction suggested that either (or both) an immune reaction or an infectious process were involved in pathogenesis. This chapter will review the data supporting a prominent role for immune mechanisms in MS-related tissue destruction and also data suggesting that there may be a continuum between the changes induced by an antibrain CNS immune response and processes of tissue destruction not directly related to systemic immune system activity. The existing data do not definitively establish that MS is an autoimmune disease. Indeed, using Koch's criteria, there are several shortfalls. Immune system mediators, both cellular and humoral, are present at sites of tissue destruction but attempts at transferring disease to immunologically deficient (SCID) mice with human cells, have not been successful (Hao *et al.*, 1994; Jones *et al.*, 1995; Lavia and Rostami, 1996; Fujimura *et al.*, 1997). The strongest datum supporting at least a partial role for immune-mediated tissue destruction in MS is the fact that all currently proven treatments for MS are believed to exert their beneficial effects by modulating immune system function. The are more fully discussed in Chapter 18. However, the great heterogeneity in the course of the disease and the response to treatment raises the possibility that there also is heterogeneity of the putative immune mechanisms. The relationship between MS and 'MS-like' syndromes, such as neuromyelitis optica (Devic's syndrome) and acute disseminated encephalomyelitis (ADEM) are discussed in Chapter 13.

Is MS one disease or is it a syndrome?

Our conception of MS could well be like that of pneumonia 200 years ago. Nineteenth-century physicians classified pneumonia as a relatively homogeneous disease. Persons became ill, developed a fever, breathing difficulties, and produced large amounts of sputum. All pneumonias were, to an extent, similar and it was not until our knowledge of infectious agents increased that physicians understood the different causes of this relatively homogeneous disease entity. Could our perception of MS be similar? There are data in support of MS being a syndrome rather than a distinct disease. First is the great variation in the course of the disease. This could result from differences in genetic susceptibility and resistance genes but also could be explained by different pathogenic processes. Second there are differences in responses to treatment. Some persons with MS respond rather dramatically to treatment with immune-modulating therapies such as the beta interferons or glatiramer acetate while others with a similar pattern of disease do not. Finally, there are the intriguing observations of several groups in which brain biopsies and autopsies of MS patients were studied to look for patterns of myelin destruction (Lucchinetti *et al.*, 1996, 2000; Lassmann *et al.*, 2001; Martin *et al.*, 2001). These data, while not universally accepted at the moment, suggest that there are four patterns of myelin destruction in persons with MS and that these patterns 'run true' in each individual. Most common is a pattern of demyelination associated with an influx of T lymphocytes into the areas of myelin loss (type 1). Next most common are individuals in which myelin loss is associated with deposition of immunoglobulins into the areas of myelin loss (type 2). In types 3 and 4 there are mild inflammatory infiltrates with changes in oligodendrocytes suggesting a degenerative or apoptotic process. These observations, if confirmed, would have considerable therapeutic implications.

Genetic susceptibility to autoimmune central nervous system disease

There are a considerable number of data supporting the concept that genetic factors play an important role in susceptibility to MS, and probably in resistance to MS too. When taken to the first cousin level, 25% of individuals with MS have other family members with MS (Sadovnick *et al.*, 1996). Population gene typing studies (Olerup and Hillert, 1991; Hillert, 1994) and three genome screening studies (Sawcer *et al.*, 1996; Haines *et al.*, 1996; Ebers *et al.*, 1999) showed an association between disease occurrence and particular genes of the major histocompatibility complex (MHC). Products of these genes have important roles in determining patterns of immune responsiveness, and are described in more detail in Chapter 9. Studies of identical and fraternal twins discordant or concordant for MS indicate that identical twins have a concordance rate as high as 25–30% in contrast to fraternal twins with a concordance rate no higher than other siblings (Sadovnick *et al.*, 1996). Yet even though genetic identity considerably increases the risk for MS, it is clear that other factors (environmental?) also are important. However, within families with multiple persons with MS there are frequently striking differences both in the severity of disease and the course of disease (relapsing–remitting versus primary progressive), strongly suggesting that in addition to susceptibility genes there must also be resistance genes, or at least genes able to modify the pathogenetic processes of MS. This postulate is supported by the observation that there are relatively genetically homogeneous populations living in areas with high incidences of MS who do not develop the disease. Examples of such 'resistant groups' are Native Americans (Oger amd Lai, 1994) and Hutterites (Hader *et al.*, 1996). The nature of these 'resistance genes' is not known, but genes controlling the magnitude of cytokines secreted by immune cells are described and are being characterized in persons with and without MS (Braun *et al.*, 1996; Kantarci *et al.*, 2000, 2003). The genetics of MS are more fully described in Chapter 9.

Are there abnormalities of the CNS in MS that trigger an immune response to CNS myelin?

There are at least two ways that the CNS in MS could be altered. One is via a persistent infection (viral or bacterial) that alters the antigenicity of CNS myelin, resulting in an immune response to the altered antigens. The other is that there are modifications in CNS myelin during maturation of the CNS such that different forms of myelin are present in MS brain, leading to loss of tolerance and immune attack.

Evidence that an infectious agent plays a role in the pathogenesis of MS

The geographic distribution of MS has suggested a role for infections in the pathogenesis of this illness. MS is most prominent in northern and southern temperate zones and diminishes with proximity to the equator (Ebers and Sadovnick, 1993; Hernan *et al.*, 1999; Rosati, 2001). While these data suggest an important influence for environmental factors such as infectious agents in predisposing to the disease, the presence of resistant populations in 'high risk' zones indicates that genetic factors too play a critical role in disease susceptibility (Kurtzke *et al.*, 1979; Ebers *et al.*, 1996; Rosati, 2001) (and see Chapter 9 on the genetics of MS). However, it is well demonstrated that there are large differences in infectious flora and fauna as one moves from a temperate zone to a tropical one (Cook *et al.*, 1990; Nicholson and Mather, 1996; Gratacap-Cavallier *et al.*, 1998; Appleton *et al.*, 1999). In addition, age of exposure to infectious agents appears to be important, as suggested by studies of migration. Populations moving from high- or low-risk areas take with them the risk of their area of origin if they leave after puberty but assume the risk of their new location if they migrate before puberty (Kurtzke, 1977, 1993; Kurtzke and Bui, 1980; Kurtzke *et al.*, 1985). These data suggest that exposure to an environmental agent, most likely an infectious one, during the period of CNS myelination, plays a role in the development of MS. Additional epidemiologic support for an infectious component in MS are descriptions of 'epidemics' of MS. Among the best documented are those that were noted in the Faeroe Islands following the end of World War II. MS was presumably unknown in these relatively isolated islands off the coast of Norway prior to 1940. However, following British occupation of the islands during the war an epidemic of the disease occurred, verified by a neurologist who lived on the islands (Kurtzke and Hyllested 1979, 1987, 1988). Subsequent epidemics after intervals of years to decades followed, suggesting that the disease recurred as new generations of susceptible individuals were born (Kurtzke *et al.*, 1993, 1995).

The nature of the infectious agent or agents has been the subject of much investigation and controversy. At one point spirochetes were implicated in the etiology of MS (Gay and Dick, 1986) and today infections with the spirochete *Borrelia burgdorferi* are considered by some to mimic MS

(Halperin *et al.*, 1991) though this is disputed (Coyle 1989; Coyle *et al.*, 1993). A multitude of different viruses have been implicated, ranging from measles virus (Haase *et al.*, 1981), to retroviruses (Koprowski *et al.*, 1985; Nowak *et al.*, 1985), to herpes viruses (Challoner *et al.*, 1995). What is established is that persons with MS have increased titers of cells and antibodies reactive with a multitude of viruses both in their sera and their spinal fluids (Forghani *et al.*, 1980; Baig *et al.*, 1989; Link *et al.*, 1992). Whether these are primary to the disease process or secondary to it is not known. In addition, immune responses to measles virus (Jacobson *et al.*, 1985; Goodman *et al.*, 1989) and herpes viruses (Soldan *et al.*, 1997, 2000) are altered in persons with MS, suggesting that infection, or reactivation of latent infection, plays a role in the pathogenesis of disease. Non-viral agents also have been implicated in pathogenesis. As noted above, spirochetes were felt at one time to be important. Currently, *Chlamydia pneumoniae* is being studied as a possible infectious contributor to the demyelinating process (Sriram *et al.*, 1999; Yao *et al.*, 2001; Derfuss *et al.*, 2001). Results to date are conflicting (Pucci *et al.*, 2000; Numazaki and Chibar, 2001; Swanborg *et al.*, 2003). The continuing question with all of these studies is the primacy of process. Does an infectious agent initiate the disease? Does it amplify tissue destruction? Is it an epiphenomenon that is not at all related to the disease? Answers are not immediately forthcoming.

How could an infectious agent cause demyelination in MS? One way is by direct infection of oligodendrocytes, the cells producing CNS myelin. Examples of such infection in other diseases exist. For example, infection of oligodendrocytes by the JC virus results in the demyelinating disease, progressive multifocal leukoencephalopathy (PML) (Safak and Khalili, 2003). There is also an animal model of demyelinating disease, an encephalomyelitis caused by Theiler's virus (Dal Canto *et al.*, 1995; Friedmann and Lorch, 1985; Kim *et al.*, 2001; Tsunoda and Fujinami, 2002). This virus infects oligodendrocytes, resulting in demyelination due to both direct destruction of oligodendrocytes by the virus and an immune response to viral antigens (Miller *et al.*, 2001). While there is no direct evidence for an infection of oligodendrocytes in MS, there are data indicating that immune responses to infectious agents can cross-react with CNS myelin antigens. An early example of such cross-reactivity (coined 'molecular mimicry') is the work of Fujinami and Oldstone (1985) demonstrating immunologic cross-reactivity between hepatitis B virus polymerase and myelin basic protein (MBP). Children with post-measles encephalomyelitis have cells in their CSF that show cross-reactivity between measles and myelin antigens (Johnson *et al.*, 1984). Using computer scanning technology looking for homologous peptide sequences in proteins of infectious agents and myelin proteins, Wucherpfenning and Strominger (1995) demonstrated not only sequence homology but immunologic cross-reactivity between several of these homologous peptides. Similar data concerning cross-reacting immune responses between infectious agents and CNS proteins are described for HTLV-1 virus, group A *Streptococcus*, and corona viruses (Nagashima *et al.*, 1978, 1979; Levin *et al.*, 2002; Kirvan *et al.*, 2003). These observations support the possibility that an infectious agent could initiate an immunologically mediated demyelinating response via the mechanism of molecular mimicry in persons with MS. T cells reactive with self antigens may have escaped thymic selection because of low affinity for such antigens. They could be triggered by exposure to exogenous antigens for which they have high affinity (see Chapters 1 and 10). Immune responses to myelin antigens are well demonstrated in persons with MS (see below) and in normal individuals (Bernard and de Rosbo, 1991; Goebels *et al.*, 2000). What is not known is whether such responses resulted from an antecedent infection, from a loss of immunologic tolerance due to an intrinsic defect of the immune system, or as a result of the release of myelin antigens due to destruction of myelin by another disease process.

While persistent infections could result in expression of cell surface proteins, triggering an immune response to them, an alternative (or additional) mechanism for altered myelin antigenicity is that in MS there are alterations in the expression of myelin proteins such that fetal or related forms of myelin persist in the adult brain, resulting in immune responses to them. There are some data in support of the expression of fetal myelin in MS brain, as well as immune responses to them (Capello *et al.*, 1997). An isotype of MBP, called Golli protein, is expressed in normal thymus (Pribyl *et al.*, 1996) and is also present in cells around lesions in MS (Filipovic *et al.*, 2002). Cross-reactive immune responses to this protein are seen in MBP-responsive T cells (Tranquill *et al.*, 1996). The presence of Golli protein in the thymus suggests it may play a role in inducing (or not inducing) immunologic tolerance to MBP. While Golli protein is not *per se* abnormal, changes in expression of this protein in thymus, leading to abnormal responses to MBP, may be important in MS (see below). Using subtraction techniques with large cDNA libraries from normal and MS brains (see Chapter 1 for a description of this technique) several investigators tried to demonstrate unique differences in protein expression in MS. To date these studies are not informative regarding altered brain antigenicity (Owens *et al.*, 1996; Gilden *et al.*, 1996), but the possibility of differences in myelin protein expression in normal and MS brains is not excluded.

Are there abnormalities of the immune system that could result in immune-mediated demyelination?

As noted above, it is possible that in MS a normal immune system is responding at it should to altered or new antigens expressed on CNS myelin and/or the cells that produce it. In this section we will review data that suggest an intrinsic defect in the immune system of persons with MS. However, the reader is reminded that these two possibilities are not mutually exclusive, and that MS may not be a single disease entity; different pathogenetic processes may operate in different individuals.

Abnormalities of cellular immune responses

As described in Chapters 1 and 2, a normal immune system recognizes autologous or self antigens, most prominently autologous MHC proteins. In addition, normal individuals can generate, at least *in vitro*, immune responses to autologous antigens such as myelin proteins (Bernard and de Rosbo, 1991; Goebels *et al.*, 2000). In MS, therefore, if pathogenic immune responses to myelin are important in the development of the disease, there must be an alteration in an individual's immune system, resulting in a loss of immunologic tolerance to myelin components. There are several mechanisms for loss of tolerance to self antigens. First there can be a change in regulatory cells that normally control responses to autologous proteins. This change must be specific for antimyelin regulatory cells since there is no general dysregulation of immune responses in persons with MS. Immuno-competent cells in persons with MS may have a pattern of response to myelin antigens that is destructive rather than protective. For example, T cells responding to myelin antigens in MS may exhibit a T helper 1 (Th1) pattern of cytokine secretion rather than a Th2 pattern (see Chapter 1), leading to formation of cytotoxic T cells and activated macrophages. Another possibility is that in MS 'new' immunocompetent cells appear that are able to recognize myelin antigens, or a least respond to them with less restriction or control. Third is the possibility that immune responses to myelin antigens that are normally 'immunologically sequestered' are exposed to an MS patient's immune system, resulting in additional damage to myelin with release of additional myelin antigens, leading to the phenomenon of 'epitope spreading', a cascading of immune responses to the additional antigens. As noted below there are data in support of all of these hypotheses.

Loss of regulatory cells, in the form of suppressor cells, in persons with MS was first described by Antel *et al.* (1979) and Arnason and Antel (1978). These cells were non-antigen specific, were generated by a mitogen (concanavalin A), and were absent mainly in persons with acute and secondary progressive disease. These cells could only be assayed *in vitro* and their relationship to antigen-specific immune responses was not known. At the time of these observations much work was being done to find phenotypic cell surface markers of suppressor cells. These were unsuccessful and the concept of a 'pure' suppressor cell, that is one that subserved only suppressor activity, fell into disregard. Rather, the concept of 'context specific' suppres-

sion emerged, a concept that espoused that a particular cell can either suppress or augment an immune response dependent on the context of its interactions with other immune cells. Thus, a CD4+ cell that 'helped' a B cell mature into an antibody-producing plasma cell could lead to suppression of an immune response if the resulting antibody attached to and 'coated' antigenic sites required for recognition by cytotoxic CD8+ cells, or could augment an immune response if the resulting antibodies contributed to tissue destruction by activating complement or macrophages via antibody-dependent cell-mediated cytotoxicity (ADCC). In the 1990s investigators described cells that had surface antigen phenotypes associated with a preponderance of suppressor activity. Many of these were studied in persons with MS and found to be altered. Most recently these have included CD25+ and CD45RA+ cells (Cafaro *et al.*, 1987; Calopa *et al.*, 1995; Viglietta *et al.*, 2004) (see Chapter 2). However, the concept of a 'pure' suppressor cell is not demonstrated (Francois Bach, 2003) and the concept of a pathologically relevant loss of regulatory cells in MS has not yet been sustained (Crockard *et al.*, 1988). With the advent of disease-modulating therapies in MS (see Chapter 18), investigators studied the effects of these drugs on subpopulations of immune cells in MS. Recent work by Karandikar *et al.* (2002) suggested that at least one of these drugs, glatiramer acetate, has an effect on restoring populations of concanavalin A-inducible regulatory cells. Again the relevance of these findings to the salutary effects of the drug on the course of MS is not known. Indirect evidence that a change in regulatory cell function may play a role in MS is the well-corroborated observation that the frequency of relapses of MS is increased in the 6–9 months post-partum. During pregnancy the incidence of relapses of MS is decreased (Voskuhl, 2002), occurring in a setting when there is a general suppression of alloreactivity, caused by multiple ill-defined mechanisms, including elevated levels of ovarian hormones such as estriol and increased levels of the cytokine interferon-tau (IFN-τ). Mother Nature's intent with these actions is, we assume, to prevent the 'rejection' of the immunologically foreign fetus. Following delivery there is a decrease in both estriol and IFN-τ levels with perhaps an 'overshoot' of immune responsiveness, leading to an increased risk of MS attacks. At this time, such conjectures are just that, conjectures.

As discussed in earlier chapters, patterns of immune response to particular antigens vary greatly among individuals (Isaguliants and Ozeretskovskaya, 2003; Sarwal *et al.*, 2003; Bochud *et al.*, 2003) and during the ontogeny of the immune system (Forsthuber *et al.*, 1996; Upham *et al.*, 2002). For example, some individuals respond to particular antigens with formation of IgE antibodies, leading to the development of asthma. Others may respond to particular antigens with Th1 patterns of response and others with Th2 patterns, resulting in major differences in disease expression. The best example of this in humans is leprosy, with tuberculoid leprosy being the form of disease in persons mounting a Th1 response to the organism and lepromatous leprosy being the form of disease seen in persons mounting a Th2 response to the mycobacterium. This is in part related to a polymorphism in an innate immune system receptor (Bochud *et al.*, 2003). In MS, the patterns of response to myelin antigens are less well defined. Perhaps the strongest evidence that a Th1 response to myelin antigens is pathogenic in MS is the unexpected observation of Panitch *et al.* (1987) that administration of the Th1 cytokine interferon-gamma (IFN-γ) to persons with MS resulted in an increased frequency of relapses of disease. Less direct support for this hypothesis is offered by the observations of Balashov *et al.* (1997), Comabella *et al.* (1998), and Makhlouf *et al.* (2001), indicating that IL-12, a T-cell cytokine leading to the induction of Th1 responses, is increased in persons with MS and appears to correlate to an extent with disease activity. More indirect evidence is provided by observations in patients treated with the therapeutic agents glatiramer acetate and cyclophosphamide (Cytoxan). Immune responses to myelin antigens change with administration of glatiramer acetate, going from a predominantly Th1 response to a Th2 response (Miller *et al.*, 1998; Gran *et al.*, 2000; Chen *et al.*, 2001). Similarly, following administration of cyclophosphamide there is a significant decrease in IL-12 levels with an increase in cytokines associated with Th2 responses, such as IL-4 and transforming growth factor beta (TGF-β) (Weiner and Cohen, 2002). Again, the conundrum is the relevance of these changes to the therapeutic effects of these agents. The issue is further complicated by the observations of Lassmann *et al.* (2001) and Luchinnetti *et al.* (1996, 2000) that there may be different forms of myelin destruction in different individuals, that is that MS is not one disease but a syndrome, with myelin destruction as the final common pathway. In one described pattern of response (type 2) myelin destruction appears to be antibody mediated rather than directly T-cell mediated. Most antibody-driven immune responses to T-cell-dependent antigens result from the actions of Th2 cells, with notable exceptions. If this is the case, there is the theoretical possibility that administration of agents resulting in a Th1 to Th2 shift could, at best, be ineffective in those persons with MS having antibody-mediated myelin destruction, and at worst, increase tissue damage. Fortunately, the latter has not been observed, but unresponsiveness to treatment is all too often seen in persons with MS.

Before discussing the presence of 'new' cell types responding to myelin antigens it is informative to review the data in support of an immune reaction to myelin antigens being of pathogenic importance in MS. The search for the antigen 'triggering' the initial immune response in MS been difficult. A variety of myelin antigens are implicated in the development of MS. Most frequently mentioned is MBP. Its popularity was supported by the observation that it can induce a severe form of experimental autoimmune encephalomyelitis (EAE) in rodents and primates (Falk *et al.*, 1968; Eylar *et al.*, 1971; Jackson *et al.*, 1972). Immune responses to MBP are increased in persons with MS and more recent data indicate that there are oligoclonal expansions of both T cells (Meinl *et al.*, 1993; Vandevyver *et al.*, 1995; Babbe *et al.*, 2000; Muraro *et al.*, 2002*a*) and B cells (Qin *et al.*, 1998, 2003; Colombo *et al.*, 2000) in the CNS and CSF of persons with MS and selective expression of T cells in MS brain lesions having receptors to those responding to MBP (Oksenberg *et al.*, 1993). However, clonal expansions of T cells responding to MBP peptides has also be identified in healthy individuals (Shanmugam *et al.*, 1995). One conundrum regarding MBP is that it is an internal myelin membrane protein, not readily accessible to the immune system when myelin is intact. Thus, immune responses to MBP could be a secondary phenomenon, occurring subsequent to an antecedent myelin injury. However, myelin proteins are expressed in the fetal thymus (Pribyl *et al.*, 1996; Feng *et al.*, 2000), leading to the retention of myelin-specific T cells during the ontogeny of the immune system. Certainly by the time clinicians see persons with MS, the disease has often already been present for months and years. Other myelin antigens also are implicated in the pathogenesis of MS. These include myelin oligodendrocyte glycoprotein (MOG) (Kerlero de Rosbo *et al.*, 1993), proteolipid protein (PLP) (Trotter *et al.*, 1997), and cyclic nucleotide phosphodiesterase (CNP) (Muraro *et al.*, 2002*b*), though these observations are not found in all labs (Johnson *et al.*, 1986; Hafler *et al.*, 1987). MOG and PLP are potent inducers of EAE in rodents and primates while inducing tolerance to CNP ameliorates this disease (Birnbaum *et al.* 1996). The issue of finding the inciting antigen in MS is complicated by the phenomenon of 'epitope spreading' in which an immune response to an initiating antigen diversifies or 'spreads' to involve responses to adjacent antigens as tissues are destroyed and 'new' antigens are released. In addition, immune responses to stress proteins are described in MS (Birnbaum and Kotilink 1992, 1993; Birnbaum and Schlievert, 1992; Birnbaum *et al.*, 1993; Van Noort *et al.*, 1998; Agius *et al.* 1999), proteins that are ubiquitous in both mammalian cells and infectious organisms. Since immune responses to these 'new' antigens could play an important role in perpetuating the disease process, attempting to modify the course of MS by inducing tolerance to a single antigen may not be fully effective. On the other hand, if immune cells are induced that respond to a particular antigen by secreting 'anti-inflammatory' cytokines, such as IL-4, IL-5, or TGF-β, such cells could modulate the activity of other cells, with different antigen specificities, in their immediate environment. This phenomenon, called 'bystander suppression' (Weiner, 2001; von Herrath and Harrison, 2003), may be a mechanism of action for the drug glatiramer acetate (Yong, 2002). In any case, while there are data implicating immune responses to myelin proteins as being of pathogenic importance in MS, the 'original' inciting antigen is not known, nor is the role of the probably secondary immune responses to myelin and stress antigens known.

The question of whether persons with MS have different populations of cells responding to myelin antigens has been the subject of investigation by several researchers. Using the toxin HPRT (hypoxanthine guanine phosphoribosyltransferase) to detect cells that had divided *in vitro*, and thus were resistant to this agent, several laboratories showed that persons with MS had increased numbers of resistant cells, and that many of these cells were specific for the myelin antigens MBP and PLP (Allegretta *et al.*, 1990; Lodge *et al.*, 1994, 1996; Sriram. 1994; Trotter *et al.*, 1997). These data suggest a selective activation and proliferation of myelin antigen-specific T cells in persons with MS. In addition, when the T-cell receptors from these lines were analysed, they bore homology to the T-cell receptors used by encephalitogenic T cells in a murine model of MS, EAE (Allegretta *et al.*, 1994). However, as is often the case, a much lower incidence of HPRT-resistant cells was found in normal individuals (Lodge *et al.*, 1996), suggesting that, while myelin antigen reactive T cells are activated in MS, this may be a secondary, rather than primary, phenomenon.

Another clue as to the antigens responsible for inducing the pathogenic immune response in MS comes from studies in both animal models and humans of altered peptide ligands (APL). APL are synthetic peptides that are similar to 'naturally' occurring peptides but are altered in their amino acid sequences. Such peptides still bind to T-cell receptors specific for the naturally occurring peptide but can induce a range of responses, ranging from increased activation of the T cells ('superagonist') (Dressel *et al.*, 1997), to normal or decreased ('antagonist') responses (Gaur *et al.*, 1997). It can also shift the pattern of cytokine release from a Th1 to a Th2 pattern (Windhagen *et al.*, 1995; Crowe *et al.*, 2000; Fischer *et al.*, 2000) (see also Chapter 1). Clinical trials using an APL derived from an immunodominant epitope of MBP reported that while there was a shift in patterns of cytokine expression from Th1 to Th2 in many patients (Crowe *et al.*, 2000; Kappos *et al.*, 2000; Kim *et al.*, 2002), several individuals also receiving high-dose therapy developed increased disease activity (Bielekova *et al.*, 2000) associated with a Th1 response directed to the altered and native MBP peptide. These data indicate that immune responses to MBP and APL of MPB have pathogenic potential but do not establish that such responses are primary to the pathogenesis of MS. Indeed, immunization with whole spinal cord as part of vaccination with early rabies vaccines led to an acute demyelinating disease, but not MS, indicating the pathogenic potential of myelin reactive cells in normal individuals.

New technologies are allowing studies of unexpected antigens in MS. Among the techniques being used most extensively are gene and protein arrays (see Chapter 1). Gene arrays (also called 'gene microarrays') can screen thousands of genes to determine their expression in normal and diseased tissues. Using these techniques several investigators showed expression of unexpected proteins in acute and chronic MS lesions (Whitney *et al.*, 1999; Chabas *et al.*, 2001; Wandinger *et al.*, 2001; Zhao *et al.*, 2001; Lock *et al.*, 2002), some of them potential antigens such as titin, a giant muscle protein that induced proliferative response in a T-cell clone responsive to a dominant MBP epitope, as well as expression of unexpected inflammatory cytokines and cytokines, such as granulocyte colony-stimulating factor (GCSF) (Lock *et al.*, 2002) and osteopontin (Chabas *et al.*, 2001). Differences in the pathophysiology of MS lesions also have been suggested. For example, data from Lock *et al.* (2002) demonstrated differences in patterns of gene expression in acute versus chronic MS lesions, with acute lesions showing evidence for transcription of the GCSF gene whereas chronic lesions had increased expression of the Fcγ immunoglobulin receptor and low expression of GCSF. Work with gene arrays and proteomics (using peptides rather than nucleotides to determine the specificity of antibodies in autoimmune diseases) is still in its infancy but promises to be of great value in studying MS. Another potentially valuable technique for determining the specificity of antigen receptors in blood and lesions of persons with MS is the use of tetramer antigens. Tetramers are groups of four MHC molecules linked together that are then exposed to an antigen of interest. Binding of these tetramer–antigen complexes can be detected on the surfaces of immune cells, providing a powerful tool for analysis of antigen-specific populations both in terms of their frequencies and also the patterns of their responses to antigenic stimulation. Such techniques have already been used to study immune cells in humans (Novak *et al.*, 1999; Gebe *et al.*, 2001; Gumperz *et al.*, 2002; Kita *et al.*, 2002) and animals with EAE (Reddy *et al.*, 2003).

Immunologic abnormalities of the spinal fluid in MS

The spinal fluid in MS reflects the inflammatory changes present in the CNS parenchyma. The changes are not unique to MS. Spinal fluid protein and sugar are usually normal, despite the presence of an altered blood–brain barrier, though with very acute disease there can be mild elevations of protein. Most frequently there are increased amounts of gamma globulin present with increased IgG synthesis rates and increased IgG indices (Sharief and Thompson, 1991; Paolino *et al.*, 1996; Brasher *et al.*, 1998). The albumin index also can be elevated (Andersson *et al.*, 1994). Numbers of white blood cells (WBCs) can vary considerably and are usually normal, though with very active disease, especially spinal cord disease, numbers can be mildly elevated. Rarely are there more than 50 WBCs/mm⁶. With polyacrylamide gel electrophoresis and isoelectric focusing techniques a high percentage (>70%) of persons with MS will have oligoclonal bands (OCBs) in the IgG region of their CSF.

A great deal of work has been done trying to identify the specificity of OCBs in MS in the hope of determining the antigen(s) that induced them and thus provide a clue as to the pathogenesis of the disease. There are two schools of thought regarding the specificity of these bands. One school states that these bands bear no relation to either the disease-inciting antigens or to disease pathogenesis. Rather their presence is a result of a non-antigen-specific activation of populations of non-myelin-specific T cells and B cells recruited to, and activated in, the CNS by inflammatory cytokines. Since numbers of recruited cells is relatively small, restricted populations of antibodies are synthesized, resulting in the appearance of OCBs. Data showing differences in OCB patterns in different regions of the same MS brain support this hypothesis (Mattson *et al.*, 1980). The other school of thought states that OCBs in MS are related to important disease antigens and thus may be involved in pathogenesis. These proponents note that there are numerous precedents in other inflammatory CNS diseases for the specificity of OCBs in these illnesses both for the inciting antigen or agent and for a role for these antibodies in the pathophysiology of the disease. Examples of this are CNS Lyme disease (Kaiser and Lucking, 1993) and subacute sclerosing panencephalitis (Mehta *et al.*, 1982). In both these illnesses, the OCBs present in CSF are specific for antigens of the infecting agents with absorption of bands with the appropriate antigens. The data in MS are conflicting. Several laboratories have demonstrated increased levels of antibodies to a variety of viral antigens in MS CSF but these did not appear to be related to OCBs (Norrby and Vandvik, 1975; Mehta *et al.*, 1980; Frederiksen and Sindic, 1998; Dhib-Jalbut *et al.*, 1990). The data are further confounded by the observation that some patients with clinically and pathologically verified MS do not have OCBs in their CSF and histologic examination of their brains shows a lack of plasma cells compared with persons with MS that had OCBs in their CSF (Farrell *et al.*, 1985).

Investigators have also studied the small populations of lymphocytes in MS CSF. As noted above, numbers are limiting. In an effort to determine if there is selective expansion of particular subpopulations of cells, researchers quantitated the expression of different T-cell receptor families by the CSF T cells. Results varied. Some researchers found restricted expression of particular T-cell and B-cell receptor families, suggesting a selective, perhaps antigen-specific, activation of these cells (Shimonkevitz *et al.*, 1993; Qin *et al.*, 2003), while others showed a pattern of expression similar to that seen in peripheral blood, suggesting a relatively random recruitment of cells into the CSF (Birnbaum and van Ness, 1992). Studies of antigen specificity of CSF lymphocytes have also been performed. Again, results are mixed. Some investigators found a selective enrichment of cells in CSF specific for such antigens as MBP, MOG, and heat shock proteins (Lisak and Zweiman, 1977; Birnbaum and Kotilinek, 1991; Link *et al.*, 1992). Immune responses to both these antigens are implicated in the pathogenesis of MS. Other researchers could not confirm these findings (Hafler *et al.*, 1987). Given the potential heterogeneity of pathogenic processes in MS (Lucchinetti *et al.*, 1996, 2000; Lassmann *et al.*, 2001), it is not surprising that results vary so greatly.

Neuroimmune interactions or 'How attacked MS brain contributes to its own destruction'

Induction of an inflammatory response in the CNS results in dramatic changes in cells resident in the brain. Resident microglia (cells believed to be *in situ* macrophages) become activated and in so doing enlarge, become phagocytic (removing myelin debris), and start to secrete potentially tissue-destructive mediators such as cytokines (IL-12 and TNF-α), proteases, and excitotoxins. In addition, numbers of receptors for the constant chain of immunoglobulins (Fc receptors) increase on the surfaces of activated macrophages. When antibodies bind to these receptors, macrophages are further activated and can destroy cells to which the antibody originally bound via the antigen-specific Fab portion of the molecule. This phenomenon is called 'antibody-dependent cell-mediated cytotoxicity' or ADCC and is described in more detail in Chapter 1. In addition to secreting mediators with cytotoxic potential, activated macrophages increase their expression of Class II MHC molecules, proteins that are necessary for both the initiation and perpetuation of immune responses. They are also capable of processing and presenting antigens with appropriate co-stimulatory signals to T cells, and may thus have a very important role in continuing immune-mediated tissue destructive processes in the CNS. Activated macrophages persist for extended periods of time in MS lesions, even those that are chronic, and presumably 'inactive' (Prineas *et al.*, 2001). Astrocytes too become activated when exposed to inflammatory mediators, and while they can express Class II MHC proteins on their surfaces (Fierz *et al.*, 1985) and also process and present antigen (Fontana *et al.*, 1984), they are unable to provide the necessary co-stimulatory signals necessary for full T-cell activation (Weber *et al.*, 1994). As described in Chapter 1, T cells presented with antigen in the absence of co-stimulation become unresponsive or anergic. Indeed, these investigators described an inhibitory effect of activated astrocytes on T-cell proliferation, suggesting that astrocytes may play a role in decreasing brain inflammation (Weber *et al.*, 1994) and subsequent tissue destruction. However, activated astrocytes also secrete inflammatory mediators such as nitric oxide (Bo *et al.*, 1994; Mollace and Nistico, 1995), and while nitric oxide may contribute to tissue destruction in MS, it can also have a modulating effect on immune responses (Smith and Lassmann, 2002). Oligodendrocytes cannot process or present antigen and cannot be induced to express Class II MHC (Takiguchi and Frelinger, 1986), though data in this regard are conflicting (Horwitz *et al.*, 1999). They do express Class I MHC proteins, necessary for the recognition of antigen by cytotoxic CD8+ T cells and can thus be destroyed via this mechanism. Oligodendrocytes exposed to inflammatory cytokines also express increased Fas ligand on their surfaces, making them susceptible to apoptosis when this protein interacts with T cells expressing Fas ligand (Pouly *et al.*, 2000). Oligodendrocytes exposed to IFN-γ also express increased amounts of the TRAIL/DR4/5 protein, an additional pathway for apoptotic death triggered by interaction with T cells (Matysiak *et al.*, 2002; Wosik *et al.*, 2003). Whether such apoptic-inducing receptors play a role in augmenting demyelination in MS is uncertain since no apoptosis is observed in oligodendrocytes expressing Fas in the CNS of patients with MS (Bonetti and Raine, 1997).

How does MS change over time, or is MS more a degenerative disease than an acute inflammatory illness?

Just as a hammer sees everything as a nail, so a neuroimmunologist sees everything as immune system mediated. However, in the case of MS such myopia is limiting. As noted above, there are persuasive data suggesting that immunological mechanisms play an important role in the pathogenesis of the disease. However, what also is becoming apparent is that more than one pathophysiologic process contributes to the destruction of CNS tissue in MS, and that the preponderance of these processes in perpetuating the disease also changes.

As noted previously, Robert Carswell, Jean Cruveilhier, and Jean-Martin Charcot were the first to document the pathological lesions in MS in the 1860s and 1870s. They first described axonal and neuronal loss as an integral part of MS pathology (Bonduelle, 1994; Moreira *et al.*, 2002). While the concept of axonal loss was known for many years, with the advent of new histological and immunochemical techniques the extent and timing of axonal injury was further delineated. Recent papers (Bjartmar *et al.*, 2001, 2003; Trapp *et al.*, 1998, 1999) show persuasively that axonal transection occurs early during the inflammatory demyelinating process in acute MS plaques and the extent of axonal loss is very high (Trapp *et al.*, 1998). In addition, other investigators have demonstrated that in addition to inflammatory cytokines, acute MS lesions contain increased concentrations of the excitatory amino acid glutamate (Werner and Raine 2001). Increased levels of nitric oxide metabolites are also present in CSF during relapses (Sarchielli *et al.*, 1997; Danilov *et al.*, 2003), probably secreted by activated glial cells (Merrill *et al.*, 1993). Apoptotic neurons are also seen in the gray matter of MS brains, indicating a non-inflammatory mechanism for nerve cell death, possibly a decline in levels of trophic factors from adjacent neurons. All these observations suggest that, in addition to a major role for inflammatory and immunologic mechanisms in MS, non-immunologic 'degenerative' mechanisms contribute to the tissue destruction seen in MS, and these degenerative components appear to become predominant over time, with loss of contrast-enhancing lesions and refractoriness to the salutary effects of anti-inflammatory drugs, such as the beta interferons and glatiramer acetate. Future therapies of MS must thus be multifaceted, with the intent of altering all aspects of the pathology of MS, both the acute inflammatory ones and the degenerative ones induced by inflammation.

References

Agius, M.A., Kirvan, C.A., Schafer, A.L., Gudipati, E., and Zhu, S. (1999). High prevalence of anti-alpha-crystallin antibodies in multiple sclerosis: correlation with severity and activity of disease. *Acta Neurol Scand* 100(3): 139–147.

Allegretta, M., Nicklas, J.A., Sriram, S., and Albertini, R.J. (1990). T cells responsive to myelin basic protein in patients with multiple sclerosis. *Science* 247(4943): 718–721.

Allegretta, M., Albertini, R.J., Howell, M.D., Smith, L.R., Martin, R., McFarland, H.F. *et al.* (1994). Homologies between T cell receptor junctional sequences unique to multiple sclerosis and T cells mediating experimental allergic encephalomyelitis. *J Clin Invest* 94(1): 105–109.

Andersson, M., Alvarez-Cermeno, J., Bernardi, G., Cogato, I., Fredman, P., Frederiksen, J. *et al.* (1994). Cerebrospinal fluid in the diagnosis of multiple sclerosis: a consensus report. *J Neurol Neurosurg Psychiatry* 57(8): 897–902.

Antel, J.P., Arnason, B.G., and Medof, M.E. (1979). Suppressor cell function in multiple sclerosis: correlation with clinical disease activity. *Ann Neurol* 5(4): 338–342.

Appleton, C.C., Maurihungirire, M., and Gouws, E. (1999). The distribution of helminth infections along the coastal plain of Kwazulu-Natal province, South Africa. *Ann Trop Med Parasitol* 93(8): 859–868.

Arnason, B.G. and Antel, J. (1978). Suppressor cell function in multiple sclerosis. *Ann Immunol (Paris)* 129(2–3): 159–170.

Babbe, H., Roers, A., Waisman, A., Lassmann, H., Goebels, N., Hohlfeld, R. *et al.* (2000). Clonal expansions of CD8(+) T cells dominate the T cell infiltrate in active multiple sclerosis lesions as shown by micromanipulation and single cell polymerase chain reaction. *J Exp Med* 192(3): 393–404.

Baig, S., Olsson, O., Olsson, T., Love, A., Jeansson, S., and Link, H. (1989). Cells producing antibody to measles and herpes simplex virus in cerebrospinal fluid and blood of patients with multiple sclerosis and controls. *Clin Exp Immunol* 78(3): 390–395.

Balashov, K.E., Smith, D.R., Khoury, S.J., Hafler, D.A., and Weiner, H.L. (1997). Increased interleukin 12 production in progressive multiple sclerosis: induction by activated CD4+ T cells via CD40 ligand. *Proc Natl Acad Sci. USA* 94(2): 599–603.

Bernard, C.C. and de Rosbo, N.K. (1991). Immunopathological recognition of autoantigens in multiple sclerosis. *Acta Neurol (Napoli)* 13(2): 171–178.

Bielekova, B., Goodwin, B., Richert, N., Cortese, I., Kondo, T., Afshar, G. *et al.* (2000). Encephalitogenic potential of the myelin basic protein peptide (amino acids 83–99) in multiple sclerosis: results of a phase II clinical trial with an altered peptide ligand. *Nat Med* 6(10): 1167–1175.

Birnbaum, G. and Kotilinek, L. (1991). Immune responses to mycobacterial antigens in multiple sclerosis and other neurological diseases. *Ann Neurol* 30(2): 307.

Birnbaum, G. and Kotilinek, L. (1993). Antibodies to 70-kd heat shock protein are present in CSF and sera from patients with multiple sclerosis. *45th Annual Meeting of the American Academy of Neurology, New York, USA, April, 1993.*

Birnbaum, G. and Shlievert, P. (1992). Antibodies to mycobacterial antigens in the spinal fluids and blood from patients with multiple sclerosis and other neurological diseases. *Neurology* 42(Suppl. 3): 247.

Birnbaum, G. and van Ness, B. (1992). Quantitation of T-cell receptor V beta chain expression on lymphocytes from blood, brain, and spinal fluid in patients with multiple sclerosis and other neurological diseases. *Ann Neurol* 32(1): 24–30.

Birnbaum, G., Kotilinek, L., and Albrecht, L. (1993). Spinal fluid lymphocytes from a subgroup of multiple sclerosis patients respond to mycobacterial antigens. *Ann Neurol* 34(1): 18–24.

Birnbaum, G., Kotilinek, L., Schlievert, P., Clark, H.B., Trotter, J., Horvath, E. *et al.* (1996). Heat shock proteins and experimental autoimmune encephalomyelitis (EAE): I. Immunization with a peptide of the myelin protein 2′,3′ cyclic nucleotide 3′ phosphodiesterase that is cross-reactive with a heat shock protein alters the course of EAE. *J Neurosci. Res* 44(4): 381–396.

Bjartmar, C., Kinkel, R.P., Kidd, G., Rudick, R.A., and Trapp, B.D. (2001). Axonal loss in normal-appearing white matter in a patient with acute MS. *Neurology* 57(7): 1248–1252.

Bjartmar, C., Wujek, J.R., and Trapp, B.D. (2003). Axonal loss in the pathology of MS: consequences for understanding the progressive phase of the disease. *J Neurol Sci* 206(2): 165–171.

Bo, L., Dawson, T.M., Wesselingh, S., Mork, S., Choi, S., Kong, P.A. *et al.* (1994). Induction of nitric oxide synthase in demyelinating regions of multiple sclerosis brains. *Ann Neurol* 36(5): 778–786.

Bochud, P.Y., Hawn, T.R., and Aderem, A. (2003). Cutting edge: a Toll-like receptor 2 polymorphism that is associated with lepromatous leprosy is unable to mediate mycobacterial signaling. *J Immunol* 170(7): 3451–3454.

Bonduelle, M. (1994). [Charcot. Dates. Legend and reality]. *Hist Sci Med* 28(4): 289–95 (in French).

Bonetti, B. and Raine, C.S. (1997). Multiple sclerosis: oligodendrocytes display cell death-related molecules *in situ* but do not undergo apoptosis. *Ann Neurol* 42(1): 74–84.

Brasher, G.W., Follender, A.B., and Spiekerman, A.M. (1998). The clinical value of commonly used spinal fluid diagnostic studies in the evaluation of patients with suspected multiple sclerosis. *Am J Manag Care* 4(8): 1119–1121.

Braun, N., Michel, U., Ernst, B.P., Metzner, R., Bitsch, A., Weber, F., and Rieckmann, P. (1996). Gene polymorphism at position -308 of the tumor-necrosis-factor-alpha (TNF-alpha) in multiple sclerosis and it's influence on the regulation of TNF-alpha production. *Neurosci Lett* 215(2): 75–78.

Cafaro, A., Spadaro, M., Pandolfi, F., Tilia, G., Scarselli, E., Liberati, F., and Aiuti, F. (1987). Reduction of circulating suppressor inducer T lymphocytes in the exacerbation phase of remitting-relapse multiple sclerosis. *Riv Neurol* 57(3): 159–162.

Calopa, M., Bas, J., Mestre, M., Arbizu, T., Peres, J., and Buendia, E. (1995). T cell subsets in multiple sclerosis: a serial study. *Acta Neurol Scand* 92(5): 361–368.

Capello, E., Voskuhl, R.R., McFarland, H.F., and Raine, C.S. (1997). Multiple sclerosis: re-expression of a developmental gene in chronic lesions correlates with remyelination. *Ann Neurol* 41(6): 797–805.

Chabas, D., Baranzini, S.E., Mitchell, D., Bernard, C.C., Rittling, S.R., Denhardt, D.T. *et al.* (2001). The influence of the proinflammatory cytokine, osteopontin, on autoimmune demyelinating disease. *Science* 294(5547): 1731–1735.

Challoner, P.B., Smith, K.T., Parker, J.D., MacLeod, D.L., Coulter, S.N., Rose, T.M. *et al.* (1995). Plaque-associated expression of human herpesvirus 6 in multiple sclerosis. *Proc Natl Acad Sci U S A* 92(16): 7440–7444.

Charcot, J.M. (1887). *Lectures on Diseases of the Nervous System* (transl. G. Sigerson), pp.158–222. The New Sydenham Society, London.

Chen, M., Gran, B., Costello, K., Johnson, K., Martin, R., and Dhib-Jalbut, S. (2001). Glatiramer acetate induces a Th2-biased response and crossreactivity with myelin basic protein in patients with MS. *Mult Scler* 7(4): 209–219.

Colombo, M., Dono, M., Gazzola, P., Roncella, S., Valetto, A., Chiorazzi, N. et al. (2000). Accumulation of clonally related B lymphocytes in the cerebrospinal fluid of multiple sclerosis patients. *J Immunol* 164(5): 2782–2789.

Comabella, M., Balashov, K., Issazadeh, S., Smith, D., Weiner, H.L., and Khoury, S.J. (1998). Elevated interleukin-12 in progressive multiple sclerosis correlates with disease activity and is normalized by pulse cyclophosphamide therapy. *J Clin Invest* 102(4): 671–678.

Cook, S.M., Glass, R.I., LeBaron, C.W., and Ho, M.S. (1990). Global seasonality of rotavirus infections. *Bull World Health Organ* 68(2): 171–177.

Coyle, P.K. (1989). *Borrelia burgdorferi* antibodies in multiple sclerosis patients. *Neurology* 39(6): 760–761.

Coyle, P.K., Krupp, L.B., and Doscher, C. (1993). Significance of reactive Lyme serology in multiple sclerosis. *Ann Neurol* 34(5): 745–747.

Crockard, A.D., McNeill, T.A., McKirgan, J., and Hawkins, S.A. (1988). Determination of activated lymphocytes in peripheral blood of patients with multiple sclerosis. *J Neurol Neurosurg Psychiatry* 51(1): 139–141.

Crowe, P.D., Qin, Y., Conlon, P.J., and Antel, J.P. (2000). NBI-5788, an altered MBP83-99 peptide, induces a T-helper 2-like immune response in multiple sclerosis patients. *Ann Neurol* 48(5): 758–765.

Dal Canto, M.C., Melvold, R.W., Kim, B.S., and Miller, S.D. (1995). Two models of multiple sclerosis: experimental allergic encephalomyelitis (EAE) and Theiler's murine encephalomyelitis virus (TMEV) infection. A pathological and immunological comparison. *Microsc Res Tech* 32(3): 215–229.

Danilov, A.I., Andersson, M., Bavand, N., Wiklund, N.P., Olsson, T., and Brundin, L. (2003). Nitric oxide metabolite determinations reveal continuous inflammation in multiple sclerosis. *J Neuroimmunol* 136(1–2): 112–118.

Derfuss, T., Gurkov, R., Then, B.F., Goebels, N., Hartmann, M., Barz, C. et al. (2001). Intrathecal antibody production against *Chlamydia pneumoniae* in multiple sclerosis is part of a polyspecific immune response. *Brain* 124(7): 1325–1335.

Dhib-Jalbut, S., Lewis, K., Bradburn, E., McFarlin, D.E., and McFarland, H.F. (1990). Measles virus polypeptide-specific antibody profile in multiple sclerosis. *Neurology* 40(3, Pt 1): 430–435.

Dressel, A., Chin, J.L., Sette, A., Gausling, R., Hollsberg, P., and Hafler, D.A. (1997). Autoantigen recognition by human CD8 T cell clones: enhanced agonist response induced by altered peptide ligands. *J Immunol* 159(10): 4943–4951.

Ebers, G.C. and Sadovnick, A.D. (1993). The geographic distribution of multiple sclerosis: a review. *Neuroepidemiology* 12(1): 1–5.

Ebers, G.C., Kukay, K., Bulman, D.E., Sadovnick, A.D., Rice, G., Anderson, C. et al. (1996). A full genome search in multiple sclerosis. *Nat Genet* 13(1): 472–476.

Eylar, E.H., Westall, F.C., and Brostoff, S. (1971). Allergic encephalomyelitis. An encephalitogenic peptide derived from the basic protein of myelin. *J Biol Chem* 246(10): 3418–3424.

Falk, G.A., Kies, M.W., and Alvord, E.C. Jr (1968). Delayed hypersensitivity to myelin basic protein in the passive transfer of experimental allergic encephalomyelitis. *J Immunol* 101(4): 638–644.

Farrell, M.A., Kaufmann, J.C., Gilbert, J.J., Noseworthy, J.H., Armstrong, H.A., and Ebers, G.C. (1985). Oligoclonal bands in multiple sclerosis: clinical-pathologic correlation. *Neurology* 35(2): 212–218.

Feng, J.M., Givogri, I.M., Bongarzone, E.R., Campagnoni, C., Jacobs, E., Handley, V.W. et al. (2000). Thymocytes express the golli products of the myelin basic protein gene and levels of expression are stage dependent. *J Immunol* 165(10): 5443–5450.

Fierz, W., Endler, B., Reske, K., Wekerle, H., and Fontana, A. (1985). Astrocytes as antigen-presenting cells. I. Induction of Ia antigen expression on astrocytes by T cells via immune interferon and its effect on antigen presentation. *J Immunol* 134(6): 3785–3793.

Filipovic, R., Rakic, S., and Zecevic, N. (2002). Expression of Golli proteins in adult human brain and multiple sclerosis lesions. *J Neuroimmunol* 127(1–2): 1–12.

Fischer, F.R., Santambrogio, L., Luo, Y., Berman, M.A., Hancock, W.W., and Dorf, M.E. (2000). Modulation of experimental autoimmune encephalomyelitis: effect of altered peptide ligand on chemokine and chemokine receptor expression. *J Neuroimmunol* 110(1–2): 195–208.

Fontana, A., Fierz, W., and Wekerle, H. (1984). Astrocytes present myelin basic protein to encephalitogenic T-cell lines. *Nature* 307(5948): 273–276.

Forghani, B., Cremer, N.E., Johnson, K.P., Fein, G., and Likosky, W.H. (1980). Comprehensive viral immunology of multiple sclerosis. III. Analysis of CSF antibodies by radioimmunoassay. *Arch Neurol* 37(10): 616–619.

Forsthuber, T., Yip, H.C., and Lehmann, P.V. (1996). Induction of TH1 and TH2 immunity in neonatal mice. *Science* 271(5256): 1728–1730.

Francois Bach, J. (2003). Regulatory T cells under scrutiny. *Nat Rev Immunol* 3(3): 189–198.

Frederiksen, J.L. and Sindic, C.J. (1998). Intrathecal synthesis of virus-specific oligoclonal IgG, and of free kappa and free lambda oligoclonal bands in acute monosymptomatic optic neuritis. Comparison with brain MRI. *Mult Scler* 4(1): 22–26.

Friedmann, A. and Lorch, Y. (1985). Theiler's virus infection: a model for multiple sclerosis. *Prog Med Virol* 31: 43–83.

Fujimura, H., Nakatsuji, Y., Sakoda, S., Toyooka, K., Okuda, Y., Yoshikawa, H. et al. (1997). Demyelination in severe combined immunodeficient mice by intracisternal injection of cerebrospinal fluid cells from patients with multiple sclerosis: neuropathological investigation. *Acta Neuropathol (Berl)* 93(6): 567–578.

Fujinami, R.S. and Oldstone, M.B. (1985). Amino acid homology between the encephalitogenic site of myelin basic protein and virus: mechanism for autoimmunity. *Science* 230(4729): 1043–1045.

Gaur, A., Boehme, S.A., Chalmers, D., Crowe, P.D., Pahuja, A., Ling, N. et al. (1997). Amelioration of relapsing experimental autoimmune encephalomyelitis with altered myelin basic protein peptides involves different cellular mechanisms. *J Neuroimmunol* 74(1–2): 149–158.

Gay, D. and Dick, G. (1986). Is multiple sclerosis caused by an oral spirochaete? *Lancet* 2(8498): 75–77.

Gebe, J.A., Novak, E.J., Kwok, W.W., Farr, A.G., Nepom, G.T., and Buckner, J.H. (2001). T cell selection and differential activation on structurally related HLA-DR4 ligands. *J Immunol* 167(6): 3250–3256.

Gilden, D.H., Devlin, M.E., Burgoon, M.P., and Owens, G.P. (1996). The search for virus in multiple sclerosis brain. *Mult Scler* 2(4): 179–183.

Goebels, N., Hofstetter, H., Schmidt, S., Brunner, C., Wekerle, H., and Hohlfeld, R. (2000). Repertoire dynamics of autoreactive T cells in multiple sclerosis patients and healthy subjects: epitope spreading versus clonal persistence. *Brain* 123(3): 508–518.

Goodman, A.D., Jacobson, S., and McFarland, H.F. (1989). Virus-specific cytotoxic T lymphocytes in multiple sclerosis: a normal mumps virus response adds support for a distinct impairment in the measles virus response. *J Neuroimmunol* 22(3): 201–209.

Gran, B., Tranquill, L.R., Chen, M., Bielekova, B., Zhou, W., Dhib-Jalbut, S., and Martin, R. (2000). Mechanisms of immunomodulation by glatiramer acetate. *Neurology* 55(11): 1704–1714.

Gratacap-Cavallier, B., Bosson, J.L., Morand, P., Dutertre, N., Chanzy, B., Jouk, P.S. et al. (1998). Cytomegalovirus seroprevalence in French pregnant women: parity and place of birth as major predictive factors. *Eur J Epidemiol* 14(2): 147–152.

Gumperz, J.E., Miyake, S., Yamamura, T., and Brenner, M.B. (2002). Functionally distinct subsets of CD1d-restricted natural killer T cells revealed by CD1d tetramer staining. *J Exp Med* 195(5): 625–636.

Haase, A.T., Ventura, P., Gibbs, C.J. Jr., and Tourtellotte, W.W. (1981). Measles virus nucleotide sequences: detection by hybridization *in situ*. *Science* 212(4495): 672–675.

Hader, W.J., Seland, T.P., Hader, M.B., Harris, C.J., and Dietrich, D.W. (1996). The occurrence of multiple sclerosis in the Hutterites of North America. *Can J Neurol Sci* 23(4): 291–295.

Hafler, D.A., Benjamin, D.S., Burks, J., and Weiner, H.L. (1987). Myelin basic protein and proteolipid protein reactivity of brain- and cerebrospinal fluid-derived T cell clones in multiple sclerosis and postinfectious encephalomyelitis. *J Immunol* 139(1): 68–72.

Haines, J.L., Ter Minassian, M., Bazyk, A., Gusella, J.F., Kim, D.J., Terwedow, H. et al. (1996). A complete genomic screen for multiple sclerosis underscores a role for the major histocompatability complex. The Multiple Sclerosis Genetics Group. *Nat Genet* **13**(4): 469–471.

Halperin, J.J., Volkman, D.J., and Wu, P. (1991). Central nervous system abnormalities in Lyme neuroborreliosis. *Neurology* **41**(10): 1571–1582.

Hammond, W.A. (1871). *A Treatise on Diseases of the Nervous System*. Appleton & Co., New York.

Hao, Q., Saida, T., Nishimura, M., Ozawa, K., and Saida, K. (1994). Failure to transfer multiple sclerosis into severe combined immunodeficiency mice by mononuclear cells from CSF of patients. *Neurology* **44**(1): 163–165.

Hernan, M.A., Olek, M.J., and Ascherio, A. (1999). Geographic variation of MS incidence in two prospective studies of US women. *Neurology* **53**(8): 1711–1718.

Hillert, J. (1994). Human leukocyte antigen studies in multiple sclerosis. *Ann Neurol* **36**(Suppl): S15–S17.

Hoeber, P.B. (1992). *Multiple Sclerosis (Disseminated Sclerosis)*, Vol. 1. Association for Research in Nervous and Menbtal Disease, New York.

Horwitz, M.S., Evans, C.F., Klier, F.G., and Oldstone, M.B. (1999). Detailed in vivo analysis of interferon-gamma induced major histocompatibility complex expression in the the central nervous system: astrocytes fail to express major histocompatibility complex class I and II molecules. *Lab Invest* **79**(2): 235–242.

Isaguliants, M.G. and Ozeretskovskaya, N.N. (2003). Host background factors contributing to hepatitis C virus clearance. *Curr Pharm Biotechnol* **4**(3): 185–193.

Jackson ,J.J., Brostoff, S.W., Lampert, P., and Eylar, E.H. (1972). Allergic encephalomyelitis in monkeys induced with A-1 protein. *Neurobiology* **2**(2): 83–88.

Jacobson, S., Flerlage, M.L., and McFarland, H.F. (1985). Impaired measles virus-specific cytotoxic T cell responses in multiple sclerosis. *J Exp Med* **162**(3): 839–850.

Johnson, D., Hafler, D.A., Fallis, R.J., Lees, M.B., Brady, R.O., Quarles, R.H., and Weiner, H.L. (1986). Cell-mediated immunity to myelin-associated glycoprotein, proteolipid protein, and myelin basic protein in multiple sclerosis. *J Neuroimmunol* **13**(1): 99–108.

Johnson, R.T., Griffin, D.E., Hirsch, R.L., Wolinsky, J.S., Roedenbeck, S., Lindo, d.S., I, and Vaisberg, A. (1984). Measles encephalomyelitis—clinical and immunologic studies. *N Engl J Med* **310**(3): 137–141.

Jones, R.E., Chou, Y., Young, A., Mass, M., Vandenbark, A., Offner, H., and Bourdette, D. (1995). T cells with encephalitogenic potential from multiple sclerosis patients and Lewis rats fail to induce disease in SCID mice following intracisternal injection. *J Neuroimmunol* **56**(2): 119–126.

Kaiser, R. and Lucking, C.H. (1993). Intrathecal synthesis of specific antibodies in neuroborreliosis. Comparison of different ELISA techniques and calculation methods. *J Neurol Sci* **118**(1): 64–72.

Kantarci, O.H., Atkinson, E.J., Hebrink, D.D., McMurray, C.T., and Weinshenker, B.G. (2000). Association of two variants in IL-1beta and IL-1 receptor antagonist genes with multiple sclerosis. *J Neuroimmunol* **106**(1–2): 220–227.

Kantarci, O.H., Schaefer-Klein, J.L., Hebrink, D.D., Achenbach, S.J., Atkinson, E.J., McMurray, C.T., and Weinshenker, B.G. (2003). A population-based study of IL4 polymorphisms in multiple sclerosis. *J Neuroimmunol* **137**(1–2): 134–139.

Kappos, L., Comi, G., Panitch, H., Oger, J., Antel, J., Conlon, P., and Steinman, L. (2000). Induction of a non-encephalitogenic type 2 T helper-cell autoimmune response in multiple sclerosis after administration of an altered peptide ligand in a placebo-controlled, randomized phase II trial. The Altered Peptide Ligand in Relapsing MS Study Group. *Nat Med* **6**(10): 1176–1182.

Karandikar, N.J., Crawford, M.P., Yan, X., Ratts, R.B., Brenchley, J.M., Ambrozak, D.R. *et al.* (2002). Glatiramer acetate (Copaxone) therapy induces CD8(+) T cell responses in patients with multiple sclerosis. *J Clin Invest* **109**(5): 641–649.

Kerlero, d.R., Milo, R., Lees, M.B., Burger, D., Bernard, C.C., and Ben Nun, A. (1993). Reactivity to myelin antigens in multiple sclerosis. Peripheral blood lymphocytes respond predominantly to myelin oligodendrocyte glycoprotein. *J Clin Invest* **92**(6): 2602–2608.

Kim, B.S., Lyman, M.A., Kang, B.S., Kang, H.K., Lee, H.G., Mohindru, M., and Palma, J.P. (2001). Pathogenesis of virus-induced immune-mediated demyelination. *Immunol Res* **24**(2): 121–130.

Kim, H.J., Antel, J.P., Duquette, P., Alleva, D.G., Conlon, P.J., and Bar-Or, A. (2002). Persistence of immune responses to altered and native myelin antigens in patients with multiple sclerosis treated with altered peptide ligand. *Clin Immunol* **104**(2): 105–114.

Kirvan, C.A., Swedo, S.E., Heuser, J.S., and Cunningham, M.W. (2003). Mimicry and autoantibody-mediated neuronal cell signaling in Sydenham chorea. *Nat Med* **9**(7): 914–920.

Kita, H., Naidenko, O.V., Kronenberg, M., Ansari, A.A., Rogers, P., He, X.S. *et al.* (2002). Quantitation and phenotypic analysis of natural killer T cells in primary biliary cirrhosis using a human CD1d tetramer. *Gastroenterology* **123**(4): 1031–1043.

Koprowski, H., DeFreitas, E.C., Harper, M.E., Sandberg-Wollheim, M., Sheremata, W.A., Robert-Guroff, M. *et al.* (1985). Multiple sclerosis and human T-cell lymphotropic retroviruses. *Nature* **318**(6042): 154–160.

Kurtzke, J.F. (1977). Geography in multiple sclerosis. *J Neurol* **215**(1): 1–26.

Kurtzke, J.F. (1993). Epidemiologic evidence for multiple sclerosis as an infection. *Clin Microbiol Rev* **6**(4): 382–427.

Kurtzke, J.F. and Bui, Q.H. (1980). Multiple sclerosis in a migrant population: 2. Half-orientals immigrating in childhood. *Ann Neurol* **8**(3): 256–260.

Kurtzke, J.F. and Hyllested, K. (1979). Multiple sclerosis in the Faroe Islands: I. Clinical and epidemiological features. *Ann Neurol* **5**(1): 6–21.

Kurtzke, J.F. and Hyllested, K. (1987). Multiple sclerosis in the Faroe Islands. III. An alternative assessment of the three epidemics. *Acta Neurol Scand* **76**(5): 317–339.

Kurtzke, J.F. and Hyllested, K. (1988). Validity of the epidemics of multiple sclerosis in the Faroe Islands. *Neuroepidemiology* **7**(4): 190–227.

Kurtzke, J.F., Beebe, G.W., and Norman, J.E., Jr. (1979). Epidemiology of multiple sclerosis in U.S. veterans: 1. Race, sex, and geographic distribution. *Neurology* **29**(9, Pt 1): 1228–1235.

Kurtzke, J.F., Beebe, G.W., and Norman, J.E., Jr. (1985). Epidemiology of multiple sclerosis in US veterans: III. Migration and the risk of MS. *Neurology* **35**(5): 672–678.

Kurtzke, J.F., Hyllested, K., Heltberg, A., and Olsen, A. (1993). Multiple sclerosis in the Faroe Islands. 5. The occurrence of the fourth epidemic as validation of transmission. *Acta Neurol Scand* **88**(3): 161–173.

Kurtzke, J.F., Hyllested, K., and Heltberg, A. (1995). Multiple sclerosis in the Faroe Islands: transmission across four epidemics. *Acta Neurol Scand* **91**(5): 321–325.

Lassmann, H., Bruck, W., and Lucchinetti, C. (2001). Heterogeneity of multiple sclerosis pathogenesis: implications for diagnosis and therapy. *Trends Mol Med* **7**(3): 115–121.

Lavi, E. and Rostami, A. (1996). Demyelination following transfer of human lymphocytes into mice with severe combined immunodeficiency. *Pathobiology* **64**(3): 136–141.

Levin, M.C., Lee, S.M., Kalume, F., Morcos, Y., Dohan, F.C., Jr., Hasty, K.A. *et al.* (2002). Autoimmunity due to molecular mimicry as a cause of neurological disease. *Nat Med* **8**(5): 509–513.

Link, H., Sun, J.B., Wang, Z., Xu, Z., Love, A., Fredrikson, S., and Olsson, T. (1992). Virus-reactive and autoreactive T cells are accumulated in cerebrospinal fluid in multiple sclerosis. *J Neuroimmunol* **38**(1–2): 63–73.

Lisak, R.P. and Zweiman, B. (1977). *In vitro* cell-mediated immunity of cerebrospinal-fluid lymphocytes to myelin basic protein in primary demyelinating diseases. *N Engl J Med* **297**(16): 850–853.

Lock, C., Hermans, G., Pedotti, R., Brendolan, A., Schadt, E., Garren, H. *et al.* (2002). Gene-microarray analysis of multiple sclerosis lesions yields new targets validated in autoimmune encephalomyelitis. *Nat Med* **8**(5): 500–508.

Lodge, P.A., Johnson, C., and Sriram, S. (1996). Frequency of MBP and MBP peptide-reactive T cells in the HPRT mutant T-cell population of MS patients. *Neurology* **46**(5): 1410–1415.

Lodge, P.A., Allegretta, M., Steinman, L., and Sriram, S. (1994). Myelin basic protein peptide specificity and T-cell receptor gene usage of HPRT mutant T-cell clones in patients with multiple sclerosis. *Ann Neurol* **36**(5): 734–740.

Lucchinetti, C.F., Bruck, W., Rodriguez, M., and Lassmann, H. (1996). Distinct patterns of multiple sclerosis pathology indicates heterogeneity on pathogenesis. *Brain Pathol* **6**(3): 259–274.

Lucchinetti, C., Bruck, W., Parisi, J., Scheithauer, B., Rodriguez, M., and Lassmann, H. (2000). Heterogeneity of multiple sclerosis lesions: implications for the pathogenesis of demyelination. *Ann Neurol* **47**(6): 707–717.

Makhlouf, K., Weiner, H.L., and Khoury, S.J. (2001). Increased percentage of IL-12+ monocytes in the blood correlates with the presence of active MRI lesions in MS. *J Neuroimmunol* **119**(1): 145–149.

Martin, R., Gran, B., Zhao, Y., Markovic-Plese, S., Bielekova, B., Marques, A. *et al.* (2001). Molecular mimicry and antigen-specific T cell responses in multiple sclerosis and chronic CNS Lyme disease. *J Autoimmun* **16**(3): 187–192.

Mattson, D.H., Roos, R.P., and Arnason, B.G. (1980). Isoelectric focusing of IgG eluted from multiple sclerosis and subacute sclerosing panencephalitis brains. *Nature* **287**(5780): 335–337.

Matysiak, M., Jurewicz, A., Jaskolski, D., and Selmaj, K. (2002). TRAIL induces death of human oligodendrocytes isolated from adult brain. *Brain* **125**(11): 2469–2480.

Mehta, P.D., Thormar, H., and Wisniewski, H.M. (1980). Quantitation of measles-specific IgG. Its presence in CSF and brain extracts of patients with multiple sclerosis. *Arch Neurol* **37**(10): 607–609.

Mehta, P.D., Patrick, B.A., and Thormar, H. (1982). Identification of virus-specific oligoclonal bands in subacute sclerosing panencephalitis by immunofixation after isoelectric focusing and peroxidase staining. *J Clin Microbiol* **16**(5): 985–987.

Meinl, E., Weber, F., Drexler, K., Morelle, C., Ott, M., Saruhan-Direskeneli, G. *et al.* (1993). Myelin basic protein-specific T lymphocyte repertoire in multiple sclerosis. Complexity of the response and dominance of nested epitopes due to recruitment of multiple T cell clones. *J Clin Invest* **92**(6): 2633–2643.

Merrill, J.E., Ignarro, L.J., Sherman, M.P., Melinek, J., and Lane, T.E. (1993). Microglial cell cytotoxicity of oligodendrocytes is mediated through nitric oxide. *J Immunol* **151**(4): 2132–2141.

Miller, A., Shapiro, S., Gershtein, R., Kinarty, A., Rawashdeh, H., Honigman, S., and Lahat, N. (1998). Treatment of multiple sclerosis with copolymer-1 (Copaxone): implicating mechanisms of Th1 to Th2/Th3 immune-deviation. *J Neuroimmunol* **92**(1–2): 113–121.

Miller, S.D., Katz-Levy, Y., Neville, K.L., and Vanderlugt, C.L. (2001). Virus-induced autoimmunity: epitope spreading to myelin autoepitopes in Theiler's virus infection of the central nervous system. *Adv Virus Res* **56**: 199–217.

Mollace, V. and Nistico, G. (1995). Release of nitric oxide from astroglial cells: a key mechanism in neuroimmune disorders. *Adv Neuroimmunol* **5**(4): 421–430.

Moreira, M.A., Tilbery, C.P., Lana-Peixoto, M.A., Mendes, M.F., Kaimen-Maciel, D.R., and Callegaro, D. (2002). [Historical aspects of multiple sclerosis]. *Rev Neurol* **34**(4): 379–383.

Muraro, P.A., Bonanni, L., Mazzanti, B., Pantalone, A., Traggiai, E., Massacesi, L. *et al.* (2002*a*). Short-term dynamics of circulating T cell receptor V beta repertoire in relapsing-remitting MS. *J Neuroimmunol* **127**(1–2): 149–159.

Muraro, P.A., Kalbus, M., Afshar, G., McFarland, H.F., and Martin, R. (2002*b*). T cell response to 2′,3′-cyclic nucleotide 3′-phosphodiesterase (CNPase) in multiple sclerosis patients. *J Neuroimmunol* **130**(1–2): 233–242.

Nagashima, K., Wege, H., Meyermann, R., and ter,M., V. (1978). Corona virus induced subacute demyelinating encephalomyelitis in rats: a morphological analysis. *Acta Neuropathol (Berl)* **44**(1): 63–70.

Nagashima, K., Wege, H., Meyermann, R., and ter,M., V. (1979). Demyelinating encephalomyelitis induced by a long-term corona virus infection in rats. A preliminary report. *Acta Neuropathol (Berl)* **45**(3): 205–213.

Nicholson, M.C. and Mather, T.N. (1996). Methods for evaluating Lyme disease risks using geographic information systems and geospatial analysis. *J Med Entomol* **33**(5): 711–720.

Norrby, E. and Vandvik, B. (1975). Relationship between measles virus-specific antibody activities and oligoclonal IgG in the central nervous system of patients with subacute sclerosing panencephalitis and multiple sclerosis. *Med Microbiol Immunol (Berl)* **162**(1): 63–72.

Novak, E.J., Liu, A.W., Nepom, G.T., and Kwok, W.W. (1999). MHC class II tetramers identify peptide-specific human CD4(+) T cells proliferating in response to influenza A antigen. *J Clin Invest* **104**(12): R63–R67.

Nowak, J., Januszkiewicz, D., Pernak, M., Liwen, I., Zawada, M., Rembowska, J. *et al.* (2003). Multiple sclerosis-associated virus-related pol sequences found both in multiple sclerosis and healthy donors are more frequently expressed in multiple sclerosis patients. *J Neurovirol* **9**(1): 112–117.

Numazaki, K. and Chibar, S. (2001). Failure to detect Chlamydia pneumoniae in the central nervous system of patients with MS. *Neurology* **57**(4): 746.

Oger, J. and Lai, H. (1994). Demyelination and ethnicity: experience at the University of British Columbia Multiple Sclerosis Clinic with special refer-

ence to HTLV-I-associated myelopathy in British Columbian natives. *Ann Neurol* **36**(Suppl): S22–S24.

Oksenberg, J.R., Panzara, M.A., Begovich, A.B., Mitchell, D., Erlich, H.A., Murray, R.S. *et al.* (1993). Selection for T-cell receptor V beta-D beta-J beta gene rearrangements with specificity for a myelin basic protein peptide in brain lesions of multiple sclerosis. *Nature* **362**(6415): 68–70.

Olerup, O. and Hillert, J. (1991). HLA class II-associated genetic susceptibility in multiple sclerosis: a critical evaluation. *Tissue Antigens* **38**(1): 1–15.

Owens, G.P., Burgoon, M.P., Devlin, M.E., and Gilden, D.H. (1996). Strategies to identify sequences or antigens unique to multiple sclerosis. *Mult Scler* **2**(4): 184–194.

Panitch, H.S., Hirsch, R.L., Haley, A.S., and Johnson, K.P. (1987). Exacerbations of multiple sclerosis in patients treated with gamma interferon. *Lancet* **1**(8538): 893–895.

Paolino, E., Fainardi, E., Ruppi, P., Tola, M.R., Govoni, V., Casetta, I. *et al.* (1996). A prospective study on the predictive value of CSF oligoclonal bands and MRI in acute isolated neurological syndromes for subsequent progression to multiple sclerosis. *J Neurol Neurosurg Psychiatry* **60**(5): 572–575.

Pouly, S., Becher, B., Blain, M., and Antel, J.P. (2000). Interferon-gamma modulates human oligodendrocyte susceptibility to Fas-mediated apoptosis. *J Neuropathol Exp Neurol* **59**(4): 280–286.

Pribyl, T.M., Campagnoni, C., Kampf, K., Handley, V.W., and Campagnoni, A.T. (1996). The major myelin protein genes are expressed in the human thymus. *J Neurosci Res* **45**(6): 812–819.

Prineas, J.W., Kwon, E.E., Cho, E.S., Sharer, L.R., Barnett, M.H., Oleszak, E.L. *et al.* (2001). Immunopathology of secondary-progressive multiple sclerosis. *Ann Neurol* **50**(5): 646–657.

Pucci, E., Taus, C., Cartechini, E., Morelli, M., Giuliani, G., Clementi, M., and Menzo, S. (2000). Lack of *Chlamydia* infection of the central nervous system in multiple sclerosis. *Ann Neurol* **48**(3): 399–400.

Qin, Y., Duquette, P., Zhang, Y., Talbot, P., Poole, R., and Antel, J. (1998). Clonal expansion and somatic hypermutation of V(H) genes of B cells from cerebrospinal fluid in multiple sclerosis. *J Clin Invest* **102**(5): 1045–1050.

Qin, Y., Duquette, P., Zhang, Y., Olek, M., Da, R.R., Richardson, J. *et al.* (2003). Intrathecal B-cell clonal expansion, an early sign of humoral immunity, in the cerebrospinal fluid of patients with clinically isolated syndrome suggestive of multiple sclerosis. *Lab Invest* **83**(7): 1081–1088.

Reddy, J., Bettelli, E., Nicholson, L., Waldner, H., Jang, M.H., Wucherpfennig, K.W., and Kuchroo, V.K. (2003). Detection of autoreactive myelin proteolipid protein 139–151-specific T cells by using MHC II (IAs) tetramers. *J Immunol* **170**(2): 870–877.

Rosati, G. (2001). The prevalence of multiple sclerosis in the world: an update. *Neurol Sci* **22**(2): 117–139.

Sadovnick, A.D., Ebers, G.C., Dyment, D.A., and Risch, N.J. (1996). Evidence for genetic basis of multiple sclerosis. The Canadian Collaborative Study Group. *Lancet* **347**(9017): 1728–1730.

Safak, M. and Khalili, K. (2003). An overview: Human polyomavirus JC virus and its associated disorders. *J Neurovirol* **9**(Suppl 1): 3–9.

Sarchielli, P., Orlacchio, A., Vicinanza, F., Pelliccioli, G.P., Tognoloni, M., Saccardi, C., and Gallai, V. (1997). Cytokine secretion and nitric oxide production by mononuclear cells of patients with multiple sclerosis. *J Neuroimmunol* **80**(1–2): 76–86.

Sarwal, M., Chua, M.S., Kambham, N., Hsieh, S.C., Satterwhite, T., Masek, M., and Salvatierra, O., Jr. (2003). Molecular heterogeneity in acute renal allograft rejection identified by DNA microarray profiling. *N Engl J Med* **349**(2): 125–138.

Sawcer, S., Jones, H.B., Feakes, R., Gray, J., Smaldon, N., Chataway, J. *et al.* (1996). A genome screen in multiple sclerosis reveals susceptibility loci on chromosome 6p21 and 17q22. *Nat Genet* **13**(4): 464–468.

Shanmugam, A., Copie-Bergman, C., Caillat, S., Bach, J.F., and Tournier-Lasserve, E. (1995). *In vivo* clonal expression of T lymphocytes specific for an immunodominant N-terminal myelin basic protein epitope in healthy individuals. *J Neuroimmunol* **59**(1–2): 165–172.

Sharief, M.K. and Thompson, E.J. (1991). The predictive value of intrathecal immunoglobulin synthesis and magnetic resonance imaging in acute isolated syndromes for subsequent development of multiple sclerosis. *Ann Neurol* **29**(2): 147–151.

Shimonkevitz, R., Colburn, C., Burnham, J.A., Murray, R.S., and Kotzin, B.L. (1993). Clonal expansions of activated gamma/delta T cells in recent-onset multiple sclerosis. *Proc Natl Acad Sci USA* **90**(3): 923–927.

Smith, K.J. and Lassmann, H. (2002). The role of nitric oxide in multiple sclerosis. *Lancet Neurol* **1**(4): 232–241.

Soldan, S.S., Berti, R., Salem, N., Secchiero, P., Flamand, L., Calabresi, P.A. *et al.* (1997). Association of human herpes virus 6 (HHV-6) with multiple sclerosis: increased IgM response to HHV-6 early antigen and detection of serum HHV-6 DNA. *Nat Med* **3**(12): 1394–1397.

Soldan, S.S., Leist, T.P., Juhng, K.N., McFarland, H.F., and Jacobson, S. (2000). Increased lymphoproliferative response to human herpesvirus type 6A variant in multiple sclerosis patients. *Ann Neurol* **47**(3): 306–313.

Sriram, S. (1994). Longitudinal study of frequency of HPRT mutant T cells in patients with multiple sclerosis. *Neurology* **44**(2): 311–315.

Sriram, S., Stratton, C.W., Yao, S., Tharp, A., Ding, L., Bannan, J.D., and Mitchell, W.M. (1999). *Chlamydia pneumoniae* infection of the central nervous system in multiple sclerosis. *Ann Neurol* **46**(1): 6–14.

Swanborg, R.H., Whittum-Hudson, J.A., and Hudson, A.P. (2003). Infectious agents and multiple sclerosis—are *Chlamydia pneumoniae* and human herpes virus 6 involved? *J Neuroimmunol* **136**(1–2): 1–8.

Takiguchi, M. and Frelinger, J.A. (1986). Induction of antigen presentation ability in purified cultures of astroglia by interferon-gamma. *J Mol Cell Immunol* **2**(5): 269–280.

Tranquill, L.R., Skinner, E., Campagnoni, C., Vergelli, M., Hemmer, B., Muraro, P. *et al.* (1996). Human T lymphocytes specific for the immunodominant 83–99 epitope of myelin basic protein: recognition of golli MBP HOG 7. *J Neurosci Res* **45**(6): 820–828.

Trapp, B.D., Peterson, J., Ransohoff, R.M., Rudick, R., Mork, S., and Bo, L. (1998). Axonal transection in the lesions of multiple sclerosis. *N Engl J Med* **338**(5): 278–285.

Trapp, B.D., Bo, L., Mork, S., and Chang, A. (1999). Pathogenesis of tissue injury in MS lesions. *J Neuroimmunol* **98**(1): 49–56.

Trotter, J.L., Damico, C.A., Cross, A.H., Pelfrey, C.M., Karr, R.W., Fu, X.T., and McFarland, H.F. (1997). HPRT mutant T-cell lines from multiple sclerosis patients recognize myelin proteolipid protein peptides. *J Neuroimmunol* **75**(1–2): 95–103.

Tsunoda, I. and Fujinami, R.S. (2002). Inside-Out versus Outside-In models for virus induced demyelination: axonal damage triggering demyelination. *Springer Semin Immunopathol* **24**(2): 105–125.

Upham, J.W., Lee, P.T., Holt, B.J., Heaton, T., Prescott, S.L., Sharp, M.J. *et al.* (2002). Development of interleukin-12-producing capacity throughout childhood. *Infect Immun* **70**(12): 6583–6588.

Van Noort, J.M., van Sechel, A.C., van Stipdonk, M.J., and Bajramovic, J.J. (1998). The small heat shock protein alpha B-crystallin as key autoantigen in multiple sclerosis. *Prog Brain Res* **117**: 435–452.

Vandevyver, C., Mertens, N., van den, E.P., Medaer, R., Raus, J., and Zhang, J. (1995). Clonal expansion of myelin basic protein-reactive T cells in patients with multiple sclerosis: restricted T cell receptor V gene rearrangements and CDR3 sequence. *Eur J Immunol* **25**(4): 958–968.

Viglietta, V., Baecher-Allan, C., Weiner, H.L., and Hafler, D.A. (2004). Loss of functional suppression by CD4+CD25+ regulatory T cells in patients with multiple sclerosis. *J Exp Med* **199**(7): 971–979.

Von Herrath, M.G. and Harrison, L.C. (2003). Antigen-induced regulatory T cells in autoimmunity. *Nat Rev Immunol* **3**(3): 223–232.

Voskuhl, R.R. (2002). Gender issues and multiple sclerosis. *Curr Neurol Neurosci Rep* **2**(3): 277–286.

Wandinger, K.P., Sturzebecher, C.S., Bielekova, B., Detore, G., Rosenwald, A., Staudt, L.M. *et al.* (2001). Complex immunomodulatory effects of interferon-beta in multiple sclerosis include the upregulation of T helper 1-associated marker genes. *Ann Neurol* **50**(3): 349–357.

Weber, F., Meinl, E., Aloisi, F., Nevinny-Stickel, C., Albert, E., Wekerle, H., and Hohlfeld, R. (1994). Human astrocytes are only partially competent antigen presenting cells. Possible implications for lesion development in multiple sclerosis. *Brain* **117**(1): 59–69.

Weiner, H.L. (2001). Oral tolerance: immune mechanisms and the generation of Th3-type TGF-beta-secreting regulatory cells. *Microbes Infect* **3**(11): 947–954.

Weiner, H.L. and Cohen, J.A. (2002). Treatment of multiple sclerosis with cyclophosphamide: critical review of clinical and immunologic effects. *Mult Scler* **8**(2): 142–154.

Werner, P., Pitt, D., and Raine, C.S. (2001). Multiple sclerosis: altered glutamate homeostasis in lesions correlates with oligodendrocyte and axonal damage. *Ann Neurol* **50**(2): 169–180.

Whitney, L.W., Becker, K.G., Tresser, N.J., Caballero-Ramos, C.I., Munson, P.J., Prabhu, V.V. *et al.* (1999). Analysis of gene expression in mutiple sclerosis lesions using cDNA microarrays. *Ann Neurol* **46**(3): 425–428.

Windhagen, A., Scholz, C., Hollsberg, P., Fukaura, H., Sette, A., and Hafler, D.A. (1995). Modulation of cytokine patterns of human autoreactive T cell clones by a single amino acid substitution of their peptide ligand. *Immunity* **2**(4): 373–380.

Wosik, K., Antel, J., Kuhlmann, T., Bruck, W., Massie, B., and Nalbantoglu, J. (2003). Oligodendrocyte injury in multiple sclerosis: a role for p53. *J Neurochem* **85**(3): 635–644.

Wucherpfennig, K.W. and Strominger, J.L. (1995). Molecular mimicry in T cell-mediated autoimmunity: viral peptides activate human T cell clones specific for myelin basic protein. *Cell* **80**(5): 695–705.

Yao, S.Y., Stratton, C.W., Mitchell, W.M., and Sriram, S. (2001). CSF oligoclonal bands in MS include antibodies against Chlamydophila antigens. *Neurology* **56**(9): 1168–1176.

Yong, V.W. (2002). Differential mechanisms of action of interferon-beta and glatiramer aetate in MS. *Neurology* **59**(6): 802–808.

Zhao, Y., Gran, B., Pinilla, C., Markovic-Plese, S., Hemmer, B., Tzou, A. *et al.* (2001). Combinatorial peptide libraries and biometric score matrices permit the quantitative analysis of specific and degenerate interactions between clonotypic TCR and MHC peptide ligands. *J Immunol* **167**(4): 2130–2141.

16 Imaging the immunobiology of multiple sclerosis

Douglas L. Arnold, Zografos Caramanos, Nicola De Stefano, Roger N. Gunn, and Joseph Frank

Introduction

Continuing advances in the field of neuroimaging, particularly those in magnetic resonance imaging (MRI), have made tremendous impacts on our understanding of multiple sclerosis (MS) (e.g. Matthews and Arnold, 2001). For example, conventional MRI has allowed for the *in vivo* visualization, albeit non-specifically, of both the focal inflammation and the result-ing tissue injury that occurs in MS. Furthermore, serial imaging and clinical imaging have helped to define both where and when tissue injury is occurring. Moreover, newer, 'non-conventional' quantitative MRI techniques have revealed important pathology outside the lesions of MS—pathology that involves both the normal-appearing white matter (NAWM) and the normal-appearing gray matter (NAGM). These techniques include (1) magnetization transfer imaging (MTI), which provides relatively-

Centrum Semiovale

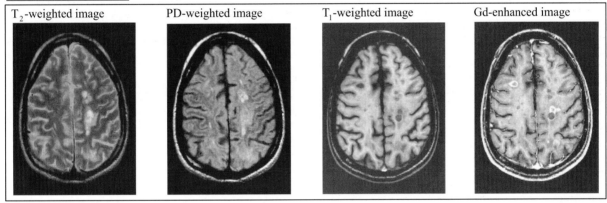

Lateral Ventricles

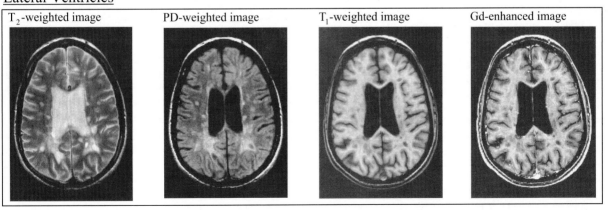

Fig. 16.1 Examples of cross-sectional slices through the centrum semiovale (top) and the lateral ventricles of a patient with multiple sclerosis (MS) as seen (from left to right) on T_2-weighted imaging, proton-density-weighted (PD) imaging, T_1-weighted, and Gd-enhanced T_1-weighted images. At the level of the centrum semiovale (top row) many of the hyperintense lesions that can be seen on the T_2- and PD-weighted images are also seen as hypointensities on the T_1-weighted images and two of these lesions are still active and inflammatory (as evidenced by the ring-like Gd-enhancement). At the level of the lateral ventricles (bottom row) it is difficult to discriminate between the periventricular lesions and cerebrospinal fluid (CSF) on the T_2-weighted image, but it is easy to discriminate between the periventricular lesions and the CSF on the PD-weighted image; the extent of T_2- and PD-weighted hyperintensity is much more extensive than the hypointensities seen on the T_1-weighted images. There are no active, inflammatory lesions at this level (as evidenced by the lack of Gd enhancement). (Images are courtesy of the Canadian MS/BMT Study Group.)

specific information on the amount and integrity of myelin; (2) diffusion-weighted imaging (DWI), which provides a localized measure of overall structural integrity of tissue; and (3) proton magnetic resonance spectroscopy (^{1}H-MRS), which provides specific information on the integrity of neurons and their axonal processes. Finally, newer techniques that are currently in development might soon be able to provide more specific information on the nature of the inflammatory infiltrates that occur in MS brain. Using combinations of these various techniques, we are now beginning to be able to observe the relationship between inflammation and injury in the myelin and the axons of both the lesional and the normal-appearing nervous tissue of patients with MS.

Conventional magnetic resonance imaging techniques

In order to understand the nature of the information provided by the different imaging techniques that are used to study patients with MS, it is useful to consider the physical basis of the signal and of the contrast in the images that they provide. The conventional MRI techniques that are used produce images that reflect the physicochemical state of protons present in the water of the tissue that is being imaged. Contrast in such images originates primarily from differences in the relaxation times, T_1 (i.e. the time constant for the recovery of magnetization in the direction of the magnetic field) and T_2 (i.e. the time constant for the decay of magnetization in the plane perpendicular to the magnetic field). For a review of MRI theory and applications see Gadian (1996).

These conventional MRI techniques include (1) T_2-weighted imaging, (2) intermediate-weighted imaging, (3) fluid-attenuated inversion-recovery imaging, (4) standard T_1-weighted imaging, and (5) gadolinium-enhanced T_1-weighted imaging—each of which is described below. Fig. 16.1 presents examples of images obtained using such techniques in patients with MS.

T_2-weighted imaging

MR images are T_2 weighted by allowing more time for signal decay to occur due to T_2 relaxation during a relatively long echo time (TE). Signals from water protons located in tissues associated with longer T_2 values decay less during a long TE than do the signals from water protons located in tissues associated with shorter T_2 values; as a result, such 'long T_2' tissues appear hyperintense on T_2-weighted images relative to tissues with shorter T_2 values.

T_2 is exquisitely sensitive to soft tissue pathology; importantly, however, it is not specific for any particular type of pathology. Thus, T_2 prolongation is associated with the many aspects of inflammation (e.g. edema, infiltration of inflammatory cells, demyelination, and tissue injury), as well as with gliosis in the white matter of the brain. For these reasons, MS lesions are hyperintense on T_2-weighted scans both in the early stages of the disease (i.e. when inflammation is most prominent) as well as in the later stages of the disease (i.e. when gliosis is more prominent).

T_2-weighted imaging of multiple sclerosis

Consistent with well-known pathological observations, the T_2-weighted MR appearance of MS is primarily one of multiple, hyperintense white-matter lesions with periventricular predominance (Li *et al.*, 2000). (See Narayanan *et al.* (1997) for an example of the probabilistic mapping of MS lesions.) Because of the exquisite sensitivity of T_2 to subtle changes in regional water content, T_2-weighted hyperintensities can identify regions of brain tissue that appear normal on gross pathology but that, nonetheless, are associated with very subtle infiltration of inflammatory cells (De Groot *et al.*, 2001).

Evolution of T_2-weighted hyperintense lesions

New lesions that are seen on T_2-weighted imaging (or on proton-density-weighted imaging—see below) have a characteristic evolution (Willoughby

et al., 1989). They reach a maximum size in approximately 4 weeks, decrease in size over the next 6 to 8 weeks, and, typically, leave a residual T_2-weighted abnormality (Li *et al.*, 2000) that is a permanent record of tissue injury (Barkhof and van Walderveen, 1999). For this reason, the total lesion volume that can be measured on T_2-weighted scans is often used as a surrogate measure of disease burden in MS. Furthermore, changes across time in the number and volume of lesions that are visible on T_2-weighted imaging can be used as indicators of disease activity and of response to treatment.

Clinical significance of T_2-weighted hyperintense lesions

Although the relationship between T_2-weighted imaging abnormalities and abnormal findings on histological examination is strong (e.g. Li *et al.*, 2000; De Groot *et al.*, 2001), the correlation between total cerebral T_2-weighted lesion load and clinical disability at any given time is only modest (e.g. Barkhof, 1999; Schreiber *et al.*, 2001). Nevertheless, the predictive value of T_2-weighted lesions for the future development of clinically definite MS is strong, particularly over the long term. For example, Brex *et al.* (2002) recently published the latest results of an ongoing, longitudinal study that had, at that point, followed a group of 71 patients for 14 years from the time of their initial episode of presumed central nervous system (CNS) demyelination. They found that clinically definite MS eventually developed in 44 of the 50 patients with T_2-weighted lesions at presentation but in only four of 21 patients that had presented with normal MRI. Furthermore, the number and the volume of T_2-weighted lesions at baseline, as well as the change in lesion volume over the first 5 years, correlated significantly with the patients' degree of long-term disability as measured by the EDSS (i.e. Kurtzke's Expanded Disability Status Scale (Kurtzke, 1983)). It should be noted, however, that the latter correlations were of only moderate strength—suggesting that, on their own, T_2-weighted lesion data cannot be used to make strong predictions about an individual patient's clinical prognosis.

The modest correlation seen between T_2-weighted lesion load and concurrent clinical disability may be explained by several factors: (1) the lack of pathological specificity of T_2-weighted abnormalities; (2) the fact that neurological disability is not easy to quantify and that the instruments used to do so (primarily the EDSS) are limited in their scope (e.g. the EDSS is based primarily on ambulatory ability); (3) the fact that lesions in different CNS locations would be expected to correlate differently with disabilities in different spheres of CNS function (e.g. cerebral lesion load would be expected to dissociate from the sensorimotor dysfunction that results from spinal cord lesions—a dissociation that increases as the MS disease process progresses (Narayanan *et al.*, 2000)); and (4) the fact that lesions may not be the only pathology responsible for disability, particularly late in the disease when a neurodegenerative process may develop (Bjartmar and Trapp, 2001). The correlation between T_2-weighted lesion volume and disability is also weakened by the potential of the brain to functionally adapt to injury (Reddy *et al.*, 2000*a,b*) and the fact that focal lesions have diffuse consequences (Narayanan *et al.*, 1997; Fu *et al.*, 1998). Thus, it may not be surprising that it has been difficult to demonstrate a strong, direct effect of the localization of cerebral T_2-weighted lesions on specific EDSS-measured functional impairments (Riahi *et al.*, 1998).

T_2-weighted hypointensity

In addition to the T_2-weighted white-matter hyperintensities that we have dealt with thus far, gray-matter hypointensities on T_2-weighted imaging of patients with MS (which is thought to reflect pathologic iron deposition and brain degeneration) have also been described (e.g. Drayer *et al.*, 1987) and related to clinical status (Bakshi *et al.*, 2000, 2001*c*, 2002).

Proton-density-weighted imaging

Because both lesions and cerebrospinal fluid (CSF) are hyperintense on T_2-weighted images, the discrimination of periventricular lesions can be difficult. One way of increasing this discrimination is to acquire intermediately weighted images that are often referred to as being 'proton-density (PD) weighted' (Butman and Frank, 2000). In fact, such images do not actually reflect the density of protons: rather, they have intermediate T_1 (see below) and T_2 weighting, such that CSF appears dark and lesions appear bright.

Fluid-attenuated inversion-recovery imaging

Another means of increasing contrast between CSF and lesions is through the use of fluid-attenuated inversion-recovery (FLAIR) imaging (Butman and Frank, 2000). This approach involves the use of an inversion pulse to suppress the signal arising from bulk water in the CSF (Gawne-Cain et al., 1997). FLAIR images provide both (1) better discrimination between ventricular CSF and the periventricular T_2-weighted-hyperintensities that are associated with MS lesions and (2) increased contrast for lesions—particularly for those that are cortical or juxtacortical (e.g. Bakshi et al., 2001a).

T_1-weighted imaging

T_1-weighted images are produced by shortening the TR (i.e. the amount of time between successive repetitions of water-proton excitation) and, thereby, allowing less time for water to regain its equilibrium magnetization. Water protons in tissues with a relatively short T_1 recover more quickly and produce more signal at relatively-short TR than do those in tissues with a longer T_1.

T_1-weighted imaging of multiple sclerosis

Protons in bulk water (e.g. in CSF, or in tissue that is associated with either extracellular edema or with a loss of structural integrity) have a long T_1 and, thus, appear hypointense on T_1-weighted sequences. T_1-weighted images are less sensitive to changes in either water content or to gliosis than are T_2-weighted images. Nevertheless, acute, inflammatory lesions can be associated with so much edema that they can show substantial T_1-weighted hypointensity. On the other hand, chronic T_1-weighted hypointensities are more specific than T_2-weighted hyperintensities for tissue destruction (van Walderveen et al., 1998; van Waesberghe et al., 1999; Barkhof et al., 2000).

The term 'black hole' has been used to describe hypointense lesions on T_1-weighted images (Truyen et al., 1996). However, given the fact that this term is typically used to imply an association with irreversible tissue destruction, the use of the term 'black hole' is probably best reserved for lesions that are chronically hypointense on T_1-weighted imaging. Importantly, only about 30% of new T_2-weighted lesions will evolve into chronic black holes (van Walderveen et al., 1999b).

Given the increased pathological specificity associated with T_1-weighted hypointensity, it is not surprising that lesions that show this feature on T_1-weighted imaging are more strongly correlated to disability in MS than lesions that are T_1 isointense (e.g. Truyen et al., 1996, Barkhof, 1999; Barkhof et al., 2000).

Gadolinium-enhanced T_1-weighted imaging

As reviewed by Rovaris and Filippi (2000), signal intensity on T_1-weighted imaging can be increased with the injection of a chelated form of gadolinium (Gd), that interacts with water so as to shorten its T_1 relaxation time. Normally, Gd does not cross the blood–brain barrier (BBB). However, focal inflammation in the CNS—as occurs during an MS attack—is associated with an 'opening' of the BBB (Rubin and Staddon, 1999). This opening allows Gd to pass through in a manner that is graded depending upon (1) the extent of the associated increase in BBB permeability, (2) the dose of Gd administered, and (3) the interval between Gd injection and T_1-weighted MR acquisition (i.e. the time available for the Gd to leak across the BBB) (Tofts and Kermode, 1991; Silver et al., 1997).

Gadolinium-enhanced T_1-weighted imaging of multiple sclerosis

The acute inflammatory process is transient. As a result, Gd only causes MS lesions to enhance for 2–6 weeks after they become detectable by conventional MRI (Silver et al., 1997; Tortorella et al., 1999). Thus, a useful role for Gd-enhanced T_1-weighted imaging is to help distinguish recently appearing, inflammatory lesions from ones that are more chronic (and no longer associated with sufficient inflammation to result in Gd enhancement). Indeed, MRI assessment of disease activity in MS is often based upon the number of Gd-enhancing lesions that are seen within a T_1-weighted scan.

Gd-based insights into disease activity

Unexpectedly, about 50% of patients with MS will have at least one Gd-enhancing lesion at any given time. In what has been called the 'clinico-radiological paradox', a large proportion of these lesions are not associated with clinical manifestations; indeed, on average, Gd-enhancing lesions occur about 10 times more frequently than clinical relapses (McFarland et al., 1992; Miller et al., 1993, 1998). Despite the striking difference between the frequency of new Gd-enhancing lesions and the frequency of clinical exacerbations, there is still, however, a strong relationship between these measures (Kappos et al., 1999). Furthermore, the number of enhancing lesions on a single scan is predictive of subsequent relapse rate and it is correlated with both subsequent enhancing-lesion activity and change in T_2-weighted lesion load (Molyneux et al., 1998).

Although the presence of one or more Gd-enhancing brain lesions is predictive of conversion to clinically definite MS (Brex et al., 1999), Gd enhancement is not a strong predictor of the development of cumulative impairment or EDSS-measured disability (Kappos et al., 1999). These findings are consistent with the hypothesis that different pathogenetic mechanisms may be responsible for the occurrence of relapses and the development of long-term disability.

Non-conventional magnetic resonance imaging techniques

The conventional MRI techniques discussed above have allowed us to image MS lesions with great sensitivity, but these techniques are not capable of fully characterizing and quantifying the extent of tissue damage in patients with MS. A number of recently developed MR techniques are better suited for such a role. These techniques include: MTI, DWI, ^{1}H-MRS, and other more experimental techniques, such as cellular imaging by MRI and by PET. Each of these are, in turn, described below.

Magnetization-transfer imaging

Magnetization transfer

Protons associated with molecules that are large and less mobile than water (e.g. the macromolecules that are 'bound' within cell membranes) have a very short T_2 and are not visible on conventional MRI; this is because their signals decay completely before conventional MRI data are acquired. The effect of these protons can, however, be observed indirectly by exploiting the phenomenon of magnetization transfer (van Buchem and Tofts, 2000). In MTI, radiofrequency pulses are applied to selectively saturate the magnetization of these bound protons. This saturation is then exchanged naturally with the relatively mobile protons of the 'free' bulk water that is found in the CSF as well as in the intracellular and the extracellular spaces (i.e. those protons that are normally observed by MRI). This reduction in the magnetization of the MRI-observable, free-water pool results in a reduction of the signal intensity from these observable protons to a degree that depends upon the nature and density of the macromolecules at a given location and their interaction with bulk water. Importantly, in CNS white matter, magnetization transfer is dominated by the large surface area and macromolecular content of myelin (Fralix et al., 1991; Dousset et al., 1995).

An important advantage of MTI is that it can be easily quantified by calculating the magnetization-transfer ratio (MTr), which is the relative MRI signal intensity measured in the absence of a saturating pulse compared with the intensity that is measured in the presence of a saturating pulse (see Fig. 16.2). A low MTr indicates less exchange of magnetization between tissue macromolecules and the surrounding water molecules.

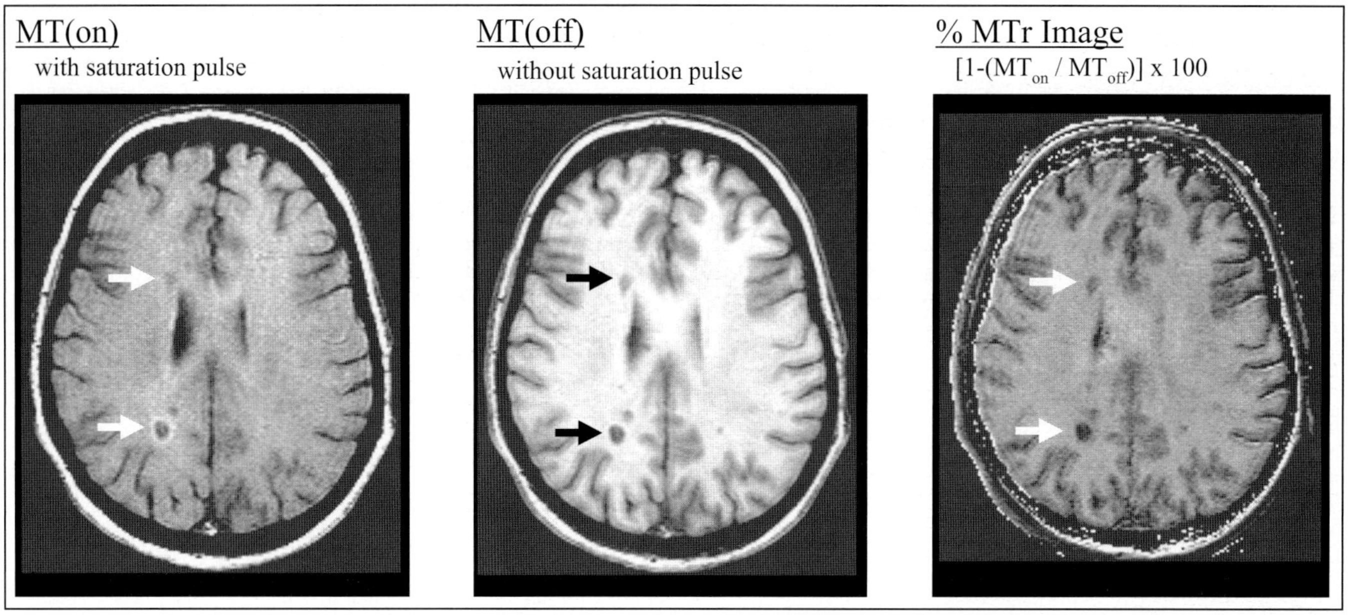

Fig. 16.2 Examples of T_1-weighted images obtained during a magnetization transfer (MT) study of a patient with multiple sclerosis. Images are obtained both with (MT(on)) and without (MT(off)) the presence of a saturation pulse, and MT ratios are calculated as shown. Note that MTr values are more reduced in lesions that are more hypointense on the standard T1-weighted image (e.g. compare top and bottom lesions). (Images are courtesy of Dr G. B. Pike.)

Magnetization-transfer imaging of multiple sclerosis

MTr values are typically reduced in MS lesions in a manner that is consistent with the degree of T_1-weighted hypointensity (Hiehle *et al.*, 1994; Loevner *et al.*, 1995*b*; van Waesberghe *et al.*, 1999), which is related to tissue destruction. Thus, lesions that are larger and more destructive generally have lower MTr values than lesions that are smaller and less destructive. Furthermore, greater reductions in MTr values are seen in lesions that are more inflammatory (Filippi *et al.*, 1998*b*).

In addition to the MTr changes observed in MS lesions, numerous studies have also reported decreased MTr in the NAWM of MS patients compared with the white matter of healthy normal controls (Hiehle *et al.*, 1994; Filippi *et al.*, 1995; Loevner *et al.*, 1995*a*; Rocca *et al.*, 1999; Pike *et al.*, 2000). Greater decreases in MTr are found in the lesions and NAWM of patients with secondary progressive (SP) MS than in patients with relapsing–remitting (RR) MS (Tortorella *et al.*, 2000; Rovaris *et al.*, 2000*a*; Filippi *et al.*, 2000*b*), and these decreases are related to both increasing EDSS-measured disability (e.g. Barkhof, 1999; Dehmeshki *et al.*, 2001) and increasing cognitive impairment (Rovaris *et al.*, 2000*b*).

MTI of lesion evolution

Longitudinal MTI studies have shown that, even before the detection of lesions is possible on proton-density- or T_2-weighted images, MTr values have begun to decline in the NAWM (Filippi *et al.*, 1998*a*; Goodkin *et al.*, 1998; Pike *et al.*, 2000). Then, as lesions begin to demonstrate Gd enhancement on T_1-weighted imaging, there is an explosive decrease in the lesional MTr values due to a combination of inflammatory edema and demyelination. This may be followed by either a stabilization of lesional MTr values at these lower levels or a recovery of lesional MTr values several weeks after the initial decrease (van Waesberghe *et al.*, 1998; Dousset *et al.*, 1998; Filippi, 1999; Richert *et al.*, 2001). Thus, MTr provides a potentially powerful tool for exploring the evolution of pathology in MS.

Diffusion-weighted imaging

As reviewed by Cercignani and Horsfield (2001), DWI allows for the *in vivo* measurement of the Brownian-motion-induced diffusion of water in the CNS. Because both the axolemma and the myelin sheath restrict water diffusion in nerve fibers (Beaulieu and Allen, 1994), pathological processes

(such as those at work in MS) that modify the integrity of such tissues can result in a loss of restricting barriers and, thereby, increase the so-called 'apparent diffusion coefficient' (ADC) of water.

The ADC is a measure of the random displacement of water molecules in a particular direction. Because of the restricting entities that are found in biological tissues, ADC values in the CNS are lower than the diffusion coefficient of pure water (hence the term 'apparent' diffusion coefficient of water). A measure of diffusion that is independent of the orientation of structures is provided by the mean diffusivity index, $\bar{D}$. Also referred to as the directionally averaged ADC (or ADC_{avg}) or the trace, $\bar{D}$ is the average of the ADCs measured in three orthogonal directions. (For a review of DWI theory and applications see, for example, Schaefer *et al.* (2000).)

As reviewed by Filippi and Inglese (2001), the pathology associated with MS modifies the water self-diffusion characteristics in the CNS by altering the geometry and/or the permeability of structural barriers that are found therein. The application of DWI techniques to the study of MS is appealing in that they can provide a quantitative estimate of the degree of fiber disruption and, thus, potentially provide information on the mechanisms that lead to irreversible disability in this disease.

Diffusion-weighted imaging of multiple sclerosis

As illustrated in Fig. 16.3, DWI studies have consistently shown that the ADC of water is higher in MS lesions than in NAWM; moreover, the ADC is higher in acute lesions than in chronic lesions (Larsson *et al.*, 1992; Christiansen *et al.*, 1993; Tievsky *et al.*, 1999). Furthermore, mean $\bar{D}$ values are increased in the NAWM of MS patients compared with those observed in the white matter of healthy normal controls—a finding that hold true in the brain (e.g. Filippi *et al.*, 2000*a*; Cercignani *et al.*, 1999; Werring *et al.*, 2001), the spinal cord (e.g. Clark *et al.*, 2000), and the NAGM (Cercignani *et al.*, 2001*a*).

$\bar{D}$ values have been shown to correlate with individual MS patients' EDSS scores (Castriota Scanderbeg *et al.*, 2000; Cercignani *et al.*, 2001*b*; Tourbah *et al.*, 2001; Wilson *et al.*, 2001) and disease duration (Castriota Scanderbeg *et al.*, 2000; Tourbah *et al.*, 2001; Wilson *et al.*, 2001). Furthermore, $\bar{D}$ values are higher in patients with SP MS than those with RR MS (Nusbaum *et al.*, 2000; Castriota Scanderbeg *et al.*, 2000), and increases in lesional $\bar{D}$ values correlate with hypointensity on T_1-weighted images (Castriota Scanderbeg *et al.*, 2000).

PD-Weighted Image

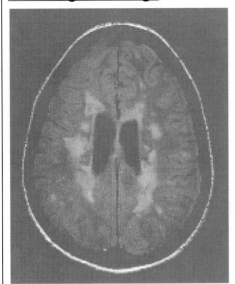

Mean Diffusivity Image

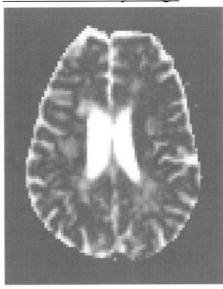

Fig. 16.3 Examples of cross-sectional slices through the lateral ventricles of a patient with multiple sclerosis as seen on proton-density-weighted (PD) and diffusion-weighted imaging. Note the lesions that are seen as hyperintensities on PD-weighted imaging and as increased mean diffusivity ($\bar{D}$) values on diffusion-weighted imaging. (Images are courtesy of J. S. W. Campbell.)

Interestingly, individual patients' $\bar{D}$ values are not significantly related to their MTr values (Cercignani *et al.*, 2000) and are only moderately related to decreases in their ¹H-MRS-measured NA/Cr values (Hagberg *et al.*, 2001) (the relevance of which is explained in the section on ¹H-MRS below). These findings suggest that these two imaging techniques (i.e. MTI and ¹H-MRS) provide information about different aspects of brain pathology in MS than does DWI.

DWI of lesion evolution

Serial DWI studies have also been used in order to investigate the changes in NAWM that precede the development of acute MS lesions. Regions of NAWM that would subsequently become Gd-enhancing lesions were found to have a significant increase in their mean $\bar{D}$ values starting 6 weeks prior to the appearance of enhancement (Rocca *et al.*, 2000). Werring *et al.* (2000) obtained monthly DWI scans over a year in MS patients and observed a steady and moderate increase in mean NAWM $\bar{D}$ values that was followed by a rapid and marked increase at the time of Gd enhancement and a slow decay after the end of enhancement. These two studies suggest that new focal lesions that are associated with an eventual breakdown of the BBB are preceded by subtle, progressive alterations in tissue integrity that are below the resolution of conventional MRI. Interestingly, Werring *et al.* (2000) also found that there was a mild increase in the mean $\bar{D}$ values of NAWM regions that were contralateral and homologous to the NAWM regions that evolved into Gd-enhancing lesions (but that themselves did not become lesional)— a finding that supports the concept that structural damage in lesions can cause disturbances in connected areas of NAWM (De Stefano *et al.*, 1999).

Proton magnetic resonance spectroscopy

Although the water-based imaging methods described above are all sensitive to MS-related pathology, none of them can provide any pathological specificity regarding injury to a particular cell type. Pathological specificity for injury to neurons and neuronal processes (i.e. axons and dendrites) can, however, be provided by ¹H-MRS quantification of the neuronal marker compound, *N*-acetylaspartate (Arnold *et al.*, 2000). This approach is fundamentally different from the water-proton-based MRI techniques that we have discussed thus far in that ¹H-MRS records signals that arise from protons in metabolites that are present in brain tissue at concentrations approximately one thousand times lower than that of tissue water (Ross and Bluml, 2001). Whereas the signal-to-noise ratio and image resolution that is possible with these metabolite-based images is much lower than that for water-based images, the resulting images can provide chemicopathological specificity that is not possible with conventional MR images. The various approaches to *in vivo* ¹H-MRS include: (1) single-voxel ¹H-MRS studies (in which proton spectra are acquired from a single volume) and (2) ¹H-MRS imaging (¹H-MRSI) studies (in which proton spectra are obtained from multiple volume elements (i.e. voxels) at the same time).

¹H-MRS metabolites of interest

As shown in Fig. 16.4, the water-suppressed, localized ¹H-MRS spectrum of the normal human brain that is recorded at relatively long echo times (usually 136–272 ms) reveals three major resonance peaks (the locations of which are expressed as the difference in parts per million (ppm) between the resonance frequency of the compound of interest and that of a standard compound (i.e. tetramethylsilane)). These peaks are commonly ascribed to the following metabolites:

(1) choline (Cho), which consists mostly of choline-containing phospholipids that participate in membrane synthesis and degradation;

(2) creatine and phosphocreatine (Cr), which are intermediates of energy metabolism; and

(3) *N*-acetyl groups (NA), which, in the CNS, arise primarily from the neuronally localized compound *N*-acetylaspartate (NAA).

A fourth peak, usually arising from either the methyl resonance of lactate (LA) or lipids (which both resonate at 1.3 ppm), is normally only barely visible above the baseline noise but can be detected in the presence of acute inflammatory infiltration (which is associated with increased presence of LA) and myelin breakdown (which is associated with increased presence of lipids). Lipids are best seen in spectra acquired at shorter echo times (e.g. 30 ms).

The resonance intensity that is ascribed to NAA is, arguably, the most important ¹H-MRS signal in the characterization of MS pathology because NAA is localized exclusively within neurons and neuronal processes such as axons and dendrites (Moffett *et al.*, 1991; Simmons *et al.*, 1991). The specificity of NAA as an axon-specific marker *in vivo* has been confirmed in a recent biochemical and immunohistochemical study of rat optic nerve transection (Bjartmar *et al.*, 2002).

NA/Cr

The ratios of within-voxel ¹H-MRSI-measured NA to CR values have been used to quantify neuronal and axonal integrity *in vivo* in the brains of

Normal Control

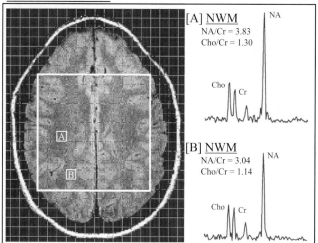

Patient with MS

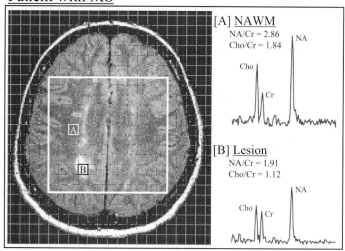

Fig. 16.4 Examples of proton-density-weighted magnetic resonance images through the centrum semiovale and the results of proton magnetic resonance spectroscopic imaging (^{1}H-MRSI) in a normal control subject (left) and in a patient with multiple sclerosis (MS) (right). The superimposed grid in each image represents individual ^{1}H-MRSI voxels, and the large, thick, white box represents the entire ^{1}H-MRSI volume of interest for that individual. The smaller, labeled boxes represent voxels of normal-appearing white matter (NAWM) and lesional brain tissue in the patient and normal white matter (NWM) in the normal control subject. The ^{1}H-MRSI spectra from within each of these voxels is shown to the right of each image. The areas under the NA and Cho peaks (normalized to Cr) are shown above each spectrum. The spectra have been scaled so that the Cr peak in each of them has the same height. Note the decrease in NA/Cr values from the patient's NAWM voxel relative to the NWM voxels in the control subject, the even greater decrease in lesional NA/Cr, and the increased Cho/Cr in the patient's NAWM voxel, which may be predictive of the imminent appearance of a lesion in that location.

patients with MS for over a decade now (e.g. Arnold *et al.*, 1990). MRS studies have shown that NA/Cr values are low in lesions and, to a lesser extent, are also low in NAWM (Matthews *et al.*, 1991; De Stefano *et al.*, 1995; Fu *et al.*, 1998). Furthermore, patients with SP MS are more affected than those with RR MS (Fu *et al.*, 1998; De Stefano *et al.*, 2001). Interestingly, this latter finding seems to be related more to NA/Cr differences in the NAWM than in lesions (Fu *et al.*, 1998). Just as with MTI and DWI, ^{1}H-MRSI-measured values of NA/Cr within the cortical NAGM of patients with MS have also been shown to be decreased relative to those in the cortical gray matter of healthy normal controls (Kapeller *et al.*, 2001; Sharma *et al.*, 2001).

Decreases in MS patients' periventricular-NA/Cr values are strongly related to both their disease duration and their EDSS scores (De Stefano *et al.*, 2001). Importantly, the correlation between patients' EDSS scores and their periventricular NA/Cr values is as strong, or stronger, than that of any other MRI measure (e.g., Mainero *et al.*, 2001)—a relationship that becomes even stronger when EDSS scores are correlated with estimates of NA/Cr in pure periventricular NAWM (Fu *et al.*, 1998; Caramanos *et al.*, 2002). In addition to correlating with patients' EDSS scores (which are greatly influenced by a patients' ambulatory status), periventricular NA/Cr values in MS patients have also been shown to be strongly related to their cognitive abilities (Pan *et al.*, 2001).

Other metabolites

^{1}H-MRS-observed Cho and lipid peaks are thought to provide important information regarding myelin breakdown in the MS disease process (Arnold *et al.*, 1992; Narayana *et al.*, 1998; Tartaglia *et al.*, 2002) and myoinositol has been proposed as a marker of glial cells (Kapeller *et al.*, 2001)

Temporal evolution of lesions on ^{1}H-MRS

As with MTI and DWI, the earliest abnormalities that are visible on ^{1}H-MRS occur months before the appearance of Gd-enhanced or T_2-weighted lesions. For example, regions of NAWM that will go on to become lesions have been shown to be associated with locally increased levels of both Cho (Tartaglia *et al.*, 2002) and of lipids (Narayana *et al.*, 1998)—both of which are markers of abnormality in cell membranes. As newly developing lesions

become detectable on conventional MRI, they are associated with focal inflammation, demyelination, and axonal injury—pathological processes that result in (1) decreases to NA/Cr values (Arnold *et al.*, 1992; Mader *et al.*, 2000, 2001; Simone *et al.*, 2001), (2) further increases to Cho/Cr values (Arnold *et al.*, 1992; Mader *et al.*, 2000, 2001; Simone *et al.*, 2001), and (3) acutely increased LA/Cr values (Arnold *et al.*, 1992)

Importantly, the NA-related decreases may persist chronically—particularly in the core of chronic lesions (Arnold *et al.*, 1992). On the other hand, the presence of LA is more common in lesions that are Gd enhancing (Simone *et al.*, 2001) and seems to resolve within weeks (Arnold *et al.*, 1992). Increases in Cho/Cr are pronounced in Gd-enhancing lesions (Simone *et al.*, 2001; Mader *et al.*, 2001) and may remain elevated for years (Arnold *et al.*, 1992), but eventually return to normal (Arnold *et al.*, 1992; van Walderveen *et al.*, 1999a).

Spatial distribution of ^{1}H-MRSI pathology

Changes in ^{1}H-MRSI metabolites are greatest in the core of lesions and decrease with increasing distance from their center (Arnold *et al.*, 1992). Importantly, they do not end at the edge of the T_2-weighted abnormality but extend into the surrounding NAWM (Arnold *et al.*, 1992). For example, in the hyperacute phase of the lesion (i.e. when it is still expanding), both the decrease in NA/Cr and the increase in Cho/Cr can be found in the NAWM around the lesion well beyond the expanding T_2-weighted abnormality. It is still not clear if the NAWM abnormalities in patients with MS represent the sum of the remote effects of focal, lesional pathology or an independent process that is more diffuse.

MR-based assessment of regional and global brain atrophy

Atrophy of the brain or spinal cord at post-mortem examination is one of the pathological hallmarks of irreversible CNS damage. As reviewed by Simon (2000), with the advent of MRI, it is now possible to assess CNS atrophy *in vivo* using a variety of measures that include, for example, ventricu-

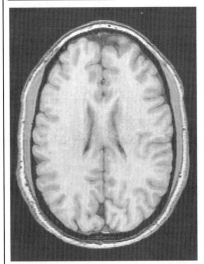
Normal Control

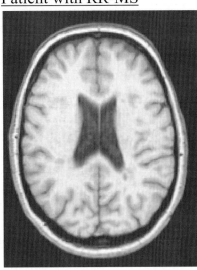
Patient with RR-MS

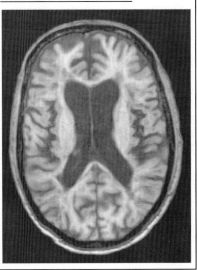
Patient with SP-MS

Fig. 16.5 Examples of cross-sectional slices through the lateral ventricles of a normal control subject, a patient with relapsing–remitting multiple sclerosis (RR-MS), and a patient with secondary progressive multiple sclerosis (SP-MS). as seen on *T*2-weighted imaging. Note the high degree of atrophy seen even in the early stage of the disease (as evidenced visually by the ventricular enlargement in the RR-MS patient as compared with the control subject) and the even greater atrophy that is seen in the secondary progressive stage of the disease (as evidenced visually by the sulcal enlargement, the decreased volume of the white- and gray-matter, and the further-increased ventricular enlargement in the SP-MS patient).

lar enlargement, gray- and white-matter volumes, and the use of global measures such as the brain parenchymal fraction (BPF, i.e. the ratio of brain parenchymal volume to the total volume within the surface contour of the brain) (Rudick *et al.*, 1999) or BICCR (i.e. the ratio of brain parenchymal volume within the surface contour of the inner table of the skull) (Collins *et al.*, 2000; Smith *et al.*, 2001, 2002).

Atrophy in multiple sclerosis

CNS atrophy in patients with MS has been documented since the original autopsy examinations of such individuals—with atrophy having been shown to reflect injury and loss of both neurons and their processes and oligodendrocytes and the myelin that they produce, as well as changes in the supporting matrix that result from the contraction of glial tissue (Simon, 2000). Until recently, such atrophy has generally been thought of as an event occurring late in the disease; this view has changed, however, with the development of neuroimaging techniques capable of demonstrating atrophy in the majority of patients with MS (see Fig. 16.5)—even at very early stages of the disease (Rudick *et al.*, 1999; Brex *et al.*, 2000; Simon, 2001).

Rate of atrophy

Brain atrophy develops at a remarkably high rate in patients with MS (Simon, 2000). For instance, Simon *et al.* (1999) studied 85 RR MS patients with mild-to-moderate disability over the course of 2 years and found that the volume of the lateral ventricles increased at a rate of 5.5% per year and the area of the corpus callosum decreased at a rate of 4.9% per year. Importantly, the course of cerebral atrophy in these patients was related to prior inflammatory disease activity as indicated by the presence of Gd-enhancing T_1-weighted lesions at baseline. Analysis of a subset of these patients ($n = 72$) found a yearly decrease of 0.61% in their BPF, which translates to a yearly loss of approximately 8 cm³ per year (Rudick *et al.*, 1999). Fox *et al.* (2000) showed that the yearly rate of cerebral atrophy in their MS group (0.8% per year) was over twice that of controls (0.3%) and the yearly rate of ventricular enlargement in patients was almost five times greater than in the controls (1.6 versus 0.3 cm³ per year).

There is some preliminary evidence to suggest that the rate of atrophy in patients with RR MS differs from that in patients with SP MS in a region-

specific manner (Bakshi *et al.*, 2001*b*; Chen *et al.*, 2001). For example, SP MS patients seem to have a significantly faster rate of atrophy around the ventricles than patients with RR MS—suggesting a greater relative volume change along the long projection tracts (Chen *et al.*, 2001). On the other hand, the rate of spinal cord atrophy has been reported to be faster in patients with RR MS (Stevenson *et al.*, 1998). These findings suggest that CNS atrophy may not be a uniform process and that different regions may have distinct responses to disease progression.

Potential techniques with more immunological specificity

Cellular imaging

Methods for imaging cell-trafficking patterns in health and disease are useful in the study and development of novel cellular therapies, but have been hampered by toxicity of cell labels and limitations of the detectability of small numbers of cells. Nevertheless, a few imaging techniques have been used to monitor the temporal spatial migration of T cells and macrophages across the BBB and into the parenchyma of the brain and spinal cord in experimental allergic encephalomyelitis (EAE) models of MS.

Nuclear medicine techniques

Nuclear medicine techniques have used ^{111}In-oxine to label peripheral blood mononuclear cells following apheresis and to monitor the trafficking of lymphocytes into tumors and autoimmune diseases (Pozzilli *et al.*, 1983; Griffith *et al.*, 1989; Read *et al.*, 1990). For example, Yeager *et al.* (2000) have performed biodistribution studies with ^{111}In radiolabeled T cells in an EAE rat model and have demonstrated a marked increase in lymphocyte localization in cervical and lumbar spinal cord tissue samples as compared with control animals up to 111 hr following the infusion of labeled T cells. Moreover, these authors observed a significant increase in radiolabeled T cells detected in the cerebellum and cerebral cortex compared with control animals that did not receive the labeled cells.

This approach has not yet been used in the evaluation or the monitoring of T-cell migration in MS patients, in part due to the inherent limitations of this technique: for example, the relatively short half-life of the radio-isotope, the inherent low resolution of nuclear medicine imaging, and the potential damage to cellular DNA from ionizing radiation (Griffith *et al.*, 1989; Read *et al.*, 1990).

Optical imaging techniques

Certain optical imaging techniques show some potential promise. For example, Costa *et al.* (2001) transfected myelin basic protein-specific CD4+ T cells with green fluorescent protein (GFP) and luciferase and, using low-light imaging cameras, were able to demonstrate the bioluminescent lymphocytes trafficking into the CNS of EAE mice. GFP–luciferase labeled T cells were detected in the lower spinal cord approximately 8 days following disease induction and prior to the development of clinical disease. In EAE mice with acute disease, optical imaging was able to identify lesions presumed to be in the brainstem 3 days after introducing the GFP–luciferase labeled T cells. In addition, the authors noted that labeled cells that had trafficked into the CNS persisted for up to 50 days. It should be noted, however, that whereas optical imaging techniques are highly sensitive research technique for detecting low numbers of transfected cells, the technique suffers from relatively poor spatial resolution and would be difficult to translate into clinical use.

Cellular MRI techniques

At present there are no high-resolution clinical imaging techniques to monitor the temporal and spatial migration of unlabeled cells into tissues. Furthermore, whereas Gd-enhanced conventional MRI can determine BBB disruption due to inflammation, it cannot classify the cellular environment within diseased CNS tissue. On the other hand, cellular MRI is a relatively new technique that is based on the labeling of cells *ex vivo* with gadolinium chelates or modified dextran-coated superparamagnetic iron oxide (SPIO) nanoparticles; importantly, these two MR contrast agents can provide researchers with the ability to monitor the migration of these cells by MR imaging (Bulte *et al.*, 1999, 2001; Dodd *et al.*, 2001; Lewin *et al.*, 2000; Josephson *et al.*, 1999).

Use of superparamagnetic iron oxide nanoparticles

SPIO and ultrasmall SPIO (USPIO) nanoparticles are MR contrast agents that have been approved by the Food and Drug Administration for use in imaging hepatic reticuloendothelial cells and are in phase III clinical trials for their use as blood pooling agents during lymphography (Harisinghani *et al.*, 1999; Semelka and Helmberger, 2001; Mack *et al.*, 2002). In their native, unmodified form (Bulte *et al.*, 1999; Josephson *et al.*, 1999; Dodd *et al.*, 1999, 2001; Lewin *et al.*, 2000) these contrast agents cannot be used *in vitro* to efficiently label cells (Bulte *et al.*, 1996; Sipe *et al.*, 1999); importantly, by conjugating antigen-specific internalizing monoclonal antibodies to the dextran coat, cells can be magnetically labeled during their normal expansion in culture (Bulte *et al.*, 1999). Other approaches have involved the synthesis and modification of USPIO particles (e.g. MION-46L) by cross-linking the dextran and conjugating with short HIV-transactivator transcription proteins (e.g. MION-Tat or CLIO-Tat), thereby facilitating their incorporation into the cells (Josephson *et al.*, 1999; Lewin *et al.*, 2000; Dodd *et al.*, 2001;).

Ex vivo MRI performed within 3 days following transplantation with CLIO-Tat labeled cells has demonstrated *in vivo* migration in tissue (Lewin *et al.*, 2000). For example, Dodd *et al.* (2001) have shown that T cells labeled with CLIO-Tat exhibited normal activation and activation-induced cell death responses when stimulated with anti-CD3 and IL-2. Furthermore, Moore and colleagues (Moore *et al.*, 2002) used CLIO-Tat to label cytotoxic lymphocytes sensitized to pancreatic beta cells in an autoimmune adoptive transfer murine model of type 1 diabetes mellitus. The authors were able to demonstrate the homing of the sensitized lymphocytes to the pancreas, the induction of disease in non-obese diabetic/severe combined immunodeficient (SCID) mice, and the presence of these labeled cells on both fluorescent microscopy and *ex vivo* high-resolution MR microscopy. These results suggest that it may be possible to track pathogenic immune cells in diabetes mellitus and to further the understanding of the relation-ship between autoimmune phenomena and disease onset. One potential limitation of CLIO-Tat, however, is that the Tat protein has an affinity for the nucleus; thus, it is possible that during biodegradation of the CLIO-Tat particle, reactive iron species may be temporarily released into the nucleus and damage the DNA.

Use of magnetodendrimers

By labeling differentiated stem cells with dendrimer-coated SPIO (i.e. magnetodendrimers), Bulte and colleagues (Bulte *et al.*, 2001, 2002) labeled rat oligodendroglial progenitor cells and, following transplantation into the lateral ventricles, were able to monitor the migration of these cells *in vivo* for up to 6 weeks in a dysmyelinated rodent model. This was the first *in vivo* demonstration of cellular imaging and the ability to monitor the migration of magnetically labeled cells at a clinically relevant MR field strength. Magnetodendrimers have also been used to label mouse embryonic stem cells that were implanted intraventricularly into the brains of Lewis rats with active EAE (Bulte *et al.*, 2003). On high-resolution, *ex vivo* MRI, the magnetically labeled embryonic stem cells were found to have migrated greater distances away from the implantation site and deeper into the periventricular white matter of EAE rats as compared with control animals. These preliminary results suggest that such labeled embryonic cells have the potential of migrating into EAE lesions. It should be noted, however, that one of the limitations of magnetodendrimers is that they are custom-made contrast agents that require a dedicated synthesis mechanism and, therefore, are not readily available to the scientific community for use as cellular contrast agents.

Use of transfection agents

Recently, Frank and colleagues (Frank *et al.*, 2002, 2003; Arbab *et al.*, 2003) have developed a novel technique to efficiently label mammalian cells by complexing, via electrostatic interactions, Feridex® (a negatively charged, FDA-approved SPIO nanoparticle) to transfection agents (TA), thereby facilitating the detection of the labeled cells' migration by MRI. Transfection agents are macromolecules possessing an electrostatic charge and are used for non-viral transfection of DNA into the nucleus. The major limitations in using this approach to chaperone DNA into the cells are endosomal capture of DNA-TA and inefficient release of the targeted material into the nucleus. By taking advantage of these inherent limitations of TAs, Feridex® was complexed to the polycationic transfection agent, poly-L-lysine (PLL). When the resulting Feridex®–PLL complex is co-incubated with cells, it sticks to the cell membrane and is captured in endosomes by endocytosis. Importantly, Feridex®–PLL labeling does not interfere with necessary cell-to-cell binding or cell-to-receptor interactions since the iron is incorporated into endosomes. When compared with unlabeled cells, Feridex®–PLL labeling of stem cells and lymphocytes had no adverse effects on cell viability, production of reactive oxygen species, or rates of apoptosis or iron metabolism. Importantly, labeling efficiency has been reported as >95%.

Anderson *et al.* (2004) labeled encephalitogenic T cells sensitized to proteolipid protein with Feridex®–PLL and used these cells to adoptively transfer and induce EAE in an SJL mouse model. *In vivo* MR microscopy at 7 T performed at times of clinical exacerbations and remissions detected areas of diffuse and focal hypointense lesions in the thoracic and lumbar spinal cord of the EAE mice. Correlation of MRI to histology revealed co-localization of Feridex®–PLL-labeled T-cells with Prussian blue staining in the lesions, in the perivascular spaces, and in the NAWM of the EAE animals. These results suggest a means for detecting the temporospatial migration of encephalitogenic T cells into the brain and spinal cord of EAE animals and a means for furthering our understanding of the role that sensitized cells play in the development of new lesions—lesions that may or may not contribute to clinical disease. T_2^*-weighted MRI (T_2^* differing from T_2 in that it incorporates the effects of field inhomogeneities as well as intrinsic relaxation effects) is the most sensitive imaging technique for detecting changes in magnetic fields. The presence of SPIO-labeled cells within a tissue results in changes to the local magnetic fields that results in regions of localized decreased signal intensity (*i.e.*, hypointensities) on T_2^*-weighted MRI. Thus, the labeling of cells with Feridex®–PLL in combination with high-field, T_2^*-weighted MRI may eventually aid in the development of novel clinical trials aimed at, for example, determining whether or not cells have migrated into tissue or whether or not repeated administrations of genetically engineered cells are needed to reach a specific therapeutic outcome.

Positron emission tomography

Positron emission tomography (PET) is an *in vivo* functional brain imaging technique which utilizes radiotracers that target specific biological processes (Phelps, 2000*a*). The interest in PET imaging for MS stems from the increase in molecular specificity over conventional MR methods. PET radiotracers are labeled with short-lived radioactive isotopes, which necessitates an on-site cyclotron for their production. After intravenous administration of a PET radiotracer, the time course of the radioactivity concentration in individual brain regions can be measured for a period of hours using a PET scanner. It is this kinetic information which allows for the application of biological models to derive quantitative estimates of the biological parameters of interest. Current clinical PET scanners typically have a resolution of approximately 4 mm and state-of-the-art research scanners are now approaching a resolution of 2 mm. A variety of radiotracers have been synthesized as probes for different biological applications which include the measurement of blood flow, metabolism, receptors, and gene expression. These latter two application areas offer the most promise for imaging of MS with PET.

Receptor binding

By measuring the time course of the binding of particular radioligands to specific receptor sites in tissues of interest it is possible to generate quantitative images of receptor parameters by applying appropriate biomathematical models (Gunn *et al.*, 2001). For example, [11C]PK11195 is one such PET radioligand that has been developed for the *in vivo* investigation of neuroinflammation (Vowinckel *et al.*, 1997; Banati *et al.*, 2000; Banati, 2002; Cagnin *et al.*, 2002). [11C]PK11195 binds to the peripheral benzodiazepine site and, importantly, this receptor is expressed on activated microglia, which have been shown to be an important component of ongoing inflammation in MS and are probably responsible for most of the cortical pathology (Trapp *et al.*, 1999).

Whereas this PET radioligand was first produced at the beginning of the 1990s, it has taken advances in scanner sensitivity and resolution (Spinks *et al.*, 2000), MRI–PET co-registration (Studholme *et al.*, 1997), and kinetic modeling (Gunn *et al.*, 1997) to produce a technique that is capable of reliably measuring neuroinflammation in humans (Banati *et al.*, 2000; Banati, 2002). These advances have enabled studies in MS which demonstrate focal binding of [11C]PK11195 that co-localize with acute symptomatic lesions in white matter (Vowinckel *et al.*, 1997) and visualize widespread microglial activation outside of lesions visible on MRI (Banati *et al.*, 2000; Banati, 2002)—findings that are both consistent with post-mortem pathological studies of MS patients.

Gene expression

An emerging application of PET involves the fusion of imaging and molecular biology to produce a technique capable of measuring gene expression *in vivo* (Phelps, 2000*b*; Blasberg, 2002). Such a technique can be targeted at endogenous genes or at externally administered genes (i.e. transgene expression). Imaging of endogenous genes may be achieved by targeting either the transcription of genes into mRNA or the translation of mRNA into a protein.

To date, methods have concentrated on the transcription route using radiolabeled antisense oligodeoxynucleotides coded with a complement for the single strand of mRNA (Gambhir *et al.*, 1999*a*). This technique is still in its infancy, and work still needs to be done in order to address such issues as how to achieve sufficiently high specific activity of the tracer and whether or not suitable signal and image contrast can be achieved using this approach. Nevertheless, if these obstacles can be overcome, the use of mRNA as a target will provide a general approach to measuring endogenous expression of any gene (Phelps, 2000*b*).

Imaging of transgene expression is generally accepted as being easier than imaging of gene transcription. In this approach, a gene of interest is transferred into the subject using a vehicle such as an adenovirus. The aim is, therefore, to develop an imaging technique that is capable of following the expression of this gene both spatially and temporally. The PET approach to this problem is based on the extension of traditional reporter gene/reporter probe techniques (Misteli and Spector, 1997). A PET reporter gene is linked to the therapeutic gene of interest by a common promoter which initiates transcription of the gene. When the therapeutic gene is promoted to transcription of mRNA the same happens to the PET reporter gene and the resulting proteins offer a suitable target for the PET reporter probe. To date, this process has been achieved in animals with two different protein products—one being an enzyme (Blasberg and Tjuvajev, 1999; Gambhir *et al.*, 1999*b*) and the other a receptor (MacLaren *et al.*, 1999). The quantification of these protein products using appropriate PET reporter probes allows for the measurement of gene expression. What such an approach could eventually tell us about the disease process in MS remains to be seen.

Summary and conclusions

As we have seen, our understanding of the pathology and pathophysiology of MS has been greatly advanced by information obtained using MRI. For example, the conventional MRI techniques that were described above have greatly increased the sensitivity with which lesions can be detected. In addition, they have also provided us with a great deal of *in vivo* information regarding the spatial distribution, temporal dynamics, and clinical significance of these lesions. The newer, non-conventional methods of MR acquisition and analysis have allowed us to quantify *in vivo* the microscopic and molecular pathology, the biochemical changes, and the progressive atrophy that may occur in the brain and spinal cord of patients with MS. Importantly, whereas contrast in currently used conventional and non-conventional MR techniques is generally not specific for different aspects of the immune response, novel approaches based on cellular imaging and molecular imaging hold the promise of our being able to image *in vivo* specific aspects of inflammation as they relate to the MS disease process.

References

Anderson, S.A., Shukaliak-Quandt, J., Jordan, E.K., *et al.* (2004). Magnetic resonance imaging of labeled T-cells in a mouse model of multiple sclerosis. *Ann Neurol*, **55**: 654–9.

Arbab, A.S., Bashaw, L.A., Miller, B.R., *et al.* (2003). Characterization of biophysical and metabolic properties of cells labeled with superparamagnetic iron oxide nonoparticles and transfection agent for cellular MR imaging. *Radiology*, **229**, 838–46.

Arnold, D.L., Matthews, P.M., Francis, G., and Antel, J. (1990). Proton magnetic resonance spectroscopy of human brain in vivo in the evaluation of multiple sclerosis: assessment of the load of disease. *Magn Reson Med* **14**: 154–159.

Arnold, D.L., Matthews, P.M., Francis, G.S., O'Connor, J., and Antel, J.P. (1992). Proton magnetic resonance spectroscopic imaging for metabolic characterization of demyelinating plaques. *Ann Neurol* **31**: 235–241.

Arnold, D.L., De Stefano, N., Narayanan, S., and Matthews, P.M. (2000). Proton MR spectroscopy in multiple sclerosis. *Neuroimaging Clin N Am* **10**: 789–798, ix–x.

Bakshi, R., Shaikh, Z.A., and Janardhan, V. (2000). MRI T2 shortening ('black T2') in multiple sclerosis: frequency, location, and clinical correlation. *Neuroreport* **11**: 15–21.

Bakshi, R., Ariyaratana, S., Benedict, R.H., and Jacobs, L. (2001*a*). Fluid-attenuated inversion recovery magnetic resonance imaging detects cortical and juxtacortical multiple sclerosis lesions. *Arch Neurol* **58**: 742–748.

Bakshi, R., Benedict, R.H., Bermel, R.A., and Jacobs, L. (2001*b*). Regional brain atrophy is associated with physical disability in multiple sclerosis: semiquantitative magnetic resonance imaging and relationship to clinical findings. *J Neuroimaging* **11**: 129–136.

Bakshi, R., Dmochowski, J., Shaikh, Z.A., and Jacobs, L. (2001c). Gray matter T2 hypointensity is related to plaques and atrophy in the brains of multiple sclerosis patients. *J Neurol Sci* 185: 19–26.

Bakshi, R., Benedict, R.H., Bermel, R.A., *et al.* (2002). T2 Hypointensity in the Deep Gray Matter of Patients With Multiple Sclerosis: A Quantitative Magnetic Resonance Imaging Study. *Arch Neurol* 59: 62–68.

Banati, R.B. (2002). Visualising microglial activation in vivo. *Glia* 40: 206–217.

Banati, R.B., Newcombe, J., Gunn, R.N., *et al.* (2000). The peripheral benzodiazepine binding site in the brain in multiple sclerosis: quantitative in vivo imaging of microglia as a measure of disease activity. *Brain* 123(11): 2321–2337.

Barkhof, F. (1999). MRI in multiple sclerosis: correlation iwth expanded disability status scale (EDSS). *Mult Scler* 5: 283–286.

Barkhof, F., Karas, G.B., and van Walderveen, M.A. (2000). T1 hypointensities and axonal loss. *Neuroimaging Clin N Am* 10: 739–752.

Barkhof, F. and van Walderveen, M. (1999). Characterization of tissue damage in multiple sclerosis by nuclear magnetic resonance *Phil Trans R Soc Lond B Biol Sci* 354: 1675–1686.

Beaulieu, C. and Allen, P.S. (1994). Water diffusion in the giant axon of the squid: implications for diffusion-weighted MRI of the nervous system. *Magn Reson Med* 32: 579–583.

Bjartmar, C. and Trapp, B.D. (2001). Axonal and neuronal degeneration in multiple sclerosis: mechanisms and functional consequences. *Curr Opin Neurol* 14: 271–278.

Bjartmar, C., Battistuta, J., Terada, N., Dupree, E., and Trapp, B.D. (2002). N-acetylaspartate is an axon-specific marker of mature white matter in vivo: A biochemical and immunohistochemical study on the rat optic nerve. *Ann Neurol* 51: 51–58.

Blasberg, R. (2002). Imaging gene expression and endogenous molecular processes: molecular imaging. *J Cereb Blood Flow Metab* 22: 1157–1164.

Blasberg, R.G. and Tjuvajev, J.G. (1999). Herpes simplex virus thymidine kinase as a marker/reporter gene for PET imaging of gene therapy. *Q J Nucl Med* 43: 163–169.

Brex, P.A., O'Riordan, J.I., Miszkiel, K.A., *et al.* (1999). Multisequence MRI in clinically isolated syndromes and the early developnment of MS. *Neurology* 53: 1184–1190.

Brex, P.A., Jenkins, R., Fox, N.C., *et al.* (2000). Detection of ventricular enlargement in patients at the earliest clinical stage of MS. *Neurology* 54: 1689–1691.

Brex, P.A., Ciccarelli, O., O'Riordan, J.I., Sailer, M., Thompson, A.J., and Miller, D.H. (2002). A longutudinal study of abnormalities on MRI and disability from multiple sclerosis. *N Engl J Med* 346: 158–164.

Bulte, J.W., Laughlin, P.G., Jordan, E.K., Tran, V.A., Vymazal, J., and Frank, J.A. (1996). Tagging of T cells with superparamagnetic iron oxide: uptake kinetics and relaxometry. *Acad Radiol*, 3 Suppl. 2, S301–S303.

Bulte, J.W., Zhang, S., van Gelderen, P., *et al.* (1999). Neurotransplantation of magnetically labeled oligodendrocyte progenitors: magnetic resonance tracking of cell migration and myelination. *Proc Natl Acad Sci USA* 96: 15256–15261.

Bulte, J.W., Douglas, T., Witwer, B., *et al.* (2001). Magnetodendrimers allow endosomal magnetic labeling and in vivo tracking of stem cells. *Nat Biotechnol* 19: 1141–1147.

Bulte, J.W., Duncan, I.D., and Frank, J.A. (2002). In vivo magnetic resonance tracking of magnetically labeled cells after trasplantation. *J Cereb Blood Flow Metab* 22: 899–907.

Bulte, J.W.M., Ben-Hur, T., Miller, B.R., *et al.* (2003). MR microscopy of magnetically labeled neurospheres transplanted into the Lewis EAE rat brain. *Magn Reson Med* 50, 201–5.

Butman, J.A. and Frank, J.A. (2000). Overview of imaging in multiple sclerosis and white matter disease. *Neuroimaging Clin N Am* 10: 669–687.

Cagnin, A., Gerhard, A., and Banati, R.B. (2002). In vivo imaging of neuroinflammation. *Eur Neuropsychopharmacol* 12: 581–586.

Caramanos, Z., Campbell, J.S.W., Narayanan, S., *et al.* (2002). Axonal integrity and fractional anisotropy in the normal-appearing white mater of patients with multiple sclerosis: Relationship to cerebro-functional reorganization and clinical disability [abstract]. *Proc Int Soc Magn Res Med* 10: 590.

Castriota Scanderbeg, A., Tomaiuolo, F., Sabatini, U., Nocentini, U., Grasso, M.G., and Caltagirone, C. (2000). Demyelinating plaques in relapsing-remitting and secondary-progressive multiple sclerosis: assessment with diffusion MR imaging. *Am J Neuroradiol* 21: 862–868.

Cercignani, M. and Horsfield, M.A. (2001). The physical basis of diffusion-weighted MRI. *J Neurol Sci* 186: S11–S14.

Cercignani, M., Iannucci, G., and Filippi, M. (1999).Diffusion-weighted imaging in multiple sclerosis. *Ital J Neurol Sci* 20: S246–S249.

Cercignani, M., Iannucci, G., Rocca, M.A., Comi, G., Horsfield, M.A., and Filippi, M. (2000). Pathologic damage in MS assessed by diffusion-weighted and magnetization transfer MRI. *Neurology* 54: 1139–1144.

Cercignani, M., Bozzali, M., Iannucci, G., Comi, G., and Filippi, M. (2001a). Magnetisation transfer ratio and mean diffusivity of normal appearing white and grey matter from patients with multiple sclerosis. *J Neurol Neurosurg Psychiatry* 70: 311–317.

Cercignani, M., Inglese, M., Pagani, E., Comi, G., and Filippi, M. (2001b). Mean diffusivity and fractional anisotropy histograms of patients with multiple sclerosis. *Am J Neuroradiol* 22: 952–958.

Chen, J.T., Matthews, P.M., Arnold, D.L., Zhang, Y., and Smith, S.M. (2001). Regional brain atrophy in multiple sclerosis: increasing sensitivity to differences in relapsing-remitting and secondary-progressive disease [abstract]. *Proc Int Soc Magn Res Med* 9: 265.

Christiansen, P., Gideon, P., Thomsen, C., Stubgaard, M., Henriksen, O., and Larsson, H.B. (1993). Increased water self-diffusion in chronic plaques and in apparently normal white matter in patients with multiple sclerosis. *Acta Neurol Scand* 87: 195–199.

Clark, C.A., Werring, D.J., and Miller, D.H. (2000). Diffusion imaging of the spinal cord in vivo: estimation of the principal diffusivities and application to multiple sclerosis. *Magn Reson Med* 43: 133–138.

Collins, L.D., Narayanan, S., Caramanos, Z., De Stefano, N., Tartaglia, M.C., and Arnold, D.L. (2000). Relation of cerebral atrophy in multiple sclerosis to severity of disease and axonal injury [abstract]. *Neurology* 54: A17.

Costa, G.L., Sandora, M.R., Nakajima, A., *et al.* (2001). Adoptive immunotherapy of experimental autoimmune encephalomyelitis via T cell delivery of the IL-12 p40 subunit. *J Immunol*, 167, 2379–87.

De Groot, C.J., Bergers, E., Kamphorst, W., *et al.* (2001). Post-mortem MRI-guided sampling of multiple sclerosis brain lesions: increased yield of active demyelinating and (p)reactive lesions. *Brain* 124: 1635–1645.

De Stefano, N., Matthews, P.M., Antel, J.P., Preul, M., Francis, G., and Arnold, D.L. (1995). Chemical pathology of acute demyelinating lesions and its correlation with disability. *Ann Neurol* 38: 901–909.

De Stefano, N., Narayanan, S., Matthews, P.M., Francis, G.S., Antel, J.P., and Arnold, D.L. (1999). In vivo evidence for axonal dysfunction remote from focal cerebral demyelination of the type seen in multiple sclerosis. *Brain* 122: 1933–1939.

De Stefano, N., Narayanan, S., Francis, G.S., *et al.* (2001). Evidence of axonal damage in the early stages of multiple sclerosis and its relevance to disability. *Arch Neurol* 58: 65–70.

Dehmeshki, J., Ruto, A.C., Arridge, S., Silver, N.C., Miller, D.H., and Tofts, P.S. (2001). Analysis of MTR histograms in multiple sclerosis using principal components and multiple discriminant analysis. *Magn Reson Med* 46: 600–609.

Dodd, C.H., Hsu, H.C., Chu, W.J., *et al.* (2001). Normal T-cell response and in vivo magnetic resonance imaging of T cells loaded with HIV transactivator-peptide-derived superparamagnetic nanoparticles. *J Immunol Methods* 256: 89–105.

Dodd, S.J., Williams, M., Suhan, J.P., Williams, D.S., Koretsky, A.P., and Ho, C. (1999). Detection of single mammalian cells by high-resolution magnetic resonance imaging. *Biophys J* 76: 103–109.

Dousset, V., Brochet, B., Vital, A., *et al.* (1995). Lysolecithin-induced demyelination in primates: preliminary in vivo study with MR and magnetization transfer. *Am J Neuroradiol* 16: 225–231.

Dousset, V., Gayou, A., Brochet, B., and Caille, J.M. (1998). Early structural changes in acute MS lesions assessed by serial magnitizationtransfer studies. *Neurology* 51: 1150–1155.

Drayer, B.P., Burger, P., Hurwitz, B., *et al.* (1987). Magnetic resonance imaging in multiple sclerosis: decreased signal in thalamus and putamen. *Ann Neurol* 22: 546–550.

Filippi, M. (1999). Magnetization transfer imaging to monitor the evolution of individual multiple sclerosis lesions. *Neurology* 53(5): S18–S22.

Filippi, M., Campi, A., Dousset, V., *et al.* (1995). A magnetization transfer imaging study of normal-appearing white matter in multiple sclerosis. *Neurology* 45: 478–482.

Filippi, M., Rocca, M.A., Martino, G., Horsfield, M.A., and Comi, G. (1998*a*). Magnetization transfer changes in the normal appearing white matter precede the appearance of enhancing lesions in patients with multiple sclerosis. *Ann Neurol* 43: 809–814.

Filippi, M., Rocca, M.A., Rizzo, G., *et al.* (1998*b*). Magnetization transfer ratios in multiple sclerosis lesions enhancing after different doses of gadolium. *Neurology* 50: 1289–1293.

Filippi, M., Iannucci, G., Cercignani, M., Assunta Rocca, M., Pratesi, A., and Comi, G. (2000*a*). A quantitative study of water diffusion in multiple sclerosis lesions and normal-appearing white matter using echo-planar imaging. *Arch Neurol* 57: 1017–1021.

Filippi, M., Inglese, M., Rovaris, M., *et al.* (2000*b*). Magnetization transfer imaging to monitor the evolution of MS: a 1-year follow-up study. *Neurology* 55: 940–946.

Fox, N.C., Jenkins, R., Leary, S.M., *et al.* (2000). Progressive cerebral atrophy in MS: a serial study using registered, volumetric MRI. *Neurology* 54: 807–812.

Fralix, T.A., Ceckler, T.L., Wolff, S.D., Simon, S.A., and Balaban, R.S. (1991). Lipid bilayer and water proton magnetization transfer: effect of cholesterol. *Magn Reson Med* 18: 214–223.

Frank, J.A., Zywicke, H., Jordan, E.K., *et al.* (2002). Magnetization intracellular labeling of mammalian cells by combining (FDA-approved) superparamagnetic iron oxide MR contrast agents and commonly used transfection agents. *Acad Radiol* 9(Suppl. 2): S484–S487.

Frank, J.A., Miller, B.R., Arbab, A.S., *et al.* (2003). Clinically applicable labeling of mammalian and stem cells by combining superparamagnetic iron oxides and transfection agents. *Radiology*, 228, 480–7.

Fu, L., Matthews, P.M., De Stefano, N., *et al.* (1998). Imaging axonal damage of normal-appearing white matter in multiple sclerosis. *Brain* 121: 103–113.

Gadian, D.G.(1996). *NMR and its Applications to Living Systems.* Oxford University Press, Oxford.

Gambhir, S.S., Barrio, J.R., Herschman, H.R., and Phelps, M.E. (1999*a*). Imaging gene expression: principles and assays. *J Nucl Cardiol* 6: 219–233.

Gambhir, S.S., Barrio, J.R., Phelps, M.E., *et al.* (1999*b*). Imaging adenoviral-directed reporter gene expression in living animals with positron emission tomography. *Proc Natl Acad Sci USA* 96: 2333–2338.

Gawne-Cain, M.L., O'Riordan, J.I., Thompson, A.J., Moseley, I.F., and Miller, D.H. (1997). Multiple sclerosis lesion detection in the brain: a comparison of fast fluid-attenuated inversion recovery and conventional T2-weighted dual spin echo. *Neurology* 49: 364–370.

Goodkin, D.E., Rooney, W.D., Sloan, R., *et al.* (1998). A serial study of new MS lesions and the white matter from which they arise. *Neurology* 51: 1689–1697.

Griffith, K.D., Read, E.J., Carrasquillo, J.A., *et al.* (1989). In vivo distribution of adoptively transferred indium-111-labeled tumor infiltrating lymphocytes and peripheral blood lymphocytes in patients with metastatic melanoma. *J Natl Cancer Inst* 81: 1709–1717.

Gunn, R.N., Lammertsma, A.A., Hume, S.P., and Cunningham, V.J. (1997). Parametric imaging of ligand-receptor binding in PET using a simplified reference region model. *Neuroimage* 6: 279–287.

Gunn, R.N., Gunn, S.R., and Cunningham, V.J. (2001). Positron emission tomography compartmental models. *J Cereb Blood Flow Metab* 21: 635–652.

Hagberg, G., Valancherry, J., Fasano, F., *et al.* (2001). Co-localization of changes in ADC, T1-relaxation time and 1 H-metabolite concentrations in MS-lesions [abstract]. *Proc Int Soc Magn Reson Med* 9: 153.

Harisinghani, M.G., Saini, S., Weissleder, R., *et al.* (1999). MR lymphangiography using ultrasmall superparamagnetic iron oxide in patients with primary abdominal and pelvic malignancies: radiographic-pathologic correlation. *Am J Roentgenol* 172: 1347–1351.

Hiehle, J.F. Jr, Lenkinski, R.E., Grossman, R.I., *et al.* (1994). Correlation of spectroscopy ad magnetization transfer imaging in the evaluation of demyelinating lesions and normal appearing white mater in multiple sclerosis. *Magn Reson Med* 32: 285–293.

Josephson, L., Tung, C.H., Moore, A., and Weissleder, R. (1999). High-efficiency intracellular magnetic labeling with novel superparamagnetic-Tat peptide conjugates. *Bioconjug Chem* 10: 186–191.

Kapeller, P., McLean, M.A., Griffin, C.M., *et al.* (2001). Preliminary evidence for neuronal damage in cortical grey matter and normal appearing white matter in short duration relapsing-remitting multiple sclerosis: a quantitative MR spectroscopic imaging study. *J Neurol* 248: 131–138.

Kappos, L., Moeri, D., Radue, E.W., *et al.* (1999). Predictive value of gadolinium-enhanced magnetic resonance imaging for relapse rate and changes in disability or impairment in multiple sclerosis: a meta-analysis. Gadolinium MRI Meta-analysis Group. *Lancet* 353: 964–949.

Kurtzke, J.F. (1983). Rating neurologic impairment in multiple sclerosis: an expanded disability status scale (EDSS). *Neurology* 33: 1444–1452.

Larsson, H.B., Thomsen, C., Frederiksen, J., Stubgaard, M., and Henriksen, O. (1992). In vivo magnetic resonance diffusion measurement in the brain of patients with multiple sclerosis. *Magn Reson Imaging* 10: 7–12.

Laule, C., Vavasour, I.M., Whittall, K.P., Oger, J., MacKay, A.L., Paty, D.W., *et al.* (2001). *Mult Scler* 7: P-298.

Le, D.A. and Lipton, S.A. (2001). *Drugs Aging* 18: 717–724.

Lewin, M., Carlesso, N., Tung, C.H., *et al.* (2000). Tat peptide-derived magnetic nanoparticles allow in vivo tracking and recovery of progenitor cells.. *Nat Biotechnol* 18: 410–414.

Li, D.K., Zhao, G., and Paty, D.W. (2000). T2 hyperintensities: findings and significance. *Neuroimaging Clin N Am* 10: 717–738, ix.

Loevner, L.A., Grossman, R.I., Cohen, J.A., Lexa, F.J., Kessler, D. ,and Kolson, D.L. (1995*a*). Microscopic disease in normal-appearing white matter on conventional MR images in patients with multiple sclerosis: assessment with magnetization-transfer measurements. *Radiology* 196: 511–515.

Loevner, L.A., Grossman, R.I., McGowan, J.C., Ramer, K.N., and Cohen, J.A. (1995*b*). Characterization of multiple sclerosis plaques with T1-weighted MR and quantitative magnetization transfer. *Am J Neuroradiol* 16: 1473–1479.

Mack, M.G., Balzer, J.O., Straub, R., Eichler, K., and Vogl, T.J. (2002). Superparamagnetic iron oxide-enhanced MR imaging of head and neck lymph nodes. *Radiology* 222: 239–244.

MacLaren, D.C., Gambhir, S.S., Satyamurthy, N., *et al.* (1999). Repetitive,non-invasive imaging of the dopamine D2 receptor as a reporter gene in living animals. *Gene Ther* 6: 785–791.

Mader, I., Roser, W., Kappos, L., *et al.* (2000). Serial spectroscopy of contrast-enhancing multiple sclerosis plaques: absolute metabolic values over 2 years during a clinical pharmacological study. *Am J Neuroradiol* 21: 1220–1227.

Mader, I., Seeger, U., Weissert, R., *et al.* (2001). Proton MR spectroscopy with metabolite-nulling reveals elevated macromolecules in acute multiple sclerosis. *Brain* 124: 953–961.

Mainero, C., De Stefano, N., Iannucci, G., *et al.* (2001). Correlates of MS disability assessed in vivo using aggregates of MR quantities. *Neurology* 56: 1331–1334.

Matthews, P.M. and Arnold, D.L. (2001). Magnetic resonance imaging of multiple sclerosis: new insights linking pathology to clinical evolution. *Curr Opin Neurol* 14: 279–287.

Matthews, P.M., Francis, G., Antel, J., and Arnold, D.L. (1991). Proton magnetic resonance spectroscopy for metabolic characterization of plaques in multiple sclerosis [published erratum appears in Neurology 1991 Nov;41(11):1828]. *Neurology* 41: 1251–1256.

McFarland, H.F., Frank, J.A., Albert, P.S., *et al.* (1992). Using gadolinium-enhanced magnetic resonance imaging lesions to monitor disease activity in multiple sclerosis. *Ann Neurol* 32: 758–766.

Miller, D.H., Barkhof, F., and Nauta, J.J. (1993). Gadolinium enhancement increases the sensitivity of MRI in detecting disease activity in multiple sclerosis. *Brain* 116: 1077–1094.

Miller, D.H., Grossman, R.I., Reingold, S.C., and McFarland, H.F. (1998). The role of magnetic resonance techniques in understanding and managing multiple sclerosis. *Brain* 121: 3–24.

Misteli, T. and Spector, D.L. (1997). Applications of the green fluorescent protein in cell biology and biotechnology. *Nat Biotechnol* 15: 961–964.

Moffett, J.R., Namboodiri, M.A., Cangro, C.B., and Neale, J.H. (1991). Immuno-histochemical localization of N-acetylaspartate in rat brain. *Neuroreport* 2: 131–134.

Molyneux, P.D., Filippi, M., Barkhof, F., *et al.* (1998). Correlations between monthly enhanced MRI lesion rate and changes in T2 lesion volume in multiple sclerosis. *Ann Neurol* 43: 332–339.

Moore, A., Sun, P.Z., Cory, D., Hogemann, D., Weissleder, R., and Lipes, M.A. (2002). MRI of insulitis in autoimmune diabetes. *Magn Reson Med* **47**: 751–758.

Narayana, P.A., Doyle, T.J., Lai, D., and Wolinsky, J.S. (1998). Serial proton magnetic resonance spectroscopic imaging, contrast-enhanced magnetic resonance imaging, and quantitative lesion volumetry in multiple sclerosis. *Ann Neurol* **43**: 56–71.

Narayanan, S., De Stefano, N., Francis, G.S., Tartaglia, M.C., Arnaoutelis, R., and Arnold, D.L. (2000). Disease duration influences the relationship between brain axonal injury, spinal cord atrophy, and disability in multiple sclerosis [abstract]. *Proc Int Soc Magn Reson Med* **1**: 297.

Narayanan, S., Fu, L., Pioro, E., *et al.* (1997). Imaging of axonal damage in multiple sclerosis: spatial distribution of magnetic resonance imaging lesions. *Ann Neurol* **41**: 385–391.

Nusbaum, A.O., Tang, C.Y., Wei, T., Buchsbaum, M.S., and Atlas, S.W. (2000). Whole-brain diffusion MR histograms differ between MS subtypes. *Neurology* **54**: 1421–1427.

Pan, J.W., Krupp, L.B., Elkins, L.E., and Coyle, P.K. (2001). Cognitive dysfunction lateralizes with NAA in multiple sclerosis. *Appl Neuropsychol* **8**: 155–160.

Phelps, M.E. (2000*a*). Inaugural article: positron emission tomography provides molecular imaging of biological processes. *Proc Natl Acad Sci USA* **97**: 9226–9233.

Phelps, M.E. (2000*b*). PET: the merging of biology and imaging into molecular imaging. *J Nucl Med* **41**: 661–681.

Pike, G.B., De Stefano, N., Narayanan, S., *et al.* (2000). Multiple sclerosis: magnetization transfer MR imaging of white matter before lesion appearance on T2-weighted images. *Radiology* **215**: 824–830.

Pozzilli, P., Pozzilli, C., Pantano, P., Negri, M., Andreani, D., and Cudworth, A.G. (1983). Tracking of indium-111-oxine labelled lymphocytes in autoimmune thyroid disease. *Clin Endocrinol* **19**: 111–116.

Read, E.J., Keenan, A.M., Carter, C.S., Yolles, P.S., and Davey, R.J. (1990). In vivo traffic of indium-111-oxine labeled human lymphocytes collected by automated apheresis. *J Nucl Med* **31**: 999–1006.

Reddy, H., Narayanan, S., Arnoutelis, R., *et al.* (2000*a*). Evidence for adaptive functional changes in the cerebral cortex with axonal injury from multiple sclerosis. *Brain* **123**: 2314–2320.

Reddy, H., Narayanan, S., Matthews, P.M., *et al.* (2000*b*). Relating axonal injury to functional recovery in MS. *Neurology* **54**: 236–239.

Riahi, F., Zijdenbos, A., Narayanan, S., *et al.* (1998). Improved correlation between scores on the expanded disability status scale and cerebral lesion load in relapsing-remitting multiple sclerosis. *Brain* **121**: 1305–1312.

Richert, N.D., Ostuni, J.L., Bash, C.N., Leist, T.P., McFarland, H.F., and Frank, J.A. (2001). Interferon beta-1b and intravenous methylprednisolone promote lesion recovery in multiple sclerosis. **7**: 49–58.

Rocca, M.A., Mastronardo, G., Rodegher, M., Comi, G. ,and Filippi, M. (1999). Long-term changes of magnetization transfer-derived measures from patients with relapsing-remitting and secondary progressive multiple sclerosis. *Am J Neuroradiol* **20**: 821–827.

Rocca, M.A., Cercignani, M., Iannucci, G., Comi, G., and Filippi, M. (2000). Weekly diffusion-weighted imaging of normal-appearing white matter in MS. *Neurology* **55**: 882–884.

Ross, B. and Bluml, S. (2001). Magnetic resonance spectroscopy of the human brain. *Anat Rec (New Anat)* **265**: 54–84.

Rovaris, M. and Filippi, M. (2000). Contrast enhancement and the acute lesion in multiple sclerosis. *Neuroimaging Clin N Am* **10**: 705–716, viii–ix.

Rovaris, M., Bozzali, M., Santuccio, G., *et al.* (2000*a*). Relative contributions of brain and cervical cord pathology to multiple sclerosis disability: a study with magnetisation transfer ratio histogram analysis. *J Neurol Neurosurg Psychiatry* **69**: 723–727.

Rovaris, M., Filippi, M., Minicucci, L., *et al.* (2000*b*). Cortical/subcortical disease burden and cognitive impairment in patients with multiple sclerosis. *Am J Neuroradiol* **21**: 402–408.

Rubin, L.L. and Staddon, J.M. (1999). The cell biology of the blood-brain barrier. *Annu Rev Neurosci* **22**: 11–28.

Rudick, R.A., Fisher, E., Lee, J.C., Simon, J., and Jacobs, L. (1999). Use of the brain parenchymal fractionto measure whole brain atrophy in relapsing-remitting MS. Multiple Sclerosis Collaborative Research Group. *Neurology* **53**: 1698–1704.

Schaefer, P.W., Grant, P.E., and Gonzalez, R.G. (2000). Diffusion-weighted MR imaging of the brain. *Radiology* **217**: 331–345.

Schreiber, K., Sorensen, P.S., Koch-Henriksen, N., *et al.* (2001). Correlations of brain MRI parameters to disability in multiple sclerosis. *Acta Neurol Scand* **104**: 24–30.

Semelka, R.C. and Helmberger, T.K. (2001). Contrast agents for MR imaging of the liver. *Radiology* **218**: 27–38.

Sharma, R., Narayana, P.A., and Wolinsky, J.S. (2001). Grey matter abnormalities in multiple sclerosis: proton magnetic resonance spectroscopic imaging. *Mult Scler* **7**: 221–226.

Silver, N.C., Good, C.D., Barker, G.J., *et al.* (1997). Sensivity of contrast enhanced MRI in multiple sclerosis. Effects of gadolinium dose, magnetization transfer contast and delayed imaging. *Brain* **120**: 1149–1161.

Simmons, M.L., Frondoza, C.G., and Coyle, J.T. (1991). *Neuroscience* **45**: 37–45.

Simon, J.H. (2000). Brain and spinal cord atrophy in multiple sclerosis. *Neuroimaging Clin N Am* **10**: 753–770, ix.

Simon, J.H. (2001). Brain and spinal cord atrophy in multiple sclerosis: role as a surrogate measure of disease progression. *CNS Drugs* **15**: 427–436.

Simon, J.H., Jacobs, L.D., Campion, M.K., *et al.* (1999). A longitudinal study of brain atrophy in relapsing multiple sclerosis. The Multiple Sclerosis Collaborative Research Group (MSCRG). *Neurology* **53**: 139–148.

Simone, I.L., Tortorella, C., Federico, F., *et al.* (2001). Axonal damage in multiple sclerosis plaques: a combined magnetic resonance imaging and 1H-magnetic resonance spectroscopty study. *J Neurol Sci* **182**: 143–150.

Sipe, J.C., Filippi, M., Martino, G., *et al.* (1999). Method for intracellular magnetic labeling of human mononuclear cells using approved iron contrast agents. *Magn Reson Imaging* **17**: 1521–1523.

Smith, S.M., De Stefano, N., Jenkinson, M., and Matthews, P.M. (2001). Normalized accurate measurement of longitudinal brain change. *J Comput Assist Tomogr* **25**: 466–475.

Smith, S.M., Zhang, Y., Jenkinson, M., *et al.* (2002). Accurate, robust, and automated longitudinal and cross-sectional brain change analysis. *Neuroimage* **17**: 479–489.

Spinks, T.J., Jones, T., Bloomfield, P.M., *et al.* (2000). Physical characteristics of the ECAT EXACT3D positron tomograph. *Phys Med Biol* **45**: 2601–2618.

Stevenson, V.L., Leary, S.M., Losseff, N.A., *et al.* (1998). Spinal cord atrophy and disability in MS: a longitudinal study. *Neurology* **51**: 234–238.

Studholme, C., Hill, D.L., and Hawkes, D.J. (1997). Automated three-dimensional registration of magnetic resonance and positron emission tomography brain images by multiresolution optimization of voxel similarity measures. *Med Phys* **24**: 25–35.

Tartaglia, M.C., Narayanan, S., Stefano, N.D., *et al.* (2001). Choline is increased in pre-lesional normal appearing white mattter in multiple sclerosis [abstract]. *Neurol* **56**: Suppl 3, A460.

Tievsky, A.L., Ptak, T., and Farkas, J. (1999). Investigation of apparent diffusion coefficient and diffusion tensor anisotrophy in acute and chronic multiple sclerosis lesions. *Am J Neuroradiol* **20**: 1491–1499.

Tofts, P.S. and Kermode, A.G. (1991). Measurement of the blood-brain barrier permeability and leakage space using dynamic MR imaging. 1. Fundamental concepts. *Magn Reson Med* **17**: 357–367.

Tortorella, C., Codella, M., Rocca, M.A., *et al.* (1999). Disease activity in multiple sclerosis studied by weekly triple-dose magnetic resonance imaging. *J Neurol* **246**: 689–692.

Tortorella, C., Viti, B., Bozzali, M., *et al.* (2000). A magnetization transfer histogram study of normal-appearing brain tissue in MS. *Neurology* **54**: 186–193.

Tourbah, A., Stievenart, J.L., Abanou, A., Fontaine, B., Cabanis, E.A., and Lyon-Caen, O. (2001). Correlating multiple MRI parameters with clinical features: an attempt to define a new strategy in multiple sclerosis. *Neuroradiology* **43**: 712–720.

Trapp, B.D., Bo, L., Mork, S., and Chang, A. (1999). Pathogenesis of tissue injury in MS lesions 14. *J Neuroimmunol* **98**: 49–56.

Truyen, L., van Waesberghe, J.H., van Walderveen, M.A., *et al.* (1996). Accumulation of hypointense lesions ("black holes") on spin-echo MRI correlates with disease progression in multiple sclerosis. *Neurology* **47**: 1469–1476.

van Buchem, M.A. and Tofts, P.S. (2000). Magnetization transfer imaging. *Neuroimaging Clin N Am* **10**: 771–788.

van Waesberghe, J.H., van Walderveen, M.A., Castelijns, J.A., *et al.* (1998). Patterns of lesion development in muliple sclerosis: longitudinal observaions with T1-weighted spin-echo and magnetization transfer MR. *Am J Neuroradiol* **19**: 675–683.

van Waesberghe, J.H., Kamphorst, W., De Groot, C.J., *et al.* (1999). Axonal loss in multiple sclerosis lesions: magnetic resonance imaging insights into substrates of disability. *Ann Neurol* **46**: 747–754.

van Walderveen, M.A., Kamphorst, W., Scheltens, P., *et al.* (1998). Histopathologic correlate of hypointense lesions on T1-weighted spin-echo MRI in multiple sclerosis. *Neurology* **50**: 1282–1288.

van Walderveen, M.A., Barkhof, F., Pouwels, P.J., van Schijndel, R.A., Polman, C.H., and Castelijns, J.A. (1999*a*). Neuronal damage in T1-hypointense multiple sclerosis lesions demonstated in vivo using proton magnetic resonance spectroscopy. *Ann Neurol* **46**: 79–87.

van Walderveen, M.A., Truyen, L., van Oosten, B.W., *et al.* (1999*b*). Development of hypointense lesions on T1-weighted spin-echo magnetic resonance images in multiple sclerosis: relation to inflammatory activity. *Arch Neurol* **56**: 345–351.

Vowinckel, E., Reutens, D., Becher, B., *et al.* (1997). PK11195 binding to the peripheral benzodiazepine receptor as a marker of microglia activation in multiple sclerosis and experimental autoimmune encephalomyelitis. *J Neurosci Res* **50**: 345–353.

Werring, D.J., Brassat, D., Droogan, A.G., *et al.* (2000). The pathogenesis of lesions and normal-appearing white matter changes in multiple sclerosis: a serial diffusion MRI study. *Brain* **123**: 1667–1676.

Werring, D.J., Clark, C.A., Droogan, A.G., Barker, G.J., Miller, D.H., and Thompson, A.J. (2001). Water diffusion is elevated in widespread regions of normal-appearing white matter in multiple sclerosis and correlates with diffusion in focal lesions. *Mult Scler* **7**: 83–89.

Willoughby, E.W., Grochowski, E., Li, D.K., Oger, J., Kastrukoff, L.F., and Paty, D.W. (1989). Serial magnetic resonance scanning in multiple sclerosis: a second prospective study in relapsing patients. *Ann Neurol* **25**: 43–49.

Wilson, M., Morgan, P.S., Lin, X., Turner, B.P., and Blumhardt, L.D. (2001). Quantitative diffusion weighted magnetic resonance imaging, cerebral atrophy, and disability in multiple sclerosis. *J Neurol Neurosurg Psychiatry* **70**: 318–322.

Yeager, M.P., DeLeo, J.A., Hoopes, P.J., Hartov, A., Hildebrandt, L., and Hickey, W.F. (2000). Trauma and inflammation modulate lymphocyte localization in vivo: quantitation of tissue entry and retention using indium-111-labeled lymphocytes. *Crit Care Med* **28**: 1477–1482.

17 Multiple sclerosis: effects of immune mediators on neurophysiological function

Richard M. Evans and Kenneth J. Smith

Introduction

Multiple sclerosis (MS) has historically been thought of as a demyelinating disease in which the major symptoms arise primarily from conduction block due to demyelination, and in which the symptoms resolve when conduction is restored, either to demyelinated axons or to axons that have been remyelinated. However, although these events undoubtedly play an important role, they do not explain how the symptoms of MS can sometimes arise and resolve over a day or two, a period that is too short for demyelination and remyelination to occur. Several observations now suggest that, in addition to the events above, neurophysiological function can be directly affected by inflammation and immune mediators. These factors may contribute not only to brief exacerbations, but also to the more prolonged impairments that typically accompany the formation of inflammatory demyelinating lesions in clinically eloquent pathways.

Evidence for an effect of immune mediators on neurophysiological function in MS

The belief that inflammation and immune mediators can impair neurological function and cause symptoms in MS arises from three groups of observations. Firstly, the symptoms of MS can sometimes arise and resolve rapidly; secondly, animal models show that a neurological deficit can arise in circumstances where demyelination is absent, but inflammation is prominent; and thirdly, clinical studies suggest that symptom expression in MS is sometimes poorly correlated with the presence of demyelination, and that a role for inflammation is likely.

The severity of symptoms in MS can change rapidly

The symptoms experienced by a patient with MS can vary dramatically within an interval of a few hours to days, including both rapid onset and rapid resolution of the neurological deficit. Such dynamic changes in deficit are well illustrated in a clinical trial for the efficacy of leukocyte depletion in MS by the antibody Campath-1H (Moreau *et al.*, 1996). Campath-1H is a monoclonal humanized antibody against the CD52 cell surface marker, which is carried by all lymphocytes and some macrophages. Within hours of the start of Campath-1H infusion patients with MS unexpectedly experienced a rehearsal of previous symptoms. For example, one patient who had suffered diplopia and numbness on the left side on two previous occasions, re-expressed these symptoms 3 hr after Campath-1H administration. Symptoms typically arose within 2–4 hr of the start of infusion and had resolved in most patients 12 hr later. The rapid fluctuation of symptoms cannot be explained by a mechanism involving demyelination and remyelination because although electrophysiological deficits due to demyelination can appear promptly, it takes days before demyelinated axons can regain the ability to conduct (at least in experimental situations), and even longer before compact myelin is formed during repair by remyelination.

In two patients, pre-treatment with corticosteroids was able to prevent both the rehearsal of symptoms and the surge in serum cytokine levels, ruling out a direct effect of the Campath-1H antibody on neurophysiological function. Interestingly, serum levels of the cytokines tumour necrosis factor-alpha (TNF-α), interferon-gamma (IFN-γ), and interleukin (IL)-6 were monitored following the start of Campath-1H infusion and were 'very substantially increased' within 4 hr, returning to baseline after 8 hr. However, whether these cytokines are directly involved in the exacerbation is uncertain. A subsequent study found that Campath-1H therapy was still able to evoke neurological exacerbation when selective blockade of TNF-α was achieved using the soluble receptor for this cytokine (Coles *et al.*, 1999). Furthermore the peak level of IL-6 was reached after those of TNF-α and IFN-γ, and after the onset of symptoms, suggesting that it plays a minor role, if any, in the rehearsal of symptoms (Moreau *et al.*, 1996). The observations with Campath-1H clearly demonstrate the speed with which symptoms may fluctuate, and also indicate that previously lesioned parts of the central nervous system (CNS) are especially vulnerable, because earlier symptoms are rehearsed rather than new symptoms appearing.

Animal models show that a neurological deficit can arise in circumstances where demyelination is absent, but inflammation is prominent

Experimental autoimmune encephalitis (EAE) is an animal model of MS that provides the opportunity to examine the serial changes in pathology throughout the development of an MS-like lesion, whereas in MS itself examination of tissues is typically only possible either post mortem, when MS pathology is advanced and usually historic, or in rare biopsy specimens. EAE studies have revealed that the onset of neurological deficits, such as hindlimb paralysis, often coincides with vasogenic oedema, indicative of inflammation and blood–brain barrier (BBB) breakdown, but not with demyelination (Kerlero de Rosbo *et al.*, 1985). Such observations support an interpretation that the neurological deficit in EAE can arise from inflammatory CNS lesions in the absence of CNS demyelination (Berger *et al.*, 1997), but it has also been suggested that such deficits might arise primarily from demyelinating lesions in the spinal roots (Pender, 1986). Although demyelination in MS occurs almost exclusively within the CNS, in several models of EAE there is also demyelination in the spinal roots, and this has typically been overlooked. The studies of Pender and his colleagues have been important in pointing out a common oversight, but although his observations may help to explain the origin of the neurological deficit in some models there nonetheless remains evidence to support a view that inflammation *per se* can result in profound neurological deficit. Thus the presence of neurological deficit, in the absence of peripheral or central demyelination, has been shown in a chronic model of EAE (Lorentzen *et al.*, 1995). In this model an initial attack occurs at around 10 days after inoculation, followed by a second attack, or relapse, at about 18–20 days. Although demyelination is found in the spinal cord at the time of the *second* attack, it is reportedly absent during the first episode (Tanuma *et al.*, 2000). The Lorentzen model therefore appears to provide good evidence that inflammation can result in a neurological deficit in the absence of demyelination.

Clinical studies suggest a role for inflammation in the expression of symptoms in MS

Optic neuritis, a condition often encountered in MS patients, involves inflammation and often demyelination of the optic nerves. Youl *et al.* (1991) studied 18 patients with acute optic neuritis in whom inflammation was detected by the leakage of gadolinium diethylene triamine pentacetic acid (Gd-DTPA) from the vasculature upon MRI examination, and deficits in conduction in the optic nerve were measured by monitoring changes in the visual evoked potential (VEP). A reduced VEP amplitude was interpreted as indicating conduction block, and an increased VEP latency as indicating delayed conduction. Youl *et al.* (1991) found that, during acute optic neuritis, vision was poor, lesions were characterized by gadolinium leakage/enhancement, and VEP examination showed a reduction in the amplitude and an increase in the latency of the VEP. Clinical recovery was associated with the resolution of the inflammation (i.e. lesions no longer showed Gd-DTPA leakage) and an improvement in the amplitude of the VEP. However, the VEP latency remained increased, suggesting the presence of successful conduction in axons that remained demyelinated. Whilst the evidence from this study is necessarily indirect and inconclusive, the neurological deficit correlated better with the presence of inflammation than with the presence of demyelination. This interpretation is also supported by findings from a recent biopsy study (from a single case of Marburg's type MS) that concluded that in MS 'inflammation alone may be sufficient to cause significant clinical deficits without demyelination' (Bitsch *et al.*, 1999).

For completeness, it should be noted that although we have reviewed evidence that inflammation can directly result in significant neurological deficits in MS, it is also true that in most patients the deficits are likely to arise from inflammation and demyelination acting in concert, rather than in isolation.

How might immune mediators alter neurophysiological function?

The information above provides quite convincing evidence that factors associated with inflammation can impair neurophysiological function to the extent of causing a demonstrable neurological deficit. Two processes that underlie all normal motor and sensory function are axonal conduction and synaptic transmission; and we now discuss how immune mediators might act on these processes to affect neurophysiological function in MS.

Impaired axonal conduction

With regard to axons, it is worth considering the vulnerability of the different types of axon that are present in the CNS of patients with MS. Normal axons, and the portions of lesioned axons that lie outside of the lesion, are almost certainly the least vulnerable to disturbance by inflammatory mediators because they conduct securely, i.e. they have a high safety factor for conduction. The safety factor for conduction is obtained by dividing the amount of current available to depolarize a given node of Ranvier by the amount of current required to do so. Normal myelinated axons have a safety factor of three to five and so they have a sufficient excess of depolarizing current available to conduct impulses securely despite limited deleterious changes in the environment of the axons. In spite of their secure conduction, the observations in EAE (see above) suggest that conduction in normal axons is nonetheless sufficiently vulnerable that inflammation can result in severe conduction deficits. The mechanism of block is uncertain, and perhaps it is the case that inflammation causes a subtle morphological change in the seemingly normal axons that is functionally important, but difficult to detect by microscopy. Whether normal axons are vulnerable to conduction block in MS remains uncertain.

Although normal axons have a high safety factor, demyelinated axons have a safety factor near unity, and so they are balanced 'on a knife's edge' between successful conduction and conduction failure (Smith and

McDonald, 1999). Such axons are very vulnerable to even subtle changes in their environment that may reduce their safety factor to below unity, and so they are expected to be the most vulnerable to inflammatory mediators. It is known, for example, that low doses of sodium channel blockers can exacerbate or unmask symptoms in MS (Sakurai *et al.*, 1992), presumably by reducing the inward nodal sodium current that is ultimately required to depolarize the adjacent, demyelinated axolemma to its firing threshold. Demyelinated axons that have been repaired by remyelination regain a relatively high safety factor (Felts and Smith, 1992) despite the fact that the remyelinated internodes are thinner and shorter than normal. Providing remyelinated axons do not retain any specific targets for inflammatory mediators it is likely that they will effectively be as resistant to conduction block as normal axons.

The brief exacerbations due to Campath-1H administration appear to support the idea that axons previously affected by the disease are selectively vulnerable, because old symptoms are rehearsed rather than new ones appearing. However, although this explanation implies that demyelinated axons may be involved, it is also possible that the vulnerability lies not with the axons but rather in the fact that the previously affected pathways are likely to contain residual inflammatory cells that can respond promptly to the effects of the Campath-1H antibody and impair axonal function. The possibility that normal or remyelinated axons are involved in the rehearsal of symptoms therefore remains a possibility.

If inflammatory mediators affect conduction, it seems intuitively likely that they would impair it, encouraging conduction block and resulting in the negative symptoms of MS such as paralysis, blindness, and numbness, but it is also possible that they could provoke hyperexcitability. If so, the mediators could contribute to the generation of the spontaneous trains of ectopic impulses that are believed to underlie the generation of positive symptoms (e.g. tingling sensations and pain) sometimes experienced by patients with MS (Smith *et al.*, 1997).

Synaptic impairment

Although MS is usually described as a disease of the white matter, it is known that lesions occur, and are in fact common, in grey matter, namely a location with a high density of synapses (Kidd *et al.*, 1999). Apart from contributing to motor and sensory disturbance, impairment of synaptic transmission would be expected to cause cognitive and neuropsychological dysfunction, and indeed some degree and form of cognitive difficulty is detectable in 45–65% of patients with MS (DeSousa *et al.*, 2002). However, Jeffery *et al.* (2000) have pointed out that abnormalities referred to cortical lesions can arise from subcortical white matter pathology, and thus that the contribution of grey matter pathology to the cognitive dysfunction in MS may be overestimated. If synaptic impairment truly is a feature of MS then this may explain why the potentiation of synaptic transmission, the likely consequence of 4-aminopyridine therapy, is an effective symptomatic treatment in many patients with MS (van Diemen *et al.*, 1992; Smith *et al.*, 2000a).

Identity of immune mediators influencing neurophysiological function in MS

If, as appears likely, inflammation can affect neurophysiological function, which factors might be involved? Several factors have been identified and their effects have been studied in isolation, but it should be remembered that inflammatory factors normally act within an interwoven cascade with other mediators and events, and these wider considerations may significantly affect the action of the factors. For example, a cytokine studied in isolation may appear to have few effects, but this may simply be because the inflammatory cells upon which it acts (e.g. macrophages or lymphocytes) may not be present within the laboratory model under investigation, which is often composed of normal tissue. However, in the remainder of this chapter we discuss factors that are expected to be present at sites of inflammation and that can have direct effects on neurophysiological function.

Nitric oxide

Nitric oxide (NO) is a free radical involved in neuronal signalling, the regulation of blood flow, and immune defence. NO is produced by the enzyme nitric oxide synthase (NOS) which exists in three main isoforms, two of which are constitutive (endothelial and neuronal NOS; eNOS and nNOS) and produce transient (calcium dependent) concentrations of NO probably in the nanomolar range. The third isoform, inducible NOS (iNOS), produces NO continuously in a calcium-independent manner, resulting in higher concentrations that perhaps reach the micromolar range. iNOS is not usually expressed in the CNS but it is induced in astrocytes and activated microglia in response to inflammatory mediators, particularly the pro-inflammatory cytokines TNF-α and IFN-γ.

Levels of nitric oxide are increased in MS

There is abundant evidence that NO is present in raised concentrations in the CNS in MS. For example, the concentration of NO metabolites (e.g. nitrite and nitrate) is increased in both the serum and the CSF of patients with MS (reviewed in Smith and Lassmann (2002)). The presence of the biochemical apparatus for NO synthesis has been demonstrated in the brains of patients with MS post mortem by immunohistochemistry for both iNOS mRNA and protein (Bo *et al.*, 1994; Oleszak *et al.*, 1998) and by the demonstration of functional NOS activity using NADPH diaphorase staining, namely a histochemical technique that allows localization of the catalytic activity of NOS isoforms (Bo *et al.*, 1994).

Nitric oxide can block axonal conduction

The presence of NO within the CNS in MS may be important because experimental studies have shown that NO can block conduction both *in vitro* (Redford *et al.*, 1997; Shrager *et al.*, 1998) and *in vivo* (Redford *et al.*, 1997), and that demyelinated axons are particularly susceptible to this effect (see Fig. 17.1) (Redford *et al.*, 1997). The particular susceptibility of demyelinated axons to NO may explain why some exacerbations selectively involve previously affected pathways (see observations on Campath-1H above).

The mechanism(s) by which NO blocks conduction are not yet clear, although the available data suggest several possibilities. One observation is that NO can cause depolarization, an effect that is proposed to cause the conduction block observed when the NO donor PAPA NONOate is applied to optic nerves *in vitro* (Garthwaite *et al.*, 2002). Interestingly, the addition of tetrodotoxin (TTX), a toxin that blocks sodium channels, prevented NO from causing conduction-block-associated depolarization, indicating a role for voltage-gated sodium channels in the mechanism. Patch clamp studies have shown that NO can directly interact with ion channels, including both blocking and, in other studies, opening sodium channels (Ahern *et al.*, 2000; Renganathan *et al.*, 2002). Clearly, by affecting sodium channels NO could have profound effects on axonal conduction. The effects of NO on ion channels are not restricted to sodium channels, however, and NO can also activate BK-type, and inhibit A-type, potassium channels or currents (Ahern *et al.*, 1999).

Apart from effects on ion channels, NO has also been shown to exert several effects on mitochondria by interfering with the electron transport chain (Borutaite *et al.*, 2000). Mitochondria play a crucial role in generating the energy required to maintain the ionic gradients on which axonal conduction relies, and so it is easy to understand why mitochondrial impairment could impair conduction. Indeed, the conduction block caused by the NO donor PAPA NONOate mentioned above was accompanied by a 50% reduction in ATP (Garthwaite *et al.*, 2002). This reduction was prevented by application of TTX, suggesting that sodium channels may be involved in the manifestation of block, even though they may not be the primary target.

Nitric oxide and synaptic impairment

Given the demonstrable interactions of NO with a range of ion channels it is not surprising that NO has been shown to affect synaptic function, acting both on the regulation of transmitter release and at post-synaptic NMDA-type glutamate receptors (Pineda *et al.*, 1996; Mang and Kilbinger, 2000). It

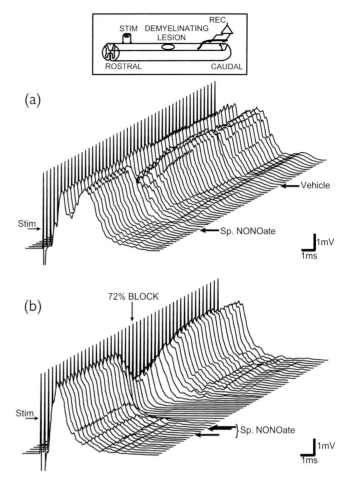

Fig. 17.1 Plots show a series of averaged compound action potentials (CAPs) recorded from a rat dorsal column over time, and offset in the z-plane. The Inset shows the recording arrangement. In (a) the conduction pathway includes a demyelinating lesion and each CAP is composed of an early component representing conduction in normal axons and a late component representing conduction in demyelinated axons. At the time indicated, a compound releasing nitric oxide (spermine-NONOate) was injected into the lesion and this resulted in conduction block in many of the demyelinated axons, but conduction in the normal axons was not noticeably affected. The records in (b) are from non-lesioned tissue, but a higher dose of the nitric oxide-releasing compound was employed. This dose was sufficient to block conduction in the healthy axons. (Redrawn from Redford *et al.* (1997) with permission from Oxford University Press.

is also predictable that the high NO concentrations resulting from iNOS expression could disturb the delicately balanced physiological function of NO at some synapses. Because synapses are found at high density in grey matter it is reasonable to suggest that NO may play a role in mediating the cortical and neuropsychological deficits of MS mentioned earlier (see section 'Synaptic impairment').

Nitric oxide and pain

Pain is not uncommon in MS patients, and although the pain can sometimes be attributed to phenomena such as spasticity it is likely that some pain is generated by events within the CNS and in which NO may be involved. A role for NO in nociception, for example in contributing to a state of allodynia (Minami *et al.*, 1995), is well established, and although firm data are not available it seems reasonable to propose that the increased production of NO within the CNS of the MS patient may contribute to painful sensations.

Certain studies have suggested that low concentrations of NO may in fact be antinociceptive, but the prevailing effect as NO concentrations are increased is to generate or intensify pain (Sousa and Prado, 2001). Low concentrations of NO have been suggested to reduce pain through a mechanism involving activation of guanylate cyclase, whilst higher concentrations, such as those anticipated in MS pathology, may intensify pain through a guanylate cyclase-independent pathway (Prado *et al.*, 2002).

NO inhibition and therapy

From the discussion above it might be predicted that the inhibition of NO production would improve neurophysiological function in EAE and MS, but the findings from studies in EAE have been confusing (Willenborg *et al.*, 1999) in that NOS inhibition can sometimes be beneficial and sometimes deleterious. Very broadly, it seems that iNOS inhibition in the periphery can be deleterious because it reduces the immunosuppressive actions of NO, whereas iNOS inhibition in the CNS can be beneficial because it reduces the toxic effects of NO on nerve tissue. However, this simple interpretation does not explain all the findings from experimental studies, and until the role of NO in MS is better understood iNOS inhibition in patients with MS may have unexpected consequences. Nonetheless it is interesting to note in this context that one of the many effects of IFN-β, a common therapy for MS, is an inhibition of the expression of iNOS (Hua *et al.*, 1998).

The role of nitric oxide in MS has recently been reviewed by Smith and Lassmann (2002).

Neuroelectric blocking factors

The possibility that factors circulating in the vasculature could cause conduction block was proposed in the 1960s, when it was reported in a small study that sera taken during an EAE or MS exacerbation could block neuroelectric activity in culture (Bornstein and Crain, 1965). Later studies confirmed that sera could block neuroelectric activity, but found that the effect was not specific to MS pathology and that it could also be shown with healthy sera. There appeared to be more than one blocking factor in human sera, and whilst some factors were thermolabile, others were heat stable, and yet others were complement-dependant (Seil *et al.*, 1976).

Interestingly, in an *in vitro* frog spinal cord model, Schauf and Davis (1981) demonstrated that the magnitude of neuroelectric block induced by sera from patients with MS correlated with disease activity, both between patients and over time in the same individuals. The same authors showed that plasmapheresis could reduce the ability of sera from patients with MS to block neuroelectric activity *in vitro*, although plasmapheresis evoked no clinical improvement in a small group of patients with progressive MS (Stefoski *et al.*, 1982). It has been suggested that plasmapheresis may have more relevance in certain MS subtypes than others, which may explain why Stefoski *et al.* (1982) saw no effect in their cohort of progressive MS (Bitsch and Bruck, 2002). The evidence for the efficacy of plasmapheresis in MS has been equivocal to date, perhaps for the same reason.

The range of different experimental techniques employed in the study of putative neuroelectric blocking factors has complicated the interpretation of the results. Studies have used both mammalian and non-mammalian preparations, and techniques ranging from *in vitro* isolated nerve preparations to tissue culture. The factors were also not precisely characterized, and sera were often tested with methods that actually measured effects on synaptic transmission, whilst the relevant literature deals with axonal conduction block. In fact, when sera described as having potent blocking activity were tested on myelinated and demyelinated axons, no effect was detected (Schauf and Davis, 1981). In summary, the role of neuroelectric blocking factors in MS remains unclear, but it is not unlikely that factors present in the vasculature could be deleterious to axonal conduction, particularly when axons are demyelinated (Smith, 1994).

QYNAD/endocaine

Some studies have demonstrated an effect of the cerebrospinal fluid (CSF) from patients with MS on the neuronal sodium current, using a variety of *in vitro* preparations (Brinkmeier *et al.*, 1993; Koller *et al.*, 1996). In particular Brinkmeier *et al.* (2000) have reported that a specific pentapeptide with potent sodium channel blocking activity has an increased expression in the CSF of patients with MS or Guillain–Barré syndrome (GBS; an inflammatory and often demyelinating disease of peripheral axons), versus controls. The pentapeptide has the amino acid sequence QYNAD and has been termed 'endocaine' because of the similarity of its channel blocking activity to local anaesthetics, such as lignocaine (lidocaine). Indeed, the effects of QYNAD at the levels detected in the CSF of MS patients (10–30 μM) are reportedly comparable to those of 50 μM lignocaine. A plasma concentration of only 10 μM lignocaine was able to provoke clinical symptoms in patients with MS (Sakurai et al., 1992) suggesting that, at the CSF concentrations reported, QYNAD would be likely to contribute to the symptoms of MS patients (Weber *et al.*, 2002).

Because QYNAD potentially plays a very important role in the symptomatology of inflammatory demyelinating disease it is especially concerning that a detailed subsequent study has failed to find evidence to support the initial observations, even when using QYNAD at higher concentrations (Cummins *et al.*, 2003)*.

Cytokines

We discuss the potential roles of individual cytokines below, but as noted earlier it is important to remember that cytokines are typically expressed as part of a cascade, and it may be that combinations of cytokines will exhibit effects that are different from the sum of their individual actions, or that their most important effects may be mediated by parts of the cascade that may not occur if the cytokines are studied in isolation. For example, combinations of pro-inflammatory cytokines, particularly TNF-α and IFN-γ, can act synergistically to result in the formation of iNOS and thence the release of NO, the potent effects of which have been discussed above.

TNF-α

TNF-α protein is found at higher levels in the CSF from MS patients than from controls with other neurological disease (Hauser *et al.*, 1990). Furthermore, in the lesions themselves, TNF-α mRNA is found in a significantly higher number of cells in active demyelinating lesions than in inactive lesions or controls (Bitsch *et al.*, 2000). Voltage-clamp studies of *Onchidium* neurons have demonstrated that both TNF-α and IL-1 can cause hyperpolarization by blocking sodium conductance and activating the sodium pump (Mimura *et al.*, 1994). If axons are similarly affected, the resulting hyperpolarization would be expected to impair conduction in demyelinated axons by reducing the safety factor.

A role for TNF-α in pain, perhaps through an effect on nociceptive fibres, has been proposed. Sorkin *et al.* (1997) found that, in an *in vitro* model, low concentrations of TNF-α increased impulse activity in normal, peripheral Aδ and C fibres. Consequently an effect of TNF-α may be the induction of a low rate of ectopic firing in nociceptive axons that could be perceived as pain, either directly or through wind-up in dorsal horn neurons. Higher TNF-α concentrations reduced firing in the same fibres (Sorkin *et al.*, 1997) and, in a separate study, intrathecal injection of either TNF-α or IL-1α was found to be analgesic (Bianchi *et al.*, 1992) suggesting that TNF-α may generate or ameliorate pain depending on the concentration present.

Interestingly, one putative MS therapy is a compound whose mode of action is thought to include an effect on TNF-α. Pentoxifylline is a phosphodiesterase inhibitor which has been shown to inhibit TNF-α production and to be active in EAE (Nataf et al., 1993).

IFN-γ

A role for IFN-γ in MS is indicated by the observations that IFN-γ mRNA is increased five-fold in whole blood samples taken during MS relapses compared with healthy controls (Kahl *et al.*, 2002), and that the administration of recombinant IFN-γ (rIFN-γ) to MS patients increases the frequency of exacerbations (Panitch et al., 1987). Interestingly, such exacerbations are clinically similar, if not identical, to those experienced previously in the disease

(Panitch *et al.*, 1987), a finding in common with the observations made following Campath-1H therapy (see section 'The severity of symptoms in MS can change rapidly').

IFN-γ has been reported to impair synaptic function by an inhibitory effect on the mechanisms of synaptic potentiation (both short and long-term: STP and LTP) (D'Arcangelo *et al.*, 1991). However, the very prompt onset of symptoms seen following Campath-1H therapy is not seen following the administration of rIFN-γ, perhaps indicating that, with regard to symptom production, IFN-γ might act synergistically with other immune mediators.

Interleukins

Interleukins 1 (IL-1) and 2 (IL-2) have the potential to affect neurophysiological function in MS since mRNA for both interleukins can be detected in tissue from the CNS of patients with MS (Woodroofe and Cuzner, 1993), and the production of IL-1β is known to be increased in active MS disease compared with inactive MS or controls with other neurological diseases (Hauser *et al.*, 1990). In voltage-clamp studies on *Onchidium* neurons IL-1 caused membrane hyperpolarization by both reducing the sodium conductance and activating the sodium pump (Mimura *et al.*, 1994), and it was shown to impair synaptic function in a brain-slice model by binding to a pre-synaptic site and activating a chloride conductance (Yu and Shinnick-Gallagher, 1994). IL-1α has also been shown to be analgesic when administered intrathecally to rats (Bianchi *et al.*, 1992).

IL-2 has been reported to have a direct inhibitory effect on sodium channels in muscle, suggesting that it may also inhibit sodium channels at other sites, and to impair transmission in central sensory afferents (Brinkmeier *et al.*, 1992; Park *et al.*, 1995). Therefore both IL-1 and IL-2 may affect either axonal conduction or synaptic transmission and, were they to do so in patients with MS, could have the inevitable consequences on neurophysiological function, as discussed in the section on 'How might immune mediators alter neurophysiological function?'.

Antibodies

Although there is little evidence for a direct effect of antibodies on neurophysiological function in MS, it is not unreasonable to suppose that such an effect might exist (Waxman, 1995). Indeed, antibodies were suggested to be the 'neuroelectric blocking factor' discussed above, although early studies did not identify either a likely antibody or antigen (Bornstein and Crain, 1965; Seil *et al.*, 1976). The intrathecal production of immunoglobulins is, however, increased in over 90% of patients with MS, including IgG, IgM,

IgD, and IgA; and IgG and IgM occur as oligoclonal bands in the CSF of MS patients (Cross *et al.*, 2001). A role for antibodies in impairing neurophysiological function is supported by the association of a more benign course of MS with the absence of oligoclonal bands, but the evidence is rather weak as the absence of these antibodies may be simply a consequence, not a cause, of the less aggressive disease process (Zeman *et al.*, 1996).

Antiganglioside antibodies (particularly anti-GM1) have been proposed in some (although not all) studies as potential modulators of conduction in GBS (Takigawa *et al.*, 1995), but the presence of anti-GM1 antibodies has not been reported in MS. In other non-MS models, antibodies have been shown to induce epileptiform activity when injected into the sensorimotor cortex of rats (Karpiak *et al.*, 1982), and to interfere with neuromuscular transmission, potentially resulting in symptoms of muscle weakness (Buchwald *et al.*, 2001). Thus the clear potential for antibodies to have diverse effects on neurophysiological function means that a direct action in MS would be unsurprising, albeit unidentified so far.

Glutamate

Among the plethora of compounds released by activated microglia and leucocytes are neurotransmitters, such as glutamate (Piani *et al.*, 1991). It seems likely that such release could have an adverse effect on function by binding to the receptors at which the transmitters normally exert their physiological effects. Indeed, blockade of the AMPA/KA type of glutamate receptor has been found to ameliorate the neurological signs of EAE by a pathway that was not simply a reduction in inflammation (Pitt *et al.*, 2000; Smith *et al.*, 2000b).

T lymphocytes, direct effects

As well as potentially exerting effects on neurophysiological function by the release of immune mediators, T lymphocytes may also directly affect axonal function. Yarom *et al.* (1983) found that the addition of T lymphocytes reactive to myelin basic protein (MBP) to isolated optic nerve could directly block axonal conduction. Interestingly the block was reversible if the period of block was less than 2 hr (see Fig. 17.2) and block did not occur when allogeneic optic nerve, or syngeneic peripheral nerve, was used. Underlying this effect is presumably an immune interaction between the T lymphocytes and CNS myelin antigens, although the precise mechanism is not known.

In addition to this reversible effect on axonal conduction, cytotoxic T lymphocytes have been reported to directly and selectively disrupt the cytoskeleton of neurites in murine neuronal cultures (Medana *et al.*, 2001). In

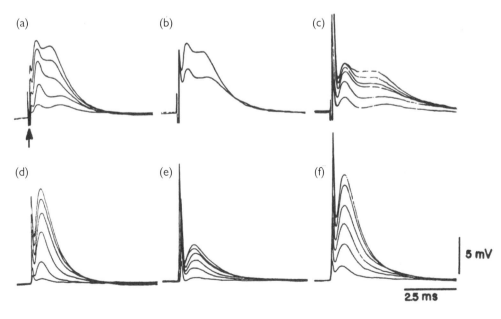

(a) (b) (c)

(d) (e) (f)

5 mV

2.5 ms

Fig. 17.2 Conduction block in isolated optic nerve mediated by exposure of the nerve to a T cell line specific for myelin basic protein. (a)–(c) Compound action potentials (CAPs) recorded before and after exposure to T cells. (a) CAPs in response to graded stimuli delivered before T-cell exposure. (b) CAPs in response to similar stimuli before and 40 min after T-cell exposure. (c) CAPs recorded in a similar way to (a) except they were recorded after exposure to T cells. The amplitude of the responses was significantly reduced by exposure to T cells. (d)–(f) Compound action potentials recorded from another nerve in response to graded stimuli delivered (d) before, (e) during (after 60 min) and (f) after exposure to T cells. (Reprinted from Yarom *et al.* (1983) by permission from *Nature*, copyright (1983) Macmillan Publishers Ltd.)

patients with MS such axonal degeneration would obviously result in a loss of neurophysiological function. Axonal degeneration in MS is reviewed in Chapter 14[†].

Mast cells

Although the role of mast cells in MS is not clear, it is known that mast cells are found in the CNS of patients with MS more frequently than in the CNS of controls (Toms *et al.*, 1990), and there is evidence that components of the mast cell's arsenal can affect neurophysiological function. Both 5-hydroxytryptamine (5-HT or serotonin) and histamine are released by mast cells and these agents can increase the permeability of the blood–brain barrier (Abbott, 2000), whilst 5-HT may also interfere with serotonergic transmission. Release of histamine from mast cells can affect NMDA receptors (Skaper *et al.*, 2001) which could presumably contribute to neurophysiological dysfunction by promoting excessive synaptic activity as well as promoting excitotoxicity. Mast cells are also able to express a variety of cytokines, the potential effects of some of which are discussed above.

It is interesting to note that mast cells can express a peripheral cannabinoid receptor (CB2) that, on binding its agonist, exerts a negative regulatory influence on mast cell activation (Facci *et al.*, 1995). Cannabinoids are potentially therapeutic in MS (Pertwee, 2002), and perhaps the mechanisms for this effect include a reduction in mast cell activation and thus a reduction in the release of mediators with potentially adverse neurophysiological effects. Alternatively, because the administration of cannabinoids to patients is most commonly associated with the relief of pain and spasticity, perhaps the effects are best explained by a direct action on the CNS.

Integrity of the blood–brain barrier

The effects of inflammation on the blood–brain barrier (BBB) have been comprehensively reviewed (Abbott, 2000; Ballabh *et al.*, 2004) so we will focus here on the potential consequences of BBB impairment on neurophysiological function.

The permeability of the brain endothelium increases in response to a variety of inflammatory mediators, including 5-HT, histamine, interleukins (IL-1, IL-1β, IL-2), and NO (Abbott, 2000). Correspondingly, lesions on MRI scans in patient with MS often show Gd-DTPA enhancement, demonstrating that BBB impairment is common in MS, because enhancement signals the increased leakage of Gd-DTPA from the vasculature. Once the BBB has been impaired it appears to be more sensitive to subsequent impairment (Hawkins *et al.*, 1991), a feature that may contribute to the effects produced by Campath-1H therapy, discussed earlier.

The composition of the extracellular fluid around central axons and neurons is normally finely regulated, but this delicate balance is lost upon disruption of the BBB, and this effect will be exacerbated if the normal buffering role of the glia is also perturbed. Indeed astrocyte numbers are known to be diminished in some lesions (Barnes *et al.*, 1991) and the loss of astrocytes in other circumstances has been shown to be deleterious for ion homeostasis, synaptic transmission, and neuron survival (Largo *et al.*, 1996). An alteration in the normal balance of sodium, potassium, and calcium ions can be expected and this is likely to affect neurophysiological function, for example by affecting the excitability of cells and perhaps evoking positive symptoms through the generation of ectopic impulses and the presence of ephaptic transmission (Smith and McDonald, 1999).

Breakdown of the BBB may also allow circulating factors (e.g. the putative neuroelectric blocking factors discussed above) to enter the CNS and exert their effect: in this way factors that are not necessarily immune mediators may have the opportunity to impair neurophysiological function.

Endnotes

[*] Since this chapter was written (early 2003) another publication has echoed the caution expressed by Cummins *et al.* (2003), as it found no effect of QYNAD on Nav1.6 and Nav1.8 sodium channels, or on axonal

conduction in rat sciatic nerve (Quasthoff *et al.*, 2003). However, yet other studies have found that QYNAD can affect at least Nav1.2 sodium channels (Meuth *et al.*, 2003; Padmashri *et al.*, 2004), although this channel subtype was amongst the types studied by Cummins *et al* (2003) and which QYNAD was found to have no effect on. The cause of this variability in effect remains unknown.

[†] Since submission of this chapter, Devaux and colleagues (Devaux *et al.*, 2003) have used a similar *in vitro* protocol to Yarom *et al.*, but they failed to reproduce the earlier findings, even though their T cells were able to induce lethal experimental autoimmune encephalomyelitis when applied *in vivo*. Devaux *et al.* concluded that other factors present in intact animals, bt not *in vitro*, were required to effect conduction block.

References

Abbott, N.J. (2000). Inflammatory mediators and modulation of blood-brain barrier permeability. *Cell Mol Neurobiol* **20**(2). 131–147.

Ahern, G.P., Hsu, S.F., and Jackson, M.B. (1999). Direct actions of nitric oxide on rat neurohypophysial K+ channels. *J Physiol* **520**(1): 165–176.

Ahern, G.P., Hsu, S.F., Klyachko, V.A., and Jackson, M.B. (2000). Induction of persistent sodium current by exogenous and endogenous nitric oxide. *J Biol Chem* **275**(37): 28810–28815.

Ballabh, P., Braun, A. and Nedergaard, M. (2004). The blood–brain barrier: an overview: structure, regulation, and clinical implications. *Neurobiol Dis* **16**: 1–13.

Barnes, D., Munro, P.M., Youl, B.D., Prineas, J.W., and McDonald, W.I. (1991). The longstanding MS lesion. a quantitative MRI and electron microscopic study. *Brain* **114**(3): 1271–1280.

Berger, T., Weerth, S., Kojima, K., Linington, C., Wekerle, H., and Lassmann, H. (1997). Experimental autoimmune encephalomyelitis: the antigen specificity of T lymphocytes determines the topography of lesions in the central and peripheral nervous system. *Lab Invest* **76**(3): 355–364.

Bianchi, M., Sacerdote, P., Ricciardi-Castagnoli, P., Mantegazza, P., and Panerai, A.E. (1992). Central effects of tumor necrosis factor alpha and interleukin-1 alpha on nociceptive thresholds and spontaneous locomotor activity. *Neurosci Lett* **148**(1–2): 76–80.

Bitsch, A. and Bruck, W. (2002). Differentiation of multiple sclerosis subtypes: implications for treatment. *CNS Drugs* **16**(6): 405–418.

Bitsch, A., Kuhlmann, T., Da Costa, C., Bunkowski, S., Polak, T., and Bruck, W. (2000). Tumour necrosis factor alpha mRNA expression in early multiple sclerosis lesions: correlation with demyelinating activity and oligodendrocyte pathology. *Glia* **29**(4): 366–375.

Bitsch, A., Wegener, C., Da Costa, C., Bunkowski, S., Reimers, C.D., Prange, H.W., *et al.* (1999). Lesion development in Marburg's type of acute multiple sclerosis: from inflammation to demyelination. *Mult Scler* **5**(3): 138–146.

Bo, L., Dawson, T.M., Wesselingh, S., Mork, S., Choi, S., Kong, P.A., *et al.* (1994). Induction of nitric oxide synthase in demyelinating regions of multiple sclerosis brains. *Ann Neurol* **36**(5): 778–786.

Bornstein, M.B. and Crain, S.M. (1965). Functional studies of cultured brain tissues as related to 'demyelinative disorders'. *Science* **148**: 1242–1244.

Borutaite, V., Budriunaite, A., and Brown, G.C. (2000). Reversal of nitric oxide-, peroxynitrite- and S-nitrosothiol-induced inhibition of mitochondrial respiration or complex I activity by light and thiols *Biochim Biophys Acta* **1459**(2–3): 405–412.

Brinkmeier, H., Kaspar, A., Wietholter, H., and Rudel, R. (1992). Interleukin-2 inhibits sodium currents in human muscle cells. *Pflugers Arch* **420**: 621–623.

Brinkmeier, H., Wollinsky, K.H., Seewald, M.J., Hulser, P.J., Mehrkens, H.H., Kornhuber, H.H., *et al.* (1993). Factors in the cerebrospinal fluid of multiple sclerosis patients interfering with voltage-dependent sodium channels. *Neurosci Lett* **156**(1–2): 172–175.

Brinkmeier, H., Aulkemeyer, P., Wollinsky, K.H., and Rudel, R. (2000). An endogenous pentapeptide acting as a sodium channel blocker in inflammatory autoimmune disorders of the central nervous system [see comments]. *Nat Med* **6**(7): 808–811.

Buchwald, B., Bufler, J., Carpo, M., Heidenreich, F., Pitz, R., Dudel, J., *et al.* (2001). Combined pre- and postsynaptic action of IgG antibodies in Miller Fisher syndrome. *Neurology* **56**(1): 67–74.

Coles, A.J., Wing, M.G., Molyneux, P., Paolillo, A., Davie, C.M., Hale, G., *et al.* (1999). Monoclonal antibody treatment exposes three mechanisms underlying the clinical course of multiple sclerosis. *Ann Neurol* **46**(3): 296–304.

Cross, A.H., Trotter, J.L., and Lyons, J. (2001). B cells and antibodies in CNS demyelinating disease. *J Neuroimmunol* **112**(1–2): 1–14.

Cummins, T.R., Renganathan, M., Stys, P.K., Herzog, R.I., Scarfo, K., Horn, R., *et al.* (2003). The pentapeptide QYNAD does not block voltage-gated sodium channels. *Neurology* **60**: 224–229.

D'Arcangelo, G., Grassi, F., Ragozzino, D., Santoni, A., Tancredi, V., and Eusebi, F. (1991). Interferon inhibits synaptic potentiation in rat hippocampus. *Brain Res* **564**: 245–248.

DeSousa, E.A., Albert, R.H., and Kalman, B. (2002). Cognitive impairments in multiple sclerosis: a review. *Am J Alzheimers Dis Other Demen* **17**(1): 23–29.

Devaux, J., Forni, C., Beeton, C., Barbaria, J., Beraud, E., Gola, M., *et al.* (2003). Myelin basic protein-reactive T-cells induce conduction failure in vivo but not in vitro. *Neuroreport* **14**: 317–320.

Facci, L., Dal Toso, R., Romanello, S., Buriani, A., Skaper, S.D., and Leon, A. (1995). Mast cells express a peripheral cannabinoid receptor with differential sensitivity to anandamide and palmitoylethanolamide. *Proc Natl Acad Sci USA* **92**(8): 3376–3380.

Felts, P.A. and Smith, K.J. (1992). Conduction properties of central nerve fibers remyelinated by Schwann cells. *Brain Res* **574**(1–2): 178–192.

Garthwaite, G., Goodwin, D.A., Batchelor, A.M., Leeming, K., and Garthwaite, J. (2002). Nitric oxide toxicity in CNS white matter: an *in vitro* study using rat optic nerve. *Neuroscience* **109**(1): 145–155.

Hauser, S.L., Doolittle, T.H., Lincoln, R., Brown, R.H., and Dinarello, C.A. (1990). Cytokine accumulations in CSF of multiple sclerosis patients: frequent detection of interleukin-1 and tumor necrosis factor but not interleukin-6. *Neurology* **40**(11): 1735–1739.

Hawkins, C.P., Mackenzie, F., Tofts, P., du Boulay, E.P., and McDonald, W.I. (1991). Patterns of blood–brain barrier breakdown in inflammatory demyelination. *Brain* **114**: 801–810.

Hua, L.L., Liu, J.S., Brosnan, C.F., and Lee, S.C. (1998). Selective inhibition of human glial inducible nitric oxide synthase by interferon-beta: implications for multiple sclerosis. *Ann Neurol* **43**(3): 384–387.

Jeffery, D.R., Absher, J., Pfeiffer, F.E., and Jackson, H. (2000). Cortical deficits in multiple sclerosis on the basis of subcortical lesions. *Mult Scler* **6**(1): 50–55.

Kahl, K.G., Kruse, N., Toyka, K.V., and Rieckmann, P. (2002). Serial analysis of cytokine MRNA profiles in whole blood samples from patients with early multiple sclerosis. *J Neurol Sci* **200**(1–2): 53–55.

Karpiak, S.E., Huang, Y.L., and Rapport, M.M. (1982). immunological model of epilepsy. epileptiform activity induced by fragments of antibody to GM1 ganglioside. *J Neuroimmunol* **3**(1): 15–21.

Kerlero de Rosbo, N., Bernard, C.C., Simmons, R.D., and Carnegie, P.R. (1985). Concomitant detection of changes in myelin basic protein and permeability of blood-spinal cord barrier in acute experimental autoimmune encephalomyelitis by electroimmunoblotting. *J Neuroimmunol* **9**: 349–361.

Kidd, D., Barkhof, F., McConnell, R., Algra, P.R., Allen, I.V., and Revesz, T. (1999). Cortical lesions in multiple sclerosis. *Brain* **122**(1): 17–26.

Koller, H., Buchholz, J., and Siebler, M. (1996). Cerebrospinal fluid from multiple sclerosis patients inactivates neuronal Na+ current. *Brain* **119**(2): 457–463.

Largo, C., Cuevas, P., Somjen, G.G., Martin del Rio, R., and Herreras, O. (1996). The effect of depressing glial function in rat brain in situ on ion homeostasis, synaptic transmission, and neuron survival. *J Neurosci* **16**(3): 1219–1229.

Lorentzen, J.C., Issazadeh, S., Storch, M., Mustafa, M.I., Lassman, H., Linington, C., *et al.* (1995). Protracted, relapsing and demyelinating experimental autoimmune encephalomyelitis in DA rats immunized with syngeneic spinal cord and incomplete Freund's adjuvant. *J Neuroimmunol* **63**(2): 193–205.

Mang, C.F. and Kilbinger, H. (2000). Modulation of acetylcholine release in the guinea-pig trachea by the nitric oxide donor, S-nitroso-N-acetyl-DL-denicillamine (SNAP). *Br J Pharmacol* **131**(1): 94–98.

Medana, I., Martinic, M.A., Wekerle, H., and Neumann, H. (2001). Transection of major histocompatibility complex class I-induced neurites by cytotoxic T lymphocytes. *Am J Pathol* **159**(3): 809–815.

Meuth, S.G., Budde, T., Duyar, H., Landgraf, P., Broicher, T., Elbs, M., *et al.* (2003). Modulation of neuronal activity by the endogenous pentapeptide QYNAD. *Eur J Neurosci* **18**: 2697–2706.

Mimura, Y., Gotow, T., Nishi, T., and Osame, M. (1994). Mechanisms of hyperpolarization induced by two cytokines, HTNF alpha and HIL-1 alpha in neurons of the mollusc, *Onchidium*. *Brain Res* **653**(1–2): 112–118.

Minami, T., Onaka, M., Okuda-Ashitaka, E., Mori, H., Ito, S., and Hayaishi, O. (1995). L-NAME, an inhibitor of nitric oxide synthase, blocks the established allodynia induced by intrathecal administration of prostaglandin E2. *Neurosci Lett* **201**(3): 239–242.

Moreau, T., Coles, A., Wing, M., Isaacs, J., Hale, G., Waldmann, H., *et al.* (1996). Transient increase in symptoms associated with cytokine release in patients with multiple sclerosis. *Brain* **119**(1): 225–237.

Nataf, S., Louboutin, J.P., Chabannes, D., Feve, J.R., and Muller, J.Y. (1993). Pentoxifylline inhibits experimental allergic encephalomyelitis. *Acta Neurol Scand* **88**(2): 97–99.

Oleszak, E.L., Zaczynska, E., Bhattacharjee, M., Butunoi, C., Legido, A., and Katsetos, C.D. (1998). Inducible nitric oxide synthase and nitrotyrosine are found in monocytes/macrophages and/or astrocytes in acute, but not in chronic, multiple sclerosis. *Clin Diagn Lab Immunol* **5**(4): 438–445.

Padmashri, R. Chakrabarti, K.S., Sahal, D., Mahalakshmi, R., Sarma, S.P. and Sikdar, S.K. (2004). Functional characterization of the pentapeptide QYNAD on rNav1.2 channels and its NMR structure. *Pflugers Arch* **447**: 895–907.

Panitch, H.S., Hirsch, R.L., Schindler, J., and Johnson, K.P. (1987). Treatment of multiple sclerosis with gamma interferon: exacerbations associated with activation of the immune system. *Neurology* **37**(7): 1097–1102.

Park, H.J., Won, C.K., Pyun, K.H., and Shin, H.C. (1995). Interleukin 2 suppresses afferent sensory transmission in the primary somatosensory cortex. *Neuroreport* **6**(7): 1018–1020.

Pender, M.P. (1986). Conduction block due to demyelination at the ventral root exit zone in experimental allergic encephalomyelitis. *Brain Res* **367**(1–2): 398–401.

Pertwee, R. (2002). Cannabinoids and multiple sclerosis. *Pharmacol Ther* **95**(2). 165–174.

Piani, D., Frei, K., Do, K.Q., Cuenod, M., and Fontana, A. (1991). Murine brain macrophages induced NMDA receptor mediated neurotoxicity *in vitro* by secreting glutamate. *Neurosci Lett* **133**(2): 159–162.

Pineda, J., Kogan, J.H., and Aghajanian, G.K. (1996). Nitric oxide and carbon monoxide activate locus coeruleus neurons through a CGMP-dependent protein kinase: involvement of a nonselective cationic channel. *J Neurosci* **16**(4): 1389–1399.

Pitt, D., Werner, P., and Raine, C.S. (2000). Glutamate excitotoxicity in a model of multiple sclerosis [see comments]. *Nat Med* **6**(1): 67–70.

Prado, W.A., Schiavon, V.F., and Cunha, F.Q. (2002). Dual effect of local application of nitric oxide donors in a model of incision pain in rats. *Eur J Pharmacol* **441**(1–2): 57–65.

Quasthoff, S., Pojer, C., Mori, A., Hofer, D., Liebmann, P., Kieseier, B.C., *et al.* (2003). No blocking effects of the pentapeptide QYNAD of Na+ channel subtypes expressed in *Xenopus* oocytes or action potential conduction in isolated rat sural nerve. *Neurosci Lett* **352**: 93–96.

Redford, E.J., Kapoor, R., and Smith, K.J. (1997). Nitric oxide donors reversibly block axonal conduction: demyelinated axons are especially susceptible. *Brain* **120**(12): 2149–2157.

Renganathan, M., Cummins, T.R., and Waxman, S.G. (2002). Nitric oxide blocks fast, slow, and persistent Na(+) channels in C-type DRG neurons by S-nitrosylation. *J Neurophysiol* **87**(2): 761–775.

Sakurai, M., Mannen, T., Kanazawa, I., and Tanabe, H. (1992). Lidocaine unmasks silent demyelinative lesions in multiple sclerosis. *Neurology* **42**(11): 2088–2093.

Schauf, C.L. and Davis, F.A. (1981). Circulating toxic factors in multiple sclerosis: a perspective. *Adv Neurol* **31**: 267–280.

Seil, F.J., Leiman, A.L., and Kelly, J.M. (1976). Neuroelectric blocking factors in multiple sclerosis and normal human sera. *Arch Neurol* **33**: 418–422.

Shrager, P., Custer, A.W., Kazarinova, K., Rasband, M.N., and Mattson, D. (1998). Nerve conduction block by nitric oxide that is mediated by the axonal environment. *J Neurophysiol* **79**(2): 529–536.

Skaper, S.D., Facci, L., Kee, W.J., and Strijbos, P.J. (2001). Potentiation by histamine of synaptically mediated excitotoxicity in cultured hippocampal
neurones: a possible role for mast cells. *J Neurochem* **76**(1): 47–55.

Smith, K.J. (1994). Conduction properties of central demyelinated and remyelinated axons, and their relation to symptom production in demyelinating
disorders. *Eye* **8**(2): 224–237.

Smith, K.J. and Lassmann, H. (2002). The role of nitric oxide in multiple sclerosis. *Lancet Neurol* **1**(4): 232–241.

Smith, K.J. and McDonald, W.I. (1999). The pathophysiology of multiple sclerosis: the mechanisms underlying the production of symptoms and the natural history of the disease. *Phil Trans R Soc Lond B Biol Sci* **354**(1390):
1649–1673.

Smith, K.J., Felts, P.A., and Kapoor, R. (1997). Axonal hyperexcitability: mechanisms and role in symptom production in demyelinating diseases.
The Neuroscientist **3**(4): 237–246.

Smith, K.J., Felts, P.A., and John, G.R. (2000*a*). Effects of 4-aminopyridine on
demyelinated axons, synapses and muscle tension. *Brain* **123**(1): 171–184.

Smith, T., Groom, A., Zhu, B., and Turski, L. (2000*b*). Autoimmune encephalomyelitis ameliorated by AMPA antagonists [see comments]. *Nat Med* **6**(1):
62–66.

Sorkin, L.S., Xiao, W.H., Wagner, R., and Myers, R.R. (1997). Tumour necrosis
factor-alpha induces ectopic activity in nociceptive primary afferent fibres.
Neuroscience **81**(1): 255–262.

Sousa, A.M. and Prado, W.A. (2001). The dual effect of a nitric oxide donor in
nociception. *Brain Res* **897**(1–2): 9–19.

Stefoski, D., Schauf, C.L., McLeod, B.C., Haywood, C.P., and Davis, F.A. (1982).
Plasmapheresis decreases neuroelectric blocking activity in multiple sclerosis. *Neurology* **32**(8): 904–907.

Takigawa, T., Yasuda, H., Kikkawa, R., Shigeta, Y., Saida, T., and Kitasato, H.
(1995). Antibodies against GM1 ganglioside affect K+ and Na+ currents in
isolated rat myelinated nerve fibers. *Ann Neurol* **37**(4): 436–442.

Tanuma, N., Shin, T., and Matsumoto, Y. (2000). Characterization of acute versus
chronic relapsing autoimmune encephalomyelitis in DA rats. *J Neuroimmunol* **108**(1–2): 171–180.

Toms, R., Weiner, H.L., and Johnson, D. (1990). Identification of IgE-positive
cells and mast cells in frozen sections of multiple sclerosis brains. *J Neuroimmunol* **30**(2–3): 169–177.

van Diemen, H.A., Polman, C.H., van Dongen, T.M., van Loenen, A.C., Nauta,
J.J., Taphoorn, M.J., *et al.* (1992). The effect of 4-aminopyridine on clinical
signs in multiple sclerosis: a randomized, placebo-controlled, double-blind,
cross-over study. *Ann Neurol* **32**(2): 123–130.

Waxman, S.G. (1995). Sodium channel blockade by antibodies: a new mechanism
of neurological disease? *Ann Neurol* **37**(4): 421–423.

Weber, F., Rudel, R., Aulkemeyer, P., and Brinkmeier, H. (2002). The endogenous
pentapeptide QYNAD induces acute conduction block in the isolated rat
sciatic nerve. *Neurosci Lett* **317**(1): 33–36.

Willenborg, D.O., Staykova, M.A., and Cowden, W.B. (1999). Our shifting understanding of the role of nitric oxide in autoimmune encephalomyelitis: a
review. *J Neuroimmunol* **100**(1–2): 21–35.

Woodroofe, M.N. and Cuzner, M.L. (1993). Cytokine MRNA expression in
inflammatory multiple sclerosis lesions: detection by non-radioactive in situ
hybridization. *Cytokine* **5**(6): 583–588.

Yarom, Y., Naparstek, Y., Lev-Ram, V., Holoshitz, J., Ben Nun, A., and Cohen, I.R.
(1983). Immunospecific inhibition of nerve conduction by T lymphocytes
reactive to basic protein of myelin. *Nature* **303**(5914): 246–247.

Youl, B.D., Turano, G., Miller, D.H., Towell, A.D., MacManus, D.G., Moore, S.G.,
et al. (1991). The pathophysiology of acute optic neuritis. an association of
gadolinium leakage with clinical and electrophysiological deficits. *Brain* **114**:
2437–2450.

Yu, B. and Shinnick-Gallagher, P. (1994). Interleukin-1 beta inhibits synaptic
transmission and induces membrane hyperpolarization in amygdala neurons.
J Pharmacol Exp Therap **271**: 590–600.

Zeman, A.Z., Kidd, D., McLean, B.N., Kelly, M.A., Francis, D.A., Miller, D.H.,
et al. (1996). A study of oligoclonal band negative multiple sclerosis. *J Neurol
Neurosurg Psychiatry* **60**(1): 27–30.

18 Multiple sclerosis—immune-directed therapy

Bernhard Hemmer, Olaf Stüve, Bernd C. Kieseier, and Hans-Peter Hartung

Multiple sclerosis (MS) is a chronic inflammatory and demyelinating disease of the central nervous system (CNS). Although the immune system is certain to play an important role in the pathogenesis of disease, specific pathways and target antigens are still uncertain. However, recent studies have added to our understanding of the disease process, broadening our view on possible scenarios for disease initiation and progression. Here we review the role of the immune system in the manifestation and progression of MS and discuss different pathogenetic concepts. Based on these considerations we review immunomodulatory therapies, some of which have proved effective and others that have failed in clinical trials. Furthermore, we discuss future immune-directed treatment strategies, which are currently being explored in pre-clinical and clinical studies.

Introduction

MS was first described almost 150 years ago. Since shortly after the early histopathological descriptions, the presence of immune cells, antibodies, and immune mediators at the site of CNS damage led clinicians and scientists to believe that the immune system may play a crucial role in the disease process. Within the last decades the first immune-directed therapies have been developed which proved to be efficient, at least during the early, inflammatory phase of the disease. To understand how these therapies may act in MS, and to rationally design future therapies, an intimate knowledge of the etiology and pathogenesis of MS is required.

Pathogenetic basis for immune intervention strategies

Immunopathology of the MS lesion

MS is a heterogeneous disorder, in which predominantly, but not exclusively, myelinated areas of the brain and spinal cord are affected. Most lesions are periventricularly located around small blood vessels (Lassmann et al., 1998). In acute MS lesions, demyelination, activation of microglia, and infiltration of immune cells are the key features. These infiltrates mostly consist of T cells, B cells, and macrophages. Eosinophilic granulocytes are sometimes found, whereas other immune cells such as granulocytes, γ/δ T cells or natural killer (NK) T cells are largely absent from lesions. Among different T-cell phenotypes, CD8+ T cells seem to outnumber CD4+ T cells in the parenchyma. CD4+ T cells are found more frequently in cuffs and meninges (Gay et al., 1997). In line with this observation, CD8+ T cells in the lesion and cerebrospinal fluid (CSF) are more often due to clonal expansion than CD4+ T cells (Babbe et al., 2000; Jacobsen et al., 2002). Similarly, clonal expansion of B cells occurs within the tissue lesions and CSF of MS patients (summarized in Cross et al. (2001)). Intrathecally produced antibodies in MS consist predominantly of immunoglobulin (Ig)G1 and IgG3 isotypes, suggesting that the humoral immune response targets protein antigens (Losy et al., 1990). A large number of different lymphokines are expressed in acute lesions including T helper 1 (Th1) and T helper 2 (Th2) cytokines, as well as a broad range of chemokines (Cannella and Raine, 1995; Baranzini et al., 2000).

Acute lesions seem to differ significantly with regard to their composition between individual patients (Lassmann et al., 2001). Work performed by Lucchinetti and co-workers suggests that at least four distinct pattern of acute demyelinating lesions are found (Lucchinetti et al., 2000). These patterns are primarily defined by oligodendrocyte pathology, the extent of remyelination, and immunopathological features. Two particular patterns are most prevalent, one characterized by significant antibody deposits and remyelination, the other by oligodendrocyte loss without remyelination. Furthermore, Devic's disease, an acute fulminant form of CNS demyelination that affects primarily the optic nerve and the cervical spinal cord, seems to be distinct from the other four histopathological patterns in that it is characterized by eosinophilic infiltration and extensive antibody deposits (Lucchinetti et al., 2002). Together with the variable clinical findings, these histopathological studies further suggest heterogeneity in the pathogenesis of MS.

Although Charcot observed axonal loss in his early histopathological description of MS, the notion that neurodegeneration may occur relatively early during the course of disease is relatively recent (Trapp et al., 1998). In acute lesions, the extent of axonal damage correlates with inflammation, especially the infiltration of macrophages and CD8+ T cells. This observation may suggest that both cell types are directly involved in neurodegeneration (Bitsch et al., 2000). However, neurodegeneration may sometimes occur in the absence of inflammation even in early lesions, raising the possibility of additional immune-independent mechanisms of neurodegeneration (Barnett and Prineas, 2004).

Compared with acute MS lesions, significantly less is known about the immunology of the chronic active or silent lesions. Chronic active lesions are characterized by ongoing inflammation, demyelination, and neurodegeneration. The extent of inflammation is usually less pronounced than in acute lesions. Gliosis and permanent neuronal and oligodendroglial damage dominate in the silent lesions with little evidence of cellular infiltrates and activation of immune mediators (Prineas et al., 2001).

Current concepts of disease pathogenesis

Based on findings in genetic, epidemiological, and experimental studies, three major components may underlie the disease pathogenesis in MS, either in individually or in concert (Hemmer et al., 2002). These include a primary autoimmune, an infectious, or a primary neurodegenerative etiology of MS. Considering the clinical and pathological heterogeneity of this disorder, it seems possible that the primary cause may vary between patients, and that more than one mechanism may be operative in individual patients during the course of the disease.

Autoimmune hypothesis

The focus of the immune response in MS is the myelinated areas of the CNS. The observation that there are striking clinical and histopathological similarities to acute disseminated encephalomyelitis following the administration of live rabies vaccine contaminated with CNS tissue further suggests an underlying autoimmune process. Basic immune mechanisms in CNS inflammation have been studied in the experimental autoimmune encephalomyelitis (EAE) model of MS. In this model, immunization of animals with myelin antigens, or adoptive transfer of CNS antigen-specific encephalitogenic T cells, leads to acute or chronic demyelinating encephalomyelitis (Wekerle *et al.*, 1994). Based on findings in the EAE model, the concept of molecular mimicry was established: T cells which may initially respond to an infectious agent and later cross-react with structurally homologous myelin antigens in the CNS cause acute damage (Wucherpfennig and Strominger, 1995; Hemmer *et al.*, 1997; Fujinami and Oldstone, 1985). The release of antigens from the brain further perpetuates the autoimmune response by recruiting additional immune cells, which eventually leads to chronic CNS inflammation (Lehmann *et al.*, 1993; Vanderlugt and Miller, 2002). In the EAE model, CD4+ myelin-specific T cells secreting Th1 cytokines are the main mediator of the autoimmune disease (Zamvil and Steinman, 1990). Under certain conditions, however, autoreactive CD8+ T cells can also cause an inflammatory disease of the CNS, which is characterized by massive neuronal and oligodendroglial damage (Huseby *et al.*, 2001; Sun *et al.*, 2001). Myelin-specific antibodies seem to enhance the disease process and particularly play a role in the chronic disease phase (Linington *et al.*, 1988). In EAE, several encephalitogenic myelin epitopes have been identified, which are often strain-specific and MHC-restricted (Kuchroo *et al.*, 2002). In humans, the situation is less clear. Although T cells specific for different myelin antigens are found in MS patients, a clear correlation between the frequency and function of myelin-specific T cells and disease onset or progression has not been established (Martin *et al.*, 1992). However, a recent study suggested that activation of myelin-specific T cells during therapy with altered peptide ligands (APLs) that mimic myelin peptide may be associated with disease activity in some MS patients (Bielekova *et al.*, 2000).

Infectious disease hypothesis

Infectious agents can cause acute and chronic inflammatory disorders of the CNS. In humans, infection with HTLV-1 or measles virus is associated with chronic neurological disease (Stohlman and Hinton, 2001). The occurrence of MS epidemics (e.g. on the Faeroe Islands), the epidemiological differences in ethnically homogeneous populations, the impact of migration on susceptibility, and the association of viral infection with relapses argue for the role of one or several infectious agents in the pathogenesis of MS (Sibley *et al.*, 1985; Hammond *et al.*, 1988; Kurtzke, 2000). This view was further strengthened by findings in infectious animal models. In mice, several viruses induce inflammatory demyelination, among them the mouse hepatitis virus (MHV) and Theiler's virus (TMEV) (Stohlman and Hinton, 2001; Haring and Perlman, 2001). In both models, viral infection of the CNS is required. In contrast to the autoimmune models, the immune response in these infectious encephalomyelitides is beneficial to the host in that it initially prevents a fatal outcome. In MHV and TMEV infection, cytolytic activity of the CD8+ T cells and release of interferon-gamma (IFN-γ) are crucial for partially containing the virus. CD4+ T cells are also important, but their detailed role during acute MHV and TMEV infection has still not been defined. During the subacute and chronic phase of disease, the humoral immune response is essential to control virus replication (Ramakrishna *et al.*, 2002). Although the immune response is crucial for controlling viral replication it also contributes to CNS damage. Likewise, MHV-induced demyelination does not occur in immunosuppressed animals or IFN-γ knockout mice. A similar observation was made in experimental Borna virus infection of the CNS, which in itself causes few clinical symptoms, as long as the immune response is suppressed or tolerized (Carbone *et al.*, 2001). Mounting an immune response, however, results in rapid development of inflammatory disease of the CNS and clinical symptoms. Therefore, although the immune system is important to clear or control infection of the CNS it can also contribute to tissue injury. The damage induced by the immune system may even exceed the damage induced by the pathogen and immunosuppression is a strongly advocated therapeutic option in this model.

Many features of the animal models reflect findings in MS, but the role of a specific infectious agent in the pathogenesis of MS has not been established. For decades, researchers have been looking for a causative infectious agent in MS leading to a long list of possible candidates. However, thus far it has been impossible to establish a definite association between any particular agent and MS.

Neurodegeneration hypothesis

Inflammation is not exclusively seen in infection and autoimmunity but also following any traumatic or degenerative tissue damage in the nervous system. This view, established in the animal models, has promoted the idea that the primary event in MS could be a neurodegenerative process followed by an inadequate response of the immune system at the site of neurodegeneration. The extensive neurodegeneration observed in active MS lesions further supports this view (Trapp *et al.*, 1998; Bitsch *et al.*, 2000). The role of the immune response in neurodegenerative disease models is less defined than its role in autoimmune or infectious models. Depending on the model, the immune system can add to the damage or even play a neuroprotective role by actively supporting neuroregeneration (Moalem *et al.*, 1999; Jones *et al.*, 2004). This view is not only supported by animal models in which autoreactive T cells can protect from secondary neurodegeneration but also the observation that T cells in MS lesions can release neurotrophins which are possibly important for neuroregeneration (Kerschensteiner *et al.*, 1999; Stadelmann *et al.*, 2002).

Although this concept fits some of the features of MS, a deregulated immune system needs to be present that explains the extent of inflammatory responses in MS lesions. In contrast to autoimmune models, the immune response in primary degenerative models may have quite distinct functions, which may even include neuroprotective and neuroregenerative properties.

For the development of immunomodulatory therapies it is essential to keep in mind that we still do not know which model best reflects the human disease. Therapies which work in one of the models may be detrimental in others. Each therapy based on the wrong concept may fail or even worsen the course of MS. Even when the disease is mainly immune-mediated continuous immunosuppression may not be appropriate since it may lead to selection of autoreactive immunocompetent cells (King *et al.*, 2004).

Status of immunomodulatory treatment in MS

Within the last decade, MS treatment options have changed dramatically. With the introduction of interferon-beta (IFN-β), the first therapy was established which affects relapse rates and MRI changes in MS patients (Paty and Li, 1993; IFNB Multiple Sclerosis Study Group, 1993). So far, three immunomodulatory therapies have been approved by European, US, and other drug administrations for use in relapsing–remitting and relapsing–progressive MS. In contrast, many other promising drugs failed in clinical trials.

Approved treatments

IFN-β

Interferons were initially introduced for treatment in MS due to their antiviral properties. The first trial with IFN-γ was stopped when a large number of relapses occurred following treatment (Panitch *et al.*, 1987a). Based on positive treatment effects observed in small trials, IFN-β was tested in a large phase III trial. The drug not only reduced the frequency of relapses but also had dramatic effects on the MRI changes including reduction of contrast-enhancing lesions and T_2 lesion load (IFNB Multiple Sclerosis Study Group, 1993; Paty and Li, 1993). Since then a number of excellent clinical trials have been performed with IFN-β using different application schemes and doses as well as preparations (Table 18.1) (Jacobs *et al.*, 1996; European Study Group on Interferon beta-1b in Secondary Progressive MS, 1998; PRISMS

Table 18.1 Immune-directed therapies with evidence from class I and II studies. The results of all class I and II trials with drugs which have proved efficacy in MS. The studies and results are displayed according to the review published by O'Connor (2002). The grading of the studies (quality) was performed following the guidelines of Goodin et al. (2002). The outcome grading was A = active, B = probably active, C = possibly active, D = inactive (conflicting). Numbers needed to treat (NNT) for 1 year are displayed for the primary outcome measurement. Gradings for secondary outcomes are displayed in parenthesis.

Phase	Substance	Dose/application	EDSS/duration	Primary endpoint	Secondary endpoint	Quality	Outcome (NNT)	Ref	RR	Prog	MRI	Reference
Clinical isolated syndrome	IFN-β1a (Avonex®)[a]	30 µg IM 1/week vs placebo	0/18 months	Development of CDMS	MRI parameters	Class I	A, 20.1	Not done	(A)			Jacobs et al. (2000)
	IFN-β1a (Rebif®)[a]	22 µg SC 1/week vs placebo	0/2 yr	Development of CDMS	MRI parameters	Class I	A, 18.2	Not done	(A)			Clanet et al. (2002)
Relapsing–remitting MS	IFN-β1b (Betaseron®)[a]	1.6/8 MIU SC vs placebo	0–5.5/2 yr	Annual relapse rate, proportion of relapse free patients	MRI parameters	Class I	A, –/4.6	Not done	(A)			IFNB Multiple Sclerosis Study Group (1993), Paty et al. (1993)
	IFN-β1a (Avonex®)[a]	30 µg IM 1/week vs placebo	1–3.5/2 yr	Time to confirmed progression	Relapse rate, MRI parameters	Class I	(A)	A, 15.7	(A)			Jacobs et al. (1996)
	IFN-β1a (Rebif®)[a]	22/44 µg SC 3/week vs placebo	0–5/2–4 yr	Annual relapse rate	Time to confirmed progression, MRI parameters	Class I	A, 4.6/4.8	(A), (18/24)	(A)			SPECTRIMS Study Group (2001), PRISMS Study Group (1998)
	Glatiramer acetate (Copaxone®)[a]	20 mg SC once daily vs placebo	0–5.5/2 yr	Annual relapse rate	MRI parameters[d]	Class I	A, 5.4	Not done	(A)			Johnson et al. (1995), Comi et al. (2001a)
	IFN-β1b (Betaseron®) vs IFN-β1a (Avonex®)	8 MIU SC every second day vs 30 µg IM 1/week	1–3.5/24 wk	Numbers of patients who remained relapse free	Time to confirmed progression, MRI parameters	Class III (clinics). Class I (MRI)	(A), (7)	(A)	A			Duda et al. (2000)
	IFN-β1a (Rebif®) vs IFN-β1a (Avonex®)	44 µg SC 3/week vs 30 µg IM 1/week	0–5.5/2 yr	Numbers of patients who remained relapse free	–	(Class I)	(A), 10	Not done	(A)			Panitch et al. (2002)
	IFN-β1a (Avonex®)	30 vs 60 µg IM 1/week	3.5–6.5/2 yr	Change in MSFC	Annual relapse rate	(Class I)	(A)	(B)	n.a.			Carbone et al. (2001)
Secondary progressive MS	Mitoxantrone (Novantrone®)[b]	5/12 mg/m² IV vs placebo every 3 months	3–6/2 yr	Composite index (EDSS, AI, relapses)	Annual relapse rate, MRI parameters	(Class II)	(A)	B	(A)			Hartung et al. (2002)
	IFN-β1a (Rebif®)	22/44 µg SC z3/week vs placebo	3–6.5/3 yr	Time to confirmed progression	Annual relapse rate, MRI parameters	Class I	(A)	C	(A)			Once Weekly Interferon for MS Study Group (1999)
	IFN-β1b (Betaferon®)[c]	8 MIU SC vs placebo	3–6.5/3 yr	Time to confirmed progression	Annual relapse rate, MRI parameters	Class I	(A)	A, 27.6	(A)			European Study Group on Interferon Beta-1b in Secondary Progressive MS (1998)
	IFN-β1b (Betaseron®)	5/8 MIU SC vs placebo	3–6.5/3 yr	Time to confirmed progression	Annual relapse rate, MRI parameters	Class I	(A)	D	(A)			–

IM, intramuscular; SC, subcutaneous, RR, relapse rate; Prog, progression; MRI, MRI parameters; Ref, Reference; AI, ambulation index.

[a]Drugs are approved for this indication.
[b]Approved also for worsening or progressive relapsing MS.
[c]Only in Europe.
[d]MRI was studied in a second trial (Comi et al., 2001a).

Study Group, 1998; Once Weekly Interferon for MS Study Group, 1999; Jacobs *et al.*, 2000; Secondary Progressive Efficacy Clinical Trial of Recombinant Interferon-beta-1a in MS (SPECTRIMS) Study Group, 2001; PRISMS Study Group and the University of British Columbia MS/MRI Analysis Group, 2001; Comi *et al.*, 2001*a*; Panitch *et al.*, 2002; Durelli *et al.*, 2002; Clanet *et al.*, 2002). Most studies have demonstrated that interferons significantly decrease relapse rates and inflammatory MRI changes throughout the disease course. This suggests that the treatment interferes with the inflammatory component of the disease. Recently, several trials have addressed the question of dose and application of interferons (Panitch *et al.*, 2002; Durelli *et al.*, 2002). Although different modes of application cannot be studied in double-blinded trials, these studies suggest that frequent application of interferons may have beneficial effects on relapse rates and MRI changes. How much dose influences disease activity is still controversial. In the PRISMS trial an impact of higher dose was seen (PRISMS Study Group and the University of British Columbia MS/MRI Analysis Group, 2001a), whereas no significant differences were seen with different doses of IFN-β once weekly (Clanet *et al.*, 2002). Finally, recent studies also demonstrate that some patients develop neutralizing antibodies which may interfere with treatment efficacy (Rice, 2001; Bertolotto *et al.*, 2002; Sorensen *et al.*, 2003).

Although disease progression seems to be influenced by IFN-β in some of the studies, the effects during a 2-year observation period are at best marginal. At present it seems that interferons do not have any measurable effects on the disease course when progression occurs in the absence of clinical relapses. The findings of the interferon trials were recently reviewed and the results of the review are summarized in Table 18.1 (O'Connor, 2002).

Although the impact of IFN-β on inflammation in MS is evident, the mode of action is still not understood. In principle, IFN-β has known antiviral and immunomodulatory properties (Yong, 2002). The antiviral effects include inhibition of viral protein synthesis, increase of major histocompatibility complex (MHC) Class I expression and induction of Mx proteins. The immunomodulatory effects include increased production of a variety of cytokines, inhibition of matrix metalloproteinases and inhibition of antiapoptotic proteins. Thus, the possible mechanisms of action of interferons do not allow us to draw conclusions about the pathogenesis of MS.

Glatiramer acetate

Glatiramer actetate (GA) was initially developed to target myelin-specific T cells. The drug is composed of large random polypeptides based on the four amino acids which are most prevalent in CNS myelin (alanine, lysine, glutamic acid, tyrosine). The drug proved efficacy in the EAE model. After several small trials in MS patients, the positive impact of GA on relapse rates was demonstrated in a large phase III trial (Johnson *et al.*, 1995) (Table 18.1). A positive impact on MRI activity was found in a recent trial. In comparison to IFN-β, the impact of GA on MRI seems less pronounced and delayed (Comi *et al.*, 2001*b*). So far, no study has addressed whether GA therapy influences long-term progression in MS.

The mode, how GA influences disease activity in MS, is at present not completely understood. Initially, based on findings in the EAE model, it was believed that the drug directly acts on myelin-specific T cells in MS. Immunization with the polypeptides also leads to the generation and expansion of GA-specific T cells. These T cells, which secrete Th2 cytokines, are believed to cross-react with myelin antigens and mediate anti-inflammatory activity when encountering myelin antigens (Neuhaus *et al.*, 2000; Duda *et al.*, 2000; Gran *et al.*, 2000). This view, however, is questioned by the observation that GA is also efficient in other inflammatory disease models (i.e. uveoretinitis models), in which myelin antigens are not present at the site of inflammation.

Alternatively, GA may interfere with antigen presentation due to its high binding affinity to several HLA molecules including the MS-associated HLA-DR2 alleles (Fridkis-Hareli *et al.*, 1999). More recently GA was shown to restore CD8+ T-cell responses with possible immunoregulatory properties (Karandikar *et al.*, 2002). Furthermore, recent *in vivo* findings suggest that GA may also have neuroprotective properties. Likewise, administration

of the drug inhibits secondary neurodegeneration in the axotomy model (Kipnis *et al.*, 2000). Given many other possible mechanisms for how GA may influence disease activity (Weber *et al.*, 2004; Aharoni *et al.*, 2003; Jung *et al.*, 2004), it is difficult to envision which of the possible mechanisms is responsible for the clinical activity of the drug.

Mitoxantrone

Recently, mitoxantrone, an antineoplastic drug that inhibits T cells, B cells, and monocytes, was studied for its efficacy in progressive MS using a modern trial design (Hartung *et al.*, 2002). In patients with frequent relapses or secondary progressive MS, mitoxantrone significantly decreased relapse rates and MRI changes (Table 18.1). In addition, a positive effect was observed for the primary endpoint, although an unconventional combined outcome measurement was used to determine disease progression. Given the fact that most of the secondary endpoints measuring clinical progression were positive in this trial, it is likely that mitoxantrone influences disease progression at least within the 2-year observation period. Similar to interferons, the impact on disease progression is at best marginal.

Although we do not know whether mitoxantrone has additional immunomodulatory properties it is certainly a powerful immunosuppressant. The positive treatment effects obtained with this drug suggest that immunosuppression in certain instances has a positive influence on disease activity, supporting the view that the immune system at least contributes to the damage in MS.

Alternative treatment strategies (as opposed to approved therapies)

Immunomodulatory drugs

Intravenous immunoglobulins (IV Ig) have been widely used for therapy of neuroimmunological diseases. The mode of action of IV Ig is still unclear. Several early and long-term effects are considered, such as blockade of Fc receptors, neutralization of circulating antibodies, or increased clearance of immune complexes. Which of these plays a role in the treatment of neurological disease is still unknown. IV Ig have also been used in MS, although their therapeutic efficacy is still controversial. While one study in patients with relapsing–remitting MS reported a positive impact on relapse rates, the larger ESIMS study in secondary progressive patients did show any treatment response in all primary and secondary outcome measures (Fazekas *et al.*, 1997). At present a large trial in relapsing–remitting MS is needed to clarify the role of IV Ig in the treatment of MS.

Immunosuppressive drugs

Immunosuppressants have been widely used in MS for more than two decades. Initially, based on small studies, azathioprine, cyclosporine, methotrexate, and cyclophosphamide were introduced for the treatment of MS (Rudge *et al.*, 1989; Canadian Cooperative Multiple Sclerosis Study Group, 1991; Yudkin *et al.*, 1991; Ellison *et al.*, 1994; Goodkin *et al.*, 1995, 1996). Larger studies that set out to evaluate the effectiveness of these drugs were conducted in the early 1990s, often using trial designs that do not adhere to current trial standards, and only partially provided conclusive results. Most of the drugs influenced relapse rates but did not show major impact on disease progression. MRI data are not available for most of these substances.

Failed treatment strategies

Immunosuppressants

Newer immunosuppressants have been tested in larger trials including MRI. Except mitoxantrone, all these drugs failed either due inefficacy (paclitaxel, sulfasalzine, desoxyspergualin, cladribine) or due to side-effects (linomide) (Table 18.2). Given these findings, it is unlikely that solely immunosuppressive drugs will have a major impact on long-term prognosis of MS.

Table 18.2 Failed immune-directed therapies. Therapies, which have failed in clinical trials or were discontinued due to side-effects

Mechanism	Substance	Brand name	Proposed mechanism	Study	Impact on MS	Reason of failure
Immunosuppression	Paclitaxel	PAXCEED	Immunosuppression	II	No significant effect	Inefficiency
	Linomide	Roquinimex	Inhibition of IFN-β and TNF-α	III	Positive effects on clinical and MRI parameters	Cardiopulmonary side-effects
	Sulfasalazine	–	Anti-inflammatory	III	No effect after 2 years	Inefficiency
	Desoxyspergualine	Gusperimus	Immunosuppressive agent probably affecting predominantly	III	No significant effect on relapse rates	Inefficiency
	Cladribine	–	Inhibition of lymphocytes	III	Clinically no effect (possible MR effects)	Inefficiency
Immunomodulation	Soluble TNF receptor	Lenercept	Accelerates elimination of TNF-α receptor	III	Increased exacerbation rate	May have negative effect on disease activity
	MAb against TNF-α	Infliximab	Accelerates elimination of TNF-α	I	Increased MRI activity	May have negative effect on disease activity
	TGF-β2	–	Inhibitory and modulatory effects on immune cells	II	No significant effect	Renal side-effects
	IL-10	–	Stimulates B-cell growth and differentiation, inhibits T-cell responses	I	No significant effect	Side-effects
	IL-4	BAY36–1677	Promotes Th2 T-cell response and Ig isotype switch	I	No significant effect	Inefficiency
	CD40L	IDEC-131	Inhibits B cell help by CD4 T cells	II	No significant effect	Renal side-effects
Specific immune intervention	Altered peptide ligand	Tiplimotide	Alteration of myelin-specific T cells, induction of immunomodulatory APL-specific T cells	II	3 patients worsened	May have negative effect on disease activity
	Altered peptide ligand	Tiplimotide		II	No significant effect on relapse rate or MRI	Skin reactions
	T-cell vaccination	–	Induction of immune responses against MBP-specific T cells	II	No significant effect	Inefficiency
	Oral myelin	AI-100	Tolerance induction of myelin-specific T cells, bystander suppression	III	No significant effect	Inefficiency
	Soluble DR2: MBP complexes	AG284	Anergy induction of MHC-specific T cells	I	No significant effect	Inefficiency
	TCR peptide vaccination	ATM-027	Suppression of T cells with TCRBV5 expression	II	No significant effect	Inefficiency

TNF, tumor necrosis factor; IFN, interferon; MBP, myelin basic protein; MAb, monoclonal antibody; TCR, T-cell receptor.

Cytokines and their modulators

Based on many findings in the EAE models, immunomodulatory drugs were considered highly promising during the last decade. In most EAE models disease is mediated by a Th1 T-cell response. Inhibition of pro-inflammatory (e.g. tumor necrosis factor-α (TNF-α)) and Th1 cytokines (e.g. IFN-γ) positively influences the course of EAE. In contrast, administration of Th2 cytokines exhibits positive effects in EAE. Application of this concept to the human disease was strongly supported by the initial IFN-γ study, which demonstrated that exogenous administration of the Th1 cytokine exacerbates MS (Table 18.2) (Panitch et al., 1987b). These observations prompted several studies in MS patients mainly targeting TNF-α or driving the immune response from Th-1 to Th-2. Surprisingly, two drugs inhibiting TNF-α or its receptor exacerbated MS (Lenercept Multiple Sclerosis Study Group and The University of British Columbia MS/MRI Analysis Group, 1999). Similarly, administration of cytokines with Th2 or anti-inflammatory activity such as IL-4, IL-10, or transforming growth factor-beta2 (TGF-β2) was not successful either due to side-effects (IL-10), inefficiency (IL-4), or both (TGF-β2). Although all the cytokine modulators were only tested in relatively small MRI-controlled trials with a short treatment phase it is quite likely that the drugs do not have a major positive impact on disease activity. Why these drugs failed is still not understood. However, these studies clearly pointed out that therapies which ameliorate EAE may not only be infective but may also exhibit opposite effects in MS.

Specific immune intervention

With major progress in basic immunology, specific modulation of antigen-specific T cells became an attractive approach to the treatment of chronic inflammatory diseases. Elegant studies in EAE demonstrated that disease can be ameliorated by selective elimination or functional alteration of encephalitogenic T cells. These strategies included oral administration of myelin antigens, immunization with altered peptide ligands, random peptide mixtures (such as GA), and application of soluble HLA–peptide complexes. Alternatively, immunization with myelin-specific T cells or T-cell receptor peptides thereof was performed to raise an immune response against the autoreactive T cells. When these antigen or T-cell based therapies were applied to humans, none of the substances, except GA, had a significant impact on disease activity. Moreover, administration of an APL peptide seemed to exacerbate disease in single patients although a general negative effect of the drug was not confirmed in second phase III trial (Bielekova *et al.*, 2000; Kappos *et al.*, 2000). The reason why all these highly specific approaches failed is uncertain. Limited access of the drug to the immune system, the wrong timing, an inadequate dose, and the wrong target antigen are possible explanations. On the other hand, these studies also raise questions about the autoimmune hypothesis on which all these approaches were based.

Future perspective

General considerations

Two main strategies will dominate the next years in the development of immune-directed therapies. One will be the combination of established therapies similar to strategies which have been successfully applied in cancer therapy. Indeed a number of phase II and III trials are under way which are investigating whether the combination of immunomodulatory drugs (i.e. interferons or GA) with immunosuppressive agents provides an advantage over single treatment regimes. Although this may enhance therapeutic potency in MS, it is unlikely that such combination therapies will have a major impact on disease progression. Therefore it is necessary that

new drugs are developed and tested in clinical trials. All new treatment strategies, however, face the problem that the etiology of MS and its pathogenetic pathways are uncertain. Furthermore, the mechanisms of approved drugs in MS are still poorly defined. Any new strategy which is based on the wrong pathogenetic concepts may not only be inefficient but also bears the risk of worsening disease. Nevertheless, identifying new drugs which significantly alter the course of disease is the major task in MS research and their identification will be the final approval of any pathogenetic hypothesis. Several immune-directed treatment strategies are currently under investigation in pre-clinical and clinical studies. Almost all these strategies are based on the autoimmune concept. Accordingly, new treatment approaches focus on suppression or alteration of immune responses or inhibition of immune cell migration to the CNS (Fig. 18.1).

Immunoablative strategies

These strategies are based on the hypothesis that the immune system is causative in MS or has an overall negative impact on the course of MS. Accordingly, the approaches focus on global inhibition or reconstitution of the immune system (Table 18.3).

Immune reconstitution

One of the most promising approaches in this field is hematopoetic stem cell /bone marrow transplantation (SCT) after total immune ablation. Theoretically, both autologous and allogeneic SCT are possible treatment options in MS. Autologous SCT does not have an impact on the immunogenetic predisposition to MS, but is supposed to result in an exchange of the entire B- and T-cell repertoire after maturation of hematopoetic bone mar-

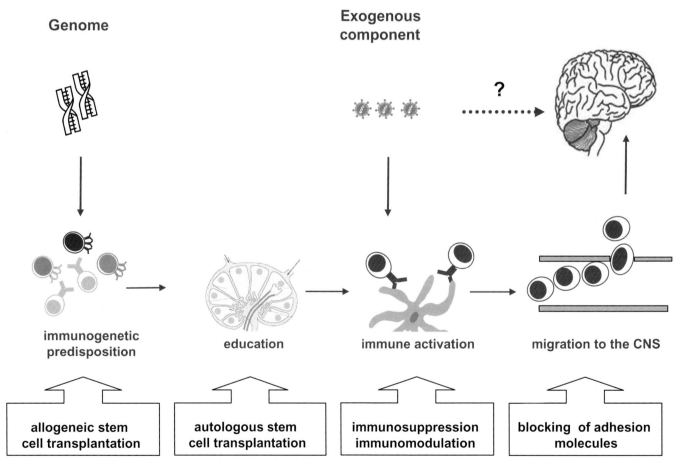

Fig. 18.1 Possible role of the immune system in the pathogenesis of MS. Summary of the possible events leading to tissue damage in multiple sclerosis and therapeutic intervention strategies.

Table 18.3 Immune-directed therapies in clinical or pre-clinical (PC) studies

Mechanism	Substance	Proposed mechanism	Pros	Cons	Phase
Immunoreconstitution	Autologous SCT	New maturation of the acquired immune system	New treatment concept. Profound alteration of T- and B-cell repertoire	Serious side-effects (mortality ~5–10%). Immunogenetic predisposition not influenced	II
	Allogeneic SCT	Alteration of immune genetic predisposition, new maturation of the acquired immune system	New treatment concept. Alteration of genetic predisposition	Serious side-effects (mortality >20%)	PC
	Genetically engineered SCT	Specific alteration of immune genetic predisposition	New treatment concept. Alteration of genetic predisposition	Genetic susceptibility factors still largely unknown. Unpredictable side-effects possible	PC
Immuno-suppression	Mycophenolate mofetil (Cell cept®)	Cytostatic effects on lymphocytes	Approved drug	May cause severe side-effects such as lymphoproliferative disorders	II
	Laquinimod (SAIK-MS)	Similar to linomide	Linomide showed positive effects	May have similar cardiopulmonary side-effects	II
	Teriflunomide (HMRI1726, similar to ARAVA®)	Inhibition of activated T cells	Similar drug approved for treatment of RA	Immunosuppression	II
	MAb against CD20 (Rituxan®)	Binds to CD20 and specifically depletes B cells	Approved drug	Can cause severe side-effects. Affects only B cells	II
	MAb against CD25 (Zenapax ®)	Blocks the high-affinity IL-2 receptor and interferes with T cell activation	No serious side-effects in small clinical trials	May have profound impact on the immune system	II
	MAb against CTLA4 (BMS 188667)	Blocks co-stimulation of T cells	Selectively affects T cells	Negative results of a phase II trial	III
	MAb against CD52 (Compath®)	Binds to CD52 (expressed leukocytes and endothelial cells). and leads cell depletion	Approved drug. Positive results in phase II trial	Can cause severe side-effects including death	II
Immunomodulation	Anti IL-12 (CNTO-1275)	Skews T-cell responses towards Th2	Interferes with most potent Th1-promoting cytokines	Unpredictable side-effects	II
	Mesopram	PDE-4 inhibitor, affects cytokine milieu	Oral drug	Gastrointestinal side-effects	II
	Rolipram	PDE-4 inhibitor, affects cytokine milieu	Oral drug. Antidepressant	Gastrointestinal side-effects	II
	Interferon-tau	Antiviral and anti-inflammatory activity	Oral drug. Type I interferon	Non-human protein	II
	FTY 720	Spingosin I-phosphate receptor agonist alters homing of immune cells	Oral drug	May have unpredicted side-effects	II
	CCI 779 (sirolimus)	Cell cycle arrest at G_1	Oral drug	Immunosuppression. May cause neoplasia	IIb
	Statins	Anti-inflammatory, immunmodulatory	Oral drug. Low side-effect profile		II
	Fumaric acid esters (Dimethylfumarate)	Anti-inflammatory activity	Oral drug. Approved drug	Few pre-clinical data	II
	TCR vaccination	Depletion of myelin-specific T cells from the repertoire	So far no serious side-effects	Negative results with similar approaches	II
Inhibiton of cell migration	Anti LFA-1 (Antegren®)	Blocks T-cell migration to the brain. Possible impact on T-cell maturation	Promising results in phase II trial. New therapeutic concept	Probably continuous administration required	III
	CCR-1 antagonist	Blocks T-cell migration	Oral drug. New therapeutic concept	May have unpredicted side-effects	II

SCT, stem cell transplantation; MAb, monoclonal antibody; RA, rheumatoid arthritis; TCR, T-cell receptor; LFA-1, leukocyte function-associated antigen 1.

row precursor cells. Autoreactive encephalitogenic lymphocytes are eliminated and replaced by naïve cells. Initial small MRI-controlled studies or larger retrospective trials in MS patients suggested that SCT may decrease MRI activity and disease progression. Small trials have shown that autologous SCT is, similar to its use in cancer and other inflammatory disorders, associated with a significant mortality of 5 to 10% (Fassas *et al.*, 2002; Nash *et al.*, 2003). Therefore, at present, this therapy should only be applied in specialized centres with a study protocol to patients who progress rapidly and have no other treatment option. Allogeneic transplantation is the more radical approach as it additionally affects immune-genetic predisposition. Single patients with MS and simultaneously occurring neoplastic disease were treated by allogeneic SCT. Due to the high mortality associated with this procedure, and the lack of sufficient clinical evidence SCT does currently not qualify as a clinical treatment approach for MS unless neoplastic disease occurs concomitantly. Transplantation of autologous SCT, which have been genetically modified, have been studied in EAE. In theory, these transplants can be modified to include disease-modifying genes (e.g. neurotrophins, Th2 cytokines) or can be depleted for possible susceptibility genes. However, this approach still has many unresolved technical problems and in the absence of promising candidates to modify, genetic alteration of SCTs will not enter clinical trials in the near future.

Immunosuppression

The low success rate of drugs that affect the immune system broadly has led to more specific strategies of immunosuppression. These focus on inhibition of a defined population of immune cells (e.g. B cells) or cells with a particular phenotype (e.g. activated T cells). Such therapies are often based on humanized monoclonal antibodies, which specifically affect immune cells bearing a particular immune receptor. The current approaches involve humanized antibodies specific for CD25 (expressed on activated T cells, B cells, and NK cells), CD20 (expressed on B cells), CD52 (expressed on lymphocytes and epithelium cells), and CTLA-4 (expressed on activated B cells, T cells, monocytes, and endothelial cells) (Cross *et al.*, 1999; Bielekova *et al.*, 2004; Rastetter *et al.*, 2004). A different mechanism targeting immunocompetent cells is mediated by FTY720, a sphingosine analogue, that promotes T-cell migration from peripheral blood into secondary lymphoid organs (Fujino *et al.*, 2003). These drugs are tested in MRI-controlled phase II trials and may enter phase III if positive results are obtained. Furthermore, additional immunosuppressive drugs (mycophenolate mofetil, teriflunomide, rapamycin, pixatrone), which were shown to be effective in the treatment of other chronic inflammatory disorders, are being tested in phase II trials for their efficacy in MS. Another ongoing trial investigates the impact of laquinimod on the course of MS. This drug shares a therapeutic mechanism with linomide, and may exhibit similar positive effects on MS without the cardiopulmonary side-effects, which have been observed in the linomide trial (Brunmark *et al.*, 2002). Overall, the future of immunosuppressive treatment will largely depend on whether any of these strategies demonstrate efficacy in clinical trials.

Immunomodulation

Despite the negative results of previous trials, immune modulation is still a highly promising treatment option in MS. In contrast to immunosuppression, immunomodulation may allow us to change the quality of an immune response without the side-effects of higher susceptibility for infections and cancer. Highly selective intervention strategies will become available within the near future for the treatment of human disease. Although high specificity without side-effects is the final goal of all therapeutic strategies, a detailed knowledge about etiology and mechanisms of disease is inevitable for these approaches. In addition it is import to keep in mind that as therapies become more specific the greater their chance of failing when they are based on vague pathogenic concepts.

Cytokine and lymphokine modulators

These approaches focus on global alteration of the inflammatory milieu based on findings in the EAE model. Desired effects are skewing immune responses from Th1 to Th2 or delivery of anti-inflammatory activity. Currently, treatment with an anti-IL-12 antibody is being studied in a small trial. IL-12 is the most important cytokine for priming Th1 responses and its inhibition strongly favors Th2 development. Inhibition of the pro-inflammatory activity mediated by IL-1 is targeted by an IL-1 receptor antagonist. Based on positive effects in rheumatoid arthritis, the drug is now being analysed for its potency to treat MS in a phase II trial. Similarly, IFN-τ, an ovine type I interferon with both anti-inflammatory and antiviral activity, which can be administered orally, is being analysed in a small phase II trial. Besides cytokine-based therapies, targeting chemokines may be another option in the future. Since some of the chemokines are highly differentially expressed they may allow selective inhibition of inflammatory responses in the CNS.

Since direct administration of cytokines often elicited intolerable side-effects, current strategies also focus on small compounds which indirectly affect the cytokine milieu. Two substances (rolipram, mesopram) that are currently being tested in phase II trials, inhibit phosphodiesterase type IV activity, directly affecting cAMP levels and cytokine release (predominantly TNF-α) (Sommer *et al.*, 1995). At least rolipram also acts as an antidepressant, which may provide additional effects on the quality of life in these patients.

Another new strategy involves statins, which have strong immunomodulatory properties. These drugs are highly efficient in EAE and were shown to be safe in two recently published small trials. A randomized, placebo-controlled trial that anticipates enrolling 152 MS patients was planned to start in summer 2004. This phase II trial will evaluate whether treatment with high-dose atorvastatin (80 mg) in patients that have experienced their first demyelinating attack (a 'clinically isolated syndrome', CIS) will decrease the risk of developing MS activity.(Youssef *et al.*, 2002; O'Connor *et al.*, 2004).

The advances in drug discovery technology will certainly lead to the discovery of additional small compounds with good pharmacological properties, which may allow highly specific intervention in the immune system without major systematic side-effects.

Antigen- or T-cell-based therapies

The unknown etiology of MS makes specific depletion of antigen-specific immune cells from the repertoire or their phenotypic alteration a difficult choice. The mostly negative results of the antigen- or T-cell-specific approaches in the past have rendered highly specific approaches less attractive. Only the least specific antigen-based approach with GA had an impact on the disease. Accordingly, it seems most attractive to follow this less specific but possibly antigen-specific approach and design similar peptide drugs. Such studies are under way but have not reached the clinics (Fridkis-Hareli *et al.*, 2002). Approaches that focus on one myelin antigen or one T-cell receptor are at this point highly likely not to work in MS.

Besides the development of these drugs, it is important to further evaluate antigen-based treatment strategies in animal models to provide strategies for highly selective intervention in MS. Those include new vaccination strategies, including the use of DNA vaccines to be prepared for emerging new target antigens in MS.

Inhibition of immune cell migration

One key to the pathogenesis of MS is the migration of immune cells through the blood–brain barrier and the infiltration of the CNS compartment. Specific inhibition of adhesion and migration would not affect systemic immune responses but would impair immune responses in the CNS. After successful studies in the EAE model, this approach has entered preclinical and clinical trials. Treatment with an anti-VLA-4 antibody, which specifically inhibits T-cell and monocyte migration to the CNS, was tested in two MRI-controlled phase II trials (Miller *et al.*, 2003). During treatment, MRI activity significantly decreased, although the effect was not sustained after discontinuing the drug in one of the trials. The drug is now being tested in a phase III trial to clarify the clinical impact of this therapy. Recently, minocycline, a broad-spectrum inhibitor of matrix metalloproteinases, was reported to reduce lymphocyte access to the CNS, as demonstrated on MRI (Metz *et al.*, 2004). Furthermore, blockade of specific chemokine receptors, such as CCR1, is currently under clinical investigation. Other drugs, among them other monoclonal antibodies, are in preclinical studies (Matsui *et al.*, 2002).

Future prospects of immune-targeting therapies

Recent studies have pointed out that the immune system may not only have detrimental effects in autoimmune and neurodegenerative disorders but may also promote neuroregeneration (Kerschensteiner *et al.*, 2003). This view is not only supported by experimental animal studies but also by the finding that immune cells in MS lesions produce neurotrophic factors such as brain-derived neurotrophic factor. These observations raise the question of whether the immune system can be used to deliver therapies to the site of tissue damage. Theoretically, antigen-specific T cells, B cells, and antibodies can be used to target drugs to the CNS. Likewise, myelin basic protein-specific T cells transfected with the nerve growth factor gene do not mediate but ameliorate EAE (Flugel *et al.*, 2001). Other genes can be introduced into immune cells (i.e. monocytes, T cells, B cells), which may allow specific delivery of the drug to the site of inflammation. Although this fascinating concept has proven efficacy in the animal models, many technical and ethical problems have to be overcome before such approaches could be feasible in humans. In addition, inflammation and neuroregeneration are highly complex processes which need an orchestrated release of a variety of molecules. Delivery of a single molecule by the transgenic approach may be over-simplified. Therefore, these strategies are certainly not applicable to MS within the next years, but may again be a highly selective, minimally invasive therapy in MS for the more distant future.

Concluding remarks

Further knowledge about the etiology and pathogenesis of MS will certainly lead to the development of new treatment strategies. Models which have been widely used for the development of MS therapeutics have not provided a solid basis for estimating the impact on human disease. Besides developing new treatment strategies on hypothetical concepts, it is necessary to put a major effort into dissecting the pathogenesis of MS. Only on the basis of a valid pathogenetic concept will we finally succeed in developing drugs that may significantly alter the long-term prognosis of MS. Furthermore, we need to use cutting-edge techniques (i.e. transcriptomics, genomics, metabolics, proteomics) to monitor treatment responses in patients. It may not be too long until pharmacotherapy can be tailored to individual patients based on their genetic makeup

Acknowledgements

We thank all our MS patients for their continuous support. Bernhard Hemmer is a Heisenberg Fellow of the Deutsche Forschungsgemeinschaft (DFG). The work was supported by the DFG 2382/4–1 and 4–2.

References

Aharoni, R., Kayhan, B., Eilam, R., *et al.* (2003) Glatiramer acetate-specific T cells in the brain express T helper 2/3 cytokines and brain-derived neurotrophic factor *in situ*. *Proc Natl Acad Sci USA* **100**: 14157–14162.

Babbe, H., Roers, A., Waisman, A., *et al.* (2000) Clonal expansions of CD8(+) T cells dominate the T cell infiltrate in active multiple sclerosis lesions as shown by micromanipulation and single cell polymerase chain reaction. *J Exp Med* **192**, 393–404.

Baranzini, S.E., Elfstrom, C., Chang, S.Y., *et al.* (2000). Transcriptional analysis of multiple sclerosis brain lesions reveals a complex pattern of cytokine expression. *J Immunol* **165**: 6576–6582.

Barnett, M.H. and Prineas, J.W. (2004). Relapsing and remitting multiple sclerosis: pathology of the newly forming lesion. *Ann Neurol* **55**: 458–468.

Bertolotto, A., Malucchi, S., Sala, A., *et al.* (2002). Differential effects of three interferon betas on neutralising antibodies in patients with multiple sclerosis: a follow up study in an independent laboratory. *J Neurol Neurosurg Psychiatry* **73**: 148–153.

Bielekova, B., Goodwin, B., Richert, N., *et al.* (2000). Encephalitogenic potential of the myelin basic protein peptide (amino acids 83–99). in multiple sclerosis: results of a phase II clinical trial with an altered peptide ligand. *Nat Med* **6**: 1167–1175.

Bielekova, B., Richert, N., Howard, T., *et al.* (2004). Humanized anti-CD25 (daclizumab). inhibits disease activity in multiple sclerosis patients failing to respond to interferon beta. *Proc Natl Acad Sci USA* **101**: 8705–8708.

Bitsch, A., Schuchardt, J., Bunkowski, S., *et al.* (2000). Acute axonal injury in multiple sclerosis. Correlation with demyelination and inflammation. *Brain* **123**: 1174–1183.

Brunmark, C., Runstrom, A., Ohlsson, L., *et al.* (2002). The new orally active immunoregulator laquinimod (ABR-215062). effectively inhibits development and relapses of experimental autoimmune encephalomyelitis. *J Neuroimmunol* **130**: 163–172.

Canadian Cooperative Multiple Sclerosis Study Group (1991). The Canadian cooperative trial of cyclophosphamide and plasma exchange in progressive multiple sclerosis. *Lancet* **337**: 441–446.

Cannella, B. and Raine, C.S. (1995). The adhesion molecule and cytokine profile of multiple sclerosis lesions. *Ann Neurol* **37**: 424–435.

Carbone, K.M., Rubin, S.A., Nishino, Y., *et al.* (2001). Borna disease: virus-induced neurobehavioral disease pathogenesis. *Curr Opin Microbiol* **4**: 467–475.

Clanet, M., Radue, E.W., Kappos, L., *et al.* (2002). A randomized, double-blind, dose-comparison study of weekly interferon beta-1a in relapsing MS. *Neurology* **59**: 1507–1517.

Comi, G., Filippi, M., Barkhof, F., *et al.* (2001*a*). Effect of early interferon treatment on conversion to definite multiple sclerosis: a randomised study. *Lancet* **357**: 1576–1582.

Comi, G., Filippi, M., and Wolinsky, J.S. (2001*b*). European/Canadian multicenter, double-blind, randomized, placebo-controlled study of the effects of glatiramer acetate on magnetic resonance imaging-measured disease activity and burden in patients with relapsing multiple sclerosis. European/Canadian Glatiramer Acetate Study Group. *Ann.Neurol* **49**: 290–297.

Cross, A.H., San, M., Keeling, R.M., *et al.* (1999). CTLA-4-Fc treatment of ongoing EAE improves recovery, but has no effect upon relapse rate. Implications for the mechanisms involved in disease perpetuation. *J Neuroimmunol* **96**: 144–147.

Cross, A.H., Trotter, J.L., and Lyons, J. (2001). B cells and antibodies in CNS demyelinating disease. *J Neuroimmunol* **112**: 1–14.

Duda, P.W., Schmied, M.C., Cook, S.L., *et al.* (2000). Glatiramer acetate (Copaxone). induces degenerate, Th2-polarized immune responses in patients with multiple sclerosis. *J Clin Invest* **105**: 967–976.

Durelli, L., Verdun, E., Barbero, P., *et al.* (2002). Every-other-day interferon beta-1b versus once-weekly interferon beta-1a for multiple sclerosis: results of a 2-year prospective randomised multicentre study (INCOMIN). *Lancet* **359**: 1453–1460.

Ellison, G.W., Myers, L.W., Leake, B.D., *et al.* (1994). Design strategies in multiple sclerosis clinical trials. The Cyclosporine Multiple Sclerosis Study Group. *Ann Neurol* **36**(Suppl.): S108–S112.

European Study Group on Interferon Beta-1b in Secondary Progressive MS (1998). Placebo-controlled multicentre randomised trial of interferon beta-1b in treatment of secondary progressive multiple sclerosis. *Lancet* **352**: 1491–1497.

Fassas, A.S., Passweg, J.R., Anagnostopoulos, A., *et al.* (2002). Hematopoietic stem cell transplantation for multiple sclerosis. A retrospective multicenter study. *J Neurol* **249**: 1088–1097.

Fazekas, F., Deisenhammer, F., Strasser-Fuchs, S., *et al.* (1997). Treatment effects of monthly intravenous immunoglobulin on patients with relapsing-remitting multiple sclerosis: further analyses of the Austrian Immunoglobulin in MS study. *Mult Scler* **3**: 137–141.

Flugel, A., Matsumuro, K., Neumann, H., *et al.* (2001). Anti-inflammatory activity of nerve growth factor in experimental autoimmune encephalomyelitis: inhibition of monocyte transendothelial migration. *Eur J Immunol* **31**: 11–22.

Fridkis-Hareli, M., Neveu, J.M., Robinson, R.A., *et al.* (1999). Binding motifs of copolymer 1 to multiple sclerosis- and rheumatoid arthritis-associated HLA-DR molecules. *J Immunol* **162**: 4697–4704.

Fridkis-Hareli, M., Santambrogio, L., Stern, J.N., *et al.* (2002). Novel synthetic amino acid copolymers that inhibit autoantigen-specific T cell responses and suppress experimental autoimmune encephalomyelitis. *J Clin Invest* **109**: 1635–1643.

Fujinami, R.S. and Oldstone, M.B. (1985). Amino acid homology between the encephalitogenic site of myelin basic protein and virus: mechanism for autoimmunity. *Science* **230**: 1043–1045.

Fujino, M., Funeshima, N., Kitazawa, Y., *et al.* (2003). Amelioration of experimental autoimmune encephalomyelitis in Lewis rats by FTY720 treatment. *J Pharmacol Exp Ther* **305**: 70–77.

Gay, F.W., Drye, T.J., Dick, G.W., *et al.* (1997). The application of multifactorial cluster analysis in the staging of plaques in early multiple sclerosis.

Identification and characterization of the primary demyelinating lesion. *Brain* **120**: 1461–1483.

Goodkin, D.E., Rudick, R.A., VanderBrug, M.S., *et al.* (1995). Low-dose (7.5 mg). oral methotrexate reduces the rate of progression in chronic progressive multiple sclerosis. *Ann Neurol* **37**: 30–40.

Goodkin, D.E., Rudick, R.A., VanderBrug, M.S., *et al.* (1996). Low-dose oral methotrexate in chronic progressive multiple sclerosis: analyses of serial MRIs. *Neurology* **47**: 1153–1157.

Gran, B., Tranquill, L.R., Chen, M., *et al.* (2000). Mechanisms of immuno-modulation by glatiramer acetate. *Neurology* **55**: 1704–1714.

Hammond, S.R., McLeod, J.G., Millingen, K.S., *et al.* (1988). The epidemiology of multiple sclerosis in three Australian cities: Perth, Newcastle and Hobart. *Brain* **111**: 1–25.

Haring, J. and Perlman, S. (2001). Mouse hepatitis virus. *Curr Opin Microbiol* **4**: 462–466.

Hartung, H.P., Gonsette, R.E., König, N., *et al.* (2002). Mitoxantrone in pro-gressive multiple sclerosis: a placebo-controlled double-blind, randomized, multicentre trial.

Hemmer, B., Fleckenstein, B.T., Vergelli, M., *et al.* (1997). Identification of high potency microbial and self ligands for a human autoreactive class II-restricted T cell clone. *J Exp Med* **185**: 1651–1659.

Hemmer, B., Archelos, J.J., and Hartung, H.P. (2002). New concepts in the immunopathogenesis of multiple sclerosis. *Nat Rev Neurosci* **3**: 291–301.

Huseby, E.S., Liggitt, D., Brabb, T., *et al.* (2001). A pathogenic role for myelin-specific CD8(+). T cells in a model for multiple sclerosis. *J Exp Med* **194**: 669–676.

IFNB Multiple Sclerosis Study Group (1993). Interferon beta-1b is effective in relapsing-remitting multiple sclerosis. I. Clinical results of a multicenter, randomized, double-blind, placebo-controlled trial. *Neurology* **43**: 655–661.

Jacobs, L.D., Cookfair, D.L., Rudick, R.A., *et al.* (1996). Intramuscular interferon beta-1a for disease progression in relapsing multiple sclerosis. The Multiple Sclerosis Collaborative Research Group (MSCRG). *Ann Neurol* **39**: 285–294.

Jacobs, L.D., Beck, R.W., Simon, J.H., *et al.* (2000). Intramuscular interferon beta-1a therapy initiated during a first demyelinating event in multiple sclerosis. CHAMPS Study Group. *N Engl J Med* **343**: 898–904.

Jacobsen, M., Cepok, S., Quak, E., *et al.* (2002). Oligoclonal expansion of mem-ory CD8+ T cells in the cerebrospinal fluid from multiple sclerosis patients. *Brain* **125**: 538–550.

Johnson, K.P., Brooks, B.R., Cohen, J.A., *et al.* (1995). Copolymer 1 reduces relapse rate and improves disability in relapsing-remitting multiple sclerosis: results of a phase III multicenter, double-blind placebo-controlled trial. The Copolymer 1 Multiple Sclerosis Study Group. *Neurology* **45**: 1268–1276.

Jones, T.B., Ankeny, D.P., Guan, Z., *et al.* (2004). Passive or active immunization with myelin basic protein impairs neurological function and exacerbates neuropathology after spinal cord injury in rats. *J Neurosci* **24**: 3752–3761.

Jung, S., Siglienti, I., Grauer, O., *et al.* (2004). Induction of IL-10 in rat peritoneal macrophages and dendritic cells by glatiramer acetate. *J Neuroimmunol* **148**: 63–73.

Kappos, L., Comi, G., Panitch, H., *et al.* (2000). Induction of a non-encephalito-genic type 2 T helper-cell autoimmune response in multiple sclerosis after administration of an altered peptide ligand in a placebo-controlled, ran-domized phase II trial. The Altered Peptide Ligand in Relapsing MS Study Group. *Nat Med* **6**: 1176–1182.

Karandikar, N.J., Crawford, M.P., Yan, X., *et al.* (2002). Glatiramer acetate (Copaxone). therapy induces CD8(+). T cell responses in patients with mul-tiple sclerosis. *J Clin Invest* **109**: 641–649.

Kerschensteiner, M., Gallmeier, E., Behrens, L., *et al.* (1999). Activated human T cells, B cells, and monocytes produce brain-derived neurotrophic factor in vitro and in inflammatory brain lesions: a neuroprotective role of inflamma-tion? *J Exp Med* **189**: 865–870.

Kerschensteiner, M., Stadelmann, C., Dechant, G., *et al.* (2003). Neurotrophic cross-talk between the nervous and immune systems: implications for neurological diseases. *Ann Neurol* **53**: 292–304.

King, C., Ilic, A., Koelsch, K., *et al.* (2004). Homeostatic expansion of T cells during immune insufficiency generates autoimmunity. *Cell* **117**: 265–277.

Kipnis, J., Yoles, E., Porat, Z., *et al.* (2000). T cell immunity to copolymer 1 con-fers neuroprotection on the damaged optic nerve: possible therapy for optic neuropathies. *Proc Natl Acad Sci USA* **97**: 7446–7451.

Kuchroo, V.K., Anderson, A.C., Waldner, H., *et al.* (2002). T cell response in experimental autoimmune encephalomyelitis (EAE): role of self and cross-reactive antigens in shaping, tuning, and regulating the autopathogenic T cell repertoire. *Annu Rev Immunol* **20**: 101–123.

Kurtzke, J.F. (2000). Epidemiology of multiple sclerosis. Does this really point toward an etiology? Lectio Doctoralis. *Neurol Sci* **21**: 383–403.

Lassmann, H., Raine, C.S., Antel, J., *et al.* (1998). Immunopathology of multiple sclerosis: report on an international meeting held at the Institute of Neurology of the University of Vienna. *J Neuroimmunol* **86**: 213–217.

Lassmann, H., Bruck, W., and Lucchinetti, C. (2001). Heterogeneity of multiple sclerosis pathogenesis: implications for diagnosis and therapy. *Trends Mol Med* **7**: 115–121.

Lehmann, P.V., Sercarz, E.E., Forsthuber, T., *et al.* (1993). Determinant spreading and the dynamics of the autoimmune T-cell repertoire. *Immunol Today* **14**: 203–208.

Lenercept Multiple Sclerosis Study Group and The University of British Columbia MS/MRI Analysis Group (1999). TNF neutralization in MS: results of a randomized, placebo-controlled multicenter study. *Neurology* **53**: 457–465.

Linington, C., Bradl, M., Lassmann, H., *et al.* (1988). Augmentation of demyel-ination in rat acute allergic encephalomyelitis by circulating mouse mono-clonal antibodies directed against a myelin/oligodendrocyte glycoprotein. *Am J Pathol* **130**: 443–454.

Losy, J., Mehta, P.D., and Wisniewski, H.M. (1990). Identification of IgG subclasses' oligoclonal bands in multiple sclerosis CSF. *Acta Neurol Scand* **82**: 4–8.

Lucchinetti, C., Bruck, W., Parisi, J., *et al.* (2000). Heterogeneity of multiple scler-osis lesions: implications for the pathogenesis of demyelination. *Ann Neurol* **47**: 707–717.

Lucchinetti, C.F., Mandler, R.N., McGavern, D., *et al.* (2002). A role for humoral mechanisms in the pathogenesis of Devic's neuromyelitis optica. *Brain* **125**: 1450–1461.

Martin, R., McFarland, H.F., and McFarlin, D.E. (1992). Immunological aspects of demyelinating diseases. *Annu Rev Immunol* **10**: 153–187.

Matsui, M., Weaver, J., Proudfoot, A.E., *et al.* (2002). Treatment of experimental autoimmune encephalomyelitis with the chemokine receptor antagonist Met-RANTES. *J Neuroimmunol* **128**: 16–22.

Metz, L.M., Zhang, Y., Yeung, M., *et al.* (2004). Minocycline reduces gadolinium-enhancing magnetic resonance imaging lesions in multiple sclerosis. *Ann Neurol* **55**: 756.

Miller, D.H., Khan, O.A., Sheremata, W.A., *et al.* (2003). A controlled trial of natalizumab for relapsing multiple sclerosis. *N Engl J Med* **348**: 15–23.

Moalem, G., Leibowitz-Amit, R., Yoles, E., *et al.* (1999). Autoimmune T cells pro-tect neurons from secondary degeneration after central nervous system axotomy. *Nat Med* **5**: 49–55.

Nash, R.A., Bowen, J.D., McSweeney, P.A., *et al.* (2003). High-dose immuno-suppressive therapy and autologous peripheral blood stem cell transplanta-tion for severe multiple sclerosis. *Blood* **102**: 2364–2372.

Neuhaus, O., Farina, C., Yassouridis, A., *et al.* (2000). Multiple sclerosis: com-parison of copolymer-1- reactive T cell lines from treated and untreated subjects reveals cytokine shift from T helper 1 to T helper 2 cells. *Proc Natl Acad Sci USA* **97**: 7452–7457.

O'Connor, P.W. (2002). Key issues in the diagnosis and treatment of multiple sclerosis: an overview. S1–S33.

O'Connor, P.W., Goodman, A., Willmer-Hulme, A.J., *et al.* (2004). Randomized multicenter trial of natalizumab in acute MS relapses: clinical and MRI effects. *Neurology* **62**: 2038–2043.

Once Weekly Interferon for MS Study Group (1999). Evidence of interferon beta-1a dose response in relapsing-remitting MS: the OWIMS Study. *Neurology* **53**: 679–686.

Panitch, H.S., Hirsch, R.L., Haley, A.S., *et al.* (1987*a*). Exacerbations of multiple sclerosis in patients treated with gamma interferon. *Lancet* **1**: 893–895.

Panitch, H.S., Hirsch, R.L., Schindler, J., *et al.* (1987*b*). Treatment of multiple sclerosis with gamma interferon: exacerbations associated with activation of the immune system. *Neurology* **37**: 1097–1102.

Panitch, H., Goodin, D.S., Francis, G., *et al.* (2002). Randomized, comparative study of interferon beta-1a treatment regimens in MS: the EVIDENCE Trial. *Neurology* **59**: 1496–1506.

Paty, D.W. and Li, D.K. (1993). Interferon beta-1b is effective in relapsing-remitting multiple sclerosis. II. MRI analysis results of a multicenter, randomized, double-blind, placebo-controlled trial. UBC MS/MRI Study Group and the IFNB Multiple Sclerosis Study Group. *Neurology* **43**: 662–667.

Prineas, J.W., Kwon, E.E., Cho, E.S., *et al.* (2001). Immunopathology of secondary-progressive multiple sclerosis. *Ann Neurol* **50**: 646–657.

PRISMS Study Group (1998). Randomised double-blind placebo-controlled study of interferon beta-1a in relapsing/remitting multiple sclerosis. PRISMS (Prevention of Relapses and Disability by Interferon beta-1a Subcutaneously in Multiple Sclerosis). Study Group. *Lancet* **352**: 1498–1504.

PRISMS Study Group and the University of British Columbia MS/MRI Analysis Group (2001). PRISMS-4: long-term efficacy of interferon-beta-1a in relapsing MS. *Neurology* **56**: 1628–1636.

Ramakrishna, C., Stohlman, S.A., Atkinson, R.D., *et al.* (2002). Mechanisms of central nervous system viral persistence: the critical role of antibody and B cells. *J Immunol* **168**: 1204–1211.

Rastetter, W., Molina, A., and White, C.A. (2004). Rituximab: expanding role in therapy for lymphomas and autoimmune diseases. *Annu Rev Med* **55**: 477–503.

Rice, G. (2001). The significance of neutralizing antibodies in patients with multiple sclerosis treated with interferon beta. *Arch Neurol* **58**: 1297–1298.

Rudge, P., Koetsier, J.C., Mertin, J., *et al.* (1989). Randomised double blind controlled trial of cyclosporin in multiple sclerosis. *J Neurol Neurosurg Psychiatry* **52**: 559–565.

Secondary Progressive Efficacy Clinical Trial of Recombinant Interferon-beta-1a in MS (SPECTRIMS) Study Group (2001). Randomized controlled trial of interferon- beta-1a in secondary progressive MS: clinical results. *Neurology* **56**: 1496–1504.

Sibley, W.A., Bamford, C.R., and Clark, K. (1985). Clinical viral infections and multiple sclerosis. *Lancet* **1**: 1313–1315.

Sommer, N., Loschmann, P.A., Northoff, G.H., *et al.* (1995). The antidepressant rolipram suppresses cytokine production and prevents autoimmune encephalomyelitis. *Nat Med* **1**: 244–248.

Sorensen, P.S., Ross, C., Clemmesen, K.M., *et al.* (2003). Clinical importance of neutralising antibodies against interferon beta in patients with relapsing-remitting multiple sclerosis. *Lancet* **362**: 1184–1191.

Stadelmann, C., Kerschensteiner, M., Misgeld, T., *et al.* (2002). BDNF and gp145trkB in multiple sclerosis brain lesions: neuroprotective interactions between immune and neuronal cells? *Brain* **125**: 75–85.

Stohlman, S.A. and Hinton, D.R. (2001). Viral induced demyelination. *Brain Pathol* **11**: 92–106.

Sun, D., Whitaker, J.N., Huang, Z., *et al.* (2001). Myelin antigen-specific CD8+ T cells are encephalitogenic and produce severe disease in C57BL/6 mice. *J Immunol* **166**: 7579–7587.

Trapp, B.D., Peterson, J., Ransohoff, R.M., *et al.* (1998). Axonal transection in the lesions of multiple sclerosis. *N Engl J Med* **338**: 278–285.

Vanderlugt, C.L. and Miller S.D. (2002). Epitope spreading in immune-mediated diseases: implications for immunotherapy. *Nat Rev Immunol* **2**: 85–95.

Weber, M.S., Starck, M., Wagenpfeil, S., *et al.* (2004). Multiple sclerosis: glatiramer acetate inhibits monocyte reactivity *in vitro* and *in vivo*. *Brain* **127**: 1370–1378.

Wekerle, H., Kojima, K., Lannes-Vieira, J., *et al.* (1994). Animal models. *Ann Neurol* **36**(Suppl.): S47–S53.

Wucherpfennig, K.W. and Strominger, J.L. (1995). Molecular mimicry in T cell-mediated autoimmunity: viral peptides activate human T cell clones specific for myelin basic protein. *Cell* **80**: 695–705.

Yong, V.W. (2002). Differential mechanisms of action of interferon-beta and glatiramer acetate in MS. *Neurology* **59**: 802–808.

Youssef, S., Stuve, O., Patarroyo, J.C., *et al.* (2002). The HMG-CoA reductase inhibitor, atorvastatin, promotes a Th2 bias and reverses paralysis in central nervous system autoimmune disease. *Nature* **420**: 78–84.

Yudkin, P.L., Ellison, G.W., Ghezzi, A., *et al.* (1991). Overview of azathioprine treatment in multiple sclerosis. *Lancet* **338**: 1051–1055.

Zamvil, S.S. and Steinman, L. (1990). The T lymphocyte in experimental allergic encephalomyelitis. *Annu Rev Immunol* **8**: 579–621.

19 Guillain–Barré syndrome and chronic inflammatory demyelinating polyradiculoneuropathy

Bernd C. Kieseier and Hans-Peter Hartung

Guillain–Barré syndrome (GBS), which is now recognized as a group of conditions with diverse pathology and pathogenesis, represents a prototypic immune-mediated peripheral neuropathy. In most instances the clinical picture develops within days to some weeks and reaches its nadir by 4 weeks, when after a plateau phase most patients start to recover. By arbitrary definition chronic inflammatory demyelinating polyneuropathy (CIDP) evolves over a time interval of at least 8 weeks, but much more frequently chronically over months and years. A similar immunopathological heterogeneity may be exhibited in CIDP (Kieseier et al., 2004; Köller et al., 2005). The gap between GBS and CIDP is bridged by a disease entity defined by some authors as subacute inflammatory demyelinating polyneuropathy (SIDP) (Oh et al., 2003). Most of the present knowledge about mechanisms involved in the pathogenesis of immune-mediated demyelination and putative autoantigens has been obtained through studies in the animal model, experimental autoimmune neuritis (EAN), which has been described in detail in Chapter 12.

Guillain–Barré syndrome

Clinical spectrum

GBS is the most common cause of acute flaccid paralysis in the Western hemisphere and probably world-wide, with an average incidence rate of about 1.5 per 100 000 (Hartung et al., 1995; Govoni and Granieri, 2001). GBS is clinically defined as a rapidly progressive ascending polyradiculoneuropathy, with involvement of cranial nerves in a significant proportion of cases (Hahn, 1998). By arbitrary definition, the nadir is reached within 4 weeks, followed by a plateau phase of variable duration and, eventually, by gradual recovery.

During recent years it has been recognized that GBS comprises several subtypes with specific clinical, electrophysiological, and pathological features, rather than being a single disease entity (Hughes, 1995). Thus, new diagnostic and classification criteria have been proposed (Van der Meché et al., 2001). Some authors subdivide GBS into five distinct forms (Hughes, 1995):

1. The classic acute demyelinating type, designated acute inflammatory demyelinating neuropathy (AIDP) representing the great majority of cases in Europe and North America.

2. A pure motor axonal type, called acute motor axonal neuropathy (AMAN), the most prevalent form in China where it occurs in summer epidemics in children and young adults.

3. An axonal variant involving both motor and sensory fibers, called acute motor and sensory axonal neuropathy (AMSAN), which is distinguished by significant sensory involvement and associated with a more severe course and poorer prognosis (Feasby, 1994).

4. The Miller–Fisher syndrome (MFS), characterized by ophthalmoplegia, ataxia, and areflexia (Willison and O'Hanlon, 1999), which in a

proportion of cases transitions to generalized GBS (Ter Bruggen et al., 1998); and perhaps

5. Acute pandysautonomia, characterized by the rapid onset of combined sympathetic and parasympathetic failure without sensory and motor involvement.

Moreover, a number of other well-characterized but uncommon regional variants occur, including pure ataxic GBS (Kusunoki et al., 1999; Ichikawa et al., 2001), pharyngeal–cervical–brachial GBS (Ropper, 1986; Koga et al., 1998), and isolated bulbar palsy (O'Leary et al., 1996).

Using novel electrophysiological approaches, differences in the axonal excitability, as measured by threshold tracking, were determined in patients with AIDP and AMAN, indicating that the predominantly distal targets of the immune attack differ in these two subgroups of GBS (Kuwabara et al., 2002). The patterns and speeds of progression differ in AMAN and AIDP, with AMAN exhibiting a rapid progression and an early nadir, whereas patients with AIDP in most cases have a long progression (Hiraga et al., 2003).

Morphology

Multifocal inflammatory demyelination of the peripheral nervous system (PNS) is the pathological hallmark of classic GBS. The spectrum of pathological changes can range from focal or extensive demyelination in the presence or absence of cellular infiltration, to axonal degeneration with or without demyelination or inflammatory infiltrates. Pathological alterations can be found at all levels along the peripheral nerve, from the roots to the most distal intramuscular motor nerve endings. However, the majority of the lesions are detectable along the ventral roots, proximal spinal nerves, and lower cranial nerves. Demyelination is found primarily at the nodes of Ranvier where clustering of macrophages, cells known to strip off and phagocytose compact myelin, can be detected.

The varied histopathological features mirror the clinical diversity of GBS. Whereas AIDP is characterized by macrophage-mediated demyelination and intense T-cell infiltration, AMAN and AMSAN exhibit signs of a macrophage-mediated axonal neuropathy and lymphocytic infiltrates are scarce (Griffin et al., 1995, 1996)

A recent autopsy study revealed inflammatory infiltrates in the spinal cord of some GBS cases, as well as focal infiltrates of the meninges pointing to the potential of CNS involvement (Muller et al., 2003).

Immunopathology

Under physiological conditions, a well-balanced network of immunocompetent cells and soluble factors meticulously regulates the immune system within the local tissue compartment, with the ultimate goal of providing maximum protection. The maintenance of self-tolerance, i.e. prevention of immune responses to host/self antigens, is a key requisite in this setting. In autoimmune diseases, however, self-tolerance breaks down, and autoreactive T and B cells that are part of the normal immune repertoire are unleashed and can initiate organ-specific damage. Why and how autoreactivity escapes the regulatory mechanisms is still unclear in most immune-mediated disorders.

A theory which is highly relevant to autoimmune neuropathies is based on the concept of 'molecular mimicry'. This term refers to a process in which the host generates an immune response to an inciting factor, most often an infectious organism, that shares epitopic determinants with the host's affected tissue (see Chapter 8). In GBS, at least in some of its forms, shared epitopes between the bacterial species *Campylobacter jejuni* (Yuki *et al.*, 2004) and *Haemophilus influenzae* (Ju *et al.*, 2004), or cytomegalovirus (CMV), and nerve fibers have been identified as targets for aberrant cross-reactive immune responses (reviewed in Gold *et al.* (1999) and Yuki (2001)). Nevertheless, laboratory findings and the clinical spectrum of this disorder cannot be explained solely by this hypothesis. Present evidence is incomplete and the pathogenetic scenario within the affected PNS is of much higher complexity than initially expected. Therefore, GBS should be considered as an organ-specific immune-mediated disorder emerging from a synergistic interaction of cell-mediated and humoral immune responses to still incompletely characterized peripheral nerve antigens.

Cellular immunity

The demonstration of inflammatory infiltrates in nerves (see Fig. 19.2) and the critical pathogenic role of neuritogenic T lymphocytes in the animal model of human GBS, experimental autoimmune neuritis (EAN), support the notion that disordered cellular immunity is of critical importance in the pathogenesis of this disease (see Chapter 8).

T-cell activation within the periphery, indicated by an enhanced expression of antigens, major histocompatibility complex (MHC) Class II and co-stimulatory molecules, various pro-inflammatory cytokines such as interferon-gamma (IFN-γ) and tumor necrosis factor-alpha (TNF-α), and

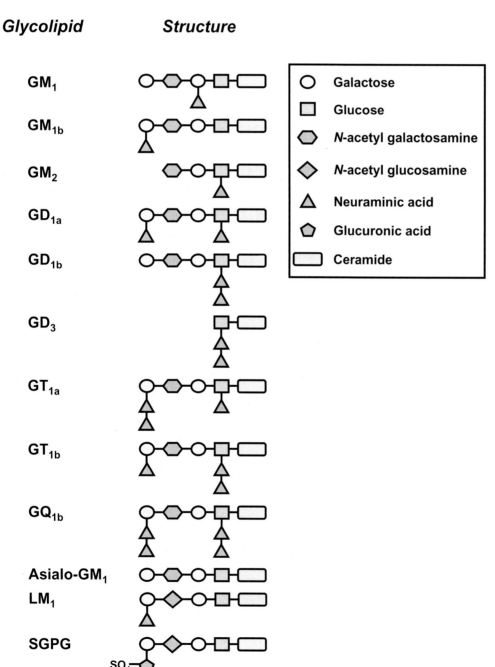

Fig. 19.1 Structure of glycolipids to which antibody responses have been detected in Guillain–Barré syndrome (adapted from Kieseier *et al.* (2004)).

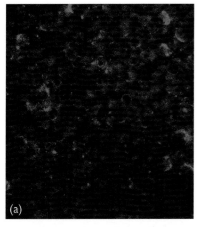

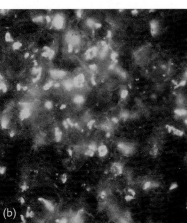

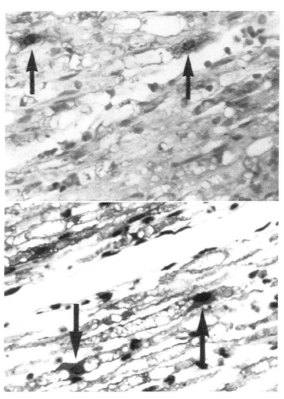

Plate 1 Expression of matrix metalloproteinases (MMPs) in the inflamed nerve. Metalloproteinases mediate tissue invasion of inflammatory cells into the peripheral nervous system. Proteolytic activity of gelatinases. such as MMP-2 and MMP-9, can be visualized by *in situ* zymography in the sciatic nerve of animals with experimental autoimmune neuritis. In control animals only background fluorescence is observable (a), whereas in animals with maximum clinical disease severity strong proteolytic activity can be found within the inflamed nerve (b). (See also Chapter 8, Fig. 8.4.)

Plate 2 Schwann cell apoptosis in experimental autoimmune neuritis. Schwann cells are detected by anti-S100 immunocytochemistry with morphological signs of apoptosis (arrows in upper figure). In double-labelling studies with the TUNEL technique apoptotic Schwann cells exhibit black nuclei (arrows in lower figure). (See also Chapter 8, Fig. 8.7.)

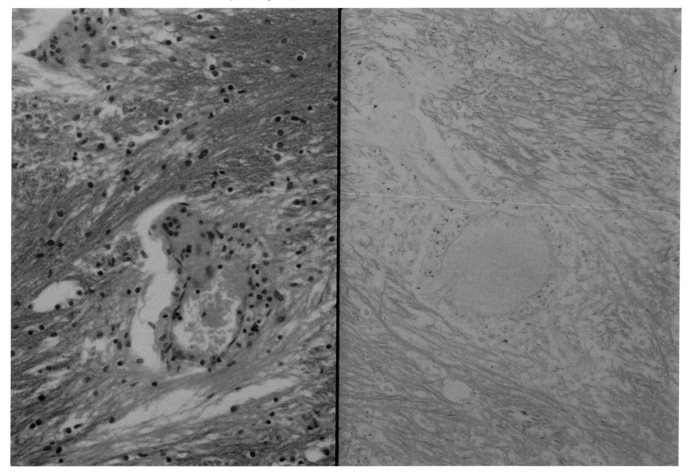

Plate 3 Acute disseminated encephalomyelitis in a human patient. Left figure shows myelin staining absent immediately around a small venule (H&E stain.) The right figure shows relative preservation of axons surrounding a venule in adjacent section, although there is some rarefaction immediately around the venule, possibly due to edema (Bielschowsky stain.) (See also Chapter 13, Fig. 13.3.)

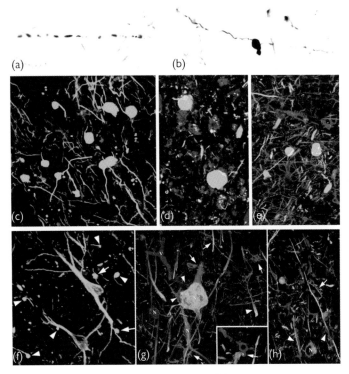

Plate 4 Characteristics of axonal pathology in white matter MS lesions (a)–(e) and neuronal pathology in cortical MS lesions (f)–(h) with associated activated microglia and macrophages. (a, b). Discontinuous staining for non-phosphorylated neurofilaments (a) with constricted and dilated axons containing large swellings (b). (c) stacked confocal image showing terminal axonal ovoids with single or dual axonal connections. Macrophages (d in red) and microglia (e in red) surround and engulf terminal axonal swellings (c and d in green). In cortical lesions, neurofilament-positive ovoids representing terminal ends of neurites were abundant in cortical lesions (f). Activated microglia (g and h in red) extend processes to neurites and neurofilament positive (g and h in green) neurons in the cortex. (See also Chapter 14, Fig. 14.2.)

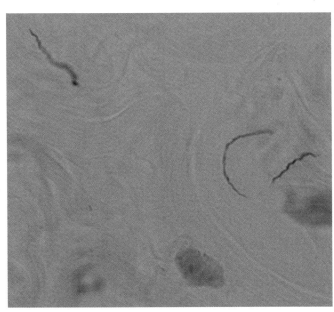

Plate 5 *B. burgdorferi* in the brachial plexus of an infected non-humnan primate stained by immunohistochemistry. (See also Chapter 24, Fig. 24.2.)

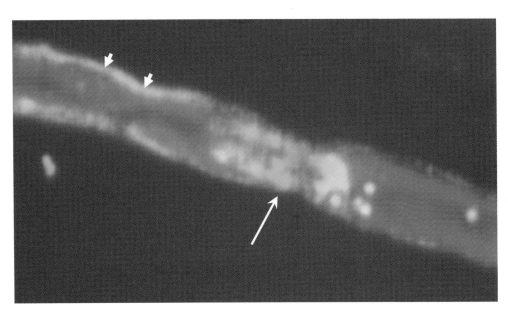

Plate 6 Confocal microscopic picture of a myelinated fiber of a sural nerve biopsy from a 63-year-old patient with anti-MAG neuropathy. Red fluorescence shows the compact myelin detected by an antibody against protein zero (P_O). Green fluorescence shows the accumulation of IgM deposits. Note the IgM deposits at the node of Ranvier (arrow) and along the fiber (arrowheads). The thickness of the fiber is approximately 8 μm. (See also Chapter 26, Fig. 26.2.)

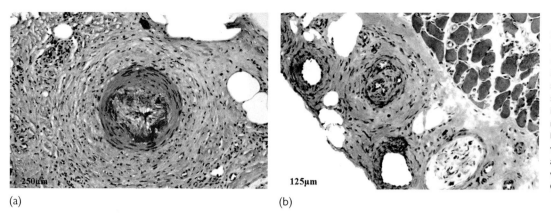

(a)

250μm

(b)

125μm

Plate 7 Nerve and muscle biopsy of a patient with non-systemic PNS vasculitis. Cross-section of a paraffin-embedded specimen; hemotoxylin–eosin staining: (a) acute vasculitic inflammation—fibrinoid necrosis, cellular infiltration and lumen occlusion; (b) chronic vasculitic changes—obliteration and recanalization of the vascular lumen. (See also Chapter 30, Fig. 30.1.)

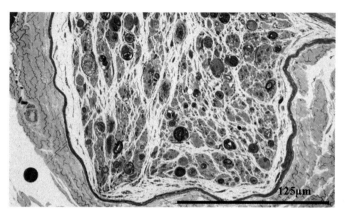

125μm

Plate 8 Nerve biopsy of a patient with non-systemic PNS vasculitis. Cross-section of a plastic-embedded nerve specimen; toluidine blue staining. Note the degeneration of all nerve fibers. (See also Chapter 30, Fig. 30.2.)

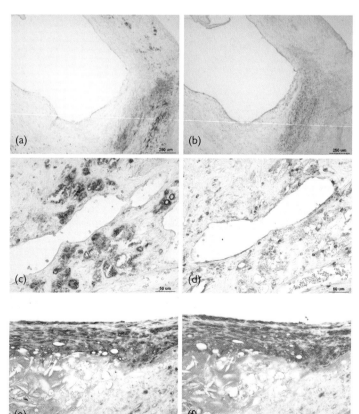

(a)

(b)

250 μm

(c)

(d)

50 μm

(e)

(f)

Plate 9 Inflammation and atherosclerosis. Endarterectomy specimens from symptomatic high-grade internal carotid artery stenosis stained for macrophages (a, higher magnification c), T cells (b, higher magnification d), pro-thrombotic tissue factor (TF) (e), and collagen-degrading matrix metalloproteinase (MMP) (f). Note that inflammation is located in the atheromatous core of the lesion and the fibrous cap from which TF and MMP expression extends to the luminal surface.(See also Chapter 32, Fig. 32.1.)

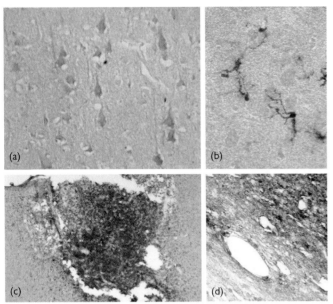

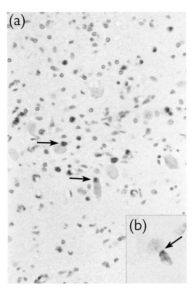

Plate 10 Cytokines in experimental cerebral ischemia. Localization of TNF (a), IL-1β (b), IL-18 (c), and TGF-β1 (d) by immunocytochemistry, and gene expression profiles of TNF, IL-1β, and inducible NO synthase (iNOS) as revealed by semiquantitative reverse transcriptase polymerase chain reaction. Note that TNF, IL-1β, and iNOS mRNA peak within 24 hours after focal ischemia. On the cellular level TNF is mainly expressed by neurons (a), IL-1 β by microglia (b), while IL-18 (c) and TGF-β1 (d) are induced with a delay and are mainly expressed by macrophages and microglia. (See also Chapter 32, Fig. 32.3.)

Plate 11 Immunohistochemical findings in Rasmussen's encephalitis. A: CD8+ lymphocytes infiltrate the right hippocampus of a 7-year-old boy undergoing right-sided hemispherectomy (seizures and progressive left-sided hemiparesis since 15 months). Note the T cells that lie in close apposition to neurons (arrows). Original magnification ×246. B: Same patient as in A. A granzyme B+ lymphocyte in apposition to a neuron. Note the polarization of the granzyme B+ granules towards the neuron (arrow). Original magnification ×990 Courtesy of Dr Christian G. Bien, University of Bonn, Department of Epileptology, Bonn, Germany and Dr Jan Bauer, University of Vienna, Brain Research Institute, Division of Neuroimmunology, Vienna, Austria. (See also Chapter 33, Fig. 33.2.)

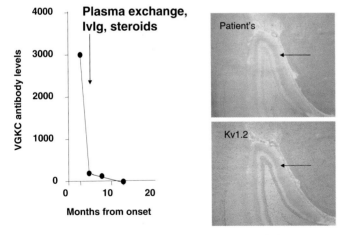

Plate 12 Antibodies to voltage-gated potassium channels in a CNS disease. Left: VGKC antibodies are found in some patients with limbic encephalitis (memory loss, disorientation, seizures, personality change). The VGKC antibodies fall markedly following treatments such as intravenous immunoglobulin, plasma exchange, and steroids, associated with substantial improvement in the patient. Right: serum from these patients bind to the neuronal processes in the dentate gyrus of the hippocampus (upper panel), in a distribution similar to that of rabbit antibodies to the VGKC Kv1.2 subtype (lower panel). Immunohistochemistry courtesy of Dr Camilla Buckley Department of Clinical Neurology, University of Oxford (See also Chapter 33, Fig. 33.3.)

cytokine receptors, can be found in the blood of GBS patients (Hartung and Toyka, 1990). However, studies to identify nerve antigens to which aberrant T-cell responses are mounted, as well as attempts to establish specific T-cell lines from affected patients, have yielded controversial results. In GBS, an increased usage of Vβ15 T-cell receptor chains has been demonstrated, pointing to a potentially restricted T-cell response to a common antigen, or a role for an as yet undefined superantigen in the pathogenesis of GBS (Khalili-Shirazi et al., 1997a). Using the complementarity-determining region (CDR)-3 spectratyping method, oligoclonal expansion of T cells bearing specific Vβ or Vδ T-cell receptor genes could be identified, however, the predominant phenotypes varied even within subgroups of GBS patients (Koga et al., 2003a). The observation of γδ T lymphocytes in nerve biopsies from affected patients points to potential involvement of this cell population in the inflamed PNS (Khalili-Shirazi et al., 1997b). An unusual Vγ8/δ1 T-cell receptor chain usage was defined in a γδ T-cell line obtained from a sural nerve biopsy of a patient with demyelinating GBS, suggesting that gut-associated lymphocytes are critically involved in the pathogenesis of this disorder (Cooper et al., 2000). However, other groups suggest a non-responsiveness of γδ T cells inducing a defective regulation of antibody production and promoting an immune response against ganglioside-like epitopes on peripheral nerve (Van Rhijn et al., 2003).

Although systemic immune activation appears to be present in GBS patients, the specificity of this immune reactivity remains elusive. In order to generate inflammatory lesions in the peripheral nerve, activated T cells need to cross the blood–nerve barrier. The complex process of homing, adhesion, and transmigration has been studied in EAN in great detail. In GBS patients, increased serum or CSF levels of soluble adhesion molecules (Previtali et al., 1998, 2001), chemokines (Hartung et al., 2002; Kieseier et al., 2002; Press et al., 2003), and matrix metalloproteinases can be detected (Kieseier et al., 1998), reflecting active T-cell migration across the blood–nerve barrier.

The potential role of a cytotoxic T-cell response in myelin damage in GBS was established by demonstrating a high number of CD8+ T lymphocytes in nervous tissue (Wanschitz et al., 2003).

Ubiquitous transcription factors such as NF-κB may play a critical role in mediating the inflammatory reaction within the PNS as their activity increases the rate of specific gene transcriptions. In sural nerve biopsies from GBS patients, NF-κB was found to be up-regulated and expressed by macrophages within the inflamed tissue (Andorfer et al., 2001; Mazzeo et al., 2004), pointing to a key position of NF-κB in the signaling cascade of various pro-inflammatory mediators, such cytokines and prostaglandins (Hu et al., 2003), during ongoing inflammation within the PNS. Studies in the peripheral venous blood of GBS patients demonstrated an early elevation of T cells with an anti-inflammatory cytokine pattern, suggesting that a shift in the systemic distribution of the T-cell pattern towards so-called T helper 2 (Th2)-type T lymphocytes may account for the self-limiting course of the disease (Press et al., 2002).

Humoral immune response

Various observations suggest that humoral factors are of critical importance in the pathogenesis of GBS: (1) plasmapheresis and intravenous immunoglobulin (IV Ig) result in clinical improvement (Hartung, 1995); (2) circulating antibodies targeting structures on peripheral nerve tissue are detectable in sera from GBS patients (Wessig et al., 2001), and (3) deposition of immunoglobulins and complement has been demonstrated on myelinated fibers in nerve biopsies as well as CSF samples from affected patients (Hartung et al., 1987; Hafer-Macko et al., 1996). Theoretically, antibodies directed against epitopes on the outermost surface of the Schwann cell or axolemma could bind complement, resulting in sublytic complement activation and the development of membrane pores formed by terminal complement components. The specific target of such antibodies remains elusive. Whether gangliosides and other glycolipids represent autoantigens is uncertain at present. Gangliosides are widely distributed within the nervous system. Numerous gangliosides, such as GM$_1$, are present at the nodes of Ranvier and as such would represent particularly sus-

ceptible targets for autoimmune attacks (Fig. 19.1). GQ$_{1b}$ is enriched in oculomotor nerves, suggesting an explanation for the regional involvement in MFS that is almost invariably associated with anti-GQ$_{1b}$ antibodies (Chiba et al., 1993). Moreover, recent data suggest that neuropathogenic antiganglioside autoantibodies can arise from the natural autoantibody repertoire (Boffey et al., 2004).

In several in vitro studies, sera from GBS patients have been added to cell cultures in order to ascertain the potential to produce demyelination or Schwann cell damage. However, divergent results were obtained, in that in some studies myelin disintegration was reported even with sera from patients with other neurological diseases or healthy controls. How such observations mirror clinically relevant pathomechanisms is difficult to judge since various variables need to be taken into account. The ganglioside GM$_2$ provides an interesting example of the difficulties encountered in investigating these issues. In cytotoxicity studies, for example, using sera from patients with demyelinating dysimmune neuropathies and high titers of anti-GM$_2$ IgM, Cavanna and co-workers were able to induce complement-mediated lysis of neuroblastoma cells (Cavanna et al., 2001). However, in studies looking at the effects of antibody and complement complexes on neuronal physiology, rabbit GM$_2$ antibodies had no effect on voltage-gated sodium channels whereas anti-GM$_1$ antibodies reduced sodium current by about one half (Weber et al., 2000). Furthermore, sera with high-titer anti-GM$_2$ antibodies did not bind to human or rodent peripheral nerve sections, despite previous biochemical evidence demonstrating GM$_2$ in peripheral nerve (O'Hanlon et al., 2000).

The electrophysiological effects of sera from patients with MFS and GQ$_{1b}$ antibodies have been studied by various groups. Although GQ$_{1b}$ antibodies did not alter the electrophysiological properties of mouse sciatic nerve preparations despite binding to nodes of Ranvier (Paparounas et al., 1999), profound effects were observable at the neuromuscular junction. Using a mouse hemidiaphragm model, an α-latrotoxin-like complement-dependent effect was found, resulting in massive quantal release of acetylcholine and subsequent failure of neuromuscular transmission (Plomp et al., 1999). Similar observations were made with IgM monoclonal antibodies directed against disialylated gangliosides, thus confirming that the effect was due to the antiganglioside antibody rather than other unidentified serum factors. This effect was complement-dependent and associated with extensive deposits of IgM and C3c at nerve terminals (Goodyear et al., 1999). Using electron microscopy, accompanying destruction of axonal terminals was noted (O'Hanlon et al., 2001). Using preparations from MFS cases, others demonstrated a reversible inhibition of pre-synaptic quantal release, as well as reduced post-synaptic quantal amplitudes following incubation with serum or purified IgG from MFS patients but not healthy controls. This effect, however, was not dependent on the presence of GQ$_{1b}$ antibodies or complement, and thus the antigenic target remains unidentified (Buchwald et al., 1998a,b). Electron microscopy revealed binding of IgG from MFS patients on both pre- and post-synaptic membranes of the neuromuscular junction (Wessig et al., 2001). Using an outside-out patch-clamp technique, an independent effect of MFS IgG on post-synaptic currents was demonstrated (Buchwald et al., 2001).

In vivo studies are beginning to clarify some of the pathogenic mechanisms involved in nerve injury mediated by antiglycolipid antibodies. Many conflicting results have been obtained in studies trying to transfer disease passively by injecting patient sera or antibodies into animals. Immunization of rabbits with GD$_{1b}$ and GM$_1$, respectively, resulted in models of sensory ataxic neuronopathy and motor axonopathy with clinical deficits (Kusunoki et al., 1996). In the studies on GM$_1$, pathological analysis revealed an axonal neuropathy with only little if any inflammation in the peripheral nerve, similar to AMAN (Yuki et al., 2001). On the other hand, others failed to exacerbate EAN by injecting sera from GBS patients and antibodies against gangliosides, raising some doubts about the pathogenic relevance of antibodies in GBS sera (Hadden et al., 2001a). Thus, a critical issue is clearly the choice of experimental model used to investigate these putative pathogenic relationships.

Peripheral nerve demyelination may be the result of serum constituents other than myelin-specific antibodies, such as cytokines, complement, or other inflammatory mediators. Similarly, it remains possible that GBS sera contain substrates that might produce conduction block without necessarily causing demyelination or evoke failure of neuromuscular transmission. Apparently, there is a link between the humoral and the cellular immune response. Anti-GM$_1$ IgG antibodies obtained from GBS patients were demonstrated to activate leukocyte inflammatory functions, such as degranulation and phagocytosis, underlining the complexity of the immunopathogenesis of GBS (van Sorge et al., 2003).

In patients with GBS circulating antibodies binding to peripheral nerve antigens or purified myelin have been detected with varying frequency; however, such antibodies can also be found in other neurological disorders and even in healthy controls (O'Leary and Willison, 2000). Between 5 and 50% of sera were reported to contain antibodies to the myelin proteins P0, P2, and PMP22 (Gabriel et al., 2000); these data, though, could not be confirmed by others (Kwa et al., 2001). Specific attention has focused on humoral immune responses to the glycoconjugate antigens. Increased titers of antiglycolipid antibodies in series of GBS cases have ranged from 5 to 60%, reflecting many variables including the patient population, the cross-reactivities of these antibodies, and differences in the sensitivities and definitions of normal ranges of the various assays used (reviewed in Willison and Yuki (2002)). The presence of these antibodies varies partly according to the clinical phenotype, and titers tend to decline after the acute phase of the disease. Cross-reactivity of antiganglioside antibodies with related structures is a critical aspect (Koga et al., 2001a; Susuki et al., 2001). Therefore, autoreactivity against a particular ganglioside moiety present on several different gangliosides, rather than autoreactivity against a single ganglioside species, may trigger a broad autoimmune response. It is thus equally important to recognize that any single serum commonly contains multiple antibodies of differing specificities and cross-reactivity patterns.

Despite tremendous effort, no characteristic pattern of antiganglioside antibodies has been established in AIDP. Anti-GM$_1$ antibodies are found in AIDP as well as in AMAN, and this association seems to be higher in patients with serologic evidence of a preceding infection with C. jejuni (Jacobs et al., 1996; Yuki et al., 2000; Ang et al., 2001a,b). Nevertheless, the prognostic value of anti-GM$_1$ antibodies is still under debate. In AMAN, the primary target appears to be the axon rather than the Schwann cell or myelin, and some evidence suggests that axon-specific target epitopes could be contained in axonal gangliosides, at least in some cases. In these forms of GBS, some authors described particularly strong associations with anti-GM$_1$, anti-GD$_{1a}$, and anti-GalNAc-GD$_{1a}$ IgG antibodies (Yuki et al., 2000). In Chinese patients a much stronger association was reported with anti-GD$_{1a}$ antibodies (Yuki et al., 1999a). Several studies have extended observations on the association between anti-GM$_1$, anti-GalNAc-GD$_{1a}$, and anti-GM$_{1ab}$ antibodies and the acute motor axonal variant (Yuki et al., 1990; Hao et al., 1999; Ogawara et al., 2003). A morphological study revealed a staining pattern for anti-GalNAc-GD1a antibodies along the inner part of compact myelin and additionally a periaxonal–axolemma-related portion in the ventral roots, small-diameter dorsal root fibers, and motor nerves (Kaida et al., 2003). Thus, in AMAN a much clearer relationships can be defined compared with AIDP, the former being associated with antibodies to either GM$_1$, GD$_{1a}$, GM$_{1b}$, or GalNAc-GD$_{1a}$ in a high proportion of cases. In the acute motor and sensory axonal variant (AMSAN), only a few patients have been studied and anti-GM$_1$, anti-GM$_{1b}$, and anti-GD$_{1a}$ IgG antibodies have been described (Yuki et al., 1999b). In the Miller–Fisher variant, increased serum titers of antibodies to GQ$_{1b}$ and GT$_{1a}$ are consistently found in 90–100% of patients (Chiba et al., 1992), including acute oropharyngeal palsy and GBS cases with prominent bulbar involvement (Koga et al., 1999; Yoshino et al., 2000; Odaka et al., 2001).

A number of studies have tried to match antibodies to clinical syndromes. The hypothesis that the regional and topographical distribution, and function, of glycolipids in different areas of the human nervous system may play a role in defining the pathophysiological features of their autoantibody-associated disease is the driving force for many studies. For example, in human ocular muscle nerves GQ$_{1b}$ is enriched, which may account for the vulnerability of these nerves to immune-mediated attack in the MFS (Chiba et al., 1992). However, the distribution pattern of GQ$_{1b}$ does not correlate entirely with the lesions expected based on clinical and neurophysiological observations in this GBS variant. Therefore, other factors, such as antibody access and glycolipid membrane topography, appear to also be important in mediating the clinical picture.

Studies have been undertaken to determine whether specific antiganglioside antibodies might be involved in GBS (Annunziata et al., 2003). In a recent study on 42 GBS patients positive for the anti-GM$_1$ antibody, the IgG1 subclass of anti-GM$_1$ antibody appeared to be a major subtype indicative of slow recovery, whereas isolated elevation of IgG$_3$ subclass antibody titer was indicative of rapid recovery. Variation in subclass patterns may depend on which pathogen precipitates GBS (Koga et al., 2003b).

Preceding infections

Antiglycolipid antibodies are frequently found at low levels in normal sera, indicating that these antibodies are part of a naturally occurring autoantibody repertoire. A trigger is needed to raise the this threshold and specifically shape a B-cell response in GBS patients. Microbial polysaccharide antigens such as lipopolysaccharides containing repetitive sugar sequences can activate B cells and drive the antiglycolipid response in many patients. Increased serum levels of antiglycolipid antibodies have been associated with a preceding infection. A number of infective agents are now firmly linked to the pathogenesis of GBS (Jacobs et al., 1998). These include C. jejuni in particular, as well as CMV, Epstein–Barr virus (EBV), Mycoplasma pneumoniae, and H. influenzae. Since AIDP and AMAN have been recognized as separate entities, more detailed studies have attempted to define differences in preceding events for these two conditions.

Campylobacter jejuni

C. jejuni is a genetically highly variable spiral, flagellated bacillus. Based on its antigenicity or direct DNA comparison, a large number of strains can be differentiated. Infections with C. jejuni precede GBS in up to two-thirds of cases, with a lower incidence in European patients compared with Asian studies. However, technical considerations should be taken into account, and in a recent study measuring patient samples in both a Japanese and a Dutch laboratory, no significant difference was found (Koga et al., 2001b). C. jejuni is strongly but not exclusively associated with AMAN both in European (Rees et al., 1993, 1995; Rees and Hughes, 1994; Jacobs et al., 1996) and Chinese patients (Ho et al., 1995). Furthermore, C. jejuni infection was relatively more common in GBS patients with pure motor symptoms or axonal electrophysiology compared with other GBS cases in a large cohort, but the majority of GBS cases with preceding C. jejuni infection still had the demyelinating phenotype (Hadden et al., 2001b). However, it is only a small proportion of patients with C. jejuni enteritis that develop subsequent GBS (van Belkum et al., 1995). In a Swedish study, nine GBS cases were detected amongst nearly 30 000 cases of C. jejuni infection, raising the risk to suffer GBS by about 100 (McCarthy and Giesecke, 2001). It appears that specific serotypes of C. jejuni may trigger GBS. In Japan for example, GBS was found to be associated with C. jejuni serotype HS:19 (Nishimura et al., 1997), whereas no such association has been reported in Europe so far. Further analysis of HS:19 isolates from GBS patients has revealed that the majority of strains but not all isolates belonged to a single clone which, however, was also found in uncomplicated enteritis (Nachamkin et al., 2001). Studies in strains other than HS:19 or unselected C. jejuni isolates failed to detect clonality of C. jejuni strains associated with GBS (Engberg et al., 2001). Therefore it can be assumed that despite some clustering of certain strains in some series, present evidence argues against the association of distinct strains of C. jejuni with GBS. Precise genetic comparisons of isolates using nucleotide sequence data confirm that C. jejuni strains associated with GBS are of diverse genetic lineage, serotype, and flagella type (Endtz et al., 2000; Dingle et al., 2001). In a recently conducted microarray analysis significant heterogeneity among C. jejuni strains associated with GBS could be confirmed (Leonard et al., 2004).

The *C. jejuni* lipopolysaccharide fraction contains sidechains with the same structures as some of the gangliosides, especially GM_1, GD_{1a}, GD_3 and GT_{1a} (Willison and Yuki, 2002). Many studies support the view that molecular mimicry between *C. jejuni* lipopolysaccharides and gangliosides plays a key role in the induction of antiganglioside antibodies and neurological symptoms in patients with GBS and some of its variants. The heterogeneity in the lipopolysaccharide structure apparently determines the specificity of the antiglycolipid response and thereby the clinical features in patients with a post-*Campylobacter* neuropathy (Ang *et al.*, 2002; Annunziata *et al.*, 2003). However, only half of the GBS patients with anti-GM_1 antibodies have had a preceding infection with *C. jejuni*, so that there must be other environmental triggers for the production of the antiganglioside antibodies (Willison and Yuki, 2002).

Other infectious agents

In 8–13 % of GBS patients serological evidence for a preceding CMV infection has been documented. These patients were younger, had severe sensorimotor involvement, and usually exhibited the demyelinating phenotype (Hadden *et al.*, 2001*b*).

An antecedent EBV infection can be established in 2–10% of GBS patients. These patients generally have higher CSF cell counts and a higher incidence of respiratory failure, but are clinically otherwise indistinguishable from other GBS cases (Jacobs *et al.*, 1998; Hadden *et al.*, 2001*b*).

Evidence for a preceding *M. pneumoniae* infection has been obtained in 5% of GBS patients. These patients are typically younger but in other respects do not differ from other GBS cases (Jacobs *et al.*, 1998).

Whereas no association has been associated in European patients so far (Jacobs *et al.*, 1998), preceding *H. influenzae* infection has been found in up to 13% of Japanese GBS patients (Mori *et al.*, 2000).

Immunogenetic factors

Disease heterogeneity and varying associations of preceding infections, antibody responses, and neurological damage may be secondary to immunogenetic factors that direct the host immune response. Attempts to identify an immunogenetic susceptibility factor have largely focused on the HLA system, but no reproducible association between any of the common serologically defined HLA Class I and II antigens and GBS and its variants has been established so far. Although some studies have suggested a positive relationship within homogeneous subgroups it has not been possible to reliably identify immune susceptibility genes in GBS at present. One complicating factor in seeking susceptibility determinants in the HLA system is that humoral immune responses to carbohydrate structures are largely T-cell independent and thus not Class I or II antigen restricted.

Therapy

Plasmapheresis and IV Ig are the mainstay of immunomodulatory treatment of GBS at present. Both treatments have proven to exhibit beneficial effects in various controlled trials in favorably altering the natural course of the disease (Guillain–Barré Syndrome Study Group, 1985; French Cooperative Group on Plasma Exchange in Guillain–Barré Syndrome, 1987; van der Meché and Schmitz, 1992; Ropper 1992; Bril *et al.*, 1996; Raphael *et al.*, 2001; Hughes *et al.*, 2001*a*; Cheng *et al.*, 2003). In a large controlled trial, combined treatment with plasmapheresis followed by IV Ig did not provide significant additional benefit. The number of plasma exchanges required for effective treatment was determined in a large prospective study: two exchanges were sufficient to shorten the disease in mildly affected patients, whereas four exchanges were appropriate for patients with moderate to severe GBS, and further exchanges did not provide any additional benefit (French Cooperative Group on Plasma Exchange in Guillain–Barré Syndrome, 1997).

In contrast to other autoimmune diseases, glucocorticoids have no rational place in the treatment of GBS at present (Hughes and van Der Meche, 2000). In a recently published Dutch study, patients receiving a combination of IV Ig and glucocorticoids did not recover faster than patients receiving IV Ig alone (van Koningsveld *et al.*, 2004).

Filtration of CSF was investigated in a small prospective study of GBS patients and found to be equally safe and effective compared with conventional plasmapheresis (Wollinsky *et al.*, 2001). This study supports the concept that soluble pathogenetic factors present particularly in the CSF, possibly including a small pentapeptide with sodium channel-blocking properties (Brinkmeier *et al.*, 2000), are of paramount importance in the pathogenesis of GBS. However, the pathology of GBS is not restricted to the CSF compartment, raising questions about the rationale of this treatment. Furthermore, serious methodological concerns have been expressed (Feasby and Hartung, 2001).

Various reports suggest that IV Ig is superior to plasma exchange, especially in GBS patients with a preceding *C. jejuni* infection, an axonal and predominantly motor syndrome, GM_1 or GM_{1b} antibodies (Visser *et al.*, 1995; Jacobs *et al.*, 1996; Yuki *et al.*, 2000). However, none of these correlations is absolute, and testing for ganglioside antibodies and preceding infections to guide therapeutic decisions may not be warranted in routine clinical situations (Hadden *et al.*, 2001*b*). Nevertheless, IV Ig is now considered the treatment of first choice by many authorities, given its efficacy, ease of administration, and the low incidence of side-effects of this drug.

Since only around 60% of GBS patients respond to plasma exchange or IV Ig, the search for other treatments is clearly warranted. Anecdotal observations suggest IFN-β1a is a useful adjunctive therapy (Créange *et al.*, 1998; Schaller *et al.*, 2001). Various approaches have been tested in the animal model so far; however, their clinical relevance still needs to be studied in great detail.

Chronic inflammatory demyelinating neuropathy

Clinical characteristics

Chronic inflammatory demyelinating polyneuropathy (CIDP) is an acquired immune-mediated peripheral neuropathy, clinically characterized in its course as steadily progressive, stepwise progressive, chronic monophasic, or recurrent (Dyck *et al.*, 1993). Recent surveys report a prevalence of 1.9

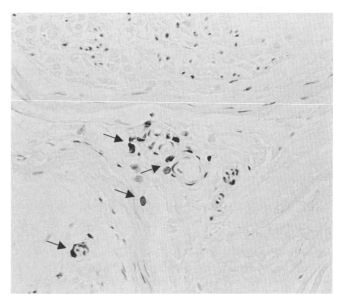

Fig. 19.2 T-cell infiltration in a sural nerve from a patient diagnosed with Guillain–Barré syndrome. In a cross-section invading CD3+ T cells can primarily be localized to perivascular infiltrates (arrows) in the epi- and perineurium by immunohistochemistry. Original magnification ×120.

and 7.7 per 100 000 (McLeod *et al.*, 1999; Mygland and Monstadt, 2001), but these numbers are probably an underestimate, most probably due to under-reporting and uncertainty in making the diagnosis. Most patients exhibit involvement of both motor and sensory fibers, but some show predominant motor or sensory neuropathy. There is a tendency to symmetric involvement, and both proximal and distal muscles may be affected. Cranial nerves and respiratory muscles are sometimes involved, though clearly much less frequently than in GBS. However, recent observations underline that many patients do not conform to these classical features of the disease, exhibiting predominantly distal distribution, pure sensory neuropathy, marked asymmetries, associated demyelinating disease, or predominant cranial nerve involvement (Rotta *et al.*, 2000). In order to include the broad spectrum of clinical presentations of CIDP and define the requirement of diagnostic procedures for establishing definite, probable, and possible CIDP, different definitions and modifications, especially of the electrodiagnostic criteria, have been proposed (Saperstein *et al.*, 2001; Hughes *et al.*, 2001*b*; Sander and Latov, 2003).

Morphology and immunopathology

Histopathologically CIDP is characterized by multifocal, predominantly proximal, inflammatory demyelination, affecting chiefly spinal nerve roots, spinal nerves, major plexuses, or proximal nerve trunks, with lesions extending throughout the PNS including, in some cases, the intramuscular nerves, sympathetic trunks, and terminal autonomic nerves (Dyck *et al.*, 1993). Sural nerve biopsies, still an important tool in confirming the clinical diagnosis, typically show endoneurial edema, ongoing or recurrent demyelination, Schwann cell proliferation with onion-bulb formation, inflammatory infiltrates, axonal degeneration, and axonal loss (Prineas, 1994; Kiefer *et al.*, 1998). Lymphocytes are found in the endoneurium, and may be observed within the basement membrane of fibers in contact with macrophages. However, myelin degradation appears to be initiated by macrophages, as no consistent changes have been identified in fibers not in contact with these cells. These morphological observations underline the key role of the immune system in the pathogenesis of CIDP (Fig. 19.3).

As in GBS, molecular mimicry has also been proposed as key mechanism in the immunopathogenesis of the disease. Whereas in GBS several epitopes shared between bacterial species and nerve fibers could be identified as putative targets for aberrant cross-reactive immune responses, such evidence has not been obtained for CIDP. A preceding illness, mostly a non-specific upper respiratory or gastrointestinal tract infection, or vaccination 6 months prior to disease onset has been observed in 32% of cases (McCombe *et al.*, 1987). Others have reported that 16% of patients noted an infectious event within 6 weeks of the first neurological manifestations (Bouchard *et al.*, 1999). Further evidence supporting the concept of molecular mimicry is based on the association of CIDP with melanoma (Bird *et al.*, 1996; Weiss *et al.*, 1998). This observation is of specific interest since melanoma and Schwann cells derive from neural crest tissues and share common antigens. A number of carbohydrate epitopes expressed on human melanoma or melanomatous cell lines, including gangliosides GM_3, GM_2, GD_3, and GD_2, have been implicated in human neuropathies (Tsuchida *et al.*, 1989). Furthermore, monoclonal antibodies raised against melanoma cells react with myelin-associated glycoprotein, other myelin glycoproteins, and sulphate-3-glucuronyl paragloboside (Noronha *et al.*, 1986).

Cellular immune response

By analogy to GBS, the presence of inflammatory infiltrates in the affected nerve suggests that disordered cellular immunity is critically involved in the pathogenesis of CIDP (Gold *et al.*, 2000). However, studies to identify nerve antigens to which aberrant T-cell responses are mounted, as well as attempts to establish specific T-cell lines from affected patients, have not met with success.

Mechanisms for the induction of inflammatory lesions in the peripheral nerve, with disruption of the blood–nerve barrier and reactivation within the PNS, are similar to those described in GBS. As in GBS, elevated serum or CSF levels of soluble adhesion molecules (Previtali *et al.*, 1998, 2001), chemokines (Kieseier *et al.*, 2002), and matrix metalloproteinases (Kieseier *et al.*, 1998; Leppert *et al.*, 1999) can be detected in CIDP patients. In nerve biopsies, reactivated T lymphocytes exerting various effects by generating and emanating differentiation and proliferation signals, such as TNF-α, IFN-γ, or IL-2, have been found (Mathey *et al.*, 1999). Apart from the initiation and perpetuation of the inflammatory cascade that culminates in demyelination and axonal degeneration, T lymphocytes may also execute salutary actions. Specialized subpopulations of T cells may terminate the acute immunoinflammatory process by the secretion of down-regulatory cytokines, such as IL-4, IL-10, or TGF-β, or other molecules. On the mRNA level, the expression of anti-inflammatory cytokines, such as IL-6, as well as of various neurotrophic factors, including nerve growth factor (NGF), glial cell line-derived neurotrophic factor (GDNF), and leukemia inhibitory factor (LIF), and their concomitant receptors were found to be up-regulated in the nerve lesion of CIDP (Yamamoto *et al.*, 2002), suggestive that these molecules might be involved in nerve regeneration. Moreover, LIF has been shown to be involved in an auotcrine signaling cascade amplifying Schwann cell-derived chemotactic signaling (Tofaris *et al.*, 2002).

Observations on the role of macrophages in CIDP are similar to those described in GBS (Hartung *et al.*, 2002).

Humoral immune response

A major role in pathogenesis has been attributed to antibodies, especially since a majority of patients respond to plasma exchange therapy (Toyka and Hartung, 1996; Hahn *et al.*, 1996*a*). Furthermore, immunoglobulins (IgM and IgG) and complement deposition have been reported in nerve biopsies of CIDP patients (Dalakas and Engel, 1980; Hays *et al.*, 1988). An emerging body of evidence points to gangliosides and other glycolipids as putative target antigens. In one study (Hughes 1995) 15% of the 40 CIDP patients studied had detectable serum IgM antibodies against GM1 (Melendez-Vasquez *et al.*, 1997). In 5%, IgM antibodies against LM_1, the predominant ganglioside in the human peripheral nerve myelin, and in 10% IgG were observed. However, in another study the presence of anti-LM_1 antibodies in CIDP patients was reported to be much lower (Yako *et al.*, 1999). The pathogenetic relevance of such autoantibodies was demonstrated by the observation that anti-GM_1 antiserum from a CIDP patient suppressed significantly Na^+ currents in single myelinated nerve fibers of rat (Takigawa *et al.*, 2000).

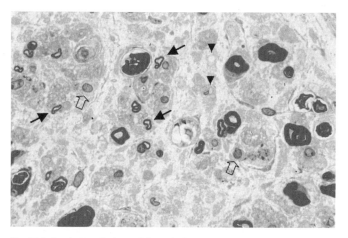

Fig. 19.3 Sural nerve findings of chronic inflammatory demyelinating polyneuropathy (CIDP). Cross-section of a sural nerve revealing typical features of CIDP: In semithin sections the extent of the inflammatory process is reflected by the loss of myelin (arrow heads indicating demyelinated axons, arrows pointing to the remains of thinly myelinated fibers), and invading macrophages (open arrows) can be visualized. Original magnification ×200.

Peripheral nerve demyelination and conduction block may be the result of serum constituents other than myelin-specific antibodies such as cytokines, complement, or other inflammatory mediators. Similarly, it remains possible that CIDP sera contain substrates that might produce conduction block without necessarily causing demyelination or evoke failure of neuromuscular transmission. Furthermore, conduction in demyelinated axons appears susceptible to a range of small variations in the internal environment, such as perturbations causing either axonal hyperpolarization or depolarization precipitating conduction block (Cappelen-Smith *et al.*, 2002). The low frequency of specific antibodies observed in patients so far makes it likely that different antibodies and separate mechanisms are critically involved in different patients (Pollard, 2002).

Axonal loss

Although by name and definition a demyelinating neuropathy, CIDP is associated with a concomitant axonal loss attributed to the primary demyelinating process (Bouchard *et al.*, 1999; Dalakas, 1999). The clinical long-term prognosis in CIDP depends on the magnitude of axonal loss rather than on demyelination.

Therapy

CIDP responds well to several treatment modalities including steroids, plasma exchange, IV Ig, and immunosuppressant drugs. The efficacy of plasma exchange correlated with significant improvement of nerve conduction parameters in several studies (Dyck *et al.*, 1986; Hahn *et al.*, 1996*a*) Clinical improvement was observed both in patients with a progressive or a relapsing course of the disease. IV Ig is very potent and a beneficial effect was also observed patients who were non-responsive to steroids and plasma exchange (van Doorn *et al.*, 1990; Cornblath *et al.*, 1991; Hahn *et al.*, 1996*a,b*; Mendell *et al.*, 2001; Hughes *et al.*, 2001*b*; van Schaik *et al.*). At present, IV Ig is commonly accepted as the first-line treatment for CIDP.

Among immunomodulatory treatments, beneficial effects have been seen with azathioprine (McCombe *et al.*, 1987) and cyclosporine (Hodgkinson *et al.*, 1990). Moreover, anecdotal reports have provided evidence that IFN-β is therapeutically effective in CIDP (Martina *et al.*, 1999). However, a randomized trial revealed that IFN-β is safe but not effective in patients with CIDP resistant to other treatment modalities (Hadden *et al.*, 1999). Mycophenolate, however, did not show any clinically significant benefit in otherwise treatment-resistant CIDP (Umapathi and Hughes, 2002). A recent Cochrane database analysis concludes that there is inadequate evidence to decide whether IFN-β, azathioprine, or any other immunosuppressive drug are beneficial in CIDP (Hughes *et al.*, 2003).

References

Andorfer, B., Kieseier, B.C., Mathey, E., Armati, P., Pollard, J., Oka, N., *et al.* (2001). Expression and distribution of transcription factor NF-kappaB and inhibitor IkappaB in the inflamed peripheral nervous system. *J Neuroimmunol* 116: 226–232.

Ang, C.W., Koga, M., Jacobs, B.C., Yuki, N., van der Meche, F.G., and van Doorn, P.A. (2001*a*). Differential immune response to gangliosides in Guillain–Barre syndrome patients from Japan and The Netherlands. *J Neuroimmunol* 121: 83–87.

Ang, C.W., De Klerk, M.A., Endtz, H.P., Jacobs, B.C., Laman, J.D., van der Meche, F.G., *et al.* (2001*b*). Guillain–Barre syndrome- and Miller Fisher syndrome-associated *Campylobacter jejuni* lipopolysaccharides induce anti-GM1 and anti-GQ1b antibodies in rabbits. *Infect Immun* 69: 2462–2469.

Ang, C.W., Laman, J.D., Willison, H.J., Wagner, E.R., Endtz, H.P., De Klerk, M.A., *et al.* (2002). Structure of *Campylobacter jejuni* lipopolysaccharides determines antiganglioside specificity and clinical features of Guillain–Barre and Miller Fisher patients. *Infect Immun* 70: 1202–1208.

Annunziata, P., Figura, N., Galli, R., Mugnaini, F., and Lenzi, C. (2003). Association of anti-GM1 antibodies but not of anti-cytomegalovirus, *Campylobacter jejuni* and *Helicobacter pylori* IgG, with a poor outcome in Guillain–Barre syndrome. *J Neurol Sci* 213: 55–60.

Bird, S.J., Brown, M.J., Shy, M.E., and Scherer, S.S. (1996). Chronic inflammatory demyelinating polyneuropathy associated with malignant melanoma. *Neurology* 46: 822–824.

Boffey, J., Nicholl, D., Wagner, E.R., Townson, K., Goodyear, C., Furukawa, K., *et al.* (2004). Innate murine B cells produce anti-disialosyl antibodies reactive with *Campylobacter jejuni* LPS and gangliosides that are polyreactive and encoded by a restricted set of unmutated V genes. *J Neuroimmunol* 152: 98–111.

Bouchard, C., Lacroix, C., Plante, V., Adams, D., Chedru, F., Guglielmi, J.M., *et al.* (1999). Clinicopathologic findings and prognosis of chronic inflammatory demyelinating polyneuropathy. *Neurology* 52: 498–503.

Bril, V., Ilse, W.K., Pearce, R., Dhanani, A., Sutton, D., and Kong, K. (1996). Pilot trial of immunoglobulin versus plasma exchange in patients with Guillain–Barre syndrome. *Neurology* 46: 100–103.

Brinkmeier, H., Aulkemeyer, P., Wollinsky, K.H., and Rudel, R. (2000). An endogenous pentapeptide acting as a sodium channel blocker in inflammatory autoimmune disorders of the central nervous system. *Nat Med* 6: 808–811.

Buchwald, B., Weishaupt, A., Toyka, K.V., and Dudel, J. (1998*a*). Pre- and postsynaptic blockade of neuromuscular transmission by Miller-Fisher syndrome IgG at mouse motor nerve terminals. *Eur J Neurosci* 10: 281–290.

Buchwald, B., Dudel, J., and Toyka, K.V. (1998*b*). Neuromuscular blockade by immunoglobulin G from patients with Miller Fisher syndrome. *Ann N Y Acad Sci* 841: 659–669.

Buchwald, B., Bufler, J., Carpo, M., Heidenreich, F., Pitz, R., Dudel, J., *et al.* (2001). Combined pre- and postsynaptic action of IgG antibodies in Miller Fisher syndrome. *Neurology* 56: 67–74.

Cappelen-Smith, C., Lin, C.S., Kuwabara, S., and Burke, D. (2002). Conduction block during and after ischaemia in chronic inflammatory demyelinating polyneuropathy. *Brain* 125: 1850–1858.

Cavanna, B., Jiang, H., Allaria, S., Carpo, M., Scarlato, G., and Nobile-Orazio, E. (2001). Anti-GM(2) IgM antibody-induced complement-mediated cytotoxicity in patients with dysimmune neuropathies. *J Neuroimmunol* 114: 226–231.

Cheng, B.C., Chang, W.N., Chen, J.B., Chee, E.C., Huang, C.R., Lu, C.H., *et al.* (2003). Long-term prognosis for Guillain–Barre syndrome: evaluation of prognostic factors and clinical experience of automated double filtration plasmapheresis. *J Clin Apheresis* 18: 175–180.

Chiba, A., Kusunoki, S., Shimizu, T., and Kanazawa, I. (1992). Serum IgG antibody to ganglioside GQ1b is a possible marker of Miller Fisher syndrome. *Ann Neurol* 31: 677–679.

Chiba, A., Kusunoki, S., Obata, H., Machinami, R., and Kanazawa, I. (1993). Serum anti-GQ1b IgG antibody is associated with ophthalmoplegia in Miller Fisher syndrome and Guillain–Barre syndrome: clinical and immunohistochemical studies. *Neurology* 43: 1911–1917.

Cooper, J.C., Ben-Smith, A., Savage, C.O., and Winer, J.B. (2000). Unusual T cell receptor phenotype V gene usage of gamma delta T cells in a line derived from the peripheral nerve of a patient with Guillain–Barre syndrome. *J Neurol Neurosurg Psychiatry* 69: 522–524.

Cornblath, D.R., Chaudry, V., and Griffin, J.W. (1991). Treatment of chronic inflammatory demyelinating polyneuropathy with intravenous immunoglobulin. *Ann Neurol* 30: 104–106.

Créange, A., Lerat, H., Meyrignac, C., Degos, J.-D., Gherardi, R.K., and Cesaro, P. (1998). Treatment of Guillain–Barré syndrome with interferon-β. *Lancet* 352: 368–369.

Dalakas, M.C. (1999). Advances in chronic inflammatory demyelinating polyneuropathy: disease variants and inflammatory response mediators and modifiers. *Curr Opin Neurol* 12: 403–409.

Dalakas, M.C. and Engel, W.K. (1980). Immunoglobulin and complement deposits in nerves of patients with chronic relapsing polyneuropathy. *Arch Neurol* 37: 637–640.

Dingle, K.E., Van Den Braak, N., Colles, F.M., Price, L.J., Woodward, D.L., Rodgers, F.G., *et al.* (2001). Sequence typing confirms that *Campylobacter jejuni* strains associated with Guillain–Barre and Miller-Fisher syndromes are of diverse genetic lineage, serotype, and flagella type. *J Clin Microbiol* 39: 3346–3349.

Dyck, P.J., Daube, J., O'Brien, P., Pineda, A., Low, P., Windebank, A.J., *et al.* (1986). Plasma exchange in chronic inflammatory demyelinating polyradiculoneuropathy. *N Engl J Med* 314: 461–465.

Dyck, P.J., Prineas, J., and Pollard, J. (1993). Chronic inflammatory demyelinating polyradiculoneuropathy. In: *Peripheral Neuropathy* (ed. P.J. Dyck, *et al.*), pp. 1498–1517. W. B. Saunders, Philadelphia, PA.

Endtz, H.P., Ang, C.W., van Den Braak, N., Duim, B., Rigter, A., Price, L.J., *et al.* (2000). Molecular characterization of *Campylobacter jejuni* from patients with Guillain–Barre and Miller Fisher syndromes. *J Clin Microbiol* **38**: 2297–2301.

Engberg, J., Nachamkin, I., Fussing, V., McKhann, G.M., Griffin, J.W., Piffaretti, J.C., *et al.* (2001). Absence of clonality of *Campylobacter jejuni* in serotypes other than HS:19 associated with Guillain–Barre syndrome and gastroenteritis. *J Infect Dis* **184**: 215–220.

Feasby, T.E. (1994). Axonal Guillain–Barré syndrome. *Muscle Nerve* **17**: 678–679.

Feasby, T.E. and Hartung, H.P. (2001). Drain the roots: a new treatment for Guillain–Barre syndrome? *Neurology* **57**: 753–754.

French Cooperative Group on Plasma Exchange in Guillain–Barré Syndrome (1987). Efficacy of plasma exchange in Guillain–Barré Syndrome. *Ann Neurol* **22**: 753–761.

French Cooperative Group on Plasma Exchange in Guillain–Barré Syndrome (1997). Appropriate number of plasma exchanges in Guillain–Barré syndrome. *Ann Neurol* **41**: 298–306.

Gabriel, C.M., Gregson, N.A., and Hughes, R.A. (2000). Anti-PMP22 antibodies in patients with inflammatory neuropathy. *J Neuroimmunol* **104**: 139–146.

Gold, R., Archelos, J.J., and Hartung, H.-P. (1999). Mechanisms of immune regulation in the peripheral nervous system. *Brain Pathol* **9**: 343–360.

Gold, R., Hartung, H.P., and Toyka, K.V. (2000). Animal models for autoimmune demyelinating disorders of the nervous system. *Mol Med Today* **6**: 88–91.

Goodyear, C.S., O'Hanlon, G.M., Plomp, J.J., Wagner, E.R., Morrison, I., Veitch, J., *et al.* (1999). Monoclonal antibodies raised against Guillain–Barre syndrome-associated *Campylobacter jejuni* lipopolysaccharides react with neuronal gangliosides and paralyze muscle-nerve preparations. *J Clin Invest* **104**: 697–708.

Govoni, V. and Granieri, E. (2001). Epidemiology of the Guillain–Barre syndrome. *Curr Opin Neurol* **14**: 605–613.

Griffin, J.W., Li, C.Y., Ho, T.W., Tian, M., Gao, C.Y., Xue, P., *et al.* (1996). Pathology of the motor-sensory axonal Guillain–Barre syndrome. *Ann Neurol* **39**: 17–28.

Griffin, J.W., Li, C.Y., Ho, T.W., Xue, P., Macko, C., Gao, C.Y., *et al.* (1995). Guillain–Barre syndrome in northern China. The spectrum of neuropathological changes in clinically defined cases. *Brain* **118**(3): 577–595.

Guillain–Barré Syndrome Study Group (1985). Plasmapheresis and acute Guillain–Baré syndrome. *Neurology* **35**: 1096–1104.

Hadden, R., Sharrack, B., Bensa, S., Soudain, S., and Hughes, R. (1999). Randomized trial of interferon beta-1a in chronic inflammatory demyelinating polyradiculoneuropathy. *Neurology* **53**: 57–61.

Hadden, R.D., Gregson, N.A., Gold, R., Willison, H.J., and Hughes, R.A. (2001*a*). Guillain–Barre syndrome serum and anti-*Campylobacter* antibody do not exacerbate experimental autoimmune neuritis. *J Neuroimmunol* **119**: 306–316.

Hadden, R.D., Karch, H., Hartung, H.P., Zielasek, J., Weissbrich, B., Schubert, J., *et al.* (2001*b*). Preceding infections, immune factors, and outcome in Guillain–Barre syndrome. *Neurology* **56**: 758–765.

Hafer-Macko, C.E., Sheikh, K.A., Li, C.Y., Ho, T.W., Cornblath, D.R., McKhann, G.M., *et al.* (1996). Immune attack on the Schwann cell surface in acute inflammatory demyelinating polyneuropathy. *Ann Neurol* **39**: 625–635.

Hahn, A.F. (1998). Guillain–Barré syndrome. *Lancet* **352**: 635–641.

Hahn, A.F., Bolton, C.F., Pillay, N., Chalk, C., Benstead, T., Bril, V., *et al.* (1996*a*). Plasma-exchange therapy in chronic inflammatory demyelinating polyneuropathy. A double-blind, sham-controlled, cross-over study. *Brain* **119**(4): 1055–1066.

Hahn, A.F., Bolton, C.F., Zochodne, D., and Feasby, T.E. (1996*b*). Intravenous immunoglobulin treatment in chronic inflammatory demyelinating polyneuropathy. A double-blind, placebo-controlled, cross-over study. *Brain* **119**(4): 1067–1077.

Hao, Q., Saida, T., Yoshino, H., Kuroki, S., Nukina, M., and Saida, K. (1999). Anti-GalNAc-GD1a antibody-associated Guillain–Barre syndrome with a predominantly distal weakness without cranial nerve impairment and sensory disturbance. *Ann Neurol* **45**: 758–768.

Hartung, H.-P. (1995). Pathogenesis of inflammatory demyelination: implications for therapy. *Curr Opin Neurol* **8**: 191–199.

Hartung, H.P. and Toyka, K.V. (1990). T-cell and macrophage activation in experimental autoimmune neuritis and Guillain–Barre syndrome. *Ann Neurol* **27**(Suppl.): S57–S63.

Hartung, H.P., Schwenke, C., Bitter-Suermann, D., and Toyka, K.V. (1987). Guillain–Barre syndrome: activated complement components C3a and C5a in CSF. *Neurology* **37**: 1006–1009.

Hartung, H.-P., Pollard, J.D., Harvey, G.K., and Toyka, K.V. (1995). Invited review—immunopathogenesis and treatment of the Guillain–Barré syndrome, Part I and II. *Muscle Nerve* **18**: 137–164.

Hartung, H.-P., Willison, H., and Kieseier, B.C. (2002). Acute immunoinflammatory neuropathy: update on Guillain–Barré Syndrome. *Curr Opin Neurol* **15**: 571–577.

Hays, A.P., Lee, S.S., and Latov, N. (1988). Immune reactive C3d on the surface of myelin sheaths in neuropathy. *J Neuroimmunol* **18**: 231–244.

Hiraga, A., Mori, M., Ogawara, K., Hattori, T., and Kuwabara, S. (2003). Differences in patterns of progression in demyelinating and axonal Guillain–Barre syndromes. *Neurology* **61**: 471–474.

Ho, T.W., Mishu, B., Li, C.Y., Gao, C.Y., Cornblath, D.R., Griffin, J.W., *et al.* (1995). Guillain–Barre syndrome in northern China. Relationship to *Campylobacter jejuni* infection and anti-glycolipid antibodies. *Brain* **118**(3): 597–605.

Hodgkinson, S., Pollard, J., and McLeod, J. (1990). Cyclosporin A in the treatment of chronic demyelinating polyneuropathy (CIDP): a double-blind, placebo controlled, cross-over study. *J Neurol Neurosurg Psychiatry* **53**: 327–330.

Hu, W., Mathey, E., Hartung, H.P., and Kieseier, B.C. (2003). Cyclo-oxygenases and prostaglandins in acute inflammatory demyelination of the peripheral nerve. *Neurology* **61**: 1774–1779.

Hughes, R.A.C. (1995). The concept and classification of Guillain–Barré syndrome and related disorders. *Rev Neurol (Paris)* **151**: 291–294.

Hughes, R.A. and van Der Meche, F.G. (2000). Corticosteroids for treating Guillain–Barre syndrome. *Cochrane Database Syst Rev* CD001446.

Hughes, R.A., Raphael, J.C., Swan, A.V., and van Doorn, P.A. (2001*a*). Intravenous immunoglobulin for Guillain–Barre syndrome (Cochrane Review). *Cochrane Database Syst Rev* **2**: CD002063.

Hughes, R., Bensa, S., Willison, H., van den Bergh, P., Comi, G., Illa, I., *et al.* (2001*b*). Randomized controlled trial of intravenous immunoglobulin versus oral prednisolone in chronic inflammatory demyelinating polyradiculopathy. *Ann Neurol* **50**: 195–201.

Hughes, R.A., Swan, A.V., and van Doorn, P.A. (2003). Cytotoxic drugs and interferons for chronic inflammatory demyelinating polyradiculoneuropathy. *Cochrane Database Syst Rev* CD003280.

Ichikawa, H., Susuki, K., Yuki, N., and Kawamura, M. (2001). Ataxic form of Guillain–Barre syndrome associated with anti-GD1b IgG antibody. *Rinsho Shinkeigaku* **41**: 523–525 (in Japanese).

Jacobs, B.C., van Doorn, P.A., Schmitz, P.I., Tio-Gillen, A.P., Herbrink, P., Visser, L.H., *et al.* (1996). *Campylobacter jejuni* infections and anti-GM1 antibodies in Guillain–Barre syndrome. *Ann Neurol* **40**: 181–187.

Jacobs, B.C., Rothbarth, P.H., van der Meche, F.G., Herbrink, P., Schmitz, P.I., de Klerk, M.A., *et al.* (1998). The spectrum of antecedent infections in Guillain–Barre syndrome: a case-control study. *Neurology* **51**: 1110–1115.

Ju, Y.Y., Womersley, H., Pritchard, J., Gray, I., Hughes, R.A., and Gregson, N.A. (2004). *Haemophilus influenzae* as a possible cause of Guillain–Barre syndrome. *J Neuroimmunol* **149**: 160–166.

Kaida, K., Kusunoki, S., Kamakura, K., Motoyoshi, K., and Kanazawa, I. (2003). GalNAc-GD1a in human peripheral nerve: target sites of anti-ganglioside antibody. *Neurology* **61**: 465–470.

Khalili-Shirazi, A., Gregson, N.A., Hall, M.A., Hughes, R.A., and Lanchbury, J.S. (1997*a*). T cell receptor V beta gene usage in Guillain–Barre syndrome. *J Neurol Sci* **145**: 169–176.

Khalili-Shirazi, A., Gregson, N., and Hughes, R. (1997*b*). CD1 expression in human peripheral nerve of GBS patients. *Biochem Soc Trans* **25**: 172S.

Kiefer, R., Kieseier, B.C., Brück, W., Toyka, K.V., and Hartung, H.-P. (1998). Macrophage differentiation antigens in acute and chronic autoimmune polyneuropathies. *Brain* **121**: 469–479.

Kieseier, B.C., Kiefer, R., Clements, J.M., Miller, K., Wells, G.M., Schweitzer, T., et al. (1998). Matrix metalloproteinase-9 and -7 are regulated in experimental autoimmune encephalomyelitis. *Brain* 121(1): 159–166.

Kieseier, B.C., Tani, M., Mahad, D., Oka, N., Ho, T., Woodroofe, N., et al. (2002). Chemokines and chemokine receptors in inflammatory demyelinating neuropathies: a central role for IP-10. *Brain* 125: 823–834.

Kieseier, B.C., Kiefer, R., Gold, R., Hemmer, B., Willison, H., and Hartung, H.-P. (2004). Advances in understanding and treatment of immune-mediated disorders of the peripheral nervous system. *Muscle Nerve* 30: 131–156.

Koga, M., Yuki, N., Ariga, T., Morimatsu, M., and Hirata, K. (1998). Is IgG anti-GT1a antibody associated with pharyngeal-cervical-brachial weakness or oropharyngeal palsy in Guillain–Barre syndrome? *J Neuroimmunol* 86: 74–79.

Koga, M., Yuki, N., Takahashi, M., Saito, K., and Hirata, K. (1999). Are *Campylobacter curvus* and *Campylobacter upsaliensis* antecedent infectious agents in Guillain–Barre and Fisher's syndromes? *J Neurol Sci* 163: 53–57.

Koga, M., Ang, C.W., Yuki, N., Jacobs, B.C., Herbrink, P., van der Meche, F.G., et al. (2001a). Comparative study of preceding *Campylobacter jejuni* infection in Guillain–Barre syndrome in Japan and The Netherlands. *J Neurol Neurosurg Psychiatry* 70: 693–695.

Koga, M., Yuki, N., and Hirata, K. (2001b). Antecedent symptoms in Guillain–Barre syndrome: an important indicator for clinical and serological subgroups. *Acta Neurol Scand* 103: 278–287.

Koga, M., Yuki, N., Hirata, K., Morimatsu, M., Mori, M., and Kuwabara, S. (2003). Anti-GM1 antibody IgG subclass: a clinical recovery predictor in Guillain–Barre syndrome. *Neurology* 60: 1514–1518.

Koga, M., Yuki, N., Tsukada, Y., Hirata, K., and Matsumoto, Y. (2003). CDR3 spectratyping analysis of the T cell receptor repertoire in Guillain–Barre and Fisher syndromes. *J Neuroimmunol* 141: 112–117.

Köller, H., Kieseier, B.C., Sander, S., and Hartung, H.P. (2005). Chronic inflammatory demyelinating neuropathy. *N Engl J Med* 353: 1343–1356.

Kusunoki, S., Shimizu, J., Chiba, A., Ugawa, Y., Hitoshi, S., and Kanazawa, I. (1996). Experimental sensory neuropathy induced by sensitization with ganglioside GD1b. *Ann Neurol* 39: 424–431.

Kusunoki, S., Chiba, A., and Kanazawa, I. (1999). Anti-GQ1b IgG antibody is associated with ataxia as well as ophthalmoplegia. *Muscle Nerve* 22: 1071–1074.

Kuwabara, S., Ogawara, K., Sung, J.Y., Mori, M., Kanai, K., Hattori, T., et al. (2002). Differences in membrane properties of axonal and demyelinating Guillain–Barre syndromes. *Ann Neurol* 52: 180–187.

Kwa, M.S., van Schaik, I.N., Brand, A., Baas, F., and Vermeulen, M. (2001). Investigation of serum response to PMP22, connexin 32 and P(0) in inflammatory neuropathies. *J Neuroimmunol* 116: 220–225.

Leonard, E.E. 2nd, Tompkins, L.S., Falkow, S., and Nachamkin, I. (2004). Comparison of *Campylobacter jejuni* isolates implicated in Guillain–Barre syndrome and strains that cause enteritis by a DNA microarray. *Infect Immun* 72: 1199–1203.

Leppert, D., Hughes, P., Huber, S., Erne, B., Grygar, C., Said, G., et al. (1999). Matrix metalloproteinase upregulation in chronic inflammatory demyelinating polyneuropathy and nonsystemic vasculitic neuropathy. *Neurology* 53: 62–70.

Martina, I., van Doorn, P., Schmitz, P., Meulstee, J., and van der Meché, F. (1999). Chronic motor neuropathies: response to interferon-b1a after failure of conventional therapies. *J Neurol Neurosurg Psychiatry* 66: 197–201.

Mathey, E.K., Pollard, J.D., and Armati, P.J. (1999). TNF alpha, IFN gamma and IL-2 mRNA expression in CIDP sural nerve biopsies. *J Neurol Sci* 163: 47–52.

Mazzeo, A., Aguennouz, M., Messina, C., and Vita, G. (2004). Immunolocalization and activation of transcription factor nuclear factor kappaB in dysimmune neuropathies and familial amyloidotic polyneuropathy. *Arch Neurol* 61: 1097–1102.

McCarthy, N. and Giesecke, J. (2001). Incidence of Guillain–Barre syndrome following infection with *Campylobacter jejuni*. *Am J Epidemiol* 153: 610–614.

McCombe, P.A., Pollard, J.D., and McLeod, J.G. (1987). Chronic inflammatory demyelinating polyradiculoneuropathy. A clinical and electrophysiological study of 92 cases. *Brain* 110(6): 1617–1630.

McLeod, J.F., Pollard, J., Macaskill, P., Mohamed, A., Spring, P., and Khurana, V. (1999). Prevalence of chronic inflammatory demyelinating neuropathy in New South Wales, Australia. *Ann Neurol* 46: 910–913.

Melendez-Vasquez, C., Redford, J., Choudhary, P.P., Gray, I.A., Maitland, P., Gregson, N.A., et al. (1997). Immunological investigation of chronic inflammatory demyelinating polyradiculoneuropathy. *J Neuroimmunol* 73: 124–134.

Mendell, J.R., Barohn, R.J., Freimer, M.L., Kissel, J.T., King, W., and Negaraja, H.N. (2001). Randomized controlled trial of IVIg in untreated chronic inflammatory demeylinating polyradiculoneuropathy. *Neurology* 56: 445–449.

Mori, M., Kuwabara, S., Miyake, M., Noda, M., Kuroki, H., Kanno, H., et al. *Haemophilus influenzae* infection and Guillain–Barre syndrome. *Brain* 123(10): 2171–2178.

Muller, H.D., Beckmann, A., and Schroder, J.M. (2003). Inflammatory infiltrates in the spinal cord of patients with Guillain–Barre syndrome. *Acta Neuropathol (Berlin)* 106: 509–517.

Mygland, A. and Monstadt, P. (2001). Chronic polyneuropathies in Vest-Agder, Norway. *Eur J Neurol* 8: 157–165.

Nachamkin, I., Engberg, J., Gutacker, M., Meinersman, R.J., Li, C.Y., Arzate, P., et al. (2001). Molecular population genetic analysis of *Campylobacter jejuni* HS:19 associated with Guillain–Barre syndrome and gastroenteritis. *J Infect Dis* 184: 221–226.

Nishimura, M., Nukina, M., Kuroki, S., Obayashi, H., Ohta, M., Ma, J.J., et al. (1997). Characterization of *Campylobacter jejuni* isolates from patients with Guillain–Barre syndrome. *J Neurol Sci* 153: 91–99.

Noronha, A.B., Harper, J.R., Ilyas, A.A., Reisfeld, R.A., and Quarles, R.H. (1986). Myelin-associated glycoprotein shares an antigenic determinant with a glycoprotein of human melanoma cells. *J Neurochem* 47: 1558–1565.

Odaka, M., Yuki, N., and Hirata, K. (2001). Anti-GQ1b IgG antibody syndrome: clinical and immunological range. *J Neurol Neurosurg Psychiatry* 70: 50–55.

Ogawara, K., Kuwabara, S., Mori, M., Hattori, T., Koga, M., and Yuki, N. (2000). Axonal Guillain–Barre syndrome: relation to anti-ganglioside antibodies and *Campylobacter jejuni* infection in Japan. *Ann Neurol* 48: 624–631.

Ogawara, K., Kuwabara, S., Koga, M., Mori, M., Yuki, N., and Hattori, T. (2003). Anti-GM1b IgG antibody is associated with acute motor axonal neuropathy and *Campylobacter jejuni* infection. *J Neurol Sci* 210: 41–45.

Oh, S.J., Kurokawa, K., de Almeida, D.F., Ryan, H.F. Jr., and Claussen, G.C. (2003). Subacute inflammatory demyelinating polyneuropathy. *Neurology* 61: 1507–1512.

O'Hanlon, G.M., Veitch, J., Gallardo, E., Illa, I., Chancellor, A.M., and Willison, H.J. (2000). Peripheral neuropathy associated with anti-GM2 ganglioside antibodies: clinical and immunopathological studies. *Autoimmunity* 32: 133–144.

O'Hanlon, G.M., Plomp, J.J., Chakrabarti, M., Morrison, I., Wagner, E.R., Goodyear, C.S., et al. (2001). Anti-GQ1b ganglioside antibodies mediate complement-dependent destruction of the motor nerve terminal. *Brain* 124: 893–906.

O'Leary, C.P. and Willison, H.J. (2000). The role of antiglycolipid antibodies in peripheral neuropathies. *Curr Opin Neurol* 13: 583–588.

O'Leary, C.P., Veitch, J., Durward, W.F., Thomas, A.M., Rees, J.H., and Willison, H.J. (1996). Acute oropharyngeal palsy is associated with antibodies to GQ1b and GT1a gangliosides. *J Neurol Neurosurg Psychiatry* 61: 649–651.

Paparounas, K., O'Hanlon, G.M., O'Leary, C.P., Rowan, E.G., and Willison, H.J. (1999). Anti-ganglioside antibodies can bind peripheral nerve nodes of Ranvier and activate the complement cascade without inducing acute conduction block *in vitro*. *Brain* 122(5): 807–816.

Plomp, J.J., Molenaar, P.C., O'Hanlon, G.M., Jacobs, B.C., Veitch, J., Daha, M.R., et al. (1999). Miller Fisher anti-GQ1b antibodies: alpha-latrotoxin-like effects on motor end plates. *Ann Neurol* 45: 189–199.

Pollard, J. (2002). Chronic inflammatory demyelinating polyradiculoneuropathy. *Curr Opin Neurol* 15: 279–283.

Press, R., Ozenci, V., Kouwenhoven, M., and Link, H. (2002). Non-T(H)1 cytokines are augmented systematically early in Guillain–Barre syndrome. *Neurology* 58: 476–478.

Press, R., Pashenkov, M., Jin, J.P., and Link, H. (2003). Aberrated levels of cerebrospinal fluid chemokines in Guillain–Barre syndrome and chronic inflammatory demyelinating polyradiculoneuropathy. *J Clin Immunol* 23: 259–267.

Previtali, S.C., Archelos, J.J., and Hartung, H.P. (1998). Expression of integrins in experimental autoimmune neuritis and Guillain–Barre syndrome. *Ann Neurol* 44: 611–621.

Previtali, S.C., Feltri, M.L., Archelos, J.J., Quattrini, A., Wrabetz, L., and Hartung, H. (2001). Role of integrins in the peripheral nervous system. *Prog Neurobiol* **64**: 35–49.

Prineas, J.W. (1994). Pathology of inflammatory demyelinating neuropathies. *Baillieres Clin Neurol* **3**: 1–24.

Raphael, J.C., Chevret, S., Hughes, R.A., and Annane, D. (2001). Plasma exchange for Guillain–Barre syndrome (Cochrane Review). *Cochrane Database Syst Rev* **2**: CD001798.

Rees, J.H. and Hughes, R.A. (1994). *Campylobacter jejuni* and Guillain–Barre syndrome. *Ann Neurol* **35**: 248–249.

Rees, J.H., Gregson, N.A., Griffiths, P.L., and Hughes, R.A. (1993). *Campylobacter jejuni* and Guillain–Barre syndrome. *Q J Med* **86**: 623–634.

Rees, J.H., Soudain, S.E., Gregson, N.A., and Hughes, R.A. (1995). *Campylobacter jejuni* infection and Guillain–Barre syndrome. *N Engl J Med* **333**: 1374–1379.

Ropper, A.H. (1986). Unusual clinical variants and signs in Guillain–Barre syndrome. *Arch Neurol* **43**: 1150–1152.

Ropper, A.H. (1992). The Guillain–Barre syndrome. *N Engl J Med* **326**: 1130–1136.

Rotta, F.T., Sussman, A.T., Bradley, W.G., Ram Ayyar, D., Sharma, K.R., and Shebert, R.T. (2000). The spectrum of chronic inflammatory demyelinating polyneuropathy. *J Neurol Sci* **173**: 129–139.

Sander, H.W. and Latov, N. (2003). Research criteria for defining patients with CIDP. *Neurology* **60**: S8–S15.

Saperstein, D.S., Katz, J.S., Amato, A.A., and Barohn, R.J. (2001). Clinical spectrum of chronic acquired demyelinating polyneuropathies. *Muscle Nerve* **24**: 311–324.

Schaller, B., Radziwill, A.J., and Steck, A. (2001). Successful treatment of Guillain–Barré syndrome with combined administration of interferon-β-1a and intravenous immunoglobulin. *Eur Neurol* **46**: 167–168.

Susuki, K., Yuki, N., and Hirata, K. (2001). Fine specificity of anti-GQ1b IgG and clinical features. *J Neurol Sci* **185**: 5–9.

Takigawa, T., Yasuda, H., Terada, M., Haneda, M., Kashiwagi, A., Saito, T., *et al.* (2000). The sera from GM1 ganglioside antibody positive patients with Guillain–Barre syndrome or chronic inflammatory demyelinating polyneuropathy blocks Na+ currents in rat single myelinated nerve fibers. *Intern Med* **39**: 123–127.

Ter Bruggen, J.P., van der Meche, F.G., de Jager, A.E., and Polman, C.H. (1998). Ophthalmoplegic and lower cranial nerve variants merge into each other and into classical Guillain–Barre syndrome. *Muscle Nerve* **21**: 239–242.

Tofaris, G.K., Patterson, P.H., Jessen, K.R., and Mirsky, R. (2002). Denervated Schwann cells attract macrophages by secretion of leukemia inhibitory factor (LIF) and monocyte chemoattractant protein-1 in a process regulated by interleukin-6 and LIF. *J Neurosci* **22**: 6696–6703.

Toyka, K.V. and Hartung, H.P. (1996). Chronic inflammatory polyneuritis and neuropathies. *Curr Opin Neurol* **9**: 240–250.

Tsuchida, T., Saxton, R.E., Morton, D.L., and Irie, R.F. (1989). Gangliosides of human melanoma. *Cancer* **63**: 1166–1174.

Umapathi, T. and Hughes, R. (2002). Mycophenolate in treatment-resistant inflammatory neuropathies. *Eur J Neurol* **9**: 683–685.

van Belkum, A., van Den Braak, N., Godschalk, P., Ang, W., Jacobs, B.C., Gilbert, M., *et al.* (1995). A *Campylobacter jejuni* gene associated with immune-mediated neuropathy. *Nat Med* **7**: 752–753.

van der Meché, F.G. and Schmitz, P.I. (1992). A randomized trial comparing intravenous immune globulin and plasma exchange in Guillain–Barre syndrome. Dutch Guillain–Barre Study Group. *N Engl J Med* **326**: 1123–1129.

van der Meché, F.G., van Doorn, P.A., Meulstee, J., and Jennekens, F.G. (2001). Diagnostic and classification criteria for the Guillain–Barre syndrome. *Eur Neurol* **45**: 133–139.

van Doorn, P., Brand, A., Strengers, P., Meulstee, J., and Vermeulen, M. (1990). High-dose intravenous immunoglobulin treatment in chronic inflammatory demyelinating polyneuropathy: a double-blind, placebo-controlled, crossover study. *Neurology* **40**: 209–212.

van Koningsveld, R., Schmitz, P.I., Meche, F.G., Visser, L.H., Meulstee, J., and van Doorn, P.A. (2004). Effect of methylprednisolone when added to standard treatment with intravenous immunoglobulin for Guillain–Barre syndrome: randomised trial. *Lancet* **363**: 192–196.

Van Rhijn, I., Logtenberg, T., Ang, C.W., and Van Den Berg, L.H. (2003). Gammadelta T cell non-responsiveness in *Campylobacter jejuni*-associated Guillain–Barre syndrome patients. *Neurology* **61**: 994–996.

van Schaik, I.N., Winer, J.B., de Haan, R., and Vermeulen, M. (2002). Intravenous immunoglobulin for chronic inflammatory demyelinating polyradiculoneuropathy: a systematic review. *Lancet Neurol* **1**: 491–498.

van Sorge, N.M., van den Berg, L.H., Geleijns, K., van Strijp, J.A., Jacobs, B.C., van Doorn, P.A., *et al.* (2003). Anti-GM1 IgG antibodies induce leukocyte effector functions via Fcgamma receptors. *Ann Neurol* **53**: 570–579.

Visser, L.H., Van der Meche, F.G., Van Doorn, P.A., Meulstee, J., Jacobs, B.C., Oomes, P.G., *et al.* (1995). Guillain–Barre syndrome without sensory loss (acute motor neuropathy). A subgroup with specific clinical, electrodiagnostic and laboratory features. Dutch Guillain–Barre Study Group. *Brain* **118**(9): 841–847.

Wanschitz, J., Maier, H., Lassmann, H., Budka, H., and Berger, T. (2003). Distinct time pattern of complement activation and cytotoxic T cell response in Guillain–Barre syndrome. *Brain* **126**: 2034–2042.

Weber, F., Rudel, R., Aulkemeyer, P., and Brinkmeier, H. (2000). Anti-GM1 antibodies can block neuronal voltage-gated sodium channels. *Muscle Nerve* **23**: 1414–1420.

Weiss, M.D., Luciano, C.A., Semino-Mora, C., Dalakas, M.C., and Quarles, R.H. (1998). Molecular mimicry in chronic inflammatory demyelinating polyneuropathy and melanoma. *Neurology* **51**: 1738–1741.

Wessig, C., Buchwald, B., Toyka, K.V., and Martini, R. (2001). Miller Fisher syndrome: immunofluorescence and immunoelectron microscopic localization of IgG at the mouse neuromuscular junction. *Acta Neuropathol (Berlin)* **101**: 239–244.

Willison, H.J. and O'Hanlon, G.M. (1999). The immunopathogenesis of Miller Fisher syndrome. *J Neuroimmunol* **100**: 3–12.

Willison, H.J. and Yuki, N. (2002). Peripheral neuropathies and anti-glycolipid antibodies. *Brain* **125**: 2591–2625.

Wollinsky, K.H., Hulser, P.J., Brinkmeier, H., Aulkemeyer, P., Bossenecker, W., Huber-Hartmann, K.H., *et al.* (2001). CSF filtration is an effective treatment of Guillain–Barre syndrome: a randomized clinical trial. *Neurology* **57**: 774–780.

Yako, K., Kusunoki, S., and Kanazawa, I. (1999). Serum antibody against a peripheral nerve myelin ganglioside, LM1, in Guillain–Barre syndrome. *J Neurol Sci* **168**: 85–99.

Yamamoto, M., Ito, Y., Mitsuma, N., Li, M., Hattori, N., and Sobue, G. (2002). Parallel expression of neurotrophic factors and their receptors in chronic inflammatory demyelinating polyneuropathy. *Muscle Nerve* **25**: 601–604.

Yoshino, H., Harukawa, H., and Asano, A. (2000). IgG antiganglioside antibodies in Guillain–Barre syndrome with bulbar palsy. *J Neuroimmunol* **105**: 195–201.

Yuki, N. (2001). Infectious origins of, and molecular mimicry in, Guillain–Barré and Fisher syndromes. *Lancet Infect Dis* **1**: 29–37.

Yuki, N., Yoshino, H., Sato, S., and Miyatake, T. (1990). Acute axonal poly neuropathy associated with anti-GM1 antibodies following *Campylobacter* enteritis. *Neurology* **40**: 1900–1902.

Yuki, N., Ho, T.W., Tagawa, Y., Koga, M., Li, C.Y., Hirata, K., *et al.* (1999a). Autoantibodies to GM1b and GalNAc-GD1a: relationship to *Campylobacter jejuni* infection and acute motor axonal neuropathy in China. *J Neurol Sci* **164**: 134–8.

Yuki, N., Kuwabara, S., Koga, M., and Hirata, K. (1999b). Acute motor axonal neuropathy and acute motor-sensory axonal neuropathy share a common immunological profile. *J Neurol Sci* **168**: 121–126.

Yuki, N., Ang, C.W., Koga, M., Jacobs, B.C., van Doorn, P.A., Hirata, K., *et al.* (2000). Clinical features and response to treatment in Guillain–Barre syndrome associated with antibodies to GM1b ganglioside. *Ann Neurol* **47**: 314–321.

Yuki, N., Yamada, M., Koga, M., Odaka, M., Susuki, K., Tagawa, Y., *et al.* (2001). Animal model of axonal Guillain–Barré syndrome induced by sensitization with GM1 ganliosides. *Ann Neurol* **49**: 712–720.

Yuki, N., Susuki, K., Koga, M., Nishimoto, Y., Odaka, M., Hirata, K., *et al.* (2004). Carbohydrate mimicry between human ganglioside GM1 and *Campylobacter jejuni* lipooligosaccharide causes Guillain–Barre syndrome. *Proc Natl Acad Sci USA* **101**: 11404–11409.

20 Antibody-mediated disorders of the neuromuscular junction

Angela Vincent

The neuromuscular junction (NMJ) has long been considered the archetypal synapse, being both relatively simple in its function and easy to study. It remains the most accessible synapse in the nervous system and is very susceptible to circulating factors, notably neurotoxins and specific autoantibodies. This chapter will briefly describe the structure and function of the NMJ, and then discuss the clinical, pathologic, and immunologic features of five autoimmune disorders of neuromuscular transmission: myasthenia gravis (MG), myasthenia gravis with MuSK antibodies, the Lambert–Eaton myasthenic syndrome, acquired neuromyotonia, and acquired autonomic neuropathy. Each of these is caused by autoantibodies to a receptor or ion channel.

The neuromuscular junction and neuromuscular transmission

To understand the pathophysiology of autoimmune disorders of the NMJ it is necessary to be familiar with its molecular structure and function (see Hall and Sanes 1993; Sanes *et al.* 1998). The terminal portions of the motor nerve axons are devoid of myelin sheath and expand into 'boutons'. These lie in close apposition to infoldings of the muscle membrane surface called post-synaptic or junctional folds. Schwann cell extensions form a protective layer around the boutons. The pre-synaptic nerve terminal is distinguished by the large number of mitochondria and small spherical vesicles (synaptic vesicles) that contain the neurotransmitter acetylcholine (ACh). These are mainly concentrated just inside the pre-synaptic membrane, particularly close to 'active zones' (AZs). AZs are defined by the presence, in freeze-fracture representations, of double parallel rows of particles that are thought to be voltage-gated calcium channels (VGCCs). The AZs are opposite the entrance to the secondary synaptic clefts between the junctional folds. Around the synaptic vesicles are cytoplasmic densities that represent a network of filaments and specific proteins that are involved in exocytosis. Between the pre-synaptic and post-synaptic membranes is a gap of 55 Å filled with a deceptively amorphous-looking basal lamina. This contains collagen IV, heparan sulfate, laminin, and other specific components, and is where the enzyme acetylcholinesterase (AChE) is anchored by its collagen tail, ColQ. The peaks of the post-synaptic folds are electron dense corresponding to the distribution of the highly concentrated ($10\ 000/\mu m^2$) AChRs. On the cytoplasmic face of the AChR-containing membrane, post-synaptic densities represent the web of proteins that anchor the AChR and other functional proteins. Some of the features are summarized in Fig. 20.1(a).

The nerve action potential is propagated along the nerve by the opening of voltage-gated sodium channels at the nodes of Ranvier. When the action potential invades the motor nerve terminals, the depolarization opens the VGCCs at the AZs, resulting in a transient and very localized increase in cytoplasmic Ca^{2+}. This causes fusion of synaptic vesicles with the motor nerve terminal membrane and release of ACh into the synaptic space, a process called exocytosis. ACh diffuses rapidly to the post-synaptic membrane and binds to the AChRs, leading to opening of the AChR-associated ion channel. Cations, mainly Na^+, diffuse through the channel, leading to a localized depolarization called the endplate potential (EPP). If the depolarization exceeds a certain threshold, voltage-gated sodium channels that lie at the bottom of the post-synaptic folds are opened. This generates the muscle action potential that propagates along the muscle fibre and activates contraction. The action of ACh is terminated by its dissociation from the AChR; the AChR ion channel closes spontaneously after 1 to 4 ms, and ACh is hydrolyzed by AChE.

Spontaneous release of single vesicles or 'quanta' of ACh occurs in the absence of nerve impulses and results in a small depolarization called the miniature endplate potential (MEPP). The number of quanta released per nerve impulse, the quantal content, can be calculated by measuring the amplitude of the EPP and dividing this by the amplitude of the MEPPs (with correction for non-linear summation). The quantal content is very sensitive to changes in extracellular Ca^{2+} or the effect of drugs or other substances on the VGCCs. The amplitude of the MEPPs is sensitive to substances that affect the number or function of the post-synaptic AChRs, or to those that increase the concentration and duration of action of ACh. AChE inhibitors, for instance, increase the amplitude and prolong the time course of both the MEPP and the EPP. Fig. 20.1(a) shows the relative size of the MEPP and EPPs at a normal human endplate.

The action potential in nerve and muscle is terminated by the spontaneous inactivation of sodium channels and the opening of potassium channels. Efflux of potassium from the cell through these channels brings the membrane potential back to its resting values (around -80 mV). The ouabain-sensitive Na^+/K^+ exchanger is responsible for restoring the concentration gradient for Na^+ and K^+.

Vulnerability of the neuromuscular junction to circulating factors including neurotoxins

The venoms of many species of snake, scorpion, spiders, fish, fish-eating snails, and other creatures contain alkaloid and polypeptide toxins that bind with high affinity to specific proteins at the NMJ and can rapidly cause paralysis, respiratory failure, and death in their prey. These neurotoxins have provided us with an astonishing library of tools for investigation and purification of the proteins involved in neuromuscular transmission (NMT) (Harris, 1984). For instance, α-bungarotoxin (α-BuTx) binds irreversibly to muscle AChRs, blocking the ACh binding site. Radioiodinated α-BuTx can be used to label AChRs in whole tissue and to tag AChR after detergent extraction for use in immunoprecipitation assays; neurotoxins specific for calcium and potassium channels are used in a similar manner (see below).

The accessibility of the NMJ to circulating factors is well illustrated by the rapid, potentially fatal, respiratory failure produced by some of the venomous species mentioned above, particularly in smaller mammals, but also in humans. There is also ample evidence that circulating autoantibodies can bind to antigenic targets at the NMJ, as illustrated by the conditions described in this chapter.

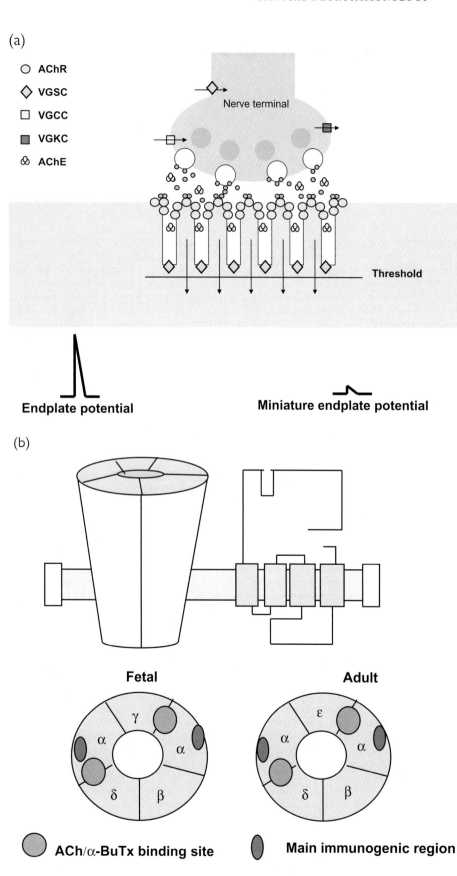

(a)

○ AChR
◇ VGSC
□ VGCC
■ VGKC
⊗ AChE

Nerve terminal

Threshold

Endplate potential

Miniature endplate potential

(b)

Fetal

Adult

γ   α   α

α   ε   α

δ   β

δ   β

⬤ **ACh/α-BuTx binding site**

⬤ **Main immunogenic region**

Developing muscle

NMJ

Fig. 20.1 The neuromuscular junction (NMJ) and acetylcholine receptors. (a) Diagrammatic representation of the NMJ with the ion channels, muscle-specific kinase (MuSK), and acetylcholine esterase (AchE) that are essential for its normal function. Below are shown examples of endplate potential (EPP) and miniature endplate potential (MEPP) that can be detected by an intramuscular microelectrode placed in the muscle fibre. The EPP must reach the firing threshold to initiate a muscle action potential. (b) The acetylcholine receptor is a pentameric membrane protein that occurs in an adult and fetal isoform. Acetylcholine (ACh) and α-bungarotoxin (α-BuTx) bind to sites on the interfaces between the α and adjacent subunits. Many of the antibodies in myasthenia bind to a main immunogenic region on the two α subunits.

Myasthenia gravis

Clinical and pathophysiologic features

Myasthenia gravis (MG) is an acquired autoimmune disorder in which autoantibodies to the post-synaptic AChRs are reduced in number or function, leading to muscle fatigue and weakness. The weakness often starts in the eye muscles, resulting in double vision and ptosis (drooping eyelids), but may involve any muscle group. Typically, the weakness varies in distribution and severity from day to day, is often worse at the end of the day, increases with stress, and tends to improve with rest. MG is frequently associated with thymic abnormalities, so-called thymic hyperplasia, in about 60% and thymoma in around 10% of patients. The clinical features are reviewed by Drachman (1994) and Vincent et al. (2001).

The diagnosis is made by a positive anti-AChR antibody titre (Lindstrom et al., 1976; Vincent and Newsom Davis, 1985), which is present in 85 to 90% of patients. Patients also show a transient clinical response to the intravenous AChE inhibitor edrophonium. A decrement in the compound muscle action potential is typically revealed on low-frequency nerve stimulation studies and, in virtually all patients, increased 'jitter' is apparent on single-fibre electromyography studies.

Treatment

Anti-AChE drugs are the first line of treatment, but most patients require further help. Plasma exchange, by removing circulating antibodies, provides short-term improvement. Thymectomy is performed in most seropositive patients who are young (<40 years) at disease onset, resulting in remission in about 25% and improvement in 50%, although the efficacy of thymectomy has not been formally demonstrated (Gronseth and Barohn, 2000). Removal of a thymoma is essential, because of the risk of local infiltration, but seldom leads to clinical improvement. Immunosuppression with corticosteroids or azathioprine, or both, is usually required in thymoma cases, and often in non-thymoma cases. It is the first choice treatment in older patients (Drachman, 1994; Vincent et al., 2001).

Autoimmunity

The occurrence of MG in young females, its association with other autoimmune diseases, the presence of thymic pathology, and the transfer of MG from mothers to their neonates, 'neonatal MG', led Simpson (1960) to propose that MG is an autoimmune disease with antibodies directed against an 'endplate' protein. Nastuk et al. (1960) also proposed an autoimmune basis. Simpson's theory was validated in 1973 when Patrick and Lindstrom (1973) showed that immunization against affinity-purified AChRs could induce weakness and paralysis in rabbits that, like MG, was responsive to edrophonium. This condition, termed experimental autoimmune myasthenia gravis (EAMG), has since been induced in many species by immunization with affinity-purified AChRs from a variety of sources (see below).

The acetylcholine receptor and antibodies

The AChR is an oligomeric membrane protein that consists of five subunits: α_2, β, γ, and δ in embryonic or denervated muscle, and α_2, β, δ, and ε at the adult endplate (see Fig. 20.1(b)). Each subunit has four transmembrane domains. Each of the two α subunits has a binding site for ACh that is shared with the neurotoxin α-BuTx (Karlin and Akabas, 1995). Isolated α subunits, and synthetic peptides representing α 185–199, bind α-BuTx but the binding is several orders of magnitude less than that to the native molecule, suggesting that other sequences and tertiary structures are essential for the high-affinity neurotoxin binding (Vincent et al., 1998a). The AChR has not been purified and crystallized for structural studies, but studies by Unwin and his colleagues have demonstrated many of the features of the molecule (Unwin et al., 2000).

Anti-AChR is measured by immunoprecipitation of ^{125}I-α-BuTx labelled AChR extracted from ischaemic human muscle, from the rhabdomyosarcoma cell line TE671, or preferably from a mixture of fetal and adult AChRs (Beeson et al., 1996). Anti-AChR titres are highly variable among MG patients, ranging from 0 to more than 1000 nm/l, and between individuals titres do not correlate well with clinical severity. The antibodies are polyclonal and mostly in the IgG1 and IgG3 subclasses. Many bind to a main immunogenic region (MIR) on the α subunits (Fig. 20.1b) but others bind to other epitopes (Tzartos et al., 1980; 1982; 1998; Whiting et al., 1986; Jacobson et al., 1999a). (However, positive values are extremely rare in healthy subjects, and the level of antibody within an individual correlates well with clinical scores after plasma exchange (Newsom Davis et al., 1978), thymectomy (Vincent et al., 1983; Kuks et al., 1991), or immunosuppressive treatments.

Pathophysiology of MG

In MG, the MEPPs are substantially reduced (Fambrough et al., 1973) owing to a reduction in the number of functional AChRs at the NMJ, as measured by binding of ^{125}I-, peroxidase-, or fluorescent-α-BuTx. The EPP is moderately reduced in amplitude but the quantal content is normal or even raised. In fact, a more recent study suggested that a compensatory increase in quantal content results from a positive-feedback mechanism in both MG and EAMG (Plomp et al., 1995).

Electron microscopy shows an essentially normal nerve terminal but the post-synaptic membrane lacks junctional folds and there are reduced areas of contact between the pre-synaptic nerve terminal and the muscle membrane (diagrammatically represented in Fig. 20.2(a)). There is also considerable debris within the synaptic cleft. The lack of post-junctional folds suggests that the voltage-gated sodium channels, which are located at the depths of the folds, may be reduced in MG, and this was demonstrated in one study (Ruff and Lennon, 1998). By increasing the threshold for activation of the muscle action potential, the reduction in sodium channels could make an important contribution to the pathophysiology of MG, and may explain why the compensatory increase in quantal content (Plomp et al., 1995) is insufficient to restore normal function.

Pathologic role and pathogenic mechanisms of anti-AChR antibodies

The presence of anti-AChR antibody is diagnostic for MG, and the levels reflect the severity of the disease within an individual, but by itself this does not prove that the antibodies cause the disease. Several approaches illustrate the pathogenic role of anti-AChR. Firstly, EAMG can be induced by the immunization of rabbits with purified AChR from the electric organ of the electric ray (Patrick and Lindstrom, 1973). Secondly, MG can be passively transferred to experimental animals by injection of MG IgG (Toyka et al., 1975), and EAMG can be transferred to naïve litter mates by injection of EAMG serum (Lindstrom et al., 1976b). Thirdly, Engel et al. (1977) showed that IgG and complement components are present at the NMJ, both on the post-synaptic membrane and in the synaptic debris; the distribution of IgG corresponds well to the distribution of AChRs as shown by peroxidase α-BuTx binding; and the amount of membrane attack complex is inversely related to the number and density of AChRs (Engel and Arahata, 1987). Thus, MG fulfils the criteria of Witbesky: the presence of antibodies to a defined antigen, the ability to induce the disease experimentally by immunization with the purified antigen and to transfer it by experimental and patient's serum, and the demonstration that these antibodies are involved in the pathology of the human disease (see Rose and Bona, 1993). The beneficial effects of plasma exchange and immunosuppression provide further confirmation. These criteria are summarized in Tables 20.1 and 20.2.

Complement-mediated damage to the NMJ is not the only mechanism by which anti-AChR reduces the numbers of AChRs. Drachman et al. (1978) and Stanley and Drachman (1978a,b) clearly demonstrated crosslinking of AChRs by divalent antibodies, resulting in an increased rate of internalization and degradation of the AChRs, and reducing the half-life for AChRs from about 10 days to about 5 days. This in itself would lead to a steady-state reduction in the numbers of AChRs to about 40%. However, there may be a compensatory increase in AChR synthesis, as shown in experimental studies of AChR turnover (Wilson et al., 1983) and in raised

(a)

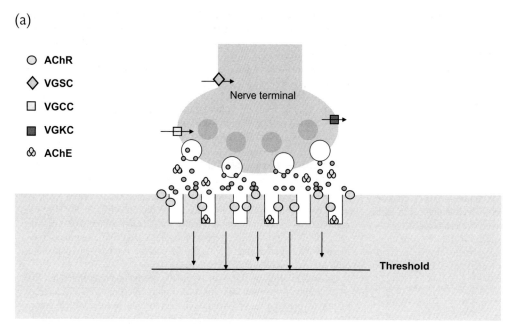

○ AChR
◇ VGSC
□ VGCC
■ VGKC
⚭ AChE

Nerve terminal

Threshold

Fig. 20.2 Pathology of myasthenia gravis. (a) In myasthenia, the number of AChRs and the depth of the post-synaptic folds are reduced. As a result the MEPPs and EPPs are reduced in amplitude and the EPP does not reach the firing threshold. (b) AChR antibody levels in myasthenia gravis are measured by immunoprecipitation of ^{125}I-α-bungarotoxin-labelled AChRs. There is a wide range of antibody titres. Negative values are found principally in patients with purely ocular MG and with normal or atrophic thymus pathology. Patients with thymic tumours (thymoma) always have AChR antibodies.

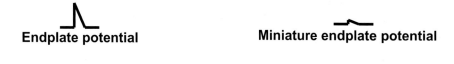

Endplate potential   **Miniature endplate potential**

(b)

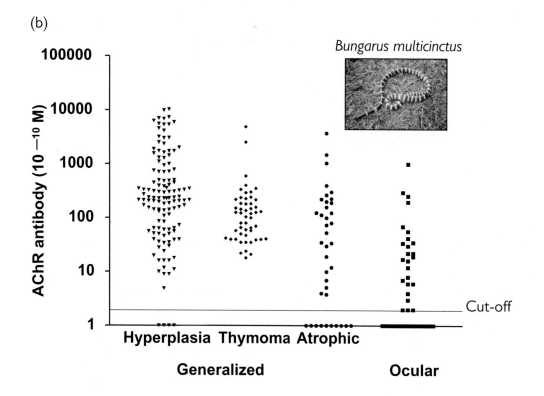

Bungarus multicinctus

AChR antibody (10^{-10} M)

100000
10000
1000
100
10
1

Cut-off

Hyperplasia Thymoma Atrophic

Generalized   **Ocular**

Table 20.1 Modified Koch's postulates for autoimmune disease in general (Rose and Bona, 1993)

Transfer of disease by placental transfer of antibodies to the baby

Transfer of disease by injection of immunoglobulins into mice

Transfer of disease by T cells into SCID mice

Induction of disease by immunization against the antigen and transfer of this disease by antibody or T cells to naïve animals

Identification of antibody or T cells in the target organ

Presence of autoantibodies or self-reactive T cells

Table 20.2 Postulates for antibody-mediated disease

Antibodies to extracellular domain of functionally-important protein

Plasma exchange produces marked clinical improvement

Transfer of disease by injection of immunoglobulins into mice

Demonstration of functional effects of antibodies using appropriate cell lines *in vitro*

messenger RNA (mRNA) levels for AChR subunits in MG (Guyon *et al.*, 1994) and in EAMG (Asher *et al.*, 1990). Thus, the importance of this mechanism in ongoing disease is not clear.

Direct inhibition of AChR function by antibodies appears to be less common. Only a few investigators have described direct functional effects of serum or an IgG preparation on the amplitudes of MEPPs *in vitro* (Burges *et al.*, 1990), although MG sera can acutely reduce AChR function in cultured human cells (Lang *et al.*, 1988). Antibodies specifically inhibiting fetal AChRs were found in two mothers with a history of recurrent fetal arthrogryposis (see below).

There have been few reports of monoclonal antibodies derived from immortalized AChR-specific MG cells, owing to low precursor frequencies and to the difficulty in obtaining stable IgG-secreting, rather than IgM-secreting, hybrids or Epstein–Barr virus (EBV)-transformed lines. Those that have been produced do not appear to recognize AChR in solution, suggesting that they may not be representative of patients' anti-AChRs. Phase display techniques, by contrast, offer the opportunity to identify specific antibodies in an MG patient library. Some preliminary success was achieved using TE671 cells for panning (Graus *et al.*, 1997) or ^{125}I-α-BuTx-labelled AChR to identify plaques containing specific Fabs (Farrar *et al.*, 1997). The latter approach produced Fab clones of more diverse origin, whereas the panning approach appears to select a restricted repertoire.

Idiotypes and molecular mimicry

Dwyer *et al.* (1983) described an extensive network of idiotype/anti-idiotypes. The network included antibodies specific for bacterial α 1–3 dextrans, and they found antidextran antibodies in about 40% of MG patients,

suggesting that anti-AChR antibodies might arise as a secondary result of an antibacterial response. In experimental rats, however, injection of an anti-dextran monoclonal antibody reduced the subsequent antibody response to AChR (Tong and Dwyer, 1990).

Other evidence for involvement of micro-organisms is the cross-reaction between the *Torpedo* AChR α subunit and microbial proteins (Stefansson *et al.*, 1985), and between human AChR α 157–170 and herpes simplex glycoprotein D (Schwimmbeck *et al.*, 1989). However, it seems unlikely that cross-reacting antibodies could demonstrate the heterogeneity, high affinity, and specificity that characterize MG anti-AChR (Vincent *et al.*, 1987), and it is noteworthy that no further developments in this area have been reported. Nevertheless, such a cross-reaction could be an initiating event that leads subsequently to autosensitization against the muscle AChR by a process of determinant spreading (see below).

Clinical heterogeneity and immunogenetics of MG

Myasthenia is not a single disease and patients can be divided into subgroups (Table 20.3) based on HLA association, thymic involvement, AChR antibody status, and particularly age at onset (Compston *et al.*, 1980). Surveys of AChR antibodies have shown a striking increase in incidence after the age of about 60 years, peaking in the late 70s (Somnier *et al.*, 1991; Robertson *et al.*, 1998; Poulas *et al.*, 2001; Vincent *et al.*, 2003b). The different groups should be considered separately when considering aetiological factors and treatments.

Ocular myasthenia gravis

Ocular MG, defined by symptoms that remain restricted to extraocular muscles for at least 2 years, has often been considered a distinct condition (although there may be electrophysiologic defects in other muscle groups). Anti-AChR levels are generally low or undetectable in about 50% of affected patients. The thymus gland is often normal, in the few patients examined, and most studies show no apparent HLA association. Most patients are treated with corticosteroids which are often effective (Sommer *et al.*, 1997). Ocular myasthenia is reviewed critically by Sommer *et al.* (1993).

It has been suggested that ocular muscle AChR is antigenically different from the AChR of other muscles; it is known that ocular muscle contains some multiply innervated fibres of the slow twitch type, and serum antibodies from patients with ocular MG bind to multiply innervated endplates as demonstrated by immunohistochemistry (Oda and Shibasaki, 1988). Horton *et al.* (1994) showed that ocular muscle contains the fetal-specific γ subunit of the AChR, but the adult-specific ε subunit is expressed even more strongly (MacLennan *et al.*, 1997). The heterogeneous muscle fibre types are a mixture of singly innervated and multiply innervated fibres; many of these express both fetal and adult AChRs (Kaminski *et al.*, 1996; reviewed in Kaminski *et al.*, 2002). Recent expression profiling of extra-ocular and limb muscles from mice suggest that they do differ in certain features (Khanna *et al.*, 2003). Ocular weakness is often the presenting symptom in neurotoxin poisoning, e.g. botulism, *Bungarus krait* envenoming; it may be that physiologic factors or accessibility of the ocular muscle

Table 20.3 Subtypes of antibody-mediated myasthenia gravis (MG)

| | AChR antibody seropositive | | | | AChR antibody seronegative | | |
| | Generalized | | Ocular | | | Generalized | |
	Early-onset MG	Late-onset MG	Thymoma-associated MG	Seropositive ocular MG	Seronegative ocular MG	MuSK antibody associated	Non-MuSK antibody associated
Age range (years)	<40 by definition	>40 by definition	2–80+	2–100	2–80+	<60	2–80+
Male:Female	1:3	3:2	1:1	3:2	3:1	5:1	3:2
HLA association	HLA B8 DR3	HLA B7 DR2 (males > females)	No clear association	None known	None known	None known	None known
Thymic pathology	Hyperplasia	Atrophy	Thymoma	Not known	Not known	Often normal for age	Often normal for age

The information is summarized from clinical data of Professor John Newsom-Davis, FRS, and from unpublished observations on seronegative MG (Vincent, Bowen, Faruggia, Newsom-Davis, 2003).

endplates to circulating factors underlie their susceptibility to clinical involvement. All of these observations suggest that ocular muscles may be physiologically distinct and more susceptible to neuromuscular junction defects than limb muscles.

Generalized myasthenia gravis

In the majority of MG patients, generalized weakness develops after puberty, without, obvious precipitating factors, and the levels of anti-AChRs are also increased. The patients can be divided into three groups on the basis of their thymic pathology and age at onset (see Table 20.3). There are only subtle differences in the amount (Fig. 20.2(b)) or characteristics of the anti-AChR between the patients (Vincent and Newsom Davis, 1982a,b), and it seems likely that the distinguishing clinical and pathologic features reflect a difference in the factors involved in the initiation of the disease, rather than an intrinsic difference in patients' immune responses to a single precipitating factor. Involvement with a particular AChR α subunit microsatellite, that is, a non-coding region of the gene, has also been reported (Garchon et al., 1994) and this may be associated with the high-susceptibility HLA gene DRB1*0301 (Djabiri et al., 1997). Therefore, it is possible that polymorphisms in gene regulatory sequences alter AChR expression and that presentation of altered AChR to a susceptible immune system underlies disease susceptibility. However, there is as yet no direct evidence in support of this hypothesis.

An important provoking factor in a minority of patients is treatment with D-penicillamine, usually for rheumatoid arthritis. About 2% of treated patients develop anti-AChR antibodies and clinical signs of MG that usually resolve after they stop taking the drug. This interesting form of MG is associated with HLA DR1 rather than DR4 (Garlepp et al., 1983), as expected in rheumatoid arthritis, or DR3 as typical in MG patients. The antibodies are of slightly lower avidity and less heterogeneous, but this may reflect their relatively short duration (Vincent and Newsom Davis, 1982b). T-cell responses to D-penicillamine suggest that the drug modifies peptides resident in surface DR1 molecules (Hill et al., 1999b).

Early onset

There is a 3:1 female male ratio for patients who develop MG in early adult life, usually defined as under 40 years at onset. The thymus gland is often hyperplastic (see below) and the patients respond well to thymectomy. In northern Europeans there is a very strong association with the HLA A1, B8, DRB1*0301, DRB*0101, DQB1*0201, DQA1*0501 ancestral haplotype (Carlsson et al., 1990; Viera et al., 1993).

Although the pathogenic autoantibodies depend on Class II restricted helper T cells, the associations are stronger with B8 than with DR3 (Compston et al., 1980). This suggests that some other predisposing gene between the Class II and Class I region may be responsible. Various possibilities, such as genes for tumour necrosis factor (TNF), heat shock proteins, and transporter proteins associated with antigen processing (TAP), have been considered (Janer et al., 1999). In addition, several groups have identified associations between MG and polymorphisms in cytokine and other immune response genes (e.g. Hjelmstrom et al., 1997, 1998).

In young-onset MG the thymus gland is often hyperplastic with many T-cell areas in the medulla, some containing lymphoid follicles (for reviews see Levine and Rosai (1978) and Hohlfeld and Wekerle (1994)). The expression of accessory molecules like CD28/B7 is normal in hyperplastic thymus (Marx et al., 1994), but a recent report claims that the expression of the apoptosis-related antigen Fas is reduced in these lymphoid follicles, suggesting that the regulation of lymphocyte survival may be abnormal (Masunaga et al., 1994). Interleukin (IL)-1 production is increased in the hyperplastic MG thymus (Aime et al., 1991), and expression of IL-2, IL-6, and interferon (IFN)-γ is up-regulated in perifollicular areas (Emilie et al., 1991). It is not clear whether any of these changes are causative or merely a predictable feature of a lymph node type infiltrate.

Lymphocytes cultured from the thymus gland synthesize anti-AChR antibody (Scadding et al., 1981), and serum anti-AChR levels frequently decline slowly after the operation (Vincent et al., 1983). Germinal centres of the MG thymus contain polyclonal activated B cells expressing a range of V_H and V_K genes, similar to that in the peripheral blood lymphocytes (Guigou et al., 1991) and somatic hypermutation of B cells occurs in thymic germinal centres (Sims et al., 2001). AChR has been demonstrated in muscle-like cells grown from thymus (Wekerle and Ketelsen, 1977; Kao and Drachman, 1977) or 'myoid' cells found in situ between the epithelial cells in both normal and MG thymic medullae (Schluep et al., 1987); myoid cells are clearly not in the lymph node type areas. Some workers (Kirchner et al., 1988) found myoid cells to be the focus of antigen-presenting cells (APCs) and T cells in MG, but it is not yet clear whether this is a primary event in MG. The thymic epithelia are hyperplastic in the MG thymus and express epidermal growth factor and integrins (Roxanis et al., 2001). The results of extensive histopathology suggest that the myoid cells are targets for autoantibody attack and that this provokes germinal centre formation (Roxanis et al., 2002).

The presence of AChR in the thymus suggests that it may be involved in inducing T-cell tolerance in normal individuals or in breaking tolerance in MG. There is expression of different AChR subunits and isoforms in MG thymuses (Andreetta et al., 1997). However, AChR may be expressed not only in the myoid cells but also in thymic epithelia, as shown by studies with transgenic mice (Salmon et al., 1998).

It is widely believed that the thymus generates AChR-specific T cells that direct antibody synthesis by B cells both in the germinal centres in the hyperplastic thymus and elsewhere. A number of attempts have been made to generate T-cell lines and clones, either with AChR peptides or with recombinant or purified AChR. Many T-cell responses have been identified against AChR peptides of each of the subunits, and there are certain peptides that appear to bind well to the relevant Class II molecules and to be relatively immunodominant (Protti et al., 1993; Manfredi et al., 1993; Moiola et al., 1994a,b; Conti-Fine et al., 1998; Wang et al., 1998a,b). Alternatively, T cells can be generated against recombinant AChR subunits, expressed usually in Escherichia coli, and the peptide epitopes mapped with synthetic peptides (Ong et al., 1991; Hawke et al., 1996; Hill et al., 1999a). There is some disagreement in the field as to the best method. T cells raised against AChR subunit peptides are relatively easy to raise but may not recognize purified AChR processed and presented by antigen-presenting cells (Matsuo et al., 1995). Conversely, T cells generated against recombinant AChR subunits are very difficult to raise, but when this is achieved they appear to be highly specific for certain peptide epitopes, and to be able to recognize naturally processed AChR.

The ability of T cells to recognize AChR in small amounts would appear to be a necessary prerequisite for an autoimmune response against this highly segregated antigen. These responses can be generated either by addition of purified AChR to the cultures or by using cell lines engineered to express both AChR and the appropriate Class II molecules. For instance, T-cell clones specific for AChR α subunit sequence 144–163 recognized AChR endogenously presented by the TE671 muscle cell line after it was transfected with DNA for the α and β chains of DR4 Dw4.2, or by human myotube cultures stimulated with IFN-γ (Baggi et al., 1993; Curnow et al., 2001). The responding T cells showed only modest proliferation, but bound to the presenting cells, secreted IFN-γ and killed the presenting cells.

This raises the issue of whether muscle cells themselves, and/or the myoid cells in the thymus, could initiate the immune response. Muscle does not normally express Class II, but there is evidence that Class II can be induced by viral infections in vivo (Bao et al., 1992) or by IFN-γ in vitro (Hohlfeld and Engel, 1990). Indeed, Class II expression in vitro does not always require IFN-γ (Cifuentes-Diaz et al., 1992). It is possible that the ability to up-regulate Class II on the muscle is controlled by genes within the MHC, and that once MHC is expressed, the muscle could present autoantigens to specific T cells. However, myoblasts cultured from human biopsies did not appear to express Class II molecules once they were differentiated (Mantegazza et al., 1996).

Late onset

Although the overall prevalence of late-onset MG is lower than that of early-onset MG, the annual incidence is actually higher. Surveys of AChR antibodies have shown a striking increase in incidence after the age of about 60 years, peaking in the late 70s (Somnier, 1996; Robertson *et al.*, 1998; Poulas *et al.*, 2001; Vincent *et al.*, 2003b). Nevertheless, when the declining numbers of the population are taken into account, there is a fall-off in diagnosis of MG after the age of 75 years (Vincent *et al.*, 2003), which suggests that MG is being underdiagnosed in the elderly.

In patients who present with symptoms of MG after the age of 40 years, the thymus is mainly atrophic or involuted and there are weak biases toward males and HLA B7, DR2 (Compston *et al.*, 1980) or DR4, DQw8 (Carlsson *et al.*, 1990). These patients do not have a thymoma (by definition) but nevertheless are often positive for antibodies to titin, ryanodine receptor, and cytokines (Meager *et al.*, 1997; Buckley *et al.*, 2001b; Somnier and Engel, 2002). The cause of the disease is entirely unknown, and given the increasing incidence, more efforts should be directed towards defining immunogenetic and environmental factors that might predispose to the development of this form of MG.

Thymoma-associated myasthenia gravis

Thymoma, which occurs in about 10% of patients in previous studies (although this may need to be revised with the increasing number of older patients) can arise at any age, although most patients with MG and thymoma present between the ages of 30 and 60 years. The thymus gland is usually removed, but the myasthenia rarely improves (Palmisani *et al.*, 1994; Somnier, 1994), anti-AChR levels seldom fall (Kuks *et al.*, 1991), and immunosuppressive therapy is often required. An HLA association has been difficult to demonstrate, although a reduced incidence of HLA B8 and DR3, and an association with DQB1*0604 (Viera *et al.*, 1993) and with DRw15 Dw2 in female patients (Carlsson *et al.*, 1990) have been found. Immunoglobulin allotypes have not generally been informative in MG, but associations in Japanese thymoma patients (Nakao *et al.*, 1980) and in White patients (Gilhus *et al.*, 1990) have been reported. Thymomas associated with MG are epithelial in origin, perhaps derived from a stem cell common to both cortical and subcapsular epithelium, and corresponding mainly to the WHO type B1 and B2 (see Muller-Hermelink and Marx, 2000).

One of the characteristic features of thymoma-associated MG is the presence of antibodies to muscle antigens that are much less frequent in early-onset MG (although this is not necessarily the case in late-onset MG). More than 90% of patients with thymoma have antibodies to antigens of striated and cardiac muscle (Aarli, 2001). These include myosin, actin, α actinin, ryanodine receptor, and a particular epitope on the giant structural protein titin (Aarli *et al.*, 1990; Ohta *et al.*, 1991; Gautel *et al.*, 1993). Morevoer, antibodies to IFN-α and IL-12 are also present in both thymoma-related MG patients and older MG patients (Meager *et al.*, 1997) and may predict the recurrence of a thymoma (Buckley *et al.*, 2001b). Both titin and ryanodine receptor epitopes are expressed in cortical thymomas (Mygland *et al.*, 1995; Marx *et al.*, 1996; Romi *et al.*, 2002) although there is some question as to their relevance (Kusner *et al.*, 1998). Equally, the cytokines IFN-α and IL-12 are both expressed by immune cells in thymoma, B cells from thymoma tissue can synthesize IFN-α antibodies, and IFN-α specific IgG Fabs can be cloned and expressed by combinatorial library techniques from B cells present in thymoma tissue (Shiono *et al.*, 2003). By contrast, AChR-specific IgG Fabs were very rarely obtained from thymomas. These observations support the idea that the thymoma is initiating and sustaining the B-cell response to certain antigens, but suggests that the AChR B-cell response must take place elsewhere. Understanding how this takes place is a major challenge in the field.

Cultured neoplastic epithelial cells from thymomas express epidermal growth factor receptor and Ki67, indicative of their growth potential (Gilhus *et al.*, 1995a). There is no increased expression of p53 or bcl-2. Interestingly, CD28/B7 expression is high in thymoma epithelial cells in comparison with those in normal cortex, indicating the potential for these cells to activate T-cell responses. Moreover, these cells can process and present antigens to Class IL restricted T cells (Gilhus *et al.*, 1995b), indicating that they express both the appropriate Class II molecule and the necessary processing apparatus and accessory molecules. However, functional AChR

does not appear to be present in thymoma tissue; the AChR α subunit is present but only at very low levels in the thymoma tissue itself, as identified by polymerase chain reaction (PCR) (Hara *et al.*, 1991; Geuder *et al.*, 1992a,b). An AChR-like epitope on a 153 kDa cytoplasmic protein in cortical epithelium was identified by binding of monoclonal antibodies specific for AChR α subunit sequence 373–380 (Marx *et al.*, 1989). Its presence correlates well with MG or the cortical epithelial tumour with which it associates (see above); however, neither T-cell nor antibody responses in thymoma patients are directed against this epitope (Nagvekar *et al.*, 1998a), making it unlikely that it is involved in initiating MG. It now appears that an epitope that cross-reacts with α subunit sequence 370–380 is expressed on neurofilament protein in cortical epithelium (Marx *et al.*, 1996), but there is no hard evidence that it is involved in the induction of AChR autoimmunity.

The typical MG thymoma contains large numbers of polyclonal developing T lymphocytes, many double positive for CD4 and CD8 and others with the single markers of maturing T cells (Fujii *et al.*, 1990). The number of T cells is often drastically depleted owing to preceding steroid therapy (Willcox, 1989). The remaining lymphocytes might either escape deletion in the grossly disorganized cortex, or be specifically sensitized to antigens presented and expressed by the thymoma epithelium. The adjacent thymus is typically hyperplastic, though not in thymoma patients without MG (Yoshitake *et al.*, 1994), and a few B cells are present in thymoma tissue (Kornstein and Kay, 1990). However, anti-AChR synthesis by thymoma cells is rare (see above), contrasting with that which occurs in early-onset hyperplastic thymuses.

There have been relatively few successful attempts to clone AChR-specific T cells from thymoma tissue or from the peripheral blood cells of thymoma MG patients. One highly specific clone, raised from a young man with thymoma and MG, was restricted to HLA DP14, and recognized the α subunit sequence 75–90. Another clone from an older patient recognized the α subunit sequence 149–158 in the context of DR52a (Nagvekar *et al.*, 1998b). Interestingly, both these thymoma-associated clones, that responded to very small amounts of purified human AChR illustrating their specificity and sensitivity, secreted IL-4 as well as IFN-γ indicating a Th0 phenotype. Although studies on specific T cells have been difficult, there is no doubt that the thymoma does generate potentially functional T cells. The proportion of both CD4 and CD8 T cells containing Trecs (T-cell receptor excision circles), which gives an indication of the number of recently emigrated T cells in the periphery, is greatly raised in thymoma MG cases and falls after thymomectomy (Buckley *et al.*, 2001a). Moreover, Trecs rise again if the tumour recurs. On the other hand, double negative CD4–/CD8– T cells were not abnormal in thymoma cases and did not change after surgery (Reinhardt and Melms, 2000).

Neonatal myasthenia gravis and arthrogryposis multiplex congenita

A proportion of babies born to MG mothers have transient respiratory and feeding difficulties, owing to placental transfer of maternal anti-AChR (Morel *et al.*, 1988). These problems may be more common in the offspring of mothers who have a high proportion of antibodies reactive with fetal type AChR (Vernet der Garabedian *et al.*, 1994), although the fetal form is thought to be replaced by the adult form from around 33 weeks' gestation (Hesselmans *et al.*, 1993). Occasionally neonatal MG occurs without maternal disease, or when the mother is anti-AChR negative.

A few cases of severe arthrogryposis multiplex congenita, a condition consisting of fixed joint contractures associated with inadequate development of jaws and lungs, have been found in a number of consecutive pregnancies in mothers with MG. One mother was diagnosed as having MG only after her fourth affected pregnancy (Barnes *et al.*, 1995), and one remains completely symptom free (Brueton *et al.*, 2001). Maternal anti-AChR antibodies that even at high dilution completely inhibited the function of fetal AChR in an *in vitro* assay but had no affect on adult AChR function were present in these mothers (for review see Polizzi *et al.* (2000)). These antibodies appeared to be responsible for the complete loss of fetal movement *in utero* and subsequent deformities that were incompatible with survival after birth. An animal model of this condition has been induced by injecting the maternal plasmas into pregnant mice; the offspring were found to be paralysed and to exhibit fixed joint contractures (Jacobson *et al.*, 1999*b*). To investigate further, combinatorial B-cell libraries were made from the thymuses of two women with MG and affected babies. AChR-specific Fabs were relatively easy to select from the libraries and were highly specific for fetal AChR; only one of 40 bound equally to fetal and adult AChR (Matthews *et al.*, 2002).

Maternal antibodies to fetal AChR are not the main cause of this syndrome. In a study of over 180 sera from mothers of babies with this condition only three symptom-free mothers were found to have antibodies to fetal AChRs (Dalton and Vincent, in preparation). Nevertheless, antibodies to other fetal antigens (muscle, nerve, cartilage) were found in about 10% of the maternal sera, suggesting that maternal antibodies should be considered as a possible cause in some cases of arthrogryposis and possibly of other developmental disorders (see also Chapter 33).

Seronegative myasthenia gravis

About 10 to 15% of all MG patients with generalized symptoms do not have detectable anti-AChRs by current laboratory methods; they appear to represent a distinct population from the majority of MG patients. Seronegative MG (SNMG) patients have symptoms and distribution of weakness similar to those of patients with seropositive generalized MG, but proportionately more develop MG before the age of puberty (Vincent *et al.*, 1993). There are some T-cell areas in the thymic medulla, but lymphoid follicles are few, and thymus histology is almost 'normal' (Willcox *et al.*, 1991; Verma and Oger, 1992). Thymoma is never found, and no HLA association has been identified. Thus on clinical and pathologic grounds, the disease appears to have several unusual features.

SNMG is associated with some reduction in ^{125}I-α-BuTx binding to AChRs at the NMJ and reduced MEPP amplitudes in patients' biopsies, as typically found in seropositive MG, but there have been no systematic studies. Seronegative patients respond well to plasma exchange and their immunoglobulins passively transfer a defect in neuromuscular transmission to mice; but the numbers of AChRs, as measured by ^{125}I-α-BuTx binding, are not substantially reduced in these animals (Mossman *et al.*, 1986; Burges *et al.*, 1994). These observations suggest that there is a humoral immune factor but that it may not be directed at the AChR.

There are at least two, and perhaps three, such factors (reviewed in Vincent *et al.* (2003*a*). Firstly, it was found that IgG antibodies from SNMG patients bound to a muscle-like cell line that expresses AChRs but not to a non-muscle cell line transfected with cRNAs for AChR (Blaes *et al.*, 2000). Since both lines expressed AChRs, this implied that the antibodies were binding to another, muscle-specific, target. A candidate antigen was the muscle-specific kinase, MuSK. This is a receptor tyrosine kinase that plays a crucial role during development of the neuromuscular junction. Antibodies to MuSK are present in up to 70% of SNMG patients (Hoch *et al.*, 2001; Scuderi *et al.*, 2002; McConville *et al.*, 2004). These antibodies are IgG and not found in patients with AChR antibody-positive MG or in other control groups; thus they define a distinct form of MG (Fig. 20.3(a)). They are not found in patients with purely ocular myasthenia (see above). In preliminary studies they appear to be found often in patients with marked combined ocular and bulbar symptoms (Scuderi *et al.*, 2002; Evoli *et al.*, 2003) or with neck extensor weakness (Sanders *et al.*, 2003). Thymic germinal centres are very rare (Lauriola *et al.* 2005; Leite *et al.* 2005). How these antibodies affect neuromuscular transmission is not clear, but since MuSK is part of the agrin-induced pathway that clusters AChRs (see Liyanage *et al.* (2002) for a review, and Fig. 20.3(b)), it is likely that they interfere with some aspect of MuSK signalling. This may involve changes in AChR synthesis (Poea *et al.*, 2000).

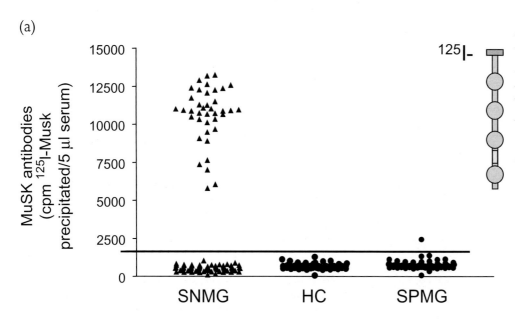

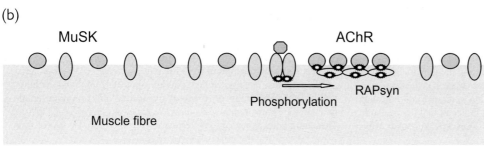

Fig. 20.3 Muscle-specific kinase (MuSK) antibodies and seronegative MG. (a) MuSK antibodies measured by immunoprecipitation of ^{125}I-MuSK are detected in about 50% of patients without AChR antibodies and not in patients with AChR antibodies or in healthy individuals. (b) During development, agrin, released from the motor nerve, interacts with MuSK to induce clustering of RAPsyn (receptor aggregating protein at the synapse) and AChRs. MuSK antibodies inhibit this process in culture models, but it is not yet clear what they do at the mature neuromuscular junction.

Secondly, many seronegative MG plasmas, and IgM-containing fractions, inhibit AChR function in the muscle like TE671 cell line, again without reducing ^{125}I-α-BuTx binding (Yamamoto *et al.*, 1991); and SNMG plasmas reduce ACh-induced currents in whole cell clamped TE671 cells (Barrett-Jolley *et al.*, 1994). The mechanism of action is still unclear, but electrophysiological observations point to enhanced desensitization of the AChR, probably acting by binding to another membrane receptor (Plested *et al.*, 2002) but possibly by binding of low-affinity IgM antibodies to the AChR itself (Spreadbury *et al.*, 2005). Finally, a direct but reversible effect of patients' IgG on AChR function was demonstrated in one study (Bufler *et al.*, 1998), but it is not clear whether this is related to the IgG MuSK antibodies, to the IgM-containing fraction described above, or to other IgG antibodies.

Experimental autoimmune myasthenia gravis (EAMG) as a model for MG

Immunization against AChRs

The induction of EAMG in experimental animals was a major contribution to demonstrating the role of AChR antibodies in MG, and the model has been helpful in elucidating the pathogenic mechanisms of the disease. The model is only reviewed briefly here (for a comprehensive review see Lindstrom (2000)). The proportion of antibodies that cross-react between the immunizing protein and the recipient's muscle AChR depends on the closeness of the species, being only about 1% between *Torpedo* and rodent AChR. Nevertheless, the animals have reduced AChR numbers at the muscle endplates, reduced amplitudes of MEPPs and EPPs, and show either overt signs of weakness or marked sensitivity to the neuromuscular blocking drug D-tubocurarine. The clinical effects of immunization depend partly on the susceptibility of the immunized strain to changes in AChR numbers. For instance, whereas New Zealand white rabbits become severely weak within 4 to 6 weeks of a single immunization, rats or mice are much more varied in their response. The AChR is very immunogenic. Rats (Lindstrom *et al.*, 1976a,b) and mice (Jermy *et al.*, 1993) can show an immune response to syngeneic AChR, even in the absence of adjuvant (Jermy *et al.*, 1993). Some features of animal models of MG are reviewed by Christadoss *et al.* (2002).

When animals are immunized against denatured α subunits, the antibody response to the cytoplasmic region of the AChR usually dominates the response. However, a few investigators have demonstrated production of anti-AChR antibodies in experimental animals immunized with peptides representing extracellular sequences of the AChR α subunit or recombinant α subunit, although few animals showed clinical signs of EAMG. For instance, three peptides spanning the human AChR sequence α 138–199 induced antipeptide antibodies, followed in most rabbits by the presence of anti-AChRs and severe muscle weakness. The anti-AChR antibodies were directed against the MIR and α-BuTx binding site on rabbit AChRs, and could be separated from the antipeptide antibodies, suggesting that they arose as a result of determinant spreading. It is possible that this represents a mechanism by which low-affinity, perhaps cross-reacting, antibodies lead to secondary high-affinity anti-AChRs.

Several investigators (e.g. Meinl *et al.*, 1991) found only minimal thymic changes in EAMG. These observations suggest that thymic changes in MG are not the secondary result of the immune response against the AChR.

It is relatively easy to measure T-cell responses to *Torpedo* AChR, which can be purified in milligramme quantities, and to map the responses using synthetic peptides (see Pachner *et al.*, 1989). A large number of epitopes, some specific to particular mouse strains, have been identified. Similarly, anti-AChR antibodies can be shown to bind to synthetic peptides. However, these approaches do not define the epitopes that are crucial in the auto anti-AChR response. In Lewis rats, the main T-cell epitope is α 100–116. B cells from rats primed with native AChR induce T-cell proliferative responses to intact AChR, and in turn can be stimulated to produce anti-AChR (Fujii and Lindstrom, 1988). Thus, this epitope fulfils the criteria for pathogenicity. This epitope is also a useful target for specific immunosuppression via a Class II–peptide complex (Spack *et al.*, 1995).

T- and B-cell reactivity toward AChR can also be detected via ELI spot assays based on IFN-γ or IgG secretion, respectively (Wang *et al.*, 1995), and such reactivity is reduced in rats orally tolerized toward AChR. Transforming growth factor (TGF)-β secretion is increased. Depletion of CD8+ T cells may suppress EAMG in Lewis rats, associated with lower proliferative responses and lower anti-AChR titres (Zhang *et al.*, 1995). Class I genes may make a substantial contribution to the induction or maintenance of the immune response, as proposed for MG (Shenoy *et al.*, 1994).

Studies on inbred rodents demonstrated the importance of immunogenetic factors in the susceptibility to EAMG. C57B1/6 mice and AKR mice are the most susceptible laboratory mouse strains correlating with H-2^b and Ig-1^b, whereas BALB/c strains are relatively resistant (Christadoss *et al.*, 1979; Berman and Patrick, 1980). Lewis rats are much more likely to become weak after immunization than are Wistar Furth rats (Biesecker and Koffler, 1988). The basis for these differences in susceptibility, however, is still not clear. It does not relate to the serum antibody levels (Berman and Patrick, 1980), nor to intrinsic muscle factors. The I-A^{bm12} mutation in C57B1/6 mice confers resistance to EAMG, probably by changing the T-cell repertoire and preventing recognition of α 146–162, a dominant T-cell epitope (Biesecker and Koffler, 1988). Detailed analysis of the role of Class II and T-cell receptor genes in EAMG is provided elsewhere (Kaul *et al.*, 1994). Recently, EAMG has been induced in mice deficient for cytokines or accessory molecules, or treated with soluble forms of these substances. In general, the results demonstrate the involvement of T helper 1 (Th1) dependent mechanisms in the pathogenic immune response to AChR. For instance, not surprisingly, these studies have shown that CD28–B7 and CD40L–CD40 interactions are important, and that IFN-γ is essential for the full immune response, whereas IL-4 does not play a major role. Mice deficient in IL-6, by contrast, are less likely to develop EAMG and showed less germinal centre formation (see Christadoss *et al.*, 2000).

The experimental model continues to be used for testing approaches to specific treatments for MG, despite the fact that the relevance of the animal model to the human disease must be limited. Many of these approaches are reviewed elsewhere (Drachman *et al.*, 1993; Christados *et al.*, 2000; Vincent and Drachman, 2002).

Severe combined immunodeficient mice

Schonbeck *et al.* (1992) found that injection of dissociated MG thymic cells into severe combined immunodeficient (SCID) mice led to transient anti-AChR production, but implantation of thymus tissue beneath the kidney capsule produced a more sustained anti-AChR response, perhaps because myogenesis was evident in the thymic transplants (Spuler *et al.*, 1994). IgG was identified at the NMJ of the mice, indicating that the antibody was able to react with AChRs *in situ*. This model was also used to investigate the role of specific T-cell subsets. AChR antibodies in the mice and AChR loss in their muscles was prevented when the MG thymic lymphocytes were deleted for Vβ5.1 T cells before transfer (Aissaoui *et al.*, 1999).

The SCID model does hold some potential for testing methods of tolerance induction of specific immunotherapy that could be used in humans, and several studies of tolerance induction are being pursued (Stacy *et al.*, 2002). In addition, mice transgenic for human T cells and human Class II molecules may provide the models that are needed for the future (Raju *et al.*, 2001; Yang *et al.*, 2002) both with respect to understanding better the role of immune factors in disease susceptibility (Yang *et al.*, 2002), and to examining the effects of strategies to induce tolerance to AChR.

Conclusions

MG is an autoantibody-mediated disease and the studies on MG have demonstrated most effectively the criteria required for an antibody-mediated disease (Table 20.2). The autoantigen muscle nicotinic AChR has been cloned and sequenced, and a great deal is known about its localization and expression. The antibodies are of high affinity and specific for human AChR, suggesting that sensitization against the AChR itself has taken place, but it is still unclear as to what initiates the disease. The origins and roles of antibodies to other antigens at the NMJ or in muscle, particularly those shared with thymoma tissue, need to be investigated. The role of the thymus, and the involvement of specific T cells that provide help for antibody production, are still under investigation. There is an animal model induced by immunization against AChR that faithfully reproduces many aspects of the disease, but no spontaneous model in laboratory animals. The new SCID or humanized mouse models may offer some hope for the future. In spite of the enormous amount of research that has led to these insights, the aetiology of the disease and the goal of specific immunotherapy are still elusive.

The Lambert–Eaton myasthenic syndrome

In 1957 Lambert and Eaton described a myasthenic syndrome that was electrophysiologically distinct from MG (Eaton and Lambert, 1957). There was a greatly reduced compound muscle action potential (CMAP) amplitude following supramaximal nerve stimulation that became smaller at low rates of repetitive nerve stimulation (<10/s), but that increased during stimulation at higher rates, or following a few seconds of voluntary contraction. These findings contrasted with those in MG where the CMAP is not usually reduced initially and fails to show an increment following high-frequency stimulation. Lambert–Eaton myasthenic syndrome (LEMS) is often associated with small cell lung cancer (SCLC), and is also sometimes found with paraneoplastic cerebellar degeneration and paraneoplastic encephalomyelitis. Thus, LEMS is a member of the expanding family of paraneoplastic autoimmune conditions. However, about 50% of patients never develop a tumour and have an acquired autoimmune disease of unknown aetiology.

Clinical features

A full review of the clinical and electrophysiologic features of LEMS can be found elsewhere (O'Neill et al., 1988). LEMS is more common in males than females. Weakness involves predominantly proximal muscles of the limbs and nearly always affects the legs first. Strength may increase during the first few seconds of a voluntary contraction. Ocular symptoms are far less common than in MG. Reflexes are absent or depressed but can show post-tetanic potentiation. The disease can occur at any age but the age at onset is lower in patients without detectable cancer (NCD LEMS). Autonomic symptoms (dry mouth, constipation, impotence) are present in many patients, suggesting that the target antigen may be present in the autonomic systems (Khurana et al., 1988).

LEMS is diagnosed by the combination of weakness, reduced tendon reflexes, improvement following voluntary contraction, and the typical electromyographic (EMG) findings mentioned already. The diagnosis can now be confirmed by identification of serum anti-VGCC antibodies, which are positive in more than 90% of patients.

Treatment

Pharmacologic treatment includes anti-acetylcholinesterase drugs that prolong the action of acetylcholine (ACh), and aminopyridines that increase the release of ACh by prolonging the depolarization of the motor nerve terminal (Murray and Newsom-Davis, 1981). In cancer-detected (CD) LEMS, treatment of the primary cancer often leads to clinical improvement (Chalk et al., 1990). In both CD and NCD LEMS, neurologic symptoms can be temporarily ameliorated by plasma exchange, and long-term improvement achieved with immunosuppression using prednisolone or azathioprine, or both. Intravenous immunoglobulin therapy resulted in the improvement of several parameters of strength, and an associated decline in specific antibody, in a double-blind crossover trial in eight LEMS patients (Bain et al., 1996).

Pathophysiology

In vitro recordings from biopsied intercostal muscle revealed normal miniature endplate potentials (MEPPs) but very small endplate potentials (EPPs), indicating that the quantal content (the number of packets of ACh released per nerve impulse) was reduced (Lambert and Elmqvist, 1971). The EPPs increased during repetitive stimulation, and also in response to

increases in extracellular calcium concentration. During high-frequency stimulation, Ca^{2+} accumulates in the nerve terminal, overcoming the reduced Ca^{2+} entry.

Freeze fracture electron microscopic studies of motor nerve terminals in healthy human muscle biopsy samples reveal, as in other species, double parallel rows of intramembranous particles (each about 10^{-2} nm in diameter). These particle arrays are associated with the pre-synaptic active zones that are known to be close to the site of exocytosis of the transmitter. The particles themselves (active zone particles) appear to represent VGCCs (see above). A highly significant reduction in the number of active zone particles and the number of particles per active zone was found in LEMS patients, and an increase in the number of clusters of particles (reviewed by Engel (1991)). Fig. 20.4(a) illustrates the neuromuscular junction and electrophysiology of LEMS.

Autoimmunity in LEMS

Many LEMS patients have other autoimmune disorders, such as thyroid disease, vitiligo, pernicious anaemia, coeliac disease, and juvenile onset diabetes mellitus. Lennon et al. (1982) found one or more organ-specific autoantibodies in almost half of their series of 64 patients. The incidence was higher in patients without a tumour. A study of 30 LEMS patients found an increased association with HLA B8, particularly in the NCD LEMS group, in whom there was also an increased frequency of IgG heavy chain markers (Willcox et al., 1985; Demaine et al., 1988). Taken together, these clinical studies strongly suggest involvement of the immune system in the aetiology of LEMS.

The evidence for an antibody-mediated pathogenesis is now overwhelming. Plasma exchange, a procedure that removes circulating factors including autoantibodies (Lang et al., 1981; Dau and Denys, 1982), leads to clinical improvement associated with an increase in CMAP amplitudes, with the maximal response occurring about 10 days after the treatment. Moreover, as mentioned already, most patients respond to immunosuppressive drugs or intravenous immunoglobulin therapy.

The passive transfer of patients' plasma or immunoglobulins into experimental animals was crucial in leading to the recognition that MG is an antibody-mediated disorder (Toyka et al., 1975). Daily injection of LEMS plasmas, or IgG fractions, into mice reproduced the principal neurophysiologic changes of LEMS (Lang et al., 1983; Kim, 1985). Interestingly, complement did not seem to be involved as C3-deficient mice were as susceptible as normal mice (Prior et al., 1985), and purified IgG was as effective as plasma. None of the mice showed signs of weakness, probably because of the extent to which the EPP normally exceeds the threshold for activation of the muscle action potential ('the safety factor') in rodents.

The reduction in quantal content followed the level of human IgG in the mouse serum during long-term daily injections (Prior et al., 1985), with the time to half maximal effect being about 36 hours for both the 'on' effect and the 'off' effect; however, in most cases acute incubation in LEMS sera or IgG (1–3 hours) did not affect quantal content, indicating that the antibodies did not inhibit function directly.

Quantitative freeze-fracture electron microscopy in mice injected daily for 52 to 69 days with LEMS IgG showed reductions in the number of active zones (Fukunaga et al., 1983) that were very similar to those seen at the nerve terminals of LEMS patients. These studies lent support to the view that LEMS IgG interferes with ACh release by targeting the channels themselves or structures very closely related to them. The clustering of the active zone particles was preceded by a reduction in the distance between particles, suggesting that the divalent antibodies were acting by cross-linking adjacent particles (Fukuoka et al., 1987a,b). Motor nerve terminals exposed to monovalent F(ab') LEMS IgG showed no changes, whereas F(ab')$_2$ was as effective as the native molecule in demonstrating morphologic and electrophysiologic changes (Peers et al., 1993). Because the F(ab)$_2$ molecule does not fix complement, these results provide further evidence that the morphologic and electrophysiologic effects of LEMS IgG do not require the complement system.

(a)

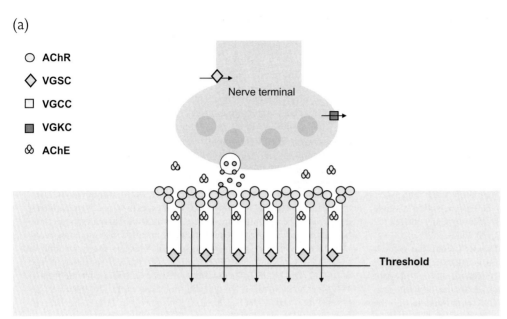

Fig. 20.4 Antibodies in Lambert–Eaton myasthenic syndrome (LEMS). (a) Antibodies reduce the number of functional voltage-gated calcium channels (VGCC) at the neuromuscular junction leading to reduced Ach release, with reduced amplitude of the endplate potentials. (b) The antibodies reduce the number of α_{1A} (P/Q-type) VGCCs in cultured cell lines but have no effects on α_{1B} (N-type) VGCC subtypes. (From Pinto et al. (1998) with permission.)

(b)

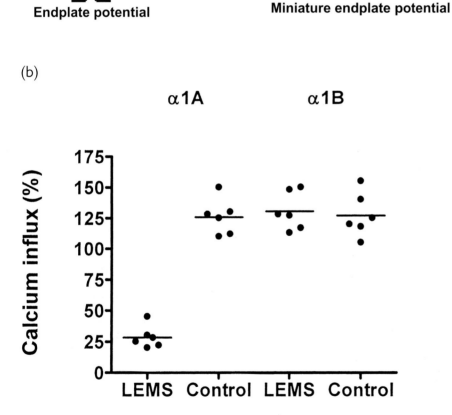

Using a sensitive immunoelectron microscopy technique, Engel and colleagues (Fukuoka *et al.*, 1987*b*; Engel *et al.*, 1989) localized IgG at the sites of pre-synaptic active zones in mice that had received multiple intraperitoneal doses of LEMS IgG. The amount and distribution of IgG were small, reflecting the low number of active zone particles and their restricted localization.

Voltage-gated calcium channel antibodies

The physiologic and morphologic passive transfer studies clearly pointed to an effect of LEMS IgG on nerve terminal VGCCs or to structures closely associated with them. SCLC cells can generate Ca²⁺ spikes that are blocked by calcium channel blockers. Roberts *et al.* (1985) showed that the function of these cells is reduced when they are grown in the presence of LEMS IgG. Others obtained similar results in SCLC lines raised from non-LEMS and from LEMS patients (De Aizpurua *et al.*, 1988), and in rat cortical synaptosomes at 37°C (Meyer *et al.*, 1986).

VGCC subtypes are transmembrane proteins comprising α_1, β, and α_2/δ subunits. The α_1 subunit is thought to contain the central Ca²⁺ conducting channel, and appears to be the principal determinant of the functional properties of the particular subtype, and to contain the ligand binding sites. Several VGCC subtypes are known and may be present within a single neuron (Tsien *et al.*, 1987), making it difficult to identify in any one cell the VGCC subtypes being targeted by LEMS autoantibodies.

The use of ω toxins derived from snail and spider venoms has made it possible to define the subtype of VGCC present in intact neurons, in cell lines, and at the neuromuscular junction. The cone snail-derived toxin ω-conotoxin (ω-CmTx) MVIIC and the spider venom-derived toxin ω-agatoxin (ω-Aga) IVA (Protti and Uchitel, 1997) both interfere with the EPP at the mouse neuromuscular junction, indicating that P- or Q-type VGCCs mediate ACh release. There is evidence for several different subtypes of VGCCs in SCLC cell lines. Johnston *et al.* (1994), using an SCLC cell line (MB) derived from a patient with LEMS, found that ω-Aga IVA and ω-CmTx MVIIC inhibited flux by about 80%, suggesting that the dominant VGCC in this SCLC cell line was the P or Q type. Since pre-incubation of the SCLC cell line in LEMS IgG produced a reduction in stimulated Ca²⁺ flux, these channels are the likely target for the antibodies in LEMS.

Solubilized VGCCs pre-labelled with ¹²⁵I neurotoxins can be immunoprecipitated by LEMS serum. Early results using N-type VGCCs labelled with ω-CgTx GVIA showed positive antibodies in a proportion of LEMS patients, but also in patients with SCLC without LEMS (Sher *et al.*, 1989). By contrast, Motomura *et al.* (1995) found that 56 (85%) of 66 LEMS serum samples immunoprecipitated ω-CmTx MVIIC-labelled P/Q-type VGCCs, extracted from rabbit or human cerebellums, and this assay was highly specific for LEMS. Lennon *et al.* (1995) reported very similar results, but also found positive results in a proportion of patients with paraneo-

plastic disorders without LEMS; these may have had paraneoplastic cerebellar syndromes (Clouston *et al.* (1992)).

An inverse relationship between the anti-VGCC antibody titre and clinical severity was found in a longitudinal study on individuals receiving immunosuppressive therapy (Bird, 1992), and after intravenous immunoglobulin treatment. In a double-blind crossover trial of eight LEMS patients, intravenous immunoglobulin reduced anti-VGCC levels by about 40%. The effect was not seen at 1 week but was evident at 2 weeks, by which time total serum IgG levels were within the normal range. The decline in specific antibody persisted until 6 to 8 weeks (Bain *et al.*, 1996). This is one of the few studies in which the effect of intravenous immunoglobulin on specific serum antibodies has been carefully studied, and it suggests that the clinical improvement and delayed fall in VGCC antibodies is unlikely to be the result of 'anti-idiotype' antibodies in the injected immunoglobulins.

The binding sites of the anti-VGCC antibodies have not been mapped in detail. Since the α_1 subunit appears to determine the channel subtype, antibodies that interfere with neuromuscular transmission presumably recognize the extracellular domain of this subunit. This was shown by applying the LEMS IgG to cultured HEK 293 cells transfected with the different types of VGCC. The LEMS IgG substantially reduced calcium currents through VGCCs expressing the α_1 subtype, but not those expressing the other subtypes (Pinto *et al.*, 1998; Fig. 20.4(b)). Takamori *et al.* (1997) showed evidence for LEMS IgG binding to the S5–S6 linker peptide sequences, in domains II and IV, that form part of the extracellular domain of the VGCC α_1 subunit. Some LEMS sera also recognize the intracellular VGCC β subunit on Western blots (Rosenfeld *et al.*, 1993), but these antibodies are not likely to be pathogenic. Antibodies binding to synaptotagmin, a synaptic vesicle protein, have also been detected, mainly in patients with high levels of anti-N-type VGCC (Leveque *et al.*, 1992). It may be that antibodies to N-type VGCC, β subunit, and synaptotagmin are associated, and represent a secondary antibody response following the primary attack on VGCC-containing cells.

The main mechanism by which LEMS antibodies interfere with calcium channel function is through cross-linking and internalization, causing a reduction in the number of functional channels. There seems to be no evidence for a complement-mediated effect, nor is there any evidence for denervation as would be expected if motor nerve terminals are being destroyed by a complement-dependent process. A study on cerebellar neurons showed that LEMS IgG reduced the number of P/Q-type VGCCs in both Purkinje cells and granule cells (Pinto *et al.*, 1998) after 15–22 hours'

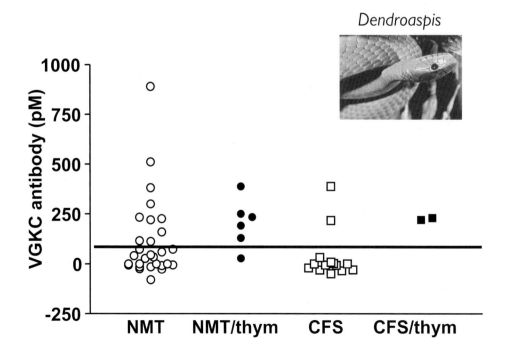

Dendroaspis

Fig. 20.5 Antibodies to voltage-gated potassium channels (VGKC) in neuromyotonia. VGKC antibodies are measured by immunoprecipitation of ¹²⁵I-dendrotoxin-labelled VGKCs extracted from rabbit brain. They are found in a proportion of patients with neuromyotonia or cramp fasciculation syndrome, including patients who have thymomas. These antibodies are also found at high titre in some patients with a form of limbic encephalitis (see Chapter 33).

incubation. At the same time there appeared to be a compensatory up-regulation of an 'R-type' VGCC. Similar compensatory changes may occur at the neuromuscular junction.

Autonomic dysfunction is common in LEMS, suggesting that LEMS IgG may interfere with neurotransmission at autonomic synapses. Multiple subtypes of VGCC are involved in the release of neurotransmitter at mouse bladder muscle and the vas deferens (Waterman, 1996) including P, Q, N, and R types. Mice injected with LEMS IgG show reduced muscle tension generated at high frequency and this was due to reduced activity through P-type VGCCs with relatively little change in N-type VGCCs (Waterman et al., 1997). However, there was no obvious clinical effect and it would be interesting to know more about the role of these channels in normal autonomic functions.

Animal models of LEMS

One of the criteria for establishing the autoimmune nature of a disease is the induction of an experimental form of the disease by immunization of experimental animals with the purified antigen (as shown for MG using affinity-purified AChR). This has not been easy for LEMS. Takamori et al. (1994) immunized rats with synthetic peptides from the N-terminus of synaptotagmin, a synaptic vesicle protein to which antibodies have been reported in LEMS (Leveque et al., 1992; Takamori et al., 2000). The animals did not become weak, but showed reduced EPP amplitudes with normal MEPP amplitudes. Since synaptotagmin is only exposed on the surface of the motor nerve terminal following exocytosis and release of ACh, one might expect antibodies to synaptotagmin to interfere with the recycling of synaptic vesicles. The physiologic evidence in this study was insufficient to define the mechanism involved. An alternative approach was to immunize against synthetic peptides representing the VGCC α_1 subunit (Kornai et al., 1999).

Conclusions

LEMS is an autoimmune disease in which antibodies to the P/Q-type VGCCs, involved in the control of neurotransmitter release at the motor nerve terminal, lead to a reduction in the number of channels and reduced calcium-dependent ACh release. The antibodies can be measured by a radioimmunoprecipitation assay employing ^{125}I-ω-conotoxin as a radioactive label for solubilized calcium channel protein. LEMS is associated with SCLC and is thus one of a growing number of paraneoplastic disorders in which an autoantibody response against a tumour leads to neuronal dysfunction.

Acquired neuromyotonia

Neuromyotonia (NMT), or Isaacs' syndrome, is a syndrome of spontaneous and continuous muscle fibre contraction resulting from hyperexcitability of motor nerves. The diagnosis largely rests on a combination of clinical and EMG findings. It is relatively rare, and the clinical presentation is heterogeneous not only in terms of severity, but also in its association with a variety of other diseases (Newsom-Davis and Mills, 1993).

Some patients have a genetic form of the disease, in some associated with mutations in the gene for a voltage-gated potassium channel (VGKC) on chromosome 12 (Browne et al., 1994). The acquired form, however, is the most prevalent and until recently has been regarded as idiopathic. However, there is now good evidence for a pathogenic role of antibodies to VGKCs.

Clinical features

These include muscle stiffness, cramps, myokymia (visible undulation of the muscle), and weakness, most prominent in the limbs and trunk. Increased sweating is common. Myokymia characteristically continues during sleep and general anaesthesia. Pseudomyotonia, a slow relaxation of muscles after contraction, may also be present. The syndrome usually follows a chronic course although spontaneous remissions have been reported.

The acquired form most commonly presents between the ages of 25 and 60 years. For detailed reviews of the clinical and electrophysiologic findings see Newsom-Davis and Mills (1993) and Hart et al. (2002). A minority of patients have sensory symptoms, including transient or continuous para-esthesia, dysaesthesia, and numbness, that may be present even when there is no peripheral neuropathy. Central nervous system symptoms such as insomnia, hallucinations, delusions, and personality change may also be present. Cramp fasciculation syndrome, that was formerly thought to be a different disorder, may represent another aspect of neuromyotonia (Hart et al., 2002).

The abnormal muscle activity may be generated at different sites throughout the length of the nerve. In most cases these sites are principally distal, but in others they may be proximal, perhaps even including the anterior horn cell (see Vincent, 2000). Diagnosis is confirmed by electromyography. The typical finding is the occurrence of spontaneous motor unit discharges that occur in distinctive doublets, triplets, or longer runs (Newsom-Davis and Mills, 1993). These neuromyotonic discharges have a high (40–300/s) intraburst frequency usually occurring at irregular intervals of 1 to 30 s. In one-third of patients there may also be evidence of damage to nerve fibres. Occasionally, the characteristic physiologic abnormalities are associated with either acute or chronic inflammatory demyelinating polyneuropathy. To date there have been no studies of motor nerve conduction or neuromuscular transmission in muscle biopsy specimens from NMT patients.

Treatment

At present the symptoms of NMT can be improved by use of the anticonvulsant drugs carbamazepine and phenytoin. Their mechanism of action may be related to their ability to reduce sodium conductance in axonal membranes and thereby to dampen down nerve hyperexcitability. Plasma exchange can be effective (Sinha et al., 1991) and intravenous immunoglobulins have also been found useful in some patients.

Autoimmunity and antibodies to VGKC in NMT

As in MG and LEMS, NMT may be associated with other autoimmune diseases or other autoantibodies. In patients with acquired NMT, cerebrospinal fluid analysis occasionally shows a raised total IgG level or oligoclonal bands, suggesting that there is intrathecal IgG synthesis (Newsom-Davis and Mills, 1993). There is one report of a patient with rheumatoid arthritis who developed NMT after treatment with penicillamine; the muscle overactivity stopped after this drug was withdrawn (Reeback et al., 1979). Penicillamine has also been implicated in triggering other autoimmune diseases, including myasthenia gravis and dermatomyositis (Fernandes et al., 1980).

Thymoma was found in 10 patients with NMT, equivalent to about 20% of all of the patients with NMT reported in the past 20 years (Hart et al., 2002). Thymoma has long been associated with MG (see Chapter 21) and with other immunologically mediated conditions (Souadjian et al., 1974). Seven of the NMT patients with thymoma had MG and two others had raised anti-AChR antibody titres (Halbach et al., 1987). In addition, a few patients with bronchial carcinoma have developed NMT. At least one tumour was a SCLC.

There is now clinical evidence that a humoral factor is involved in the pathogenesis of acquired NMT. Plasma exchange, which depletes circulating immunoglobulins, resulted in clinical improvement and a reduction in the frequency of the abnormal muscle discharges on EMG (Bady et al., 1991; Sinha et al., 1991). Plasma or IgG from patients with NMT was injected into mice. The mice did not have any signs of muscle overactivity, nor was there any evidence of spontaneous nerve discharges. However, phrenic nerve diaphragm preparations from animals treated with NMT IgG showed increased β-tubocurarine resistance at the neuromuscular junction (Sinha et al., 1991), and a moderate increase in the quantal content of the EPP (i.e. there were more ACh quanta released per nerve impulse (Shillito et al., 1995). Moreover, purified IgG injected into mice led to prolonged sensory nerve action potentials, and when incubated overnight with dorsal root ganglia cultures caused repetitive action potentials. The results were very similar to those obtained with low concentrations of the voltage-gated potassium channel (VGKC) blockers, 4-amino-pyridine or 3,4-diaminopyridine (Shillito et al., 1995).

The most likely target for the autoantibodies, therefore, was a potassium channel. After generation of a nerve action potential, the sodium channels are inactivated and the resting membrane potential is restored through the action of VGKCs in the motor nerve membrane. Drugs that lead to delayed inactivation of sodium channels can cause repetitive activity in the nerve. VGKC blockers, aminopyridines, tetraethylammonium, or specific toxins such as α-dendrotoxin (Harvey and Anderson, 1985), cause the axon membrane to become more excitable and generate spontaneous bursts of action potentials. A functional VGKC consists of four-transmembrane β subunits that combine as homomultimeric and heteromultimeric (Wang et al., 1993) tetramers to interact with intracellular α subunits (Rettig et al., 1994), which are also thought to group as a tetramer. At least eight different VGKC a subunits have been identified, each is encoded by a different gene. VGKCs of the subtypes Kv1.1 and 1.2 are highly expressed in the peripheral nervous system (and also in the CNS, see Chapter 33).

Immunoprecipitation of VGKCs by neuromyotonia sera

Antibodies to VGKCs can be detected in about 40% of NMT patients by immunoprecipitation of ^{125}I α-dendrotoxin-labelled VGKCs extracted from human frontal cortex (Shillito et al., 1995; Hart et al., 2002), and the level of this antibody is reduced by immunosuppressive treatment. The 60% of sera negative for these antibodies may contain antibodies to some other peripheral nerve or motor nerve terminal protein. Attempts to improve the positivity using different neurotoxins, for instance, have not been successful.

An alternative approach was to use immunohistochemistry on frozen sections of Xenopus oocytes that were transfected with cRNAs for VGKC subunits (Hart et al., 1997). The advantages of this method are the high concentration of the individual subunit that can be expressed in the oocyte cytoplasm and the lack of solubilization or labelling required. With this assay, antibodies to Kv1.2 α-subunit proteins were detected in 13 of 14 NMT sera, and to Kv1.1 and Kiv1.6 in some of the sera. An alternative approach that has not yet been applied systematically is to express the VGKCs in mammalian cell lines, and use fluorescence-activated cell sorting to detect antibody binding. This approach has been useful in demonstrating the existence of human antibodies to other neuronal antigens, for instance MuSK (McConville et al., 2004).

As in the other diseases considered in this chapter, there is no clear information regarding the aetiology of. neuromyotonia. However, there are anecdotal reports of the condition occurring in association with infections (e.g. Maddison et al., 1998) and some patients seem to have a monophasic illness that recovers spontaneously within 1 to 2 years. Theses observations suggest that there may be specific conditions, probably infections, that can predispose to development of these antibodies.

Conclusions

NMT is a condition in which muscle hyperactivity stems from peripheral nerve hyperexcitability. Some patients have other immunologic disorders and at least two tumours are frequently associated with autoimmune disease. Patients with acquired NMT have autoantibodies that bind to some subtypes of VGKC and these antibodies may play an important role in the pathogenesis of the nerve hyperexcitability that characterizes NMT. Further electrophysiologic and immunologic characterization of the effect of these antibodies and identification of the region-specific expression of VGKCs may eventually throw light on the clinical diversity of the condition, and the predisposing conditions.

Autonomic neuropathy

There are many forms of peripheral neuropathy and only a subgroup of these disorders are immune mediated. The peripheral nerve disorders are covered in Chapter 19. Idiopathic autonomic neuropathy is rare disorder which is presumed to be autoimmune because of its subacute, usually adult, onset. One form is associated with paraneoplastic antibodies and various forms of cancer (see Chapter 25). A recent report showed that around 41% of patients had antibodies to the ganglionic acetylcholine receptor $\alpha_2\beta_4$ detected by immunoprecipiatation of ^{125}I-epibatidine binding sites. Epibatidine binds to the ganglioinic form of AChR. Titres of antibody ranged from 90 pM to 17, 180 pM, an extremely high range but not dissimilar to that found in myasthenia gravis. The majority of patients had an abnormal pupillary response to light, dry eyes and mouth, gastrointestinal symptoms, usually constipation, urinary retention, and areas of absent sweating. All of these symptoms can be explained by a defect in ganglionic transmission in the parasympathetic nervous system. Symptoms tended to improve with immunological treatments, with an associated fall in ganglionic receptor antibody titres, but in some cases there was spontaneous improvement suggesting a monophasic illness. These new findings are reviewed in Vernino et al. (2000) and Klein et al. (2003).

The response to treatment is consistent with an antibody-mediated condition. Another feature in favour of this hypothesis is the response of rabbits to immunization against ganglionic AChRs. The rabbits developed gastrointestinal hypomotility, dilated pupils, impaired light response, and distended bladders (Lennon et al., 2003).

References

Aarli, J.A. (2001). Titin, thymoma, and myasthenia gravis. Arch Neurol 58: 869–870.

Aarli, J.A., Stefansson, K., Marton, L.S., and Wollmann, R.L. (1990). Patients with myasthenia gravis and thymoma have in their sera IgG autoantibodies against titin. Clin Exp Immunol 82: 284–288.

Aime, C., Cohen-Kaminsky, S., and Berrih-Aknin, S. (1991). In vitro interleukin-1 (IL-1) production in thymic hyperplasia and thymoma from patients with myasthenia gravis. J Clin Immunol 11: 268–278.

Aissaoui, A., Klingel-Schmitt, I., Couderc, J., et al. (1999). Prevention of autoimmune attack by targeting specific T-cell receptors in a severe combined immunodeficiency mouse model of myasthenia gravis. Ann Neurol 46: 559–567.

Andreetta, F., Baggi, F., Antozzi, C., et al. (1997). Acetylcholine receptor alpha-subunit isoforms are differentially expressed in thymuses from myasthenic patients. Am J Pathol 150: 341–348.

Asher, O., Neumann, D., Witzemann, V., and Fuchs, S. (1990). Acetylcholine receptor gene expression in experimental autoimmune myasthenia gravis. FEBS Lett 267: 231–235.

Bady, B., Chauplannaz, G., and Vial, C. (1991). Autoimmune aetiology for acquired neuromyotonia. Lancet 338: 1330.

Baggi, F., Nicolle, M., Vincent, A., et al. (1993). Presentation of endogenous acetylcholine receptor epitope by an MHC class II-transfected human muscle cell line to a specific CD4+ T cell clone from a myasthenia gravis patient. J Neuroimmunol 46: 57–65.

Bain, P.G., Motomura, M., Newsom-Davis, J., et al. (1996). Effects of intravenous immunoglobulin on muscle weakness and calcium-channel autoantibodies in the Lambert-Eaton myasthenic syndrome. Neurology 47: 678–683.

Bao, S., King, N.J., and Dos Remedios, C.G. (1992). Flavivirus induces MHC antigen on human myoblasts: a model of autoimmune myositis? Muscle Nerve 15: 1271–1277.

Barnes, P.R., Kanabar, D.J., Brueton, L., et al. (1995). Recurrent congenital arthrogryposis leading to a diagnosis of myasthenia gravis in an initially asymptomatic mother. Neuromuscul Disord 5: 59–65.

Barrett-Jolley, R., Byrne, N., Vincent, A., and Newsom-Davis, J. (1994). Plasma from patients with seronegative myasthenia gravis inhibit nAChR responses in the TE671/RD cell line. Pflugers Arch 428: 492–498.

Beeson, D., Jacobson, L., Newsom-Davis, J., and Vincent, A. (1996). A transfected human muscle cell line expressing the adult subtype of the human muscle acetylcholine receptor for diagnostic assays in myasthenia gravis. *Neurology* 47: 1552–1555.

Berman, P.W. and Patrick, J. (1980). Linkage between the frequency of muscular weakness and loci that regulate immune responsiveness in murine experimental myasthenia gravis. *J Exp Med* 152: 507–520.

Biesecker, G. and Koffler, D. (1988). Resistance to experimental autoimmune myasthenia gravis in genetically inbred rats. Association with decreased amounts of in situ acetylcholine receptor-antibody complexes. *J Immunol* 140: 3406–3410.

Bird, S.J. (1992). Clinical and electrophysiologic improvement in Lambert-Eaton syndrome with intravenous immunoglobulin therapy. *Neurology* 42: 1422–1423.

Blaes, F., Beeson, D., Plested, P., et al. (2000). IgG from 'seronegative' myasthenia gravis patients binds to a muscle cell line, TE671, but not to human acetylcholine receptor. *Ann Neurol* 47: 504–510.

Browne, D.L., Gancher, S.T., Nutt, J.G., et al. (1994). Episodic ataxia/myokymia syndrome is associated with point mutations in the human potassium channel gene, KCNA1. *Nat Genet* 8: 136–140.

Brueton, L.A., Huson, S.M., Cox, P.M., et al. (2000). Asymptomatic maternal myasthenia as a cause of the Pena-Shokeir phenotype. *Am J Med Genet* 92: 1–6.

Buckley, C., Douek, D., Newsom-Davis, J., et al. (2001a). Mature, long-lived CD4+ and CD8+ T cells are generated by the thymoma in myasthenia gravis. *Ann Neurol* 50: 64–72.

Buckley, C., Newsom-Davis, J., Willcox, N., and Vincent, A. (2001b). Do titin and cytokine antibodies in MG patients predict thymoma or thymoma recurrence? *Neurology* 57: 1579–1582.

Bufler, J., Pitz, R., Czep, M., et al. (1998). Purified IgG from seropositive and seronegative patients with mysasthenia gravis reversibly blocks currents through nicotinic acetylcholine receptor channels. *Ann Neurol* 43: 458–464.

Burges, J., Wray, D.W., Pizzighella, S., et al. (1990). A myasthenia gravis plasma immunoglobulin reduces miniature endplate potentials at human endplates in vitro. *Muscle Nerve* 13: 407–413.

Burges, J., Vincent, A., Molenaar, P.C., et al. (1994). Passive transfer of seronegative myasthenia gravis to mice. *Muscle Nerve* 17: 1393–1400.

Carlsson, B., Wallin, J., Pirskanen, R., et al. (1990). Different HLA DR-DQ associations in subgroups of idiopathic myasthenia gravis. *Immunogenetics* 31: 285–290.

Chalk, C.H., Murray, N.M., Newsom-Davis, J., et al. (1990). Response of the Lambert–Eaton myasthenic syndrome to treatment of associated small-cell lung carcinoma. *Neurology* 40: 1552–1556.

Christadoss, P., Lennon, V.A., and David, C. (1979). Genetic control of experimental autoimmune myasthenia gravis in mice. I. Lymphocyte proliferative response to acetylcholine receptors is under H-2-linked Ir gene control. *J Immunol* 123: 2540–2543.

Christadoss, P., Poussin, M., and Deng, C. (2000). Animal models of myasthenia gravis. *Clin Immunol* 94: 75–87.

Cifuentes-Diaz, C., Delaporte, C., Dautreaux, B., et al. (1992). Class II MHC antigens in normal human skeletal muscle. *Muscle Nerve* 15: 295–302.

Clouston, P.D., Saper, C.B., Arbizu, T., et al. (1992). Paraneoplastic cerebellar degeneration. III. Cerebellar degeneration, cancer, and the Lambert–Eaton myasthenic syndrome. *Neurology* 42: 1944–1950.

Compston, D.A., Vincent, A., Newsom-Davis, J., and Batchelor, J.R. (1980). Clinical, pathological, HLA antigen and immunological evidence for disease heterogeneity in myasthenia gravis. *Brain* 103: 579–601.

Conti-Fine, B.M., Navaneetham, D., Karachunski, P.I., et al. (1998). T cell recognition of the acetylcholine receptor in myasthenia gravis. *Ann N Y Acad Sci* 841: 283–308.

Curnow, J., Corlett, L., Willcox, N., and Vincent, A. (2001). Presentation by myoblasts of an epitope from endogenous acetylcholine receptor indicates a potential role in the spreading of the immune response. *J Neuroimmunol* 115: 127–134.

Dau, P.C. and Denys, E.H. (1982). Plasmapheresis and immunosuppressive drug therapy in the Eaton-Lambert syndrome. *Ann Neurol* 11: 570–575.

De Aizpurua, H.J., Lambert, E.H., Griesmann, G.E., et al. (1988). Antagonism of voltage-gated calcium channels in small cell carcinomas of patients with and without Lambert-Eaton myasthenic syndrome by autoantibodies omega-conotoxin and adenosine. *Cancer Res* 48: 4719–4724.

Demaine, A., Willcox, N., Welsh, K., and Newsom-Davis, J. (1988). Associations of the autoimmune myasthenias with genetic markers in the immunoglobulin heavy chain region. *Ann N Y Acad Sci* 540: 266–268.

Djabiri, F., Caillat-Zucman, S., Gajdos, P., et al. (1997). Association of the AChRalpha-subunit gene (CHRNA), DQA1*0101, and the DR3 haplotype in myasthenia gravis. Evidence for a three-gene disease model in a subgroup of patients. *J Autoimmun* 10: 407–413.

Drachman, D.B. (1994). Myasthenia gravis. *N Engl J Med* 330: 1797–1810.

Drachman, D.B., Angus, C.W., Adams, R.N., and Kao, I. (1978a). Effect of myasthenic patients' immunoglobulin on acetylcholine receptor turnover: selectivity of degradation process. *Proc Natl Acad Sci USA* 75: 3422–3426.

Drachman, D.B., Angus, C.W., Adams, R.N., et al. (1978b). Myasthenic antibodies cross-link acetylcholine receptors to accelerate degradation. *N Engl J Med* 298: 1116–1122.

Drachman, D.B., McIntosh, K.R., Reim, J., and Balcer, L. (1993). Strategies for treatment of myasthenia gravis. *Ann N Y Acad Sci* 681: 515–528.

Dwyer, D.S., Bradley, R.J., Urquhart, C.K., and Kearney, J.F. (1983). Naturally occurring anti-idiotypic antibodies in myasthenia gravis patients. *Nature* 301: 611–614.

Eaton, L.M. and Lambert, E.H. (1957). Electromyography and electric stimulation of nerves in diseases of motor unit; observations of myasthenic syndrome associated with malignant tumors. *J Am Med Assoc* 163(13): 1117–24.

Emilie, D., Crevon, M.C., Cohen-Kaminsky, S., et al. (1991). *In situ* production of interleukins in hyperplastic thymus from myasthenia gravis patients. *Hum Pathol* 22: 461–468.

Engel, A.G. (1991). Review of evidence for loss of motor nerve terminal calcium channels in Lambert–Eaton myasthenic syndrome. *Ann N Y Acad Sci* 635: 246–258.

Engel, A.G. and Arahat,a K. (1987). The membrane attack complex of complement at the endplate in myasthenia gravis. *Ann N Y Acad Sci* 505: 326–332.

Engel, A.G., Lindstrom, J.M., Lambert, E.H., and Lennon, V.A. (1977). Ultrastructural localization of the acetylcholine receptor in myasthenia gravis and in its experimental autoimmune model. *Neurology* 27: 307–315.

Engel, A.G., Nagel, A., Fukuoka, T., et al. (1989). Motor nerve terminal calcium channels in Lambert–Eaton myasthenic syndrome. Morphologic evidence for depletion and that the depletion is mediated by autoantibodies. *Ann N Y Acad Sci* 560: 278–290.

Evoli, A., Tonali, P.A., Padua, L., et al. (2003). Clinical correlates with anti-MuSK antibodies in generalized seronegative myasthenia gravis. *Brain* 126: 2304–2311.

Fambrough, D.M., Drachman, D.B., and Satyamurti, S. (1973). Neuromuscular junction in myasthenia gravis: decreased acetylcholine receptors. *Science* 182: 293–295.

Farrar, J., Portolano, S., Willcox, N., et al. (1997). Diverse Fab specific for acetylcholine receptor epitopes from a myasthenia gravis thymus combinatorial library. *Int Immunol* 9: 1311–1318.

Fernandes, L., Berry, H., Hamilton, E. (1980). Historical perspectives on penicillamine. *Cah Haut Marnais* 14: 130–136.

Fujii, Y. and Lindstrom, J. (1988). Regulation of antibody production by helper T cell clones in experimental autoimmune myasthenia gravis. *J Immunol* 141: 3361–3369.

Fujii, Y., Hayakawa, M., Inada, K., and Nakahara, K. (1990). Lymphocytes in thymoma: association with myasthenia gravis is correlated with increased number of single-positive cells. *Eur J Immunol* 20: 2355–2358.

Fukunaga, H., Engel, A.G., Lang, B., et al. (1983). Passive transfer of Lambert–Eaton myasthenic syndrome with IgG from man to mouse depletes the presynaptic membrane active zones. *Proc Natl Acad Sci USA* 80: 7636–7640.

Fukuoka, T., Engel, A.G., Lang, B., et al. (1987a). Lambert–Eaton myasthenic syndrome: I. Early morphological effects of IgG on the presynaptic membrane active zones. *Ann Neurol* 22: 193–199.

Fukuoka, T., Engel, A.G., Lang, B., et al. (1987b). Lambert–Eaton myasthenic syndrome: II. Immunoelectron microscopy localization of IgG at the mouse motor end-plate. *Ann Neurol* 22: 200–211.

Garchon, H.J., Djabiri, F., Viard, J.P., *et al.* (1994). Involvement of human muscle acetylcholine receptor alpha-subunit gene (CHRNA) in susceptibility to myasthenia gravis. *Proc Natl Acad Sci USA* **91**: 4668–4672.

Garlepp, M.J., Dawkins, R.L., and Christiansen, F.T. (1983). HLA antigens and acetylcholine receptor antibodies in penicillamine induced myasthenia gravis. *Br Med J (Clin Res Educ)* **286**: 338–340.

Gautel, M., Lakey, A., Barlow, D.P., *et al.* (1993). Titin antibodies in myasthenia gravis: identification of a major immunogenic region of titin. *Neurology* **43**: 1581–1585.

Geuder, K.I., Marx, A., Witzemann, V., *et al.* (1992*a*). Genomic organization and lack of transcription of the nicotinic acetylcholine receptor subunit genes in myasthenia gravis-associated thymoma. *Lab Invest* **66**: 452–458.

Geuder, K.I., Marx, A., Witzemann, V., *et al.* (1992*b*). Pathogenetic significance of fetal-type acetylcholine receptors on thymic myoid cells in myasthenia gravis. *Dev Immunol* **2**: 69–75.

Gilhus, N.E., Pandey, J.P., Gaarder, P.I. and Aarli, J.A., (1990). Immunoglobin allotypes in myasthenia gravis patients with a thymoma. *J Autoimmun* **3**(3): 299–305.

Gilhus, N.E., Jones, M., Turley, H., *et al.* (1995*a*). Oncogene proteins and proliferation antigens in thymomas: increased expression of epidermal growth factor receptor and Ki67 antigen. *J Clin Pathol* **48**: 447–455.

Gilhus, N.E., Willcox, N., Harcourt, G., *et al.* (1995*b*). Antigen presentation by thymoma epithelial cells from myasthenia gravis patients to potentially pathogenic T cells. *J Neuroimmunol* **56**: 65–76.

Graus, Y.F., de Baets, M.H., Parren, P.W., *et al.* (1997). Human anti-nicotinic acetylcholine receptor recombinant Fab fragments isolated from thymus-derived phage display libraries from myasthenia gravis patients reflect predominant specificities in serum and block the action of pathogenic serum antibodies. *J Immunol* **158**: 1919–1929.

Gronseth, G.S. and Barohn, R.J. (2000). Practice parameter: thymectomy for autoimmune myasthenia gravis (an evidence-based review): report of the Quality Standards Subcommittee of the American Academy of Neurology. *Neurology* **55**: 7–15.

Guigou, V., Emilie, D., Berrih-Aknin, S., *et al.* (1991). Individual germinal centres of myasthenia gravis human thymuses contain polyclonal activated B cells that express all the Vh and Vk families. *Clin Exp Immunol* **83**: 262–266.

Guyon, T., Levasseur, P., Truffault, F., *et al.* (1994). Regulation of acetylcholine receptor alpha subunit variants in human myasthenia gravis. Quantification of steady-state levels of messenger RNA in muscle biopsy using the polymerase chain reaction. *J Clin Invest* **94**: 16–24.

Halbach, M., Homberg, V., and Freund, H.J. (1987). Neuromuscular, autonomic and central cholinergic hyperactivity associated with thymoma and acetylcholine receptor-binding antibody. *J Neurol* **234**: 433–436.

Hall, Z.W. and Sanes, J.R. (1993). Synaptic structure and development: the neuromuscular junction. *Cell* **72**(Suppl.): 99–121.

Hara, Y., Ueno, S., Uemichi, T., *et al.* (1991). Neoplastic epithelial cells express alpha-subunit of muscle nicotinic acetylcholine receptor in thymomas from patients with myasthenia gravis. *FEBS Lett* **279**: 137–140.

Harris, J.B. (1984). Polypeptides from snake venoms which act on nerve and muscle. *Prog Med Chem* **21**: 63–110.

Hart, I.K., Waters, C., Vincent, A., *et al.* (1997). Autoantibodies detected to expressed K⁺ channels are implicated in neuromyotonia. *Ann Neurol* **41**: 238–246.

Hart, I.K., Maddison, P., Newsom-Davis, J., *et al.* (2002). Phenotypic variants of autoimmune peripheral nerve hyperexcitability. *Brain* **125**: 1887–1895.

Harvey, A.L. and Anderson, A.J. (1985). Dendrotoxins: snake toxins that block potassium channels and facilitate neurotransmitter release. *Pharmacol Ther* **31**: 33–55.

Hawke, S., Matsuo, H., Nicolle, M., *et al.* (1996). Autoimmune T cells in myasthenia gravis: heterogeneity and potential for specific immunotargeting. *Immunol Today* **17**: 307–311.

Hesselmans, L.F., Jennekens, F.G., Van den Oord, C.J., *et al.* (1993). Development of innervation of skeletal muscle fibers in man: relation to acetylcholine receptors. *Anat Rec* **236**: 553–562.

Hill, M., Beeson, D., Moss, P., *et al.* (1999*a*). Early-onset myasthenia gravis: a recurring T-cell epitope in the adult-specific acetylcholine receptor epsilon subunit presented by the susceptibility allele HLA-DR52a. *Ann Neurol* **45**: 224–231.

Hill, M., Moss, P., Wordsworth, P., *et al.* (1999*b*). T cell responses to D-penicillamine in drug-induced myasthenia gravis: recognition of modified DR1:peptide complexes. *J Neuroimmunol* **97**: 146–153.

Hjelmstrom, P., Giscombe, R., Lefvert, A.K., *et al.* (1997). TAP polymorphisms in Swedish myasthenia gravis patients. *Tissue Antigens* **49**: 176–179.

Hjelmstrom, P., Peacock, C.S., Giscombe, R., *et al.* (1998). Myasthenia gravis with thymic hyperplasia is associated with polymorphisms in the tumor necrosis factor region. *Ann N Y Acad Sci* **841**: 368–370.

Hoch, W., McConville, J., Helms, S., *et al.* (2001). Auto-antibodies to the receptor tyrosine kinase MuSK in patients with myasthenia gravis without acetylcholine receptor antibodies. *Nat Med* **7**: 365–368.

Hohlfeld, R. and Engel, A.G. (1990). Induction of HLA-DR expression on human myoblasts with interferon-gamma. *Am J Pathol* **136**: 503–508.

Hohlfeld, R. and Wekerle, H. (1994). The role of the thymus in myasthenia gravis. *Adv Neuroimmunol* **4**: 373–386.

Horton, R.M., Conti-Tronconi, B.M., and Manfredi, A.A. (1994). ACh receptor in ocular MG. *Neurology* **44**: 778–779.

Jacobson, L., Beeson, D., Tzartos, S., and Vincent, A. (1999*a*). Monoclonal antibodies raised against human acetylcholine receptor bind to all five subunits of the fetal isoform. *J Neuroimmunol* **98**: 112–120.

Jacobson, L., Polizzi, A., Morriss-Kay, G., and Vincent, A. (1999*b*). Plasma from human mothers of fetuses with severe arthrogryposis multiplex congenita causes deformities in mice. *J Clin Invest* **103**: 1031–1038.

Janer, M., Cowland, A., Picard, J., *et al.* (1999). A susceptibility region for myasthenia gravis extending into the HLA-class I sector telomeric to HLA-C. *Hum Immunol* **60**: 909–917.

Jermy, A., Beeson, D., and Vincent, A. (1993). Pathogenic autoimmunity to affinity-purified mouse acetylcholine receptor induced without adjuvant in BALB/c mice. *Eur J Immunol* **23**: 973–976.

Johnston, I., Lang, B., Leys, K., and Newsom-Davis, J. (1994). Heterogeneity of calcium channel autoantibodies detected using a small-cell lung cancer line derived from a Lambert–Eaton myasthenic syndrome patient. *Neurology* **44**: 334–338.

Kaminski, H.J., Kusner, L.L., and Block, C.H. (1996).Expression of acetylcholine receptor isoforms at extraocular muscle endplates. *Invest Ophthalmol Vis Sci* **37**: 345–351.

Kaminski, H.J., Richmonds, C.R., Kusner, L.L., and Mitsumoto, H. (2002). Differential susceptibility of the ocular motor system to disease. *Ann N Y Acad Sci* **956**: 42–54.

Kao, I. and Drachman, D.B. (1977). Thymic muscle cells bear acetylcholine receptors: possible relation to myasthenia gravis. *Science* **195**: 74–75.

Karlin, A. and Akabas, M.H. (1995). Toward a structural basis for the function of nicotinic acetylcholine receptors and their cousins. *Neuron* **15**: 1231–1244.

Kaul, R., Shenoy, M., Goluszko, E., and Christadoss, P. (1994). Major histocompatibility complex class II gene disruption prevents experimental autoimmune myasthenia gravis. *J Immunol* **152**: 3152–3157.

Khanna, S., Richmonds, C.R., Kaminski, H.J., and Porter, J.D. (2003). Molecular organization of the extraocular muscle neuromuscular junction: partial conservation of and divergence from the skeletal muscle prototype. *Invest Ophthalmol Vis Sci* **44**: 1918–1926.

Khurana, R.K., Koski, C.L. and Mayer, R.F. (1998). Autonomic dysfunction in Lambert-Eaton myasthenic syndrome. *J Neurol Sci* **85**(1): 77–86.

Kim, Y.I. (1985). Passive transfer of the Lambert–Eaton myasthenic syndrome: neuromuscular transmission in mice injected with plasma. *Muscle Nerve* **8**: 162–172.

Kirchner, T., Hoppe, F., Schalke, B., and Muller-Hermelink, H.K. (1988). Microenvironment of thymic myoid cells in myasthenia gravis. *Virchows Arch B Cell Pathol Incl Mol Pathol* **54**: 295–302.

Klein, C.M., Vernino, S., Lennon, V.A., *et al.* (2003). The spectrum of autommune autonomic neuropathies. *Ann Neurol* **53**: 752–758.

Komai, K., Iwasa, K., and Takamori, M. (1999). Calcium channel peptide can cause an autoimmune-mediated model of Lambert–Eaton myasthenic syndrome in rats. *J Neurol Sci* **166**: 126–130.

Kornstein, M.J. and Kay, S., (1990). B cells in thymomas. *Mod Pathol* **3**(1): 61–3.

Kuks, J.B., Oosterhuis, H.J., Limburg, P.C., and The, T.H. (1991). Anti-acetylcholine receptor antibodies decrease after thymectomy in patients with myasthenia gravis. Clinical correlations. *J Autoimmun* **4**: 197–211.

Kusner, L.L., Mygland, A., and Kaminski, H.J. (1998). Ryanodine receptor gene expression thymomas. *Muscle Nerve* 21: 1299–1303.

Lambert, E.H. and Elmqvist, D. (1971). Quantal components of end-plate potentials in the myasthenic syndrome. *Ann N Y Acad Sci* 183: 183–199.

Lang, B., Newsom-Davis, J., Wray, D., *et al.* (1981). Autoimmune aetiology for myasthenic (Eaton–Lambert) syndrome. *Lancet* 2: 224–226.

Lang, B., Newsom-Davis, J., Prior, C., and Wray, D. (1983). Antibodies to motor nerve terminals: an electrophysiological study of a human myasthenic syndrome transferred to mouse. *J Physiol* 344: 335–345.

Lang, B., Richardson, G., Rees, J., *et al.* (1988). Plasma from myasthenia gravis patients reduces acetylcholine receptor agonist-induced Na⁺ flux into TE671 cell line. *J Neuroimmunol* 19: 141–148.

Lauriola, L., Ranelletti, F., Maggiano, N., Guerriero, M., Punzi, C., Marsili, F., Bartoccioni, E., Evoli, A., (2005) Thymus changes in anti-MuSK-positive and -negative myasthenia gravis. *Neurology* 64: 536–8.

Leite, M. I., Strobel, P., Jones, M., Micklem, K., Moritz, R., Gold, R. *et al.* (2005) Fewer thymic changes in MuSK-antibody-positive than in MuSK-antibody-negative MG. *Ann Neurol* 57: 444–8.

Lennon, V.A., Lambert, E.H., Whittingham, S., and Fairbanks, V. (1982). Autoimmunity in the Lambert–Eaton myasthenic syndrome. *Muscle Nerve* 5: S21–S25.

Lennon, V.A., Kryzer, T.J., Griesmann, G.E., *et al.* (1995). Calcium-channel antibodies in the Lambert–Eaton syndrome and other paraneoplastic syndromes. *N Engl J Med* 332: 1467–1474.

Lennon, V.A., Ermilov, L.G., Szurszewski, J.H., and Vernino, S. (2003). Immunization with neuronal nicotinic acetylcholine receptor induces neurological autoimmune disease. *J Clin Invest* 111: 907–913.

Leveque, C., Hoshino, T., David, P., *et al.* (1992). The synaptic vesicle protein synaptotagmin associates with calcium channels and is a putative Lambert–Eaton myasthenic syndrome antigen. *Proc Natl Acad Sci USA* 89: 3625–3629.

Levine, G.D. and Rosai, J. (1978). Thymic hyperplasia and neoplasia: a review of current concepts. *Hum Pathol* 9: 495–515.

Lindstrom, J.M. (2000). Acetylcholine receptors and myasthenia. *Muscle Nerve* 23: 453–477.

Lindstrom, J.M., Einarson, B.L., Lennon, V.A., and Seybold, M.E. (1976a). Pathological mechanisms in experimental autoimmune myasthenia gravis. I. Immunogenicity of syngeneic muscle acetylcholine receptor and quantitative extraction of receptor and antibody-receptor complexes from muscles of rats with experimental autoimmune myasthenia gravis. *J Exp Med* 144: 726–738.

Lindstrom, J.M., Engel, A.G., Seybold, M.E., *et al.* (1976b). Pathological mechanisms in experimental autoimmune myasthenia gravis. II. Passive transfer of experimental autoimmune myasthenia gravis in rats with anti-acetylcholine receptor antibodies. *J Exp Med* 144: 739–753.

Lindstrom, J.M., Seybold, M.E., Lennon, V.A., *et al.* (1976c). Antibody to acetylcholine receptor in myasthenia gravis. Prevalence, clinical correlates, and diagnostic value. *Neurology* 26: 1054–1059.

Liyanage, Y., Hoch, W., Beeson, D., and Vincent, A. (2002). The agrin/muscle-specific kinase pathway: new targets for autoimmune and genetic disorders at the neuromuscular junction. *Muscle Nerve* 25: 4–16.

MacLennan, C., Beeson, D., Buijs, A.M., *et al.* (1997). Acetylcholine receptor expression in human extraocular muscles and their susceptibility to myasthenia gravis. *Ann Neurol* 41: 423–431.

Maddison, P., Lawn, N., Mills, K.R., *et al.* (1998). Acquired neuromyotonia in a patient with spinal epidural abscess. *Muscle Nerve* 21: 672–674.

Manfredi, A.A., Protti, M.P., Dalton, M.W., *et al.* (1993). T helper cell recognition of muscle acetylcholine receptor in myasthenia gravis. Epitopes on the gamma and delta subunits. *J Clin Invest* 92: 1055–1067.

Mantegazza, R., Gebbia, M., Mora, M., *et al.* (1996). Major histocompatibility complex class II molecule expression on muscle cells is regulated by differentiation: implications for the immunopathogenesis of muscle autoimmune diseases. *J Neuroimmunol* 68: 53–60.

Marx, A., O'Connor, R., Tzartos, S., *et al.* (1989). Acetylcholine receptor epitope in proteins of myasthenia gravis-associated thymomas and non-thymic tissues. *Thymus* 14: 171–178.

Marx, A., Schomig, D., Schultz, A., *et al.* (1994). Distribution of molecules mediating thymocyte-stroma-interactions in human thymus, thymitis and thymic epithelial tumors. *Thymus* 23: 83–93.

Marx, A., Wilisch, A., Schultz, A., *et al.* (1996). Expression of neurofilaments and of a titin epitope in thymic epithelial tumors. Implications for the pathogenesis of myasthenia gravis. *Am J Pathol* 148: 1839–1850.

Mason, W.P., Graus, F., Lang, B., *et al.* (1997). Small-cell lung cancer, paraneoplastic cerebellar degeneration and the Lambert–Eaton myasthenic syndrome. *Brain* 120(8): 1279–1300.

Masunaga, A., Arai, T., Yoshitake, T., *et al.* (1994). Reduced expression of apoptosis-related antigens in thymuses from patients with myasthenia gravis. *Immunol Lett* 39: 169–172.

Matsuo, H., Batocchi, A.P., Hawke, S., *et al.* (1995). Peptide-selected T cell lines from myasthenia gravis patients and controls recognize epitopes that are not processed from whole acetylcholine receptor. *J Immunol* 155: 3683–3692.

Matthews, I., Farrar, J., McLachlan, S., *et al.* (1998). Production of Fab fragments against the human acetylcholine receptor from myasthenia gravis thymus lambda and kappa phage libraries. *Ann N Y Acad Sci* 841: 418–421.

Matthews, I., Sims, G., Ledwidge, S., *et al.* (2002). Antibodies to acetylcholine receptor in parous women with myasthenia: evidence for immunization by fetal antigen. *Lab Invest* 82: 1407–1417.

McConville, J., Farrugia, M.E., Beeson, D., *et al.* (2004). Detection and characterization of MuSK antibodies in seronegative myasthenia gravis. *Ann Neurol* 55(4):580–584.

Meager, A., Vincent, A., Newsom-Davis, J., and Willcox, N. (1997). Spontaneous neutralising antibodies to interferon–alpha and interleukin-12 in thymoma-associated autoimmune disease. *Lancet* 350: 1596–1597.

Meinl, E., Klinkert, W.E., and Wekerle, H. (1991). The thymus in myasthenia gravis. Changes typical for the human disease are absent in experimental autoimmune myasthenia gravis of the Lewis rat. *Am J Pathol* 139: 995–1008.

Melms, A., Schalke, B.C., Kirchner, T., *et al.* (1988). Thymus in myasthenia gravis. Isolation of T-lymphocyte lines specific for the nicotinic acetylcholine receptor from thymuses of myasthenic patients. *J Clin Invest* 81: 902–908.

Meyer, E.M., Momol, A.E., Kramer, B.S., *et al.* (1986). Effects of serum-fractions from patients with Eaton-Lambert syndrome on rat cortical synaptosomal [3H]acetylcholine release. *Biochem Pharmacol* 35: 3412–3414.

Moiola, L., Karachunski, P., Protti, M.P., *et al.* (1994a). Epitopes on the beta subunit of human muscle acetylcholine receptor recognized by CD4+ cells of myasthenia gravis patients and healthy subjects. *J Clin Invest* 93: 1020–1028.

Moiola, L., Protti, M.P., McCormick, D., *et al.* (1994b). Myasthenia gravis. Residues of the alpha and gamma subunits of muscle acetylcholine receptor involved in formation of immunodominant CD4+ epitopes. *J Immunol* 152: 4686–4698.

Morel, E., Eymard, B., Vernet der Garabedian, B., *et al.* (1988). Neonatal myasthenia gravis: a new clinical and immunologic appraisal on 30 cases. *Neurology* 38: 138–142.

Mossman, S., Vincent, A., and Newsom-Davis, J. (1986). Myasthenia gravis without acetylcholine-receptor antibody: a distinct disease entity. *Lancet* 1: 116–119.

Motomura, M., Johnston, I., Lang, B., *et al.* (1995). An improved diagnostic assay for Lambert-Eaton myasthenic syndrome. *J Neurol Neurosurg Psychiatry* 58: 85–87.

Muller-Hermelink, H.K. and Marx, A. (2000). Towards a histogenetic classification of thymic epithelial tumours? *Histopathology* 36: 466–469.

Murray, N.M. and Newsom-Davis, J. (1981). Treatment with oral 4-aminopyridine in disorders of neuromuscular transmission. *Neurology* 31(3): 265–71.

Mygland, A., Kuwajima, G., Mikoshiba, K., *et al.* (1995). Thymomas express epitopes shared by the ryanodine receptor. *J Neuroimmunol* 62: 79–83.

Nagvekar, N., Jacobson, L.W., Willcox, N., and Vincent, A. (1998a). Epitopes expressed in myasthenia gravis (MG) thymomas are not recognized by patients' T cells or autoantibodies. *Clin Exp Immunol* 112: 17–20.

Nagvekar, N., Moody, A.M., Moss, P., *et al.* (1998b). A pathogenetic role for the thymoma in myasthenia gravis. Autosensitization of IL-4- producing T cell clones recognizing extracellular acetylcholine receptor epitopes presented by minority class II isotypes. *J Clin Invest* 101: 2268–2277.

Nakao, Y., Matsumoto, H., Miyazaki, T., *et al.* (1980). Gm allotypes in myasthenia gravis. *Lancet* 1: 677–680.

Nastuk, W.L., Plescia, O.J. and Osserman, K.E. (1960). Changes in serum complement activity in patients with myasthenia gravis. *Proc Soc exp Biol Med* 105: 177–184.

Newsom-Davis, J. and Mills, K.R. (1993). Immunological associations of acquired neuromyotonia (Isaacs' syndrome). Report of five cases and literature review. *Brain* 116(2): 453–469.

Newsom-Davis, J., Pinching, A.J., Vincent, A., and Wilson, S.G. (1978). Function of circulating antibody to acetylcholine receptor in myasthenia gravis: investigation by plasma exchange. *Neurology* 28: 266–272.

Oda, K. and Shibasaki, H. (1988). Antigenic difference of acetylcholine receptor between single and multiple form endplates of human extraocular muscle. *Brain Res.* 449: 337–340.

Ohta, M., Itoh, M., Hara, H., *et al.* (1991). Anti-skeletal muscle and anti-acetylcholine receptor antibodies in patients with thymoma without myasthenia gravis: relation to the onset of myasthenia gravis. *Clin Chim Acta* 201: 201–205.

O'Neill, J.H., Murray, N.M., and Newsom-Davis, J. (1988). The Lambert–Eaton myasthenic syndrome. A review of 50 cases. *Brain* 111(3): 577–596.

Ong, B., Willcox, N., Wordsworth, P., *et al.* (1991). Critical role for the Val/Gly86 HLA-DR beta dimorphism in autoantigen presentation to human T cells. *Proc Natl Acad Sci USA* 88: 7343–7347.

Pachner, A.R., Kantor, F.S., Mulac-Jericevic, B., and Atassi, M.Z. (1989). An immunodominant site of acetylcholine receptor in experimental myasthenia mapped with T lymphocyte clones and synthetic peptides. *Immunol Lett* 20: 199–204.

Palmisani, M.T., Evoli, A., Batocchi, A.P., *et al.* (1994). Myasthenia gravis and associated autoimmune diseases. *Muscle Nerve* 17: 1234–1235.

Patrick, J. and Lindstrom, J. (1973). Autoimmune response to acetylcholine receptor. *Science* 180: 871–2.

Peers, C., Johnston, I., Lang, B., and Wray, D. (1993). Cross-linking of presynaptic calcium channels: a mechanism of action for Lambert–Eaton myasthenic syndrome antibodies at the mouse neuromuscular junction. *Neurosci Lett* 153: 45–48.

Pinto, A., Gillard, S., Moss, F., *et al.* (1998). Human autoantibodies specific for the alpha1A calcium channel subunit reduce both P-type and Q-type calcium currents in cerebellar neurons. *Proc Natl Acad Sci USA* 95: 8328–8333.

Plested, C.P., Tang, T., Spreadbury, I., *et al.* (2002). AChR phosphorylation and indirect inhibition of AChR function in seronegative MG. *Neurology* 59: 1682–1688.

Plomp, J.J., Van Kempen, G.T., De Baets, M.B., *et al.* (1995). Acetylcholine release in myasthenia gravis: regulation at single end-plate level. *Ann Neurol* 37: 627–636.

Poea, S., Guyon, T., Bidault, J., *et al.* (2000). Modulation of acetylcholine receptor expression in seronegative myasthenia gravis. *Ann Neurol* 48: 696–705.

Polizzi, A., Huson, S.M., and Vincent, A. (2000). Teratogen update: maternal myasthenia gravis as a cause of congenital arthrogryposis. *Teratology* 62: 332–341.

Poulas, K., Tsibri, E., Kokla, A., *et al.* (2001). Epidemiology of seropositive myasthenia gravis in Greece. *J Neurol Neurosurg Psychiatry* 71: 352–356.

Prior, C., Lang, B., Wray, D., and Newsom-Davis, J. (1985). Action of Lambert–Eaton myasthenic syndrome IgG at mouse motor nerve terminals. *Ann Neurol* 17: 587–592.

Protti, D.A. and Uchitel, O.D. (1997). P/Q-type calcium channels activate neighboring calcium-dependent potassium channels in mouse motor nerve terminals. *Pflugers Arch* 434: 406–412.

Protti, M.P., Manfredi, A.A., Horton, R.M., *et al.* (1993). Myasthenia gravis: recognition of a human autoantigen at the molecular level. *Immunol Today* 14: 363–368.

Raju, R., Navaneetham, D., Protti, M.P., *et al.* (1997). TCR V beta usage by acetylcholine receptor-specific CD4+ T cells in myasthenia gravis. *J Autoimmun* 10: 203–217.

Raju, R., Spack, E.G., and David, C.S. (2001). Acetylcholine receptor peptide recognition in HLA DR3-transgenic mice: *in vivo* responses correlate with MHC-peptide binding. *J Immunol* 167: 1118–1124.

Raju, R., Marietta, E., Vinasco, J., *et al.* (2002). Cryptic determinants and promiscuous sequences on human acetylcholine receptor: HLA-dependent dichotomy in T-cell function. *Hum Immunol.* 63 :237–247.

Reeback, J., Benton, S., Swash, M., and Schwartz, M.S. (1979). Penicillamine-induced neuromyotonia. *Br Med J* 1: 1464–1465.

Reinhardt, C. and Melms, A. (2000). Normalization of elevated CD4–/CD8– (double-negative) T cells after thymectomy parallels clinical remission in myasthenia gravis associated with thymic hyperplasia but not thymoma. *Ann Neurol* 48: 603–608.

Rettig, J., Heinemann, S.H., Wunder, F., *et al.* (1994). Inactivation properties of voltage-gated K+ channels altered by presence of beta-subunit. *Nature* 369: 289–294.

Riemersma, S., Vincent, A., Beeson, D., *et al.* (1996). Association of arthrogryposis multiplex congenita with maternal antibodies inhibiting fetal acetylcholine receptor function. *J Clin Invest* 98: 2358–2363.

Roberts, A., Perera, S., Lang, B., *et al.* (1985). Paraneoplastic myasthenic syndrome IgG inhibits 45Ca^{2+} flux in a human small cell carcinoma line. *Nature* 317: 737–739.

Robertson, N.P., Deans, J., and Compston, D.A. (1998). Myasthenia gravis: a population based epidemiological study in Cambridgeshire, England. *J Neurol Neurosurg Psychiatry* 65: 492–496.

Romi, F., Bo, L., Skeie, G.O., *et al.* (2002). Titin and ryanodine receptor epitopes are expressed in cortical thymoma along with costimulatory molecules. *J Neuroimmunol* 128: 82–89.

Rose, N.R. and Bona, C. (1993). Defining criteria for autoimmune diseases (Witebsky's postulates revisited). *Immunol Today* 14(9): 426–430.

Rosenfeld, M.R., Wong, E., Dalmau, J., *et al.* (1993). Sera from patients with Lambert–Eaton myasthenic syndrome recognize the beta-subunit of Ca^{2+} channel complexes. *Ann N Y Acad Sci* 681: 408–411.

Roxanis, I., Micklem, K., and Willcox, N. (2001). True epithelial hyperplasia in the thymus of early-onset myasthenia gravis patients: implications for immunopathogenesis. *J Neuroimmunol* 112: 163–173.

Roxanis, I., Micklem, K., McConville, J., *et al.* (2002). Thymic myoid cells and germinal center formation in myasthenia gravis; possible roles in pathogenesis. *J Neuroimmunol* 125: 185–197.

Ruff, R.L. and Lennon, V.A. (1998). End-plate voltage-gated sodium channels are lost in clinical and experimental myasthenia gravis. *Ann Neurol* 43: 370–379.

Salmon, A.M., Bruand, C., Cardona, A., *et al.* (1998). An acetylcholine receptor alpha subunit promoter confers intrathymic expression in transgenic mice. Implications for tolerance of a transgenic self-antigen and for autoreactivity in myasthenia gravis. *J Clin Invest* 101: 2340–2350.

Sanders, D.B., El-Salem, K., Massey, J.M., *et al.* (2003). Clinical aspects of MuSK antibody positive seronegative MG. *Neurology* 60: 1978–1980.

Sanes, J.R., Apel, E.D., Burgess, R.W., *et al.* (1998). Development of the neuromuscular junction: genetic analysis in mice. *J Physiol Paris* 92: 167–172.

Scadding, G.K., Vincent, A., Newsom-Davis, J., and Henry, K. (1981). Acetylcholine receptor antibody synthesis by thymic lymphocytes: correlation with thymic histology. *Neurology* 31: 935–943.

Schluep, M., Willcox, N., Vincent, A., *et al.* (1987). Acetylcholine receptors in human thymic myoid cells *in situ*: an immunohistological study. *Ann Neurol* 22: 212–222.

Schonbeck, S., Padberg, F., Hohlfeld, R., and Wekerle, H. (1992). Transplantation of thymic autoimmune microenvironment to severe combined immunodeficiency mice. A new model of myasthenia gravis. *J Clin Invest* 90: 245–250.

Schwimmbeck, P.L., Dyrberg, T., Drachman, D.B., and Oldstone, M.B. (1989). Molecular mimicry and myasthenia gravis. An autoantigenic site of the acetylcholine receptor alpha-subunit that has biologic activity and reacts immunochemically with herpes simplex virus. *J Clin Invest* 84: 1174–1180.

Scuderi, F., Marino, M., Colonna, L., *et al.* (2002). Anti-p110 autoantibodies identify a subtype of 'seronegative' myasthenia gravis with prominent oculobulbar involvement. *Lab Invest* 82: 1139–1146.

Serratrice, G. and Azulay, J.P. (1994). [What is left of Morvan's fibrillary chorea?]. *Rev Neurol (Paris)* 150: 257–265 (in French).

Shenoy, M., Kaul, R., Goluszko, E., *et al.* (1994). Effect of MHC class I and CD8 cell deficiency on experimental autoimmune myasthenia gravis pathogenesis. *J Immunol* 153: 5330–5335.

Sher, E., Comola, M., Nemni, R., *et al.* (1990). Calcium channel autoantibody and non-small-cell lung cancer in patients with Lambert–Eaton syndrome. *Lancet* 335: 413.

Shillito, P., Molenaar, P.C., Vincent, A., *et al.* (1995). Acquired neuromyotonia: evidence for autoantibodies directed against K+ channels of peripheral nerves. *Ann Neurol* 38: 714–722.

Shiono, H., Wong, Y.L., Matthews, I., *et al.* (2003). Spontaneous production of anti-IFN-alpha and anti-IL-12 autoantibodies by thymoma cells from myasthenia gravis patients suggests autoimmunization in the tumor. *Int Immunol* 15: 903–913.

Simpson, J.A. (1960). Myasthenia gravis, a new hypothesis. *Scott Med J* 5: 419–436.

Sims, G.P., Shiono, H., Willcox, N., and Stott, D.I. (2001). Somatic hypermutation and selection of B cells in thymic germinal centers responding to acetylcholine receptor in myasthenia gravis. *J Immunol* 167: 1935–1944.

Sinha, S., Newsom-Davis, J., Mills, K., *et al.* (1991). Autoimmune aetiology for acquired neuromyotonia (Isaacs' syndrome). *Lancet* 338: 75–77.

Sommer, N., Willcox, N., Harcourt, G.C., and Newsom-Davis, J. (1990). Myasthenic thymus and thymoma are selectively enriched in acetylcholine receptor-reactive T cells. *Ann Neurol* 28: 312–319.

Sommer, N., Melms, A., Weller, M., and Dichgans, J. (1993). Ocular myasthenia gravis. A critical review of clinical and pathophysiological aspects. *Doc Ophthalmol* 84: 309–333.

Sommer, N., Sigg, B., Melms, A., *et al.* (1997). Ocular myasthenia gravis: response to long-term immunosuppressive treatment. *J Neurol Neurosurg Psychiatry* 62: 156–162.

Somnier, F.E. (1994). Exacerbation of myasthenia gravis after removal of thymomas. *Acta Neurol Scand* 90: 56–66.

Somnier, F.E. and Engel, P.J. (2002). The occurrence of anti-titin antibodies and thymomas: a population survey of MG 1970–1999. *Neurology* 59: 92–98.

Somnier, F.E., Keiding, N., and Paulson, O.B. (1991). Epidemiology of myasthenia gravis in Denmark. A longitudinal and comprehensive population survey. *Arch Neurol* 48: 733–739.

Somnier, F.E. (1996). Myasthenia gravis. *Dan Med Bul* 43(1): 1–10. Review.

Souadjian, J.V., Enriquez, P., Silverstein, M.N., and Pepin, J.M. (1974). The spectrum of diseases associated with thymoma. Coincidence or syndrome? *Arch Intern Med* 134: 374–379.

Spack, E.G., McCutcheon, M., Corbelletta, N., *et al.* (1995). Induction of tolerance in experimental autoimmune myasthenia gravis with solubilized MHC class II: acetylcholine receptor peptide complexes. *J Autoimmun* 8: 787–807.

Spreadbury, I., Kishre, U., Beeson, D. and Vincent, A. (2005). Inhibition of acetylcholine receptor function by seronegative myasthenia gravis non-IgG factor correlates with desensitization. *J Neuroimmunol* 162: 149–56.

Spuler, S., Marx, A., Kirchner, T., *et al.* (1994). Myogenesis in thymic transplants in the severe combined immunodeficient mouse model of myasthenia gravis. Differentiation of thymic myoid cells into striated muscle cells. *Am J Pathol* 145: 766–770.

Spuler, S., Sarropoulos, A., Marx, A., *et al.* (1996). Thymoma-associated myasthenia gravis. Transplantation of thymoma and extrathymomal thymic tissue into SCID mice. *Am J Pathol* 148: 1359–1365.

Stacy, S., Gelb, B.E., Koop, B.A., *et al.* (2002). Split tolerance in a novel transgenic model of autoimmune myasthenia gravis. *J Immunol* 169: 6570–6579.

Stanley, E.F. and Drachman, D.B. (1978). Effect of myasthenic immunoglobulin on acetylcholine receptors of intact mammalian neuromuscular junctions. *Science* 200: 1285–1287.

Stefansson, K., Dieperink, M.E., Richman, D.P., *et al.* (1985). Sharing of antigenic determinants between the nicotinic acetylcholine receptor and proteins in *Escherichia coli, Proteus vulgaris,* and *Klebsiella pneumoniae.* Possible role in the pathogenesis of myasthenia gravis. *N Engl J Med* 312: 221–225.

Strobel, P., Helmreich, M., Kalbacher, H., *et al.* (2001). Evidence for distinct mechanisms in the shaping of the CD4 T cell repertoire in histologically distinct myasthenia gravis-associated thymomas. *Dev Immunol* 8: 279–290.

Takamori, M., Hamada, T., Komai, K., *et al.* (1994). Synaptotagmin can cause an immune-mediated model of Lambert–Eaton myasthenic syndrome in rats. *Ann Neurol* 35: 74–80.

Takamori, M., Iwasa, K., and Komai, K. (1997). Antibodies to synthetic peptides of the alpha1A subunit of the voltage-gated calcium channel in Lambert–Eaton myasthenic syndrome. *Neurology* 48: 1261–1265.

Takamori, M., Komai, K., and Iwasa, K. (2000). Antibodies to calcium channel and synaptotagmin in Lambert–Eaton myasthenic syndrome. *Am J Med Sci* 319: 204–208.

Tong, Z. and Dwyer, D.S. (1990). Alteration of the humoral immune response against muscle acetylcholine receptor by timed administration of alpha (1–3)dextran. *Eur J Immunol* 20: 1627–1634.

Toyka, K.V., Brachman, D.B., Pestronk, A., and Kao, I. (1975). Myasthenia gravis: passive transfer from man to mouse. *Science* 190: 397–399.

Truffault, F., Cohen-Kaminsky, S., Khalil, I., *et al.* (1997). Altered intrathymic T-cell repertoire in human myasthenia gravis. *Ann Neurol* 41: 731–741.

Tsien, R.W., Fox, A.P., Hess, P., *et al.* (1987). Multiple types of calcium channel in excitable cells. *Soc Gen Physiol Ser* 41: 167–187.

Tzartos, S.J. and Lindstrom, J.M. (1980). Monoclonal antibodies used to probe acetylcholine receptor structure: localization of the main immunogenic region and detection of similarities between subunits. *Proc Natl Acad Sci USA* 77: 755–759.

Tzartos, S.J., Seybold, M.E., and Lindstrom, J.M. (1982). Specificities of antibodies to acetylcholine receptors in sera from myasthenia gravis patients measured by monoclonal antibodies. *Proc Natl Acad Sci USA* 79: 188–192.

Tzartos, S.J., Barkas, T., Cung, M.T., *et al.* (1998). Anatomy of the antigenic structure of a large membrane autoantigen, the muscle-type nicotinic acetylcholine receptor. *Immunol Rev* 163: 89–120.

Unwin, N. (2000). The Croonian Lecture 2000. Nicotinic acetylcholine receptor and the structural basis of fast synaptic transmission. *Phil Trans R Soc Lond B Biol Sci* 355: 1813–1829.

Verma, P.K. and Oger, J.J. (1992). Seronegative generalized myasthenia gravis: low frequency of thymic pathology. *Neurology* 42: 586–589.

Vernet der Garabedian, B., Lacokova, M., Eymard, B., *et al.* (1994). Association of neonatal myasthenia gravis with antibodies against the fetal acetylcholine receptor. *J Clin Invest* 94: 555–559.

Vernino, S., Low, P.A., Fealey, R.D., *et al.* (2000). Autoantibodies to ganglionic acetylcholine receptors in autoimmune autonomic neuropathies. *N Engl J Med* 343: 847–855.

Viera, M.L., Caillat-Zucman, S., Gajdos, P., *et al.* (1993). Identification by genomic typing of non-DR3 HLA class II genes associated with myasthenia gravis. *J Neuroimmunol* 47: 115–122.

Vincent, A.. (2000). Understanding neuromyotonia. *Muscle Nerve* 23: 655–657.

Vincent, A. and Drachman, D.B. (2002). Myasthenia gravis. *Adv Neurol* 88: 159–188.

Vincent, A. and Newsom-Davis, J. (1982a). Acetylcholine receptor antibody characteristics in myasthenia gravis. II. Patients with penicillamine-induced myasthenia or idiopathic myasthenia of recent onset. *Clin Exp Immunol* 49: 266–272.

Vincent, A. and Newsom-Davis, J. (1982b). Acetylcholine receptor antibody characteristics in myasthenia gravis. I. Patients with generalized myasthenia or disease restricted to ocular muscles. *Clin Exp Immunol* 49: 257–265.

Vincent, A. and Newsom-Davis, J. (1985). Acetylcholine receptor antibody as a diagnostic test for myasthenia gravis: results in 153 validated cases and 2967 diagnostic assays. *J Neurol Neurosurg Psychiatry* 48: 1246–1252.

Vincent, A., Newsom-Davis, J., Newton, P., and Beck, N. (1983). Acetylcholine receptor antibody and clinical response to thymectomy in myasthenia gravis. *Neurology* 33: 1276–1282.

Vincent, A., Whiting, P.J., Schluep, M., *et al.* (1987). Antibody heterogeneity and specificity in myasthenia gravis. *Ann N Y Acad Sci* 505: 106–120.

Vincent, A., Li, Z., Hart, A., *et al.* (1993). Seronegative myasthenia gravis. Evidence for plasma factor(s) interfering with acetylcholine receptor function. *Ann N Y Acad Sci* 681: 529–538.

Vincent, A., Jacobson, L., and Curran, L. (1998a). Alpha-bungarotoxin binding to human muscle acetylcholine receptor: measurement of affinity, delineation of AChR subunit residues crucial to binding, and protection of AChR function by synthetic peptides. *Neurochem Int* 32: 427–433.

Vincent, A., Willcox, N., Hill, M., *et al.* (1998b). Determinant spreading and immune responses to acetylcholine receptors in myasthenia gravis. *Immunol Rev* 164: 157–168.

Vincent, A., Palace, J., and Hilton-Jones, D. (2001). Myasthenia gravis. *Lancet* 357: 2122–2128.

Vincent, A., Bowen, J., Newsom-Davis, J., and McConville, J. (2003a). Seronegative generalised myasthenia gravis: clinical features, antibodies, and their targets. *Lancet Neurol* 2: 99–106.

Vincent, A., Clover, L., Buckley, C., *et al.* (2003*b*). Evidence of underdiagnosis of myasthenia gravis in older people. *J Neurol Neurosurg Psychiatry* **74**: 1105–1108.

Wakkach, A., Guyon, T., Bruand, C., *et al.* (1996). Expression of acetylcholine receptor genes in human thymic epithelial cells: implications for myasthenia gravis. *J Immunol* **157**: 3752–3760.

Wang, H., Kunkel, D.D., Martin, T.M., *et al.* (1993). Heteromultimeric K⁺ channels in terminal and juxtaparanodal regions of neurons. *Nature* **365**: 75–79.

Wang, Z.Y., He, B., Qiao, J. and Link, H. (1995). Suppression of experimental autoimmune myasthenia gravis and experimental allergic encephalomyelitis by oral administration of acetylcholine receptor any myelin basic protein: double tolerance. *J Neuroimmunol* **63**(1): 79–86.

Wang, Z.Y., Okita, D.K., Howard, J. Jr, and Conti-Fine, B.M. (1997). Th1 epitope repertoire on the alpha subunit of human muscle acetylcholine receptor in myasthenia gravis. *Neurology* **48**: 1643–1653.

Wang, Z.Y., Okita, D.K., Howard, J. Jr, and Conti-Fine, B.M. (1998*a*). T-cell recognition of muscle acetylcholine receptor subunits in generalized and ocular myasthenia gravis. *Neurology* **50**: 045–1054.

Wang, Z.Y., Okita, D.K., Howard, J.F. Jr, and Conti-Fine, B.M. (1998*b*). T-cell repertoire on the epsilon subunit of muscle acetylcholine receptor in myasthenia gravis. *J Neuroimmunol* **91**: 33–42.

Wang, Z.Y., Karachunski, P.I., Howard, J.F. Jr, and Conti-Fine, B.M. (1999), Myasthenia in SCID mice grafted with myasthenic patient lymphocytes: role of CD4+ and CD8+ cells. *Neurology* **52**: 484–497.

Waterman, S.A. (1996). Multiple subtypes of voltage-gated calcium channel mediate transmitter release from parasympathetic neurons in the mouse bladder. *J Neurosci* **16**: 4155–4161.

Waterman, S.A., Lang, B., and Newsom-Davis, J. (1997). Effect of Lambert–Eaton myasthenic syndrome antibodies on autonomic neurons in the mouse. *Ann Neurol* **42**: 147–156.

Wekerle, H. and Ketelsen, U.P. (1977). Intrathymic pathogenesis and dual genetic control of myasthenia gravis. *Lancet* **1**: 678–680.

Whiting, P.J., Vincent, A., and Newsom-Davis, J. (1986). Myasthenia gravis: monoclonal antihuman acetylcholine receptor antibodies used to analyze antibody specificities and responses to treatment. *Neurology* **36**: 612–617.

Willcox, N., Demaine, A.G., Newsom-Davis, J., *et al.* (1985). Increased frequency of IgG heavy chain marker Glm(2) and of HLA-B8 in Lambert–Eaton myasthenic syndrome with and without associated lung carcinoma. *Hum Immunol* **14**: 29–36.

Wilcox, N., Schluep, M., Sommer, N., Campana, D., Janossy, G., Brown, A.N., *et al.* (1989). Variable corticosteriod sensitivity of thymic cortex and medullary peripheral-type lymphoid tissue in myasthenia gravis patients: structural and functional effects. *Q J Med* **73**(271): 1071–87.

Willcox, N., Schluep, M., Ritter, M.A., and Newsom-Davis, J. (1991). The thymus in seronegative myasthenia gravis patients. *J Neurol* **238**: 256–261.

Wilson, S., Vincent, A., and Newsom-Davis, J. (1983). Acetylcholine receptor turnover in mice with passively transferred myasthenia gravis. II. Receptor synthesis. *J Neurol Neurosurg Psychiatry* **46**: 383–387.

Yamamoto, T., Vincent, A., Ciulla, T.A., *et al.* (1991). Seronegative myasthenia gravis: a plasma factor inhibiting agonist-induced acetylcholine receptor function copurifies with IgM. *Ann Neurol* **30**: 550–557.

Yang, H., Goluszko, E., David, C., *et al.* (2002). Mapping myasthenia gravis-associated T cell epitopes on human acetylcholine receptors in HLA transgenic mice. *J Clin Invest* **109**: 1111–1120.

Yoshitake, T., Masunaga, A., Sugawara, I., *et al.* (1994). A comparative histological and immunohistochemical study of thymomas with and without myasthenia gravis. *Surg Today* **24**: 1044–1049.

Zhang, G.X., Ma, C.G., Xiao, B.G., *et al.* (1995). Depletion of CD8+ T cells suppresses the development of experimental autoimmune myasthenia gravis in Lewis rats. *Eur J Immunol* **25**: 1191–1198.

21 Immune-mediated mechanisms in inflammatory myopathies

Marinos C. Dalakas

Introduction

The inflammatory myopathies comprise three major and distinct subsets: polymyositis (PM), dermatomyositis (DM), and inclusion-body myositis (IBM) (Askanas and Engel, 1988; Karpati and Carpenter, 1988; Dalakas, 1991, 1995, 1998; Sekul and Dalakas, 1993; Engel *et al.*, 1994; Hohlfeld and Engel, 1994). The diseases are clinically important because they represent the largest group of acquired and potentially treatable myopathies both in children and adults. Although unique clinical, immunopathologic, and histologic criteria along with different prognoses and response to therapies characterize each subset, all of them share three dominant histological features which are ultimately responsible for the clinical signs of muscle weakness—inflammation, fibrosis, and loss of muscle fibers.

The cause of PM, DM, and IBM still remains unknown but an auto-immune pathogenesis is strongly implicated, as discussed below. Progress in the cellular and molecular pathology of these disorders has advanced our understanding of the T-cell activation, recognition of muscle antigens, myofiber cell loss, and fibrosis. In DM, the endomysial inflammation and muscle fiber destruction is preceded by activation of complement and deposition of membranolytic attack complex on the endomysial capillaries (Kissel *et al.*, 1986; Dalakas, 1991, 1995*a*; Engel *et al.*, 1994; Hohlfeld and Engel, 1994). In PM and IBM, activated CD8+ T cells are clonally expanded and reach the endomysial parenchyma to recognize muscle antigen(s) associated with up-regulation of major histocompatibility complex (MHC) Class I antigen on the muscle fibers (Karpati and Carpenter, 1988; Dalakas, 1991, 1995*a*, 1998; Engel *et al.*, 1994; Hohlfeld and Engel, 1994). The auto-invasive T cells, probably driven by specific stimuli, exhibit gene rearrangement of their T-cell receptors (TCRs) and restricted amino acid sequences in the CDR3 region (Mantegazza *et al.*, 1993; O'Hanlon *et al.*, 1994; Bender *et al.*, 1995, 1998; Fyhr *et al.*, 1997; Amemiya *et al.*, 2000*a*), as discussed later. In IBM, in addition to specifically driven T cells that invade intact fibers, there exist vacuolated muscle fibers containing β-amyloid and amyloid-related proteins. Because vacuolated fibers are almost never associated with T-cell infiltrates, it seems that in IBM two parallel processes co-exist, a primary immune response and a degenerative process.

Clinical features

General clinical features

The incidence of PM, DM, and IBM is approximately 1 in 100 000. Dermatomyositis affects both children and adults, and females more often than males, whereas polymyositis is seen after the second decade of life and very rarely in childhood. Inclusion body myositis is three times more frequent in men than in women, is more common in Whites than in Blacks, and is most likely to affect persons over the age of 50 years.

All three forms have in common a myopathy characterized by proximal and often symmetric muscle weakness that develops relatively slowly (weeks to months) and occasionally insidiously, as in inclusion body myositis, but rarely acutely (Dalakas, 1991; Engel *et al.*, 1994). Patients usually report increasing difficulty with everyday tasks predominantly requiring the use of proximal muscles, such as getting up from a chair, climbing steps, stepping onto a curb, lifting objects, or combing their hair. Fine motor movements that depend on the strength of distal muscles, such as buttoning a shirt, sewing, knitting, or writing, are affected only late in the course of DM and PM, but earlier in IBM. Falling is common among patients with IBM because of early involvement of the quadriceps muscle and buckling of the knees. Ocular muscles remain normal, even in advanced, untreated cases, and if these muscles were affected, the diagnosis of inflammatory myopathy would be in doubt. Facial muscles also remain normal except, rarely, in advanced cases. Mild facial muscle weakness, however, is seen in up to 60% of patients with sporadic IBM (s-IBM) (Sekul and Dalakas, 1993). The pharyngeal and neck flexor muscles are often involved, causing dysphagia or fatigue and difficulty in holding up the head. In advanced cases and rarely in acute cases, respiratory muscles may also be affected. Severe weakness is almost always associated with muscular wasting. Sensation remains normal. The tendon reflexes are preserved but may be absent in severely weakened or atrophied muscles, especially in s-IBM where atrophy of the quadriceps and the distal muscles is common. Weakness in PM and DM progresses over a period of weeks or months, in contrast with the much slower progression of limb-girdle dystrophies from which they sometimes need to be differentiated. However, IBM may progress slowly for years, and its clinical features may simulate those of limb-girdle muscular dystrophy or peroneal muscular atrophy.

Dermatomyositis

Dermatomyositis occurs in both children and adults. It is a distinct clinical entity identified by a characteristic rash accompanying, or more often preceding, the muscle weakness. The skin manifestations include a heliotrope rash (blue-purple discoloration) on the upper eyelids with edema, a flat red rash on the face and upper truck, and erythema of the knuckles with a raised violaceous scaly eruption (Gottron rash) that later results in scaling of the skin. The erythematous rash can also occur on other body surfaces, including the knees, elbows, malleoli, neck, and anterior chest (often in a V sign), or back and shoulders (shawl sign), and may be exacerbated after exposure to the sun. In some patients the rash is pruritic especially in the scalp, chest, and back. Dilated capillary loops at the base of the finger nails are also characteristic of DM. The cuticles may be irregular, thickened, and distorted, and the lateral and palmar areas of the fingers may become rough and cracked, with irregular, 'dirty' horizontal lines, resembling mechanic's hands. The degree of weakness can be mild, moderate, or severe leading to quadraparesis. At times, the muscle strength appears normal, hence the tern 'dermatomyositis sine myositis'. When muscle biopsy is performed in such cases, however, significant perivascular and perimysial inflammation is seen. In children, DM resembles the adult disease except for more frequent extramuscular manifestations, as discussed later. A common early abnormality in children is 'misery', defined as an irritable child that feels uncomfortable, has a red flush on the face, is fatigued, does not feel well enough to socialize, and has a varying degree of proximal muscle weakness. A tip-toe gait due to flexion contracture of the ankles is also common.

Dermatomyositis usually occurs alone, but may overlap with systemic sclerosis, and mixed connective tissue disease (Dalakas, 1991, 1998). Fasciitis and skin changes similar to those found in DM have occurred in patients with the eosinophilia–myalgia syndrome associated with the ingestion of contaminated L-tryptophan (Dalakas, 1991, 1998). The diagnosis of DM is often clear from the characteristic clinical picture. The serum creatine kinase (CK) level is elevated or normal, needle electromyography (EMG) shows active myopathy and the muscle biopsy shows characteristic features, as described later.

Polymyositis

Patients with PM do not present with any unique clinical feature that heralds the diagnosis. Unlike in DM, in which the rash secures early recognition, the actual onset of PM cannot be easily determined. Patients present with subacute onset of proximal muscle weakness and myalgia that may exist for several months before they seek medical advice. In our judgment, the diagnosis of PM is one of exclusion. It is best diagnosed and defined as an inflammatory myopathy that develops subacutely, usually over weeks to months, progresses steadily, and occurs in adults who *do not* have a rash, involvement of the extraocular and facial muscles (mild facial weakness is seen in IBM but not in PM), family history of a neuromuscular disease, history of exposure to myotoxic drugs or toxins, endocrinopathy, neurogenic disease, dystrophy, biochemical muscle disorder, or IBM, as determined by muscle enzyme histochemistry and biochemistry.

Polymyositis can be viewed as a syndrome of diverse causes that may occur separately or in association with systemic autoimmune or connective tissue diseases and certain known viral or bacterial infections. Other than D-penicillamine and zidovudine (AZT), in which the myopathy has endomysial inflammation, myotoxic drugs, such as emetine, chloroquine, steroids, cimetidine, ipecac, and lovostatin, do not cause PM. Instead, they elicit a *toxic non-inflammatory* myopathy that is histologically different from PM and does not require immunosuppressive therapy (Dalakas, 1991, 1998).

Several animal parasites, such as protozoa (*Toxoplasma*, *Trypanosoma*), cestodes (cysticerci), and nematodes (trichinae), may produce a focal or diffuse inflammatory myopathy known as parasitic polymyositis. A suppurative myositis, known as *tropical* polymyositis or *pyomyositis* may be produced by *Staphylococcus aureus*, *Yersinia*, *Streptococcus*, or other anaerobes. Pyomyositis, a previous rarity in the West, can now be seen in rare patients with acquired immunodeficiency syndrome (AIDS). Certain bacteria, such as *Borrelia burgdorferi* of Lyme disease and *Lefionella pneumophila* of Legionnaire's disease may infrequently be the cause of polymyositis.

Inclusion-body myositis

Inclusion-body myositis is the commonest of the inflammatory myopathies. It affects men more often than women and it is most frequent above the age of 50 years. It is the most common acquired myopathy in men over 50 years old. Although IBM is commonly suspected when a patient with presumed polymyositis does not respond to therapy, involvement of distal muscles, especially foot extensors and deep finger flexors, in almost all the cases, may be a clue to the early clinical diagnosis (Askanas and Engel, 1988; Karpati and Carpenter, 1988; Dalakas, 1991; Engel *et al.*, 1994; Griggs *et al.*, 1995). Some patients present with falls because their knees collapse due to early weakness of the quadriceps muscles. Others present with weakness in the small muscles of the hands, especially finger flexors, and complain of inability to hold certain objects such as golf clubs, play the guitar, turn on keys, or tie knots. The weakness and the accompanied atrophy can be asymmetric with selective involvement of the quadriceps, iliopsoas, triceps, biceps, and finger flexors in the forearm. Dysphagia is common, occurring in up to 60% of patients, especially late in the disease. Because of the distal, and at times asymmetric, weakness and atrophy and the early loss of the patellar reflex owing to severe weakness of the quadriceps muscle, a lower motor neuron disease is often suspected, especially when the serum CK is not elevated. Sensory examination is generally normal except for a mildly diminished vibratory sensation at the ankles, presumably related to the patient's age. Contrary to early suggestions, the distal weakness does not represent neurogenic involvement but it is part of the distal myopathic process, as we have confirmed with macro EMG (Luciano and Dalakas, 1997). The diagnosis is always made by the characteristic findings on the muscle biopsy, as discussed later.

Inclusion-body myositis can be associated with systemic autoimmune or connective tissue diseases in at least 20% of the cases. An increased frequency, in up to 75% of patients, of DRb_10301 and DQb_10201 alleles associated with DR and DQ phenotypes has been documented (Koffman *et al.*, 1998). There is a subset of patients with familial IBM with the typical phenotype of sporadic IBM and histological and immunopathological features identical to the sporadic form, designated as 'familial inflammatory inclusion-body myositis' (Sivakumar *et al.*, 1997). These cases are different from those with the hereditary form of IBM, a group of various, ill-defined, vacuolar, distal greater than proximal, myopathies of recessive or dominant inheritance with a clinical profile different from the one described above for the sporadic disease. There is, however, a distinct subset of hereditary IBM with sparing of the quadriceps muscle which was originally described in Iranian Jews. This entity is not limited to Iranian Jews but occurs in many ethnic groups (Sivakumar and Dalakas, 1996) and it is a distinct genetic, non-inflammatory, vacuolar myopathy with a gene locus on chromosome 9p1 (Mitrani-Rosenbaum *et al.*, 1996).

Progression of IBM is slow but steady. The degree of disability in relation to the duration of the disease has not been systematically studied. Review of the course of 14 randomly chosen patients with symptoms for more than 5 years revealed that 10 of them required a cane or support for ambulation by the fifth year after onset of disease while 3 of 5 patients with symptoms for 10 years or more were using wheelchairs for ambulation (Askanas and Engel, 1988). Recent data from 86 consecutively studied patients have shown that progression is faster when the disease begins later in life. Patients whose disease begins in their 60s may require an assistive device many years later than those patients whose disease begins in their 70s, presumably due to lesser reserves (Peng *et al.*, 2000).

The diagnosis is made based on the characteristic clinical features mentioned above and the muscle biopsy which, if typical, is diagnostic even at the light microscopy level.

Extramuscular manifestations

In addition to the primary disturbance of the skeletal muscles, extramuscular manifestations may be prominent in patients with inflammatory myopathies. These include:

1. Dysphagia, most prominent in IBM and DM, due to involvement of the oropharyngeal striated muscles and distal esophagus.

2. Cardiac abnormalities consisting of atrioventricular conduction defects, tachyarrythmias, low ejection fraction and dilated cardiomyopathy either from the disease itself or from hypertension associated with long-term steroid use.

3. Pulmonary involvement, as the result of primary weakness of the thoracic muscles, drug-induced pneumonitis (e.g. from methotrexate), or interstitial lung disease. Interstitial lung disease may precede the myopathy or occur early in the disease and develops in up to 10% of patients with PM or DM, the majority of whom have anti-Jo-1 antibodies. Fatality related to adult respiratory distress syndrome has been noted in PM patients with anti-Jo-1 antibodies (Clawson and Oddis, 1995), emphasizing the diagnostic importance of these antibodies. Pulmonary capillaritis with varying degrees of diffuse alveolar hemorrhage has been also described (Schwarz *et al.*, 1995).

4. Subcutaneous calcifications, sometimes extruding onto the skin and causing ulcerations and infections, are found in patients with DM, not only children but also in some adults (Dalakas, 1995*b*).

5. Gastrointestinal ulcerations, seen more often in the past, in childhood DM, due to vasculitis and infection.

6. Contractures of the joints especially in childhood DM.

7. General systemic disturbances, such as fever, malaise, weight loss, arthralfia, and Raynaud's phenomenon, when the inflammatory myopathy is associated with a connective tissue disorder.

8. An increase incidence of malignancies in patients with DM, but not PM or IBM. Because tumors are usually uncovered not by a radiologic blind search but by abnormal findings on their medical history and physical examination, it is our practice to recommend only a complete annual physical examination, with breast, pelvic, and rectal examinations, urinalysis, complete blood-cell count, blood chemistry tests, and a chest X-ray film.

Diagnosis

The clinically suspected diagnosis of PM, DM, or IBM is established or confirmed by elevated activity of the muscle-derived serum enzymes, electromyographic findings, and muscle biopsy.

Muscle-derived serum enzyme levels

The most sensitive enzyme is creatine kinase (CK), which, in the presence of active disease, can be elevated by as much as 50 times above the normal level. Although CK usually parallels the disease activity, it can be normal in active DM and rarely even in active PM. In IBM, CK is not usually elevated more than 10-fold, and in some cases may be normal even from the beginning of the illness. CK may also be normal in patients with untreated, even active, childhood DM and in some patients with PM or DM associated with a connective tissue disease, reflecting the restriction of the pathologic process to the intramuscular vessels and perimysium. Along with the CK, the serum glutamic-oxaloacetic transaminase (SGOT), serum glutamate pyruvate transaminase (SGPT), lactate dehydrogenase (LDH), and aldolase may be elevated.

Electromyography

Needle electromyography (EMG) shows myopathic motor unit potentials characterized by short-duration, low-amplitude polyphasic units on voluntary activation, and increased spontaneous activity with fibrillations, complex repetitive discharges, and positive sharp waves. This electromyographic pattern also occurs in a variety of acute, toxic, and active myopathic processes and should not be considered diagnostic for the inflammatory myopathies. Mixed myopathic and neurogenic potentials (polyphasic units of short and long duration) are more often seen in IBM but they can be seen in both PM and DM as a consequence of muscle fiber regeneration and chronicity of the disease. Contrary to previous reports, our findings using macro-EMG have failed to show a neurogenic pattern of involvement in IBM patients (Luciano and Dalakas, 1997) even though histologic evidence of an axonal neuropathy may be present in some cases. Electromyographic studies, thus, are generally useful for excluding primary neurogenic disorders in such cases.

Muscle biopsy

Muscle biopsy shows characteristic features for each subset. In DM, the hallmark histological findings consist of perivascular and interstitial inflammation, necrosis, phagocytosis, and degeneration of muscle fibers around the fascicle or within a muscle fasciculus in a wedge-like shape due to microinfarcts within the muscle, and perifascicular atrophy which can be seen even without inflammation. In PM, the muscle biopsy shows endomysial infiltrates scattered in several foci consisting of lymphocytes invading healthy muscle fibers and phagocytosis of the necrotic fibers. In IBM, the histological hallmarks are:

1. Basophilic granular inclusions distributed around the edge of slit-like vacuoles (rimmed vacuoles).

2. Angulated or round fibers, scattered or in small groups.

3. Eosinophilic cytoplasmic inclusions.

4. Primary endomysial inflammation with T cells invading muscle fibers in a pattern identical to (but often more severe) than the one seen in PM.

5. Tiny deposits of Congo-red- or crystal-violet-positive amyloid within or next to some vacuoles. The amyloid, seen in approximately 80% of our patients, immunoreacts with β-amyloid protein, the type of amyloid sequenced from the amyloid fibrils of blood vessels of patients with Alzheimer's disease (Mendell et al., 1991; Askanas et al., 1992a,b).

6. Characteristic filamentous inclusions seen by electron microscopy in the cytoplasm or myonuclei, prominent in the vicinity of the rimmed vacuoles. Although demonstration of the filaments by electron microscopy was initially essential for the diagnosis of IBM, we do not feel that this is now necessary if all the characteristic light microscopic features including the amyloid deposits are fulfilled. Further, such filaments are not unique to IBM; they can be seen in other vacuolar myopathies. The cytoplasmic tubulofilaments within the vacuolated muscle fibers immunoreact strongly with tau, ubiquitin, chymotrypsin, and prion (Askanas et al., 1992a).

7. Abnormal mitochondria seen as ragged-red fibers which are often negative with cytochrome oxidase and contain mitochondrial DNA deletions (Santorelli et al., 1996).

Immune-mediated mechanisms

Immunopathology of dermatomyositis

The primary antigenic targets in DM are components of the vascular endothelium of the endomysial blood vessels and the capillaries. The earliest pathological alterations are changes in the endothelial cells consisting of pale and swollen cytoplasm with microvacuoles and undulating tubules in the smooth endoplasmic reticulum followed by obliteration, vascular necrosis, and thrombi (Banker, 1975; Carpenter et al., 1976). Such alterations in the microvasculature occur early in the disease by the C5b-9 membranolytic attack complex (MAC), the lytic component of the complement pathway, which is deposited on the capillaries before the onset of inflammatory or structural changes in the muscle fibers (Emslie-Smith and Engel, 1990). MAC and the active fragments of the early complement components C3b and C4b, are increased in patients' serum (Basta and Dalakas, 1994). Further, patients with active, but not chronic, DM, have very high C3 uptake in their serum, based on the C3 consumption by sensitized erythrocytes (Basta and Dalakas, 1994). The activation of complement, perhaps by putative anti-endothelial cell antibodies (Cervera et al., 1991; Stein et al., 1993), is believed to be responsible for the induction of cytokines (Stein and Dalakas, 1993; Lundberg et al., 1995; Tews and Goebel, 1996) which, in turn, up-regulate the expression of vascular cell adhesion molecule (VCAM)-1 and intracellular adhesion molecule (ICAM)-1 on the endothelial cells and facilitate the exit of activated lymphoid cells to the perimysial and endomysial spaces.

Sequentially, the disease begins when putative antibodies directed against endothelial cells of the endomysium (Cervera et al., 1991; Stein et al., 1993) activate complement C3 that forms C3b and C4b fragments and leads to formation and deposition of MAC on the endomysial microvasculature. The deposition of MAC leads through osmotic lysis of the endothelial cells to necrosis of the capillaries, perivascular inflammation, ischemia, and muscle fiber destruction, often resembling microinfarcts (Dalakas, 1995a). The perifascicular atrophy often seen in more chronic stages is a reflection of the endofascicular hypoperfusion which is prominent distally. Finally there is marked reduction in the number of capillaries per muscle fiber with dilatation of the remaining capillaries in an effort to compensate for the impaired perfusion (Dalakas, 1995a). The presence of systemic features, with involvement of myocardium, pericardium, lungs, and the gut suggests that the MAC-mediated microvascular injury may be widespread and the target antigen may be a ubiquitous component of the endothelium of the blood vessels.

Immunophenotypic analysis of the lymphocytic infiltrates in the muscle biopsies of patients with DM demonstrates that B cells and CD4+ cells are the predominant cells in the perimysial and perivascular regions, supporting the view of a humoral-mediated process, as described above (Arahata and Engel, 1986; Dalakas, 1991; Engel *et al.*, 1994; Hohlfeld and Engel, 1994). In the perifascicular areas, however, the infiltrates are mostly CD8+ cells and macrophages and invade MHC Class I antigen expressing muscle fibers, a sign of a co-existing T-cell-mediated and MHC Class I-restricted cytotoxic process.

In spite of the progress made a number of uncertainties exist in the pathogenesis of DM, namely:

1. What triggers complement activation?

2. Do the endomysial B cells produce antibodies? If so, what is the target antigen?

3. Is there a role for T-cell-mediated cytotoxicity?

4. Does the triggering agent recognize common antigens in skin and muscle that explain their concurrent involvement?

5. What factors (cytokines, transforming growth factor (TGF)-β, other?) drive the excessive fibrosis seen in the disease?

6. Do certain factors share common antigens with endothelial cells of muscle (?molecular mimicry) that explains the high incidence of cancer in DM?

7. What triggers the formation of calcinosis?

Immunopathology of polymyositis and inclusion body myositis

Cytotoxic T cells

In PM and IBM, there is evidence not of microangiopathy and muscle ischemia, as in DM, but of an antigen-directed cytotoxicity mediated by

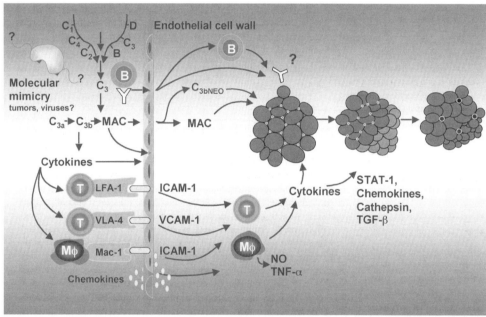

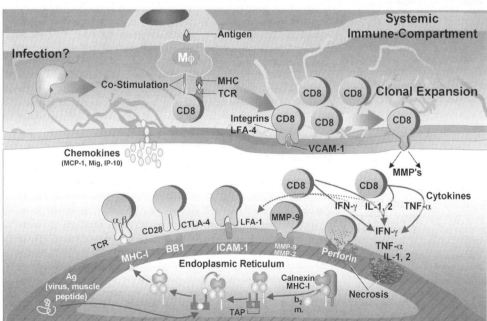

Fig. 21.1 Molecules, receptors, and their ligands involved in movement of the T cells through the endothelial cell wall and recognition of muscle antigens on the surface of muscle fibers. Sequentially, the LFA-1/ICAM-1 binding anchors the cytoskeletal molecules in the nascent immunological synapse. This allows the interaction of TCR/MHC with the sampling of MHC–peptide complexes and the engagement of BB1 and CD40 co-stimulatory molecules with their ligands CD28, CTLA, and CD40L, the prerequisites for antigen recognition. Metalloproteinases facilitate the attachment of the T cell to the muscle surface. Muscle fiber necrosis occurs via the perforin granules released by the autoinvasive T cells. A direct myocytotoxic effect exerted by the released IFN-γ, IL-1 or TNF-α may also take place. Muscle fiber cell death is mediated through necrosis and not apoptosis, presumably because of the counterbalancing effect or protection by the anti-apoptotic molecules Bcl-2, hILP, and FLIP which are up-regulated in PM and IBM muscles. Fas is also expressed, but it does not mediate apoptosis, in the muscle. The up-regulated NCAM on degenerating muscle fibers may enhance regeneration. (See text for abbreviations.)

cytotoxic T cells (Dalakas, 1991, 1995a, 1998; Hohlfeld et al., 1993; Engel et al., 1994; Hohlfeld and Engel, 1994). This conclusion is supported by the presence of CD8+ cells, which along with macrophages initially surround healthy, but MHC Class I expressing, non-necrotic muscle fibers that eventually invade and destroy. These T cells are activated, as evidenced by their expression of ICAM-1 and MHC Class I and II antigens on their surface, and exert a cytotoxic effect against muscle fibers. The T-cell-mediated myocytotoxicity is supported by the following:

1. Cell cytotoxicity. Cell lines established from muscle biopsies of PM patients exert cytotoxicity to their autologous myotubes in vitro (Hohlfeld and Engel, 1991). By immunoelectron microscopy, CD8+ cells and macrophages can be seen to send spike-like processes into non-necrotic muscle fibers, which traverse the basal lamina and focally displace or compress the muscle fibers (Arahata and Engel, 1986).

2. Perforin. The cytotoxic autoinvasive CD8+ T cells contain perforin and granzyme granules (Goebel et al., 1996) which are directed towards the surface of the fibers and upon release induce cell destruction by necrosis, but not apoptosis, as described later (Fig. 21.1).

3. TCR gene rearrangement of the endomysial T cells. The T cells recognize an antigen by the TCR, a heterodimer of two α and β chains, encoded by multiple gene families in the V (variable), D (diversity), J (joining), and C (constant) regions of the TCR. The part of the TCR that recognizes an antigen is the CDR3 region, which is encoded by genes in the V–J and V–D–J segments of the TCR gene. If the endomysial T cells are selectively recruited by a muscle-specific autoantigen, the use of the V and J genes of the TCR should be restricted, and the amino acid sequence in their CDR3 region should be conserved. In patients with PM and IBM, but not in those with DM, only certain T cells of specific TCRα and TCRβ families are recruited to the muscle from the circulation (Mantegazza et al., 1993; O'Hanlon et al., 1994; Bender et al., 1995). Cloning and sequencing of the amplified endomysial or autoinvasive TCR gene families has demonstrated a restricted use of the Jβ gene with a conserved amino acid sequence in the CDR3 region indicating that CD8+ cells are specifically selected and clonally expanded in situ by muscle-specific autoantigens (Mantegazza et al., 1993; O'Hanlon et al., 1994; Bender et al., 1995). This is true not only in PM but also in IBM, where immunocytochemistry combined with polymerase chain reaction (PCR) and sequencing of the most prominent TCR families has shown that the autoinvasive, but not the perivascular, CD8+ endomysial cells are also clonally expanded (Fyhr et al., 1997; Bender et al., 1998). Sequential muscle biopsy specimens obtained during a 19–22 month period in three patients with IBM has further shown a persistent clonal restriction of the same Vβ families among the autoinvasive CD8+ cells (Amemiya et al., 2000a). The most frequently detected gene families were again the Vβ3, Vβ5.1, Vβ6.7, and Vβ13, while several of the autoinvasive CD8+ T cells persistently expressed the Vβ6.7 and Vβ5.1 genes. Further, the autoinvasive T cells in these biopsies exhibited restricted usage of certain Vβ gene families and a persistent amino acid sequence homology in the complementary CDR3-determining region (Amemiya et al., 2000a). Of interest, in the CDR3 region only a small number of amino acids was found (Amemiya et al., 2000a), suggesting that the MHC Class I expressing muscle fibers present limited number of antigenic peptides to the autoinvasive CD8+ T cells during the course of the disease. These latest findings support the clonal restriction of the T cells in IBM muscles and suggest that the endomysial T cells appear driven continuously by the same antigen(s). Consistent with the above is the universal observation that the endomysial inflammatory response in IBM remains prominent, even late in the disease. Although such a strong immunological signal may be surprising because patients with IBM do not respond to immunotherapies and their muscle biopsies contain prominent degenerative features, it is surmised that the immunopathology of IBM is more complex.

4. The CD45RO+ memory T cells predominate among the endomysial infiltrates, exceeding the number seen in normal blood. Such an observation implies that memory cells may be primed to putative muscle-specific target antigens. The up-regulation of the inducible co-stimulator ligand (ICOS-L), often associated with memory T cells, as described later, supports this view.

5. γ/β T cells, a subset of cytotoxic T cells, have mediated cytotoxicity in one patient with PM. A restricted profile of γ/β TCR gene expression was also demonstrated in this case. When the γ/β TCR of these cells were transfected into a TCR-deficient hybridoma cell line, the transfectants could be stimulated with human myoblasts indicating that the γ/β T cells from this case of polymyositis recognize a heretofore unidentified muscle autoantigen.

MHC expression for antigen presentation

Muscle fibers do not normally express detectable amount of MHC Class I or II antigens. In PM and IBM, however, widespread overexpression of MHC is an early event that can be seen even in areas remote from the inflammation (Karpati et al., 1988). Based on in vitro data, MHC Class I is induced by cytokines such as interferon (IFN)-γ and tumor necrosis factor (TNF)-α (Bao et al., 1990; Hohlfeld and Engel, 1990; Mantegazza et al., 1991; Roy et al., 1991; Michaelis et al., 1993) and at least two of these cytokines are detected at a given time in the muscle biopsy tissue of patients with active PM (Lundberg et al., 1995; Tews and Goebel, 1996; Dalakas, 1998; De et al., 1999).

It has recently been hypothesized, based on observations in transgenic mice overexpressing MHC Class I molecules, that prolonged expression of MHC Class I on the surface of muscle fibers may be sufficient by itself to act as an inciting event to trigger myositis independent of a specific stimulus (Nagaraju et al., 2000a). This concept, however, does not appear applicable to human PM because up-regulation of MHC Class I, without a concomitant T-cell autoinvasion, is not associated with muscle fiber destruction nor does it trigger a T-cell response (Dalakas, in press a). This has been confirmed in patients with chronic PM and inactive disease following therapy, where the muscles continue to express MHC Class I molecules but do not exhibit signs of inflammation (Nyberg et al., 2000), indicating that up-regulation of MHC by itself, without concurrent invasion by activated T cells driven by non-MHC-related stimuli, does not engage the muscle fibers in antigen presentation or cell destruction.

Another MHC molecule of some interest in inflammatory myopathy may be HLA-G which was found expressed on muscle fibers of patients with PM and IBM, but not in dystrophies (Wiendl et al., 2000). The expression of HLA-G in vivo and in vitro parallels that of MHC Class I and it is up-regulated by cytokines, especially IFN-γ, at the protein and mRNA level. Although the exact role of HLA-G has not yet been determined, it is conceivable that in PM some bacterial, viral, or muscle antigens may be presented to a subset of CD8+ T cells via up-regulated HLA-G antigens. It is also conceivable that the HLA-G expression may have a protective role, as in the trophoblast, where it prevents maternal lymphocytes from attacking fetal tissue. Whether the co-expression of HLA-G and MHC Class I exerts a counterbalancing or an additive immunogenic effect remains unclear.

Co-stimulatory molecules

For the activation of T cells and antigen recognition, the presence of co-stimulatory molecules and their counter-receptors is fundamental (Reiser and Stadecker, 1996). As mentioned, in PM and IBM muscle there is evidence that the autoinvasive CD8+ T cells are preferentially recruited and clonally expanded in situ, most likely by small, muscle-specific antigenic peptides, presented by the MHC Class I molecule expressed on muscle fibers (Dalakas, 1991, 1995a, 1998; Engel et al., 1994; Hohlfeld and Engel, 1994). For antigen presentation, however, the MHC Class I expressing muscle fibers should co-express the B7 family of co-stimulatory molecules (B7-1, B7-2, or BB1) while the autoinvasive CD8+ T cells express the counter-receptors CD28 and CTLA-4 (Boussiotis et al., 1993). At least two studies have now confirmed that among the B7 family of molecules, the BB1 (CD80) is expressed on MHC Class-I-positive muscle fibers and make cell-to-cell contact with their CD28 or CTLA-4 ligand on the autoinvasive

CD8+ T cells (Behrens *et al.*, 1998; Murata and Dalakas, 1999) (Fig. 21.1). Further, the BB1 which is induced by IFN-γ on human myoblasts, is a functional molecule playing a role in antigen presentation and T-cell differentiation (Behrens *et al.*, 1998). The co-stimulatory molecule CD40, is also up-regulated on muscle fibers in patients with PM, while the CD40 ligand (CD40L) is expressed on the infiltrating T cells (Sugiura *et al.*, 2000). Because CD40 ligation induces CD80 (BB1) (van Kooten and Banchereau, 1996), the CD40/CD40L interaction in PM may enhance not only T-cell activation but also antigen presentation. The B7-related co-stimulatory molecule ICOS-L (inducible co-stimulator ligand) is also up-regulated on the muscle fibers of patients with PM and IBM while ICOS, which is expressed also by the memory T cells, is overexpressed on the endomysial T cells.

The important role of these up-regulated molecules lies in their potential for therapeutic manipulation. Humanized monoclonal antibodies against the counter-receptors CD28, CTLA4 or against CD40L are strong inhibitors of T-cell activation (Reiser and Stadecker, 1996), opening the avenue for applying semi-specific molecular immunotherapies in patients with PM, DM, and IBM.

Cytokines, cytokine signaling, chemokines, metalloproteinases, and adhesion molecules

After binding to their receptors on the cell surface, cytokines induce dimerization and phosphorylation of the Janus kinase (JAK) family of kinases, followed by phosphorylation of the signal transduction and activation of a transducer family of proteins that translocate to the nucleus for gene transcription and cell proliferation. In the muscle biopsy specimens of patients with PM, DM, and IBM, there is an overexpression of signal transduction and activation of type I transducers, indicative of cytokine up-regulation (Illa *et al.*, 1997). Polymerase chain reaction studies of muscle tissue have confirmed a varying degree of amplification of messenger RNA of the various cytokines including interleukins (IL)-1, IL-2, TNF-α, IFN-γ, TGF-β, granulocyte–macrophage colony-stimulating factor (GM-CSF), IL-6, and IL-10 (Arahata and Engel, 1986; Dalakas, 1995a, 1998; Lundberg *et al.*, 1995).

Some cytokines also exert a direct cytotoxic effect on the muscle fibers. Transgenic mice, overexpressing IFN-γ develop a necrotizing inflammatory myopathy with macrophages and calcium deposits in the necrotic fibers, resembling human PM (Shelton *et al.*, 1999). Further, IL-1β and TNF-α can be toxic to human myotubes *in vitro* (Leon-Monzon and Dalakas, 1994; Kalovidouris and Plotkin, 1995). TNF-α may also participate in the initiation of myocytotoxicity *in vivo*, as evidenced by the selective increase of TNF-α mRNA and protein in the CD8+ autoinvasive T cells around the non-necrotic muscle fibers of PM patients (Kuru *et al.*, 2000).

Chemokines, a class of small cytokines, are known participating molecules in the leukocyte recruitment and activation at the sites of inflammation. Chemokines, such as IL-8, RANTES (regulated on activation, normal T-cell expressed and secreted), monocyte chemoattractant protein 1 (MCP-1), monokine induced by IFN-γ (MIG), and inducible protein (IP)-10, are also expressed on myoblasts after proper induction by IFN-γ (De Rossi *et al.*, 2000). *In vivo*, MCP-1 and macrophage inflammatory protein (MIP)-1a, are also expressed in the endomysial inflammatory cells and the neighboring extracellular matrix of PM, IBM, and DM muscles and may be driving or amplifying the inflammatory response by facilitating the trafficking of activated T cells to the muscle (De Rossi *et al.*, 2000; Confalonieri *et al.*, 2000). The up-regulation and possibly *in situ* synthesis of MCP-1 and MIP-1a in the extracellular matrix may have an effect in promoting tissue fibrosis in the late stages of DM and IBM. Recently, IFN-γ-induced chemokines MIG and IP-10 and their mRNA as well as their receptors CXCR3 were found up-regulated on the autoinvasive CD8+ T cells. Further, IFN-γ up-regulated the mRNA expression of MIG and IP-10 by human myoblasts in a dose-dependent manner. These observations noted in PM and IBM suggest that IFN-γ is involved in the up-regulation of these chemokines which, in turn, participate in the recruitment of activated

T cells and may contribute to the self-sustaining nature of endomysial inflammation.

Another pleiotropic cytokine produced by T cells but also by human myogenic cells that promotes chronic inflammation and facilitates fibrosis, is TGF-β (Murakami *et al.*, 1999). Such an effect of TGF-β is best evident in the muscles of patients with DM, where fibrosis is prominent and TGF-β and TGF-β mRNA are up-regulated (Amemiya *et al.*, 2000b). In the repeated muscle biopsy specimens of patients with DM who improved after successful immunotherapy, there was substantial down-regulation of TGF-β and TGF-β mRNA (Amemiya *et al.*, 2000b) along with suppression of MHC Class I antigen, VCAM, ICAM-1, endomysial inflammation, and fibrosis (Dalakas *et al.*, 1993).

Another important group of molecules facilitating the adhesion and transmigration of lymphocytes is the matrix metalloproteinases (MMPs), a family of calcium-dependent zinc endopeptidases involved in the remodeling of the extracellular matrix. Pathologically, MMPs propagate the inflammatory response by facilitating T-cell adhesion to matrices and endothelial cells and the exit of lymphoid cells from the circulation to targeted tissues. Among MMPs, MMP-9 and MMP-2 are up-regulated on the non-necrotic and MHC Class I expressing muscle fibers of patients with PM and IBM (Choi and Dalakas, 2000). Further, MMP-2 immunostains the autoinvasive CD8+ T cells which make cell-to-cell contact with muscle fibers (Fig. 21.1). Because collagen IV is prominent on the muscle membrane, the overexpression of MMPs in PM and IBM may facilitate T-cell adhesion and enhance T-cell-mediated cytotoxicity by degrading extracellular matrix proteins (Choi and Dalakas, 2000). Targeting MMPs with the newly available pharmacologic agents may offer new therapeutic options in the management of patients with PM and IBM.

ICAM and VCAM are also up-regulated on the endothelial cells, fibroblasts, and infiltrating T cells in patients with PM, DM, or IBM and facilitate the transgression of T cells across the endothelial cell wall. Varying amounts of very late antigen (VLA)-4, sialyl Lewis X (SLex), and leukocyte function-associated antigen (LFA)-1a and -1b, the respective ligands for VCAM-1, endothelial leukocyte adhesion molecule (ELAM)-1, and ICAM-1, have been consistently found increased in the muscle tissue of PM, DM, IBM.

Apoptotic or antiapoptotic molecules

Cytotoxic T cells induce cell death either through the perforin pathway or the Fas/FasL-dependent process (Shresta *et al.*, 1998). In PM and IBM, the autoinvasive activated T cells contain perforin granules which are re-oriented toward the surface of the muscle fibers and, when released, induce pores on the plasma membrane, causing osmotic cell lysis (Karpati *et al.*, 1988) (Fig. 21.1). The Fas-dependent pathway is not involved in myocytic cell death nor in the death of the autoinvasive T cells, in spite of the Fas antigen expression on the muscle fibers of patients with PM or IBM and the FasL on the autoinvasive CD8+ cells (Schneider *et al.*, 1996; Behrens *et al.*, 1997). These Fas/FasL interactions do not cause apoptosis in the muscle fibers, even in patients with myositis associated with human immuno-deficiency virus (HIV) infection where apoptosis of CD8+ cells takes place in the circulation (Schneider *et al.*, 1999). The Fas-positive muscle fibers co-express the regenerating neural cell adhesion molecule (NCAM) as well as the death suppressor molecule Bcl-2, a 26 kDa anti-apoptotic proto-onco-gene protein, both of which may counteract a putative apoptotic process (Fig. 21.1).

Two additional strong anti-apoptotic molecules have recently been found to be expressed in the muscle fibers. One is the FLICE (Fas-associated death domain-like IL-1-converting enzyme)-inhibitory protein (FLIP), which inhibits Fas death receptor signaling and is expressed on the muscle fibers and infiltrating lymphocytes of PM and IBM muscle (Nagaraju *et al.*, 2000b). Because inhibition of FLIP mRNA expression facilitates apoptosis of muscle cells *in vitro*, there is a convincing argument that FLIP confers resistance of muscle to Fas-mediated apoptosis. The second relevant anti-apoptotic molecule is the human inhibitor of apoptosis (IAP)-like protein (hILP), an evolutionary conserved cell death suppressor, that exerts major anti-apoptotic effects by inhibiting the executioner caspases. In s-IBM and PM, hILP is expressed on the sarcolemmal region (Li and Dalakas, 2000a) and may act as an anti-apoptotic shield by inhibiting the caspase activation cascade initiated extracellularly by the auto-invasive CD8+ T cells. The presence of hILP and FLIP provides sufficient justification for the resistance of muscle to apoptosis.

Association with viral infections

Several viruses, including coxsackieviruses, influenza, paramyxoviruses, cytomegalovirus (CMV), and Epstein–Barr virus (EBV) have been indirectly associated with chronic and acute myositis (Leff et al., 1992). A possible molecular mimicry phenomenon has been proposed with the coxsakie-viruses because of structural homology between the Jo-1, a histidyl-transfer RNA synthetase mentioned later, and the genomic RNA of an animal picornavirus, the encephalomyocarditis virus. Our very sensitive PCR studies, however, have repeatedly failed to confirm the presence of such viruses in these patients' muscle biopsies suggesting that it is unlikely, although not impossible, for these viruses to replicate in the muscles of patients with PM, DM, and IBM (Leff et al., 1992; Leon-Monzon and Dalakas, 1992).

The best evidence of a viral connection in PM and IBM is with retroviruses which have been associated with inflammatory myopathy in monkeys infected with the simian immunodeficiency virus (SIV) (Dalakas et al., 1986a), and in humans infected with HIV and HTLV-I (Dalakas et al., 1986b; Morgan et al., 1989). In HIV-positive patients, an inflammatory myopathy (HIV-PM) can occur either as an isolated clinical phenomenon, being the first clinical indication of HIV infection, or concurrently with other manifestations of the acquired immune deficiency syndrome (AIDS) (Dalakas et al., 1986b; Dalakas and Pezeshkpour, 1988). HIV seroconversion can also coincide with myoglobulinuria and acute myalgia, suggesting that myotropism for HIV may be symptomatic early in the infection. In addition, HTLV-I does not only cause a myeloneuropathy—referred to as tropical spastic paraparesis (TSP)—but also polymyositis, which may coexist with TSP or may be the only clinical manifestation of HTLV-I infection (Morgan et al., 1989; Leon-Monzon et al., 1994). Of interest, IBM can also occur in a setting of HIV or HTLV-I infection (Cupler et al., 1996). Using in situ hybridization, PCR, immunocytochemistry, and electron microscopy we could not detect viral antigens within the muscle fibers of these patients' muscle biopsies but only in occasional endomysial macrophages (Illa et al., 1991; Leon-Monzon et al., 1994; Cupler et al., 1996). We have interpreted these observations to suggest that in HIV-1 and HTLV-I PM and IBM there is no evidence of persistent infection of the muscle fiber with the virus or viral replication within the muscle. The predominant endomysial cell in HIV-1 and HTLV-I PM and IBM are CD8+, non-viral-specific, cytotoxic T cells which along with macrophages invade or surround MHC Class I antigen expressing non-necrotic muscle fibers. Because this immunopathological pattern is identical to the one described earlier for retroviral-negative PM and IBM, a T-cell-mediated and MHC Class I restricted cytotoxic process appears to be a common pathogenetic mechanism in both retroviral-negative and retroviral-positive PM and IBM. In the retroviral-positive patients, however, viral-induced cyokines may be the triggering factors for T-cell activation and MHC up-regulation.

Future investigations

In spite of the progress made, a number of missing links need to be identified, most importantly, the nature of the antigenic peptide bound by the MHC Class I molecules for presentation to CD8+ T cells. Whether this is an endogenous self-protein synthesized within the muscle fiber or is an endogenous peptide, i.e. a virus, is unclear. The failure to amplify viruses within the muscle fibers does not exclude involvement of viruses that 'hit and run'. In IBM, the mystery of the inflammation is disturbing because in spite of its similarities to PM, the disease remains resistant to immuno-therapies, as discussed later.

Degenerative features in s-IBM and interrelationship between amyloid, cytokines, and inflammation

In IBM, the presence of amyloid-positive deposits within some of the vacuolated muscle fibers, and the finding of abnormal mitochondria, has generated reasonable concerns that, in addition to the autoimmune components mentioned earlier, there is also a degenerative process (Askanas and Engel, 1988; Mendell et al., 1991; Askanas et al., 1992a,b; Barohn et al., 1995; Sivakumar and Dalakas, 1996, 1997; Santorelli et al., 1996). The latter is supported by the resistance of IBM to immunotherapies and the observation that vacuoles increase with chronicity of the disease (Barohn et al., 1995). Of interest, vacuoles are almost always present in muscle fibers not invaded by T cells; in contrast, the muscle fibers undergoing T-cell invasion are seemingly healthy but never vacuolated.

The amyloid in IBM is accompanied by all the other proteins seen in the β-amyloid of Alzheimer's disease, including β-APP, chymotrypsin, apoE, and phosphorylated tau (Askanas and Engel, 1988; Mendell et al., 1991; Askanas et al., 1992a,b). Whether these deposits are secondarily related to the chronicity of the disease or they are generated de novo and contribute to disease pathogenesis remains unclear. The mitochondrial abnormalities and the mitochondrial DNA deletions appear to be secondary, perhaps augmented by the up-regulated cytokines, because similar changes are seen in the normal aging muscle. Also, they do not seem to contribute to muscle dysfunction because ^{31}P magnetic resonance spectroscopy has shown normal muscle oxidative metabolism during recovery from exercise (Argov et al., 1998).

The vacuolated muscle fibers express mitogen activated protein kinases (MAPKs), and more specifically the active P42 MAPK, indicating abnormal intracellular protein phosphorylation (Li and Dalakas, 2000b). The chaperone aB crystallin stress protein is specifically up-regulated in apparently healthy, non-vacuolated muscle fibers. Whether this is a sign of a stressor effect before vacuolar formation, or it serves as a putative autoantigen, remains to be determined (Banwell and Engel, 2000).

A link between β-APP and inflammation may be via IL-1, TNF-α, and MMP-2, all of which are up-regulated on the amyloid deposits (Dalakas, 1998). In IBM, the noted excess of IL-1β may be derived not only from the abundant endomysial macrophages and T cells but also by the β-APP, which is a known enhancer of IL-1β production. In turn, IL-1β up-regulates β-APP and β-APP gene expression and closes the loop, as follows: IL1β ↔ β-APP ↔ IL1β ↔ inflammation (Dalakas, 1998). Treatment trials with agents that deplete inflammation or break the amyloid deposits may tell us which of the two is the main culprit in IBM.

Presence of autoantibodies

Various autoantibodies against nuclear (antinuclear antibodies) and cytoplasmic antigens are found in up to 20% of patients with inflammatory myopathies (Dalakas, 1991, 1998; Engel et al., 1994; Plotz et al., 1989; Targoff, 1990). The antibodies to cytoplasmic antigens are directed against cytoplasmic ribonucleoproteins which are involved in translation and protein synthesis. They include antibodies against various synthetases, translation factors, and proteins of the signal-recognition particles. The antibody directed against the histidyl-transfer RNA synthetase, called anti-Jo-1, accounts for 75% of all the antisynthetases and it is clinically useful because up to 80% of patients with anti-Jo-1 antibodies have interstitial lung disease. In general, these antibodies may be non-muscle specific because: (1) they are directed against ubiquitous targets and may represent epiphenomena of no pathogenic significance; (2) they occur in all three subtypes (PM, DM, and rarely in IBM), in spite of their clinical and immunopathologic differences; and (3) they are almost always associated with interstitial lung disease even in patients who do not have active myositis. No benefit of intravenous immunoglobulin (IV Ig) was found (Dalakas et al., 2001).

Treatment

Because the specific target antigens in DM, PM, and IBM are unknown, the immunosuppressive therapies are not selectively targeting the autoreactive T cells or the complement-mediated process on the intramuscular blood vessels. Instead, they are inducing a non-selective immunosuppression or immunomodulation. Further, many of these therapies are empirical, and mostly uncontrolled (Dalakas, 1989, 1992, 1994a,b). The goal of therapy in the inflammatory myopathies is to improve the function in activities of daily living as the result of improvement in muscle strength. Although when the strength improves the serum CK falls concurrently the reverse is not always true, because most of the immunosuppressive therapies can result in decrease of serum muscle enzymes without necessarily improving muscle strength. The following agents are used in the treatment of PM and DM:

1. Corticosteroids. Prednisone is the first-line drug of this empirical treatment. Its action is unclear, but it may exert a beneficial effect by inhibiting recruitment and migration of lymphocytes to the areas of muscle inflammation and interfering with the production of lymphokines.

   Our preference has been to start with a high-dose prednisone, 80–100 mg/day, from early in the disease. After an initial period of 3–4 weeks, prednisone is tapered over a 10-week period to 80–100 mg single daily/alternate-day by gradually reducing an alternate 'off day' dose by 10 mg per week, or faster if necessitated by side-effects, though this carries a greater risk of breakthrough of disease. Although almost all the patients with bona fide PM or DM respond to steroids to some degree and for some period of time, a number of them fail to respond or become steroid-resistant. The decision to start an immunosuppressive drug in PM or DM patients is based on the following factors: (a) need for its 'steroid-sparing' effect, when in spite of steroid responsiveness the patient has developed significant complications; (b) attempts to lower a high steroid dosage have repeatedly resulted in a new relapse; (c) adequate dose of prednisone for at least a 2–3 month period has been ineffective; and (d) rapidly progressive disease with evolving severe weakness and respiratory failure. The preference for selecting the next in line immunosuppressive therapy is, however, empirical. The choice is usually based on our own prejudices, our personal experience with each drug, and our own assessment of the relative efficacy/safety ratio. The following immunosuppressive agents are then used.

2. Azathioprine. This is a derivative of 6-mercaptopurine and it is given orally. Although lower doses (1.5–2 mg/kg) are commonly used, we prefer higher doses, up to 3 mg/kg for effective immunosuppression.

3. Methotrexate. This is an antagonist of folate metabolism. It has a faster action than azathioprine. It is given orally starting at 7.5 mg weekly for the first 3 weeks (given in a total of three doses, 2.5 mg every 12 hours), increasing it gradually by 2.5 mg/week up to a total of 25 mg weekly. A relevant side-effect is methotrexate pneumonitis which can be difficult to distinguish from the interstitial lung disease of the primary myopathy, often associated with Jo-1 antibodies, as described above.

4. Cyclophosphamide. This alkylating agent is given intravenously or orally, at doses of 2.0–2.5 mg/kg, usually 50 mg orally three times a day. Cyclophosphamide has not been ineffective in our hands (Cronin et al., 1989) in spite of occasional promising results reported by others (Bombardieri et al., 1989).

5. Chlorambucil. This is an antimetabolite that has been tried in some patients with variable results (Sinoway and Callen, 1993).

6. Ciclosporin. Although the toxicity of the drug can now be monitored by measuring optimal trough serum levels (which vary between 100 and 250 ng/ml), its effectiveness in PM and DM is uncertain. A report that low doses of ciclosporin could be of benefit in children with DM needs confirmation (Heckmatt et al., 1989). The advantage of ciclosporin is that it is faster acting than azathioprine or methotrexate (Grau et al., 1994).

7. Mycophenolate mofetil is emerging as an interesting, promising, and well-tolerated drug at doses up to 2 g per day.

8. Plasmapheresis was not helpful in a double-blind, placebo-controlled study that we have conducted (Miller et al., 1992).

9. Total lymphoid irradiation. This has been helpful in rare patients and may have long-lasting benefit. The long-term side-effects of this treatment, however, should be seriously considered before deciding on this experimental and rather extreme approach. Total lymphoid irradiation has been ineffective in IBM (Kelly et al., 1986).

10. Intravenous immunoglobulin (IV Ig). In uncontrolled studies, IV Ig was effective (Cherin et al., 1991; Lang et al., 1991; Jan et al., 1992). In the first double-blind study conducted for DM, we have demonstrated that IV Ig is effective in patients with refractory DM. Not only does strength improves but the underlying immunopathology may resolve (Dalakas et al., 1993). The improvement begins after the first IV Ig infusion but it is clearly evident by the second monthly infusion. The benefit is short-lived (not more than 8 weeks) requiring repeated infusions every 6–8 weeks to maintain improvement. A controlled double-blind study for PM has never been completed. However, the drug has been effective in up to 80% of the patients in uncontrolled series.

    The mechanism of action of IV Ig in DM may be by inhibiting the deposition of activated complement fragment on the capillaries, by suppressing cytokines especially ICAM-1, or by saturating Fc receptors and interfering with the action of macrophages (Soueidan and Dalakas, 1993; Dalakas, 1997). IV Ig has also exerted some benefit, although not statistically significant, in up to 30% of patients with IBM in a controlled double-blind study we conducted (Dalakas et al., 1997). Although the improvement was not dramatic, it made a difference to these patients' life styles. A second controlled study showed similar effects (Walter et al., 2000). A third controlled study that investigated if IV Ig in combination with prednisone is better than prednisone alone showed no benefit of IV Ig (Dalakas et al., 2001).

Future immunotherapies

Although the immunosuppressive therapies in DM and PM are not antigen-specific, they induce significant improvement in most of patients for a period of time.

For IBM, treatment decisions are difficult. If mild, we may do nothing or add low-dose steroids combined with CoQ10 and an exercise program. If the disease is rapidly worsening and dysphagia is life-threatening, we try IV Ig. The value of mycophenolate has not been studied. Recent progress in molecular immunology will allow the application of more rational therapeutic approaches (Dalakas, in press a).

Blockade of the signal transduction in T lymphocytes

Selective inhibition of TCR signaling pathways induces selective immunosuppression. Upon TCR ligation, there is activation of several tyrosin kinases, which leads to transcriptional activation of the cytoplasmic serine phosphatase calcineurin (Halloran, 2000). Calcineurin leads to activation of IL-2 promoter. Two immunosuppressive drugs, FK506 and ciclosporin inhibit the calcineurin phosphatase activity (Halloran, 2000) and appear promising in difficult cases. Rapamycin, which acts via a calcineurin-independent pathway to prevent the translation of mRNA for key cytokines, is another promising drug. Further, the co-stimulatory molecules CD28 and CTLA-4 which are up-regulated in PM and IBM, may become specific targets for immunotherapy. The currently available monoclonal antibodies against CD28/CTLA-4 which induce anergy by blocking co-stimulation, may be considered.

Agents against immunomodulating cytokines

There are two approaches:

1. Anti-TNF-α strategies: TNF-α is not only up-regulated in vivo in PM and IBM muscle but it is also toxic to myotubes in vitro. The currently

available monoclonal antibodies against TNF-α may be considered for future trials.

2. β-Interferons. These agents, currently used in multiple sclerosis, may be also applicable for trials in inflammatory myopathies.

Agents against adhesion molecules and receptors (anticellular 'glues')

1. Matrix metalloproteinases (MMPs). These are endopeptidases that play a fundamental role in T-cell attachment to the endothelial cell wall and muscle fibers. Among them MMP-2 and MMP-9 are up-regulated in PM and IBM muscles. Currently available drugs that block the activity of MMPs may be considered for future trials.

2. Integrins and their receptors. Integrins integrate the activation of extracellular matrix and cytoskeleton and facilitate cell-to-cell and cell-to-matrix communication. Among them, β$_2$ integrins/VCAM receptors, β$_1$ integrins/ICAM-1, and α$_2$ and β$_4$ integrins/LFA-1, are up-regulated in PM, DM, and IBM muscles and facilitate T-cell transport across the blood vessel wall. Available agents against integrins and their receptors may be considered in future trials.

References

Amemiya, K., Granger, R.P., and Dalakas, M.C. (2000*a*). Clonal restriction of T-cell receptor expression by infiltrating lymphocytes in inclusion body myositis persists over time: studies in repeated muscle biopsies. *Brain* 123: 2030–2039.

Amemiya, K., Semino-Mora, C., Granger, R.P., and Dalakas, M.C. (2000*b*). Downregulation of TGF-β1 mRNA and protein in the muscles of patients with inflammatory myopathies after treatment with high-dose intravenous immunoglobulin. *Clin Immunol* 94: 99–104.

Arahata, K. and Engel, A.G. (1986). Monoclonal antibody analysis of mononuclear cells in myopathies III. Immunoelectron microscopy aspects of cell-mediated muscle fiber injury. *Ann Neurol* 19: 112–125.

Argov, Z., Taivassalo, T., De Stefano, N., Genge, A., Karpati, G., and Arnold, D.L. (1998). Intracellular phosphates in inclusion body myositis—a ^{31}P magnetic resonance imaging study. *Muscle Nerve* 21: 1523–1525.

Askanas V. and Engel, W.K. (1988). Sporadic inclusion body myositis and hereditary inclusion-body myopathies. *Arch Neurol* 55: 915–920.

Askanas, V., Serdaroglu, P., Engel, W.K., and Alvarez, R.B. (1992*a*). Immunocytochemical localization of ubiquitin in inclusion body myositis allows its light-microscopic distinction from polymyositis. *Neurology* 42: 460–461.

Askanas, V., Engel, W.K., Alvarez, R.B., and Glenner, G.G. (1992*b*). β-amyloid protein immunoreactivity in muscle of patients with inclusion-body myositis. *Lancet* 339: 560–561.

Banker, B.Q. (1975). Dermatomyositis of childhood. Ultrastructural alterations of muscle and intramuscular blood vessels. *J Neurop Exp Neurol* 35: 46–75.

Banwell, B.L. and Engel, A.G. (2000). AB-crystallin immunolocalization yields new insights into inclusion body myositis. *Neurology* 54: 1033.

Bao, S.S., King, N.J., and dos Remedios, C.G. (1990). Elevated MHC class I and II antigens in cultured human embryonic myoblasts following stimulation with gamma-interferon. *Immunol Cell Biol* 68: 235–241.

Barohn, R.J., Amato, A.A., Sahenk, Z., Kissel, J.T., and Mendell, J.R. (1995). Inclusion body myositis; explanation for poor response to immunosuppressive therapy. *Neurology* 45: 1302–1304.

Basta, M. and Dalakas, M.C. (1994). High-dose intravenous immunoglobulin exerts its beneficial effect in patients with dermatomyositis by blocking endomysial deposition of activated complement fragments. *J Clin Invest* 94: 1729–1735.

Behrens, L., Bender, A., Johnson, M.A., and Hohlfeld R. (1997). Cytotoxic mechanisms in inflammatory myopathies: co-expression of Fas and protective Bcl-2 in muscle fibres and inflammatory cells. *Brain* 120: 929.

Behrens, L., Kerschensteiner, M., Misgeld, T., Goebels, N., Wekerle, H., and Hohlfeld R. (1998). Human muscle cells express a functional costimulatory molecule distinct from B7.1 (CD80) and B7.2 (CD86) *in vitro* and in inflammatory lesions. *J Immunol* 161: 5943–5951.

Bender, A., Behrens, L., Engel, A.G., and Hohlfeld R. (1998). T-cell heterogeneity in muscle lesions of inclusion body myositis. *J Neuroimmunol* 84: 86–91.

Bender, A., Ernst, N., Iglesias, A., Dornmair, K., Wekeria, H., and Hohlfeld R. (1995). T cell receptor repertoire in polymyositis: clonal expansion of autoaggresive CD8 T cells. *J Exp Med* 181: 1863–1868.

Bombardieri, S., Hughes, G.R.V., Neri, R., Del Bravo, P., and Del Bono L. (1989). Cyclophosphamide in severe polymyositis. *Lancet* 1: 1138–1139.

Boussiotis, V.A., Freeman, G.J., Gribben, J.G., Daley, J., Gray, G., and Nadler, L.M. (1993). Activated human B lymphocytes express three CTLA-4 counter-receptors that costimulate T cell activation. *Proc Natl Acad Sci USA* 90: 11059–11063.

Carpenter, S., Karpati, G., Rothman, S., and Walters G. (1976). The childhood type of dermatomyositis. *Neurology* 26: 952–962.

Cervera, R., Ramires, G., Fernandez-Sola J., *et al.* (1991). Antibodies to endothelial cells in dermatomyositis: association with interstitial lung diseases. *Br Med J* 302: 880–882.

Cherin, P., Herson, S., Wechsler, B., *et al.* (1991). Efficacy of intravenous immunoglobulin therapy in chronic refractory polymyositis and dermatomyositis. An open study with 20 adult patients. *Am J Med* 91: 162–168.

Choi, Y.C. and Dalakas, M.C. (2000). Expression of matrix metalloproteinases in the muscle of patients with inflammatory myopathies. *Neurology* 54: 65–71.

Clawson, K. and Oddis, C.V. (1995). Adult respiratory distress syndrome in polymyositis patients with the anti-Jo-I antibody. *Arthritis Rheum* 38: 1519–1523.

Confalonieri, P., Bernasconi, P., Megna, P., Galbiati, S., Cornelio, F., and Mantegazza R. (2000). Increased expression of beta-chemokines in muscle of patients with inflammatory myopathies. *J Neuropathol Exp Neurol* 59: 164–169.

Cronin, M.E., Miller, F.W., Hicks, J.E., Dalakas, M., and Plotz, P.H. (1989). The failure of intravenous cyclophosphamide therapy in refractory idiopathic inflammatory myopathy. *J Rheumatol* 16: 1225–1228.

Cupler, E.J., Leon-Monzon, M., Miller, J., Semino-Mora, C., Anderson, T.L., and Dalakas, M.C. (1996). Inclusion body myositis in HIV-I and HTLV-I infected patients. *Brain* 119: 1887–1893.

Dalakas, M.C. (1989). Treatment of polymyositis and dermatomyositis. *Curr Opin Rheumatol* 1: 443–449.

Dalakas, M.C. (1991). Polymyositis, dermatomyositis and inclusion-body myositis. *N Engl J Med* 325: 1487–1498.

Dalakas, M.C. (1992). Inflammatory myopathies: In: *Handbook of Clinical Neurology, Vol. 18 (62): Myopathies* (ed. L.P. Rowland and S. DiMauro), pp. 369–390. Elsevier Science Publishers, Amsterdam.

Dalakas, M.C. (1994*a*). How to diagnose and treat the inflammatory myopathies. *Semin Neurol* 14: 137–145.

Dalakas, M.C. (1994*b*). Current treatment of the inflammatory myopathies. *Curr Opin Rheumatol* 6: 595–601.

Dalakas, M.C. (1995*a*). Immunopathogenesis of inflammatory myopathies. *Ann Neurol* 37(Suppl. 1): S74–S86.

Dalakas, M.C. (1995*b*). Images in clinical medicine. Calcifications in dermatomyositis. *N Engl J Med* 333: 978.

Dalakas, M.C. (1997). Intravenous immunoglobulin therapy for neurological diseases. *Ann Intern Med* 126: 721–730.

Dalakas, M.C. (1998). Molecular immunology and genetics of inflammatory muscle diseases. *Arch Neurol* 55: 1509–1512.

Dalakas, M.C. The molecular and cellular pathology of inflammatory muscle diseases. *Curr Opin Pharmacol* (in press a).

Dalakas, M.C. Progress in inflammatory myopathies: good but not good enough. Editorial. *J Neurol Neurosurg Psychiatry* (in press b).

Dalakas, M.C. and Pezeshkpour, G.H. (1988). Neuromuscular diseases associated with human immunodeficiency virus infection. *Ann Neurol* 23(Suppl.): 38–48.

Dalakas, M.C., London, W.T., Gravell, M., and Sever, J.L. (1986*a*). Polymyositis in an immunodeficiency disease in monkeys induced by a type D retrovirus. *Neurology* 36: 569–572.

Dalakas, M.C., Pezeshkpour, G.H., Gravell, M., and Sever, J.L. (1986*b*). Polymyositis in patients with AIDS. *J Am Med Assoc* 256: 2381–2383.

Dalakas, M.C., Illa, I., Dambrosia, J.M., Soueidan, S.A., Stein, D.P., Otero, C., et al. (1993). A controlled trial of high-dose intravenous immunoglobulin infusions as treatment for dermatomyositis. N Engl J Med 329: 1993–2000.

Dalakas, M.C., Sekul, E.A., Cupler, E.J., and Sivakumar K. (1997). The efficacy of high dose intravenous immunoglobulin (IVIg) in patients with inclusion-body myositis (IBM). Neurology 48: 712–716.

Dalakas, M.C., Koffman, B., Fujii, M., Spector, S., Sivakumar, K., and Cupler E. (2001). A controlled study of intravenous immunoglobulin combined with prednisone in the treatment of IBM. Neurology 56: 323–327.

De Bleecker, J.L., Meire, V.I., Declercq, W., and Van Aken, H.E. (1999). Immunolocalization of tumor necrosis factor-alpha and its receptors in inflammatory myopathies. Neuromusc Disord 9: 239.

De Rossi, M., Bernasconi, P., Bagfi, F., de Waal Maleft, R., and Mantegazza R. (2000). Cytokines and chemokines are both expressed by human myoblasts: possible relevance for the immune pathogenesis of muscle inflammation. Int Immunol 12: 1329–1335.

Emslie-Smith, A.M. and Engel A.G. (1990). Microvascular changes in early and advanced dermatomyositis: a quantitative study. Ann. Neurol 27: 343–356.

Engel, A.G., Hohfeld, R., and Banker, B.Q. (1994). The polymyositis and dermatomyositis syndromes. In: Myology, 2nd edn (ed. A.G. Engel and C. Franzini-Armstrong), pp. 1335–1383. McGraw-Hill, New York.

Fyhr, I.M., Moslemi, A.R., Mosavi, A.A., Lindberg, C., Tarkowski, A., and Oldfors A. (1997). Oligoclonal expansion of muscle infiltrating T cells in inclusion body myositis. J Neuroimmunol 79: 185–189.

Goebel, N., Michaelis, D., Engelhardt, M., Huber, S., Bender, A., et al. (1996). Differential expression of perforin in muscle-infiltrating T cell in polymyositis and dermatomyositis. J Clin Invest 97: 2905.

Grau, J.M., Herrero, C., Casademont, J., et al. (1994). Cyclosporine A as first choice for dermatomyositis. J Rheumatol 21: 381–382.

Griggs, R.C., Askanas, V., Di Mauro, S., et al. (1995). Inclusion body myositis and myopathies. Ann Neurol 38: 705–713.

Halloran, P.F. (2000). Sirolimus and ciclosporin for renal transplantation. Lancet 356: 179–180.

Heckmatt, J., Hasson, N., Saunders, C., et al. (1989). Cyclosporin in juvenile dermatomyositis. Lancet 1: 1063–1066.

Hohlfeld, R. and Engel, A.G. (1991). Coculture with autologous myotubes of cytotoxic T cells isolated from muscle in inflammatory myopathies. Ann Neurol 29: 498–507.

Hohlfeld, R. and Engel, A.G. (1990). Induction of HLA-DR expression on human myoblasts with interferon-gamma. Am J Pathol 136: 503.

Hohlfeld, R. and Engel, A.G. (1994). The immunobiology of muscle. Immunol Today 15: 269–274.

Hohlfeld, R., Goebels, N., and Engel A.G. (1993). Cellular mechanisms in inflammatory myopathies. In: Bailliere's Clinical Neurology (ed. F. L. Mastaglia), pp. 617–636. W.B. Saunders, London.

Illa, I., Nath, A., and Dalakas, M.C. (1991). Immunocytochemical and virological characteristics of HIV-associated inflammatory myopathies: similarities with seronegative polymyositis. Ann Neurol 29: 474–481.

Illa, I., Gallardo, E., Gimeno, R., Serrano, C., Ferrer, I., and Juarez C. (1997). Signal transducer and activator of transcription 1 in human muscle: implications in inflammatory myopathies. Am J Pathol 151: 81–88.

Jan, S., Beretta, S., Mogfio, M., Alobbati, L., and Pellegrini G. (1992). High-dose intravenous human immunoglobulin in polymyositis resistant to treatment. J Neurol Neurosug Psych 55: 60–64.

Kalovidouris, A.E. and Plotkin Z. (1995). Synergistic cytotoxic effect of interferon γ and tumor necrosis factor α on cultured human muscle cells. J Rheumatol 22: 1698–1703.

Karpati, G. and Carpenter S. (1988). Idiopathic inflammatory myopathies. Curr Opin. Neurol Neurosurg 1: 806–814.

Karpati, G., Pouliot, Y., and Carpenter S. (1988). Expression of immunoreactive major histocapability complex products in human skeletal muscles. Ann Neurol 23: 64–72.

Kelly, J.J. Jr, Madoc-Jones, H., Adelman, L.S., Andres, P.L., and Munsat, T.L. (1986). Total body irradiation not effective in inclusion body myositis. Neurology 36: 1264–1266.

Kissel, J.T., Mendell, J.R., and Rammohan, K.W. (1986). Microvascular deposition of complement membrane attack complex in dermatomyositis. N Engl J Med 314: 329–334.

Koffman, B.M., Sivakumar, K., Simonis, T., Stroncek, D., and Dalakas, M.C. (1998). HLA allele distribution distinguishes sporadic inclusion body myositis from hereditary inclusion body myopathies. J Neuroimmunol 84: 139–142.

Kuru, S., Inukai, A., Liang, Y., Doyu, M., Takano, A., and Sobue G. (2000). Tumor necrosis factor-a expression in muscles of polymyositis and dermatomyositis. Acta Neuropathol 99: 585–588.

Lang, B., Laxer, R.M., Murphy, G., et al. (1991). Treatment of dermatomyositis with intravenous immunoglobulin. Am J Med 91: 169–172.

Leff, R.L., Love, L.A., Miller, F.W., Greenberg, S.J., Klein, E.A., Dalakas, M.C., et al. (1992). Viruses in the idiopathic inflammatory myopathies: absence of candidate viral genomes in muscle. Lancet 339: 1192–1195.

Leon-Monzon, M. and Dalakas, M.C. (1992). Absence of persistent infection with enteroviruses in muscles of patients with inflammatory myopathies. Ann Neurol 32: 219–222.

Leon-Monzon, M. and Dalakas, M.C. (1994). Interleukin-1 (IL-1) is toxic to human muscle. Neurology 44(Suppl.): 132.

Leon-Monzon, M., Illa, I., and Dalakas, M.C. (1994). Polymyositis in patients infected with HTLV-I: the role of the virus in the cause of the disease. Ann Neurol 36: 643–649.

Li, M. and Dalakas, M.C. (2000a). Expression of human IAP-like protein in skeletal muscle: an explanation for the rare incidence of muscle fiber apoptosis in T-cell mediated inflammatory myopathies. J Neuroimmunol 106: 1–5.

Li, M. and Dalakas, M.C. (2000b). The muscle mitogen-activated protein kinase is altered in sporadic inclusion body myositis. Neurology 54: 1665–1670.

Luciano, C.A. and Dalakas, M.C. (1997). A macro-EMG study in inclusion-body myositis: no evidence for a neurogenic component. Neurology 48: 29–33.

Lundberg, I., Brengman, J.M., and Engel, A.G. (1995). Analysis of cytokine expression in muscle in inflammatory myopathies, Duchenne's dystrophy and non-weak controls. J Neuroimmunol 63: 9–16.

Mantegazza, R., Hughes, S.M., Mitchell D, Travis, M., Blau, H.M., and Steinman L. (1991). Modulation of MHC class II antigen expression in human myoblasts after treatment with IFN-gamma. Neurology 41: 1128.

Mantegazza, R., Andreetta, F., Bernasconi, P., et al. (1993). Analysis of T cell receptor repertoire of muscle infiltrating T lymphocytes in polymyositis: restricted V α/β rearrangements may indicated antigen-driven selection. J Clin Invest 91: 2880–2886.

Mendell, J.R., Sahenk, Z., Gales, T., and Paul L. (1991). Amyloid filaments in inclusion body myositis. Arch Neurol 48: 1229–1234.

Metcalf, D., Di Rago, L., Mifsud, S., Hartley, L., and Alexander, W.S. (2000). The development of fatal myocarditis and Polymyositis in mice heterozygous for IFN-g and lacking the SOCS-1 gene. Proc Natl Acad Sci USA 97: 9174–9179.

Michaelis, D., Goebels, N., and Hohlfeld R. (1993). Constitutive and cytokine-induced expression of human leukocyte antigens and cell adhesion molecules by human myotubes. Am J Pathol 143: 1142.

Miller, F.W., Leitman, S.F., Cronin, M.E., et al. (1992). A randomized double-blind controlled trial of plasma exchange and leukapheresis in patients with polymyositis and dermatomyositis. N Engl J Med 326: 1380–1384.

Mitrani-Rosenbaum, S., Argov, Z., Blumenfeld, A., Seidmen, C.E., and Seidman, J.G. (1996). Hereditary inclusion body myopathy maps to chromosome 9p1-a1. Hum Mol Genet 5: 159–163.

Morgan, O. St C., Rodgers-Johnson, P., Mora, C., and Char G. (1989). HTLV-1 and polymyositis in Jamaica. Lancet ii: 1184–1187.

Murakami, N., McLennan, I.S., Nonaka, I., Koishi, K., Baker, C., and Tooke-Hammond G. (1999). Transforming growth factor-b2 is elevated in skeletal muscle disorders. Muscle Nerve 22: 889–898.

Murata, K. and Dalakas, M.C. (1999). Expression of the costimulatory molecule BB-1, the ligands CTLA-4 and CD28 and their mRNA in inflammatory myopathies. Am J Pathol 155: 453–460.

Nagaraju, K., Raben, N., Loeffler, L., Parker, T., Rochon, P.J., Lee, E., et al. (2000a). Conditional up-regulation of MHC class I in skeletal muscle leads to self-sustaining autoimmune myositis and myositis-specific autoantibodies. Proc Natl Acad Sci USA 97: 9209–9214.

Nagaraju, K., Casciola-Rosen, L., Rosen, A., Thompson, C., Loeffler, L., Parker, T., et al. (2000b). The inhibition of apoptosis in myositis and in normal muscle cells. J Immunol 164: 5459–5465.

Nyberg, P., Wikman, A.L., Nennesmo, I., and Lundberg I. (2000). Increased expression of interleukin 1a and MHC Class I in muscle tissue of patients with chronic, inactive polymyositis and dermatomyositis. J Rheumatol 27: 940–948.

O'Hanlon, T.P., Dalakas, M.C., Plotz, P.H., and Miller, F.W. (1994). Predominant I T cell receptor variable and joining gene expression by muscle-infiltrating lymphocytes in the idiopathic inflammatory myopathies. J Immunol 152: 2569–2576.

Peng, A., Koffman, B.M., Malley, J.D., and Dalakas, M.C. (2000). Diseases progression in sporadic inclusion body Myositis (s-IBM): observation in 78 patients. Neurology 55: 296–298.

Plotz, P.H., Dalakas, M., Leff, R.L., Love, L.A., Miller, F.W., and Cronin, M.E. (1989). Current concepts in the idiopathic inflammatory myopathies: polymyositis, dermatomyositis and related disorders. Ann Intern Med 111: 143–157.

Reiser, H. and Stadecker, M.J. (1996). Costimulatory B7 molecules in the pathogenesis of infectious and autoimmune diseases. N Engl J Med 335: 1369–1377.

Roy, R., Danserau, G., Tremblay, J.P., Belles-Isles, M., Huard, J., Labrecque, C., et al. (1991). Expression of major histocompatibility complex antigens on human myoblasts. Transplant Proc 23: 799.

Santorelli, F.M., Sciacco, M., Tanji, K., et al. (1996). Multiple mitochondrial DNA deletions in sporadic inclusion body myositis: a study of 56 patients. Ann Neurol 39: 789–795.

Schneider, C., Gold, R., Dalakas, M.C., Schmied, M., Lassmann, H., Toyka, K.V., et al. (1996). MHC class I mediated cytotoxicity does not induce apoptosis in muscle fibers nor in inflammatory T cells: Studies in patients with polymyositis, dermatomyositis, and inclusion body myositis. J Neuropathol Exp Neurol 55: 1205–1209.

Schneider, C., Dalakas, M.C., Toyka, K.V., Said, G., Hartung, H.P., and Gold R. (1999). T cell apoptosis in inflammatory neuromuscular disorders associated with human immunodeficiency virus infection. Arch Neurol 56: 79–83.

Schwarz, M.I., Sutarik, J.M., Nick, J.A., Leff, J.A., Emlen, J.W., and Tuder, R.M. (1995). Pulmonary capillaritis and diffuse alveolar hemmorrhage: a primary manifestation of polymyositis. Am J Respir Crit Care Med 151: 2037–2040.

Sekul, E.A. and Dalakas, M.C. (1993). Inclusion body myositis: new concepts. Semin Neurol 13: 256–263.

Shelton , G.D., Calcutt, N.A., Garrett, R.S., Gu, D., Sarvetnick, N., Campana, W.M., et al. (1999). Necrotizing myopathy induced by overexpression of interferon-γ in transgenic mice. Muscle Nerve 22: 156–165.

Shresta, S., Pham, C.T., Thomas, D.A., Graubert, T.A., and Ley, T.J. (1998). How do cytotoxic lymphocytes kill their targets? Curr Opin Immunol 10: 581.

Sinoway, T.A. and Callen, J.P. (1993). Chlorambucil: an effective corticosteroid-sparing agent for patients with recalcitrant dermatomyositis. Arthritis Rheum 36: 319–324.

Sivakumar, K. and Dalakas, M.C. (1996). The spectrum of familial inclusion body myopathies in 13 families and description of a quadriceps sparing phenotype in non-Iranian Jews. Neurology 47: 977–984.

Sivakumar, K. and Dalakas, M.C. (1997). Inclusion body myositis and myopathies. Curr Opin Neurol 10: 413–420.

Sivakumar, K., Semino-Mora, and Dalakas, M.C. (1997). An inflammatory, familial, inclusion body myositis with autoimmune features and a phenotype identical to sporadic inclusion body myositis: studies in 3 families. Brain 120: 653–661.

Soueidan, S.A. and Dalakas, M.C. (1993). Treatment of inclusion-body myositis with high-dose intravenous immunoglobulin. Neurology 43: 876–879.

Starr, R., Willson, T.A., Viney, E.M., Murray, L.J., Rayner, J.R., Jenkins, B.J., et al. (1997). A family of cytokine-inducible inhibitors of signaling. Nature 387: 917–921.

Stein, D.P. and Dalakas, M.C. (1993). Intercellular adhesion molecule-i expression is upregulated in patients with dermatomyositis (DM). Ann Neurol 34: 268.

Stein, D.P., Jordan, S.C., Toyoda, M., Gallera, O., and Dalakas, M.C. (1993). Anti-endothelial cell antibodies (AECA) in dermatomyositis (DM). Neurology 43(Suppl.): 356.

Sugiura, T., Kawaguchi, Y., Harigai, M., Takagi, K., Ohta, S., Fukasawa, C., et al. (2000). Increased CD40 expression on muscle cells of polymyositis and dermatomyositis: role of CD40-CD40 ligand interaction in IL-6, IL-8, IL-15 and monocyte chemoattractant protein-1 production. J Immunol 164: 6593–6600.

Targoff, I.N. (1990). Immune mechanisms of myositis. Curr Opin Rheumatol 2: 882–888.

Tews, D.S. and Goebel, H.H. (1996). Cytokine expression profiles in idiopathic inflammatory myopathies. J Neuropathol Exp Neurol 55: 342–347.

van Kooten, C. and Banchereau, J. (1996). CD40-CD40 ligand: a multifunctional receptor-ligand pair. Adv Immunol 61: 1.

Walter, M.C., Lochmuller, H., Toepfer, et al. (2000). High-dose immunoglobulin therapy in sporadic inclusion body myositis: a double-blind, placebo-controlled study. J Neurol 247: 22–28.

Wiendl, H., Behrens, L., Maier, S., Johnson, M.A., Weiss, E.H., and Hohlfeld, R. (2000). Muscle fibers in inflammatory myopathies and cultured myoblasts express the nonclassical major histocompatibility antigen HLA-G. Ann Neurol 48: 679–684.

22 The neuroimmunology of HIV infection

Christopher Power and Guido van Marle

Introduction

Although the principal manifestation of human immunodeficiency virus type 1 (HIV-1) infection is immunosuppression with ensuing development of acquired immunodeficiency syndrome (AIDS), multisystem involvement including all levels of the neural axis is also part of the disease process (Power, 2001) (Fig. 22.1). HIV-related neurological disease is most common at later stages of infection, with over 95% of infected individuals exhibiting some neurological involvement by the time of death (Johnson, 1998). HIV-1 also shares the property of all lentiviruses including simian (SIV), feline (FIV), and bovine (BIV) immunodeficiency viruses (Narayan and Clements, 1989), of infecting non-dividing macrophages, which is assumed to be pivotal in the development of organ (neurological, respiratory, gastrointestinal) disease (Power and Johnson, 2001). HIV-induced immunological disease begins soon after infection, characterized by a mononucleosis-like syndrome that is accompanied by transient leucopenia, thrombocytopenia, and a burst of viral replication, which is measured as viral RNA copies per ml (load) of plasma (Weiss, 1996). A decline in viral load and a rise in CD8+ lymphocytes usually succeed these events, within weeks to months post contact. Seroconversion usually occurs 6 weeks after infection. Thereafter, an insidious progression in viral replication occurs during a relatively symptom-free period until the eventual development of the acquired immunodeficiency syndrome (AIDS), defined by fewer than 200 CD4 cells/ml in blood. In North America and western Europe, the interval between onset of AIDS and initial infection is approximately 10 years (O'Brien *et al.*, 1996). The clinical progression towards AIDS is accompanied by a rise in viral load and decline and CD4+ lymphocytes in blood. Opportunistic infections such as *Pneumocystis pneumoniae*, central nervous system (CNS) toxoplasmosis, or tumors such as Kaposi's sarcoma or CNS lymphoma are usually the cause of death. Typical of many RNA viruses, HIV-1 exhibits immense molecular diversity, which is reflected by multiple subtypes or clades identified for HIV-1. All HIV-1 clades are associated with neurological disease while HIV-2, which is closely related to SIV, appears to be less immunologically and neurologically virulent.

Clinical and neurological aspects

Primary infection of the nervous system by HIV-1 was first shown in 1985, by several groups (Ho *et al.*, 1985; Levy *et al.*, 1985) who isolated virus from the cerebrospinal fluid (CSF), brain, spinal cord, and peripheral nerves of patients dying with AIDS. Viral RNA was identified in microglial nodules in the brains of children, and viral DNA levels in brain were found to be higher than in lymph node and spleen (Shaw *et al.*, 1985). These findings were complemented by the demonstration of intrathecal synthesis of antibodies against HIV-1 (Resnick *et al.*, 1985). Early on in the epidemic, it became apparent that two general categories of neurological diseases developed as HIV infection progressed; the first group includes opportunistic infections of the CNS such as toxoplasmosis, lymphoma, and tuberculous and cryptococcal meningitis, which are complications of systemic immune suppression; the second group were primary HIV-induced syndromes such as dementia, myelopathies, and peripheral neuropathies (McArthur, 1987). Soon after primary infection, other immunologically based syndromes may present, including an acute demyelinating peripheral neuropathy, similar to Guillain–Barre syndrome, acute encephalopathy, mononeuritis multiplex, and meningitis (McArthur, 1987). However, the neurological syndromes with the greatest morbidity and prevalence are dementia, vacuolar myelopathy, and painful distal sensory polyneuropathy, which become evident with advancing immunosuppression. (Simpson and Tagliati, 1994; Lipton and Gendelman, 1995; Power and Johnson, 2001).

AIDS-related neurological syndromes

With the onset of AIDS, the three prototypic HIV-induced syndromes may present, including (1) HIV-associated dementia (HAD) that has also been termed AIDS dementia complex or HIV encephalopathy, (2) vacuolar myelopathy (VM), and (3) a distal sensory polyneuropathy (DSP) (McArthur, 1987). Estimates of HAD prevalence among patients with AIDS range from 5–20% with an annual incidence of dementia after AIDS development of 7% per year (McArthur *et al.*, 1993). HAD has been identified in all populations infected by HIV-1, regardless of viral clade (subtype) (Maj *et al.*, 1994). Among children with advanced HIV infection, the prevalence of progressive HIV encephalopathy approaches 50% and is defined by developmental delays, impaired brain growth, and abnormalities in motor function and tone (Belman, 1997). HAD is also associated with a significantly worsened survival prognosis (McArthur *et al.*, 1993). HAD dementia is characterized by progressive motor, cognitive, and behavioral abnormalities and displays diversity in its clinical phenotype (Navia *et al.*, 1986a; Mirsattari *et al.*, 1999). The newer antiretroviral drugs may influence this variation in presentation and course (Dore *et al.*, 1999; Sacktor *et al.*, 1999). Dementia is usually manifested after the development of AIDS, but dementia is an AIDS-defining illness in 3% of infected individuals. HAD has been shown to be responsive to highly active antiretroviral therapy (HAART) (Clifford, 2000), indicating that viral replication in the brain may participate in the development of this neurological syndrome.

The neuropathological hallmarks of HIV infection in the brain include multinucleated giant cells, diffuse white matter pallor, and microglial nodules (Navia *et al.*, 1986b; Vinters and Anders, 1990; Sharer, 1992). HIV encephalitis is defined by the presence of multinucleated giant cells and microglial nodules (see Fig. 22.4). Among adults with AIDS, approximately 20–80% of individuals will display multinucleated giant cells (Navia *et al.*, 1986b; Sharer *et al.*, 1986; Glass *et al.*, 1996). In cases in which multinucleated giant cells are not detectable, the presence of viral antigen has been used to confirm this neuropathological diagnosis (Wiley *et al.*, 1996). Diffuse white matter pallor with sparing of the U fibers shows relatively preserved myelin proteins, but conversely deposition of serum proteins is observed in white matter, suggesting altered permeability of the blood–brain barrier (Petito and Cash, 1992; Power *et al.*, 1993). This latter finding is complemented by studies showing apoptotic cell death in cerebral endothelia in brains of HIV-infected patients (Shi *et al.*, 1996) and MRI studies showing altered blood–brain barrier permeability (Berger *et al.*, 2000). Perivascular CNS demyelination has been reported that is reminiscent of

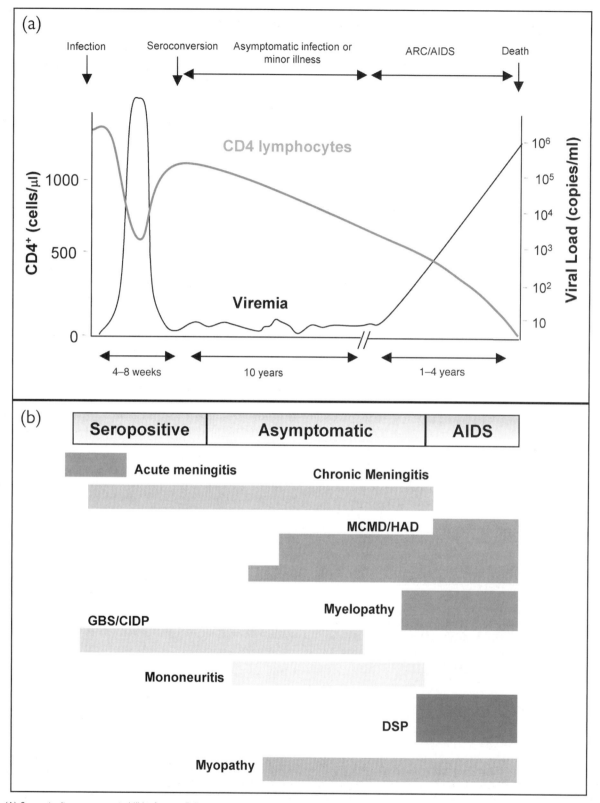

Fig. 22.1 (A) Systemic disease course in HIV infection. Following primary infection there is a rapid transient rise in plasma viremia accompanied by a decline CD4+ lymphocyte count, which resolves over time. However, viral replication continues throughout infection and escalates with the development of AIDS with a concomitant drop in CD4+ cells below 200 cells/ml in blood. (B) Neurological diseases occurring during the course of HIV infection. All levels of the neural axis may be affected by HIV infection but the individual syndromes usually emerge depending on the level of immune suppression. HIV-associated dementia (HAD), minor cognitive motor disorder (MCMD), and distal sensory polyneuropathy (DSP) present during advanced infection (GBS, Guillain–Barré syndrome; CIDP, chronic inflammatory demyelinating polyradiculoneuropathy). (After Power and Johnson (2001), with permission.).

post-infectious encephalomyelitis. Over half of adult AIDS patients with dementia do not exhibit diffuse myelin pallor or multinucleated giant cells at autopsy while microglial nodules may be present in 90% of autopsied AIDS patients (Glass *et al.*, 1995). A correlation between abundance of viral antigen and dementia has been proposed (Achim *et al.*, 1993). Other studies have shown that macrophage and microglia activation, particularly in the basal ganglia, is a stronger predictive marker for HIV dementia (Glass *et al.*, 1995). Neuronal injury and death in the cortex and deep gray matter have also been observed in the brains of patients with AIDS (Everall *et al.*, 1991; Masliah *et al.*, 1992*a*,*b*). Studies reveal neuronal loss and a reduction in neuronal cell body volume in the frontal cortex of patients who are AIDS defined (Ketzler *et al.*, 1990) and the degree of neuronal loss has been correlated with the severity of cognitive impairment (Everall *et al.*, 1999). Dendritic simplification with loss of pre-synaptic terminals in the brains of HIV-infected individuals has also been reported (Masliah *et al.*, 1992*b*). The mechanism of neuronal death remains uncertain, although both necrosis and apoptosis have been implicated in the loss of cortical and basal ganglia neurons in both children and adults. Indeed, these neuronal abnormalities are likely responsible for the phenotypic expression of HIV-associated dementia (Power, 2001).

The prevalence of clinical myelopathy is approximately 15% among AIDS-defined patients, and is characterized by progressive spasticity and weakness, loss of sensation in the legs, and bladder dysfunction (Dal Pan *et al.*, 1994). Hyperreflexia may be present in the arms, although weakness and sensory changes are not usually detected. These clinical findings are associated with vacuolization observed pathologically in the posterior and lateral columns of the spinal cord (Dal Pan and Berger, 1997). Vacuolization represents intralaminar edema within the myelin sheaths with relative preservation of the axon. Macrophages may be detected in the vacuole (Tan *et al.*, 1995). Within the posterior columns, increased numbers of macrophages and enhanced expression of activation markers on macrophages have been reported in VM (Tyor *et al.*, 1993).

The most common peripheral nerve abnormality associated with HIV infection is a distal sensory polyneuropathy (DSP) with a prevalence of 20% among AIDS patients (McArthur, 1987; de la Monte *et al.*, 1988; Simpson and Tagliati, 1994). Symptoms include sensory loss in the hands and feet, complicated by painful dyesthesias and a loss of deep tendon reflexes. Pathological studies reveal distal axonal degeneration involving myelinated and unmyelinated fibers with a loss of dorsal root ganglia neurons (Brannagan *et al.*, 1998). Macrophage infiltration and increased expression of activation markers on macrophages within the lesion have also been reported. A toxic neuropathy (TN) has become an increasing problem over the past several years due to the neurotoxic actions of several antiretroviral drugs including didanosine (ddI), zalcitabine (ddC), and stavudine (d4T) (Brannagan *et al.*, 1998). This neurotoxin-induced axonal neuropathy is dose-dependent and reversible with cessation of the drug. The clinical presentation and epidemiology of these primary HIV-induced syndromes is changing as newer and more effective drugs have become available to treat HIV infection, as evidenced by the marked decline in incidence of neurocognitive impairment and rise in prevalence of peripheral neuropathy over the past 2–5 years (Dore *et al.*, 1999; Sacktor *et al.*, 1999).

Neuropathogenesis

HIV-1 belongs to the lentiviral genus of the family of *Retroviridae*. Lentiviruses are defined by a relatively slow disease course in their natural hosts. Like all retroviruses, the HIV-1 genome structure is defined by *gag*, *pol*, and *env* genes, but HIV also contains several additional genes that influence splicing and transcriptional events, for a total of 10 open reading frames within approximately 10 kilobase pairs of the viral genome (Greene, 1991). There is extensive variation within different HIV-1 strains that is manifested both genotypically as well as phenotypically (Korber *et al.*, 1997; Levy, 1998, p.137). This variation is the result of poor fidelity during reverse transcription and recombination in the virion between the diploid RNA molecules. The vast viral molecular diversity during HIV-1 infections has significant implications because it results in many different viral varieties or quasi-species with differing properties and pathogenicity. Like all viruses infecting the CNS, the neuropathogenesis of HIV-1 can be discussed in terms of (1) *neuroinvasion*, or the ability to enter the CNS, (2) *neurotropism*, or the ability to infect brain cells, (3) *neurovirulence*, or the ability to cause disease, and (4) *neurosusceptibility*, or the vulnerability of the individual

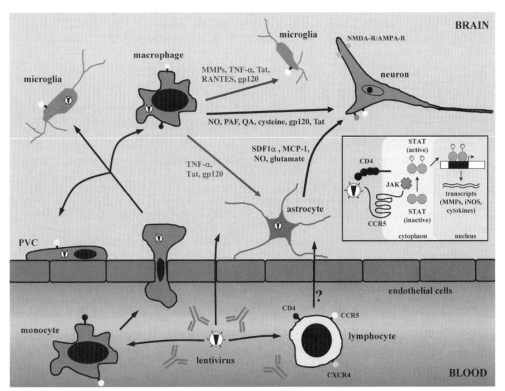

Fig. 22.2 Potential mechanisms by which HIV-1 enters the nervous system and causes neuronal injury. Macrophages and lymphocytes, expressing CD4 and CCR5 or CXCR4, are infected in the periphery and subsequently traverse the blood–brain (or blood–nerve). barrier. CCR5-dependent viruses are neutralized by antibodies in patients with HIV-associated dementia (HAD). Upon entering the nervous system, other cells of the macrophage/microglia lineage are infected or are induced to release potential neurotoxins including cytokines, chemokines, matrix metalloproteinases, quinolinic acid, glutamate, and nitric oxide. To a limited extent astrocytes are infected which also influence neuronal survival through the release of potential neurotoxins. The inset shows a potential signaling pathway in macrophage/microglia involving HIVgp120 induction of host inflammatory genes through CCR5 engagement and subsequent activation and nuclear translocation of the transcription factor, STAT-1. (After Power (2001), with permission.)

host to neurological disease, based on age and genetic background (Patrick *et al.*, 2002). HIV neuropathogenesis is largely the consequence of enhanced innate immunity mediated by monocytoid cells (macrophages and microglia) with failing adaptive immunity and ensuing immune dysregulation (Fig. 22.2).

Neuroinvasion

Neuroinvasion by HIV-1 occurs early after primary infection and is present in almost all patients at the time of death. HIV antigens and/or genome have been detected in the brains of HIV-infected patients at all stages of infection (Budka, 1991; Davis *et al.*, 1992; Bell *et al.*, 1993). The mechanism by which HIV-1 is assumed to enter the CNS is via the infection of macrophages, which cross the blood–brain barrier and infect other cells of macrophage lineage including microglia and perivascular macrophages, also termed the 'Trojan horse' hypothesis (Haase, 1986). An alternative route for entry into the CNS has been postulated to occur through the choroid plexus (Falangola *et al.*, 1995). In general it is unclear exactly how HIV-1 enters the brain, and definitive studies examining the route by which the virus enters the CNS have yet to be performed.

The viruses recovered from the brains of AIDS and pre-AIDS patients are macrophage-tropic viruses based on sequence similarities and *in vitro* tropism (Cheng-Mayer *et al.*, 1989; Power *et al.*, 1994; Reddy *et al.*, 1996). Monocyte/macrophage traffic through the CNS is limited, unless some injury or infection has occurred within the brain. Several chemokines including stromal-cell-derived factor (SDF)-1 and monocyte chemoattractant protein (MCP)-1 show enhanced expression in the brains of HIV-infected patients indicating that monocyte/macrophages (HIV-infected or uninfected) may be recruited into the CNS through a chemotactic mechanism (Letendre *et al.*, 1999). Additionally, up-regulation of adhesion molecules such as intercellular adhesion molecule (ICAM) on the luminal aspect of brain endothelial cells has been demonstrated *in vivo*, which may facilitate monocyte/macrophage adherence and subsequent CNS entry (Hurwitz *et al.*, 1994). Whether the virus found in the CSF influences the extent or pattern of infection of the brain is uncertain. As discussed below, viral load in CSF may be a predictor of severity of HIV dementia (Brew *et al.*, 1997).

Neurotropism

HIV antigens and genome (DNA and RNA) are found primarily in microglia and perivascular macrophages (Koenig *et al.*, 1986; Wiley *et al.*, 1986) and in astrocytes, albeit less frequently (Takahashi *et al.*, 1996). Infected cells are principally localized in the central white matter and the deep gray matter structures (Kure *et al.*, 1990). Unlike many other retroviruses, lentiviruses including HIV are capable of infecting and replicating in terminally differentiated cells. Viral phenotypes have been defined in terms of cell tropism: most HIV strains are either macrophage- or T-cell-tropic but dual tropic viruses have also been described (Collman *et al.*, 1992). Human to human transmission is usually characterized by macrophage-tropic strains, which predominates in blood early after infection (McNearney *et al.*, 1992). HIV-1 cell tropism is chiefly defined by which chemokine receptor the individual strain uses as a co-receptor, together with CD4, for viral entry (Deng *et al.*, 1996). It is clear from both viral sequence analyses, *in vitro* studies, and studies of autopsied or biopsied brain that HIV infection of the CNS principally involves cells of macrophage lineage, although other cell types including astrocytes and possibly neurons are infected (Power, 2001). Among HIV-infected children there appears to greater infection of astrocytes and differential expression of antigens with enhanced expression of HIV Nef (Saito *et al.*, 1994). *In situ* hybridization with and without PCR amplification confirm these immunocytochemical findings (Shaw *et al.*, 1985; Nuovo *et al.*, 1994; Bagasra *et al.*, 1996; Takahashi *et al.*, 1996). To date endothelia and oligodendrocytes have not been shown to be infected *in vivo*, although *in vitro* studies indicate that these cell types are permissive to some strains of HIV-1 (Gyorkey *et al.*, 1987; Moses *et al.*, 1993). The question of *in vivo* infection of neurons remains controversial: Nuovo *et al.* (1994) have reported the viral genome in neurons by *in situ* PCR and this

finding has been confirmed by other groups (Bagasra *et al.*, 1996). However, *in vivo* productive infection of neurons has not been shown to date, although *in vitro* productive infection of neuronal cell lines has been demonstrated. Recent studies using laser capture microdissection of brain tissue suggest that HIV genome is present in neurons (Torres-Munoz *et al.*, 2001).

HIV infection has been shown to be mediated by CD4 as the principal viral receptor on lymphocytes and macrophages (Levy, 1998). However, CD4 expression is comparatively low in the brain. Several chemokine receptors on blood-derived cells serve as viral co-receptors such as CCR5 on macrophages and CXCR4 on lymphocytes (Alkhatib *et al.*, 1996; Feng *et al.*, 1996). Other co-receptors have been reported (Deng *et al.*, 1996) although their roles are less well defined. In the brain, CCR5 and CCR3 have been postulated as potential receptors on microglia (He *et al.*, 1997). This observation has been confirmed by *in vitro* studies showing that infectious recombinant HIV clones containing brain-derived envelope sequences use CCR5 and CCR3 to a lesser extent (Chan *et al.*, 1999). CXCR4 has been also demonstrated on microglia, in addition to cells such as neurons and astrocytes (Sanders *et al.*, 1998). The failure of T-cell-tropic HIV-1 strains to establish productive infection of microglia, despite the presence of CXCR4, is enigmatic and may reflect a requirement for interaction between multiple co-receptors for infection and post-entry factors (Kaul and Lipton, 1999). Nonetheless, the role of CXCR4 as a co-receptor in HIV neuropathogenesis remains intriguing because it may have important implications in mediating neuronal injury and death (Zheng *et al.*, 1999). Other HIV receptors in the brain have been reported, including galactosyl ceramide (Harouse *et al.*, 1991) and a 260 kDa astrocyte cell membrane protein (Ma *et al.*, 1994). Hence, the mechanisms of viral entry into brain cells remain uncertain and may differ from blood cells.

Cell tropism or infectivity of a retrovirus is determined by multiple viral genes that influence events during infection, including viral entry, reverse transcription, integration, transport of viral proteins and genome to the cell surface, and budding of virions (Levy, 1998). Hence, several genes found within HIV are likely to influence its tropism. HIV entry appears to be modulated by different regions of the viral envelope protein, which mediates receptor and co-receptor binding (Chesebro *et al.*, 1991; Westervelt *et al.*, 1992). The V3 hypervariable region of the viral envelope protein surface unit (SU or gp120) has attracted the most attention in terms of influencing tropism and it is also the virus' principal neutralizing determinant (Hwang *et al.*, 1991). The control of viral infectivity by the gp120 V3 region appears to be dependent on distinct sequences and specific amino acids that are necessary for macrophage tropism and its interaction with co-receptors such as CCR5 (Cocchi *et al.*, 1996). The V1 and V2 hypervariable regions of gp120 have also been implicated in regulating tropism (Koito *et al.*, 1994; Toohey *et al.*, 1995; Power *et al.*, 1998*b*). Repeated passages of HIV in cultured microglia can result in mutations in the envelope that resemble mutations identified in brain-derived sequences, suggesting that the virus adapts to the brain (Strizki *et al.*, 1996). Studies of other viral genes and their ability to influence neurotropism indicate that the long terminal repeats (LTRs) gag (Morris *et al.*, 1999) and tat (Mayne *et al.*, 1998) contain distinct sequences which may influence neurotropism. Other groups using transgenic mice have shown that the HIV-1 LTRs may be important for expression in the brain (Corboy *et al.*, 1992). Reverse transcriptase (Wong *et al.*, 1997) and envelope (Morris *et al.*, 1999) sequences from brain, blood, and spleen cluster separately by phylogenetic analyses, suggesting that different organs may exert differing selective pressures on viral replication and evolution.

Neurovirulence

Viral diversity and viral proteins

Among several animal lentiviruses including SIV (Zink *et al.*, 1997), FIV (Power *et al.*, 1998*a*), and visna/maedi virus (VMV) (Andresson *et al.*, 1993), it is clear that specific viral strains are associated with the development of neurological disease (Patrick *et al.*, 2002). In addition, it has been reported that the HIV–SIV chimeric (SHIV) viruses may also cause neurological disease in monkeys (Liu *et al.*, 1999). There are extensive *in vitro* data indicating that HIV-1 strains differ in tropism, and cytotoxicity (Power, 2001). Among many RNA viruses, molecular differences between viral strains, viral diversity, and specific mutations can influence viral pathogenesis dramatically (Domingo and Holland, 1999). Genetic diversity within specific HIV-1 genes also has an impact on *in vivo* neurovirulence (Johnston *et al.*, 2001).

By studying a well-characterized prospective cohort of AIDS patients with and without HAD that came to autopsy, our group has shown that specific mutations within the V3 (Power *et al.*, 1994) and V1 (Power *et al.*, 1998*b*) domains of brain-derived HIV-1 envelope sequences differed between AIDS patients with and without dementia. In addition, conditioned media from HIV-infected macrophages caused varying levels of neuronal death when applied to human neuronal cultures; neurotoxicity induced by recombinant viruses derived from patients with HAD was higher than neurotoxicity caused by viruses derived from non-demented patients (Power *et al.*, 1998*b*). Other groups have found that T-cell-tropic strains of HIV-1 induced the highest levels of neuronal injury when tested in an *in vitro* model of neuronal death, possibly through activation of CXCR4 expressed on neurons (Ohagen *et al.*, 1999). Because of the immense molecular diversity within HIV-1, it has been difficult to identify strain-specific HIV-related syndromes. Similarly, we have not found mutations in Tat and reverse transcriptase sequences that differentiated patients with and without HIV dementia in the same cohort, although phylogenetic comparisons showed some clustering of Tat sequences from patients with dementia (Bratanich *et al.*, 1998).

There is a rapidly expanding literature implicating several different viral proteins in HIV-1 neuropathogenesis (Nath and Geiger, 1998). HIV-1 gp120 has been shown to be directly and indirectly neurotoxic *in vitro* and *in vivo* (Dreyer *et al.*, 1990; Kaiser *et al.*, 1990; Barks *et al.*, 1997). Specific domains within gp120 have been implicated as especially neuropathogenic including the CD4 binding (Giulian *et al.*, 1993) and the V3 regions (Pattarini *et al.*, 1998). The underlying mechanism appears to be related to accumulation of intracellular calcium in neurons following activation of glutamate receptors and voltage-operated calcium channels (Lipton and Gendelman, 1995). Other neurotransmitters may be affected by gp120-induced activation of NMDA receptors such as impaired dopamine transport as demonstrated in dopaminergic neurons cultured from rat midbrain (Bennett *et al.*, 1995). Dawson *et al.* (1993) have also shown that nitric oxide may be influencing gp120 neurotoxicity. Transgenic mice expressing HIV-1 gp120 in astrocytes display neuropathological findings including astrogliosis, neuronal loss, and dendritic vacuolizations, resembling HIV encephalitis (Toggas *et al.*, 1994). This model used a gp120 sequence from a T-cell-tropic strain of HIV-1; initial studies did not show protein expression but later studies disclosed gp120 protein detection and corresponding neurophysiological changes (Krucker *et al.*, 1998). gp120 has also been shown to affect intracellular signaling that controls the expression of different cell adhesion molecules and cytokines and perhaps nitric oxide through the JAK–STAT pathway (Shrikant *et al.*, 1996; Johnston *et al.*, 2000). The above *in vitro* and *in vivo* findings support the hypothesis that gp120 is involved in the pathogenesis of HIV-induced neurological injury.

Other HIV proteins including Tat, the transmembrane region of the envelope protein (gp41), and Nef have been shown to be neurotoxic *in vitro* (Adamson *et al.*, 1996; Nath *et al.*, 1996). The transactivating protein, Tat, has attracted extensive attention in neuropathogenesis studies because of early studies showing that it was neurotoxic, released from infected lymphocytes, and was taken up by cells and could in turn transactivate host genes such as TNF-α (Chen *et al.*, 1997) and IL-1β (Nath *et al.*, 1999). As with gp120, several domains have been found to be especially neurotoxic, including the basic region and the RGD (arginine–glycine–aspartic acid) residues in the second exon, while other groups have shown that the entire first exon is necessary for neurotoxicity. Conant *et al.* (1998) have shown that Tat induces the expression MCP-1 in astrocytes, which may influence macrophage trafficking in the CNS. Other groups have shown that multiple glial-derived proteins including cytokines and chemokines can be induced by treatment with Tat through several intracellular signaling pathways.

Immune selection and neurovirulence

As described above, genetic diversity within viral genes influences neurovirulence by differential activation of cell signaling pathways and responses. The host immune system is a pivotal factor controlling HIV diversity and pathogenesis in systemic disease; differences in humoral and cellular immune responses could potentially select for or against viruses that infect the CNS and cause neurological damage. Since the viruses present in the CNS enter via the bloodstream, differences in the neutralization ability of antibodies in the serum may influence viral evolution of HIV-1 in the blood and might also determine which viruses infect the CNS. Differences in viral neutralization have been reported between sera from AIDS patients with and without neurological disease (Beilke *et al.*, 1991; van Marle *et al.*, 2002). Recently, we have been able to demonstrate the relationship between viral sequence diversity and neutralization (van Marle *et al.*, 2002). CCR5-dependent viruses were less efficiently neutralized by sera from patients with HAD compared with non-demented (ND) HIV/AIDS patients, which was dependent on the C2V3 region of the HIV-1 envelope protein and corresponded to increased molecular diversity in this envelope region among patients with HAD compared with ND patients (Fig. 22.3). A similar pattern in viral diversity and evolution was also observed in C2V3 sequences derived from brains of a different cohort, with a preference for amino-acid-changing substitutions in the V3 envelope region in HAD patients relative to ND patients. These observations indicate that the viruses found in each patient group are subjected to differing selection pressures, which is associated with differences in the humoral immune response.

In addition to the humoral immunity, failing adaptive cellular immunity may directly participate in the development of neurological disease. The cellular immune response in HIV-1 infection is directed against the majority of the HIV-1 genes (Walker and Goulder, 2000; Altfeld *et al.*, 2001; Addo *et al.*, 2002). Many observations suggest a role for cytotoxic T lymphocyte (CTL) escape in systemic disease progression in HIV (Carrington *et al.*, 1999; Evans *et al.*, 1999; Goulder and Walker, 1999; Goulder *et al.*, 2001; McMichael and Rowland-Jones, 2001; Barouch *et al.*, 2002). The influence of the cellular immune response on viral evolution could affect HIV-1 neurological disease in several ways. An inefficient cellular immune response would allow for increased replication and viral diversity due to fewer restraints by the immune system. Viral diversity may also emerge through replication in immune-privileged tissue compartments (CNS) or drug resistance. This increased viral diversity enhances the probability of amino acid substitutions that allow for viral escape and potential emergence of neuropathogenic virus strains. A robust and broad cellular immune response would minimize viral escape. However, viral escape leading to disease progression has been observed even after years of successful immune control (Goulder *et al.*, 1997). The cellular and humoral immune responses can direct viral evolution by applying positive selection pressure, resulting in more amino acid changing mutations (Overbaugh and Bangham, 2001). Increased amino acid substitution rates have been observed in the sequences found in the CNS and the periphery of patients with neurological disease (Kuiken *et al.*, 1995; Bratanich *et al.*, 1998; Huang *et al.*, 2002; van Marle *et al.*, 2002), which could be mediated by the cellular immune response. This raises the intriguing possibility that the immune system would select for rather than against more pathogenic viral species that infect the CNS. Indeed, a recent study using an HIV-infected SCID mouse model showed that an enhanced T-lymphocyte response reduced HIV infection of the brain (Poluektova *et al.*, 2002). Such immune selection would explain the increased risk of HIV-1 systemic disease associated with certain HLA types (Kaslow *et al.*, 1996; Carrington *et al.*, 1999; Migueles *et al.*, 2000).

Viral load

Studies of plasma virus levels indicate that viral replication and 'load' in blood are extremely high in persons with HIV-1 infection (Perelson *et al.*, 1997). However, the role of viral load in brain in relation to the development of neurological disease is uncertain. Viral load in cerebrospinal fluid is usually several orders less than plasma but correlated to some extent with the presence of dementia (McArthur, 1987). Quantitative PCR studies of

(a)

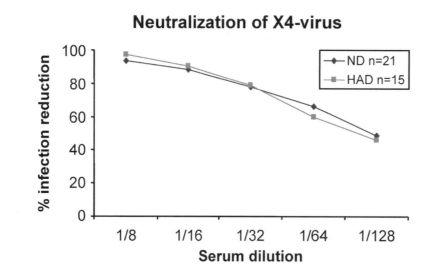

(b)

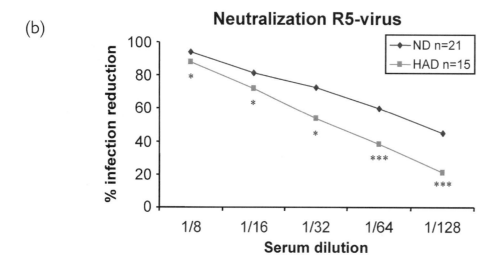

(c)

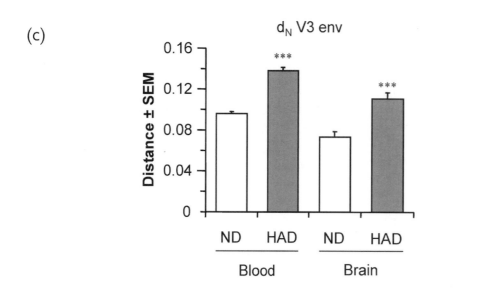

Fig. 22.3 Neutralization of X4- and R5-dependent HIV-1 strains by sera from HIV-associated dementia (HAD; $n = 15$) or non-demented (ND; $n = 21$) AIDS patients. While no differences were observed in neutralization ability of an X4 virus (NL4-3) between groups (A), the ND-derived sera neutralized the R5 virus (YU-2) more efficiently than the HAD-derived sera (B). (C) Analysis of viral molecular diversity, as indicated by non-synonymous nucleotide substitutions (dN, amino acid changing mutations). Greater diversity was apparent within the gp120 V3 hypervariable domain (the principal neutralizing determinant). in viruses derived from both blood and brain of HAD patients compared with viruses from ND patients, permitting the potential emergence of escape mutants in the HAD group. (*$p < 0.05$, **$p < 0.01$, ***$p < 0.001$). (Adapted from van Marle et al. (2002), with permission.)

brain-derived viral mRNA and provirus in brain indicate no significant difference in levels between AIDS patients with and without HIV dementia (Johnson *et al.*, 1996; Lazarini *et al.*, 1997). In contrast, viral protein and RNA levels detected in CSF (Royal *et al.*, 1994; Brew *et al.*, 1997) and brain, detected by immunocytochemistry (Brew *et al.*, 1995; Glass *et al.*, 1995) show modestly elevated levels in patients with HAD, compared to non-demented AIDS controls. Other studies suggest that CSF viral load is correlated with neuropsychological abnormalities (Ellis *et al.*, 1997) but the relationship of plasma viral load to CSF viral load is dependent on the level of immune suppression (McArthur *et al.*, 1997). Viral load in the brain measured by immunostaining or quantitative molecular methods is closely associated with the extent of pathological change accompanying HIV encephalitis (Vazeux *et al.*, 1992). Several studies have also suggested that levels of unintegrated viral DNA in brain macrophages is associated with the development of HIV dementia (Pang *et al.*, 1991; Teo *et al.*, 1997) implying that increased viral genome levels in select cell populations may be important determinants of disease in the brain.

Specific drug resistance conferring mutations in the reverse transcriptase and protease encoding genes have been identified in viruses from patients who show high viral loads despite HAART (Hirsch *et al.*, 1998; Harrigan and Alexander, 1999). Several reports suggest that brain-derived viruses have fewer drug-resistant sequences than matched blood-derived HIV, which may reflect poor CNS penetration of the drug and/or limited replication in the brain and hence, a restricted potential for drug-resistant mutations to emerge (Wong *et al.*, 1997; Bratanich *et al.*, 1998; McClernon *et al.*, 2001). Nonetheless, drug resistance is becoming an increasingly important issue and has resulted in at least one clinical trial failing to show clinical benefit among AIDS patients with dementia who received a drug with high CNS penetration, underlining the importance of ongoing viral replication as an important factor in the development of neurological disease (Brew, personal communication).

Host molecules/neuroinflammation

Excess production of host-encoded inflammatory molecules by microglia, perivascular macrophages, and perhaps astrocytes has been proposed as a chief cause of damage within the brain in a number of (CNS) diseases including Alzheimer's disease, stroke, and HIV-associated dementia (Kolson and Pomerantz, 1996) (Table 22.1). This hypothesis is predicated on data derived from *in vitro* and animal models and studies of autopsied tissues. In HIV neuropathogenesis, this hypothesis is supported by the consistent observation that microglia and astrocytes are the principal cells infected by HIV-1.

In 1990, Giulian and colleagues showed that HIV-infected monocytoid cell lines secreted diffusible molecules that killed several different neuronal cell types by a presumed excitotoxic mechanism, mediated by NMDA receptors (Giulian *et al.*, 1990). Pulliam *et al.* (1991) also reported that HIV-infected macrophages produced a neurotoxic compound(s) causing cytopathic effects in cultured cell aggregates from human fetal brain tissue.

Table 22.1 Neurotoxic molecules implicated in HIV neuropathogenesis

Host factors	Cytokines: TNF-α, IL-1α, IL-6, GM-CSF, IFN-α
	Chemokines: MCP-1, RANTES, MIP-1α, SDF-1α
	Low molecular weight toxic factors: quinolinic acid, Ntox, NO, super anion
	Arachidonic acid metabolites: prostaglandins and leukotrienes
	Platelet-activating factor
	Matrix metalloproteinases
Viral proteins	Tat, Nef, gp41, gp120, Vpr, Rev

GM-CSF, granulocyte-macrophage colony-stimulating factor; IFN, interferon; IL, interleukin; TNF, tumor necrosis factor; SDF, stromal cell-derived factor; MIP, macrophage inflammatory protein; MCP, monocyte chemoattractant protein; RANTES, regulated on activation, normal T-cell expressed and secreted.

Apart from the viral neurotoxins, several potential host neurotoxins released upon HIV-1 infection or exposure of cells to HIV-1 proteins have been identified and characterized *in vitro* and *in vivo*.

Cytokines

Multiple cytokines have been shown to be elevated in the brains and CSF of patients with HIV dementia (Tyor *et al.*, 1992; Wesselingh *et al.*, 1993; Gelbard *et al.*, 1994), which include tumor necrosis factor-alpha (TNF-α), interleukin-1 (IL-1), interleukin-6 (IL-6), and transforming growth factor-beta (TGF-β). Although almost all cells in the CNS can produce cytokines, the chief sources of these small soluble molecules are activated glial cells that include macrophages, microglia, and astrocytes. TNF-α is a pro-inflammatory cytokine that has received extensive attention for its potential neurotoxic effects in HIV infection and ability to influence the release of other cytokines (Barna *et al.*, 1990; Benveniste, 1994). It has been shown to be released by microglia and astrocytes (Tyor *et al.*, 1992; Wilt *et al.*, 1995) in HIV infection and prevent uptake of glutamate (Fine *et al.*, 1996). Several studies have shown that TNF-α mRNA and protein levels are increased in the brains and CSF of patients with HIV infection. Notably, Wesselingh *et al.* (1993), showed that TNF-α mRNA levels were increased in patients with HAD compared with AIDS patients without dementia or non-infected controls; furthermore, the level of mRNA was correlated with the severity of dementia. These *in vivo* studies are supported by *in vitro* studies showing neurotoxic and gliotoxic effects of TNF-α, often at low concentrations in conjunction with other potentially neurotoxic molecules (Westmoreland *et al.*, 1996). TNF-α expression may be dependent on the simultaneous action of other molecules to produce neurological disease (Chao and Hu, 1994). IL-6 has also been reported to be increased in the brains of patients with HIV infection (Tyor *et al.*, 1992; Sippy *et al.*, 1995). *In vitro* studies suggest that IL-6 may mediate neurotoxicity indirectly (Gruol *et al.*, 1998). TGF-α, IL-1β, and nerve growth factor (NGF) have reported to be over-expressed in HIV-infected brains (Boven *et al.*, 1999b). These three molecules have some neurotropic properties and hence, their increased production may reflect a host defense response to the neurotoxic actions of HIV. It is also likely that the increased expression of inflammatory cytokines in the brain may indirectly mediate neurological injury during HIV infection by enhancing the permeability of the blood–brain barrier. Inflammatory cytokines such as TNF-α increase blood–brain barrier permeability, as shown for other CNS diseases (Quagliarello *et al.*, 1991). In addition, increased blood–brain barrier permeability may permit the influx of potential neurotoxins from the systemic circulation.

Arachidonic acid

Cells of macrophage lineage are major producers of arachidonic acid and its metabolites (Triggiani *et al.*, 1995). These metabolites have been shown to influence neuronal NMDA and non-NMDA receptor action and cell survival. Griffin *et al.* (1994) reported that prostaglandin E_2 and F_{2a}, and thromboxane B_2 were elevated in CSF from patients with AIDS dementia compared with patients without dementia. Other groups have shown elevated levels of arachidonic acid metabolites including platelet-activating factor (PAF) in HIV-infected macrophages, although most of the products were produced through the lipoxygenase pathway (Genis *et al.*, 1992). It maybe that arachidonic acid metabolites influence neurotoxicity indirectly, such as by regulating the expression of glutamate uptake by astrocytes as has been shown *in vitro* (Rothstein *et al.*, 1993, 1996). As potential mediators of neuronal survival they are likely to be involved in the neuropathogenesis of HIV infection.

Quinolinic acid and other macrophage products

Quinolinic acid (QA) is produced by macrophages following different types of stimulation and as a product of tryptophan metabolism (Saito and Heyes, 1996). By binding to NMDA receptors, QA has been shown to have neurotoxic properties, following acute or chronic exposure (Moroni, 1999). The source of QA in the brain is not clear as it has been shown to cross the blood–brain barrier. QA has been shown to be elevated in CSF and brains from patients with HIV dementia as well as in CSF from macaques infected with SIV compared with controls (Heyes *et al.*, 1990. 1991). In addition, QA levels in CSF appear to correlate with the severity of dementia (Heyes *et al.*, 1991; Sei *et al.*, 1995). Like TNF-α, another product of macrophages, QA levels are increased in other neurological diseases in which macrophages or microglia are activated (Flanagan *et al.*, 1995; Heyes *et al.*, 1997). Whether QA is directly neurotoxic or is merely a marker of macrophage activation remains to be demonstrated among patients with HIV-associated dementia.

Other products of macrophage and microglia have been shown to be a potential neurotoxins in several neurological conditions including HIV infection (Gendelman *et al.*, 1997). For example, increased levels of inducible nitric oxide synthase (iNOS) have been reported in the brains of patients with severe HAD, implicating nitric oxide as a potential neurotoxin (Boven *et al.*, 1999*c*; Rostasy *et al.*, 1999). iNOS levels were also highly correlated with the levels of HIV gp41 expression in brain (Adamson *et al.*, 1996). These findings are supported recent studies showing that metabolites of NO are also increased in the brains of patients with HIV dementia compared with non-demented controls. An intriguing report described a novel neurotoxin, Ntox, which is released by activated microglial cells although full characterization of the molecule is pending (Giulian *et al.*, 1996). Other molecules produced by activated macrophages include neopterin (Griffin *et al.*, 1991) and β² microglobulin (Brew *et al.*, 1996) and have been shown to be increased in the CSF of patients with HIV infection. To some extent, these levels are correlated with the severity of dementia, although a direct relationship between the activity of these molecules and pathogenic mechanism is unclear at present (Brew *et al.*, 1990; McArthur *et al.*, 1992).

Matrix metalloproteinases (MMP)

MMPs have been shown to have both neuropathogenic but also neuroreparative properties in the CNS and PNS (Yong *et al.*, 2001). MMP-2 and -7 levels are increased in the CSF of patients with HAD (Conant *et al.*, 1999). HIV and FIV infections increase MMP-2 and -9 expression in cultured macrophages, which is correlated with increased expression of both MMPs during lentivirus CNS infections (Johnston *et al.*, 2000). HIV Tat also selectively induces MMP-2 with ensuing neurotoxicity, which is blocked by the MMP inhibitor, prinomastat (Johnston *et al.*, 2001, 2002). The precise mechanism by which MMP-2 is neurotoxic remains uncertain.

Chemokines

With the increased understanding in the role of chemokine receptors as co-receptors for HIV infection, there has also been a concomitant expanding interest in the actions of chemokines in the nervous system in the context of HIV infection and other neurological diseases (Ransohoff and Tani, 1998). Several chemokines have been shown to be increased in the spinal fluids and brains of patients with HIV infection. (Kelder *et al.*, 1998; Sanders *et al.*, 1998; Letendre *et al.*, 1999), including macrophage inflammatory protein-1β (MIP-1β) and macrophage inflammatory protein-1α (MIP-1β), regulated upon activation normal T-cell suppressed and secreted (RANTES) and inflammatory protein-10 (IP-10). Other groups have shown that monocyte chemoattractant protein-1 (MCP-1) levels are increased in the cerebrospinal fluids and brains of patients with HIV dementia (Conant *et al.*, 1998). The exact role of these chemokines remains uncertain because several groups have shown *in-vitro* that MIP-1α and RANTES are able to block gp120-induced neuronal death (Kaul and Lipton, 1999). These studies are supported by other studies showing that different chemokines affect calcium signaling in neurons and demonstrate chemokine receptors which have shown to be expressed on neurons, thereby directly influencing neuronal survival. The exact mechanisms by which chemokines induce signaling events in macrophages and/or neurons remain uncertain.

Autoimmunity

Dysregulation of the immune system is a cardinal feature of HIV infection, resulting in both systemic immune suppression and activation. Within the CNS during HIV infection, increased expression of Class I and II antigens on glia and the release of inflammatory molecules reflects immune activation. However, activation of autoimmune mechanisms may also participate in the development of HIV-induced neurological disease. These potential mechanisms include (1) the expression of superantigens, (2) molecular mimicry, and (3) polyclonal B-cell activation.

Although a superantigen expressed by HIV has not been demonstrated to date, other retroviruses such as mouse mammary tumor virus (MMTV) (Acha-Orbea *et al.*, 1999) and a human endogenous retrovirus (Conrad *et al.*, 1997) have been proposed to express superantigens that have been implicated in pathogenesis. A superantigen would explain some features of HIV infection including activation and T-cell depletion. This is supported by a limited repertoire of T-cell receptor Vβ sequences among some HIV-infected individuals. Conflicting data exhibiting MHC-restricted immune responses have also been reported, thus leaving the role of superantigens open for further analysis. Molecular mimicry has also been proposed as a possible mechanism by which neurological disease develops during HIV infection. Autoreactive antibodies from HIV-infected individuals that recognize HIV gp41 have been shown to bind an astrocyte-derived protein, although a pathogenic role for these antibodies has not been demonstrated (Yamada *et al.*, 1991). Regions of homology between HIV gp160 and specific HLA domains, IL-2, and human IgA have also suggested that molecular mimicry may participate HIV pathogenesis.

Polyclonal B-cell activation has been posited as the explanation for the increased levels of immunoglobulins in the blood and CSF of HIV-infected persons. These include IgG, IgA, IgM, and IgD of which approximately 20–50% target HIV-encoded antigens. Nonetheless, the remaining fraction are viewed as polyclonal or oligoclonal immunoglobulins which may target specific pathogens or host antigens. Antibodies directed to antigens such as phospholipids (Rubbert *et al.*, 1994) have been reported in HIV infection and may be involved in the neuropathogenesis of HIV infection.

Host neurosusceptibility

Like many other infectious diseases, apart from the intrinsic pathogenic properties of the infecting HIV-1 strain, the neurosusceptibility of the infected individual, i.e.their genetic background and age, seem to dictate HIV-1 neurovirulence (Power *et al.*, 1994, 1998*a*; Corder *et al.*, 1998; Boven *et al.*, 1999*a*; Van Rij *et al.*, 1999; Quasney *et al.*, 2001) Recent studies indicate that several genetic polymorphisms may influence the clinical presentation of HAD. The Δ32 mutation with chemokine receptor CCR5 appears to reduce the risk of developing HAD (Boven *et al.*, 1999*a*; Van Rij *et al.*, 1999) but also reduces the risk of infection by HIV-1. Conversely, single nucleotide polymorphisms (SNP) in the TNF-α (Quasney *et al.*, 2001) and MCP-1 (Gonzalez *et al.*, 2002) promoters increase the risk of developing HAD. The apolipoprotein E e4 allele, which is a risk factor for Alzheimer's disease, also appears to confer greater susceptibility to HAD and DSP (Corder *et al.*, 1998). Finally, the age of the host has significant impact on clinical presentation. The risk of dementia or encephalopathy during HIV infection is greatest in elderly adults and children, respectively, probably reflecting diminished immune competence at these extremes of life. These factors determine how the host reacts to the infection by HIV-1, and hence, disease onset could be accelerated by inefficient or inappropriate host responses.

Summary

Like many lentiviruses, HIV-1 causes both immune suppression and neurological disease. Neurological disease may occur at any stage of HIV infection but is most apparent with severe immune suppression. Cognitive impairment, manifested as HIV-associated dementia, has attracted intense interest since the outset of the HIV epidemic, and understanding of its pathogenesis has been spurred on by the emergence of several hypotheses outlining potential pathogenic mechanisms. The release of inflammatory molecules by HIV-infected microglia and macrophages and the concurrent neuronal damage play a central role in the conceptualization of HIV neuropathogenesis. Many inflammatory molecules appear to contribute to the pathogenic cascade and their individual roles remain undefined. At the same time, the abundance of virus in the brain and type or strain of virus found in the brain may also be important co-determinants of neurological disease, as shown for other neurotropic viruses. Co-receptor use by HIV found in the brain appears to closely mirror what has been reported in systemic macrophages. The impact of HAART on viral genotype and phenotype found in the brain and its relationship to clinical disease remains uncertain.

Acknowledgements

The authors thank Belinda Ibrahim and Linda Mills for assistance with the preparation of the manuscript. GvM is a Canadian Institutes of Health Research (CIHR) and Alberta Heritage Foundation for Medical Research (AHFMR) Fellow. CP is an AHFMR Scholar and CIHR Investigator.

References

Acha-Orbea, H., Finke, D., Attinger, A., et al. (1999). Interplays between mouse mammary tumor virus and the cellular and humoral immune response. *Immunol Rev* **168**: 287–303.

Achim, C.L., Heyes, M.P., and Wiley, C.A. (1993). Quantitation of human immunodeficiency virus, immune activation factors, and quinolinic acid in AIDS brains. *J Clin Invest* **91**: 2769–2775.

Adamson, D.C., Wildemann, B., Sasaki, M., et al. (1996). Immunologic NO synthase: elevation in severe AIDS dementia and induction by HIV-1 gp41. *Science* **274**: 1917–21.

Addo, M.M., Altfeld, M., Rathod, A., et al. (2002). HIV-1 Vpu represents a minor target for cytotoxic T lymphocytes in HIV-1-infection. *AIDS* **16**: 1071–1073.

Alkhatib, G., Combadiere, C., Broder, C.C., et al. (1996). CC CKR5: a RANTES, MIP-1alpha, MIP-1beta receptor as a fusion cofactor for macrophage-tropic HIV-1. *Science* **272**: 1955–1958.

Altfeld, M., Rosenberg, E.S., Shankarappa, R., et al. (2001). Cellular immune responses and viral diversity in individuals treated during acute and early HIV-1 infection. *J Exp Med* **193**: 169–180.

Andresson, O.S., Elser, J.E., Tobin, G.J., et al. (1993). Nucleotide sequence and biological properties of a pathogenic proviral molecular clone of neurovirulent visna virus. *Virology* **193**: 89–105.

Bagasra, O., Lavi, E., Bobroski, L., et al. (1996). Cellular reservoirs of HIV-1 in the central nervous system of infected individuals: identification by the combination of *in situ* polymerase chain reaction and immunohistochemistry. *AIDS* **10**: 573–585.

Barks, J.D., Liu, X.H., Sun, R., and Silverstein, F.S. (1997). gp120, a human immunodeficiency virus-1 coat protein, augments excitotoxic hippocampal injury in perinatal rats. *Neuroscience* **76**: 397–409.

Barna, B.P., Estes, M.L., Jacobs, B.S., Hudson, S., and Ransohoff, R.M. (1990). Human astrocytes proliferate in response to tumor necrosis factor alpha. *J Neuroimmunol* **30**: 239–243.

Barouch, D.H., Kunstman, J., Kuroda, M.J., et al. (2002). Eventual AIDS vaccine failure in a rhesus monkey by viral escape from cytotoxic T lymphocytes. *Nature* **415**: 335–339.

Beilke, M.A., Minagawa, H., Stone, G., Leon-Monzon, M., and Gibbs, C.J. Jr (1991). Neutralizing antibody responses in patients with AIDS with neurologic complications. *J Lab Clin Med* **118**: 585–588.

Bell, J.E., Busuttil, A., Ironside, J.W., et al. (1993). Human immunodeficiency virus and the brain: investigation of virus load and neuropathologic changes in pre-AIDS subjects. *J Infect Dis* **168**: 818–824.

Belman, A. (1997). Infants, children and adolescents. In: *AIDS and the Nervous System*, 2nd edn (ed. J.L. Berger and R.M. Levy), pp. 223–253. Lippincott-Raven, Philadelphia, PA.

Bennett, B.A., Rusyniak, D.E., and Hollingsworth, C.K. (1995). HIV-1 gp120-induced neurotoxicity to midbrain dopamine cultures. *Brain Res* **705**: 168–176.

Benveniste, E.N. (1994). Cytokine circuits in brain: implications for AIDS dementia complex. In: *HIV, AIDS, and the Brain* (ed. R.W. Price and S.W. Perry), pp. 71–88. Raven Press, New York.

Berger, J.R., Nath, A., Greenberg, R.N., et al. (2000). Cerebrovascular changes in the basal ganglia with HIV dementia. *Neurology* **54**: 921–926.

Boven, L.A., van der Bruggen, T., Sweder van Asbeck, B., Marx, J.J., and Nottet, H.S. (1999a). Potential role of CCR5 polymorphism in the development of AIDS dementia complex. *FEMS Immunol Med Microbiol* **26**: 243–247.

Boven, L.A., Middel, J., Portegies, P., Verhoef, J., Jansen, G.H., and Nottet, H.S. (1999b). Overexpression of nerve growth factor and basic fibroblast growth factor in AIDS dementia complex. *J Neuroimmunol* **97**: 154–162.

Boven, L.A., Gomes, L., Hery, C., et al. (1999c). Increased peroxynitrite activity in AIDS dementia complex: implications for the neuropathogenesis of HIV-1 infection. *J Immunol* **162**: 4319–4327.

Brannagan, T.H., McAlarney, T., Latov, N. (1998). Peripheral neuropathy in HIV-1 infection. In: *Immunological and Infectious Diseases of the Peripheral Nerves* (ed. N. Latov, J.H. Wokke, and J.J. Kelly), pp. 285–307. Cambridge University Press, Cambridge.

Bratanich, A.C., Liu, C., McArthur, J.C., et al. (1998). Brain-derived HIV-1 tat sequences from AIDS patients with dementia show increased molecular heterogeneity. *J Neurovirol* **4**: 387–393.

Brew, B.J., Bhalla, R.B., Paul, M., et al. (1990). Cerebrospinal fluid neopterin in human immunodeficiency virus type 1 infection. *Ann Neurol* **28**: 556–560.

Brew, B.J., Rosenblum, M., Cronin, K., and Price, R.W. (1995). AIDS dementia complex and HIV-1 brain infection: clinical-virological correlations. *Ann Neurol* **38**: 563–570.

Brew, B.J., Dunbar, N., Pemberton, L., and Kaldor J. (1996). Predictive markers of AIDS dementia complex: CD4 cell count and cerebrospinal fluid concentrations of beta 2-microglobulin and neopterin. *J Infect Dis* **174**: 294–298.

Brew, B.J., Pemberton, L., Cunningham, P., and Law, M.G. (1997). Levels of human immunodeficiency virus type 1 RNA in cerebrospinal fluid correlate with AIDS dementia stage. *J Infect Dis* **175**: 963–966.

Budka, H. (1991). Neuropathology of human immunodeficiency virus infection. *Brain Pathol* **1**: 163–175.

Carrington, M., Nelson, G.W., Martin, M.P., et al. (1999). HLA and HIV-1: heterozygote advantage and B*35-Cw*04 disadvantage. *Science* **283**: 1748–1752.

Chan, S.Y., Speck, R.F., Power, C., Gaffen, S.L., Chesebro, B., and Goldsmith, M.A. (1999). V3 recombinants indicate a central role for CCR5 as a co-receptor in tissue infection by human immunodeficiency virus type 1. *J Virol* **73**: 2350–2358.

Chao, C.C. and Hu, S. (1994). Tumor necrosis factor-alpha potentiates glutamate neurotoxicity in human fetal brain cell cultures. *Dev Neurosci* **16**: 172–179.

Chen, P., Mayne, M., Power, C., and Nath, A. (1997). The Tat protein of HIV-1 induces tumor necrosis factor-alpha production. Implications for HIV-1-associated neurological diseases. *J Biol Chem* **272**: 22385–22388.

Cheng-Mayer, C., Weiss, C., Seto, D., Levy, J.A. (1989). Isolates of human immunodeficiency virus type 1 from the brain may constitute a special group of the AIDS virus. *Proc Natl Acad Sci USA* **86**: 8575–8579.

Chesebro, B., Nishio, J., Perryman, S., et al. (1991). Identification of human immunodeficiency virus envelope gene sequences influencing viral entry into CD4-positive HeLa cells, T-leukemia cells, and macrophages. *J Virol* **65**: 5782–5789.

Clifford, D.B. (2000). Human immunodeficiency virus-associated dementia. *Arch Neurol* **57**: 321–324.

Cocchi, F., DeVico, A.L., Garzino-Demo, A., Cara, A., Gallo, R.C., and Lusso, P. (1996). The V3 domain of the HIV-1 gp120 envelope glycoprotein is critical for chemokine-mediated blockade of infection. *Nat Med* **2**: 1244–1247.

Collman, R., Balliet, J.W., Gregory, S.A., et al. (1992). An infectious molecular clone of an unusual macrophage-tropic and highly cytopathic strain of human immunodeficiency virus type 1. *J Virol* **66**: 7517–7521.

Conant, K., Garzino-Demo, A., Nath, A., et al. (1998). Induction of monocyte chemoattractant protein-1 in HIV-1 Tat-stimulated astrocytes and elevation in AIDS dementia. *Proc Natl Acad Sci USA* **95**: 3117–3121.

Conant, K., McArthur, J.C., Griffin, D.E., Sjulson, L., Wahl, L.M., and Irani, D.N. (1999). Cerebrospinal fluid levels of MMP-2, 7, and 9 are elevated in association with human immunodeficiency virus dementia. *Ann Neurol* **46**: 391–398.

Conrad, B., Weissmahr, R.N., Boni, J., Arcari, R., Schupbach, J., and Mach B. (1997). A human endogenous retroviral superantigen as candidate autoimmune gene in type I diabetes. *Cell* **90**: 303–313.

Corboy, J.R., Buzy, J.M., Zink, M.C., and Clements, J.E. (1992). Expression directed from HIV long terminal repeats in the central nervous system of transgenic mice. *Science* **258**: 1804–1808.

Corder, E.H., Robertson, K., Lannfelt, L., *et al.* (1998). HIV-infected subjects with the E4 allele for APOE have excess dementia and peripheral neuropathy. *Nat Med* **4**: 1182–1184.

Dal Pan, G.J. and Berger, J.R. (1997). Spinal cord disease in human immunodeficiency virus infection. In: *AIDS and the Nervous System*, 2nd edn (ed. J.R. Berger, R.M. Levy), pp. 173–187. Lippincott-Raven, Philadelphia, PA.

Dal Pan, G.J., Glass, J.D., and McArthur, J.C. (1994). Clinicopathologic correlations of HIV-1-associated vacuolar myelopathy: an autopsy-based case-control study. *Neurology* **44**: 2159–2164.

Davis, T.H., Morton, C.C., Miller-Cassman, R., Balk, S.P., and Kadin, M.E. (1992). Hodgkin's disease, lymphomatoid papulosis, and cutaneous T-cell lymphoma derived from a common T-cell clone. *N Engl J Med* **326**: 1115–1122.

Dawson, V.L., Dawson, T.M., Uhl, G.R., and Snyder, S.H. (1993). Human immunodeficiency virus type 1 coat protein neurotoxicity mediated by nitric oxide in primary cortical cultures. *Proc Natl Acad Sci USA* **90**: 3256–3259.

de la Monte, S.M., Gabuzda, D.H., Ho, D.D., *et al.* (1988). Peripheral neuropathy in the acquired immunodeficiency syndrome. *Ann Neurol* **23**: 485–492.

Deng, H., Liu, R., Ellmeier, W., *et al.* (1996). Identification of a major co-receptor for primary isolates of HIV-1. *Nature* **381**: 661–666.

Domingo, E. and Holland, J.J. (1999). *Origin and Evolution of Viruses*. Academic Press, New York.

Dore, G.J., Correll, P.K., Li, Y., Kaldor, J.M., Cooper, D.A., and Brew, B.J. (1999). Changes to AIDS dementia complex in the era of highly active antiretroviral therapy. *AIDS* **13**: 1249–1253.

Dreyer, E.B., Kaiser, P.K., Offermann, J.T., and Lipton, S.A. (1990). HIV-1 coat protein neurotoxicity prevented by calcium channel antagonists. *Science* **248**: 364–367.

Ellis, R.J., Hsia, K., Spector, S.A., *et al.* (1997). Cerebrospinal fluid human immunodeficiency virus type 1 RNA levels are elevated in neurocognitively impaired individuals with acquired immunodeficiency syndrome. HIV Neurobehavioral Research Center Group. *Ann Neurol* **42**: 679–688.

Evans, D.T., O'Connor, D.H., Jing, P., *et al.* (1999). Virus-specific cytotoxic T-lymphocyte responses select for amino-acid variation in simian immunodeficiency virus Env and Nef. *Nat Med* **5**: 1270–1276.

Everall, I.P., Luthert, P.J., and Lantos, P.L. (1991). Neuronal loss in the frontal cortex in HIV infection. *Lancet* **337**: 1119–1121.

Everall, I.P., Heaton, R.K., Marcotte, T.D., *et al.* (1999). Cortical synaptic density is reduced in mild to moderate human immunodeficiency virus neurocognitive disorder. HNRC Group. HIV Neurobehavioral Research Center. *Brain Pathol* **9**: 209–217.

Falangola, M.F., Hanly, A., Galvao-Castro, B., and Petito, C.K. (1995). HIV infection of human choroid plexus: a possible mechanism of viral entry into the CNS. *J Neuropathol Exp Neurol* **54**: 497–503.

Feng, Y., Broder, C.C., Kennedy, P.E., and Berger, E.A. (1996). HIV-1 entry cofactor: functional cDNA cloning of a seven-transmembrane, G protein-coupled receptor. *Science* **272**: 872–877.

Fine, S.M., Angel, R.A., Perry, S.W., *et al.* (1996). Tumor necrosis factor alpha inhibits glutamate uptake by primary human astrocytes. Implications for pathogenesis of HIV-1 dementia. *J Biol Chem* **271**: 15303–15306.

Flanagan, E.M., Erickson, J.B., Viveros, O.H., Chang, S.Y., and Reinhard, J.F. Jr (1995). Neurotoxin quinolinic acid is selectively elevated in spinal cords of rats with experimental allergic encephalomyelitis. *J Neurochem* **64**: 1192–1196.

Gelbard, H.A., Nottet, H.S., Swindells, S., *et al.* (1994). Platelet-activating factor: a candidate human immunodeficiency virus type 1-induced neurotoxin. *J Virol* **68**: 4628–4635.

Gendelman, H.E., Persidsky, Y., Ghorpade, A., *et al.* (1997). The neuropathogenesis of the AIDS dementia complex. *AIDS* **11**: S35–S45.

Genis, P., Jett, M., Bernton, E.W., *et al.* (1992). Cytokines and arachidonic metabolites produced during human immunodeficiency virus (HIV)-infected macrophage-astroglia interactions: implications for the neuropathogenesis of HIV disease. *J Exp Med* **176**: 1703–1718.

Giulian, D., Vaca, K., and Noonan, C.A. (1990). Secretion of neurotoxins by mononuclear phagocytes infected with HIV-1. *Science* **250**: 1593–1596.

Giulian, D., Wendt, E., Vaca, K., and Noonan, C.A. (1993). The envelope glycoprotein of human immunodeficiency virus type 1 stimulates release of neurotoxins from monocytes. *Proc Natl Acad Sci USA* **90**: 2769–2773.

Giulian, D., Yu, J., Li, X., *et al.* (1996). Study of receptor-mediated neurotoxins released by HIV-1-infected mononuclear phagocytes found in human brain. *J Neurosci* **16**: 3139–3153.

Glass, J.D., Fedor, H., Wesselingh, S.L., and McArthur, J.C. (1995). Immunocytochemical quantitation of human immunodeficiency virus in the brain: correlations with dementia. *Ann Neurol* **38**: 755–762.

Glass, M., Faull, R.L., Bullock, J.Y., *et al.* (1996). Loss of A1 adenosine receptors in human temporal lobe epilepsy. *Brain Res* **710**: 56–68.

Gonzalez, E., Rovin, B.H., Sen, L., *et al.* (2002). HIV-1 infection and AIDS dementia are influenced by a mutant MCP-1 allele linked to increased monocyte infiltration of tissues and MCP-1 levels. *Proc Natl Acad Sci USA* **99**: 13795–13800.

Goulder, P.J. and Walker, B.D. (1999). The great escape—AIDS viruses and immune control. *Nat Med* **5**: 1233–1235.

Goulder, P.J., Phillips, R.E., Colbert, R.A., *et al.* (1997). Late escape from an immunodominant cytotoxic T-lymphocyte response associated with progression to AIDS. *Nat Med* **3**: 212–217.

Goulder, P.J., Altfeld, M.A., Rosenberg, E.S., *et al.* (2001). Substantial differences in specificity of HIV-specific cytotoxic T cells in acute and chronic HIV infection. *J Exp Med* **193**: 181–194.

Greene, W.C. (1991). The molecular biology of human immunodeficiency virus type 1 infection. *N Engl J Med* **324**: 308–317.

Griffin, D.E., McArthur, J.C., and Cornblath, D.R. (1991). Neopterin and interferon-gamma in serum and cerebrospinal fluid of patients with HIV-associated neurologic disease. *Neurology* **41**: 69–74.

Griffin, D.E., Wesselingh, S.L., and McArthur, J.C. (1994). Elevated central nervous system prostaglandins in human immunodeficiency virus-associated dementia. *Ann Neurol* **35**: 592–597.

Gruol, D.L., Yu, N., Parsons, K.L., Billaud, J.N., Elder, J.H., and Phillips, T.R. (1998). Neurotoxic effects of feline immunodeficiency virus, FIV-PPR. *J Neurovirol* **4**: 415–425.

Gyorkey, F., Melnick, J.L., and Gyorkey P. (1987). Human immunodeficiency virus in brain biopsies of patients with AIDS and progressive encephalopathy. *J Infect Dis* **155**: 870–876.

Haase, A.T. (1986). Pathogenesis of lentivirus infections. *Nature* **322**: 130–136.

Harouse, J.M., Bhat, S., Spitalnik, S.L., *et al.* (1991). Inhibition of entry of HIV-1 in neural cell lines by antibodies against galactosyl ceramide. *Science* **253**: 320–323.

Harrigan, P.R. and Alexander, C.S. (1999). Selection of drug-resistant HIV. *Trends Microbiol* **7**: 120–123 [published erratum appears in *Trends Microbiol* **7**(7): 302].

He, J., Chen, Y., Farzan, M., *et al.* (1997). CCR3 and CCR5 are co-receptors for HIV-1 infection of microglia. *Nature* **385**: 645–649.

Heyes, M.P., Gravell, M., London, W.T., *et al.* (1990). Sustained increases in cerebrospinal fluid quinolinic acid concentrations in rhesus macaques (*Macaca mulatta*) naturally infected with simian retrovirus type-D. *Brain Res* **531**: 148–158.

Heyes, M.P., Brew, B.J., Martin, A., *et al.* (1991). Quinolinic acid in cerebrospinal fluid and serum in HIV-1 infection: relationship to clinical and neurological status. *Ann Neurol* **29**: 202–209.

Heyes, M.P., Saito, K., Chen, C.Y., *et al.* (1997). Species heterogeneity between gerbils and rats: quinolinate production by microglia and astrocytes and accumulations in response to ischemic brain injury and systemic immune activation. *J Neurochem* **69**: 1519–1529.

Hirsch, M.S., Conway, B., D'Aquila, R.T., *et al.* (1998). Antiretroviral drug resistance testing in adults with HIV infection: implications for clinical management. International AIDS Society–USA Panel. *J Am Med Assoc* **279**: 1984–1991.

Ho, D.D., Rota, T.R., Schooley, R.T., *et al.* (1985). Isolation of HTLV-III from cerebrospinal fluid and neural tissues of patients with neurologic syndromes related to the acquired immunodeficiency syndrome. *N Engl J Med* **313**: 1493–1497.

Huang, K.J., Alter, G.M., and Wooley, D.P. (2002). The reverse transcriptase sequence of human immunodeficiency virus type 1 is under positive evolutionary selection within the central nervous system. *J Neurovirol* **8**: 281–294.

Hurwitz, A.A., Berman, J.W., and Lyman, W.D. (1994). The role of the blood-brain barrier in HIV infection of the central nervous system. *Adv Neuroimmunol* **4**: 249–256.

Hwang, S.S., Boyle, T.J., Lyerly, H.K., and Cullen, B.R. (1991). Identification of the envelope V3 loop as the primary determinant of cell tropism in HIV-1. *Science* **253**: 71–74.

Johnson R. (1998). *Viral Infections of the Nervous System*, 2nd edn. Lippincott-Raven, Philadelphia, PA.

Johnson, R.T., Glass, J.D., McArthur, J.C., and Chesebro, B.W. (1996). Quantitation of human immunodeficiency virus in brains of demented and non-demented patients with acquired immunodeficiency syndrome. *Ann Neurol* **39**: 392–395.

Johnston, J.B., Jiang, Y., van Marle, G., *et al.* (2000). Lentiviral infection in the brain induce matrix metalloproteinase expression: the role of envelope diversity. *J Virol* **74**: 7211–7220.

Johnston, J.B., Zhang, K., Silva, C., *et al.* (2001). HIV-1 Tat neurotoxicity is prevented by matrix metalloproteinase inhibitors. *Ann Neurol* **49**: 230–241.

Johnston, J.B., Silva, C., and Power C. (2002). Envelope gene-mediated neurovirulence in feline immunodeficiency virus infection: induction of matrix metalloproteinases and neuronal injury. *J Virol* **76**: 2622–2633.

Kaiser, P.K., Offermann, J.T., and Lipton, S.A. (1990). Neuronal injury due to HIV-1 envelope protein is blocked by anti-gp120 antibodies but not by anti-CD4 antibodies. *Neurology* **40**: 1757–1761.

Kaslow, R.A., Carrington, M., Apple, R., *et al.* (1996). Influence of combinations of human major histocompatibility complex genes on the course of HIV-1 infection. *Nat Med* **2**: 405–411.

Kaul, M. and Lipton, S.A. (1999). Chemokines and activated macrophages in HIV gp120-induced neuronal apoptosis. *Proc Natl Acad Sci USA* **96**: 8212–8216.

Kelder, W., McArthur, J.C., Nance-Sproson, T., McClernon, D., and Griffin, D.E. (1998). Beta-chemokines MCP-1 and RANTES are selectively increased in cerebrospinal fluid of patients with human immunodeficiency virus- associated dementia. *Ann Neurol* **44**: 831–835.

Ketzler, S., Weis, S., Haug, H., and Budka H. (1990). Loss of neurons in the frontal cortex in AIDS brains. *Acta Neuropathol* **80**: 92–94.

Koenig, S., Gendelman, H.E., Orenstein, J.M., *et al.* (1986). Detection of AIDS virus in macrophages in brain tissue from AIDS patients with encephalopathy. *Science* **233**: 1089–1093.

Koito, A., Harrowe, G., Levy, J.A., and Cheng-Mayer C. (1994). Functional role of the V1/V2 region of human immunodeficiency virus type 1 envelope glycoprotein gp120 in infection of primary macrophages and soluble CD4 neutralization. *J Virol* **68**: 2253–2259.

Kolson, D. and Pomerantz R. (1996). AIDS dementia and HIV-1-induced neurotoxicity: possible pathogenic associations and mechanisms. *J Biomed Sci* **3**: 389–414.

Korber, B., Foley, B., Leitner, T., *et al.*, eds (1997). *Human Retroviruses and AIDS 1997*. Theoretical Biology and Biophysics, Los Alamos, NM.

Krucker, T., Toggas, S.M., Mucke, L., and Siggins, G.R. (1998). Transgenic mice with cerebral expression of human immunodeficiency virus type-1 coat protein gp120 show divergent changes in short- and long-term potentiation in CA1 hippocampus. *Neuroscience* **83**: 691–700.

Kuiken, C.L., Goudsmit, J., Weiller, G.F., *et al.* (1995). Differences in human immunodeficiency virus type 1 V3 sequences from patients with and without AIDS dementia complex. *J Gen Virol* **76**: 175–180.

Kure, K., Lyman, W.D., Weidenheim, K.M., and Dickson, D.W. (1990). Cellular localization of an HIV-1 antigen in subacute AIDS encephalitis using an improved double-labeling immunohistochemical method. *Am J Pathol* **136**: 1085–1092.

Lazarini, F., Seilhean, D., Rosenblum, O., *et al.* (1997). Human immunodeficiency virus type 1 DNA and RNA load in brains of demented and nondemented patients with acquired immunodeficiency syndrome. *J Neurovirol* **3**: 299–303.

Letendre, S.L., Lanier, E.R., and McCutchan, J.A. (1999). Cerebrospinal fluid beta chemokine concentrations in neurocognitively impaired individuals infected with human immunodeficiency virus type 1. *J Infect Dis* **180**: 310–319.

Levy, J. (1998). *HIV and the Pathogenesis of AIDS*, 2nd edn. American Society of Microbiology, Washington, DC.

Levy, J.A., Shimabukuro, J., Hollander, H., Mills, J., and Kaminsky L. (1985). Isolation of AIDS-associated retroviruses from cerebrospinal fluid and brain of patients with neurological symptoms. *Lancet* **2**: 586–598.

Lipton, S.A. and Gendelman, H.E. (1995). Seminars in medicine of the Beth Israel Hospital, Boston. Dementia associated with the acquired immunodeficiency syndrome. *N Engl J Med* **332**: 934–940.

Liu, Z.Q., Muhkerjee, S., Sahni, M., *et al.* (1999). Derivation and biological characterization of a molecular clone of SHIV(KU-2) that causes AIDS, neurological disease, and renal disease in rhesus macaques. *Virology* **260**: 295–307.

Ma, M., Geiger, J.D., and Nath A. (1994). Characterization of a novel binding site for the human immunodeficiency virus type 1 envelope protein gp120 on human fetal astrocytes. *J Virol* **68**: 6824–6828.

Maj, M., Satz, P., Janssen, R., *et al.* (1994). WHO Neuropsychiatric AIDS study, cross-sectional phase II. Neuropsychological and neurological findings. *Arch Gen Psychiat* **51**: 51–61.

Masliah, E., Ge, N., Achim, C.L., Hansen, L.A., and Wiley, C.A. (1992*a*). Selective neuronal vulnerability in HIV encephalitis. *J Neuropathol Exp Neurol* **51**: 585–593.

Masliah, E., Ge, N., Morey, M., DeTeresa, R., Terry, R.D., and Wiley, C.A. (1992*b*). Cortical dendritic pathology in human immunodeficiency virus encephalitis. *Lab Invest* **66**: 285–291.

Mayne, M., Bratanich, A.C., Chen, P., Rana, F., Nath, A., and Power, C. (1998). HIV-1 tat molecular diversity and induction of TNF-alpha: implications for HIV-induced neurological disease. *Neuroimmunomodulation* **5**: 184–192.

McArthur, J.C. (1987). Neurologic manifestations of AIDS. *Medicine (Baltimore)* **66**: 407–437.

McArthur, J.C., Nance-Sproson, T.E., Griffin, D.E., *et al.* (1992). The diagnostic utility of elevation in cerebrospinal fluid beta 2- microglobulin in HIV-1 dementia. Multicenter AIDS Cohort Study. *Neurology* **42**: 1707–1712.

McArthur, J.C., Hoover, D.R., Bacellar, H., *et al.* (1993). Dementia in AIDS patients: incidence and risk factors. Multicenter AIDS Cohort Study. *Neurology* **43**: 2245–2252.

McArthur, J.C., McClernon, D.R., Cronin, M.F., *et al.* (1997). Relationship between human immunodeficiency virus-associated dementia and viral load in cerebrospinal fluid and brain. *Ann Neurol* **42**: 689–698.

McClernon, D.R., Lanier, R., Gartner, S., *et al.* (2001). HIV in the brain: RNA levels and patterns of zidovudine resistance. *Neurology* **57**: 1396–1401.

McMichael, A.J. and Rowland-Jones, S.L. (2001). Cellular immune responses to HIV. *Nature* **410**: 980–987.

McNearney, T., Hornickova, Z., Markham, R., *et al.* (1992). Relationship of human immunodeficiency virus type 1 sequence heterogeneity to stage of disease. *Proc Natl Acad Sci USA* **89**: 10247–10251.

Migueles, S.A., Sabbaghian, M.S., Shupert, W.L., *et al.* (2000). HLA B*5701 is highly associated with restriction of virus replication in a subgroup of HIV-infected long term nonprogressors. *Proc Natl Acad Sci USA* **97**: 2709–2714.

Mirsattari, S.M., Berry, M.E., Holden, J.K., Ni, W., Nath, A., and Power C. (1999). Paroxysmal dyskinesias in patients with HIV infection. *Neurology* **52**: 109–114.

Moroni F. (1999). Tryptophan metabolism and brain function: focus on kynurenine and other indole metabolites. *Eur J Pharmacol* **375**: 87–100.

Morris, A., Marsden, M., Halcrow, K., *et al.* (1999). Mosaic structure of the human immunodeficiency virus type 1 genome infecting lymphoid cells and the brain: evidence for frequent *in vivo* recombination events in the evolution of regional populations. *J Virol* **73**: 8720–8731.

Moses, A.V., Bloom, F.E., Pauza, C.D., and Nelson, J.A. (1993). Human immunodeficiency virus infection of human brain capillary endothelial cells occurs via a CD4/galactosylceramide-independent mechanism. *Proc Natl Acad Sci USA* **90**: 10474–10478.

Narayan, O.J. and Clements, J.E. (1989). Biology and pathogenesis of lentiviruses. *J Gen Virol* **70**: 1617–1639.

Nath, A. and Geiger J. (1998). Neurobiological aspects of human immunodeficiency virus infection: neurotoxic mechanisms. *Prog Neurobiol* **54**: 19–33.

Nath, A., Psooy, K., Martin, C., *et al.* (1996). Identification of a human immunodeficiency virus type 1 Tat epitope that is neuroexcitatory and neurotoxic. *J Virol* **70**: 1475–1480.

Nath, A., Conant, K., Chen, P., Scott, C., and Major, E.O. (1999). Transient exposure to HIV-1 Tat protein results in cytokine production in macrophages and astrocytes. A hit and run phenomenon. *J Biol Chem* **274**: 17098–17102.

Navia, B.A., Jordan, B.D., and Price, R.W. (1986a). The AIDS dementia complex: I. Clinical features. *Ann Neurol* **19**: 517–524.

Navia, B.A., Cho, E.S., Petito, C.K., and Price, R.W. (1986b). The AIDS dementia complex: II. Neuropathology. *Ann Neurol* **19**: 525–535.

Nuovo, G.J., Gallery, F., MacConnell, P., and Braun A. (1994). *In situ* detection of polymerase chain reaction-amplified HIV-1 nucleic acids and tumor necrosis factor-alpha RNA in the central nervous system. *Am J Pathol* **144**: 659–666.

O'Brien, W.A., Hartigan, P.M., Martin, D., *et al.* (1996). Changes in plasma HIV-1 RNA and CD4+ lymphocyte counts and the risk of progression to AIDS. Veterans Affairs Cooperative Study Group on AIDS. *N Engl J Med* **334**: 426–431.

O'Hagen, A., Ghosh, S., He, J., *et al.* (1999). Apoptosis induced by infection of primary brain cultures with diverse human immunodeficiency virus type 1 isolates: evidence for a role of the envelope. *J Virol* **73**: 897–906.

Overbaugh, J. and Bangham, C.R. (2001). Selection forces and constraints on retroviral sequence variation. *Science* **292**: 1106–1109.

Pang, S., Vinters, H.V., Akashi, T., O'Brien, W.A., and Chen, I.S. (1991). HIV-1 env sequence variation in brain tissue of patients with AIDS- related neurologic disease. *J Acq Immune Def Synd* **4**: 1082–1092.

Patrick, M.K., Johnston, J.B., and Power C. (2002). Lentiviral neuropathogenesis: comparative neuroinvasion, neurotropism, neurovirulence and host neurosusceptibility. *J Virol* **76**: 7923–7231.

Pattarini, R., Pittaluga, A., and Raiteri M. (1998). The human immunodeficiency virus-1 envelope protein gp120 binds through its V3 sequence to the glycine site of N-methyl-D-aspartate receptors mediating noradrenaline release in the hippocampus. *Neuroscience* **87**: 147–157.

Perelson, A.S., Essunger, P., Cao, Y., *et al.* (1997). Decay characteristics of HIV-1-infected compartments during combination therapy. *Nature* **387**: 188–191.

Petito, C.K. and Cash, K.S. (1992). Blood-brain barrier abnormalities in the acquired immunodeficiency syndrome: immunohistochemical localization of serum proteins in postmortem brain. *Ann Neurol* **32**: 658–666.

Poluektova, L.Y., Munn, D.H., Persidsky, Y., and Gendelman, H.E. (2002). Generation of cytotoxic T cells against virus-infected human brain macrophages in a murine model of HIV-1 encephalitis. *J Immunol* **168**: 3941–3949.

Power, C. (2001). Retroviral diseases of the nervous system: pathogenic host response or viral gene-mediated neurovirulence? *Trends Neurosci* **24**: 162–169.

Power, C. and Johnson, R.T. (2001). Neurovirological and neuroimmunological aspects of HIV infection. *Adv Virus Res* **56**: 579–624.

Power, C., Kong, P.A., Crawford, T.O., *et al.* (1993). Cerebral white matter changes in acquired immunodeficiency syndrome dementia: alterations of the blood-brain barrier. *Ann Neurol* **34**: 339–350.

Power, C., McArthur, J.C., Johnson, R.T., *et al.* (1994). Demented and non-demented patients with AIDS differ in brain-derived human immunodeficiency virus type 1 envelope sequences. *J Virol* **68**: 4643–4649.

Power, C., Buist, R., Johnston, J.B., *et al.* (1998a). Neurovirulence in feline immunodeficiency virus-infected neonatal cats is viral strain specific and dependent on systemic immune suppression. *J Virol* **72**: 9109–9115.

Power, C., McArthur, J.C., Nath, A., *et al.* (1998b). Neuronal death induced by brain-derived human immunodeficiency virus type 1 envelope genes differs between demented and nondemented AIDS patients. *J Virol* **72**: 9045–9053.

Pulliam, L., Herndier, B.G., Tang, N.M., and McGrath, M.S. (1991). Human immunodeficiency virus-infected macrophages produce soluble factors that cause histological and neurochemical alterations in cultured human brains. *J Clin Invest* **87**: 503–512.

Quagliarello, V.J., Wispelwey, B., Long, W.J. Jr, and Scheld, W.M. (1991). Recombinant human interleukin-1 induces meningitis and blood-brain barrier injury in the rat. Characterization and comparison with tumor necrosis factor. *J Clin Invest* **87**: 1360–1366.

Quasney, M.W., Zhang, Q., Sargent, S., Mynatt, M., Glass, J., and McArthur J. (2001). Increased frequency of the tumor necrosis factor-alpha-308 A allele in adults with human immunodeficiency virus dementia. *Ann Neurol* **50**: 157–162.

Ransohoff, R.M., Tani M. (1998). Do chemokines mediate leukocyte recruitment in post-traumatic CNS inflammation? *Trends Neurosci* **21**: 154–159.

Reddy, R.T., Achim, C.L., Sirko, D.A., *et al.* (1996). Sequence analysis of the V3 loop in brain and spleen of patients with HIV encephalitis. *AIDS Res Hum Retroviruses* **12**: 477–482.

Resnick, L., diMarzo-Veronese, F., Schupbach, J., *et al.* (1985). Intra-blood-brain-barrier synthesis of HTLV-III-specific IgG in patients with neurologic symptoms associated with AIDS or AIDS-related complex. *N Engl J Med* **313**: 1498–1504.

Rostasy, K., Monti, L., Yiannoutsos, C., *et al.* (1999). Human immunodeficiency virus infection, inducible nitric oxide synthase expression, and microglial activation: pathogenetic relationship to the acquired immunodeficiency syndrome dementia complex. *Ann Neurol* **46**: 207–216.

Rothstein, J.D., Jin, L., Dykes-Hoberg, M., and Kuncl, R.W. (1993). Chronic inhibition of glutamate uptake produces a model of slow neurotoxicity. *Proc Natl Acad Sci USA* **90**: 6591–6595.

Rothstein, J.D., Dykes-Hoberg, M., Pardo, C.A., *et al.* (1996). Knockout of glutamate transporters reveals a major role for astroglial transport in excitotoxicity and clearance of glutamate. *Neuron* **16**: 675–686.

Royal, W. 3rd, Selnes, O.A., Concha, M., Nance-Sproson, T.E., and McArthur, J.C. (1994). Cerebrospinal fluid human immunodeficiency virus type 1 (HIV-1). p24 antigen levels in HIV-1-related dementia. *Ann Neurol* **36**: 32–39.

Rubbert, A., Bock, E., Schwab, J., *et al.* (1994). Anticardiolipin antibodies in HIV infection: association with cerebral perfusion defects as detected by 99mTc-HMPAO SPECT. *Clin Exp Immunol* **98**: 361–368.

Sacktor, N.C., Lyles, R.H., Skolasky, R.L., *et al.* (1999). Combination antiretroviral therapy improves psychomotor speed performance in HIV-seropositive homosexual men. Multicenter AIDS Cohort Study (MACS). *Neurology* **52**: 1640–1647.

Saito, K. and Heyes, M.P. (1996). Kynurenine pathway enzymes in brain. Properties of enzymes and regulation of quinolinic acid synthesis. *Adv Exp Med Biol* **398**: 485–492.

Saito, Y., Sharer, L.R., Epstein, L.G., *et al.* (1994). Overexpression of nef as a marker for restricted HIV-1 infection of astrocytes in postmortem pediatric central nervous tissues. *Neurology* **44**: 474–481.

Sanders, V.J., Pittman, C.A., White, M.G., Wang, G., Wiley, C.A., and Achim, C.L. (1998). Chemokines and receptors in HIV encephalitis. *AIDS* **12**: 1021–1026.

Sei, S., Saito, K., Stewart, S.K., *et al.* (1995). Increased human immunodeficiency virus (HIV). type 1 DNA content and quinolinic acid concentration in brain tissues from patients with HIV encephalopathy. *J Infect Dis* **172**: 638–647.

Sharer, L.R. (1992). Pathology of HIV-1 infection of the central nervous system. A review. *J Neuropathol Exp Neurol* **51**: 3–11.

Sharer, L.R., Epstein, L.G., Cho, E.S., *et al.* (1986). Pathologic features of AIDS encephalopathy in children: evidence for LAV/HTLV-III infection of brain. *Hum Pathol* **17**: 271–284.

Shaw, G.M., Harper, M.E., Hahn, B.H., *et al.* (1985). HTLV-III infection in brains of children and adults with AIDS encephalopathy. *Science* **227**: 177–182.

Shi, B., De Girolami, U., He, J., *et al.* (1996). Apoptosis induced by HIV-1 infection of the central nervous system. *J Clin Invest* **98**: 1979–1990.

Shrikant, P., Benos, D.J., Tang, L.P., and Benveniste, E.N. (1996). HIV glycoprotein 120 enhances intercellular adhesion molecule-1 gene expression in glial cells. Involvement of Janus kinase/signal transducer and activator of transcription and protein kinase C signaling pathways. *J Immunol* **156**: 1307–1314.

Simpson, D.M. and Tagliati M. (1994). Neurologic manifestations of HIV infection. *Ann Intern Med* **121**: 769–785 [published erratum appears in *Ann Intern Med* 1995 **122**(4): 317].

Sippy, B.D., Hofman, F.M., Wallach, D., and Hinton, D.R. (1995). Increased expression of tumor necrosis factor-alpha receptors in the brains of patients with AIDS. *J Acq Immune Def Synd Hum Retrovirol* **10**: 511–521.

Strizki, J.M., Albright, A.V., Sheng, H., O'Connor, M., Perrin, L., and Gonzalez-Scarano F. (1996). Infection of primary human microglia and monocyte-derived macrophages with human immunodeficiency virus type 1 isolates: evidence of differential tropism. *J Virol* **70**: 7654–7662.

Takahashi, K., Wesselingh, S.L., Griffin, D.E., McArthur, J.C., Johnson, R.T., and Glass, J.D. (1996). Localization of HIV-1 in human brain using polymerase chain reaction/*in situ* hybridization and immunocytochemistry. *Ann Neurol* **39**: 705–711.

Tan, S.V., Guiloff, R.J., and Scarvilli F. (1995). AIDS-associated vacuolar myelopathy, a morphometric study. *Brain* **118**: 1247–1261.

Teo, I., Veryard, C., Barnes, H., *et al.* (1997). Circular forms of unintegrated human immunodeficiency virus type 1 DNA and high levels of viral protein expression: association with dementia and multinucleated giant cells in the brains of patients with AIDS. *J Virol* **71**: 2928–2933.

Toggas, S.M., Masliah, E., Rockenstein, E.M., Rall, G.F., Abraham, C.R., and Mucke, L. (1994). Central nervous system damage produced by expression of the HIV-1 coat protein gp120 in transgenic mice [see comments]. *Nature* **367**: 188–193.

Toohey, K., Wehrly, K., Nishio, J., Perryman, S., and Chesebro, B. (1995). Human immunodeficiency virus envelope V1 and V2 regions influence replication efficiency in macrophages by affecting virus spread. *Virology* **213**: 70–79.

Torres-Munoz, J., Stockton, P., Tacoronte, N., Roberts, B., Maronpot, R.R., and Petito, C.K. (2001). Detection of HIV-1 gene sequences in hippocampal neurons isolated from postmortem AIDS brains by laser capture microdissection. *J Neuropathol Exp Neurol* **60**: 885–892.

Triggiani, M., Oriente, A., de Crescenzo, G., Rossi, G., and Marone, G. (1995). Biochemical functions of a pool of arachidonic acid associated with triglycerides in human inflammatory cells. *Int Arch Allergy Appl Immunol* **107**: 261–263.

Tyor, W.R., Glass, J.D., Griffin, J.W., *et al.* (1992). Cytokine expression in the brain during the acquired immunodeficiency syndrome. *Ann Neurol* **31**: 349–360.

Tyor, W.R., Glass, J.D., Baumrind, N., *et al.* (1993). Cytokine expression of macrophages in HIV-1-associated vacuolar myelopathy. *Neurology* **43**: 1002–1009.

van Marle, G., Rourke, S.B., Zhang, K., *et al.* (2002). HIV dementia patients exhibit reduced viral neutralization and increased envelope sequence diversity in blood and brain. *AIDS* **16**: 1905–1914.

Van Rij, R.P., Portegies, P., Hallaby, T., *et al.* (1999). Reduced prevalence of the CCR5 delta32 heterozygous genotype in human immunodeficiency virus-infected individuals with AIDS dementia complex. *J Infect Dis* **180**: 854–857.

Vazeux, R., Lacroix-Ciaudo, C., Blanche, S., *et al.* (1992). Low levels of human immunodeficiency virus replication in the brain tissue of children with severe acquired immunodeficiency syndrome encephalopathy. *Am J Pathol* **140**: 137–144.

Vinters, H.V. and Anders, K.H. (1990). *Neuropathology of AIDS*. CRC Press, Boca Raton, FL.

Walker, B.D. and Goulder, P.J. (2000). AIDS. Escape from the immune system. *Nature* **407**: 313–314.

Weiss, R.A. (1996). HIV receptors and the pathogenesis of AIDS. *Science* **272**: 1885–1886.

Wesselingh, S.L., Power, C., Glass, J.D., *et al.* (1993). Intracerebral cytokine messenger RNA expression in acquired immunodeficiency syndrome dementia. *Ann Neurol* **33**: 576–582.

Westervelt, P., Trowbridge, D.B., Epstein, L.G., *et al.* (1992). Macrophage tropism determinants of human immunodeficiency virus type 1 *in vivo. J Virol* **66**: 2577–2582.

Westmoreland, S.V., Kolson, D., and Gonzalez-Scarano, F. (1996). Toxicity of TNF alpha and platelet activating factor for human NT2N neurons: a tissue culture model for human immunodeficiency virus dementia. *J Neurovirol* **2**: 118–126.

Wiley, C.A., Baldwin, M., and Achim, C.L. (1996). Expression of HIV regulatory and structural mRNA in the central nervous system. *AIDS* **10**: 843–847.

Wiley, C.A., Schrier, R.D., Nelson, J.A., Lampert, P.W., and Oldstone, M.B. (1986). Cellular localization of human immunodeficiency virus infection within the brains of acquired immune deficiency syndrome patients. *Proc Natl Acad Sci USA* **83**: 7089–7093.

Wilt, S.G., Milward, E., Zhou, J.M., *et al.* (1995). *In vitro* evidence for a dual role of tumor necrosis factor-alpha in human immunodeficiency virus type 1 encephalopathy. *Ann Neurol* **37**: 381–394.

Wong, J.K., Ignacio, C.C., Torriani, F., Havlir, D., Fitch, N.J., and Richman, D.D. (1997). *In vivo* compartmentalization of human immunodeficiency virus: evidence from the examination of pol sequences from autopsy tissues. *J Virol* **71**: 2059–2071.

Yamada, M., Zurbriggen, A., Oldstone, M.B., and Fujinami, R.S. (1991). Common immunologic determinant between human immunodeficiency virus type 1 gp41 and astrocytes. *J Virol* **65**: 1370–1376.

Yong, V.W., Power, C., Forsyth, P., and Edwards D. (2001). Metalloproteinases in the biology and pathology of the nervous system. *Nat Neurosci* **2**: 502–511.

Zheng, J., Ghorpade, A., Niemann, D., *et al.* (1999). Lymphotropic virions affect chemokine receptor-mediated neural signaling and apoptosis: implications for human immunodeficiency virus type 1-associated dementia. *J Virol* **73**: 8256–8267.

Zink, M.C., Amedee, A.M., Mankowski, J.L., *et al.* (1997). Pathogenesis of SIV encephalitis. Selection and replication of neurovirulent SIV. *Am J Pathol* **151**: 793–803.

23 HTLV-I infection and the nervous system

Utano Tomaru, Yoshihisa Yamano, and Steven Jacobson

Introduction

The human T-cell lymphotropic virus type I (HTLV-I) is an exogenous human retrovirus that infects 10–20 million people worldwide (Poiesz *et al.*, 1980; de The and Bomford, 1993). This virus has been demonstrated to be the etiologic agent in adult T-cell leukemia (ATL), a progressive neurological disease called HTLV-I-associated myelopathy/tropical spastic paraparesis (HAM/TSP), and other inflammatory diseases including uveitis, arthritis, myositis, and alveolitis (Uchiyama *et al.*, 1977; Gessain *et al.*, 1985; Osame *et al.*, 1986*b*; Sugimoto *et al.*, 1987; Vernant *et al.*, 1988; Sasaki *et al.*, 1989; Ohba *et al.*, 1989; Nishioka *et al.*, 1989; Morgan *et al.*, 1989; Sato *et al.*, 1991; Mochizuki *et al.*, 1992; Higuchi *et al.*, 1993; Leon-Monzon *et al.*, 1994; Terada *et al.*, 1994). While HTLV-I persists throughout life, fewer than 5% of individuals infected with HTLV-I develop ATL or HAM/TSP, and the vast majority remains as asymptomatic carriers (Uchiyama, 1997). For nearly two decades, HTLV-I has been studied because of its association with a broad spectrum of virus-related diseases including hematological malignancies and inflammatory disorders;

however, it is still unclear how HTLV-I infection induces these different diseases in a subset of infected individuals.

This chapter will review the biology of HTLV-I and current approaches for understanding the immunopathogenesis of HTLV-I-associated neurological disease. Based on recent studies, virus–host immunological interactions, specifically cellular immune responses of HTLV-I-specific CD8+ T cells, have been suggested to play an important role in the pathogenesis of HAM/TSP. A more complete understanding of HTLV-I and host immune responses will allow for the development of immunotherapeutic strategies for the treatment of this chronic progressive neurologic disease.

Biology of HTLV-I

Genetic structure of HTLV-I

HTLV-I was the first retrovirus known to be associated with human disease. HTLV-I belongs to the *Oncoviridae* subfamily of retroviruses, which

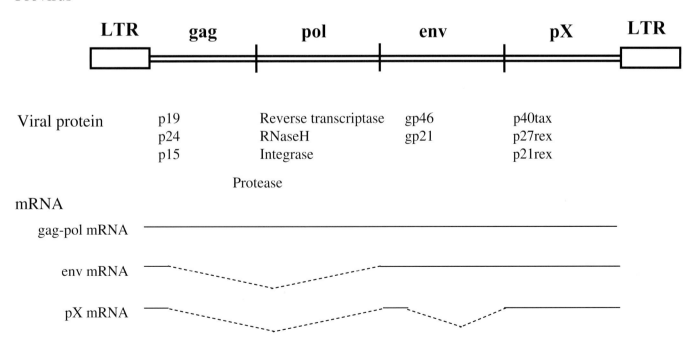

Fig. 23.1 Structure of HTLV-I. The HTLV-I proviral genome has the *gag*, *pol*, and *env* genes, flanked by long terminal repeat (LTR) sequences on both sides. A unique structure is found between *env* and the 3′-LTR, which is named the *pX* gene and encodes the regulatory proteins p40tax, p27rex, and p21rex. Three major mRNA species have been identified for HTLV-I; full-length mRNA is utilized for synthesis of gag and pol gene products and is also the genomic RNA packaged into virions. A single-spliced subgenomic mRNA encodes the env gene product. A second subgenomic mRNA has two introns removed (doubly spliced or completely spliced) and encodes the tax and rex gene products.

includes HTLV-II, bovine leukemia virus (BLV), and simian T-cell leukemia virus (STLV) (Koralnik, 1996; Brady, 1996). Similar to other retroviruses, the HTLV-I proviral genome has the group antigen (*gag*), polymerase (*pol*), and envelope (*env*) genes flanked by long terminal repeat (LTR) sequence at both ends (Fig. 23.1) (Seiki *et al.*, 1983). The characteristic feature of this retroviral group is an additional proviral sequence of regulatory genes at the 3′-end of the proviral genome (Seiki *et al.*, 1983). This sequence, called *pX* (tax) in HTLV-I, contains four open reading frames and codes for three major regulatory proteins, p40tax, p27rex and p21rex (Koralnik, 1996).

The p40tax (Tax) protein has the capacity to transactivate viral transcription through indirect action upon the Tax-responsive element to the LTR as well as numerous cellular genes through several cellular transcription factors such as cyclic AMP response element binding protein (CREB), nuclear factor-κB (NF-κB), serum response factor (SRF), and basic helix– loop–helix proteins (bHLH) (Leung and Nabel, 1988; Zhao and Giam, 1991; Fujii *et al.*, 1992; Suzuki *et al.*, 1993; Uittenbogaard *et al.*, 1994). Transactivated cellular genes include cytokines, cytokine receptors, proto-oncogenes, and adhesion molecules such as interleukin-2 (IL-2), IL-3, IL-6, tumor necrosis factor-α (TNF-α), granulocyte/macrophage colony- stimulating factor (GM-CSF), transforming growth factor-β1 (TGF-β1), nerve growth factor-β (NGF-β), IL-2 receptor (IL-2R) α-chain, c-*fos*, c-*sis*, and parathyroid hormone related protein (Brady, 1996). In contrast, the expression of certain genes such as *lck*, and the β-polymerase gene which is involved in DNA repair, are down-regulated by the Tax protein (Lemasson *et al.*, 1997; Jeang *et al.*, 1990).

Although the function of the HTLV-I p21rex protein is still unclear, like the HTLV-I Tax protein, the p27rex (Rex) protein is essential for HTLV-I replication, but unlike Tax, Rex acts at a post-transcriptional level to regulate viral gene expression. Rex has been shown to increase the expression of unspliced mRNA coding for viral structure and enzymatic proteins, Gag and Pol, and singly spliced mRNA coding for Env protein, while Rex indirectly inhibits the expression of the doubly spliced mRNA coding for Tax and Rex (Seiki *et al.*, 1988; Hidaka *et al.*, 1988; Koralnik, 1996) (Fig. 23.1). The ultimate effect of Rex is therefore to regulate the levels of expression of genes encoding virion components, and thus determining whether infectious virions are produced (Koralnik, 1996).

Genetic variation of HTLV-I

HTLV-I can be classified phylogenetically into three major groups: Cosmopolitan, Central African, and Melanesian. Because different clinical outcomes are associated with an HTLV-I infection, it is important to clarify whether a specific variant of HTLV-I is associated with a particular HTLV-I-related disease. However, despite considerable studies, there is no significant indication that specific subtypes of HTLV-I are associated with particular pathologic consequences. For example, there are no consistent differences between subgroups from patients with ATL and those from patients with HAM/TSP. Recently, Furukawa *et al.* (2000) demonstrated that there was a four nucleotide substitution in the HTLV-I *tax* gene that was associated with a high risk of the development of HAM/TSP. Although it is still unclear how this HTLV-I *tax* variant is directly related to the pathogenesis of HAM/TSP, it is possible that a variation in HTLV-I *tax* gene alters host immune function, because HTLV-I Tax protein is a strong transactivator of numerous host genes including inflammatory cytokines, and is dominant epitope recognized by HTLV-I-specific CD8+ cytotoxic T lymphocytes (CTL) (Niewiesk *et al.*, 1995).

HTLV-I infectivity

Although extensive studies have been performed, the cellular receptor for HTLV-I has not been identified. *In vitro* infection experiments suggested that the HTLV-I receptor has a wide species and cell type distribution (Clapham *et al.*, 1983; Yamamoto *et al.*, 1984; Krichbaum-Stenger *et al.*, 1987). The gene encoding the receptor was mapped to chromosome 17 and further localized to 17q23.2–25.3 (Sommerfelt *et al.*, 1988; Gavalchin *et al.*, 1995), although later studies have questioned this assignment (Okuma *et al.*, 1999; Jassal *et al.*, 2001).

HTLV-I can infect a wide range of human and non-human cells *in vitro* (Trejo and Ratner, 2000); however, as in human immunodeficiency virus

type1 (HIV-1) infection, the lymphatic organs are the major reservoir in the HTLV-I-infected individuals (Jacobson *et al.*, 1997; Kazanji *et al.*, 2000). HTLV-I has been thought to preferentially infect CD4+ T cells *in vivo* (Richardson *et al.*, 1990), and recent work using quantitative polymerase chain reaction (PCR) indicated that CD8+ T cells were also a significant *in vivo* cellular reservoir for HTLV-I (Nagai *et al.*, 2001a). There is some evidence that macrophages and dendritic cells also might be infected *in vivo* (Hoffman *et al.*, 1992; Koyanagi *et al.*, 1993; Ali *et al.*, 1993). Therefore, from 90–99% of the HTLV-I proviral DNA in peripheral blood from infected patients is found in CD4+ or CD8+ T cells (Richardson *et al.*, 1990; Hanon *et al.*, 2000; Nagai *et al.*, 2001a).

In addition to peripheral blood, there are several reports that have demonstrated viral localization in infiltrating inflammatory cells or resident cells within central nervous system (CNS) lesions (Hara *et al.*, 1994; Furukawa *et al.*, 1994; Lehky *et al.*, 1995; Moritoyo *et al.*, 1996). For example, in the affected lesions of the spinal cord, infiltrating CD4+ T cells have been shown by *in situ* PCR hybridization to have proviral DNA, and to express viral protein by *in situ* hybridization (Hara *et al.*, 1994; Moritoyo *et al.*, 1996). HTLV-I RNA has been reported to be localized in resident astrocyte populations in the affected spinal cord (Lehky *et al.*, 1995). Other potential cell types harboring HTLV-I proviral DNA in the CNS may include macrophages, microglial cells, oligodendrocytes, and neurons, however, HTLV-I proviral DNA or viral RNA and protein have not yet been conclusively demonstrated in these cell types in the CNS (Hara *et al.*, 1994; Kubota *et al.*, 1994; Lehky *et al.*, 1995; Moritoyo *et al.*, 1996).

T-cell immortalization and transformation by HTLV-I

One of the striking abilities of HTLV-I that appears to be associated with oncogenesis and immune abnormalities is immortalization and transformation of T cells. In contrast to the cytopathic effect of HIV-1 for its host CD4+ cell, HTLV-I infection is not directly cytotoxic. However, HTLV-I can activate and immortalize human T lymphocytes *in vitro*, resulting in oligoclonal or monoclonal expansion of HTLV-I-infected cells in the absence of exogenous IL-2 (Kimata and Ratner, 1991). While HTLV-I has been demonstrated to be oncogenic in humans, HTLV-I does not contain homologous sequences to any known proto-oncogenes in the viral construct. In addition, HTLV-I has been known to integrate randomly into the host genomic DNA, and there is no specific integration site where the virus can selectively up-regulate proto-oncogene expression by a *cis*-acting effect (Seiki *et al.*, 1983; Koralnik, 1996).

It has been shown that HTLV-I Tax is critical for transformation of T lymphocytes, because specific mutations of the HTLV-I *tax* gene eliminate the transforming potential of the virus (Grassmann *et al.*, 1992). HTLV-I Tax can transactivate IL-2 and IL-2R genes, the products of which have a pivotal role in T-cell proliferation and differentiation. This observation leads to the suggestion of an IL-2 autocrine model for T-cell transformation by HTLV-I (Brady, 1996; Arima *et al.*, 1986). However, while ATL cells expressed abundant IL-2R on their surface, the majority of ATL cells do not respond to IL-2 and produce undetectable levels of this cytokine, indicating that the IL-2 autocrine model does not solely account for leukemogenesis (Arya *et al.*, 1984; Kodaka *et al.*, 1989). Recently, it has been demonstrated that HTLV-I transformation is associated with constitutive activation of the Janus family of tyrosine kinases (JAK)/signal transducers and activators of transcription (STAT) pathway (Migone *et al.*, 1995).

Epidemiology of HTLV-I

HTLV-I is distributed worldwide, and 10–20 million people are infected (Poiesz *et al.*, 1980; de The and Bomford, 1993). There are small clusters of high prevalence, most notably in the southern region of Japan (Kyushu, Shikoku, Okinawa), the Caribbean (Jamaica, Trinidad, Martinique, Barbados, Haiti), the equatorial regions of Africa (Ivory Coast, Nigeria, Zaire, Kenya, Tanzania), South America (Brazil, Colombia), the Middle East (Iran), and Melanesia (Tajima and Hinuma, 1984; Levine *et al.*, 1988; Mueller, 1991; Kaplan and Khabbaz, 1993; Tajima *et al.*, 1994; Blattner and Gallo, 1994; Gessain, 1996). This highly restricted geographic seroprevalence is a remarkable feature of HTLV-I epidemiology. The seroprevalence rate in the endemic areas can exceed 30% and the majority of infected individuals are clinically asymptomatic (Gessain, 1996). In the general population of the USA, the seroprevalence of HTLV-I is as low as 0.025%, but it can be as high as 2.1% in the southeastern region of the country (Williams et al., 1988; Khabbaz et al., 1990). It is not surprising that the prevalence of HTLV-I is significantly higher in intravenous drug users and patients in clinics for sexually transmitted diseases (Khabbaz et al., 1992).

Transmission of HTLV-I

Unlike HIV-1, there is little or no cell-free HTLV-I in the plasma, therefore HTLV-I requires cell-to-cell contact to infect other cells. In vitro, efficient infection can occur by co-cultivation with HTLV-I-infected cells (Yamamoto et al., 1982; Hollsberg and Hafler, 1993), where cell-free infection is extremely inefficient. Indeed, epidemiological studies suggest that transmission of HTLV-I in vivo also requires infected cells (Okochi et al., 1984; Lairmore et al., 1989; Sandler et al., 1991). There is no evidence for the transmission of HTLV-I by cell-free blood products including factor VIII (Okochi et al., 1984; Lairmore et al., 1989; Sandler et al., 1991).

The modes of transmission include perinatal transmission, sexual transmission, and transmission by blood, either from transfusion or by contaminated needles and syringes. Mother-to-child transmission occurs mainly via breast milk, and this is the major mode of transmission in endemic areas. As breast milk is known to contain maternal HTLV-I-infected T cells, approximately 10–30% of children fed breast milk from HTLV-I-infected mothers become infected with HTLV-I (Hino et al., 1985, 1994; Ando et al., 1987; Gessain, 1996). A preventive program in which HTLV-I-infected mothers were advised not to feed their children with breast milk led to a significant decrease of mother-to-child infection, from 20–30% to 3% in an endemic area of Japan (Hino et al., 1994). A reduction in the duration of breast feeding to less than 6 months may also decrease the possibility of mother-to-child infection (Takahashi et al., 1991). Other mechanisms of transmission, such as transplacental, have been less well documented.

Sexual transmission is greater from infected men to women than from infected women to men, probably through HTLV-I-infected T cells in semen (Murphy et al., 1989; Gessain, 1996). Some studies estimate the transmission risk for HTLV-I seropositive husbands to wives as approximately 60% over 10 years, while 0.4% of husbands with HTLV-I seropositive wives can be infected in the same period (Kajiyama et al., 1986). Transmission by breast milk generally requires breast feeding for more than 7 months, and wives of seropositive husbands reach 50% seroconversion after 1 to 4 years of marriage. These finding suggest inefficient transmission of HTLV-I and the need for multiple exposures (Xu et al., 1996).

In contrast, transmission of HTLV-I after receiving a contaminated whole blood transfusion and transmission among drug abusers through shared needles is well documented. Transmission by blood appears very efficient, and 25% of the patients with HAM/TSP in Japan have had a transfusion history (Osame et al., 1990b). It has been indicated that most patients seroconvert after receiving contaminated blood and that up to 20% of those receiving contaminated blood develop a myelopathy (Gessain and Gout, 1992). This is an extraordinary percentage and suggests that an infection by this route of inoculation (with greater dosage of virus or greater numbers of infected cells) imposes particular risk for developing myelopathy or that reinfection causes activation or induces an immune response related to the development of neurologic disease. The number of new HAM/TSP patients dramatically decreased after screening for HTLV-I in blood donors was launched in Japan (Osame et al., 1986a, 1990b).

HTLV-I infection and the nervous system

Clinical features of HAM/TSP

Several neurological manifestations have been linked to HTLV-I infection, e.g. muscular atrophy, polymyositis, peripheral neuropathy, polyradiculopathy, cranial neuropathy, meningitis, encephalopathy (Osame, 1990);

however, the most common neurological disorder associated with an HTLV-I infection is HTLV-I-associated myelopathy/tropical spastic paraparesis (HAM/TSP) (Gessain et al., 1985; Osame et al., 1986b).

HAM/TSP is characterized clinically by paraparesis associated with spasticity, hyper-reflexia, and Babinski's sign of the lower extremities (Osame et al., 1987, 1990a; Osame and McArthur, 1990; McFarlin and Blattner, 1991). The main neurological symptoms of HAM/TSP include bladder dysfunction, paraesthesia, low lumber pain, and impairment of vibration sense (Osame, 1990). Less frequent neurological findings are ataxia, hand tremor, optic atrophy, deafness, nystagmus, and other cranial nerve deficits. Convulsions, cognitive impairment, and dementia are rare. Usually HAM/TSP progress slowly over many years, but rarely acute cases have been observed (Osame, 1990).

The age of onset is usually 35 to 45 years, but can be as early as 12 years of age (Osame et al., 1990b; McFarlin and Blattner, 1991). HAM/TSP is three times more prevalent in women than men (Osame and McArthur, 1990; Osame et al., 1990b). The incubation period from time of infection to onset of disease ranges typically from years to decades, but can be as short as 18 weeks following blood transfusion with HTLV-I-contaminated blood (Osame et al., 1986a, 1987, 1990b; Gout et al., 1990). A quarter of the HAM/TSP patients in Japan have a previous history of blood transfusion (Osame et al., 1986a, 1990b). In these cases, progression of symptoms appears to be more rapid than in those patients with HAM/TSP who acquired HTLV-I through vertical transmission. Familial occurrence of HAM/TSP has been reported in a total of 44 cases in Japan and in occasional tropical cases (Osame et al., 1990b).

It has been reported that several inflammatory diseases, such as Sjögren's syndrome (Vernant et al., 1988), arthropathy (Kitajima et al., 1989), alveolitis (Sugimoto et al., 1987), uveitis (Sasaki et al., 1989), and interstitial cystitis (Nomata et al., 1992), occasionally occur in conjunction with HAM/TSP. In a clinical analysis of 213 cases of HAM/TSP patients in Japan, other organ diseases were frequently observed in HAM/TSP patients, including leukoencephalopathy (69%), abnormal chest X-ray (50%), Sjögren's syndrome (25%), and arthropathy (17%) (Nakagawa et al., 1995).

Diagnostic investigations of HAM/TSP

As shown in Table 23.1, the diagnosis of HAM/TSP is based on clinical criteria in association with positive serum and cerebrospinal fluid (CSF) antibody titers to HTLV-I, as determined by enzyme-linked immunosorbent assay (ELISA), particle agglutination (PA) testing, Western blot (WB), and immunofluorescent assays (IFA) (Osame, 1990).

In HAM/TSP, anti-HTLV-I-specific antibodies (Osame et al., 1987; Gessain et al., 1988), HTLV-I proviral DNA (Puccioni-Sohler et al., 1999), and HTLV-I Tax-expressing lymphocytes (Moritoyo et al., 1999) can be detected both in peripheral blood and CSF. ATL-like cells make up approximately 1% of peripheral lymphocytes in about 50% of HAM/TSP patients (Osame et al., 1987). Furthermore, there are several additional non-specific findings in CSF which demonstrate inflammatory changes, including mild lymphocytic pleocytosis, mild protein elevation, elevated IgG synthesis and IgG index (which indicates antibody production in the CSF), oligoclonal bands (Osame et al., 1987; Ceroni et al., 1988; Link et al., 1989; Jacobson et al., 1990a; Hollsberg and Hafler, 1993), and increased neopterin levels (Nomoto et al., 1991). Neopterin is released by macrophages under stimulation by T lymphocytes, and measurement of neopterin in the CSF can be a useful marker for the differential diagnosis of HAM/TSP, specifically to rule out HAM/TSP in HTLV-I carriers suffering from other forms of chronic myelopathy, such as cervical spondylosis, spinal canal stenosis, or chronic multiple sclerosis (Nomoto et al., 1991).

MRI of the spinal cord of HAM/TSP patients may show swelling or atrophy, and MRI of the brain shows periventricular white matter lesions in as many as 50% of patients (Mattson et al., 1987; Cruickshank et al., 1989; Godoy et al., 1995; Nakagawa et al., 1995). Electrophysiologic abnormalities are frequently seen in lower-limb somatosensory evoked potentials, peripheral nerve conductions, and visual and brainstem evoked potentials (Arimura et al., 1987, 1989; Ludolph et al., 1988; Cruickshank et al., 1989).

Table 23.1 Diagnostic guidelines for human T-cell lymphotropic virus type I-associated myelopathy/tropical spastic paraparesis

Clinical criteria	The florid picture of chronic spastic paraparesis is not always seen when the patient first comes to medical attention. A single symptom or physical sign may be the only evidence of early HAM/TSP
A. Age and sex incidence	Mostly sporadic and adult, but sometimes familial: occasionally seen in childhood: female patients predominant
B. Onset	Usually insidious, but may be sudden
C. Main neurologic manifestations	1. Chronic spastic paraparesis usually slowly but sometimes remains static after progression
	2. Weakness of the lower limb occurs and is more marked proximally
	3. Bladder disturbance is usually an early feature, constipation usually occurs later, and impotence or decreased libido is common
	4. Sensory symptoms, such as tingling, pins-and-needles sensation, and burning, are more prominent than objective physical signs
	5. Low lumber pain with radiation to the legs is common
	6. Vibration sense is frequently impaired: proprioception is less often affected
	7. Hyper-reflexia of the lower limbs, often with clonus and Babinbki's sign, occurs
	8. Hyper-reflexia of the upper limbs and positive Hoffmann's and Trömner's signs are frequent; weakness may be absent
	9. Exaggerated jaw jerk is seen in some patients
D. Less frequent neurologic findings	1. Cerebellar signs, optic atrophy, deafness, nystagmus and other cranial nerve deficits, hand tremor, and absent or depressed ankle jerk are found
	2. Convulsions, cognitive impairment, dementia, and impaired consciousness are rare
E. Other neurologic manifestations that may be associated with HAM/TSP	Muscular atrophy, fasciculations (rare): polymyositis, peripheral neuropathy, polyradiculopathy, cranial neuropathy, meningitis, and encephalopathy may be noted
F. Systemic non-neurologic manifestations that may be associated with HAM/TSP	Pulmonary alveolotis, uveitis, Sjögren's syndrome, arthropathy, vasculitis, ichthyosis, cryoglobulinemia, monoclonal gammapathy, and adult T-cell leukemia/lymphoma may be found
Laboratory diagnosis	A. HTLV-I antibodies or antigens are present in blood and CSF
	B. CSF may show mild lymphocytic pleocytosis
	C. Lobulated lymphocytes may be present in blood and/or CSF
	D. Mild to moderate increase of protein concentration may be present in CSF
	E. Viral isolation when possible from blood and/or CSF

In addition, electromyographic abnormalities of lower thoracic paraspinal muscles are frequently seen and help in the diagnosis of HAM/TSP (Arimura *et al.*, 1995).

Host genetic background in HAM/TSP

As mentioned, the majority (95%) of HTLV-I-infected individuals remain asymptomatic while fewer than 5% develop clinical disease. A number of possibilities have been proposed to explain these vastly different outcomes of an HTLV-I infection, including the suggestion that the genetic background of the host is important for development of HAM/TSP and ATL. Indeed, several studies have demonstrated an association between HTLV-I-related diseases and genetic background, specifically with HLA allele typing. In patients with HAM/TSP, HLA-typing studies have shown an increased frequency of HLA-DRB1*0101 (Sonoda *et al.*, 1996). In addition, there are a few studies which have demonstrated the association of HLA-A*201 in HAM/TSP patients. Previously, it was demonstrated that HLA-A*201 was associated with reduction in both the HTLV-I proviral load and the risk of development of neurologic disease (Jeffery *et al.*, 1999), although this report has been challenged by a more recent study that showed that there was no significant difference in the frequency of HLA-A*201 in the development of HAM/TSP (Yashiki *et al.*, 2001). Vine *et al.* (2002) showed polymorphisms in TNF-α-863A, SDF-1 and IL-15 that were associated with increased risk of HAM/TSP.

Neuropathology in HAM/TSP

Neuropathological findings in HAM/TSP have demonstrated that the affected site is predominantly the spinal cord, especially the thoracic region (Izumo *et al.*, 1989; Levin and Jacobson, 1997). Inflammatory changes are most pronounced in the affected lesions and include mononuclear cellular infiltration, destruction of myelin sheaths and axons, and gliosis (Iwasaki, 1990; Umehara *et al.*, 1993).

Of interest is the observation that the neuropathology of HAM/TSP appears to change gradually during the progression of the disease. Initially, most of the infiltrating cells are CD4+ T lymphocytes, CD8+ T cells, or macrophages in the predominantly perivascular areas (Umehara *et al.*, 1993). Later in the disease, the number of CD8+ T cells in the affected lesions increases (Umehara *et al.*, 1993; Levin *et al.*, 1997). CD8+ cells, thought to represent functionally cytotoxic cells, are observed frequently in active chronic lesions and occasionally in inactive chronic lesions in HAM/TSP patients (Umehara *et al.*, 1994b). In addition to the detection of inflammatory cells in the affected lesions of HAM/TSP, the expression of pro-inflammatory cytokines (such as IL-1β, TNF-α, and IFN-γ) and adhesion molecules (Umehara *et al.*, 1996) were also detected in the spinal cord of HAM/TSP patients (Umehara *et al.*, 1994a). As the disease progresses to a more inactive chronic form, the number of inflammatory cells as well as the expression of inflammatory cytokines decreases.

To investigate the immunopathogenesis of HAM/TSP, extensive efforts have been made to localize HTLV-I in the CNS lesions of HAM/TSP patients and to determine which cells might serve as targets for inflammatory CD8+ cells in the CNS. HTLV-I *gag*, *pX*, and *pol* sequences have been reported to localize in the thoracic cord areas (Akizuki et al., 1989; Yoshioka *et al.*, 1993) and greater in areas of increased CD4+ cell infiltration. By using *in situ* hybridization, both HTLV-I proviral DNA and RNA were detected in many infiltrating CD4+ T lymphocytes (Hara *et al.*, 1994; Moritoyo *et al.*, 1996; Matsuoka *et al.*, 1998), and resident astrocytes also have been reported to be positive for HTLV-I RNA (Lehky *et al.*, 1995).

Immune responses and immune abnormalities in HAM/TSP

Although immune responses against virus are typically beneficial in eliminating infected cells and in recovery from viral infection, virus-specific immune response can also be immunopathologic and cause disease. A number of immunologic parameters have been described in HAM/TSP including HTLV-I proviral load, humoral and cellular immune response, and cytokine production. Based on a large body of evidence, it has been suggested that HTLV-I-specific immune responses and immune dysregulation contribute to the inflammatory process in the CNS of HAM/TSP patients.

Humoral immune response to HTLV-I

The humoral immune response in HTLV-I infection is mainly directed against products of HTLV-I envelope (*env*), core (*gag*), and *pX* genes (Constantine *et al.*, 1992). In general, HAM/TSP patients tend to have increased levels of HTLV-I-specific antibodies (Gessain and Gout, 1992), and antibodies against HTLV-I can be readily detected in serum (Chen *et al.*, 1989; Palker *et al.*, 1989; Ida *et al.*, 1991; Inoue *et al.*, 1992) and CSF (Gessain *et al.*, 1988; Ceroni *et al.*, 1988; McLean *et al.*, 1989; Link *et al.*, 1989; Jacobson *et al.*, 1990*a*; Nakamura *et al.*, 1991; Kitze *et al.*, 1995). Unlike other acute viral infections, seroconversion to HTLV-I does not mean that the virus has been eliminated. The first specific antibodies to appear after HTLV-I infection are directed against Gag protein and predominate in the first 2 months. Subsequently, anti-envelope antibodies appear, and finally about 50% of infected people produce detectable levels of antibodies to the Tax protein (Manns *et al.*, 1991).

An important question is the function of anti-HTLV-I antibodies in HAM/TSP. Although some peptide-specific antibodies have been shown to neutralize HTLV-I *in vitro* (Inoue *et al.*, 1992), high levels of these antibodies were found both in serum and CSF of many patients with HAM/TSP.

The titer of anti-HTLV-I antibodies correlates with the provirus load and may reach very high levels. Some studies suggested that antibody titer (particularly to HTLV-I Tax) was proportional to the severity of disease (Osame *et al.*, 1987). Therefore, it is unlikely that these antibodies have a protective effect against HTLV-I-associated CNS disease, although they may be important to initially control HTLV-I infection after transmission by transfusion or in infancy (Hino *et al.*, 1985).

Cellular immune response to HTLV-I

HTLV-I-specific cytotoxic T lymphocytes (CTL) have been investigated in the pathogenesis of HAM/TSP. CTL have an important role in the normal immunologically mediated recovery from infectious disease through recognition and subsequent elimination of foreign antigens. Utilizing their antigen-specific T-cell receptors, CTL recognize foreign proteins as short peptide fragments in association with HLA. CD8+ CTL recognize foreign antigens in the context of HLA Class I molecules while CD4+ CTL recognize slightly larger peptide fragments in association with HLA Class II molecules. Both populations have been shown to be beneficial in eliminating infected cells and in recovery from viral infection. However, it has been suggested that virus-specific CTL could also be immunopathologic. Since a characteristic feature of HAM/TSP is an accumulation of inflammatory T lymphocytes in the affected lesion, and it has been known that immunomodulatory therapies such as prednisolone can be effective in reducing clinical symptoms of HAM/TSP, it is possible that T-cell antiviral immune responses are closely related to the immunopathogenesis of HAM/TSP.

To date there has been relatively little information on the CD4+ T-cell responses against HTLV-I in patients with HAM/TSP. The HLA-DRB1* 0101 haplotype (an HLA Class II allele) is related to a higher risk of HAM/TSP (Sonoda *et al.*, 1996; Jeffery *et al.*, 1999). Immunodominant epitopes in the HTLV-I *env* gp21 and gp46 were demonstrated from CD4+ T lymphocytes in patients with HAM/TSP (Jacobson *et al.*, 1991; Kitze *et al.*, 1998). These CD4+ HTLV-I-specific CTL could only be demonstrated after

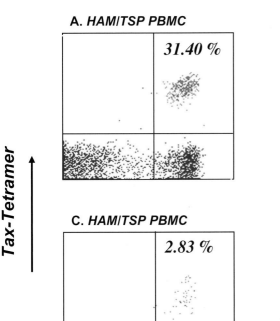

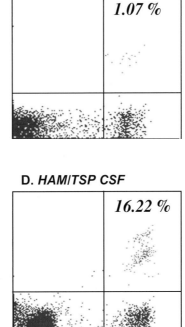

A. *HAM/TSP PBMC* 31.40 %

B. *Asymptomatic carrier PBMC* 1.07 %

C. *HAM/TSP PBMC* 2.83 %

D. *HAM/TSP CSF* 16.22 %

Tax-Tetramer

CD8

Fig. 23.2 Representative flow cytometry analysis of HTLV-I Tax 11–19-specific CD8+ T cells from peripheral blood mononuclear cells (PBMC) and cerebrospinal fluid (CSF) of HTLV-I-associated myelopathy/tropical spastic paraparesis (HAM/TSP) patients stained with HLA-A*201/Tax 11–19 tetramers and anti-CD8 antibody. An extraordinarily high frequency of HTLV-I Tax 11–19-specific CD8+ T cells is detected in PBMC of a HLA-A*201 HAM/TSP patient (A) relative to HLA-A*201 asymptomatic carrier (B). An example of patient with fewer HTLV-I Tax 11–19-specific CD8+ T cells is demonstrated in (C). These cells are selectively expanded in the CSF (D).

repeated *in vitro* antigenic stimulation. In addition, HTLV-I-specific CD4+ CTL were demonstrated from patients with HAM/TSP as well as asymptomatic HTLV-I carriers (Jacobson *et al.*, 1991; Kannagi *et al.*, 1994). Recently, Goon *et al.* (2002) demonstrated that frequencies of HTLV-I Env- and Tax-specific CD4+ T cells were greater in HAM/TSP than in asymptomatic carriers, and that HTLV-I-specific CD4+ T cells in the patients with HAM/TSP were mainly of the T helper 1 (Th1) phenotype. Although the role of CD4+ T-cell responses in the HAM/TSP is not fully understood, CD4+ T cells might be important for inducing efficient HTLV-I humoral and cellular immune responses (Ahmed and Gray, 1996).

One of the most striking features of the cellular immune responses in HAM/TSP patients is the extraordinarily increased numbers of HTLV-I-specific CD8+ T cells in peripheral blood mononuclear cells (PBMC) and CSF (Jacobson *et al.*, 1990b; Elovaara *et al.*, 1993; Kubota *et al.*, 1998; Nagai *et al.*, 2001c; Yamano *et al.*, 2002). Although HTLV-I-specific CD8+ cells are seen in PBMC of asymptomatic carriers (Parker *et al.*, 1992; Yamano *et al.*, 2002), the magnitude and frequency of these responses are higher in patients with neurologic disease (Elovaara *et al.*, 1993; Yamano *et al.*, 2002). Several experimental studies have generated strongly corroborative evidence that there is an intense CD8+ cytotoxic T-cell response against the HTLV-I Tax protein in HAM/TSP (Jacobson *et al.*, 1990b; Kannagi *et al.*, 1992; Daenke *et al.*, 1996). Specifically, the HTLV-I Tax 11–19 peptide (LLFGYPVYV) was defined as an immunodominant epitope by HLA-A2-restricted CD8+ CTL (Koenig *et al.*, 1993; Parker *et al.*, 1994). Recently, HTLV-I Tax peptide-loaded HLA-A2 (*0201) dimers and tetramers were developed and used to demonstrate HTLV-I Tax-specific HLA-A2-restricted CD8+ cells (Greten *et al.*, 1998; Bieganowska *et al.*, 1999). Using these techniques, HTLV-I Tax 11–19-specific CD8+ cells from PBMC of HLA-A2 HAM/TSP patients were found to represent an extraordinarily high proportion of the total CD8+ population (as high as 31% of CD8+ cells in some HAM/TSP patients) (Fig. 23.2) (Greten *et al.*, 1998; Nagai *et al.*, 2001b; Yamano *et al.*, 2002). In addition, the high frequency of HTLV-I-specific CD8+ cells in HAM/TSP patients correlates with the production of several cytokines such as IFN-γ, TNF-α, and IL-2 (Kubota *et al.*, 1998).

Immune dysfunction and immunological abnormalities in HAM/TSP

Abnormalities in cellular immune responses of HAM/TSP patients have also been identified. Natural killer cells tend to be diminished in both number and activity in HAM/TSP (Kitajima *et al.*, 1988). In particular, the phenomenon of spontaneous lymphoproliferation, defined as the ability of PBMC to proliferate *ex vivo* in the absence of antigenic stimulation or IL-2, has been well described in HAM/TSP PBMC, in HTLV-I asymptomatic carriers, and in HTLV-II-infected persons (Itoyama *et al.*, 1988; Kramer *et al.*, 1989). However, the magnitude of the response is typically higher in HAM/TSP patients (Wiktor *et al.*, 1991). The spontaneous lymphoproliferation of HTLV-I-infected PBMC is thought to consist of two components; proliferation of HTLV-I-infected CD4+ cells and expansion of CD8+ cells (Ijichi *et al.*, 1989; Eiraku *et al.*, 1992; Nagai *et al.*, 1995; Machigashira *et al.*, 1997). Ijichi *et al.* (1989, 1993) proposed that this *in vitro* spontaneous lymphoproliferation may epitomize the immunological events occurring in the CNS of HAM/TSP patients, where high inducibility of viral antigens and increased CD8+ cell response may induce severe inflammation.

Expression of cytokine and immune-mediated molecules in HAM/TSP

Elevated levels of several pro-inflammatory cytokines, chemokines, matrix metalloproteinase (MMP) which is implicated in extracellular matrix degradation, and adhesion molecules have been demonstrated in serum, CSF, and spinal cord lesions of HAM/TSP patients (Kuroda and Matsui, 1993; Nakamura *et al.*, 1993; Umehara *et al.*, 1994a). Patients have elevated levels of cytokines such as IFN-γ, TNF-α, and IL-6, in serum and CSF (Nishimoto *et al.*, 1990; Hollsberg and Hafler, 1993; Kuroda and Matsui, 1993; Nakamura *et al.*, 1993; Furuya *et al.*, 1999). IL-12 (p70 heterodimer) is also elevated in serum (Furuya *et al.*, 1999). Moreover, mRNA expression

of IL-1β, IL-2, TNF-α, and IFN-γ has been shown to be up-regulated in the PBMC of patients with HAM/TSP (Tendler *et al.*, 1990, 1991). The levels of MMP-9 and tissue inhibitors of metalloproteinases (TIMP)-3 in CSF of HAM/TSP patients were higher than that of HTLV-I carriers without neurological symptoms (Lezin *et al.*, 2000). HAM/TSP patients have increased levels of soluble vascular cell adhesion molecule-1 (VCAM-1) in sera and CSF (Matsuda *et al.*, 1995). In addition to the detection of these molecules from serum and CSF of patients with HAM/TSP, immunohistochemistry showed localized expression of pro-inflammatory cytokines such as IL-1β, TNF-α, and IFN-γ in the perivascular infiltrating cells (Umehara *et al.*, 1994a). MMP-2, MMP-9, and very late antigen-4 (VLA-4) were also detected in infiltrating cells (Umehara *et al.*, 1998), and the expression of VCAM-1 was demonstrated on endothelium cells in the spinal cord lesions of HAM/TSP (Umehara *et al.*, 1996). Moreover, lymphocyte function-associated antigen-1 (LFA-1), Mac-1, and monocyte chemoattractant protein-1 (MCP-1) were up-regulated in CNS lesions (Umehara *et al.*, 1996).

It has been reported that CD4+ T cells from patients with HAM/TSP can spontaneously express pro-inflammatory cytokines such as IFN-γ, TNF-α, and GM-CSF (Nishiura *et al.*, 1996). In addition, these pro-inflammatory cytokines secreted by HTLV-I-infected CD4+ T cells can induce production of MMP-2, -3, and -9 and TIMP-1, -2, and -3 in human astrocytes *in vitro* (Giraudon *et al.*, 2000). Moreover, it has been demonstrated that HTLV-I Tax 11–19-specific CD8+ CTL clones from HLA-A2 HAM/TSP patients can secrete pro-inflammatory cytokines, chemokines, and matrix metalloproteinase upon recognition of the HTLV-I Tax 11–19 peptide, including IFN-γ, TNF-α, macrophage inflammatory protein (MIP)-1α, IL-1β, IL-2, IL-6, and MMP-9 (Biddison *et al.*, 1997; Kubota *et al.*, 1998). This IFN-γ production was observed with co-cultivation with autologous CD4 cells or HTLV-I Tax 11–19 peptide-pulsed HLA-A2-matched cells, and suppressed by anti-HLA Class I antibodies. Similar to the increased frequency of HTLV-I-specific CTL in HAM/TSP (Jacobson *et al.*, 1990b; Kannagi *et al.*, 1991; Elovaara *et al.*, 1993; Koenig *et al.*, 1993), CD8+ T cells of HAM/TSP patients also have a potential to produce IFN-γ and TNF-α at a high frequency in comparison with asymptomatic carriers or healthy controls.

The recently described cytokine IL-15 has also been reported to be increased in PBMC from HAM/TSP patients (Azimi *et al.*, 2000), and may function to maintain virus-specific CD8+ T cells *in vivo* (Ku *et al.*, 2000; Azimi *et al.*, 2001).

Autoimmune responses

Although an autoimmune hypothesis had been proposed in the pathogenesis of HAM/TSP (Hollsberg and Hafler, 1993; Oger and Dekaban, 1995), to date there are only a few immunological studies which suggest that autoimmune responses may play a role in the pathogenesis of HAM/TSP. Levin *et al.* (1998) previously showed that IgG antibody from patients with HAM/TSP specifically labeled neurons in uninfected CNS, but not cells in the other organs. Antibodies to a neuronal antigen could be demonstrated in all tested patients with HAM/TSP by Western blot, but not in HTLV-I-uninfected controls. Interestingly, by Western blotting, HTLV-I Tax-specific antibodies labeled a neuronal protein with the same molecular weight to the IgG antibody from patients with HAM/TSP, suggesting that antibodies to the viral Tax protein bound to the same neuronal antigen as patient antibodies. Most recently, they identified a neuronal protein, hnRNP-A1, as a target antigen recognized by IgG antibody from patients with HAM/TSP as well as Tax-specific antibody. In addition (Levin *et al.*, 2002) they demonstrated that affinity-purified antibodies from patients and Tax antibodies inhibit neuronal function, indicating that the observed cross-reactivity with a neuronal protein may be relevant in the pathogenesis of the HTLV-I-associated neurological disease.

Hara *et al.* (1994) reported that the lymphocytes in the spinal cord lesions of HAM/TSP patients have a unique CDR3 motif, which has been demonstrated in brain lesions of multiple sclerosis and experimental autoimmune encephalomyelitis by the analysis of T-cell receptor Vβ genes, suggesting that a T-cell clone recognizing autoantigens was activated by HTLV-I and that this clone was related to the pathogenesis of HAM/TSP.

Migration of HTLV-I-infected cells into the CNS

HAM/TSP is an inflammatory disease of the spinal cord where inflammatory cells, predominantly T cells (both CD4+ and CD8+), infiltrate perivascular area (Umehara *et al.*, 1993). To understand the pathogenesis of HAM/TSP, it is important to know the process of migration of inflammatory cells from the periphery into CNS lesions.

In PBMC of patients with HAM/TSP, HTLV-I has been shown to preferentially infect CD4+ and CD8+ T cells *in vivo* (Richardson *et al.*, 1990; Nagai *et al.*, 2001*a*). Since it was demonstrated that HTLV-I-infected lymphocytes shared the same HTLV-I integration site of cellular DNA in both the peripheral blood and CSF from a HAM/TSP patient, this suggested that HTLV-I-infected cells migrate from peripheral blood to CNS *in vivo* (Cavrois *et al.*, 2000). Although the mechanism of migration of HTLV-I-infected cells to the CNS is still unclear, several possibilities have been demonstrated. In patients with HAM/TSP, CD4+ T cells (particularly HTLV-I-infected CD4+ cells) have been shown to increase adherent activity to endothelial cells and transmigrating activity through basement membranes (Ichinose *et al.*, 1992, 1994; Furuya *et al.*, 1997). In addition, it has been observed that CD4+ cells of patients with HAM/TSP have splicing variants of CD44 (v6 variants). CD44 is known as a multifunctional cell adhesion molecule as well as a lymphocyte homing receptor. Interestingly, these splicing variants of CD44 were highly detected in PBMC (especially CD4+ cells) from HAM/TSP and in some of HTLV-I-infected cells by *in situ* PCR (Matsuoka *et al.*, 2000).

As mentioned, it has been known that the number of CD8+ T cells in the affected lesions increases later in disease and infiltration of CD8+ cells is observed frequently in active chronic lesions of HAM/TSP patients (Umehara *et al.*, 1993, 1994*b*; Levin *et al.*, 1997). Indeed, it has been demonstrated that the frequency of HTLV-I-specific CD8+ T cells in CSF is much higher than in PBMC of HAM/TSP patients (Fig. 23.2) (Elovaara *et al.*, 1993; Greten *et al.*, 1998), and that this accumulation was HTLV-I-specific (Nagai *et al.*, 2001*c*). These results suggest that HTLV-I-specific CD8+ T cells may preferentially migrate into the CSF from peripheral blood and/or these cells may selectively expand in this compartment. The increased expression of T-cell activation markers has demonstrated in HTLV-I Tax-specific CD8+ T cells in the PBMC of HAM/TSP patients, suggesting that these cells may have selective advantage to migrate into the CNS of HAM/TSP patients (Nagai *et al.*, 2001*b,c*).

HTLV-I proviral load and mRNA expression in HAM/TSP

As noted, HTLV-I-specific immune responses and immune abnormalities are significantly related to the pathogenesis of HAM/TSP, specifically with regard to viral antigen-specific CD8+ T-cell responses. An important question is how HTLV-I-specific immune responses are continuously stimulated in HAM/TSP patients. There is considerable evidence to suggest that a high HTLV-I proviral load in patients with HAM/TSP may drive increased HTLV-I-specific immune responses (Fig. 23.3). In PBMC of HAM/TSP patients, it has been demonstrated that HTLV-I proviral loads are significantly higher than in asymptomatic HTLV-I carriers (Yoshida *et al.*, 1989; Gessain *et al.*, 1990*b*; Kira *et al.*, 1991; Kubota *et al.*, 1993). More recently, using newly established real-time quantitative PCR techniques, it has been reported that the level of HTLV-I proviral DNA in the PBMC of HAM/TSP patients is approximately 16-fold greater than in asymptomatic carriers (Nagai *et al.*, 1998). For example, HAM/TSP patients had usually 2–20 copies per 100 isolated PBMC (and certain HAM/TSP patients had as many as 60 copies of HTLV-I proviral DNA per 100 isolated PBMC), while the median value of HTLV-I proviral load in asymptomatic carriers was around 0.1–1 copy per 100 isolated PBMC. Moreover, analysis of HTLV-I proviral loads from lymphocytes of the CSF of HAM/TSP patients also demonstrated high levels of HTLV-I *tax* DNA (Nagai *et al.*, 2001*c*). Importantly, HTLV-I proviral levels were even higher compared with PBMC proviral loads. In HLA A201 HAM/TSP patients, the increased HTLV-I proviral DNA loads in CSF were proportional to the frequency of HTLV-I Tax 11–19-specific CD8+ T cells. These observations support the hypothesis that the HTLV-I proviral load may drive the increased HTLV-I-specific immune responses that have been suggested to be immunopathogenic in HAM/TSP (Fig. 23.3). Interestingly, the HTLV-I proviral loads of HTLV-I asymptomatic carriers in the families of HAM/TSP patients were higher than those of unrelated asymptomatic carriers, suggesting that genetic factors may also influence HTLV-I proviral levels (Nagai *et al.*, 1998, 2001*c*).

Paradoxically, even though a high proviral DNA load is characteristic of HAM/TSP patients, the expression of HTLV-I in PBMC appears to be low (Shimoyama *et al.*, 1983; Sugamura *et al.*, 1984; Tochikura *et al.*, 1985; Kinoshita *et al.*, 1989; Gessain *et al.*, 1990*a*). These observations have led a number of investigators to consider that HTLV-I may be latent in peripheral blood. Recently, using a newly established real-time quantitative RT-

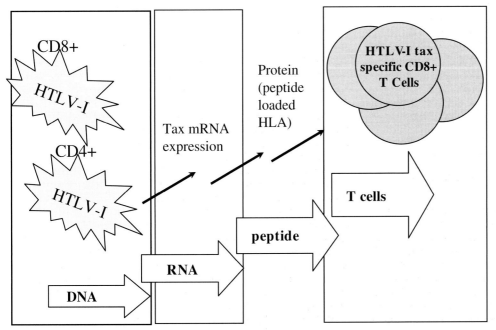

Fig. 23.3 Scheme of induction of HTLV-I-specific CD8+ T-cell responses associated with immunopathogenesis of HTLV-I-associated myelopathy/tropical spastic paraparesis (HAM/TSP). High levels of HTLV-I proviral load are observed in the patients with HAM/TSP, which is directly proportional to increased mRNA levels for HTLV-I tax. Elevated levels of HTLV-I tax mRNA lead to increased expression of HTLV-I protein that can be processed into immunodominant peptides. HTLV-I peptides (e.g. Tax 11–19). strongly bind to HLA-A*201 molecules and can stimulate virus-specific CD8+ T-cell responses (which are detected by HLA-A*201/Tax 11–19-specific tetramers). These antigen-specific responses are expanded in the cerebrospinal fluid of HAM/TSP patients and may contribute to disease progression.

PCR technique, it was demonstrated that HTLV-I mRNA load in PBMC of HAM/TSP patients appeared to be significantly higher than that in asymptomatic HTLV-I carriers (0.004–0.4% of PBMC were expressing HTLV-I mRNA in HAM/TSP patients) (Yamano et al., 2002). This is consistent with a previous study that detected HTLV-I Tax protein in PBMC and CSF cells of HAM/TSP patients by use of laser scanning cytometry (0.02–0.54% of PBMC and 0.04–1.16% of CSF cells were positive for the HTLV-I Tax protein) (Moritoyo et al., 1999). HTLV-I Tax protein expression in CSF cells was higher than that in PBMC and was more frequent in HAM/TSP patients with a shorter duration of illness. This low number of HTLV-I mRNA and Tax protein-expressing PBMC compared with the high HTLV-I proviral DNA load suggests that the majority of HTLV-I-infected cells are latent in peripheral blood, although this amount may be sufficient to continuously activate the immune system in vivo.

Animal models for HAM/TSP

The development of an animal model for HTLV-I infection would be extremely useful for investigating mechanisms of immunopathogenesis in HTLV-I-associated diseases. To date, several animal models, including HTLV-I infectious models and experimental transgenic models of HTLV-I genes, have been generated.

It has been known that HTLV-I can be successfully transmitted to rats and to rabbits by inoculation of HTLV-I-infected cells. Recently, the development of a chronic myelopathy similar to HAM/TSP has been reported in one specific strain of rats inoculated with an HTLV-I-infected cell line (Ishiguro et al., 1992). This HTLV-I-infected rat model develops paraparesis of the hind limbs after an incubation period of 15 months. In the spinal cord of infected rats, the expression of HTLV-I tax mRNA was observed (Tomaru et al., 1996), and moreover, it was demonstrated that some resident glial cells were expressing Tax protein in the CNS (Jiang et al., 2000). An increased level of neurotoxic cytokines such as TNF-α was also detected in the CSF of infected rats (Tomaru et al., 1996). Interestingly, the pathologic analysis shows demyelination centered in the thoracic cord with massive infiltration of activated macrophages/microglias and apoptosis of resident glial cells such as oligodendrocytes, while lymphocytic infiltration was not observed (Ohya et al., 1997). Although the mechanism of demyelination in HTLV-I-infected rats is still unclear, it has been suggested that the increased sensitivity to inflammatory cytokines such as TNF-α in glial cells, which may be derived from infection with HTLV-I, was related to the development of myelopathy in this rat model (Jiang et al., 2000). In addition, a rabbit model has also been used to examine HTLV-I infection, replication, cellular transformation, transmission, induced immune responses, disease manifestations, vaccine candidates, and therapeutic approaches (Ratner, 1996).

Recently, a number of transgenic models containing portions of the HTLV-I genome have been generated; however, these animals did not develop a neurologic disease like HAM/TSP but thy did manifest a number of symptoms. For example, mice carrying the HTLV-I genome or HTLV-I Tax developed chronic arthritis resembling rheumatoid arthritis (Iwakura et al., 1991). LTR-env-pX transgenic rats have been shown to develop a wide spectrum of collagen vascular and autoimmune diseases (Yamazaki et al., 1997).

Model of immunopathogenesis in HAM/TSP

The results discussed above demonstrate that virus–host immunological interactions play a pivotal role in HAM/TSP. Based on extensive experimentation, a number of possible models for the pathogenesis of this disorder have been proposed. Three major immunopathogenic models have been considered:

1. Cytotoxic model: inflammatory HTLV-I-infected T cells in the CNS or CNS resident glial cells may be presenting HTLV-I antigens and become direct targets for lysis by HTLV-I-specific CTL (Jacobson et al., 1990b).

2. Autoaggressive bystander model: HTLV-I virus-specific cellular infiltrates that have migrated into the CNS that recognize HTLV-I-infected cells may result in the release of cytokines and chemokines which may cause damage to nearby cells such as glial and neural cells (Ijichi et al., 1993).

3. Autoimmune model: activated HTLV-I-specific T cells cross-react with self antigens in the CNS (Hollsberg and Hafler, 1993) and/or virus specific immune responses lead to epitope spreading and recognition of multiple CNS antigens (Hafler, 1999).

Although it has not been proven which, if any, of these mechanisms predominate in HAM/TSP, or if one or more of these mechanisms act in concert, the large body of evidence summarized in this chapter suggests that HTLV-I-specific CD8+ T cells contribute to the inflammatory process in CNS lesions of HAM/TSP regardless of which mechanism is involved. HTLV-I-specific CD8+ T cells may kill HTLV-I antigen(s)-expressing target cells directly by a perforin-dependent mechanism (Hanon et al., 2000) as well as by the production of a large amount of matrix metalloproteinases (MMP-9), chemoattractants (MIP-1α and -1β) and pro-inflammatory cytokines (TNF-α and IFN-γ) which can induce HLA expression in neuronal cells and damage CNS tissue (Biddison et al., 1997; Greten et al., 1998; Kubota et al., 1998). High levels of HTLV-I proviral loads were observed in both CD4+ and CD8+ T-cell populations in HAM/TSP patients, and it is possible to propose that these high viral loads can drive increased levels of HTLV-I mRNA and HTLV-I protein expressions. As shown in Fig. 23.3, processing and presentation of HTLV-I-specific peptides leads to activation and expansion of antigen-specific T-cell responses. The hypothesis that HTLV-I-specific CD8+ T cells play a role in the development of HAM/TSP is supported by localization of these T cells in the CNS. Inflammatory CD8+ cells have been found in the spinal cord lesions of HAM/TSP patients (Jacobson et al., 1992) and tend to increase with disease progression. Activated T cells have been reported in the CSF of HAM/TSP patients, usually of the CD8+, CD11a+, CD45RO+, CD28− phenotype (Elovaara et al., 1995).

The precursor frequency of HTLV-I-specific CTL from CSF lymphocytes is extraordinarily high (Elovaara et al., 1993). HTLV-I-specific CD8+ T cells could recognize HTLV-I antigen-expressing target cells in the CNS and induce large amounts of pro-inflammatory cytokines and chemokines that can induce HLA expression in resident cells in the CNS and damage CNS tissue (Lehky et al., 1994). As the HTLV-I proviral load in CSF of HAM/TSP patients was more than two times higher than in PBMC (Nagai et al., 2001c), this suggests that HTLV-I-infected lymphocytes may preferentially migrate into the CSF from peripheral blood, or that HTLV-I-infected lymphocytes may selectively expand in this compartment. Indeed, the exaggerated transmigrating activity of HTLV-I-infected cells to the CNS tissue has been reported (Cavrois et al., 2000; Romero et al., 2000; Matsuoka et al., 2000; Hanon et al., 2001), and expansion of HTLV-I-infected T-cell clones has also been observed (Furukawa et al., 1992; Wattel et al., 1995; Cavrois et al., 1998; Eiraku et al., 1998). In addition, HTLV-I genomic sequences, RNA, and the HTLV-I proteins have been shown to localize in the spinal cord lesions. Therefore, all requirements for CTL recognition including viral antigen and HLA Class I expression are present in the HAM/TSP lesions, lending support to the argument that HTLV-I-specific CD8+ CTL may be immunopathogenic in this disease.

A model for HTLV-I immunopathogenesis is represented in Fig. 23.4 that encompasses many aspects of HTLV-I T-cell tropism and host immune responses to the virus. In the HAM/TSP lesions, HTLV-I-infected CD4+ and CD8+ T cells can cross the blood–brain barrier. In addition, activated CD8+ antigen-specific cells may also migrate into the CNS. These cells may recognize productively infected cells and respond by either direct lysis of the infected cells (which may also be HTLV-I-infected resident CNS cells such as glial cells) or through the release of chemokines and cytokines. These molecules can act to recruit and expand additional inflammatory cells and have been shown to be toxic to resident CNS cells. Intensive studies regarding the interaction between HTLV-I-specific CD8+ T cells and HTLV-I-infected cells will clarify the pathogenesis of HAM/TSP. This understanding will allow for directed immunotherapeutic strategies for the treatment of this disease.

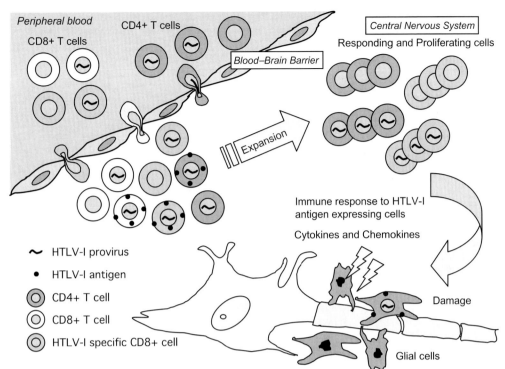

Fig. 23.4 Immunopathogenic model of HAM/TSP. Activated T cells, which may consist of HTLV-I-infected CD4+, CD8+, or antigen-specific T cells, migrate across the blood–brain barrier from the peripheral blood to the CNS. As a portion of the HTLV-I-infected cells such as infected inflammatory cells and possible resident CNS cells express HTLV-I antigens, T-cell immune responses recognize and attack these HTLV-I antigen-expressing cells. Recognition by HTLV-I-specific CD8+ cytotoxic T lymphocytes can result in lysis of infected target cells and/or the release of a cascade of inflammatory cytokines and chemokines in the CNS. HTLV-I-infected CD4+ and CD8+ T cells may also produce these immunomodulatory molecules. Cytokines such as IL-2 and IL-15 may help bystander T cells to expand, whereas IFN-γ and TNF-α may damage resident CNS cells such as glia and neurons.

Treatment

Based on a number of investigative studies on the immunopathogenesis of HAM/TSP, it has been suggested that reduction of the virus and control of excessive immune responses to the virus are important for therapeutic approaches. Although an ideal therapeutic strategy for HAM/TSP patients has still not been established, there are several reports regarding treatment focusing on both antiviral and immunomodulatory action.

For the reduction of virus in the patients with HAM/TSP, anti-IL-2R therapy has been undertaken to reduce IL-2R-expressing HTLV-I-infected cells, and the reduction of HTLV-I proviral load in PBMC has been demonstrated without exacerbation of disease (Lehky et al., 1998). Treatment with antiretroviral reagents (reverse transcriptase inhibitors) such as zidovudine and lamivudine is also under investigation, and regimens including these antiretroviral reagents have been reported to decrease HTLV-I proviral load in HTLV-I-infected subjects (Sheremata et al., 1993; Taylor et al., 1999). A preliminary trial with lamivudine has shown a decrease in both HTLV-I proviral load and HTLV-I-specific CTL responses in some HAM/TSP patients (Wodarz et al., 1999); however, an improvement in neurological symptoms was not observed. Further clinical trials are necessary to develop treatments for HAM/TSP. Since clonal expansion of HTLV-I-infected cells seems to be a major pathway for virus propagation rather than viral replication through reverse transcriptase enzymes (Wattel et al., 1996), it is suggested that therapeutic approaches to prevent clonal expansion of infected cells may be effective in reducing virus load.

Besides antiviral therapies, immunomodulatory therapies such as prednisolone, IFN-α methylprednisolone, and azathioprine, have been reported as possible treatments for HAM/TSP (Izumo et al., 1996; Nakagawa et al., 1996). Since activated immune responses to the virus are significantly observed in spinal cord lesions of HAM/TSP patients it has been suggested that immunomodulatory therapies to control harmful immune reaction against the virus may be effective for treatment. Among these therapies, it has been demonstrated that predonisolone and IFN-α may be effective in improving the clinical symptoms of HAM/TSP. For example, oral prednisolone has been reported to show a beneficial effect in 69.5% of patients with HAM/TSP, especially in patients with a short duration of illness in which active inflammation presumably occurs in the CNS (Nakagawa et al.,

1996). The treatment with IFN-α shows effective improvement in 61.5% of patients (Izumo et al., 1996). Azathioprine (22.2%), methylprednisolone (30%), and plasmapheresis and lymphocytopheresis (43.8%) also showed partial effectiveness for patients with HAM/TSP (Nakagawa et al., 1996).

Conclusion

The large body of evidence summarized in this chapter suggests that HTLV-I-specific immune responses contribute to the inflammatory process in CNS lesions of HAM/TSP. Immunological abnormalities induced by a high HTLV-I proviral load may be involved in the neuropathologic events of this disease. In this chapter, we have emphasized the role of HTLV-I-specific CD8+ cells in the development of HAM/TSP, but many questions remain. Intensive studies regarding the interaction between HTLV-I-specific T cells and HTLV-I-infected cells will clarify the pathogenesis of HAM/TSP. This understanding will allow for directed immunotherapeutic strategies for the treatment of this chronic progressive neurologic disease similar to treatments currently being evaluated in multiple sclerosis (Bielekova and Martin, 1999). These experimental therapeutic strategies include inhibition of T-cell activation, altered peptide ligand therapies, and transmigration through the blood–brain barrier.

References

Ahmed, R. and Gray, D. (1996). Immunological memory and protective immunity: understanding their relation. *Science,* 272: 54–60.

Akizuki, S., Yoshida, S., Setoguchi, M., et al. (1989). The neuropathology of human T-lymphotropic virus type I associated myelopathy. In: *HTLV-I and the Nervous System* (ed. G.C. Roman, J.C. Vernant, M. Osame, et al.), pp. 253–260. Alan R Liss, New York.

Ali, A., Patterson, S., Cruickshank, K., Rudge, P., Dalgleish, A.G., and Knight, S.C. (1993). Dendritic cells infected in vitro with human T cell leukaemia/lymphoma virus type-1 (HTLV-1); enhanced lymphocytic proliferation and tropical spastic paraparesis. *Clin Exp Immunol* 94: 32–37.

Ando, Y., Nakano, S., Saito, K., Shimamoto, I., Ichijo, M., Toyama, T., et al. (1987). Transmission of adult T-cell leukemia retrovirus (HTLV-I) from mother to child: comparison of bottle- with breast-fed babies. *Japan J Cancer Res* 78: 322–324.

Arima, N., Daitoku, Y., Ohgaki, S., Fukumori, J., Tanaka, H., Yamamoto, Y., *et al.* (1986). Autocrine growth of interleukin 2-producing leukemic cells in a patient with adult T cell leukemia. *Blood* 68: 779–782.

Arimura, K., Rosales, R., Osame, M., and Igata, A. (1987). Clinical electrophysiologic studies of HTLV-I-associated myelopathy. *Arch Neurol* 44: 609–612.

Arimura, K., Arimura, M., Yonenaga, Y., Rosales, R., and Osame, M. (1989). Clinical electrophysiologic findings in patients with HTLV-I-associated myelopathy (HAM). In: *HTLV-I and the Nervous System* (ed. G.C. Roman, J.C. Vernant, M. Osame, *et al.*), pp. 240–250. Alan R. Liss, New York.

Arimura, K., Arimura, Y., Moritoyo, H., Tokimura, Y., Takenaga, S., Sonoda, Y., *et al.* (1995). How helpful is thoracic paraspinal EMG in HAM/TSP? *Muscle Nerve* 18: 248–250.

Arya, S. K., Wong-Staal, F., and Gallo, R.C. (1984). T-cell growth factor gene: lack of expression in human T-cell leukemia-lymphoma virus-infected cells. *Science* 223: 1086–1087.

Azimi, N., Mariner, J., Jacobson, S., and Waldmann, T.A. (2000). How does interleukin 15 contribute to the pathogenesis of HTLV type 1-associated myelopathy/tropical spastic paraparesis? *AIDS Res Hum Retroviruses* 16: 1717–1722.

Azimi, N., Nagai, M., Jacobson, S., and Waldmann, T.A. (2001). IL-15 plays a major role in the persistence of Tax-specific CD8 cells in HAM/TSP patients. *Proc Natl Acad Sci USA* 98: 14559–14564.

Biddison, W.E., Kubota, R., Kawanishi, T., Taub, D.D., Cruikshank, W.W., Center, D.M., *et al.* (1997). Human T cell leukemia virus type I (HTLV-I)-specific CD8+ CTL clones from patients with HTLV-I-associated neurologic disease secrete proinflammatory cytokines, chemokines, and matrix metalloproteinase. *J Immunol* 159: 2018–2025.

Bieganowska, K., Hollsberg, P., Buckle, G.J., Lim, D.G., Greten, T.F., Schneck, J., *et al.* (1999). Direct analysis of viral-specific CD8+ T cells with soluble HLA-A2/Tax11-19 tetramer complexes in patients with human T cell lymphotropic virus-associated myelopathy. *J Immunol* 162: 1765–1771.

Bielekova, B. and Martin, R. (1999). Multiple Sclerosis: Immunotherapy. *Curr Treat Options Neurol* 1: 201–220.

Blattner, W.A. and Gallo, R.C. (1994). Epidemiology of HTLV-I and HTLV-II infections. In: *Adult T-cell Leukemia* (ed. K. Takatsuki), pp. 45–90. Oxford University Press, Oxford.

Brady, J. (1996). Biology of HTLV-I: Host cell interactions. In: *Human T-cell Lymphotropic Virus Type I* (ed. P. Hollsberg and D. Hafler), pp. 79–112. John Wiley, Chichester.

Cavrois, M., Gessain, A., Gout, O., Wain-Hobson, S., and Wattel, E. (2000). Common human T cell leukemia virus type 1 (HTLV-1) integration sites in cerebrospinal fluid and blood lymphocytes of patients with HTLV-1-associated myelopathy/tropical spastic paraparesis indicate that HTLV-1 crosses the blood-brain barrier via clonal HTLV-1-infected cells. *J Infect Dis* 182: 1044–1050.

Cavrois, M., Leclercq, I., Gout, O., Gessain, A., Wain-Hobson, S., and Wattel, E. (1998). Persistent oligoclonal expansion of human T-cell leukemia virus type 1-infected circulating cells in patients with Tropical spastic paraparesis/HTLV-1 associated myelopathy. *Oncogene* 17: 77–82.

Ceroni, M., Piccardo, P., Rodgers-Johnson, P., Mora, C., Asher, D.M., Gajdusek, D.C., *et al.* (1988). Intrathecal synthesis of IgG antibodies to HTLV-I supports an etiological role for HTLV-I in tropical spastic paraparesis. *Ann Neurol* 23: S188–S191.

Chen, Y.M., Lee, T.H., Samuel, K.P., Okayama, A., Tachibana, N., Miyoshi, I., *et al.* (1989). Antibody reactivity to different regions of human T-cell leukemia virus type 1 gp61 in infected people. *J Virol* 63: 4952–4957.

Clapham, P., Nagy, K., Cheingsong-Popov, R., Exley, M., and Weiss, R. A. (1983). Productive infection and cell-free transmission of human T-cell leukemia virus in a nonlymphoid cell line. *Science* 222: 1125–1127.

Constantine, N.T., Callahan, J.D., and Watts, D.M. (1992). *HTLV-I and HTLV-II.* CRC Press, Boca Raton, FL.

Cruickshank, J.K., Rudge, P., Dalgleish, A.G., Newton, M., McLean, B.N., Barnard, R.O., *et al.* (1989). Tropical spastic paraparesis and human T cell lymphotropic virus type 1 in the United Kingdom. *Brain* 112: 1057–1090.

Daenke, S., Kermode, A.G., Hall, S.E., Taylor, G., Weber, J., Nightingale, S., *et al.*

(1996). High activated and memory cytotoxic T-cell responses to HTLV-1 in healthy carriers and patients with tropical spastic paraparesis. *Virology* 217: 139–146.

de The, G. and Bomford, R. (1993). An HTLV-I vaccine: why, how, for whom? *AIDS Res Hum Retroviruses* 9: 381–386.

Eiraku, N., Ijichi, S., Yashiki, S., Osame, M., and Sonoda, S. (1992). Cell surface phenotype of in vitro proliferating lymphocytes in HTLV-I-associated myelopathy (HAM/TSP). *J Neuroimmunol* 37: 223–228.

Eiraku, N., Hingorani, R., Ijichi, S., Machigashira, K., Gregersen, P.K., Monteiro, J., *et al.* (1998). Clonal expansion within CD4+ and CD8+ T cell subsets in human T lymphotropic virus type I-infected individuals. *J Immunol* 161: 6674–6680.

Elovaara, I., Koenig, S., Brewah, A.Y., Woods, R.M., Lehky, T., and Jacobson, S. (1993). High human T cell lymphotropic virus type 1 (HTLV-1)-specific precursor cytotoxic T lymphocyte frequencies in patients with HTLV-1-associated neurological disease. *J Exp Med* 177: 1567–1573.

Elovaara, I., Utz, U., Smith, S., and Jacobson, S. (1995). Limited T cell receptor usage by HTLV-I tax-specific, HLA class I restricted cytotoxic T lymphocytes from patients with HTLV-I associated neurological disease. *J Neuroimmunol* 63: 47–53.

Fujii, M., Tsuchiya, H., Chuhjo, T., Akizawa, T., and Seiki, M. (1992). Interaction of HTLV-1 Tax1 with p67SRF causes the aberrant induction of cellular immediate early genes through CArG boxes. *Genes Dev* 6: 2066–2076.

Furukawa, K., Mori, M., Ohta, N., Ikeda, H., Shida, H., and Shiku, H. (1994). Clonal expansion of CD8+ cytotoxic T lymphocytes against human T cell lymphotropic virus type I (HTLV-I) genome products in HTLV-1-associated myelopathy/tropical spastic paraparesis patients. *J Clin Invest* 94: 1830–1839.

Furukawa, Y., Fujisawa, J., Osame, M., Toita, M., Sonoda, S., Kubota, R., *et al.* (1992). Frequent clonal proliferation of human T-cell leukemia virus type 1 (HTLV-1)-infected T cells in HTLV-1-associated myelopathy (HAM-TSP). *Blood* 80: 1012–1016.

Furukawa, Y., Yamashita, M., Usuku, K., Izumo, S., Nakagawa, M., and Osame, M. (2000). Phylogenetic subgroups of human T cell lymphotropic virus (HTLV) type I in the tax gene and their association with different risks for HTLV-I-associated myelopathy/tropical spastic paraparesis. *J Infect Dis* 182: 1343–1349.

Furuya, T., Nakamura, T., Shirabe, S., Nishiura, Y., Tsujino, A., Goto, H., *et al.* (1997). Heightened transmigrating activity of CD4-positive T cells through reconstituted basement membrane in patients with human T-lymphotropic virus type I-associated myelopathy. *Proc Assoc Am Physicians* 109: 228–236.

Furuya, T., Nakamura, T., Fujimoto, T., Nakane, S., Kambara, C., Shirabe, S., *et al.* (1999). Elevated levels of interleukin-12 and interferon-gamma in patients with human T lymphotropic virus type I-associated myelopathy. *J Neuroimmunol* 95: 185–189.

Gavalchin, J., Fan, N., Waterbury, P.G., Corbett, E., Faldasz, B.D., Peshick, S.M., *et al.* (1995). Regional localization of the putative cell surface receptor for HTLV-I to human chromosome 17q23.2-17q25.3. *Virology* 212: 196–203.

Gessain, A. (1996). Epidemiology of HTLV-I and associated diseases. In: *Human T-cell Lymphotropic Virus Type I* (ed. P. Hollsberg and D. Hafler), pp. 33–64. John Wiley, Chichester.

Gessain, A. and Gout, O. (1992). Chronic myelopathy associated with human T-lymphotropic virus type I (HTLV-I). *Ann Intern Med* 117: 933–946.

Gessain, A., Barin, F., Vernant, J.C., Gout, O., Maurs, L., Calender, A., *et al.* (1985). Antibodies to human T-lymphotropic virus type-I in patients with tropical spastic paraparesis. *Lancet* 2: 407–410.

Gessain, A., Caudie, C., Gout, O., Vernant, J.C., Maurs, L., Giordano, C., *et al.* (1988). Intrathecal synthesis of antibodies to human T lymphotropic virus type I and the presence of IgG oligoclonal bands in the cerebrospinal fluid of patients with endemic tropical spastic paraparesis. *J Infect Dis* 157: 1226–1234.

Gessain, A., Saal, F., Giron, M.L., Lasneret, J., Lagaye, S., Gout, O., *et al.* (1990a). Cell surface phenotype and human T lymphotropic virus type 1 antigen expression in 12 T cell lines derived from peripheral blood and cerebrospinal fluid of West Indian, Guyanese and African patients with tropical spastic paraparesis. *J Gen Virol* 71: 333–341.

Gessain, A., Saal, F., Gout, O., Daniel, M.T., Flandrin, G., de The, G., *et al.* (1990b). High human T-cell lymphotropic virus type I proviral DNA load with polyclonal integration in peripheral blood mononuclear cells of French West Indian, Guianese, and African patients with tropical spastic paraparesis. *Blood* 75: 428–433.

Giraudon, P., Szymocha, R., Buart, S., Bernard, A., Cartier, L., Belin, M.F., et al. (2000). T lymphocytes activated by persistent viral infection differentially modify the expression of metalloproteinases and their endogenous inhibitors, TIMPs, in human astrocytes: relevance to HTLV-I-induced neurological disease. *J Immunol* 164: 2718–2727.

Godoy, A.J., Kira, J., Hasuo, K., and Goto, I. (1995). Characterization of cerebral white matter lesions of HTLV-I-associated myelopathy/tropical spastic paraparesis in comparison with multiple sclerosis and collagen-vasculitis: a semi-quantitative MRI study. *J Neurol Sci* 133: 102–111.

Goon, P.K., Hanon, E., Igakura, T., Tanaka, Y., Weber, J.N., Taylor, G.P., et al. (2002). High frequencies of Th1-type CD4(+) T cells specific to HTLV-1 Env and Tax proteins in patients with HTLV-1-associated myelopathy/tropical spastic paraparesis. *Blood* 99: 3335–3341.

Gout, O., Baulac, M., Gessain, A., Semah, F., Saal, F., Peries, J., et al. (1990). Rapid development of myelopathy after HTLV-I infection acquired by transfusion during cardiac transplantation. *N Engl J Med* 322: 383–388.

Grassmann, R., Berchtold, S., Radant, I., Alt, M., Fleckenstein, B., Sodroski, J.G., et al. (1992). Role of human T-cell leukemia virus type 1 X region proteins in immortalization of primary human lymphocytes in culture. *J Virol* 66: 4570–4575.

Greten, T.F., Slansky, J.E., Kubota, R., Soldan, S.S., Jaffee, E.M., Leist, T.P., et al. (1998). Direct visualization of antigen-specific T cells: HTLV-1 Tax11-19-specific CD8(+) T cells are activated in peripheral blood and accumulate in cerebrospinal fluid from HAM/TSP patients. *Proc Natl Acad Sci USA* 95: 7568–7573.

Hafler, D.A. (1999). The distinction blurs between an autoimmune versus microbial hypothesis in multiple sclerosis. *J Clin Invest* 104: 527–529.

Hanon, E., Hall, S., Taylor, G.P., Saito, M., Davis, R., Tanaka, Y., et al. (2000). Abundant tax protein expression in CD4+ T cells infected with human T-cell lymphotropic virus type I (HTLV-I) is prevented by cytotoxic T lymphocytes. *Blood* 95: 1386–1392.

Hanon, E., Goon, P., Taylor, G.P., Hasegawa, H., Tanaka, Y., Weber, J.N., et al. (2001). High production of interferon gamma but not interleukin-2 by human T-lymphotropic virus type I-infected peripheral blood mononuclear cells. *Blood* 98: 721–726.

Hara, H., Morita, M., Iwaki, T., Hatae, T., Itoyama, Y., Kitamoto, T., et al. (1994). Detection of human T lymphotrophic virus type I (HTLV-I) proviral DNA and analysis of T cell receptor V beta CDR3 sequences in spinal cord lesions of HTLV-I-associated myelopathy/tropical spastic paraparesis. *J Exp Med* 180: 831–839.

Hidaka, M., Inoue, J., Yoshida, M., and Seiki, M. (1988). Post-transcriptional regulator (rex) of HTLV-1 initiates expression of viral structural proteins but suppresses expression of regulatory proteins. *EMBO J* 7: 519–523.

Higuchi, I., Montemayor, E.S., Izumo, S., Inose, M., and Osame, M. (1993). Immunohistochemical characteristics of polymyositis in patients with HTLV-I-associated myelopathy and HTLV-I carriers. *Muscle Nerve* 16: 472–476.

Hino, S., Yamaguchi, K., Katamine, S., Sugiyama, H., Amagasaki, T., Kinoshita, K., et al. (1985). Mother-to-child transmission of human T-cell leukemia virus type-I. *Japan J Cancer Res* 76: 474–480.

Hino, S., Katamine, S., Kawase, K., Miyamoto, T., Doi, H., Tsuji, Y., et al. (1994). Intervention of maternal transmission of HTLV-1 in Nagasaki, Japan. *Leukemia* 8(Suppl. 1): S68–S70.

Hoffman, P.M., Dhib-Jalbut, S., Mikovits, J.A., Robbins, D.S., Wolf, A.L., Bergey, G.K., et al. (1992). Human T-cell leukemia virus type I infection of monocytes and microglial cells in primary human cultures. *Proc Natl Acad Sci USA* 89: 11784–11788.

Hollsberg, P. and Hafler, D. (1993). Seminars in medicine of the Beth Israel Hospital, Boston. Pathogenesis of diseases induced by human lymphotropic virus type I infection. *N Engl J Med* 328: 1173–1182.

Ichinose, K., Nakamura, T., Kawakami, A., Eguchi, K., Nagasato, K., Shibayama, K., et al. (1992). Increased adherence of T cells to human endothelial cells in patients with human T-cell lymphotropic virus type I-associated myelopathy. *Arch Neurol* 49: 74–76.

Ichinose, K., Nakamura, T., Nishiura, Y., Nagasato, K., Ohishi, K., Watanabe, H., et al. (1994). Characterization of adherent T cells to human endothelial cells in patients with HTLV-I-associated myelopathy. *J Neurol Sci* 122: 204–209.

Ida, H., Kurata, A., Eguchi, K., Kawakami, A., Migita, K., Fukuda, T., et al. (1991). Different B-cell responses to human T-cell lymphotropic virus type I (HTLV-I) envelope synthetic peptides in HTLV-I-infected individuals. *J Clin Immunol* 11: 143–151.

Ijichi, N., Eiraku, N., Osame, M., et al. (1989). Hypothetical pathogenesis of HAM/TSP: occurrence of proliferative response of lymphocytes in the central nervous system. In: *HTLV-I and the Nervous System* (ed. G.C. Roman, J.C. Vernant, and M. Osame), pp. 242–259. Alan R Liss, New York.

Ijichi, S., Izumo, S., Eiraku, N., Machigashira, K., Kubota, R., Nagai, M., et al. (1993). An autoaggressive process against bystander tissues in HTLV-I-infected individuals: a possible pathomechanism of HAM/TSP. *Med Hypotheses* 41: 542–547.

Inoue, Y., Kuroda, N., Shiraki, H., Sato, H., and Maeda, Y. (1992). Neutralizing activity of human antibodies against the structural protein of human T-cell lymphotropic virus type I. *Int J Cancer* 52: 877–880.

Ishiguro, N., Abe, M., Seto, K., Sakurai, H., Ikeda, H., Wakisaka, A., et al. (1992). A rat model of human T lymphocyte virus type I (HTLV-I) infection. 1. Humoral antibody response, provirus integration, and HTLV-I-associated myelopathy/tropical spastic paraparesis-like myelopathy in seronegative HTLV-I carrier rats. *J Exp Med* 176: 981–989.

Itoyama, Y., Minato, S., Kira, J., Goto, I., Sato, H., Okochi, K., et al. (1988). Spontaneous proliferation of peripheral blood lymphocytes increased in patients with HTLV-I-associated myelopathy. *Neurology* 38: 1302–1307.

Iwakura, Y., Tosu, M., Yoshida, E., Takiguchi, M., Sato, K., Kitajima, I., et al. (1991). Induction of inflammatory arthropathy resembling rheumatoid arthritis in mice transgenic for HTLV-I. *Science* 253: 1026–1028.

Iwasaki, Y. (1990). Pathology of chronic myelopathy associated with HTLV-I infection (HAM/TSP). *J Neurol Sci* 96: 103–123.

Izumo, S., Usuku, K., Osame, M., Machigashira, K., Johnson, M. and Hakagawa, M. (1989). The neuropathology of HTLV-I-associated myelopathy in Japan: Report of an autopsy case and review of the literature. In *HTLV-I and the Nervous System* (ed. G.C. Roman, J.C. Vernant, and M. Osame), pp. 261–267. Alan R. Liss, New York.

Izumo, S., Goto, I., Itoyama, Y., Okajima, T., Watanabe, S., Kuroda, Y., et al. (1996). Interferon-alpha is effective in HTLV-I-associated myelopathy: a multicenter, randomized, double-blind, controlled trial. *Neurology* 46: 1016–1021.

Jacobson, S., Gupta, A., Mattson, D., Mingioli, E., and McFarlin, D.E. (1990a). Immunological studies in tropical spastic paraparesis. *Ann Neurol* 27: 149–156.

Jacobson, S., Shida, H., McFarlin, D.E., Fauci, A.S., and Koenig, S. (1990b). Circulating CD8+ cytotoxic T lymphocytes specific for HTLV-I pX in patients with HTLV-I associated neurological disease. *Nature* 348: 245–248.

Jacobson, S., Reuben, J.S., Streilein, R.D., and Palker, T.J. (1991). Induction of CD4+, human T lymphotropic virus type-1-specific cytotoxic T lymphocytes from patients with HAM/TSP. Recognition of an immunogenic region of the gp46 envelope glycoprotein of human T lymphotropic virus type-1. *J Immunol* 146: 1155–1162.

Jacobson, S., McFarlin, D.E., Robinson, S., Voskuhl, R., Martin, R., Brewah, A., et al. (1992). HTLV-I-specific cytotoxic T lymphocytes in the cerebrospinal fluid of patients with HTLV-I-associated neurological disease. *Ann Neurol* 32: 651–657.

Jacobson, S., Krichavsky, M., Flerlage, N., and Levin, M. (1997). Immuno-pathogenesis of HTLV-I associated neurologic disease: massive latent HTLV-I infection in bone marrow of HAM/TSP patients. *Leukemia* 11(Suppl. 3): 73–75.

Jassal, S.R., Pohler, R.G., and Brighty, D.W. (2001). Human T-cell leukemia virus type 1 receptor expression among syncytium-resistant cell lines revealed by a novel surface glycoprotein-immunoadhesin. *J Virol* 75: 8317–8328.

Jeang, K.T., Widen, S.G., Semmes, O.J.T., and Wilson, S.H. (1990). HTLV-I trans-activator protein, tax, is a trans-repressor of the human beta-polymerase gene. *Science* 247: 1082–1084.

Jeffery, K.J., Usuku, K., Hall, S.E., Matsumoto, W., Taylor, G.P., Procter, J., et al. (1999). HLA alleles determine human T-lymphotropic virus-I (HTLV-I) proviral load and the risk of HTLV-I-associated myelopathy. *Proc Natl Acad Sci USA* **96**: 3848–3853.

Jiang, X., Ikeda, H., Tomaru, U., Morita, K., Tanaka, Y., and Yoshiki, T. (2000). A rat model for human T lymphocyte virus type I-associated myeloneuropathy. down-regulation of bcl-2 expression and increase in sensitivity to TNF-alpha of the spinal oligodendrocytes. *J Neuroimmunol* **106**: 105–113.

Kajiyama, W., Kashiwagi, S., Ikematsu, H., Hayashi, J., Nomura, H., and Okochi, K. (1986). Intrafamilial transmission of adult T cell leukemia virus. *J Infect Dis* **154**: 851–857.

Kannagi, M., Harada, S., Maruyama, I., Inoko, H., Igarashi, H., Kuwashima, G., et al. (1991). Predominant recognition of human T cell leukemia virus type I (HTLV-I) pX gene products by human CD8+ cytotoxic T cells directed against HTLV-I-infected cells. *Int Immunol* **3**: 761–767.

Kannagi, M., Shida, H., Igarashi, H., Kuruma, K., Murai, H., Aono, Y., et al. (1992). Target epitope in the Tax protein of human T-cell leukemia virus type I recognized by class I major histocompatibility complex-restricted cytotoxic T cells. *J Virol* **66**: 2928–2933.

Kannagi, M., Matsushita, S., Shida, H., and Harada, S. (1994). Cytotoxic T cell response and expression of the target antigen in HTLV-I infection. *Leukemia* **8**(Suppl. 1): S54–S59.

Kaplan, J.E. and Khabbaz, R.F. (1993). The epidemiology of human T-lymphotropic virus types I and II. *Med Virol* **3**: 137–148.

Kazanji, M., Ureta-Vidal, A., Ozden, S., Tangy, F., de Thoisy, B., Fiette, L., et al. (2000). Lymphoid organs as a major reservoir for human T-cell leukemia virus type 1 in experimentally infected squirrel monkeys (Saimiri sciureus): provirus expression, persistence, and humoral and cellular immune responses. *J Virol* **74**: 4860–4867.

Khabbaz, R.F., Douglas, J.M. Jr, Judson, F.N., Spiegel, R.A., St Louis, M.E., Whittington, W., et al. (1990). Seroprevalence of human T-lymphotropic virus type I or II in sexually transmitted disease clinic patients in the USA. *J Infect Dis* **162**: 241–244.

Khabbaz, R.F., Onorato, I.M., Cannon, R.O., Hartley, T.M., Roberts, B., Hosein, B., et al. (1992). Seroprevalence of HTLV-1 and HTLV-2 among intravenous drug users and persons in clinics for sexually transmitted diseases. *N Engl J Med* **326**: 375–380.

Kimata, J.T. and Ratner, L. (1991). Temporal regulation of viral and cellular gene expression during human T-lymphotropic virus type I-mediated lymphocyte immortalization. *J Virol* **65**: 4398–4407.

Kinoshita, T., Shimoyama, M., Tobinai, K., Ito, M., Ito, S., Ikeda, S., et al. (1989). Detection of mRNA for the tax1/rex1 gene of human T-cell leukemia virus type I in fresh peripheral blood mononuclear cells of adult T-cell leukemia patients and viral carriers by using the polymerase chain reaction. *Proc Natl Acad Sci USA* **86**: 5620–5624.

Kira, J., Koyanagi, Y., Yamada, T., Itoyama, Y., Goto, I., Yamamoto, N., et al. (1991). Increased HTLV-I proviral DNA in HTLV-I-associated myelopathy: a quantitative polymerase chain reaction study. *Ann Neurol* **29**: 194–201.

Kitajima, I., Osame, M., Izumo, S., and Igata, A. (1988). Immunological studies of HTLV-I associated myelopathy. *Autoimmunity* **1**: 125–131.

Kitajima, I., Maruyama, I., Maruyama, Y., Ijichi, S., Eiraku, N., Mimura, Y., et al. (1989). Polyarthritis in human T lymphotropic virus type I-associated myelopathy. *Arthritis Rheum* **32**: 1342–1344.

Kitze, B., Puccioni-Sohler, M., Schaffner, J., Rieckmann, P., Weber, T., Felgenhauer, K., et al. (1995). Specificity of intrathecal IgG synthesis for HTLV-1 core and envelope proteins in HAM/TSP. *Acta Neurol Scand* **92**: 213–217.

Kitze, B., Usuku, K., Yamano, Y., Yashiki, S., Nakamura, M., Fujiyoshi, T., et al. (1998). Human CD4+ lymphocytes recognize a highly conserved epitope of human T lymphotropic virus type 1 (HTLV-1) env gp21 restricted by HLA DRB1*0101. *Clin Exp Immunol* **111**: 278–285.

Kodaka, T., Uchiyama, T., Umadome, H., and Uchino, H. (1989). Expression of cytokine mRNA in leukemic cells from adult T cell leukemia patients. *Japan J Cancer Res* **80**: 531–536.

Koenig, S., Woods, R.M., Brewah, Y.A., Newell, A.J., Jones, G.M., Boone, E., et al. (1993). Characterization of MHC class I restricted cytotoxic T cell responses to tax in HTLV-1 infected patients with neurologic disease. *J Immunol* **151**: 3874–3883.

Koralnik, I. (1996). Structure of HTLV-I. In: *Human T-cell Lymphotropic Virus Type I* (ed. P. Hollsberg and D. Hafler), pp. 79–112. John Wiley, Chichester.

Koyanagi, Y., Itoyama, Y., Nakamura, N., Takamatsu, K., Kira, J., Iwamasa, T., et al. (1993). In vivo infection of human T-cell leukemia virus type I in non-T cells. *Virology* **196**: 25–33.

Kramer, A., Jacobson, S., Reuben, J.F., Murphy, E.L., Wiktor, S.Z., Cranston, B., et al. (1989). Spontaneous lymphocyte proliferation in symptom-free HTLV-I positive Jamaicans. *Lancet* **2**: 923–924.

Krichbaum-Stenger, K., Poiesz, B.J., Keller, P., Ehrlich, G., Gavalchin, J., Davis, B.H., et al. (1987). Specific adsorption of HTLV-I to various target human and animal cells. *Blood* **70**: 1303–1311.

Ku, C.C., Murakami, M., Sakamoto, A., Kappler, J., and Marrack, P. (2000). Control of homeostasis of CD8+ memory T cells by opposing cytokines. *Science* **288**: 675–678.

Kubota, R., Fujiyoshi, T., Izumo, S., Yashiki, S., Maruyama, I., Osame, M., et al. (1993). Fluctuation of HTLV-I proviral DNA in peripheral blood mononuclear cells of HTLV-I-associated myelopathy. *J Neuroimmunol* **42**: 147–154.

Kubota, R., Umehara, F., Izumo, S., Ijichi, S., Matsumuro, K., Yashiki, S., et al. (1994). HTLV-I proviral DNA amount correlates with infiltrating CD4+ lymphocytes in the spinal cord from patients with HTLV-I-associated myelopathy. *J Neuroimmunol* **53**: 23–29.

Kubota, R., Kawanishi, T., Matsubara, H., Manns, A., and Jacobson, S. (1998). Demonstration of human T lymphotropic virus type I (HTLV-I) tax-specific CD8+ lymphocytes directly in peripheral blood of HTLV-I-associated myelopathy/tropical spastic paraparesis patients by intracellular cytokine detection. *J Immunol* **161**: 482–488.

Kuroda, Y. and Matsui, M. (1993). Cerebrospinal fluid interferon-gamma is increased in HTLV-I-associated myelopathy. *J Neuroimmunol* **42**: 223–226.

Lairmore, M.D., Jason, J.M., Hartley, T.M., Khabbaz, R.F., De, B., and Evatt, B.L. (1989). Absence of human T-cell lymphotropic virus type I coinfection in human immunodeficiency virus-infected hemophilic men. *Blood* **74**: 2596–2599.

Lehky, T.J., Cowan, E.P., Lampson, L.A., and Jacobson, S. (1994). Induction of HLA class I and class II expression in human T-lymphotropic virus type I-infected neuroblastoma cells. *J Virol* **68**: 1854–1863.

Lehky, T.J., Fox, C.H., Koenig, S., Levin, M.C., Flerlage, N., Izumo, S., et al. (1995). Detection of human T-lymphotropic virus type I (HTLV-I) tax RNA in the central nervous system of HTLV-I-associated myelopathy/tropical spastic paraparesis patients by in situ hybridization. *Ann Neurol* **37**: 167–175.

Lehky, T.J., Levin, M.C., Kubota, R., Bamford, R.N., Flerlage, A.N., Soldan, S.S., et al. (1998). Reduction in HTLV-I proviral load and spontaneous lymphoproliferation in HTLV-I-associated myelopathy/tropical spastic paraparesis patients treated with humanized anti-Tac. *Ann Neurol* **44**: 942–947.

Lemasson, I., Robert-Hebmann, V., Hamaia, S., Duc Dodon, M., Gazzolo, L., and Devaux, C. (1997). Transrepression of lck gene expression by human T-cell leukemia virus type 1-encoded p40tax. *J Virol* **71**: 1975–1983.

Leon-Monzon, M., Illa, I., and Dalakas, M.C. (1994). Polymyositis in patients infected with human T-cell leukemia virus type I: the role of the virus in the cause of the disease. *Ann Neurol* **36**: 643–649.

Leung, K. and Nabel, G.J. (1988). HTLV-1 transactivator induces interleukin-2 receptor expression through an NF-kappa B-like factor. *Nature* **333**: 776–778.

Levin, M.C. and Jacobson, S. (1997). HTLV-I associated myelopathy/tropical spastic paraparesis (HAM/TSP): a chronic progressive neurologic disease associated with immunologically mediated damage to the central nervous system. *J Neurovirol* **3**: 126–140.

Levin, M.C., Lehky, T.J., Flerlage, A.N., Katz, D., Kingma, D.W., Jaffe, E.S., et al. (1997). Immunologic analysis of a spinal cord-biopsy specimen from a patient with human T-cell lymphotropic virus type I-associated neurologic disease. *N Engl J Med* **336**: 839–845.

Levin, M.C., Krichavsky, M., Berk, J., Foley, S., Rosenfeld, M., Dalmau, J., et al. (1998). Neuronal molecular mimicry in immune-mediated neurologic disease. *Ann Neurol* **44**: 87–98.

Levin, M.C., Lee, S.M., Kalume, F., Morcos, Y., Dohan, F.C. Jr, Hasty, K.A., et al. (2002). Autoimmunity due to molecular mimicry as a cause of neurological disease. *Nat Med* **8**: 509–513.

Levine, P.H., Blattner, W.A., Clark, J., Tarone, R., Maloney, E.M., Murphy, E.M., et al. (1988). Geographic distribution of HTLV-I and identification of a new high-risk population. *Int J Cancer* **42**: 7–12.

Lezin, A., Buart, S., Smadja, D., Akaoka, H., Bourdonne, O., Perret-Liaudet, A., et al. (2000). Tissue inhibitor of metalloproteinase 3, matrix metallo-proteinase 9, and neopterin in the cerebrospinal fluid: preferential presence in HTLV type I-infected neurologic patients versus healthy virus carriers. *AIDS Res Hum Retroviruses* **16**: 965–972.

Link, H., Cruz, M., Gessain, A., Gout, O., de The, G., and Kam-Hansen, S. (1989). Chronic progressive myelopathy associated with HTLV-I: oligoclonal IgG and anti-HTLV-I IgG antibodies in cerebrospinal fluid and serum. *Neurology* **39**: 1566–1572.

Ludolph, A.C., Hugon, J., Roman, G.C., Spencer, P.S., and Schoenberg, B.S. (1988). A clinical neurophysiologic study of tropical spastic paraparesis. *Muscle Nerve* **11**: 392–397.

Machigashira, K., Ijichi, S., Nagai, M., Yamano, Y., Hall, W.W., and Osame, M. (1997). In vitro virus propagation and high cellular responsiveness to the infected cells in patients with HTLV-I-associated myelopathy (HAM/TSP). *J Neurol Sci* **149**: 141–145.

Manns, A., Murphy, E.L., Wilks, R., Haynes, G., Figueroa, J.P., Hanchard, B., et al. (1991). Detection of early human T-cell lymphotropic virus type I antibody patterns during seroconversion among transfusion recipients. *Blood* **77**: 896–905.

Matsuda, M., Tsukada, N., Miyagi, K., and Yanagisawa, N. (1995). Increased levels of soluble vascular cell adhesion molecule-1 (VCAM-1) in the cerebrospinal fluid and sera of patients with multiple sclerosis and human T lymphotropic virus type-1-associated myelopathy. *J Neuroimmunol* **59**: 35–40.

Matsuoka, E., Takenouchi, N., Hashimoto, K., Kashio, N., Moritoyo, T., Higuchi, I., et al. (1998). Perivascular T cells are infected with HTLV-I in the spinal cord lesions with HTLV-I-associated myelopathy/tropical spastic para-paresis: double staining of immunohistochemistry and polymerase chain reaction in situ hybridization. *Acta Neuropathol (Berlin)* **96**: 340–346.

Matsuoka, E., Usuku, K., Jonosono, M., Takenouchi, N., Izumo, S., and Osame, M. (2000). CD44 splice variant involvement in the chronic inflammatory disease of the spinal cord: HAM/TSP. *J Neuroimmunol* **102**: 1–7.

Mattson, D.H., McFarlin, D.E., Mora, C., and Zaninovic, V. (1987). Central-nervous-system lesions detected by magnetic resonance imaging in an HTLV-1 antibody positive symptomless individual. *Lancet* **2**: 49.

McFarlin, D.E. and Blattner, W.A. (1991). Non-AIDS retroviral infections in humans. *Annu Rev Med* **42**: 97–105.

McLean, B.N., Rudge, P., and Thompson, E.J. (1989). Viral specific IgG and IgM antibodies in the CSF of patients with tropical spastic paraparesis. *J Neurol* **236**: 351–352.

Migone, T.S., Lin, J.X., Cereseto, A., Mulloy, J.C., O'Shea, J.J., Franchini, G., et al. (1995). Constitutively activated Jak-STAT pathway in T cells transformed with HTLV-I. *Science* **269**: 79–81.

Mochizuki, M., Watanabe, T., Yamaguchi, K., Takatsuki, K., Yoshimura, K., Shirao, M., et al. (1992). HTLV-I uveitis: a distinct clinical entity caused by HTLV-I. *Japan J Cancer Res* **83**: 236–239.

Morgan, O.S., Rodgers-Johnson, P., Mora, C., and Char, G. (1989). HTLV-1 and polymyositis in Jamaica. *Lancet* **2**: 1184–1187.

Moritoyo, T., Reinhart, T.A., Moritoyo, H., Sato, E., Izumo, S., Osame, M., et al. (1996). Human T-lymphotropic virus type I-associated myelopathy and tax gene expression in CD4+ T lymphocytes. *Ann Neurol* **40**: 84–90.

Moritoyo, T., Izumo, S., Moritoyo, H., Tanaka, Y., Kiyomatsu, Y., Nagai, M., et al. (1999). Detection of human T-lymphotropic virus type I p40tax protein in cerebrospinal fluid cells from patients with human T-lymphotropic virus type I-associated myelopathy/tropical spastic paraparesis. *J Neurovirol* **5**: 241–248.

Mueller, N. (1991). The epidemiology of HTLV-I infection. *Cancer Causes Control* **2**: 37–52.

Murphy, E.L., Figueroa, J.P., Gibbs, W.N., Brathwaite, A., Holding-Cobham, M., Waters, D., et al. (1989). Sexual transmission of human T-lymphotropic virus type I (HTLV-I). *Ann Intern Med* **111**: 555–560.

Nagai, M., Ijichi, S., Hall, W.W., and Osame, M. (1995). Differential effect of TGF-beta 1 on the in vitro activation of HTLV-I and the proliferative response of CD8+ T lymphocytes in patients with HTLV-I-associated myelopathy (HAM/TSP). *Clin Immunol Immunopathol* **77**: 324–331.

Nagai, M., Usuku, K., Matsumoto, W., Kodama, D., Takenouchi, N., Moritoyo, T., et al. (1998). Analysis of HTLV-I proviral load in 202 HAM/TSP patients and 243 asymptomatic HTLV-I carriers: high proviral load strongly predisposes to HAM/TSP. *J Neurovirol* **4**: 586–593.

Nagai, M., Brennan, M.B., Sakai, J.A., Mora, C.A., and Jacobson, S. (2001a). CD8(+) T cells are an in vivo reservoir for human T-cell lymphotropic virus type I. *Blood* **98**: 1858–1861.

Nagai, M., Kubota, R., Greten, T.F., Schneck, J.P., Leist, T.P., and Jacobson, S. (2001b). Increased activated human T cell lymphotropic virus type I (HTLV-I) Tax11-19-specific memory and effector CD8+ cells in patients with HTLV-I-associated myelopathy/tropical spastic paraparesis: correlation with HTLV-I provirus load. *J Infect Dis* **183**: 197–205.

Nagai, M., Yamano, Y., Brennan, M.B., Mora, C.A., and Jacobson, S. (2001c). Increased HTLV-I proviral load and preferential expansion of HTLV-I Tax-specific CD8+ T cells in cerebrospinal fluid from patients with HAM/TSP. *Ann Neurol* **50**: 807–812.

Nakagawa, M., Izumo, S., Ijichi, S., Kubota, H., Arimura, K., Kawabata, M., et al. (1995). HTLV-I-associated myelopathy: analysis of 213 patients based on clinical features and laboratory findings. *J Neurovirol* **1**: 50–61.

Nakagawa, M., Nakahara, K., Maruyama, Y., Kawabata, M., Higuchi, I., Kubota, H., et al. (1996). Therapeutic trials in 200 patients with HTLV-I-associated myelopathy/ tropical spastic paraparesis. *J Neurovirol* **2**: 345–355.

Nakamura, M., Kuroki, M., Kira, J., Itoyama, Y., Shiraki, H., Kuroda, N., et al. (1991). Elevated antibodies to synthetic peptides of HTLV-1 envelope transmembrane glycoproteins in patients with HAM/TSP. *J Neuroimmunol* **35**: 167–177.

Nakamura, S., Nagano, I., Yoshioka, M., Shimazaki, S., Onodera, J., and Kogure, K. (1993). Detection of tumor necrosis factor-alpha-positive cells in cerebrospinal fluid of patients with HTLV-I-associated myelopathy. *J Neuroimmunol* **42**: 127–130.

Niewiesk, S., Daenke, S., Parker, C.E., Taylor, G., Weber, J., Nightingale, S., et al. (1995). Naturally occurring variants of human T-cell leukemia virus type I Tax protein impair its recognition by cytotoxic T lymphocytes and the trans-activation function of Tax. *J Virol* **69**: 2649–2653.

Nishimoto, N., Yoshizaki, K., Eiraku, N., Machigashira, K., Tagoh, H., Ogata, A., et al. (1990). Elevated levels of interleukin-6 in serum and cerebrospinal fluid of HTLV-I-associated myelopathy/tropical spastic paraparesis. *J Neurol Sci* **97**: 183–193.

Nishioka, K., Maruyama, I., Sato, K., Kitajima, I., Nakajima, Y., and Osame, M. (1989). Chronic inflammatory arthropathy associated with HTLV-I. *Lancet* **1**: 441.

Nishiura, Y., Nakamura, T., Ichinose, K., Shirabe, S., Tsujino, A., Goto, H., et al. (1996). Increased production of inflammatory cytokines in cultured CD4+ cells from patients with HTLV-I-associated myelopathy. *Tohoku J Exp Med* **179**: 227–233.

Nomata, K., Nakamura, T., Suzu, H., Yushita, Y., Kanetake, H., Sawada, T., et al. (1992). Novel complications with HTLV-1-associated myelopathy/tropical spastic paraparesis: interstitial cystitis and persistent prostatitis. *Japan J Cancer Res* **83**: 601–608.

Nomoto, M., Utatsu, Y., Soejima, Y., and Osame, M. (1991). Neopterin in cere-brospinal fluid: a useful marker for diagnosis of HTLV-I-associated myelopathy/tropical spastic paraparesis. *Neurology* **41**: 457.

Oger, J. and Dekaban, G. (1995). HTLV-I associated myelopathy: a case of viral-induced auto-immunity. *Autoimmunity* **21**: 151–159.

Ohba, N., Matsumoto, M., Sameshima, M., Kabayama, Y., Nakao, K., Unoki, K., et al. (1989). Ocular manifestations in patients infected with human T-lymphotropic virus type I. *Japan J Ophthalmol* **33**: 1–12.

Ohya, O., Tomaru, U., Yamashita, I., Kasai, T., Morita, K., Ikeda, H., et al. (1997). HTLV-I induced myeloneuropathy in WKAH rats: apoptosis and local act-ivation of the HTLV-I pX and TNF-alpha genes implicated in the patho-genesis. *Leukemia* **11**(Suppl. 3): 255–257.

Okochi, K., Sato, H., and Hinuma, Y. (1984). A retrospective study on transmis-sion of adult T cell leukemia virus by blood transfusion: seroconversion in recipients. *Vox Sang* **46**: 245–253.

Okuma, K., Nakamura, M., Nakano, S., Niho, Y., and Matsuura, Y. (1999). Host range of human T-cell leukemia virus type I analyzed by a cell fusion-dependent reporter gene activation assay. *Virology* **254**: 235–244.

Osame, M. (1990). Review of WHO Kagoshima Meeting and diagnostic guide-lines for HAM/TSP. In: *Human Retrovirology HTLV* (ed. W. Blattner), pp. 191–197. Raven Press, New York.

Osame, M. and McArthur, J.C. (1990). Neurologic manifestations of infection with human T cell lymphotropic virus type I. In: *Disease of the Nervous System: Clinical Neurobiology* (ed. A.K. Asburr, G.M. McKhann, and W.I. McDonald), pp. 1331–1339. W.B. Saunders, New York.

Osame, M., Izumo, S., Igata, A., Matsumoto, M., Matsumoto, T., Sonoda, S., *et al.* (1986a). Blood transfusion and HTLV-I associated myelopathy. *Lancet* 2: 104–105.

Osame, M., Usuku, K., Izumo, S., Ijichi, N., Amitani, H., Igata, A., *et al.* (1986b). HTLV-I associated myelopathy, a new clinical entity. *Lancet* 1: 1031–1032.

Osame, M., Matsumoto, M., Usuku, K., Izumo, S., Ijichi, N., Amitani, H., *et al.* (1987). Chronic progressive myelopathy associated with elevated antibodies to human T-lymphotropic virus type I and adult T-cell leukemialike cells. *Ann Neurol* 21: 117–122.

Osame, M., Igata, A., Matsumoto, M., Kohka, M., Usuku, K., and Izumo, S. (1990a). HTLV-I-associated myelopathy(HAM), treatment trials, retrospective survey and clinical and laboratory findings. *Hematol Rev* 3: 271–284.

Osame, M., Janssen, R., Kubota, H., Nishitani, H., Igata, A., Nagataki, S., *et al.* (1990b). Nationwide survey of HTLV-I-associated myelopathy in Japan: association with blood transfusion. *Ann Neurol* 28: 50–56.

Palker, T.J., Tanner, M.E., Scearce, R.M., Streilein, R.D., Clark, M.E., and Haynes, B.F. (1989). Mapping of immunogenic regions of human T cell leukemia virus type I (HTLV-I) gp46 and gp21 envelope glycoproteins with env-encoded synthetic peptides and a monoclonal antibody to gp46. *J Immunol* 142: 971–978.

Parker, C.E., Daenke, S., Nightingale, S., and Bangham, C.R. (1992). Activated, HTLV-1-specific cytotoxic T-lymphocytes are found in healthy seropositives as well as in patients with tropical spastic paraparesis. *Virology* 188: 628–636.

Parker, C.E., Nightingale, S., Taylor, G.P., Weber, J., and Bangham, C.R. (1994). Circulating anti-Tax cytotoxic T lymphocytes from human T-cell leukemia virus type I-infected people, with and without tropical spastic paraparesis, recognize multiple epitopes simultaneously. *J Virol* 68: 2860–2868.

Poiesz, B.J., Ruscetti, F.W., Gazdar, A.F., Bunn, P.A., Minna, J.D., and Gallo, R.C. (1980). Detection and isolation of type C retrovirus particles from fresh and cultured lymphocytes of a patient with cutaneous T-cell lymphoma. *Proc Natl Acad Sci USA* 77: 7415–7419.

Puccioni-Sohler, M., Rios, M., Bianco, C., Zhu, S.W., Oliveira, C., Novis, S.A., *et al.* (1999). An inverse correlation of HTLV-I viral load in CSF and intrathecal synthesis of HTLV-I antibodies in TSP/HAM. *Neurology* 53: 1335–1339.

Ratner, L. (1996). (STET: no insertion needed) *Animal Models of HTLV-I Infection*. John Wiley, Chichester.

Richardson, J.H., Edwards, A.J., Cruickshank, J.K., Rudge, P., and Dalgleish, A.G. (1990). In vivo cellular tropism of human T-cell leukemia virus type 1. *J Virol* 64: 5682–5687.

Romero, I.A., Prevost, M.C., Perret, E., Adamson, P., Greenwood, J., Couraud, P.O., *et al.* (2000). Interactions between brain endothelial cells and human T-cell leukemia virus type 1-infected lymphocytes: mechanisms of viral entry into the central nervous system. *J Virol* 74: 6021–6030.

Sandler, S.G., Fang, C.T., and Williams, A.E. (1991). Human T-cell lymphotropic virus type I and II in transfusion medicine. *Transfus Med Rev* 5: 93–107.

Sasaki, K., Morooka, I., Inomata, H., Kashio, N., Akamine, T., and Osame, M. (1989). Retinal vasculitis in human T-lymphotropic virus type I associated myelopathy. *Br J Ophthalmol* 73: 812–815.

Sato, K., Maruyama, I., Maruyama, Y., Kitajima, I., Nakajima, Y., Higaki, M., *et al.* (1991). Arthritis in patients infected with human T lymphotropic virus type I. Clinical and immunopathologic features. *Arthritis Rheum* 34: 714–721.

Seiki, M., Hattori, S., Hirayama, Y., and Yoshida, M. (1983). Human adult T-cell leukemia virus: complete nucleotide sequence of the provirus genome integrated in leukemia cell DNA. *Proc Natl Acad Sci USA* 80: 3618–3622.

Seiki, M., Inoue, J., Hidaka, M., and Yoshida, M. (1988). Two cis-acting elements responsible for posttranscriptional trans-regulation of gene expression of human T-cell leukemia virus type I. *Proc Natl Acad Sci USA* 85: 7124–7128.

Sheremata, W.A., Benedict, D., Squilacote, D.C., Sazant, A. and DeFreitas, E. (1993). High-dose zidovudine induction in HTLV-I-associated myelopathy: safety and possible efficacy. *Neurology* 43: 2125–2129.

Shimoyama, M., Minato, K., Tobinai, K., Nagai, M., Setoya, T., Takenaka, T., *et al.* (1983). Atypical adult T-cell leukemia-lymphoma: diverse clinical manifestations of adult T-cell leukemia-lymphoma. *Japan J Clin Oncol* 13: 165–187.

Sommerfelt, M.A., Williams, B.P., Clapham, P.R., Solomon, E., Goodfellow, P.N., and Weiss, R. A. (1988). Human T cell leukemia viruses use a receptor determined by human chromosome 17. *Science* 242: 1557–1559.

Sonoda, S., Fujiyoshi, T., and Yashiki, S. (1996). Immunogenetics of HTLV-I/II and associated diseases. *J Acquir Immune Defic Syndr Hum Retrovirol* 13: S119–S123.

Sugamura, K., Fujii, M., Kannagi, M., Sakitani, M., Takeuchi, M., and Hinuma, Y. (1984). Cell surface phenotypes and expression of viral antigens of various human cell lines carrying human T-cell leukemia virus. *Int J Cancer* 34: 221–228.

Sugimoto, M., Nakashima, H., Watanabe, S., Uyama, E., Tanaka, F., Ando, M., *et al.* (1987). T-lymphocyte alveolitis in HTLV-I-associated myelopathy. *Lancet* 2: 1220.

Suzuki, T., Fujisawa, J.I., Toita, M., and Yoshida, M. (1993). The trans-activator tax of human T-cell leukemia virus type 1 (HTLV-1) interacts with cAMP-responsive element (CRE) binding and CRE modulator proteins that bind to the 21-base-pair enhancer of HTLV-1. *Proc Natl Acad Sci USA* 90: 610–614.

Tajima, K. and Hinuma, Y. (1984). Epidemiological features of **adult T-cell** leukemia virus In: *Pathophysiological Aspects of Cancer Epidemiology* (ed. G. Mathe and P. Rizenstein), pp. 75–87. Pergamon Press, Oxford.

Tajima, K., Inoue, H., Takezaki, T., Itoh, M., and Itoh, S.I. (1994). Ethnoepidemiology of ATL in Japan with special reference to the Mongoloid dispersal. In: *Adult T-cell Leukemia* (ed. K. Takatsuki), pp. 91–112. Oxford University Press, Oxford.

Takahashi, K., Takezaki, T., Oki, T., Kawakami, K., Yashiki, S., Fujiyoshi, T., *et al.* (1991). Inhibitory effect of maternal antibody on mother-to-child transmission of human T-lymphotropic virus type I. The Mother-to-Child Transmission Study Group. *Int J Cancer* 49: 673–677.

Taylor, G.P., Hall, S.E., Navarrete, S., Michie, C.A., Davis, R., Witkover, A.D., *et al.* (1999). Effect of lamivudine on human T-cell leukemia virus type 1 (HTLV-1) DNA copy number, T-cell phenotype, and anti-tax cytotoxic T-cell frequency in patients with HTLV-1-associated myelopathy. *J Virol* 73: 10289–10295.

Tendler, C.L., Greenberg, S.J., Blattner, W.A., Manns, A., Murphy, E., Fleisher, T., *et al.* (1990). Transactivation of interleukin 2 and its receptor induces immune activation in human T-cell lymphotropic virus type I-associated myelopathy: pathogenic implications and a rationale for immunotherapy. *Proc Natl Acad Sci USA* 87: 5218–5222.

Tendler, C.L., Greenberg, S.J., Burton, J.D., Danielpour, D., Kim, S.J., Blattner, W.A., *et al.* (1991). Cytokine induction in HTLV-I associated myelopathy and adult T-cell leukemia: alternate molecular mechanisms underlying retroviral pathogenesis. *J Cell Biochem* 46: 302–311.

Terada, K., Katamine, S., Eguchi, K., Moriuchi, R., Kita, M., Shimada, H., *et al.* (1994). Prevalence of serum and salivary antibodies to HTLV-1 in Sjogren's syndrome. *Lancet* 344: 1116–1119.

Tochikura, T., Iwahashi, M., Matsumoto, T., Koyanagi, Y., Hinuma, Y., and Yamamoto, N. (1985). Effect of human serum anti-HTLV antibodies on viral antigen induction in vitro cultured peripheral lymphocytes from adult T-cell leukemia patients and healthy virus carriers. *Int J Cancer* 36: 1–7.

Tomaru, U., Ikeda, H., Ohya, O., Abe, M., Kasai, T., Yamasita, I., *et al.* (1996). Human T lymphocyte virus type I-induced myeloneuropathy in rats: implication of local activation of the pX and tumor necrosis factor-alpha genes in pathogenesis. *J Infect Dis* 174: 318–323.

Trejo, S.R. and Ratner, L. (2000).The HTLV receptor is a widely expressed protein. *Virology* 268: 41–48.

Uchiyama, T. (1997). Human T cell leukemia virus type I (HTLV-I) and human diseases. *Annu Rev Immunol* 15: 15–37.

Uchiyama, T., Yodoi, J., Sagawa, K., Takatsuki, K., and Uchino, H. (1977). Adult T-cell leukemia: clinical and hematologic features of 16 cases. *Blood* 50: 481–492.

Uittenbogaard, M.N., Armstrong, A.P., Chiaramello, A., and Nyborg, J.K. (1994). Human T-cell leukemia virus type I Tax protein represses gene expression through the basic helix-loop-helix family of transcription factors. *J Biol Chem* 269: 22466–22469.

Umehara, F., Izumo, S., Nakagawa, M., Ronquillo, A.T., Takahashi, K., Matsumuro, K., *et al.* (1993). Immunocytochemical analysis of the cellular infiltrate in the spinal cord lesions in HTLV-I-associated myelopathy. *J Neuropathol Exp Neurol* 52: 424–430.

Umehara, F., Izumo, S., Ronquillo, A.T., Matsumuro, K., Sato, E., and Osame, M. (1994a). Cytokine expression in the spinal cord lesions in HTLV-I-associated myelopathy. *J Neuropathol Exp Neurol* 53: 72–77.

Umehara, F., Nakamura, A., Izumo, S., Kubota, R., Ijichi, S., Kashio, N., *et al.* (1994b). Apoptosis of T lymphocytes in the spinal cord lesions in HTLV-I-associated myelopathy: a possible mechanism to control viral infection in the central nervous system. *J Neuropathol Exp Neurol* 53: 617–624.

Umehara, F., Izumo, S., Takeya, M., Takahashi, K., Sato, E., and Osame, M. (1996). Expression of adhesion molecules and monocyte chemoattractant protein -1 (MCP-1) in the spinal cord lesions in HTLV-I-associated myelopathy. *Acta Neuropathol* 91: 343–350.

Umehara, F., Okada, Y., Fujimoto, N., Abe, M., Izumo, S., and Osame, M. (1998). Expression of matrix metalloproteinases and tissue inhibitors of metalloproteinases in HTLV-I-associated myelopathy. *J Neuropathol Exp Neurol* 57: 839–849.

Vernant, J.C., Buisson, G., Magdeleine, J., De Thore, J., Jouannelle, A., Neisson-Vernant, C., *et al.* (1988). T-lymphocyte alveolitis, tropical spastic paresis, and Sjogren syndrome. *Lancet* 1: 177.

Vine, A.M., Witkover, A.D., Lloyd, A.L., Jeffery, K.J., Siddiqui, A., Marshall, S.E., *et al.* (2002). Polygenic control of human T lymphotropic virus type I (HTLV-I) provirus load and the risk of HTLV-I-associated myelopathy/tropical spastic paraparesis. *J Infect Dis* 186: 932–939.

Wattel, E., Vartanian, J.P., Pannetier, C., and Wain-Hobson, S. (1995). Clonal expansion of human T-cell leukemia virus type I-infected cells in asymptomatic and symptomatic carriers without malignancy. *J Virol* 69: 2863–2868.

Wattel, E., Cavrois, M., Gessain, A., and Wain-Hobson, S. (1996). Clonal expansion of infected cells: a way of life for HTLV-I. *J Acquir Immune Defic Syndr Hum Retrovirol* 13(Suppl. 1): S92–S99.

Wiktor, S.Z., Jacobson, S., Weiss, S.H., Shaw, G.M., Reuben, J.S., Shorty, V.J., *et al.* (1991). Spontaneous lymphocyte proliferation in HTLV-II infection. *Lancet* 337: 327–328.

Williams, A.E., Fang, C.T., Slamon, D.J., Poiesz, B.J., Sandler, S.G., Darr, W.F. 2nd, *et al.* (1988). Seroprevalence and epidemiological correlates of HTLV-I infection in U.S. blood donors. *Science* 240: 643–646.

Wodarz, D., Nowak, M.A., and Bangham, C.R. (1999). The dynamics of HTLV-I and the CTL response. *Immunol Today* 20: 220–227.

Xu, X., Heidenreich, O., and Nerenberg, M. (1996). HAM/TSP and ATL: persistent paradoxes and new hypotheses. *J Neurovirol* 2: 60–69.

Yamamoto, N., Okada, M., Koyanagi, Y., Kannagi, M., and Hinuma, Y. (1982). Transformation of human leukocytes by cocultivation with an adult T cell leukemia virus producer cell line. *Science* 217: 737–739.

Yamamoto, N., Chosa, T., Koyanagi, Y., Tochikura, T., Schneider, J., and Hinuma, Y. (1984) Binding of adult T-cell leukemia virus to various hematopoietic cells.. *Cancer Lett* 21: 261–268.

Yamano, Y., Nagai, M., Brennan, M., Mora, C.A., Soldan, S.S., Tomaru, U., *et al.* (2002). Correlation of human T-cell lymphotropic virus type 1 (HTLV-1) mRNA with proviral DNA load, virus-specific CD8(+) T cells, and disease severity in HTLV-1-associated myelopathy (HAM/TSP). *Blood* 99: 88–94.

Yamazaki, H., Ikeda, H., Ishizu, A., Nakamaru, Y., Sugaya, T., Kikuchi, K., *et al.* (1997). A wide spectrum of collagen vascular and autoimmune diseases in transgenic rats carrying the env-pX gene of human T lymphocyte virus type I. *Int Immunol* 9: 339–346.

Yashiki, S., Fujiyoshi, T., Arima, N., Osame, M., Yoshinaga, M., Nagata, Y., *et al.* (2001). HLA-A*26, HLA-B*4002, HLA-B*4006, and HLA-B*4801 alleles predispose to adult T cell leukemia: the limited recognition of HTLV type 1 tax peptide anchor motifs and epitopes to generate anti-HTLV type 1 tax CD8(+) cytotoxic T lymphocytes. *AIDS Res Hum Retroviruses* 17: 1047–1061.

Yoshida, M., Osame, M., Kawai, H., Toita, M., Kuwasaki, N., Nishida, Y., *et al.* (1989). Increased replication of HTLV-I in HTLV-I-associated myelopathy. *Ann Neurol* 26: 331–335.

Yoshioka, A., Hirose, G., Ueda, Y., Nishimura, Y., and Sakai, K. (1993). Neuropathological studies of the spinal cord in early stage HTLV-I-associated myelopathy (HAM). *J Neurol Neurosurg Psychiatry* 56: 1004–1007.

Zhao, L.J. and Giam, C.Z. (1991). Interaction of the human T-cell lymphotrophic virus type I (HTLV-I) transcriptional activator Tax with cellular factors that bind specifically to the 21-base-pair repeats in the HTLV-I enhancer. *Proc Natl Acad Sci USA* 88: 11445–11449.

24 Lyme neuroborreliosis

Andrew R. Pachner

Lyme disease or Lyme borreliosis (LB) is a chronic infection in which the relentless effort by the host to clear the pathogen is associated with tissue damage caused by inflammation. The disease has been called 'The new great imitator' (Pachner, 1988), in comparison to its sister disease, syphilis, the original 'great imitator', because once the spirochete disseminates, the manifestations of the infection can be protean. This chapter will focus predominantly on neurological manifestations of LB, also called Lyme neuroborreliosis or LNB. Information about LNB has been gained both from studies in humans with LNB and in experimental animals; both sources will be summarized.

Borrelia burgdorferi, the causative pathogen of Lyme borreliosis

Although Lyme disease was first described in the United States in 1977 (Steere *et al.*, 1977*a*) as an oligoarticular arthritis, with the clinical spectrum expanded early to include neurological and dermatological manifestations (Steere *et al.*, 1977*b*), the spirochete was identified 6 years later in 1983 (Steere *et al.*, 1983*a*; Benach *et al.*, 1983) as the causative agent. It is now considered a species cluster, called *B. burgdorferi sensu lato*, composed of the pathogenic species, *B. burgdorferi sensu stricto*, *B. garinii*, *B. afzelii*, and *B. japonica* (Wang *et al.*, 1999). The organism is a thin, long, spiral-shaped bacterium (Fig.24. 1), which can be readily visualized in highly infected tissue using antispirochetal antibody and immunohistochemistry (Fig. 24.2). The molecular organization of the spirochete is very unusual. The complete genomic and plasmid sequences of B31, a *B. burgdorferi sensu stricto* organism, have been determined and analysed (Casjens *et al.*, 2000). A very small

fraction, only 8%, of the genes have similarity to genes in other bacteria, and these similarities are not known bacterial virulence genes. This suggests that the spirochete interacts with its host in very different ways from better-studied bacterial pathogens. The unusual aspects of the genome(Casjens *et al.*, 2000) include such features as linear replicons, more than 20 replicons in a single bacterium(consisting of genome, linear, and circular plasmids), large tracts of directly repeated short DNA sequences, a substantial fraction of plasmid DNA that appears to be in a state of evolutionary decay, and evidence for numerous and sometimes recent exchanges of DNA sequences among the plasmids. Another distinctive aspect of the organism is the large fraction (14.5–17%) of the plasmid genes which encode for lipoprotein genes. All three pathogenic species can be found in Europe, while only *B. burgdorferi sensu stricto* is found in the United States.

The sequencing of the complete genome of *B. burgdorferi* revealed the presence of 105 putative lipoproteins, which constitute more than 8% of the coding sequence of strain B31 (Fraser *et al.*, 1997; Casjens *et al.*, 2000). The function of most of these lipoproteins is unknown. Lipoproteins of *B. burgdorferi* are 50- to 500-fold more active inducers of cytokines and mitogens of B cells than lipoproteins of *Escherichia coli* or synthetic peptides containing only the lipid moiety, tripalmitoyl-*S*-glyceryl-cysteine (Weis *et al.*, 1994). One of the most thoroughly studied of these lipoproteins is outer surface protein A (OspA) (Howe *et al.*, 1985), the lipoprotein which was used for the Lyme vaccine which was available in the early 2000s. OspA is not expressed during infection in humans (Fikrig *et al.*, 1998), in

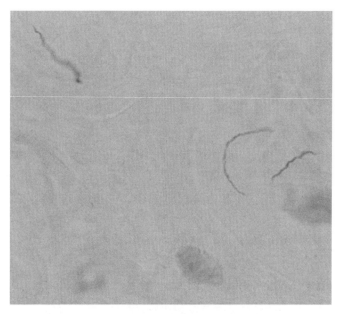

Fig. 24.2 *B. burgdorferi* in the brachial plexus of an infected non-humnan primate stained by immunohistochemistry. (see also Plate 5 of the colour plate section at the center.)

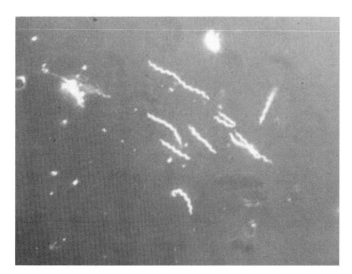

Fig. 24.1 *B. burgdorferi* in culture stained by immunofluorescence.

mice (Barthold *et al.*, 1996), or in rhesus macaques (Pachner *et al.*, 2002*b*); in this respect it is like other most other lipoproteins of *B.burgdorferi* which are highly expressed in cultured organisms, but are down-regulated *in vivo* (Liang *et al.*, 2002). In contrast, OspA is highly expressed by the spirochete when it is in the tick vector, where the protein participates in attachment to the midgut of the tick (Pal *et al.*, 2000). OspA, like most of the other outer surface proteins of *B. burgdorferi*, is encoded on extrachromosomal plasmids.

Several studies have provided direct or indirect evidence that several *B. burgdorferi* proteins are the diametric opposites of OspA; they can be considered 'in vivo expressed' since they are expressed predominantly during infection in mammalian hosts, and poorly or not at all during *in vitro* cultivation of the spirochete. These include OspC (Zhong *et al.*, 1999), Bbk32 and Bbk50 (Fikrig *et al.*, 2000), decorin binding proteins A and B (Hanson *et al.*, 1998; Cinco *et al.*, 2000), ErpT (Fikrig *et al.*, 1999), flagellin (Limbach *et al.*, 1999), pG (Wallich *et al.*, 1995), p35 and p37 (Fikrig *et al.*, 1997*b*, 1998), members of the Mlp family (Yang *et al.*, 1999), and VlsE (Zhang *et al.*, 1997).

B. burgdorferi can persist in almost any vertebrate animal studied (Barthold *et al.*, 1988, 1993*a*; Moody *et al.*, 1990*b*; Pachner and Itano, 1990; Pachner *et al.*, 1994, 1995*a*; Foley *et al.*, 1995; Zhang and Norris, 1998). Much research has been devoted to studies of how the spirochete might be able to establish persistence in such a wide host range. One of the mechanisms by which borrelias can evade the immune response is through antigenic variation. This phenomenon has been recently dubbed 'the controlled chaos of shifty pathogens' (Faguy, 2000). A complex mechanism of antigenic variation has been well characterized in the relapsing fever borrelias (Barbour, 1991). During relapsing fever, one surface-exposed lipoprotein among a family known as variable major proteins (Vmp) can be expressed at any given time from a single expression locus in a linear plasmid. Antigenic variation occurs when the expressed *vmp* gene is replaced completely or partially by one of the previously unexpressed *vmp* genes by interplasmidic recombination (Barbour *et al.*, 1991; Pennington *et al.*, 1999). The host's specific antibody response eliminates the predominant serotypes in the population, and the newly emerged serotypes proliferate and cause a relapse.

The occurrence of antigenic variation in *B. burgdorferi* has only recently been recognized (Nordstrand *et al.*, 2000). Zhang and colleagues characterized a genetic locus called *vmp*-like sequence (vls) in *B. burgdorferi* that closely resembles the *vmp* system of the relapsing fever borrelias (Zhang *et al.*, 1997). One *vls* expression site (*vlsE*) and 15 silent *vls* cassettes were identified on a 28 kb linear plasmid of virulent isolates of *B. burgdorferi*. This locus is responsible for expression of the 35 kDa surface exposed lipoprotein VlsE. During infection in mice, frequent and promiscuous recombination occurred between the *vlsE* and the silent, i.e. unexpressed, *vls*, resulting in antigenic variation and decreased reactivity to antiserum against the parental strain. Silent *vls* genes are organized head to tail as a single open reading frame, and each represents only the central third of the open reading frame. This central variable domain contains six invariable regions, IR(1) to IR(6), and six variable regions (Liang and Philipp, 1999). Unlike the invariable regions of Vmps, variant surface glycoproteins, and pilin, which are not antigenic in natural infections, there is some evidence that the most conserved of the IRs, IR6, is recognized by antisera in Lyme disease patients and in monkeys infected with *B. burgdorferi* (Liang *et al.*, 1999), and there is evidence in mice that there may be immune selection of new VlsE variants (Zhang and Norris, 1998). Other bacterial components which may be important antigens during chronic infection include phospholipids (Mackworth-Young *et al.*, 1988; Martin *et al.*, 1988; Garcia Monco *et al.*, 1993) and glycolipids(Honarvar *et al.*, 1994).

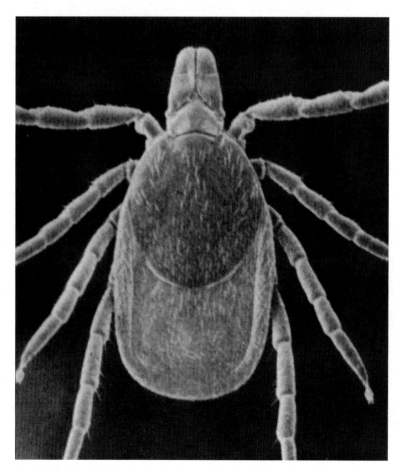
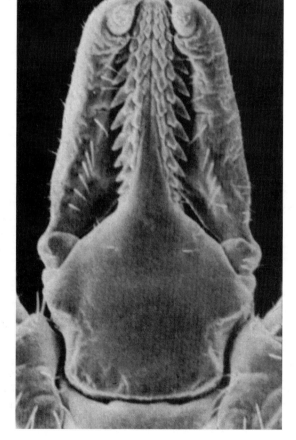

Fig. 24.3 *Ixodes scapularis*—the vector of Lyme disease in the United States.

Lyme borreliosis pathogenesis

Transmission

At this time only the ixodid tick (Fig. 24.3) is considered able to transmit the infection to humans, although a variety of animals, including field mice, rats, deer, birds, and rabbits, are reservoirs of the infection (Anderson *et al.*, 1986, 1990; Smith *et al.*, 1993; Burgess *et al.*, 1993; Bishop *et al.*, 1994; Humair *et al.*, 1998; Gern and Humair, 2000). Thus, human infection can only occur after the bite of tick infected with the spirochete. There are many open questions about tick transmission, such as how frequently ticks are co-infected with other infectious agents, how often a bite by an infected tick results in transmission of the spirochete, whether there is a spectrum of infectious and non-infectious *B. burgdorferi* strains in any particular tick, whether ticks will bite any human, etc. It seems likely that most humans who become infected clear the tick-transmitted spirochete by local or innate immate responses, since only a small percentage of patients develop erythema migrans, disseminated disease, or seronconversion after bites by infected ticks.

Spirochetemia

Within a few weeks of intradermal inoculation, *B. burgdorferi* can be found in the blood of experimental animals by polymerase chain reaction (PCR) or culture. The duration of spirochetemia appears to correlate inversely with the development of the IgG anti-*B. burgdorferi* antibody response: i.e., as the levels of IgG rise over the second, third, and fourth weeks of infection, the likelihood of finding spirochetes in the peripheral blood drops. It is felt by most investigators that the pathogen disseminates throughout the body primarily through the blood. In contrast, Straubinger *et al.* (1998, 2000) have postulated spread through tissues in addition as an important mechanism; tissue and hematogenous spread are, of course, not mutually exclusive. The duration of spirochetemia in the non-human primate, like the human, is short, a few weeks at the onset of infection; in contrast, the mouse may have extended periods of spirochetemia (Cassatt *et al.*, 1998).

Establishment of infection in tissue

The precise mechanism by which *B. burgdorferi* establishes infection in tissues is unknown. Much of the inflammation in the disease is perivascular (Museteanu *et al.*, 1991), so invasion probably occurs through binding to capillary endothelium (Szczepanski *et al.*, 1990), penetration through or between endothelial cells (Burns and Furie, 1998), and early accumulation in the perivascular space (Pachner *et al.*, 1995a). Whether *B. burgdorferi* exists *in vivo* intracellularly is still an open question; certainly, spirochetes are rarely, if ever, seen intracellularly in experimental models (Pachner *et al.*, 1995a), although there is little doubt that the spirochete can be found intracellularly in tissue culture conditions (Kurtti *et al.*, 1993; Montgomery *et al.*, 1993; Girschick *et al.*, 1996). In the non-human primate model, localization of the spirochete has consistently been to extracellular spaces. The extracellular nature of the spirochetes is also supported by the finding that the most active immune mechanism for protection is anti-*B. burgdorferi* immunoglobulin (Johnson *et al.*, 1986), primarily IgG (Pachner *et al.*, 2001a).

Lyme borreliosis in the skin

Once a tick injects an invasive strain into a susceptible human at an adequate dose of spirochetes, localized infection in the skin occurs as the first stage of the process. The initial clinical manifestation of skin infection is usually erythema migrans (EM) (Berger, 1984; Berger *et al.*, 1985), an inflammatory response of the skin to the presence of spirochetes spreading through the skin from the initial point of injection at the tick bite. This rash is a spreading red area, hence the name, but secondary lesions can appear in distant areas, presumably spread through the bloodstream. After weeks, and sometimes a few months, erythema migrans clears, even without therapy.

In Lyme borreliosis in Europe, persistent infection in the skin may lead to a chronic atrophying condition called acrodermatitis chronica atroph-

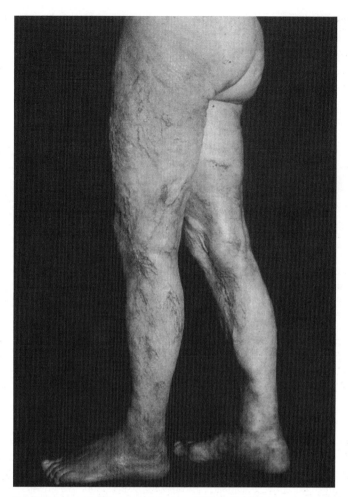

Fig. 24.4 Acrodermatitis chronica atrophicans (ACA). The lesion is inflammatory, chronic, and atrophic.

icans, or ACA (Fig. 24.4). In ACA spirochetes can be cultured from the skin years after onset of infection, a finding which provided the first direct and conclusive demonstration that the spirochete could persist for long periods despite high titers of antispirochetal antibody in the host. ACA has not been definitively reported in the United States. This clearcut difference between European and American LB may may be due to genetic differences since *B. burgdorferi sensu stricto* does not persist in the skin in the rhesus model, in contrast to *B. garinii* and *B. afzelii* strains, the dominant strains in Europe (Pachner *et al.*, unpublished results), which do persist in skin.

Disseminated Lyme borreliosis (extraneural)

B. burgdorferi, after days to weeks in the skin, disseminates to other tissues. Dissemination is thought by some investigators to be blood-borne, but others feel that direct local invasion may also have a role (Straubinger *et al.*, 1998). The two organs most commonly involved in disseminated Lyme borreliosis, other than the nervous system, are joints and the heart.

Lyme borreliosis was first described as an arthritis (Steere *et al.*, 1977a; Steere, 1997). Relapsing–remitting arthritis involving one or a few large joints, most commonly the knees, is the usual presentation (Steere *et al.*, 1987; Sigal, 1997). Spirochetes are found in joint tissue by silver stains (Johnston *et al.*, 1985) or by PCR (Nocton *et al.*, 1994a), but never by culture. Relapses of arthritis usually last for a few weeks, followed by arthritis remission. Why joint inflammation occurs suddenly, and then resolves, and subsequently recurs, is unknown. Carditis in human Lyme borreliosis, usually causing conduction disturbances, is probably very common as a subclinical phenomenon, but uncommon as a clinical problem (Steere *et al.*,

1980; Berglund *et al.*, 1995; Nagi *et al.*, 1996; Rosenfeld *et al.*, 1999); it usually presents with conduction disturbances.

Host–spirochete interaction during persistent infection

Most evidence points to humoral immunity as being the major host defense mechanism. During early dissemination, the predominant immunoglobulin isotype involved in the non-human primate anti-*B. burgdorferi* humoral immune response is IgM, which is relatively impotent at spirochete killing. As isotype switching proceeds in the third and fourth weeks of infection, more and more IgG appears in the serum, concurrent with and presumably related to spirochetes disappearing from the blood. The first month of infection can be thought of as a race between the spirochete and the host. The spirochete must grow and spread through the skin, down-regulate expression of immunogenic epitopes (Liang *et al.*, 2002), enter the bloodstream, attach to endothelium, and invade the parenchyma of target tissues such as the nervous system (Pachner, 1995; Roberts *et al.*, 1995, 1998), heart, and bladder. The host must recognize the new pathogen, and mount a strong humoral response directed against multiple *B. burgdorferi* antigens. If a strong IgG anti-*B. burgdorferi* response can be mounted quickly before the spirochete has established itself in tissues, tissue invasion will be minimal. If the IgG response is blunted or delayed, spirochetes are able to invade target tissues. As the IgG response begins to develop, the number of organisms in the blood begins to decrease. After the first month of infection, *B. burgdorferi* generally cannot be found in the blood of non-human primates or humans (Goodman *et al.*, 1995). There is no reliable information about how long it takes spirochetes to penetrate from blood, through endothelium (Szczepanski *et al.*, 1990), and into the extracellular matrix. Spirochetes which survive into this phase of infection are very different from the original strain in the tick or even spirochetes which spread through the skin, and very little is known about them. Spirochetes which were identified in hearts of infected non-human primates 3 months after infection expressed only flagellin and did not express OspA, B, or C by immunohistochemical staining (Cadavid *et al.*, 2000). Chronic infection in the non-human primate is also associated with spirochetal expression of *dbpA* and *bbk32*, two genes which encode proteins in the spirochete which bind decorin and fibronectin respectively, major components of the extracellular matrix(Pachner, unpublished results). The increasing complexity of the antibody response with time is characteristic of the late disseminated phase, and it is during this period, 3–6 weeks after infection, that the IgG response goes from being low titer and directed to a few antigens, to being high titer and directed to a large number of spirochetal antigens. This diversity of the antibody response is associated with a dramatic decrease of expression of most spirochetal genes (Liang *et al.*, 2002); they may be cause and effect. After the first 3 or 4 months of infection, new bands generally do not appear on immunoblots in the serum, indicating absence of new *B. burgdorferi* proteins recognized by the host.

Why the host, be it mouse, monkey, or human, cannot completely clear infection is unknown. The persistence of the spirochete in mice is critical for the spirochete's life cycle, and thus its survival, and the mechanisms it has developed for mice probably allow it to persist in other animals. One survival mechanism described above is the rapid down-regulation of potential immunogenic proteins. However, there must be other mechanisms operative, which allow the spirochete to express critical genes and continue to survive despite strong immune responses to the gene products. An example of such a gene is *dbpA*, coding for a decorin binding protein (DbpA) needed for persistence in the host extracellular matrix. *B. burgdorferi* expresses this gene at higher levels in chronic infection in non-human primates than during *in vitro* culture. High levels of anti-DbpA antibodies made by the rhesus macaque are unable to clear the *dbpA*-expressing spirochetes. A clue to the enigma may lie in the recent identification of proteins, labeled Erp proteins of *B. burgdorferi* (Sung *et al.*, 1998), which bind the complement inhibitor, factor H (Stevenson *et al.*, 2002). The presence of multiple Erp proteins on the surface provide the spirochete with a mechan-

ism to resist complement-mediated killing in any of the wide range of potential hosts that it might infect (Stevenson and Babb, 2002).

Lyme neuroborreliosis—clinical manifestations

Neurological manifestations represent the most frequent clinical involvement apart from the skin for Lyme disease world-wide (Ackermann *et al.*, 1984; Pachner, 1988) and can be divided into acute (first weeks after infection), subacute (weeks to months), and chronic (months to years).

Acute Lyme neuroborreliosis in the human
Non-specific symptoms associated with erythema migrans
Patients with EM often have neurological symptoms such as headache, stiff neck, or myalgia. Occasionally the severity of these symptoms prompts a lumbar puncture which is usually normal. The etiology of these symptoms is unclear and they usually resolve by the appearance of other signs.

Facial palsy
The most common focal neurological finding in LNB is unilateral or bilateral facial palsy which is often a manifestation of acute disease, but can be seen in subacute LNB. The VIIth nerve palsy of LNB cannot be clinically differentiated from Bell's palsy unless a concurrent EM lesion is present. Hence, the index of suspicion for LNB in a patient with isolated Bell's palsy in an endemic area is relatively high. Since antibody testing in early LB is commonly negative, the best way to diagnose facial palsy secondary to LNB remains controversial. The natural history of Lyme VIIth nerve palsy has been described and mimics that of idiopathic VIIth nerve palsy in that resolution of the deficit usually occurs, irrespective of treatment. Bilateral VIIth nerve palsy from LNB is relatively common, and thus bilateral facial palsy in the summer or autumn in an endemic area has a very high likelihood of being due to *B. burgdorferi* infection. The skin of patients with VIIth nerve palsy in endemic areas should always be examined for EM lesions even if the patient does not give a history of a rash; the presence of such a lesion, which is sometimes not appreciated by the patient, will make the diagnosis of LNB irrespective of any other diagnostic studies. Facial palsy due to LNB usually clears up spontaneously (Clark *et al.*, 1985), and it is unknown whether the deficit is due to direct invasion of the VIIth nerve or to a non-infectious, inflammatory etiology. Thus, the optimal diagnosis and therapy of VIIth nerve palsy is unknown. An acceptable minimalist approach would be clinical and serological follow-up of the patient and therapy with oral doxycycline 100 mg twice a day for 2 weeks (see sections on LNB diagnosis and therapy below).

Acute Lyme neuroborreliosis in the non-human primate model
The non-human primate model of Lyme borreliosis represents one of a number of animal models of this infection. Its main advantage is that it is the only animal model of the infection in which involvement of the central and peripheral nervous system has been a consistent feature (Pachner *et al.*, 1995b, 2001b; Coyle, 1995; Roberts *et al.*, 1998). The subprimate models which have provided the most information about the infection are the mouse (Pachner and Itano, 1990; Barthold *et al.*, 1993a,b; Pachner *et al.*, 1993; Yang *et al.*, 1994; Morrison *et al.*, 1999: Kumar *et al.*, 2000), the hamster (Johnson *et al.*, 1984, 1986; Schmitz *et al.*, 1988; DuChateau *et al.*, 1997), the rat (Barthold *et al.*, 1988, 1990; Moody *et al.*, 1990a), and the rabbit (Moody *et al.*, 1990a; Pachner *et al.*, 1994; Foley *et al.*, 1995; Shang *et al.*, 2000). These animals all manifest chronic infection and inflammation after infection with *B. burgdorferi*.

Beginning in 1993, we have infected 38 non-human primates intradermally with a *sensu stricto* strain of *Borrelia burgdorferi* called N40Br. This strain was originally derived from a commonly used strain in experimental Lyme borreliosis called N40 (Malawista *et al.*, 1994; Anguita *et al.*, 2000); the 'Br' refers to the fact that this strain was obtained as a brain isolate from mice infected with N40 in our laboratory in the late 1980s (Pachner and Itano, 1990). Spirochetes can be detected in the blood of the non-human primates within 1–2 weeks after intradermal injection, and then in the CSF by 3–4 weeks after injection. The inflammatory response follows shortly thereafter. Thus, the presence of spirochetes precedes the inflammatory response and the presence of antibody. Thus, a lumbar puncture which shows no cells and no antibody, should at this stage in the illness be considered negative only if the PCR and culture of the CSF are also negative. We have demonstrated that these four assays of spinal fluid (cell count, anti-*B. burgdorferi* antibody, PCR, and culture) are almost never positive in the same CSF sample in the non-human primate model; tests for the spirochete predominate early in invasion and tests for antibody are present later (Pachner *et al.*, 1998). Facial palsy has not been a feature of rhesus LNB. We have also infected rhesus macaques with European strains of *B. burgdorferi*; these experiments are in their early stages.

Subacute Lyme neuroborreliosis in humans

The most well-studied syndromes of LNB fall into this category, since these syndromes are the most common and generally are the most symptomatic as a whole.

Lyme meningitis

In the United States the most common presentation of LNB is that of a subacute, relatively low-grade basilar meningitis. Symptoms are those one would expect from such a process, and include headache, stiff neck, photophobia, malaise, fatigue, and low-grade fever. Examination is rarely contributory except for ruling out other diseases or ruling in LB by finding the remnants of an EM lesion or lesions. Thus, Kernig's sign or meningismus are usually not present, although they can be found. The headache is usually mild, almost never the 'the worst headache of my life'. Patients also very frequently complain of extra-CNS symptoms. Symptoms can be surprisingly variable, so that days of near normality can alternate with days of profound debility. At this stage in the infection, cognitive symptoms can appear, probably from a low-grade encephalopathy. Some patients complain of being inattentive, confused, unfocused, irritable, forgetful, drowsy, or mentally slow. Focal deficits other than a VIIth nerve palsy such as dysphasias, visual field deficits, parietal lobe syndromes, frontal deficits, or major personality changes are almost never seen and their presence should increase suspicion for an alternative diagnosis; seizures or involuntary movements are also almost never found. Patients with seemingly trivial complaints can have dramatic inflammation in the subarachnoid space demonstrated by LP. A triad of meningitis, cranial neuritis, and radiculoneuritis, often incomplete, is frequently seen (Pachner and Steere, 1985), and myelitis has been described (Reik *et al.*, 1979).

Lyme meningoradiculitis, including Bannwarth's syndrome; also called meningopolyneuritis(MPN)

A painful radiculitis following tick bite was described by Bannwarth (1941) and painful radiculitis in LNB is frequently called Bannwarth's syndrome. Paresis can also occur with or without pain, and was described following tick bite by Garin and Bujadoux (1922). This syndrome, sometimes called Garin–Bujadoux–Bannwarth syndrome (Ackermann *et al.*, 1984; Schmidt and Ackermann, 1985), associated with *B. burgdorferi* infection in Europe is well appreciated; in the United States it is less common, but can be seen occasionally and is sometimes confused with radiculopathy caused by intervertebral disc disease. In European Lyme meningitis cranial nerve involvement other than VII is common during subacute disease (Schmutzhard *et al.*, 1985; Stiernstedt *et al.*, 1988), in contrast to American LNB in which it occurs very rarely.

The largest and most complete study of this entity was authored by Hansen and Lebech in Denmark, in which 187 consecutive patients with intrathecal anti-*B burgdorferi* antibody production were studied (Hansen and Lebech, 1992). The use of positive intrathecal antibody production ensured that every patient indeed had LNB. Ninety-four per cent of these patients had subacute neuroborreliosis. The most common manifestation was a painful lymphocytic meningoradiculitis (Bannwarth's syndrome) either with paresis (61%) or as a radicular pain syndrome only (25%). Central nervous system (CNS) involvement in early neuroborreliosis was rare; 4% had signs of myelitis and only one patient had acute encephalitis. Meningeal findings in this group of patients were unusual. MPN, also called Garin–Bujadoux–Bannwarth syndrome, is, in contrast, not commonly seen in the United States. The reason for this difference between clinical manifestations in Europe and the United States is probably due to differences in the *in vivo* behaviour of the strains of the spirochete causing LNB, *B. garinii* and *B. afzelii* in Europe and *B. burgdorferi sensu stricto* in the United States.

Subacute Lyme neuroborreliosis in the non-human primate model

Tissue invasion is an important part of early dissemination; the spirochetes are thought to be more likely to survive in tissue if they escape the perivascular areas and penetrate deeply. Most evidence points to this process being extracellular, so that invasion through extracellular matrix is critical. *B. burgdorferi* may utilize host matrix metalloproteinases, activated via plasmin on the surface of the spirochete (Gebbia *et al.*, 2001). Decorin-binding proteins of the spirochete may also be involved in this process (Guo *et al.*, 1998).

During subacute LNB, spirochetes are found extensively in nervous system tissue (Pachner *et al.*, 2001*a*). They are predominantly found in muscles, nerves, dorsal root ganglia, nerve roots, and meninges by PCR and immunohistochemistry; there are essentially no spirochetes in CNS parenchyma (Cadavid *et al.*, 2000). In the roots and nerves, the spirochetes are in the perineurium and not in the axons themselves. Thus, since the dorsal root ganglia are the only place in which the spirochetes are close to neurons (Fig. 24.5), this localization is consistent with the syndrome of meningopolyradiculitis, the painful sensory symptoms, and the relative absence of motor involvement. In rhesus monkeys chronically infected with the JD1 strain of *B. burgdorferi* (England *et al.*, 1997*b*) five of eight infected monkeys demonstrated primarily axonal-loss-variety multifocal neuropathies on EMG studies, while only one nerve lesion exhibited findings compatible with demyelination (England *et al.*, 1997*a*). Pathology in these animals reveals multifocal axonal degeneration and regeneration and occasional perivascular inflammatory cellular infiltrates without vessel wall necrosis.

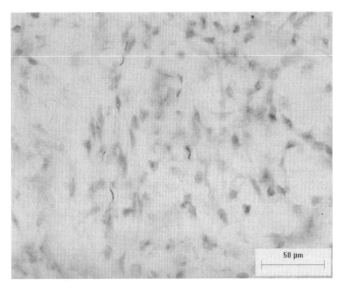

Fig. 24.5 *B. burgdorferi* in the dorsal root ganglion in a rhesus macaque with Lyme neuroborreliosis.

Analysis of the CSF reveals a pleocytosis within the first month or two of infection (Pachner *et al.*, 1995*b*) and positive measures of spirochetal presence, such as culture, PCR, and mouse infectivity (transfer of infection to mice by injection with CSF) (Pachner *et al.*, 1998). Later analysis of the CSF is dominated by the presence of antispirochetal antibody, and positive culture, PCR, and mouse infectivity are no longer present. Thus, subacute LNB represents a time period in which the host is shifting from early infection with rapid spirochetal multiplication and dissemination and only innate host immunity, to chronic infection with minimal spirochetal multiplication maintained by adaptive immunity with high levels of avid antispirochetal IgG.

Chronic Lyme neuroborreliosis in the human

Chronic neurological manifestations represent a particularly troublesome manifestation because some of the symptoms can be non-specific (Pachner and Steere, 1986; Ackermann *et al.*, 1988; Coyle, 1993; (Logigian *et al.*, 1990*a*, 1997; Fallon and Nields, 1994; Halperin, 1997). Symptoms of headache, fatigue, arm or leg numbness or tingling, low-grade fever, diffuse weakness, and decreased cognitive function can be chronic if the infection persists.

Focal and destructive neurological disease can also be a feature of chronic LNB in Europe. Ackermann *et al.* (1985) described a syndrome they called 'progressive Borrelia encephalomyelitis':

These patients presented symptoms characteristic of a disseminated disease of the CNS, with spastic pareses and evidence in the spinal fluid of chronic inflammation and disruption of CSF barriers in particular. This progressive encephalomyelitis differs from the common and spontaneously healing meningopolyneuritis (Garin–Bujadoux–Bannwarth), the usual manifestation of erythema chronicum migrans of the nervous system, in its progressive nature, its invasion of the CNS and the possible long lasting severe damage when not specifically treated.

Most of these patients had been symptomatic for years. The frequency with which untreated Lyme borreliosis progresses to chronic LNB is unknown, but is likely to be low. Some investigators feel that Bannwarth's syndrome is self-limiting, has a benign prognosis if untreated, and may not even require antibiotics (Kruger *et al.*, 1989).

The neuropsychiatric manifestations of chronic infection are controversial (Halperin *et al.*, 1989; Pachner, 1989; Burdge and O'Hanlon, 1993). There is no question that encephalopathy is in the spectrum of the disease, and that personality changes and mild cognitive disorders can occur either as a manifestation of the early meningoencephalitis (Reik *et al.*, 1979) or as a late manifestation (Ackermann *et al.*, 1985; Halperin *et al.*, 1990). This is usually manifest as memory loss, mood changes, or sleep disturbance (Pachner and Steere, 1986; Logigian *et al.*, 1990*b*; Kaplan *et al.*, 1992). These relatively mild neuropsychiatric manifestations generally overlap with fibromyalgia, although it is felt that they are probably separate disorders. More serious neurological disorders such as mania, major depression, and psychotic disorders have been reported, (Fallon *et al.*, 1995, 1998) but must be very rare. A study by Nadelman *et al.* (1997) has been instructive. These investigators prospectively screened sera for Lyme disease from adults admitted to an acute care psychiatric hospital in Westchester County, New York, a highly endemic area. The prevalence in healthy blood donors from this area was reported to be 0.7%. The prevalence of positive serologies in the psychiatric population was 1/517 or 0.2%, and the enzyme-linked immunsorbent assay (ELISA)-positive patient had a non-reactive Western blot, suggestive of a false-positive antibody test. The conclusion of the study was that routine serologic screening for Lyme disease for adult psychiatric inpatients, even in areas of the United States where this illness is endemic, was not indicated; thus, it is highly unlikely that Lyme disease can cause psychiatric disease severe enough to result in acute in-patient admission.

Chronic Lyme neuroborreliosis in the non-human primate model

Three independent lines of evidence point to the persistence of spirochetes at a low level in chronic infection in non-human primates:

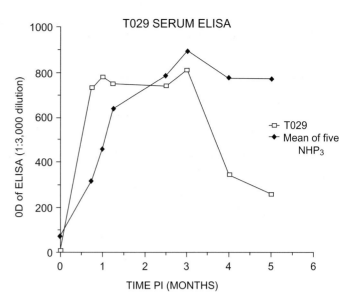

Fig. 24.6 Dropping anti-*B. burgdorferi* antibody levels after therapy in the rhesus macaque model. The *x*-axis represent months after infection with strain N40Br and the *y*-axis is optic density in a anti-*B. burgdorferi* IgG ELISA with sera at a 1:3000 dilution.

- persistence of *B. burgdorferi*-specific nucleic acid in tissue;
- persistence of high-titered specific antibody in serum and cerebrospinal fluid for years;
- rapid drop in titer of both serum and CSF anti-*B. burgdorferi* antibody after antibiotic therapy.

PCR, optimized to increase sensitivity in tissue, has consistently detected the presence of *B. burgdorferi* in multiple sites in non-human primates infected for 3–4 months. The total spirochetal load is low in the chronically infected non-human primate, probably fewer than 10^9 spirochetes. Cultures of blood, cerebrospinal fluid, and tissue in non-human primates after the first few months of infection have been consistently negative in immunocompetent animals. This fact, however, is not surprising, and is consistent with chronic low-grade infection, since the organism is notoriously difficult to culture in chronic infection; e.g. in human Lyme arthritis, synovium or synovial tissue has consistently been culture-negative despite PCR positivity (Nocton *et al.*, 1994).

We infected a group of six non-human primates with the N40Br strain for 18 months to assess the manifestations of chronic infection and inflammation. None of the animals developed clinical signs. One animal, TO29, developed a cellulitis caused by a bite and was given 5 days of antibiotics 3 months post-infection. The anti-*B. burgdorferi* antibody level in the serum and CSF dropped precipitously (see Fig. 24.6) after the treatment consistent with the hypothesis that antibody production in chronically infected animals was driven by live spirochetes, despite culture negativity of sampled tissues. These data are consistent with findings in the dog model of Lyme borreliosis (Straubinger *et al.*, 2000). None of our five non-human primates infected for 18 months or longer without antibiotic treatment developed clinical disease, and analysis of tissues at necropsy revealed barely detectable levels of spirochetal DNA. The situation in dogs and non-human primates is somewhat different from that in mice, in which, after a peak at 1 month post-infection, IgG anti-*B. burgdorferi* antibody levels drop spontaneously over time (Bockenstedt *et al.*, 2002).

The inflammatory response to infection of rhesus macaques with North American strains of *B. burgdorferi* results in signs of both localized and disseminated Lyme disease. Specific features of early disease include erythema migrans and of disseminated disease myositis, myocarditis, arthritis, meningitis, and peripheral neuritis (Cadavid *et al.*, 2000; England *et al.*, 1997*a*; Pachner *et al.*, 1995*b*; Roberts *et al.*, 1995). There is significant variability in the inflammatory response to infection when different monkeys are infected with the same strain, as expected from outbred populations.

Diagnosis of Lyme neuroborreliosis

LNB is generally easy to diagnose if there is a reasonable index of suspicion. Symptoms of the subacute illness usually occur within 1–2 months of infection, so it usually presents in the summer or autumn in an endemic area. Many patients recall the characteristic skin rash, erythema migrans, which may still be present in the Lyme patient with neurological symptoms. Erythema migrans is by far the most common clinical presentation in the United States and is a very characteristic and highly specific clinical entity (Berger, 1984; Berger et al., 1985). In recent vaccine studies, erythema migrans was the only clinical manifestation seen in more than 90% of humans with Lyme borreliosis (Sigal et al., 1998). Routine laboratory studies for confirmation of active infection during erythema migrans are sometimes not helpful because the infection is early and localized. Thus, measurement of antibody in the serum during erythema migrans is frequently negative. In a recent study, Wormser et al. (2000)ound that culturing the plasma was positive in 50% of patients with erythema migrans.

One clinical syndrome of LNB is readily recognizable. In Europe, Bannwarth's syndrome of painful radiculitis is frequently seen as a manifestation of the infection. Patients with LNB in the United States, as well as Europe, frequently get a facial palsy, either unilateral or bilateral (Clark et al., 1985). Many patients also report, frequently concurrently with their neurological symptoms, a new rash, which, on inspection, proves to be erythema migrans. The diagnosis of erythema migrans can also be made retrospectively although it is then less precise. In addition, LNB is usually detected within weeks to a few months after initial infection, so that it usually occurs in the summer or early autumn. The patient must have been in an area endemic for Lyme borreliosis, since the bite of an infected tick is the only way to contract the infection; but it must be remembered that most infected individuals do not recall a tick bite. Thus, the diagnosis will commonly either be made conclusively, or thought highly likely, after the history and neurological examination.

Symptoms consistent with meningeal irritation will frequently lead to a lumbar puncture, which almost always reveals a lymphocytic or monocytic pleocytosis and a mildly elevated protein, but generally under normal pressure. Ideally, one could identify the pathogen by culture or PCR, and this has been done in the research setting (Karlsson et al., 1990), usually within the first few weeks of infection, but the yield is generally low from the CSF. Thus, the host antibody response to the spirochete, i.e. anti-B. burgdorferi antibodies, is used as a diagnostic aid. As we have learned more about the genetics and gene expression of the spirochete, serology has become a better and better tool, especially for neurologists trying to identify LNB in the United States.

The most common form of LNB in the United States is Lyme meningitis, often associated with symptoms of radiculoneuritis and/or facial palsy; in the United States this form is almost always seropositive. However, facial palsy may be a very early manifestation and thus is frequently seronegative. There are no features of facial palsy from Lyme disease to distinguish it from Bell's palsy (Clark et al., 1985; Halperin, 1995). In facial palsy patients from endemic areas in the non-winter months who are seronegative and may have facial palsy from Lyme disease, the diagnostic and therapeutic issues are difficult because most facial palsy in these circumstances will *not* be due to Lyme disease. At a minimum, one can say that treatment of facial palsy with corticosteroids is contraindicated unless Lyme disease is highly unlikely, since the risk of worsening spirochetal infection with steroid therapy is a significant one.

Measurement of anti-*B. burgdorferi* antibodies

Serum anti-*B. burgdorferi* antibodies

The utility of a diagnostic assay, i.e. its predictive value, is based on the probability of the disease in the population being tested, as well as the test's sensitivity and specificity. Before ordering an antibody assay it is important to determine how likely Lyme borreliosis is in the particular patient. If the assay is being used as a 'rule-out' in a patient in whom a different diagnosis is likely, the assay will not work well. This point is made best by reviewing data on the HIV ELISA which has a sensitivity of >99% and a specificity of >99% and thus would be generally considered as an excellent assay. If the prevalence of HIV is 10% in the population you are screening, the assay has a predictive value of 96%. However, if the prevalence of the infection in the population you are screening is only 0.1%, the predictive value of the assay is only 18%. Since the prevalence of Lyme borreliosis in the population is less than 0.1%, and the sensitivity and specificity of the assay are much lower than 99%, the clinician needs to be selective in the type of patient for which Lyme antibody tests are ordered; otherwise, the test will have a very low predictive value.

Anti-*B. burgdorferi* antibodies are generally measured using an ELISA methodology in which proteins from sonicates of the spirochete are coated onto a plastic plate and then serum from the patient is incubated on the plate. In the United States the genetic heterogeneity of the spirochete is relatively low, and an American Lyme borreliosis patient's serum will bind to proteins from almost any *B. burgdorferi sensu stricto* isolate. However, in Europe, there is a great deal of heterogeneity of the spirochetes and the choice of the ideal strain for the ELISA is not clear (Hauser et al., 1998a, 1999; Wilske et al., 1999). Thus, optimal testing for Lyme borreliosi in Europe remains a controversial issue, while in the United States criteria for positivity have been outlined by a working group of investigators and clinical laboratory directors (CAW Group, 1995), and these standards have been widely accepted. The American approach utilizes a standard two-step approach with an initial screen by ELISA, followed by confirmation of all ELISA positives with immunoblotting (also call Western blotting). This general approach to the determination of a 'positive' antibody is used by most American clinical laboratories at this time, although not all laboratories agree on the band patterns which constitute positivity on the immunoblot; these may vary from one laboratory to the next.

The problem with serodiagnosis of Lyme disease in Europe is one of the issues which has prompted the formation of EUCALB (European Union Concerted Action on Lyme Borreliosis). A study of 224 serum specimens from European Union countries (44% of which were from patients with neuroborreliosis) led to a recommendation of using a single strain, i.e. Pko, for immunoblotting but restricted this suggestion to sera from patients in Germany (Hauser et al., 1998a,b). Some European countries use purified proteins of *B. burgdorferi* to screen patients, e.g. flagellin (Wallich et al., 1990; Jiang et al., 1992; Magnarelli et al., 1992; Kaiser et al., 1993; Hansen, 1994). However, the flagellin ELISA cannot always differentiate Lyme disease from syphilis (Robinson et al., 1993), although the clinical syndromes are generally distinct.

An important variable determining the predictive value of the ELISA in the United States or Europe is the duration of infection. Thus, patients with erythema migrans, an early manifestation of infection, have a seronegativity rate of about 50%, while patients with Lyme arthritis, a late manifestation, are rarely seronegative. Patients with MPN are intermediate; they are usually seropositive, but not with levels as high as patients with arthritis. In Europe, LNB patients may be negative for antibody in the serum, but strongly positive in the CSF (Hansen, 1994). Simultaneous determination of serum and CSF antibody, especially in European LNB, is very helpful (Kaiser and Rauer, 1998; Kaiser, 1998; Oschmann et al., 1998), as reviewed below.

The humoral response to the spirochete is generally felt to be the most potent effector arm for protection from the infection. The anti-*B. burgdorferi* antibody response is necessary for limiting the numbers of spirochetes during initial dissemination in the non-human primate, and may be important for eventually clearing the infection. Passive transfer of immune serum into naïve recipients is highly protective in the hamster and mouse models (Johnson et al., 1986; Fikrig et al., 1994; Barthold et al., 1997). There are few data, however, on how effective antibody is in clearance of established infection, and some investigators believe antibody is not effective in clearing infection once established in the mouse (Barthold et al., 1997). In the non-human primate model, specific immunoglobulin appears in the serum soon after infection. IgM antibody appears early followed by isotype switching, so that by 1 month, IgM antibody drops and IgG rises in immunocompetent non-human primates.

Increasing durations of infection are associated with a higher complexity of the anti-*B. burgdorferi* antibody immune response. More and more bands appear on serum IgG immunoblots from infected non-human primates, indicating that antigens of the spirochete are being exposed to the humoral response at variable times. This could be due to a number of reasons, including changing expression of protein by spirochetes or a variable rate of immunological processing of various proteins by the host. The *B. burgdorferi* proteins identified on immunoblots in the non-human primate model are very similar to those identified by infected humans, with prominent responses to a variety of *B. burgdorferi* proteins, including flagellin, BmpA, decorin binding protein A, and heat shock proteins.

We have also evaluated the serum antibody response to recombinant proteins of *B. burgdorferi* in the rhesus model (Pachner *et al.*, 2002a). We studied the IgM and IgG antibody response to N40 whole cell sonicate and recombinant protein using ELISA and immunoblotting with commercially available strips; quantitative densitometry of the bands was also used. Sera from four different groups of non-human primates were used: immunocompetent, transiently immunosuppressed, extended immunosuppressed, and uninfected. In immunocompetent and transiently immunosuppressed non-human primates, there was a strong IgM and IgG response. Major proteins for the early IgM response were P39 and P41 and recombinant BmpA and OspC. Major proteins for the later IgG response were P39, P41, P18, P60, P66, and recombinant BmpA and DbpA. There was no significant response in the non-human primates to recombinant OspA or to Arp, a 37 kDa protein that elicits an antibody response during infection in mice. Most antibody responses, except for that to DbpA, were markedly diminished by prolonged dexamethasone treatment. The data supported the feasibility of recent efforts by a variety of investigators to use recombinant proteins for serodiagnosis in human infection (Wilske *et al.*, 1999; Magnarelli *et al.*, 2000; Heikkila *et al.*, 2002).

CSF anti-*B. burgdorferi* antibodies

Infection within the CNS commonly results in antipathogen antibodies in the CSF (Reiber, 1998), and the diagnosis of LNB can be supported by the demonstration of anti-*B. burgdorferi* antibodies in the CSF (Stiernstedt *et al.*, 1985; Baig *et al.*, 1991; Hansson *et al.*, 1993; Tumani *et al.*, 1995). However, the simple detection of anti-*B. burgdorferi* antibodies in CSF can be seen in Lyme disease patients without neurological involvement, since IgG antibodies cross into the subarachnoid space from the serum and are detected at a level 1/300 to 1/500 that of the level in the serum. Thus, many European investigators use selective concentration of antibody in the CSF, i.e. concentrations of anti-*B. burgdorferi* antibody in the CSF higher than one would expect from the ratio of IgG in CSF/IgG in serum, as a diagnostic test for LNB (Wilske *et al.*, 1986; Hammers-Berggren *et al.*, 1993; Issakainen *et al.*, 1996). In fact, in the largest clinical study of LNB (Hansen and Lebech, 1992), the diagnosis was established in 187 Danish patients by selective intrathecal antibody concentration, which was present in all individuals.

There are three different laboratory techniques to measure intrathecal antibody production. One involves using a standard curve based on a reference serum or monoclonal antibody and calculating the number of arbitrary units relative to the reference; this value is then expressed per quantity of immunoglobulin. CSF with higher values than serum is indicative of intrathecal antibody production. A similar technique is to dilute serum to the same concentration of Ig as the CSF and compare reactivity on an ELISA; higher optical densities in CSF relative to serum defines intrathecal antibody production. The third technique is to utilize a capture assay, which uses an anti-immunoglobulin to capture a fixed and constant amount of immunoglobulin onto the ELISA plate prior to testing samples for specific anti-*B. burgdorferi* reactivity (Berardi *et al.*, 1988). Each of these three methods has its own advantages and disadvantages relative to the other techniques and none has been identified as the technique of choice. Compared with 19 American patients, 30 European patients with neuroborreliosis had significantly higher CSF:serum ratios of specific antibody, both early and late in the illness (Steere *et al.*, 1990). These data are consistent with the hypothesis that Europeans

strains, especially *B. garinii* (Marconi *et al.*, 1999), are more neuroinvasive and that European Lyme disease has a much higher percentage of patients with neurological involvement than American Lyme disease (Stiernstedt *et al.*, 1987; Stanek *et al.*, 1988).

Therapy of Lyme neuroborreliosis

B. burgdorferi is exquisitely sensitive to antibiotics both *in vitro* and *in vivo*. The combination of antibiotic administration and the human's own immunity to the spirochete will clear the spirochete in the vast majority of infected patients. The most commonly used antibiotics are doxycycline (Dattwyler *et al.*, 1997), ceftriaxone (Dattwyler *et al.*, 1997), or other cephalosporins (Skoldenberg *et al.*, 1988), and penicillin (Steere *et al.*, 1983b; Halperin, 1995; Karlsson *et al.*, 1996). The antibiotic of choice for any particular patient depends on the clinical circumstances. Since the doubling time of the spirochete is much longer than for most bacteria, i.e. many hours to a day *in vitro* and possibly longer *in vivo*, the duration of therapy ought to be relatively long also, 2 weeks to a month.

Most American physicians tend to use intravenous therapy, while oral therapy is common in Europe. In an excellent study performed in well-characterized LNB patients in Sweden and Denmark, oral doxycycline (31 patients treated with 200 mg every 24 hours) was compared with IV penicillin G (23 patients treated with 3 g every 6 hours) in a randomized study. The entry criteria were an appropriate clinical picture, and antibodies against *B. burgdorferi* in serum, CSF, or both, or a positive CSF culture. Treatment was successful in all patients, without significant differences between the two treatment groups in patient scoring, CSF analysis, or serologic and clinical follow-up during 1 year. There were no clear treatment failures, although one patient in each treatment group was retreated because of residual symptoms. It was concluded that oral doxycycline represented an excellent and cost-effective alternative to IV penicillin for the treatment of Lyme neuroborreliosis.

LNB is an inflammatory syndrome and the inflammation can be extensive including the meninges, nerve roots, nerves, and muscles(see below). Thus, treatment with anti-inflammatory medication can be very useful to treat patient's symptoms while antibiotics are clearing the infection. In addition, symptoms can frequently still be present after completion of therapy, and these tend to be very responsive to anti-inflammatory medication. Aspirin or ibuprofen are generally adequate, although other anti-inflammatories can be used.

The role of corticosteroids to treat the inflammation of LNB is controversial. There is no question that corticosteroids suppress the immune response and result in much higher spirochetal loads if given early during infection (Pachner *et al.*, 2001a). On the other hand, they may be very helpful in highly symptomatic patients, such as those with severe, painful Bannwarth's syndrome (Ragnaud *et al.*, 1995; Kaiser, 1998). Thus, there is a role for corticosteroid therapy as a potent anti-inflammatory tool in some patients with LNB, but ideally it should be delayed until substantial spirochetal killing by antibiotics has occurred, i.e. at least 2 weeks after initiation of antibiotics.

The most common cause of treatment failure is incorrect diagnosis. The American neurologist can feel fortunate in having serology as such an accurate diagnostic aid. The limited heterogeneity of American strains which cause LNB, and the extended duration of infection required to develop neurological involvement, means that almost all patients with LNB in the United States are seropositive, defined as being positive in both the ELISA and Western blot. Thus, in patients who are seronegative, alternative diagnoses must be rigorously and continuously sought; if antibiotics are used to treat, objective measures of treatment response such as clearance of CSF pleocytosis or eradication of pain should be used.

Pathology of Lyme neuroborreliosis

Human Lyme neuroborreliosis

Since LNB is a treatable, non-fatal infection which does not require tissue for diagnosis, the pathology is usually not determined. Reports of brain

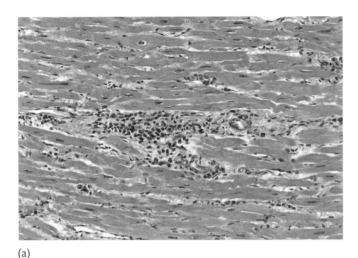

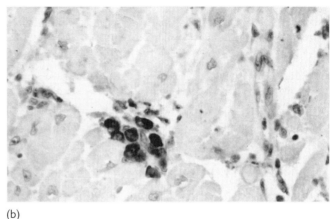

Fig. 24.7 (a) Inflammation in the heart of an infected non-human primate. H&E stain. (b) Inflammation in the heart of an infected non-human primate. Immunohistochemistry, stained for plasma cells.

pathology in the literature are rare, and are generally from clinically unusual cases and thus must be considered somewhat suspect, since, by definition, they contain features that make the diagnosis of *B. burgdorferi* alone less likely (MacDonald and Miranda, 1987; Miklossy *et al.*, 1990; Kuntzer *et al.*, 1991; Kobayashi *et al.*, 1997). Nerve or muscle biopsies have been performed more commonly (Tezzon *et al.*, 1991; Reimers *et al.*, 1993; Zifko *et al.*, 1995; Maimone *et al.*, 1997; Kindstrand *et al.*, 2000), and reveal axonal or demyelinative lesions, vasculitis, perineuritis, and myositis.

Non-human primate Lyme neuroborreliosis

Of all the organs examined from monkeys infected with the N40 strain of *B. burgdorferi*, inflammation has been most consistently observed in the heart (Cadavid *et al.*, 2000). Fifty seven per cent of 51 heart blocks from 16 immunocompetent monkeys infected for 3–24 months showed inflammation, compared with only 4% of 44 brain blocks and none of 20 spinal cord blocks. The inflammatory infiltrate was positive for T cells, B cells, macrophages, and plasma cells. Where severe inflammation was present in the heart, necrosis and fibrosis was a consistent associated feature (Fig. 24.7). The inflammation was patchy, with severely involved areas of inflammation scattered in normal-appearing tissue. Other tissues, in which spirochetes were present, had no inflammation and no tissue injury or fibrosis. Thus, what determines which organs become inflamed and how severely they are inflamed in the model is not clear. The presence of spirochete, as assessed by PCR, is a necessary but not sufficient condition for inflammation.

Skeletal myositis and neuritis have been observed commonly, particularly in younger animals. The inflammatory response has been more severe and destructive in immunosuppressed animals with high spirochetals loads than in immunocompetent animals with low spirochetal loads (Cadavid *et al.*, 2000). Patchy, mild meningitis and leptomeningeal thickening are seen, but CNS parenchymal inflammation has not been a feature of the model in our animals infected for 3 months, consistent with the very low numbers of spirochetes which enter the CNS parenchyma.

The development or resolution of cellular infiltrates within organs may differ depending on the organ involved. For instance, differences between the heart and the joint within the same system have been noted (Fikrig *et al.*, 1997a; McKisic *et al.*, 2000). For instance, antibodies to a p37 protein, called arp or arthritis-resolving protein, led to resolution of arthritis but had no effect on carditis (Feng *et al.*, 2000). Administration of IL-11 or anti-IL-11 antibodies affected arthritis, but had no effect on carditis, in infected mice (Anguita *et al.*, 1999). Local production of IFN-γ may be important in inducing changes in *B. burgdorferi* since immune sera can clear spirochetes in IFN-γ deficient, but not immunocompetent, mice 4 days after infection.

References

Ackermann, R., Horstrup, P., and Schmidt, R. (1984). Tick-borne meningo-polyneuritis (Garin-Bujadoux, Bannwarth). *Yale J Biol Med* **57**: 485–490.

Ackermann, R., Gollmer, E., and Rehse-Kupper, B. (1985). [Progressive *Borrelia* encephalomyelitis. Chronic manifestation of erythema chronicum migrans disease of the nervous system.] *Dtsch Med Wochenschr* **110**: 1039–1042 (in German).

Ackermann, R., Rehse-Kupper, B., Gollmer, E., and Schmidt, R. (1988). Chronic neurologic manifestations of erythema migrans borreliosis. *Ann N Y Acad Sci* **539**: 16–23.

Anderson, J.F., Johnson, R.C., Magnarelli, L.A., and Hyde, F.W. (1986). Involvement of birds in the epidemiology of the Lyme disease agent *Borrelia burgdorferi*. *Infect Immun* **51**: 394–396.

Anderson, J.F., Magnarelli, L.A., and Stafford, K.C.D. (1990). Bird-feeding ticks transstadially transmit *Borrelia burgdorferi* that infect Syrian hamsters. *J Wildl Dis* **26**: 1–10.

Anguita, J., Barthold, S.W., Samanta, S., Ryan, J., and Fikrig, E. (1999). Selective anti-inflammatory action of interleukin-11 in murine Lyme disease: arthritis decreases while carditis persists. *J Infect Dis* **179**: 734–737.

Anguita, J., Samanta, S., Revilla, B., Suk, K., Das, S., Barthold, S.W., *et al.* (2000). *Borrelia burgdorferi* gene expression *in vivo* and spirochete pathogenicity. *Infect Immun* **68**: 1222–1230.

Baig, S., Olsson, T., Hansen, K., and Link, H. (1991). Anti-*Borrelia burgdorferi* antibody response over the course of Lyme neuroborreliosis. *Infect Immun* **59**: 1050–1056.

Bannwarth, A. (1941). Chronische lymphocytare Meningitis, entzundliche Polyneuritis und 'Rheumatismus' Ein Beitrag zum Problem 'Allergie und Nervensystem'. *Arch Psychiat Nervenkr* **113**: 284–376.

Barbour, A.G. (1991). Molecular biology of antigenic variation in Lyme borreliosis and relapsing fever: a comparative analysis. *Scand J Infect Dis* **77**(Suppl.): 88–93.

Barbour, A.G., Burman, N., Carter, C.J., Kitten, T., and Bergstrom, S. (1991). Variable antigen genes of the relapsing fever agent *Borrelia hermsii* are activated by promoter addition. *Mol Microbiol* **5**: 489–493.

Barthold, S.W., Moody, K.D., Terwilliger, G.A., Duray, P.H., Jacoby, R.O., and Steere, A.C. (1988). Experimental Lyme arthritis in rats infected with *Borrelia burgdorferi*. *J Infect Dis* **157**: 842–846.

Barthold, S., Moody, K., and Beck, D. (1990). Susceptibility of laboratory rats to isolates of *Borrelia burgdorferi* from different geographic areas. *Am J Trop Med Hyg* **42**: 596–600.

Barthold, S.W., de Souza, M.S., Janotka, J.L., Smith, A.L., and Persing, D.H. (1993a). Chronic Lyme borreliosis in the laboratory mouse. *Am J Pathol* **143**: 959–971.

Barthold, S.W., de Souza, M.S., Janotka, J.L., Smith, A.L., and Persing, D.H. (1993b). Chronic Lyme borreliosis in the laboratory mouse. *Am J Pathol* 143: 959–972.

Barthold, S.W., de Souza, M., and Feng, S. (1996). Serum-mediated resolution of Lyme arthritis in mice. *Lab Invest* 74: 57–67.

Barthold, S.W., Feng, S., Bockenstedt, L.K., Fikrig, E., and Feen, K. (1997). Protective and arthritis-resolving activity in sera of mice infected with *Borrelia burgdorferi*. *Clin Infect Dis* 25(Suppl. 1): S9–S17.

Benach, J.L., Bosler, E.M., Hanrahan, J.P., Coleman, J.L., Habicht, G.S., Bast, T.F., et al. (1983). Spirochetes isolated from the blood of two patients with Lyme disease. *N Engl J Med* 308: 740–742.

Berardi, V.P., Weeks, K.E., and Steere, A.C. (1988). Serodiagnosis of early Lyme disease: analysis of IgM and IgG antibody responses by using an antibody-capture enzyme immunoassay. *J Infect Dis* 158: 754–760.

Berger, B.W. (1984). Erythema chronicum migrans of Lyme disease. *Arch Dermatol* 120: 1017–1021.

Berger, B.W., Kaplan, M.H., Rothenberg, I.R., and Barbour, A.G. (1985). Isolation and characterization of the Lyme disease spirochete from the skin of patients with erythema chronicum migrans. *J Am Acad Dermatol* 13: 444–449.

Berglund, J., Eitrem, R., Ornstein, K., Lindberg, A., Ringer, A., Elmrud, H., et al. (1995). An epidemiologic study of Lyme disease in southern Sweden [see comments]. *N Engl J Med* 333: 1319–1327.

Bishop, K.L., Khan, M.I., and Nielsen, S.W. (1994). Experimental infection of northern bobwhite quail with *Borrelia burgdorferi*. *J Wildl Dis* 30: 506–513.

Bockenstedt, L.K., Mao, J., Hodzic, E., Barthold, S.W., and Fish, D. (2002). Detection of attenuated, non-infectious spirochetes in *Borrelia burgdorferi*-infected mice after antibiotic treatment. *J Infect Dis* 186:1430–1437

Burdge, D.R. and O'Hanlon, D.P. (1993). Experience at a referral center for patients with suspected Lyme disease in an area of nonendemicity: first 65 patients. *Clin Infect Dis* 16: 558–560.

Burgess, E.C., Wachal, M.D., and Cleven, T.D. (1993). *Borrelia burgdorferi* infection in dairy cows, rodents, and birds from four Wisconsin dairy farms. *Vet Microbiol* 35: 61–77.

Burns, M.J. and Furie, M.B. (1998). *Borrelia burgdorferi* and interleukin-1 promote the transendothelial migration of monocytes *in vitro* by different mechanisms. *Infect Immun* 66: 4875–4883.

Cadavid, D., O'Neill, T., Schaefer, H., and Pachner, A.R. (2000). Localization of *Borrelia burgdorferi* in the nervous system and other organs in a nonhuman primate model of lyme disease. *Lab Invest* 80: 1043–1054.

Casjens, S., Palmer, N., van Vugt, R., Huang, W.M., Stevenson, B., Rosa, P., et al. (2000). A bacterial genome in flux: the twelve linear and nine circular extra-chromosomal DNAs in an infectious isolate of the Lyme disease spirochete *Borrelia burgdorferi*. *Mol Microbiol* 35: 490–516.

Cassatt, D.R., Patel, N.K., Ulbrandt, N.D., and Hanson, M.S. (1998). DbpA, but not OspA, is expressed by *Borrelia burgdorferi* during spirochetemia and is a target for protective antibodies. *Infect Immun* 66: 5379–5387.

CAW Group (1995). *Report of a CDC/ASTPHLD Working Group on Standardization of Immunoblotting for Serodiagnosis of Lyme Disease*. Centers for Disease Control, Atlanta. GA..

Cinco, M., Ruscio, M., and Rapagna, F. (2000). Evidence of Dbps (decorin binding proteins) among European strains of *Borrelia burgdorferi sensu lato* and in the immune response of LB patient sera. *FEMS Microbiol Lett* 183: 111–114.

Clark, J.R., Carlson, R., Sasaki, C.T., Pachner, A.R., and Steere, A.C. (1985). Facial paralysis in Lyme disease. *Laryngoscope* 95: 1341–1345.

Coyle, P.K. (1993). Neurologic complications of Lyme disease. *Rheum Dis Clin North Am* 19: 993–1009.

Coyle, P.K. (1995). Neurological Lyme disease: is there a true animal model? *Ann Neurol* 38: 560–562.

Dattwyler, R.J., Luft, B.J., Kunkel, M.J., Finkel, M.F., Wormser, G.P., Rush, T.J., et al. (1997). Ceftriaxone compared with doxycycline for the treatment of acute disseminated Lyme disease. *N Engl J Med* 337: 289–294.

DuChateau, B.K., Jensen, J.R., England, D.M., Callister, S.M., Lovrich, S.D., and Schell, R.F. (1997). Macrophages and enriched populations of T lymphocytes interact synergistically for the induction of severe, destructive Lyme arthritis. *Infect Immun* 65: 2829–2836.

England, J.D., Bohm, R.P. Jr, Roberts, E.D., and Philipp, M.T. (1997a). Lyme neuroborreliosis in the rhesus monkey. *Semin Neurol* 17: 53–56.

England, J.D., Bohm, R.P. Jr, Roberts, E.D., and Philipp, M.T. (1997b). Mononeuropathy multiplex in rhesus monkeys with chronic Lyme disease. *Ann Neurol* 41: 375–384.

Faguy, D.M. (2000). The controlled chaos of shifty pathogens. *Curr Biol* 10: R498–R501.

Fallon, B.A. and Nields, J.A. (1994). Lyme disease: a neuropsychiatric illness. *Am J Psychiat* 151: 1571–1583.

Fallon, B.A., Schwartzberg, M., Bransfield, R., Zimmerman, B., Scotti, A., Weber, C.A., et al. (1995). Late-stage neuropsychiatric Lyme borreliosis. Differential diagnosis and treatment. *Psychosomatics* 36: 295–300.

Fallon, B.A., Kochevar, J.M., Gaito, A., and Nields, J.A. (1998). The under-diagnosis of neuropsychiatric Lyme disease in children and adults. *Psychiatr Clin North Am* 21: 693–703, viii.

Feng, S., Hodzic, E., and Barthold, S.W. (2000). Lyme arthritis resolution with antiserum to a 37-kilodalton *Borrelia burgdorferi* protein. *Infect Immun* 68: 4169–4173.

Fikrig, E., Bockenstedt, L.K., Barthold, S.W., Chen, M., Tao, H., Ali-Salaam, P., et al. (1994). Sera from patients with chronic Lyme disease protect mice from Lyme borreliosis [see comments]. *J Infect Dis* 169: 568–574.

Fikrig, E., Barthold, S.W., Chen, M., Chang, C.H., and Flavell, R.A. (1997a). Protective antibodies develop, and murine Lyme arthritis regresses, in the absence of MHC class II and CD4+ T cells. *J Immunol* 159: 5682–5686.

Fikrig, E., Barthold, S.W., Sun, W., Feng, W., Telford, S.R. 3rd, and Flavell, R.A. (1997b). *Borrelia burgdorferi* P35 and P37 proteins, expressed *in vivo*, elicit protective immunity *Immunity* 6: 531–539. (Published erratum in *Immunity* 1998, 9(5): following 755.)

Fikrig, E., Feng, W., Aversa, J., Schoen, R.T., and Flavell, R.A. (1998). Differential expression of *Borrelia burgdorferi* genes during erythema migrans and Lyme arthritis. *J Infect Dis* 178: 1198–1201.

Fikrig, E., Chen, M., Barthold, S.W., Anguita, J., Feng, W., Telford, S.R. 3rd, et al. (1999). *Borrelia burgdorferi* erpT expression in the arthropod vector and murine host. *Mol Microbiol* 31: 281–290.

Fikrig, E., Feng, W., Barthold, S.W., Telford, S.R. 3rd, and Flavell, R.A. (2000). Arthropod- and host-specific *Borrelia burgdorferi* bbk32 expression and the inhibition of spirochete transmission. *J Immunol* 164: 5344–5351.

Foley, D.M., Gayek, R.J., Skare, J.T., Wagar, E.A., Champion, C.I., Blanco, D.R., et al. (1995). Rabbit model of Lyme borreliosis: erythema migrans, infection-derived immunity, and identification of *Borrelia burgdorferi* proteins associated with virulence and protective immunity. *J Clin Invest* 96: 965–975.

Fraser, C.M., Casjens, S., Huang, W.M., Sutton, G.G., Clayton, R., Lathigra, R., et al. (1997). Genomic sequence of a Lyme disease spirochaete, *Borrelia burgdorferi*. *Nature* 390: 580–586.

Garcia Monco, J.C., Wheeler, C.M., Benach, J.L., Furie, R.A., Lukehart, S.A., Stanek, G., et al. (1993). Reactivity of neuroborreliosis patients (Lyme disease) to cardiolipin and gangliosides. *J Neurol Sci* 117: 206–214.

Garin, C. and Bujadoux, M. (1922). Paralysie par tiques. *J Med Lyon* 71: 765–767.

Gebbia, J.A., Coleman, J.L., and Benach, J.L. (2001). *Borrelia* spirochetes up-regulate release and activation of matrix metalloproteinase gelatinase B (MMP-9) and collagenase 1 (MMP-1) in human cells. *Infect Immun* 69: 456–462.

Gern, L. and Humair, P.F. (2000). American robins as reservoir hosts for lyme disease spirochetes. *Emerg Infect Dis* 6: 657–658 (discussion 659–662).

Girschick, H.J., Huppertz, H.I., Russmann, H., Krenn, V., and Karch, H. (1996). Intracellular persistence of *Borrelia burgdorferi* in human synovial cells. *Rheumatol Int* 16: 125–132.

Goodman, J.L., Bradley, J.F., Ross, A.E., Goellner, P., Lagus, A., Vitale, B., et al. (1995). Bloodstream invasion in early Lyme disease: results from a prospective, controlled, blinded study using the polymerase chain reaction. *Am J Med* 99: 6–12. (Published erratum in *Am J Med* 1996, 101(2): 239.)

Guo, B.P., Brown, E.L., Dorward, D.W., Rosenberg, L.C., and Hook, M. (1998). Decorin-binding adhesins from *Borrelia burgdorferi*. *Mol Microbiol* 30: 711–723.

Halperin, J.J. (1995). Neuroborreliosis. *Am J Med* 98: 52S–56S (discussion 56S–59S).

Halperin, J.J. (1997). Neuroborreliosis: central nervous system involvement. *Semin Neurol* 17: 19–24.

Halperin, J.J., Luft, B.J., Anand, A.K., Roque, C.T., Alvarez, O., Volkman, D.J., et al. (1989). Lyme neuroborreliosis: central nervous system manifestations [see comments]. *Neurology* 39: 753–759.

Halperin, J., Krupp, L.B., Golightly, M.G., and Volkman, D.J. (1990). Lyme borreliosis-associated encephalopathy. *Neurology* **40**: 1340–1343.

Hammers-Berggren, S., Hansen, K., Lebech, A.M., and Karlsson, M. (1993). *Borrelia burgdorferi*-specific intrathecal antibody production in neuroborreliosis: a follow-up study. *Neurology* **43**: 169–175.

Hansen, K. (1994). Lyme neuroborreliosis: improvements of the laboratory diagnosis and a survey of epidemiological and clinical features in Denmark 1985–1990. *Acta Neurol Scand Suppl* **151**: 1–44.

Hansen, K. and Lebech, A.M. (1992). The clinical and epidemiological profile of Lyme neuroborreliosis in Denmark 1985–1990. A prospective study of 187 patients with *Borrelia burgdorferi* specific intrathecal antibody production. *Brain* **115**: 399–423.

Hanson, M.S., Cassatt, D.R., Guo, B.P., Patel, N.K., McCarthy, M.P., Dorward, D.W., *et al.* (1998). Active and passive immunity against *Borrelia burgdorferi* decorin binding protein A (DbpA) protects against infection. *Infect Immun* **66**: 2143–2153.

Hansson, L.O., Link, H., Sandlund, L., and Einarsson, R. (1993). Oligoclonal IgG in cerebrospinal fluid detected by isoelectric focusing using PhastSystem. *Scand J Clin Lab Invest* **53**: 487–492.

Hauser, U., Krahl, H., Peters, H., Fingerle, V., and Wilske, B. (1998*a*). Impact of strain heterogeneity on Lyme disease serology in Europe: comparison of enzyme-linked immunosorbent assays using different species of *Borrelia burgdorferi sensu lato*. *J Clin Microbiol* **36**: 427–436.

Hauser, U., Lehnert, G., and Wilske, B. (1998*b*). Diagnostic value of proteins of three *Borrelia* species (*Borrelia burgdorferi sensu lato*) and implications for development and use of recombinant antigens for serodiagnosis of Lyme borreliosis in Europe. *Clin Diagn Lab Immunol* **5**: 456–462.

Hauser, U., Lehnert, G., and Wilske, B. (1999). Validity of interpretation criteria for standardized Western blots (immunoblots) for serodiagnosis of Lyme borreliosis based on sera collected throughout Europe. *J Clin Microbiol* **37**: 2241–2247.

Heikkila, T., Seppala, I., Saxen, H., Panelius, J., Yrjanainen, H., and Lahdenne, P. (2002). Species-specific serodiagnosis of Lyme arthritis and neuroborreliosis due to *Borrelia burgdorferi sensu stricto*, *B. afzelii*, and *B. garinii* by using decorin binding protein A. *J Clin Microbiol* **40**: 453–460.

Honarvar, N., Schaible, U.E., Galanos, C., Wallich, R., and Simon, M.M. (1994). A 14,000 MW lipoprotein and a glycolipid-like structure of *Borrelia burgdorferi* induce proliferation and immunoglobulin production in mouse B cells at high frequencies. *Immunology* **82**: 389–396.

Howe, T.R., Mayer, L.W., and Barbour, A.G. (1985). A single recombinant plasmid expressing two major outer surface proteins of the Lyme disease spirochete. *Science* **227**: 645–646.

Humair, P.F., Postic, D., Wallich, R., and Gern, L. (1998). An avian reservoir (*Turdus merula*) of the Lyme borreliosis spirochetes. *Zentralbl Bakteriol* **287**: 521–538.

Issakainen, J., Gnehm, H.E., Lucchini, G.M., and Zbinden, R. (1996). Value of clinical symptoms, intrathecal specific antibody production and PCR in CSF in the diagnosis of childhood Lyme neuroborreliosis. *Klin Padiatr* **208**: 106–109.

Jiang, W., Luft, B.J., Schubach, W., Dattwyler, R.J., and Gorevic, P.D. (1992). Mapping the major antigenic domains of the native flagellar antigen of *Borrelia burgdorferi*. *J Clin Microbiol* **30**: 1535–1540.

Johnson, R., Marek, N., and Kodner, C. (1984). Infection of Syrian hamsters with Lyme disease spirochetes. *J Clin Microbiol* **20**: 1099–1101.

Johnson, R.C., Kodner, C., and Russell, M. (1986). Passive immunization of hamsters against experimental infection with the Lyme disease spirochete. *Infect Immun* **53**: 713–714.

Johnston, Y.E., Duray, P.H., Steere, A.C., Kashgarian, M., Buza, J., Malawista, S.E., *et al.* (1985). Lyme arthritis. Spirochetes found in synovial microangiopathic lesions. *Am J Pathol* **118**: 26–34.

Kaiser, R. (1998). Neuroborreliosis. *J Neurol* **245**: 247–255.

Kaiser, R. and Rauer, S. (1998). Analysis of the intrathecal immune response in neuroborreliosis to a sonicate antigen and three recombinant antigens of *Borrelia burgdorferi sensu stricto*. *Eur J Clin Microbiol Infect Dis* **17**: 159–166.

Kaiser, R., Rasiah, C., Gassmann, G., Vogt, A., and Lucking, C.H. (1993). Intrathecal antibody synthesis in Lyme neuroborreliosis: use of recombinant p41 and a 14-kDa flagellin fragment in ELISA. *J Med Microbiol* **39**: 290–297.

Kaplan, R.F., Meadows, M.E., Vincent, L.C., Logigian, E.L., and Steere, A.C. (1992). Memory impairment and depression in patients with Lyme encephalopathy: comparison with fibromyalgia and nonpsychotically depressed patients. *Neurology* **42**: 1263–1267.

Karlsson, M., Hovind-Hougen, K., Svenungsson, B., and Stiernstedt, G. (1990). Cultivation and characterization of spirochetes from cerebrospinal fluid of patients with Lyme borreliosis. *J Clin Microbiol* **28**: 473–479.

Karlsson, M., Hammers, S., Nilsson-Ehle, I., Malmborg, A.S., and Wretlind, B. (1996). Concentrations of doxycycline and penicillin G in sera and cerebrospinal fluid of patients treated for neuroborreliosis. *Antimicrob Agents Chemother* **40**: 1104–1107.

Kindstrand, E., Nilsson, B.Y., Hovmark, A., Nennesmo, I., Pirskanen, R., Solders, G., *et al.* (2000). Polyneuropathy in late Lyme borreliosis—a clinical, neurophysiological and morphological description. *Acta Neurol Scand* **101**: 47–52.

Kobayashi, K., Mizukoshi, C., Aoki, T., Muramori, F., Hayashi, M., Miyazu, K., *et al.* (1997). *Borrelia burgdorferi*-seropositive chronic encephalomyelopathy: Lyme neuroborreliosis? An autopsied report. *Dement Geriatr Cogn Disord* **8**: 384–390.

Kruger, H., Reuss, K., Pulz, M., Rohrbach, E., Pflughaupt, K.W., Martin, R., *et al.* (1989). Meningoradiculitis and encephalomyelitis due to *Borrelia burgdorferi*: a follow-up study of 72 patients over 27 years. *J Neurol* **236**: 322–328.

Kumar, H., Belperron, A., Barthold, S.W., and Bockenstedt, L.K. (2000). Cutting edge: CD1d deficiency impairs murine host defense against the spirochete, *Borrelia burgdorferi*. *J Immunol* **165**: 4797–4801.

Kuntzer, T., Bogousslavsky, J., Miklossy, J., Steck, A.J., Janzer, R., and Regli, F. (1991). *Borrelia* rhombencephalomyelopathy. *Arch Neurol* **48**: 832–836.

Kurtti, T.J., Munderloh, U.G., Krueger, D.E., Johnson, R.C., and Schwan, T.G. (1993). Adhesion to and invasion of cultured tick (*Acarina*: Ixodidae) cells by *Borrelia burgdorferi* (Spirochaetales: Spirochaetaceae) and maintenance of infectivity. *J Med Entomol* **30**: 586–596.

Liang, F.T. and Philipp, M.T. (1999). Analysis of antibody response to invariable regions of VlsE, the variable surface antigen of *Borrelia burgdorferi*. *Infect Immun* **67**: 6702–6706.

Liang, F.T., Alvarez, A.L., Gu, Y., Nowling, J.M., Ramamoorthy, R., and Philipp, M.T. (1999). An immunodominant conserved region within the variable domain of VlsE, the variable surface antigen of *Borrelia burgdorferi*. *J Immunol* **163**: 5566–5573.

Liang, F.T., Nelson, F.K., and Fikrig, E. (2002). Molecular adaptation of *Borrelia burgdorferi* in the murine host. *J Exp Med* **196**: 275–280.

Limbach, F.X., Jaulhac, B., Piemont, Y., Kuntz, J.L., Monteil, H., and Sibilia, J. (1999). One-step reverse transcriptase PCR method for detection of *Borrelia burgdorferi* mRNA in mouse Lyme arthritis tissue samples. *J Clin Microbiol* **37**: 2037–2039.

Logigian, E.L., Kaplan, R.F., and Steere, A.C. (1990*a*). Chronic neurologic manifestations of Lyme disease [see comments]. *N Engl J Med* **323**: 1438–1444.

Logigian, E.L., Kaplan, R.F., and Steere, A.C. (1990*b*). Chronic neurological manifestations of Lyme disease. *N Engl J Med* **323**: 1438–1444.

Logigian, E.L., Johnson, K.A., Kijewski, M.F., Kaplan, R.F., Becker, J.A., Jones, K.J., *et al.* (1997). Reversible cerebral hypoperfusion in Lyme encephalopathy. *Neurology* **49**: 1661–1670.

MacDonald, A.B. and Miranda, J.M. (1987). Concurrent neocortical borreliosis and Alzheimer's disease. *Hum Pathol* **18**: 759–761.

Mackworth-Young, C.G., Harris, E.N., Steere, A.C., Rizvi, F., Malawista, S.E., Hughes, G.R., *et al.* (1988). Anticardiolipin antibodies in Lyme disease. *Arthritis Rheum* **31**: 1052–1056.

Magnarelli, L.A., Fikrig, E., Berland, R., Anderson, J.F., and Flavell, R.A. (1992). Comparison of whole-cell antibodies and an antigenic flagellar epitope of *Borrelia burgdorferi* in serologic tests for diagnosis of Lyme borreliosis. *J Clin Microbiol* **30**: 3158–3162.

Magnarelli, L.A., Ijdo, J.W., Padula, S.J., Flavell, R.A., and Fikrig, E. (2000). Serologic diagnosis of Lyme borreliosis by using enzyme-linked immunosorbent assays with recombinant antigens. *J Clin Microbiol* **38**: 1735–1739.

Maimone, D., Villanova, M., Stanta, G., Bonin, S., Malandrini, A., Guazzi, G.C., *et al.* (1997). Detection of *Borrelia burgdorferi* DNA and complement membrane attack complex deposits in the sural nerve of a patient with chronic polyneuropathy and tertiary Lyme disease. *Muscle Nerve* **20**: 969–975.

Malawista, S.E., Barthold, S.W., and Persing, D.H. (1994). Fate of *Borrelia burgdorferi* DNA in tissues of infected mice after antibiotic treatment. *J Infect Dis* **170**: 1312–1316.

Marconi, R.T., Hohenberger, S., Jauris-Heipke, S., Schulte-Spechtel, U., LaVoie, C.P., Rossler, D., et al. (1999). Genetic analysis of *Borrelia garinii* OspA serotype 4 strains associated with neuroborreliosis: evidence for extensive genetic homogeneity. *J Clin Microbiol* **37**: 3965–3970.

Martin, R., Ortlauf, J., Sticht-Groh, V., Bogdahn, U., Goldmann, S.F., and Mertens, H.G. (1988). *Borrelia burgdorferi*–specific and autoreactive T-cell lines from cerebrospinal fluid in Lyme radiculomyelitis. *Ann Neurol* **24**: 509–516.

McKisic, M.D., Redmond, W.L., and Barthold, S.W. (2000). Cutting edge: T cell-mediated pathology in murine Lyme borreliosis. *J Immunol* **164**: 6096–6099.

Miklossy, J., Kuntzer, T., Bogousslavsky, J., Regli, F., and Janzer, R.C. (1990). Meningovascular form of neuroborreliosis: similarities between neuropathological findings in a case of Lyme disease and those occurring in tertiary neurosyphilis. *Acta Neuropathol (Berlin)* **80**: 568–572.

Montgomery, R.R., Nathanson, M.H., and Malawista, S.E. (1993). The fate of *Borrelia burgdorferi*, the agent for Lyme disease, in mouse macrophages. Destruction, survival, recovery. *J Immunol* **150**: 909–915.

Moody, K.D., Barthold, S.W., and Terwilliger, G.A. (1990*a*). Lyme borreliosis in laboratory animals: effect of host species and in vitro passage of *Borrelia burgdorferi*. *Am J Trop Med Hyg* **43**: 87–92.

Moody, K.D., Barthold, S.W., Terwilliger, G.A., Beck, D.S., Hansen, G.M., and Jacoby, R.O. (1990*b*). Experimental chronic Lyme borreliosis in Lewis rats. *Am J Trop Med Hyg* **42**: 165–174.

Morrison, T.B., Ma, Y., Weis, J.H., and Weis, J.J. (1999). Rapid and sensitive quantification of *Borrelia burgdorferi*-infected mouse tissues by continuous fluorescent monitoring of PCR. *J Clin Microbiol* **37**: 987–992.

Museteanu, C., Schaible, U.E., Stehle, T., Kramer, M.D., and Simon, M.M. (1991). Myositis in mice inoculated with *Borrelia burgdorferi*. *Am J Pathol* **139**: 1267–1271.

Nadelman, R.B., Herman, E., and Wormser, G.P. (1997). Screening for Lyme disease in hospitalized psychiatric patients: prospective serosurvey in an endemic area. *Mt Sinai J Med* **64**: 409–412.

Nagi, K.S., Joshi, R., and Thakur, R.K. (1996). Cardiac manifestations of Lyme disease: a review [see comments]. *Can J Cardiol* **12**: 503–506.

Nocton, J.J., Dressler, F., Rutledge, B.J., Rys, P.N., Persing, D.H., and Steere, A.C. (1994). Detection of *Borrelia burgdorferi* DNA by polymerase chain reaction in synovial fluid from patients with Lyme arthritis [see comments]. *N Engl J Med* **330**: 229–234.

Nordstrand, A., Barbour, A.G., and Bergstrom, S. (2000). *Borrelia* pathogenesis research in the post-genomic and post-vaccine era. *Curr Opin Microbiol* **3**: 86–92.

Oschmann, P., Dorndorf, W., Hornig, C., Schafer, C., Wellensiek, H.J., and Pflughaupt, K.W. (1998). Stages and syndromes of neuroborreliosis. *J Neurol* **245**: 262–272.

Pachner, A.R. (1988). *Borrelia burgdorferi* in the nervous system: the new 'great imitator'. *Ann N Y Acad Sci* **539**: 56–64.

Pachner, A.R. (1989). Neurologic manifestations of Lyme disease, the new 'great imitator'. *Rev Infect Dis* **11**(Suppl. 6): S1482–S1486.

Pachner, A.R. (1995). Early disseminated Lyme disease: Lyme meningitis. *Am J Med* **98**: 30S–37S (discussion 37S–43S).

Pachner, A.R. and Itano, A. (1990). *Borrelia burgdorferi* infection of the brain: characterization of the organism and response to antibiotics and immune sera in the mouse model. *Neurology* **40**: 1535–1540.

Pachner, A.R. and Steere, A.C. (1985). The triad of neurologic manifestations of Lyme disease: meningitis, cranial neuritis, and radiculoneuritis. *Neurology* **35**: 47–53.

Pachner, A.R. and Steere, A.C. (1986). CNS manifestations of third stage Lyme disease. *Zbl Bakt Hyg A* **263**: 301–306.

Pachner, A.R., Ricalton, N., and Delaney, E. (1993). Comparison of polymerase chain reaction with culture and serology for diagnosis of murine experimental Lyme borreliosis. *J Clin Microbiol* **31**: 208–214.

Pachner, A.R., Braswell, S.T., Delaney, E., Amemiya, K., and Major, E. (1994). A rabbit model of Lyme neuroborreliosis: characterization by PCR, serology, and sequencing of the OspA gene from the brain. *Neurology* **44**: 1938–1943.

Pachner, A.R., Basta, J., Delaney, E., and Hulinska, D. (1995*a*). Localization of *Borrelia burgdorferi* in murine Lyme borreliosis by electron microscopy. *Am J Trop Med Hyg* **52**: 128–133.

Pachner, A.R., Delaney, E., O'Neill, T., and Major, E. (1995*b*). Inoculation of nonhuman primates with the N40 strain of *Borrelia burgdorferi* leads to a model of Lyme neuroborreliosis faithful to the human disease. *Neurology* **45**: 165–172.

Pachner, A.R., Zhang, W.F., Schaefer, H., Schaefer, S., and O'Neill, T. (1998). Detection of active infection in nonhuman primates with Lyme neuroborreliosis: comparison of PCR, culture, and a bioassay. *J Clin Microbiol* **36**: 3243–3247.

Pachner, A.R., Amemiya, K., Bartlett, M., Schaefer, H., Reddy, K., and Zhang, W.F. (2001*a*). Lyme borreliosis in rhesus macaques: effects of corticosteroids on spirochetal load and isotype switching of anti-*Borrelia burgdorferi* antibody. *Clin Diagn Lab Immunol* **8**: 225–232.

Pachner, A.R., Cadavid, D., Shu, G., Dail, D., Pachner, S., Hodzic, E., and , et al. (2001*b*). Central and peripheral nervous system infection, immunity, and inflammation in the NHP model of Lyme borreliosis. *Ann Neurol* **50**: 330–338.

Pachner, A.R., Dail, D., Li, L., Gurey, L., Feng, S., Hodzic, E., et al. (2002*a*). Humoral immune response associated with lyme borreliosis in nonhuman primates: analysis by immunoblotting and enzyme-linked immunosorbent assay with sonicates or recombinant proteins. *Clin Diagn Lab Immunol* **9**: 1348–1355.

Pachner, A.R., Narayan, K., Price, N., Hurd, M., and Dail, D. (2002*b*). IFNβ-induced gene expression analysis in MS patients: loss of bioavailability can be caused by either binding or neutralizing antibodies, submitted.

Pal, U., de Silva, A.M., Montgomery, R.R., Fish, D., Anguita, J., Anderson, J.F., et al. (2000). Attachment of *Borrelia burgdorferi* within ixodes scapularis mediated by outer surface protein A. *J Clin Invest* **106**: 561–569.

Pennington, P.M., Cadavid, D., Bunikis, J., Norris, S.J., and Barbour, A.G. (1999). Extensive interplasmidic duplications change the virulence phenotype of the relapsing fever agent *Borrelia turicatae*. *Mol Microbiol* **34**: 1120–1132.

Ragnaud, J.M., Morlat, P., Buisson, M., Ferrer, X., Orgogozo, J.M., Julien, J., et al. (1995). [Neurologic manifestations of Lyme disease. Apropos of 25 cases]. *Rev Med Interne* **16**: 487–494 (in French).

Reiber, H. (1998). Cerebrospinal fluid–physiology, analysis and interpretation of protein patterns for diagnosis of neurological disease. *Mult Scler* **4**: 99–107.

Reik, L., Steere, A.C., Bartenhagen, N.H., Shope, R.E., and Malawista, S.E. (1979). Neurologic abnormalities of Lyme disease. *Medicine* **58**: 281–294.

Reimers, C.D., de Koning, J., Neubert, U., Preac-Mursic, V., Koster, J.G., Muller-Felber, W., et al. (1993). *Borrelia burgdorferi* myositis: report of eight patients. *J Neurol* **240**: 278–283.

Roberts, E.D., Bohm, R.P. Jr, Cogswell, F.B., Lanners, H.N., Lowrie, R.C. Jr, Povinelli, L., et al. (1995). Chronic Lyme disease in the rhesus monkey. *Lab Invest* **72**: 146–160.

Roberts, E.D., Bohm, R.P. Jr, Lowrie, R.C. Jr, Habicht, G., Katona, L., Piesman, J., et al. (1998). Pathogenesis of Lyme neuroborreliosis in the rhesus monkey: the early disseminated and chronic phases of disease in the peripheral nervous system. *J Infect Dis* **178**: 722–732.

Robinson, J.M., Pilot-Matias, T.J., Pratt, S.D., Patel, C.B., Bevirt, T.S., and Hunt, J.C. (1993). Analysis of the humoral response to the flagellin protein of *Borrelia burgdorferi*: cloning of regions capable of differentiating Lyme disease from syphilis [see comments]. *J Clin Microbiol* **31**: 629–635.

Rosenfeld, M.E., Beckerman, B., Ward, M.F., and Sama, A. (1999). Lyme carditis: complete AV dissociation with episodic asystole presenting as syncope in the emergency department. *J Emerg Med* **17**: 661–664.

Schmidt, R. and Ackermann, R. (1985). [Meningopolyneuritis (Garin–Bujadoux–Bannwarth) erythema chronicum migrans disease of the nervous system transmitted by ticks]. *Fortschr Neurol Psychiatr* **53**: 145–153 (in German).

Schmitz, J.L., Schell, R.F., Hejka, A., England, D.M., and Konick, L. (1988). Induction of Lyme arthritis in LSH hamsters. *Infect Immun* **56**: 2336–2342.

Schmutzhard, E., Stanek, G., and Pohl, P. (1985). Polyneuritis cranialis associated with *Borrelia burgdorferi*. *J Neurol Neurosurg Psychiatry* **48**: 1182–1184.

Shang, E.S., Champion, C.I., Wu, X.Y., Skare, J.T., Blanco, D.R., Miller, J.N., et al. (2000). Comparison of protection in rabbits against host-adapted and cultivated *Borrelia burgdorferi* following infection-derived immunity or immunization with outer membrane vesicles or outer surface protein A. *Infect Immun* **68**: 4189–4199.

Sigal, L.H. (1997). Lyme disease: a review of aspects of its immunology and immunopathogenesis. *Ann Rev Immunol* **15**: 63–92.

Sigal, L.H., Zahradnik, J.M., Lavin, P., Patella, S.J., Bryant, G., Haselby, R., et al. (1998). A vaccine consisting of recombinant *Borrelia burgdorferi* outer-surface protein A to prevent Lyme disease. Recombinant Outer-Surface Protein A Lyme Disease Vaccine Study Consortium [see comments]. *N Engl J Med* **339**: 216–222. (Published erratum in *N Engl J Med* 1998, **339**(8): 571.)

Skoldenberg, B., Stiernstedt, G., Karlsson, M., Wretlind, B., and Svenungsson, B. (1988). Treatment of Lyme borreliosis with emphasis on neurological disease. *Ann N Y Acad Sci* **539**: 317–323.

Smith, R.P. Jr, Rand, P.W., Lacombe, E.H., Telford S.R.D., Rich, S.M., Piesman, J., et al. (1993). Norway rats as reservoir hosts for Lyme disease spirochetes on Monhegan Island, Maine. *J Infect Dis* **168**: 687–691.

Stanek, G., Pletschette, M., Flamm, H., Hirschl, A.M., Aberer, E., Kristoferitsch, W., et al. (1988). European Lyme borreliosis. *Ann N Y Acad Sci* **539**: 274–282.

Steere, A.C. (1997). Diagnosis and treatment of Lyme arthritis. *Med Clin North Am* **81**: 179–194.

Steere, A., Malawista, S., Snydman, D., Shope, R., Andiman, W., Ross, M., et al. (1977a). Lyme arthritis: an epidemic of oligoarthritis in children and adults in three Connecticut communities. *Arthritis Rheum* **20**: 7–17.

Steere, A.C., Malawista, S.E., Hardin, J.A., Ruddy, S., Askenase, P.W., and Andiman, W.A. (1977b). Erythema chronicum migrans and Lyme arthritis: the enlarging clinical spectrum. *Ann Intern Med* **86**: 685–698.

Steere, A.C., Batsford, W.P., Weinberg, M., Alexander, J., Berger, H.J., Wolfson, S., et al. (1980). Lyme carditis: cardiac abnormalities of Lyme disease. *Ann Intern Med* **93**: 8–16.

Steere, A.C., Grodzicki, R.L., Kornblatt, A.N., Craft, J.E., Barbour, A.G., Burgdorfer, W., et al. (1983a). The spirochetal etiology of Lyme disease. *N Engl J Med* **308**: 733–740.

Steere, A.C., Pachner, A.R., and Malawista, S.E. (1983b). Successful treatment of neurologic abnormalities of Lyme disease with high-dose intravenous penicillin. *Ann Intern Med* **99**: 767–772.

Steere, A., Schoen, R., and Taylor, E. (1987). The clinical evolution of Lyme arthritis. *Ann Intern Med* **107**: 725–731.

Steere, A.C., Berardi, V.P., Weeks, K.E., Logigian, E.L., and Ackermann, R. (1990). Evaluation of the intrathecal antibody response to *Borrelia burgdorferi* as a diagnostic test for Lyme neuroborreliosis. *J Infect Dis* **161**: 1203–1209.

Stevenson, B. and Babb, K. (2002). LuxS-mediated quorum sensing in *Borrelia burgdorferi*, the Lyme disease spirochete. *Infect Immun* **70**: 4099–4105.

Stevenson, B., El-Hage, N., Hines, M.A., Miller, J.C., and Babb, K. (2002). Differential binding of host complement inhibitor factor H by *Borrelia burgdorferi* Erp surface proteins: a possible mechanism underlying the expansive host range of Lyme disease spirochetes. *Infect Immun* **70**: 491–497.

Stiernstedt, G., Granstrom, M., Hederstedt, B., and Skoldenberg, B. (1985). Diagnosis of spirochetal meningitis by enzyme-linked immunosorbent assay in serum and cerebrospinal fluid. *J Clin Microbiol* **21**: 819–825.

Stiernstedt, G., Skoldenberg, B., Garde, A., Kolmodin, G., Jorbeck, H., Svenungsson, B., et al. (1987). Clinical manifestations of *Borrelia* infections of the nervous system. *Zentralbl Bakteriol Mikrobiol Hyg A* **263**: 289–296.

Stiernstedt, G., Gustafsson, R., Karlsson, M., Svenungsson, B., and Skoldenberg, B. (1988). Clinical manifestations and diagnosis of neuroborreliosis. *Ann N Y Acad Sci* **539**: 46–55.

Straubinger, R.K., Straubinger, A.F., Summers, B.A., Jacobson, R.H., and Erb, H.N. (1998). Clinical manifestations, pathogenesis, and effect of antibiotic treatment on Lyme borreliosis in dogs. *Wien Klin Wochenschr* **110**: 874–881.

Straubinger, R.K., Straubinger, A.F., Summers, B.A., and Jacobson, R.H. (2000). Status of *Borrelia burgdorferi* infection after antibiotic treatment and the effects of corticosteroids: an experimental study. *J Infect Dis* **181**: 1069–1081.

Sung, S.Y., Lavoie, C.P., Carlyon, J.A., and Marconi, R.T. (1998). Genetic divergence and evolutionary instability in ospE-related members of the upstream homology box gene family in *Borrelia burgdorferi sensu lato* complex isolates. *Infect Immun* **66**: 4656–4668.

Szczepanski, A., Furie, M.B., Benach, J.L., Lane, B.P., and Fleit, H.B. (1990). Interaction between *Borrelia burgdorferi* and endothelium *in vitro*. *J Clin Invest* **85**: 1637–1647.

Tezzon, F., Corradini, C., Huber, R., Egarter Vigl, E., Simeoni, J., Stanek, G., et al. (1991). Vasculitic mononeuritis multiplex in patient with Lyme disease. *Ital J Neurol Sci* **12**: 229–232.

Tumani, H., Nolker, G., and Reiber, H. (1995). Relevance of cerebrospinal fluid variables for early diagnosis of neuroborreliosis. *Neurology* **45**: 1663–1670.

Wallich, R., Brenner, C., Kramer, M.D., and Simon, M.M. (1995). Molecular cloning and immunological characterization of a novel linear-plasmid-encoded gene, pG, of *Borrelia burgdorferi* expressed only *in vivo*. *Infect Immun* **63**: 3327–3335.

Wallich, R., Moter, S.E., Simon, M.M., Ebnet, K., Heiberger, A., and Kramer, M.D. The *Borrelia burgdorferi* flagellum-associated 41-kilodalton antigen (flagellin): molecular cloning, expression, and amplification of the gene. *Infect Immun* **58**: 1711–1719.

Wang, G., van Dam, A.P., Schwartz, I., and Dankert, J. (1999). Molecular typing of *Borrelia burgdorferi sensu lato*: taxonomic, epidemiological, and clinical implications. *Clin Microbiol Rev* **12**: 633–653.

Weis, J.J., Ma, Y., and Erdile, L.F. (1994). Biological activities of native and recombinant *Borrelia burgdorferi* outer surface protein A: dependence on lipid modification. *Infect Immun* **62**: 4632–4636.

Wilske, B., Schierz, G., Preac-Mursic, V., von Busch, K., Kuhbeck, R., Pfister, H.W., et al. (1986). Intrathecal production of specific antibodies against *Borrelia burgdorferi* in patients with lymphocytic meningoradiculitis (Bannwarth's syndrome). *J Infect Dis* **153**: 304–314.

Wilske, B., Habermann, C., Fingerle, V., Hillenbrand, B., Jauris-Heipke, S., Lehnert, G., et al. (1999). An improved recombinant IgG immunoblot for serodiagnosis of Lyme borreliosis. *Med Microbiol Immunol (Berlin)* **188**: 139–144.

Wormser, G.P., Bittker, S., Cooper, D., Nowakowski, J., Nadelman, R.B., and Pavia, C. (2000). Comparison of the yields of blood cultures using serum or plasma from patients with early Lyme disease. *J Clin Microbiol* **38**: 1648–1650.

Yang, L., Weis, J.H., Eichwald, E., Kolbert, C.P., Persing, D.H., and Weis, J.J. (1994). Heritable susceptibility to severe *Borrelia burgdorferi*-induced arthritis is dominant and is associated with persistence of large numbers of spirochetes in tissues. *Infect Immun* **62**: 492–500.

Yang, X., Popova, T.G., Hagman, K.E., Wikel, S.K., Schoeler, G.B., Caimano, M.J., et al. (1999). Identification, characterization, and expression of three new members of the *Borrelia burgdorferi* Mlp (2.9) lipoprotein gene family. *Infect Immun* **67**: 6008–6018.

Zhang, J.R. and Norris, S.J. (1998). Kinetics and in vivo induction of genetic variation of vlsE in *Borrelia burgdorferi*. *Infect Immun* **66**: 3689–3697.

Zhang, J.R., Hardham, J.M., Barbour, A.G., and Norris, S.J. (1997). Antigenic variation in Lyme disease borreliae by promiscuous recombination of VMP-like sequence cassettes. *Cell* **89**: 275–285. (Published erratum in *Cell* 1999, **96**(3): 447).

Zhong, W., Gern, L., Stehle, T., Museteanu, C., Kramer, M., Wallich, R., et al. (1999). Resolution of experimental and tick-borne *Borrelia burgdorferi* infection in mice by passive, but not active immunization using recombinant OspC. *Eur J Immunol* **29**: 946–957.

Zifko, U., Wondrusch, E., Machacek, E., and Grisold, W. (1995). [Inflammatory demyelinating neuropathy in neuroborreliosis]. *Wien Med Wochenschr* **145**: 188–190 (in German).

25 Paraneoplastic syndromes

Josep Dalmau and Jan Verschuuren

Cancer can affect the nervous system by one of two ways: direct spread or metastases, and indirect mechanisms, including vascular disorders, metabolic and nutritional deficits, toxic effects of treatment, and paraneoplastic or 'remote effects' of cancer on the nervous system. Therefore, *paraneoplastic neurologic disorders* (PND) are defined as neurologic disorders pathogenetically related to cancer but not ascribable to nervous system metastases or to any of the other indirect mechanisms just mentioned (Posner, 1995). Paraneoplastic syndromes are uncommon neurologic complications in patients with cancer. The exact frequency of these syndromes is unknown, and varies depending on the criteria used to define the paraneoplastic syndrome and the studies done to exclude other causes of neurologic dysfunction.

PND may affect any portion of the central or peripheral nervous system (Table 25.1) (Posner, 1995). Frequently, neurologic symptoms develop before the tumor is known to be present, and therefore, the correct identification of the disorder permits early detection of the neoplasm. The diagnosis of PND is based mainly on the degree of suspicion by the clinician, which depends on their knowledge of the statistical relationship between the development of characteristic neurologic symptoms and the presence of

a specific type of tumor. However, in many instances, even when a PND is strongly suspected, the underlying cancer is small and escapes detection despite repetitive clinical and radiologic evaluations.

This chapter reviews the pathogenesis and approach to the diagnosis and treatment of these disorders, and focuses on specific PND for which immune responses against the tumor, the nervous system, or both, have been demonstrated.

Pathogenesis

Current evidence suggests that many PND are immune-mediated (Dalmau *et al.*, 1999a). One hypothesis is that the ectopic expression of neuronal antigens by the tumor triggers an immune response against the tumor that affects the nervous system, resulting in the PND. An antibody-mediated pathogenesis has been demonstrated for the Lambert–Eaton myasthenic syndrome (LEMS) (Lang *et al.*, 1981). The IgG of these patients contains antibodies against P/Q-type voltage-gated calcium channels (VGCC) expressed by the tumor, usually a small-cell lung cancer (SCLC) (Chester

Table 25.1 Paraneoplastic syndromes of the nervous system

Paraneoplastic syndromes of the central nervous system	Paraneoplastic cerebellar degeneration
	Paraneoplastic encephalomyelitis[a] (limbic encephalitis, brainstem encephalitis, cerebellitis, myelitis)
	Paraneoplastic opsoclonus–myoclonus
	Cancer- and melanoma-associated retinopathy
	Paraneoplastic stiff-man syndrome
	Paraneoplastic necrotizing myelopathy[b]
	Motor neuron syndromes[b] (ALS, subacute motor neuronopathy)
Paraneoplastic syndromes of the peripheral nervous system	Subacute sensory neuronopathy
	Autonomic neuropathy
	Acute sensorimotor neuropathy: polyradiculoneuropathy (Guillain–Barré syndrome); brachial neuritis
	Chronic sensorimotor neuropathy: sensorimotor neuropathies associated with malignant monoclonal gammopathies
	Vasculitic neuropathy
	Neuromyotonia
Paraneoplastic syndromes of the neuromuscular junction and muscle	Lambert-Eaton myasthenic syndrome[b]
	Myasthenia gravis[b]
	Polymyositis-dermatomyositis
	Acute necrotizing myopathy[b]
	Cachectic myopathy[b]
	Carcinoid myopathy[b]

[a]Can include cerebellar symptoms, autonomic dysfunction, and sensory neuronopathy.
[b]Not discussed in this chapter; see review by Rudnicki and Dalmau (Dalmau 2000).
ALS, amyotrophic lateral sclerosis.

et al., 1988). These antibodies react with similar epitopes expressed at the pre-synaptic level of the neuromuscular junction, interfering with the release of acetylcholine and resulting in weakness and fatigue. A similar antibody-mediated mechanism directed against post-synaptic neuromuscular acetylcholine receptors has been demonstrated for myasthenia gravis (Drachman, 1994), which is triggered by the presence of a thymoma in 10 to 15% of patients. In these two disorders, passive transfer of the patients' IgG to animals reproduces the clinical, electrophysiologic, and morphological abnormalities of the disorder.

Similar immune-mediated mechanisms have been suggested for antibody-associated PND of the central nervous system (CNS). Although administration of these antibodies to animals and immunization with recombinant antigens have not reproduced the disease (Graus *et al.*, 1991; Tanaka *et al.*, 1994; Sillevis Smitt *et al.*, 1995), the immune origin of these disorders is suggested by several findings, including the presence of high titers of antibodies that react with antigens restricted to the nervous system and tumor (Dalmau *et al.*, 1990), intrathecal synthesis of antibodies and deposits of antibodies in neurons and tumor (Brashear *et al.*, 1991; Furneaux *et al.*, 1990; Graus *et al.*, 1988), and the absence of similar antibodies in other inflammatory disorders of the CNS that are associated with neuronal destruction, or with tumors that do not express the specific antigen (Anderson *et al.*, 1988b).

In addition to the presence of antineuronal antibodies, the nervous system and tumor of patients with PND of the CNS contain inflammatory infiltrates composed of CD4+ and CD8+ cytotoxic T cells (Graus *et al.*, 1990). Some studies show cytotoxic cells surrounding and indenting neurons undergoing degeneration (Wanschitz *et al.*, 1997). Interest in the T-cell responses has been bolstered by the lack of success in modeling PNS in animals using only the antibody response. The evidence that cytotoxic T-cell mechanisms play a pathogenic role is strong and provided by studies from different investigators (Tanaka *et al.*, 1998, 1999; Voltz *et al.*, 1998; Benyahia *et al.*, 1999; Albert *et al.*, 2000). However, despite several studies demonstrating specific T-cell responses against the same onconeuronal antigens recognized by the antibodies, no animal model is yet available. Because the T-cell and humoral immune responses appear to be directed against the same antigens, it is likely that PND result from the cooperation of both arms of the immune response. It is not known why only a small proportion of tumors expressing paraneoplastic antigens trigger an immune response associated with the PND. Factors related to the tumor, such as the co-expression of antigen-presenting molecules (MHC Class I and II) (Dalmau *et al.*, 1995) and factors related to the patient, such as gender and HLA haplotype (Albert *et al.*, 1998; Tanaka and Tanaka, 1996) may be involved.

Clinical diagnosis of paraneoplastic disorders

It is important to recognize that neurologic disorders that are clinically and pathologically identical to PND may occur in the absence of cancer. This, in addition to the difficulty in demonstrating the underlying tumor, complicates the diagnosis of a paraneoplastic syndrome.

The discovery of antineuronal antibodies (Table 25. 2) has modified the strategy for diagnosing PND, particularly those involving the CNS. Regardless of whether these antibodies are causal or not, they can be used as markers of the paraneoplastic origin of the neurologic symptoms and also serve as markers for the presence of specific tumor types, directing the search for the tumor to a few organs. It is important to note that all antibodies shown in Table 25.2 can also be identified (usually at low titers) in a small proportion of cancer patients without PND.

If antineuronal antibodies are not identified, the demonstration that a neurologic disorder is paraneoplastic depends on localizing the tumor using ancillary tests, such as serum tumor markers, computed tomography (CT) or magnetic resonance imaging (MRI) studies, and positron emission tomography (PET) (Rees *et al.*, 2001).

For patients in whom the presence of cancer is known, efforts should be directed to rule out metastatic complications and other non-paraneoplastic mechanisms of neuronal injury, such as side-effects of cancer treatment, coagulopathy, or infections (Posner, 1995). If metastases are not found, the detection of paraneoplastic antibodies usually establishes the paraneoplastic origin of the disorder.

If the tumor is 'atypical or unusual' for the type of paraneoplastic antibodies identified, or does not show reactivity with the serum antibodies, the presence of a second neoplasm should be considered (Graus *et al.*, 2001).

Table 25.2 Antibodies associated with paraneoplastic neurologic syndromes

Antibody	Associated cancer	Syndrome	Antigens (test to detect antibodies)
Anti-Hu	SCLC, other	Focal encephalitis, myelitis, encephalomyelitis, cerebellar degeneration, sensory neuronopathy, peripheral neuropathy	HuD, HuC, Hel-N1 (IHC, IB)
Anti-Yo	Gynecological, breast	Cerebellar degeneration	CDR34 and CDR62 (IHC, IB)
Anti-Zic	SCLC	Encephalomyelitis, cerebellar degeneration	Zic1, 2 and 4 (IHC, IB)
Anti-Ri	Breast, gynecological, SCLC	Cerebellar ataxia, opsoclonus, brainstem encephalitis	Nova 1 and 2 (IHC, IB)
Anti-Tr	Hodgkin's lymphoma	Cerebellar degeneration	Antigen unknown (IHC)
Anti-CV2 or anti-CRMP5	SCLC, other	Focal encephalitis, myelitis, encephalomyelitis, cerebellar degeneration, peripheral neuropathy chorea, uveitis	CRMP5 (IHC, IB)
Anti-Ma proteins	Testicular germ-cell tumors and other cancers	Limbic, brainstem encephalitis, cerebellar degeneration	Ma1–3 (IHC, IB)
Anti-amphiphysin	Breast, SCLC	Stiff-man syndrome, encephalomyelitis	Amphiphysin (IHC, IB)
Antiretinal antibodies	SCLC and other	Cancer-associated retinopathy (CAR)	Recoverin, tubby-like, PNR[a] (IB)
	Melanoma	Melanoma-associated retinopathy (MAR)	Unknown, expressed in bipolar cells of the retina (IHC)
Anti-VGKC[b]	Thymoma, others	Neuromyotonia. Limbic encephalitis	VGKC (IP)
Anti-P/Q type VGCC[b]	SCLC	LEMS. Cerebellar degeneration	P/Q-type VGCC (IP)
Anti-acetylcholine receptor[b]	Thymoma	Myasthenia gravis	Acetylcholine receptor (IP)

[a]Photoreceptor-specific nuclear receptor.
[b]The same antibodies are also identified in the non-paraneoplastic form of the disorder.
IHC, immunohistochemistry; IB, immunoblot; IP, immunoprecipitation; SCLC, small-cell lung cnacer; LEMS, Lambert–Eaton myasthenic syndrome.

Specific paraneoplastic syndromes of the central nervous system

Paraneoplastic cerebellar degeneration

This disorder is characterized by the subacute onset of cerebellar dysfunction that eventually stabilizes leaving the patient with severe deficits. Initial symptoms typically include dizziness, visual problems (diplopia, blurry vision, or oscillopsia), nausea, vomiting, and dysarthria (Posner, 1995). These symptoms may be considered secondary to a viral process, but in a few days (sometimes hours) the patient develops ataxia of gait and extremities often accompanied by dysphagia. The intensity and course of the symptoms, and the association with other neurologic deficits, may vary from patient to patient, but these differences are less noticeable between patients with the same type of tumor and particularly between patients with the same antineuronal antibody in serum and cerebrospinal fluid (CSF) (Table 25.2).

Post-mortem studies demonstrate near or total loss of Purkinje cells with relative preservation of other cerebellar neurons and Bergmann astrogliosis. Inflammatory infiltrates, if present, usually involve the deep cerebellar nuclei. Demyelinating changes may be present in cerebellum and dorsal spinocerebellar and posterior columns of the spinal cord (Henson and Urich, 1982).

The diagnosis of paraneoplastic cerebellar degeneration (PCD) should be suspected in any patient older than 50 years who develops subacute symptoms of cerebellar dysfunction of unknown etiology. In the early stages, examination of the CSF usually demonstrates pleocytosis, increased protein concentrations, increased IgG index, and oligoclonal bands. The detection of a well-characterized paraneoplastic antibody establishes the diagnosis and directs the search for the neoplasm (see Table 25.2). Other tests, such as MRI of the brain, do not usually demonstrate abnormalities in the acute phase of the disease; atrophy of the cerebellum may be seen several months after symptom development (Posner, 1995).

Anti-Yo-associated paraneoplastic cerebellar degeneration

This disorder is the best-characterized PCD (Peterson *et al.*, 1992). Typically, patients are post-menopausal women with no history of cancer (two-thirds of patients), or with a recent diagnosis of cancer of the breast or ovary (one-third of patients). As a result of the neurologic deficits, most of the patients are unable to read, feed themselves, or walk without assistance. Autopsy studies demonstrate total or near-total loss of Purkinje cells (Fig. 25.1) (Verschuuren *et al.*, 1996).

The anti-Yo antibodies react with 34 and 62 kDa protein antigens (CDR34 and 62) expressed in the cytoplasm of Purkinje cells and tumor

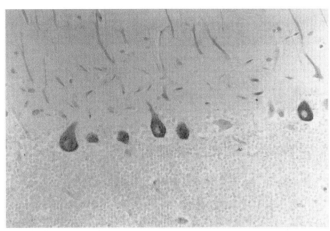

Fig. 25.2 Reactivity of anti-Yo antibodies with a section of cerebellum obtained at autopsy of a neurologically normal individual. Note the predominant granular reactivity of the anti-Yo antibodies with the cytoplasm of Purkinje cells. Section mildly counterstained with hematoxylin.

(Fig. 25.2) (Dropcho *et al.*, 1987; Sakai *et al.*, 1990; Fathallah-Shaykh *et al.*, 1991). The function of these antigens is unknown, but CDR62 contains a helix-leucine-zipper motif that interacts with and down-regulates c-Myc by sequestering it in the neuronal cytoplasm (Okano *et al.*, 1999).

Based on the strong correlation between detection of anti-Yo antibodies and the presence of breast or gynecological tumors, anti-Yo-positive patients should undergo mammography and CT scans of the pelvis and abdomen. If these tests are negative, a body PET scan often uncovers the neoplasm (Rees *et al.*, 2001). Treatment of the tumor, plasma exchange, and intravenous immunoglobulin (IV Ig) do not usually affect the course of this PND (Graus *et al.*, 1992; Uchuya *et al.*, 1996; Rojas *et al.*, 2000).

Paraneoplastic cerebellar degeneration associated with Hodgkin's disease

This disorder predominates in men, and the patients are usually younger than patients with PCD associated with other tumors. The first anti-Purkinje cell antibody identified was from the serum of a patient with Hodgkin's disease and PCD (Trotter *et al.*, 1976). This antibody, called anti-Tr, shows a dot-like pattern of reactivity with the cytoplasm of Purkinje cells and molecular layer of the cerebellum. The results of Western blot analysis with homogenates of cerebellum or Purkinje cells are usually negative, and the identity of the Tr antigen(s) remains unknown.

A series of 28 patients with anti-Tr antibodies showed that 27 patients had PCD and one had limbic encephalitis. Hodgkin's disease was identified in 25 patients and no tumor in three. Only four of 28 patients had neurologic improvement, and younger patients (<40 years) were more likely to improve than elderly patients. Different from other PND in which the tumors usually express the neuronal antigens, only one of 15 tumors examined showed expression of Tr antigens (Bernal *et al.*, 2003).

Paraneoplastic cerebellar ataxia and opsoclonus associated with anti-Ri antibodies

In some women with subacute cerebellar dysfunction, the predominant symptoms are gait difficulty, truncal ataxia, and opsoclonus. These patients may harbor an antineuronal antibody in their serum and CSF called anti-Ri (Luque *et al.*, 1991). This antibody reacts with 55 and 80 kDa proteins expressed in the nuclei of most neurons of the CNS (Fig. 25.3) as well as in the associated tumor, usually a breast or gynecologic cancer (Luque *et al.*, 1991). The Ri antigens are a family of RNA-binding proteins coded by two genes, *NOVA1* and *NOVA2* (Buckanovich *et al.*, 1993; Yang *et al.*, 1998). Nova1 binds RNA in a sequence-specific manner to regulate neuronal pre-mRNA alternative splicing of the glycine and GABA (A) inhibitory receptors (Jensen *et al.*, 2000).

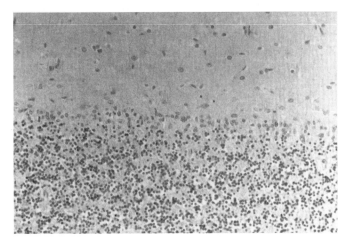

Fig. 25.1 Section of cerebellum from a patient with anti-Yo associated paraneoplastic cerebellar degeneration, demonstrating the absence of Purkinje cells and Bergmann gliosis.

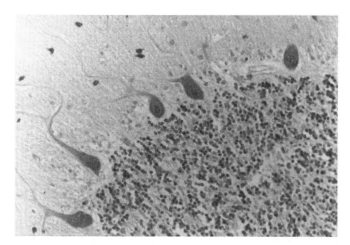

Fig. 25.3 Reactivity of anti-Ri antibodies with a section of cerebellum obtained at autopsy of a neurologically normal individual. Note that the anti-Ri antibodies react predominantly with the nuclei of all neurons (Purkinje cells and neurons of the granular and molecular layers). Section mildly counterstained with hematoxylin.

Clinical responses (usually partial) have been noted with clonazepam, triazolam, thiamine, steroids, cyclophosphamide, and treatment of the tumor (Luque *et al.*, 1991; Dropcho *et al.*, 1993).

Paraneoplastic cerebellar degeneration with other or no antineuronal antibodies

The cerebellum is a frequent target of paraneoplastic autoimmunity. Most antineuronal antibodies shown in Table 25.2 can associate with syndromes that include cerebellar dysfunction. Of these, the most frequent antibodies include CV2/CRMP5 antibodies (Honnorat *et al.*, 1996; Yu *et al.*, 2001) and antibodies to Ma and Zic proteins (Dalmau *et al.*, 1999b; Rosenfeld *et al.*, 2001; Bataller *et al.*, 2002).

The association of PCD and LEMS has suggested that antibodies to P/Q-type VGCC can be involved in the pathogenesis of some PCD (Mason *et al.*, 1997). This concept is supported by the recent finding of intrathecal synthesis of antibodies to P/Q-type VGCC in patients with PCD, with or without LEMS (Graus *et al.*, 2002).

Paraneoplastic cerebellar dysfunction can occur without identifiable antineuronal antibodies. In this setting, the neoplasms more commonly involved are SCLC and non-Hodgkin's lymphoma.

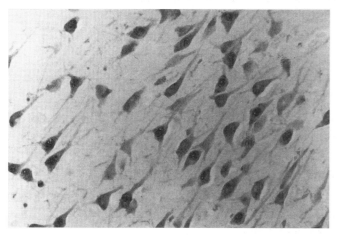

Fig. 25.4 Reactivity of anti-Hu antibodies with a section of cerebral cortex (hippocampus) obtained at autopsy of a neurologically normal individual. Note that the anti-Hu antibodies react predominantly with the nuclei of all neurons.

Paraneoplastic encephalomyelitis

Patients with this disorder develop symptoms of multifocal involvement of the nervous system, which can include dementia (limbic encephalopathy), brainstem encephalopathy, cerebellar dysfunction, myelopathy (lower motor neuron), sensory deficits due to involvement of dorsal root ganglia (DRG), and autonomic dysfunction. The distribution of symptoms as well as the pathological findings along the neuraxis are variable, giving rise to several syndromes that can occur alone or in association. The main pathologic abnormalities include interstitial and perivascular inflammatory infiltrates, neuronal degeneration, lymphocytic neuronophagic nodules (microglial nodules), and gliosis.

In 80% of patients the associated tumor is SCLC, but the disorder has been reported with almost any type of neoplasm. Most patients with paraneoplastic encephalomyelitis (PEM) and SCLC harbor high titers of anti-Hu antibodies in their serum and CSF (Dalmau *et al.*, 1990). Anti-Hu antibodies react with a family of RNA-binding proteins (HuD, Hel-N1, HuC) expressed in the nuclei, and to a lesser degree the cytoplasm of all neurons of the central and peripheral nervous systems and tumor cells (Fig. 25.4) (Szabo *et al.*, 1991; Dropcho and King, 1994). Other antineuronal antibodies associated with PEM or fragments of this disorder (i.e. limbic encephalitis, basal ganglia dysfunction, brainstem encephalitis) are shown in Table 25.2.

Limbic encephalopathy includes the presence of personality changes, irritability, depression, anxiety, sleep disturbances, and short-term memory deficits. Partial complex and general seizures may occur at the presentation. More than two-thirds of patients develop symptoms of involvement of other areas of the nervous system, indicating that the disorder is a fragment of PEM. In this situation, when SCLC is the associated tumor, the anti-Hu antibody is often present in serum and CSF. This antibody however, may be absent in patients with SCLC and 'pure' limbic encephalopathy, and is almost always absent when tumors other than SCLC are involved (Alamowitch *et al.*, 1997; Gultekin *et al.*, 2000). Another antibody associated with paraneoplastic limbic encephalopathy is CV2/CRMP5.

Antibodies to Ma proteins associate with high specificity with focal encephalitis involving the limbic region, hypothalamus, brainstem, and less frequently the cerebellum; the tumors more frequently involved include germ-cell tumors of the testis, and cancers of the lung, ovary, or colon (Rosenfeld *et al.*, 2001).

Symptoms of *cerebellar dysfunction* (see section on Paraneoplastic cerebellar degeneration) may be the presentation of PEM (Dalmau *et al.*, 1992; Lucchinetti *et al.*, 1998; Graus *et al.*, 2001). Patients with SCLC who develop symptoms of pure or predominant cerebellar dysfunction may not harbor anti-Hu antibodies. The detection of anti-Hu antibodies usually predicts that other areas of the nervous system will become involved (Mason *et al.*, 1997).

Autopsies of patients with PEM usually demonstrate inflammatory changes involving the *brainstem*, particularly the medulla (Henson *et al.*, 1965). In a series of patients with anti-Hu-associated PEM and sensory neuronopathy (PSN), symptoms of brainstem encephalopathy were identified in 32% of the patients (Dalmau *et al.*, 1992).

Motor weakness, muscle atrophy, and fasciculations are prominent in 20% of patients with PEM. Although some of these symptoms result from inflammatory involvement of motor nerve roots, the pathologic studies of these patients often demonstrate involvement of the *spinal cord* (myelitis). If spinal cord involvement is the leading and predominant dysfunction, the diagnosis of subacute motor neuron dysfunction (or atypical amyotrophic lateral sclerosis (ALS)) may be entertained until other areas of the nervous system become symptomatic.

Autonomic dysfunction, resulting from involvement of the central and peripheral nervous system, affects about 30% of patients with PEM. Symptoms include orthostatic hypotension, gastrointestinal paresis and pseudo-obstruction, erectile dysfunction, dry mouth, bladder dysfunction, abnormal pupillary responses, and sweating disturbances (Lennon *et al.*, 1991; Condom *et al.*, 1993). SCLC is the neoplasm most commonly involved; other neoplasms include carcinoma of the pancreas (Thomas and Shields, 1970) and carcinoid tumor of the lung (Veilleux et al., 1990). The autonomic dysfunction, including hypoventilation, and cardiac arrhythmias may be the cause of sudden death (Zacharias et al., 1996). Pathologic studies may show involvement of sympathetic and parasympathetic nerves, reticular formation of the medulla oblongata, and locus ceruleus (Veilleux et al., 1990).

About 75% of patients with anti-Hu-associated PEM develop an asymmetric neuropathy, as a result of inflammation of the DRG and neuronal degeneration (see section on Paraneoplastic sensory neuronopathy) (Graus et al., 2001).

Analysis of CSF obtained during the early stages of PEM demonstrates pleocytosis, increased protein concentrations, intrathecal synthesis of IgG, and oligoclonal bands. In patients with anti-Hu-associated paraneoplastic symptoms, tumors other than SCLC are extremely rare, and when detected they express the Hu antigens. If no tumor is detected, periodic (every 6 months) clinical follow-up and CT or PET studies of the chest are recommended.

The CV2/CRMP5 antibodies are also associated with PEM/PSN, chorea and uveitis. The tumors more frequently involved are SCLC and thymoma (Honnorat et al., 1996; Yu et al., 2001). There is recent evidence that antibodies to Zic proteins frequently associate to PEM/PSN and SCLC (Bataller et al., 2002). Some patients harbor several antibodies in their serum and CSF (i.e. anti-Hu, anti-CV2/CRMP5, and anti-Zic antibodies).

Except for the detection of these paraneoplastic antibodies there are no other markers of PEM/PSN, or specific diagnostic tests. MRI of the brain and spinal cord are often normal, but in patients with limbic encephalitis, T_2-weighted images show abnormalities and T_1-weighted images of the medial aspect of the temporal lobes may show foci of contrast enhancement (Dirr et al., 1990). MRI abnormalities appear to be more frequent in patients with antibodies to Ma proteins (Rosenfeld et al., 2001). The prognosis for anti-Hu-associated PEM is poor. Patients with complete tumor response to treatment are more likely to have stabilization or mild improvement of neurologic symptoms than patients with poor tumor response to treatment or untreated patients (Keime-Guibert et al., 1999). Plasma exchange and IV Ig do not modify the course of PEM, which often results in death. Patients with anti-CV2/CRMP5-associated PEM/PSN have a similar prognosis and the treatment approach is as indicated for patients with anti-Hu antibodies. Patients with antibodies against Ma2 proteins may show improvement of neurologic symptoms after prompt treatment of the tumor, steroids, and IV Ig (Rosenfeld et al., 2001).

Paraneoplastic opsoclonus–myoclonus

The opsoclonus–myoclonus syndrome consists of spontaneous, arrhythmic, large-amplitude conjugate saccades occurring in all directions of gaze, often associated with myoclonus of the head, trunk, or extremities (Leigh and Zee, 1991). Opsoclonus–myoclonus may occur as a result of viral, toxic, metabolic, and vascular disorders (Dyken and Kolar, 1968). Paraneoplastic opsoclonus–myoclonus has been described in three clinical settings: pediatric patients with neuroblastoma, adult patients with anti-Ri antibodies, usually female with breast cancer (see section on Paraneoplastic cerebellar degeneration), and adult patients with other tumors, or without anti-Ri antibodies (these patients usually have SCLC). For all these subgroups of paraneoplastic opsoclonus–myoclonus, the pathologic basis of the disorder remains unknown. Pathologic findings vary from mild to severe inflammatory infiltrates involving the brainstem, cerebellum, and leptomeninges; there may also be loss of Purkinje cells (Anderson et al., 1988a).

In children, the clinical features of paraneoplastic opsoclonus–myoclonus are similar to the non-paraneoplastic disorder that often occurs after a viral infection. Symptoms develop acutely and include irritability, vomiting, hypotonia, and ataxia (Dyken and Kolar, 1968). In most pediatric patients, these symptoms lead to the discovery of the neuroblastoma.

Between 2 and 3% of patients with neuroblastoma develop opsoclonus–myoclonus. There are no specific antibodies or markers of this disorder. Treatment with steroids or adrenocorticotropin (ACTH), or treatment of the tumor, results in neurologic improvement in one-half to two-thirds of patients. Symptoms may relapse with steroid withdrawal or during a intercurrent febrile illness. Despite an initial response to steroids or ACTH and treatment of the tumor, about two-thirds of patients are left with sleep and behavioral problems, and psychomotor retardation (Koh et al., 1994; Russo et al., 1997). It has been suggested that the presence of opsoclonus–myoclonus predicts indolent tumor behavior, independently of the age and stage of disease (Altman and Baehner, 1976; Rudnick et al., 2001). Compared with the neuroblastomas of patients without paraneoplastic symptoms, those associated with opsoclonus–myoclonus are more likely to show evidence for maturation to ganglioneuromas and contain fewer copies of N-myc (Cohn et al., 1988; Hiyama et al., 1994).

In adults, paraneoplastic opsoclonus usually develops in association with SCLC, but other tumors can be involved. Except for a subgroup of patients with breast and gynecologic cancers who harbor anti-Ri antibodies (see section on Paraneoplastic cerebellar degeneration), most adult patients with paraneoplastic opsoclonus do not have identifiable serum or CSF antibodies (Anderson et al., 1988a; Bataller et al., 2001). In these patients, the disorder may vary from opsoclonus and mild truncal ataxia to a severe clinical syndrome characterized by opsoclonus, myoclonus, ataxia, and encephalopathy that leads to stupor and death. If the tumor is not treated the neurologic symptoms rarely improve. In addition to treating the tumor, symptoms may respond to steroids and IV Ig (Bataller et al., 2001).

Paraneoplastic retinopathy

The retina can be affected as a paraneoplastic manifestation of carcinoma (cancer-associated retinopathy or CAR) or melanoma (melanoma-associated retinopathy or MAR). Patients with CAR develop subacute visual loss (Buchanan et al., 1984; Thirkill et al., 1989). Symptoms usually precede the diagnosis of the tumor, usually a SCLC, but other tumors have been identified, including gynecologic cancers and breast cancer (Keltner and Thirkill, 1998). Symptoms develop abruptly, first involving one eye, but become bilateral over days or weeks; they include, photosensitivity, light-induced glare, color vision deficits, and intermittent visual obscuration that progress to gradual loss of vision. Ophthalmologic examination demonstrates peripheral and ring-like scotomata, impaired visual acuity and color vision, and narrowing of the retinal arteries (Jacobson et al., 1990). Inflammatory cells in the vitreous can be identified with slit-lamp examination. The visual evoked responses may be normal, but electroretinography demonstrates reduced or flat photopic and scotopic responses, indicating involvement of the photoreceptors. The pathological abnormalities include loss of photoreceptors or less frequently, degeneration of ganglion cells. The inner retinal layers, optic nerves, and visual tracts are usually preserved (Sawyer et al., 1976; Buchanan et al., 1984). The presence of antibodies reacting with several retinal proteins (see Table 25.2) suggests an immune-mediated mechanism of retinal injury. The main retinal autoantigen is recoverin, a 23 kDa photoreceptor calcium-binding protein of the calmodulin family (Polans et al., 1993; Adamus et al., 1997). Other autoantigens of CAR include tubby-like protein 1 and the photoreceptor-specific nuclear receptor (Kikuchi et al., 2000; Eichen et al., 2001). There is experimental evidence that anti-recoverin antibodies cause apoptotic retinal cell death (Adamus et al., 1997).

The melanoma-associated retinopathy (MAR) syndrome affects patients with metastatic cutaneous melanoma (Boeck et al., 1997). Symptoms include acute onset of night blindness and shimmering, flickering, or pulsating photopsias, and often progress to complete visual loss. The electroretinogram demonstrates reduction in the b-wave amplitude. The target autoantigens of MAR antibodies are expressed by the bipolar cells of the retina (Milam et al., 1993).

Although the paraneoplastic retinopathies rarely improve with treatment, there are reports of responses to steroids, plasma exchange, and IV Ig (Keltner and Thirkill, 1998).

Paraneoplastic stiff-man syndrome and muscle rigidity

Stiff-man syndrome is characterized by progressive muscle rigidity and painful spasms that are triggered by different stimuli and can lead to limb deformities and fractures. Muscle stiffness primarily affects the lower trunk and legs, but it can extend to the upper limbs, shoulders, and neck (Moersch and Woltman, 1956). Symptoms improve during sleep and after local or general anesthesia. Electrophysiologic studies demonstrate continuous discharge of motor unit potentials. The tumors more commonly involved include breast cancer and SCLC (Bateman et al., 1990; Folli et al., 1993). An autoimmune basis of the disorder was initially suggested by the identification of antibodies against glutamic acid decarboxylase (GAD) in patients who had non-paraneoplastic stiff-man syndrome (Solimena et al., 1990). More recently, a subset of patients with paraneoplastic stiff-man syndrome and breast cancer were found to harbor antibodies against amphiphysin, a 128 kDa neuronal protein involved in synaptic-vesicle re-uptake and endocytosis (De Camilli et al., 1993; Folli et al., 1993). Antibodies against 125–130 kDa proteins have also been identified in patients with colon carcinoma and Hodgkin's disease (Grimaldi et al., 1993).

In patients with breast cancer, paraneoplastic stiff-man syndrome, and anti-amphiphysin antibodies, treatment of the tumor and steroids may result in neurologic improvement (Folli et al., 1993). The benefit of IV Ig has been demonstrated in patients with stiff-man syndrome and anti-GAD antibodies (Dalakas et al., 2001). Because GAD and amphiphysin are part of GABA/glycine inhibitory synapses and both are located at the pre-synaptic level, the use of IV Ig may also be considered for the paraneoplastic form of the disorder.

Muscle rigidity, myoclonus, and spasms have been reported also in patients with PEM (Whitely et al., 1976; Roobol et al., 1987).

Specific paraneoplastic syndromes of the peripheral nervous system

Paraneoplastic sensory neuronopathy (PSN)

PSN resulting from DRG dysfunction is usually a component of PEM (Dalmau et al., 1992; Graus et al., 2001). About three-quarters of patients with PEM have symptoms of PSN. The typical onset of PSN includes pain and paresthesias asymmetrically involving upper or lower limbs. These symptoms can lead to the misdiagnosis of radiculopathy or multineuropathy. Usually, symptoms progress rapidly (weeks) to involve other extremities and sometimes the face and trunk. Other cranial nerves may be affected, resulting in loss of taste and sensorineural deafness. Eventually, there is severe involvement of all modalities of sensation, which interferes with walking and movement of the extremities. Deep tendon reflexes are asymmetrically decreased or abolished. In more than 70% of patients with PSN, the associated tumor is SCLC (Dalmau et al., 1992; Graus et al., 2001). Sensory symptoms usually precede the diagnosis of the tumor. Electrophysiologic studies demonstrate decreased or abolished somatosensory evoked potentials and action potentials of sensory nerves (Chalk et al., 1992). Motor conduction is usually normal; signs of motor denervation are absent unless there is a concomitant involvement of peripheral nerves or motor neurons of the spinal cord (Graus et al., 1987; Camdessanche et al., 2002).

The pathologic hallmark of PSN is the degeneration of DRG neurons, associated with inflammatory infiltrates, and proliferation of the satellite cells (Nageotte nodules). Inflammatory infiltrates are usually not restricted to DRG, and may be found in other areas of the neuraxis (encephalomyelitis) including the anterior and posterior nerve roots, and peripheral nerves (Graus et al., 2001; Camdessanche et al., 2002).

As occurs with other components of PEM, the detection of anti-Hu antibodies in the serum or CSF should direct the search for a SCLC. Anti-

CV2/CRMP5 antibodies can be found in isolation or in association with anti-Hu antibodies in some patients (Honnorat et al., 1996; Yu et al., 2001).

For those patients with anti-Hu-associated PSN who do not develop other symptoms of CNS dysfunction (about 25% of all patients with anti-Hu-associated PND), immunosuppression may stabilize the disorder or, more rarely, result in improvement (Graus et al., 1994; Oh et al., 1997).

Sensorimotor neuropathies associated with malignant monoclonal gammopathies

Approximately 10% of patients with peripheral neuropathy of unknown origin have a monoclonal gammopathy (M protein). Malignant monoclonal gammopathies include multiple and sclerotic myeloma associated with IgG or IgA monoclonal proteins, and Waldenström's macroglobulinemia, B-cell lymphoma, and chronic B-cell lymphocytic leukemia that are associated with IgM monoclonal proteins.

The main mechanisms by which M proteins can result in neurologic dysfunction include deposition of amyloid in peripheral nerves and specific antibody activity with binding to myelin-associated glycoprotein (MAG) and gangliosides (Nobile-Orazio et al., 1994).

Patients with osteolytic multiple myeloma may develop peripheral neuropathy as a result of compression of nerve roots secondary to involvement of the spine by the disease, amyloid neuropathy, including symptoms of carpal tunnel compression, autonomic dysfunction, and pain, and paraneoplastic dysfunction. The paraneoplastic neuropathy resembles the chronic axonal sensorimotor neuropathy seen in patients with carcinoma. The incidence is 5 to 10%. Treatment of the myeloma does not result in neurologic improvement (Kelly, 1985).

Osteosclerotic myeloma is characterized by a high incidence (50%) of paraneoplastic sensorimotor neuropathy (Kelly et al., 1983). The clinical and electrophysiologic picture resembles a chronic inflammatory demyelinating polyneuropathy (CIDP), with elevated CSF protein concentrations. The serum level of M protein is relatively low, rarely more than 3 g/dl. Patients with osteosclerotic myeloma are younger than those with osteolytic myeloma, have less involvement of the bone marrow, and often have sparing of renal function. Radiologic studies typically show sclerotic lesions (plasmacytomas) in the spine, pelvic bones, and ribs. Treatment of these lesions with resection, radiation, or chemotherapy often results in improvement of the neuropathy.

Patients with osteosclerotic myeloma may develop symptoms included in the POEMS syndrome: Polyneuropathy, Organomegaly (hepatosplenomegaly, lymphadenopathy), Endocrinopathy (gynecomastia, erectile dysfunction, testicular atrophy, low serum testosterone and thyroxine levels, high serum estrogen level, hyperglycemia), M protein, and Skin changes (hirsutism, thickening of the skin, hyperpigmentation) (Miralles et al., 1992). Patients with multicentric Castleman's disease may also develop a POEMS syndrome with a severe sensorimotor neuropathy (Ku et al., 1995; Vingerhoets et al., 1995).

Between 5 and 10% of patients with Waldenström's macroglobulinemia develop a demyelinating sensorimotor neuropathy with marked slowing of nerve conduction velocities. Deposits of IgM antibodies to MAG and other antigens are common in the peripheral nerves of these patients and result in widening the distance between lamellae of myelin sheaths (Vital et al., 1982). Specific treatment of the Waldenström's macroglobulinemia along with plasma exchange may improve this type of neuropathy; other treatments include chlorambucil, cyclophosphamide, fludarabine, and rituximab (Rudnicki and Dalmau, 2000).

Brachial neuritis and acute polyradiculoneuropathy

A few studies suggest an increased incidence of brachial neuritis and acute polyradiculopathy in patients with Hodgkin's and non-Hodgkin's lymphoma (Pezzimenti et al., 1973; Lisak et al., 1977; Lachance et al., 1991; Vallat et al., 1995). The clinical picture of these disorders is similar to those observed in patients without cancer.

Patients with Hodgkin's disease and other histologic tumor types (Plante-Bordeneuve *et al.*, 1994) can develop symptoms that resemble a subacute sensory neuronopathy but these patients usually improve. This disorder is probably a variant of CIDP or a sensory variant of Guillain–Barré syndrome (Oh *et al.*, 1992).

In patients with leukemia or lymphoma, neoplastic infiltration of the peripheral nerves may mimic acute neuritis. While the diagnosis can be made by nerve biopsy or demonstration of malignant cells in the CSF, these studies are often normal (Krendel *et al.*, 1991).

Vasculitis of the nerve and muscle

This disorder is characterized by symmetric or asymmetric sensorimotor deficits, sometimes resembling a multiple mononeuropathy, and often accompanied by pain. Some patients develop proximal muscle weakness. Typically, the erythrocyte sedimentation rate (ESR) is elevated and the CSF protein concentrations are increased. The tumors more commonly involved include SCLC, adenocarcinoma of the lung, prostate, endometrium, and lymphoma (Oh, 1997). Electrophysiologic studies are compatible with an axonal neuropathy, sometimes associated with myopathic changes. Nerve and muscle biopsies show intramural and perivascular infiltrates of CD8+ T cells. Treatment of the tumor, steroids, and cyclophosphamide may result in neurologic improvement.

Peripheral nerve vasculitis may develop in association with PEM and SCLC, and some of these patients harbor anti-Hu or anti-CV2/CRMP5 antibodies (Younger *et al.*, 1994).

Peripheral nerve hyperexcitability (PNH)

This term describes a syndrome characterized by spontaneous and continuous muscle overactivity (Hart *et al.*, 2002). Symptoms of motor nerve hyperexcitability include cramps, muscle twitching (fasciculations and myokymia), stiffness, pseudomyotonia, and pseudotetany. Limb and trunk muscles are predominantly involved, but face and bulbar muscles can be affected. In addition, patients often develop paresthesias, dysesthesias, and numbness indicating hyperexcitability of sensory nerves, and hyperhydrosis suggesting autonomic dysfunction. Electromyography (EMG) may show myokymic discharges (doublet, multiplet motor unit discharges), fasciculations (single spontaneous motor unit discharges), and fibrillations (single spontaneous muscle fiber discharges). Nerve conduction studies occasionally demonstrate a mild axonal or demyelinating neuropathy. Symptoms of PNH can also occur without EMG findings (Hart *et al.*, 2002). Irrespective of EMG findings, PNH results from multiple disorders, including as a paraneoplastic manifestation of cancer. The tumors more frequently involved are thymoma and cancer of the lung (SCLC and non-SCLC) (Walsh, 1976; Garcia-Merino *et al.*, 1991; Newsom-Davis and Mills, 1993).

An immune pathogenesis of PNH is suggested by its frequent association to other immune-mediated disorders (i.e. myasthenia gravis) and the identification of several autoantibodies in patients' sera, mainly those directed against voltage-gated potassium channels (VGKC). These antibodies are identified in more than one-third of patients with paraneoplastic and non-paraneoplastic PNH. Anti-VGKC antibodies contribute to the nerve hyperexcitability by increasing the release of acetylcholine resulting in prolongation of the action potential (Newsom-Davis and Mills, 1993; Shillito *et al.*, 1995). Patients with PNH may harbor acetylcholine receptor (AChR) antibodies with or without myasthenia gravis. Patients with PNH over the age of 40 years who are seropositive for VGKC and AChR antibodies should undergo chest CT or MRI studies to rule out thymoma. Similar studies should be considered in smokers with late-onset PNH to rule out lung cancer. Neurologic symptoms may precede the tumor diagnosis by 4 years.

Symptomatic improvement has been reported with diphenylhydantoin, carbamazepine, and plasma exchange (Newsom-Davis and Mills, 1993).

Some patients with PNH develop symptoms of CNS dysfunction, including psychiatric problems, delusions, and visual hallucinations (Morvan's syndrome). The pathogenic role of VGKC antibodies in the CNS dysfunction is unclear, but these antibodies have been reported in two patients with non-paraneoplastic limbic dysfunction whose symptoms improved with plasma exchange (Buckley *et al.*, 2001).

Polymyositis and dermatomyositis

While most studies agree that there is a statistical association between cancer and dermatomyositis, the association between cancer and polymyositis is weak or questionable (Sigurgeirsson *et al.*, 1992; Hill *et al.*, 2001). The tumors more frequently involved are cancer of the breast, lung, ovary, and gastrointestinal tract. The neurologic symptoms and electrophysiologic findings of these disorders are similar to those associated with the non-paraneoplastic disorders (Dalakas, 1991). Patients develop myalgias and proximal muscle weakness; the flexor muscles of the neck, pharyngeal, and respiratory muscles may also be involved. Dysphagia occurs in at least one-third of the patients. Respiratory muscle weakness may lead to ventilatory failure and contribute to death. The serum creatine kinase level is usually, but not always, elevated. Patients with dermatomyositis develop skin changes that often precede the proximal muscle weakness; these include a purplish discoloration of the eyelids (heliotrope rash) and erythematous lesions over the knuckles.

In patients with dermatomyositis, the muscle biopsy shows varying degrees of mononuclear inflammatory infiltrates that in some patients can be virtually absent. Lymphocytes are mainly found in the interstitial and perivascular areas, with B cells and CD4+ T cells predominating (Engel *et al.*, 1994). A characteristic finding of dermatomyositis is the presence of perifascicular muscle atrophy involving type I and type II fibers, felt to result from endofascicular hypoperfusion (Dalakas, 1995).

An immune-mediated intramuscular angiopathy appears to be involved in the pathogenesis of dermatomyositis. Deposits of IgG and IgM, as well as deposits of complement (including C3, C9, and membrane attack complex) are identified in muscle blood vessels. In patients with polymyositis, however, the endomysial inflammatory infiltrates are mainly composed of CD8+ T cells and macrophages; B cells are less prominent and have a perivascular distribution (Dalakas, 1991; Engel *et al.*, 1994).

The treatment of patients with paraneoplastic polymyositis or dermatomyositis should be primarily directed to the tumor. There are no studies comparing the effects of immunosuppressants in these patients and patients without cancer, and therefore it appears reasonable to use similar strategies. These include, steroids and azathioprine for polymyositis and dermatomyositis, and IV Ig for refractory cases of dermatomyositis (Amato and Barohn, 1997; Dalakas *et al.*, 1993).

Treatment of paraneoplastic neurologic disorders

Removal or treatment of the tumor (the source of the antigen) can be effective for PND of the peripheral nervous system, particularly those involving the neuromuscular junction, such as LEMS (usually associated with SCLC) (Chalk *et al.*, 1990) and myasthenia gravis (associated with thymoma) (Drachman, 1994). Treatment of osteosclerotic myeloma can result in dramatic improvement of the sensorimotor neuropathy associated with this disorder (Kelly *et al.*, 1983). Excluding these disorders, most paraneoplastic peripheral neuropathies do not improve with tumor treatment.

Despite isolated anecdotal reports of PND of the CNS that improved dramatically after treatment of the tumor (Paone and Jeyasingham, 1980; Kearsley *et al.*, 1985), studies with large series of patients have failed to support this. A correlation was found between stabilization of neurologic deficits and complete tumor response to treatment (Keime-Guibert *et al.*, 1999). In addition to treating the tumor, there have been several endeavors to treat the immune response associated with the PND. Table 25.3 summarizes the response of PND to immunosuppressants and treatment of the tumor. For disorders in which no clear responses to any therapy have been identified, efforts should be directed to early diagnosis of the paraneoplastic

Table 25.3 Paraneoplastic disorders: response to therapy.[a] Modified from Rosenfeld and Dalmau (2003)

Type of response	Syndrome	Treatment
Syndromes that often respond to treatment	Lambert–Eaton myasthenic syndrome	3,4-diaminopyridine, IV Ig, plasma exchange, immunosuppression[b]
	Myasthenia gravis	Plasma exchange, IV Ig, immunosuppression[b]
	Dermatomyositis	Immunosuppression,[b] IV Ig
	Opsoclonus-myoclonus (pediatric)	Steroids, IV Ig, ACTH
	Neuropathy (osterosclerotic myeloma)	Radiation, chemotherapy
Syndromes that may respond to treatment	Stiff-man syndrome	IV Ig, steroids, diazepam, baclofen
	Neuromyotonia	Plasma exchange, IV Ig
	Guillain–Barré (Hodgkin's)	Plasma exchange, IV Ig
	Vasculitis of nerve and muscle	Steroids, cyclophosphamide
	Limbic encephalitis	IV Ig, steroids
	Opsoclonus–myoclonus (adults)	Steroids, protein A column, cyclophosphamide
Syndromes that do not usually respond to treatment	Cerebellar degeneration Encephalomyelitis/sensory neuronopathy/autonomic dysfunction	
	Cancer- and melanoma-associated retinopathy	
Syndromes that may improve spontaneously	Cerebellar degeneration (Hodgkin's)	
	Guillain–Barré (Hodgkin's)	
	Lower motor neuropathy (lymphoma)	
	Opsoclonus–myoclonus (pediatric/adult)	

[a]For all PNS initial treatment should focus on detecting and treating the tumor.
[b]Immunosuppression includes steroids, azathioprine or cyclosporine.
IV Ig, intravenous immunoglobulin; ACTH, adrenocorticotropin.

syndrome and, if the clinical condition allows, aggressive immunotherapy. If the deficits are caused by CNS dysfunction and have been established for several months, treatment of the tumor and the best supportive care are the main therapeutic options (Rosenfeld and Dalmau, 2003).

References

Adamus, G., Machnicki, M., and Seigel, G.M. (1997). Apoptotic retinal cell death induced by antirecoverin autoantibodies of cancer-associated retinopathy. *Invest Ophthalmol Vis Sci* **38**: 283–291.

Alamowitch, S., Graus, F., Uchuya, M., Reñé, R., Bescansa, E., and Delattre, J.Y. (1997). Limbic encephalitis and small cell lung cancer—clinical and immunological features. *Brain* **120**: 923–928.

Albert, M.L., Darnell, J.C., Bender, A., Francisco, L.M., Bhardwaj, N., and Darnell, R.B. (1998). Tumor-specific killer cells in paraneoplastic cerebellar degeneration. *Nat Med* **11**: 1321–1324.

Albert, M.L., Austin, L.M., and Darnell, R.B. (2000). Detection and treatment of activated T cells in the cerebrospinal fluid of patients with paraneoplastic cerebellar degeneration. *Ann Neurol* **47**: 9–17.

Altman, A.J. and Baehner, R.L. (1976). Favorable prognosis for survival in children with coincident opso-myoclonus and neuroblastoma. *Cancer* **37**: 846–852.

Amato, A.A. and Barohn, R.J. (1997). Idiopathic inflammatory myopathies. *Neurol Clin* **15**: 615–648.

Anderson, N.E., Budde-Steffen, C., Rosenblum, M.K., Graus, F., Ford, D., Synek, B.J., *et al.* (1988a). Opsoclonus, myoclonus, ataxia, and encephalopathy in adults with cancer: a distinct paraneoplastic syndrome. *Medicine* **67**: 100–109.

Anderson, N.E., Rosenblum, M.K., Graus, F., Wiley, R.G., and Posner, J.B. (1988b). Autoantibodies in paraneoplastic syndromes associated with small-cell lung cancer. *Neurology* **38**: 1391–1398.

Bataller, L., Graus, F., Saiz, A., and Vilchez, J. (2001). Clinical outcome in adult onset idiopathic or paraneoplastic opsoclonus-myoclonus. *Brain* **124**: 437–443.

Bataller, L., Wade, D.F., Rosenfeld, M.R., and Dalmau, J. (2002). Immunity to Zic proteins frequently associates with paraneoplastic neurologic disorders (PND) and predicts small-cell lung cancer. *Ann Neurol* **52**: S80.

Bateman, D.E., Weller, R.O., and Kennedy, P. (1990). Stiff man syndrome: a rare paraneoplastic disorder? *J Neurol Neurosurg Psych* **53**: 695–696.

Benyahia, B., Liblau, R., Merle-Béral, H., Tourani, J.M., Dalmau, J., and Delattre J-Y (1999). Cell-mediated auto-immunity in paraneoplastic neurologic syndromes with anti-Hu antibodies. *Ann Neurol* **45**: 162–167.

Bernal, F., Shamsili, S., Rojas, I., Sanchez-Valle, R., Saiz, A., Dalmau, J., *et al.* (2003). Clinical and immunological features of patients with anti-Tr antibodies. *Neurology* **60**: 230–234.

Boeck, K., Hofmann, S., Klopfer, M., Ian, U., Schmidt, T., Engst, R., *et al.* (1997). Melanoma-associated paraneoplastic retinopathy: case report and review of the literature. *Br J Dermatol* **137**: 457–460.

Brashear, H.R., Caccamo, D.V., Heck, A., and Keeney, P.M. (1991). Localization of antibody in the central nervous system of a patient with paraneoplastic encephalomyeloneuritis. *Neurology* **41**: 1583–1587.

Buchanan, T.A., Gardiner, T.A., and Archer, D.B. (1984). An ultrastructural study of retinal photoreceptor degeneration associated with bronchial carcinoma. *Am J Ophthalmol* **97**: 277–287.

Buckanovich, R.J., Posner, J.B., and Darnell, R.B. (1993). Nova, the paraneoplastic Ri antigen, is homologous to an RNA- binding protein and is specifically expressed in the developing motor system. *Neuron* **11**: 657–672.

Buckley, C., Oger, J., Clover, L., Tuzun, E., Carpenter, K., Jackson, M., *et al.* (2001). Potassium channel antibodies in two patients with reversible limbic encephalitis. *Ann Neurol* **50**: 73–78.

Camdessanche, J.P., Antoine, J.C., Honnorat, J., Vial, C., Petiot, P., Convers, P., *et al.* (2002). Paraneoplastic peripheral neuropathy associated with anti-Hu antibodies. A clinical and electrophysiological study of 20 patients. *Brain* **125**: 166–175.

Chalk, C.H., Murray, N.M., Newsom-Davis, J., O'Neill, J.H., and Spiro, S.G. (1990). Response of the Lambert–Eaton myasthenic syndrome to treatment of associated small-cell lung carcinoma. *Neurology* **40**: 1552–1556.

Chalk, C.H., Windebank, A.J., Kimmel, D.W., and McManis, P.G. (1992). The distinctive clinical features of paraneoplastic sensory neuronopathy. *Can J Neurol Sci* **19**: 346–351.

Chester, K.A., Lang, B., Gill, J., Vincent, A., and Newsom-Davis, J. (1988). Lambert–Eaton syndrome antibodies: reaction with membranes from a small cell lung cancer xenograft. *J Neuroimmunol* **18**: 97–104.

Cohn, S.L., Salwen, H., Herst, C.V., Maurer, H.S., Nieder, M.L., Morgan, E.R., *et al.* (1988). Single copies of the N-myc oncogene in neuroblastomas from children presenting with the syndrome of opsoclonus-myoclonus. *Cancer* **62**: 723–726.

Condom, E., Vidal, A., Rota, R., Graus, F., Dalmau, J., and Ferrer, I. (1993). Paraneoplastic intestinal pseudo-obstruction associated with high titres of Hu autoantibodies. *Virchows Arch A Pathol Anat Histopathol* **423**: 507–511.

Dalakas, M.C. (1991). Polymyositis, dermatomyositis, and inclusion-body myositis. *N Engl J Med* **325**: 1487–1498.

Dalakas, M.C. (1995). Immunopathogenesis of inflammatory myopathies. *Ann Neurol* **37**: S74–S75.

Dalakas, M.C., Illa, I., Dambrosia, J.M., Soueidan, S.A., Stein, D.P., Otero, C., *et al.* (1993). A controlled trial of high-dose intravenous immune globulin infusions as treatment for dermatomyositis. *N Engl J Med* **329**: 1993–2000.

Dalakas, M.C., Fujii, M., Li, M., Lutfi, B., Kyhos, J., and McElroy, B. (2001). High-dose intravenous immune globulin for stiff-person syndrome. *N Engl J Med* **345**: 1870–1876.

Dalmau, J., Furneaux, H.M., Gralla, R.J., Kris, M.G., and Posner, J.B. (1990). Detection of the anti-Hu antibody in the serum of patients with small cell lung cancer-a quantitative Western blot analysis. *Ann Neurol* **27**: 544–552.

Dalmau, J., Graus, F., Rosenblum, M.K., and Posner, J.B. (1992). Anti-Hu-associated paraneoplastic encephalomyelitis/sensory neuronopathy. A clinical study of 71 patients. *Medicine* **71**: 59–72.

Dalmau, J., Graus, F., Cheung, N.K., Rosenblum, M.K., Ho, A., Canete, A., *et al.* (1995). Major histocompatibility proteins, anti-Hu antibodies, and paraneoplastic encephalomyelitis in neuroblastoma and small cell lung cancer. *Cancer* **75**: 99–109.

Dalmau, J., Gultekin, H.S., and Posner, J.B. (1999a). Paraneoplastic neurologic syndromes: pathogenesis and physiopathology. *Brain Pathol* **9**: 275–284.

Dalmau, J., Gultekin, S.H., Voltz, R., Hoard, R., DesChamps, T., Balmaceda, C., *et al.* (1999b). Ma1, a novel neuron- and testis-specific protein, is recognized by the serum of patients with paraneoplastic neurological disorders. *Brain* **122**: 27–39.

De Camilli, P., Thomas, A., Cofiell, R., Folli, F., Lichte, B., Piccolo, G., *et al.* (1993). The synaptic vesicle-associated protein amphiphysin is the 128 kD autoantigen of stiff-man syndrome with breast cancer. *J Exp Med* **178**: 2219–2223.

Dirr, L.Y., Elster, A.D., Donofrio, P.D., and Smith, M. (1990). Evolution of brain MRI abnormalities in limbic encephalitis. *Neurology* **40**: 1304–1306.

Drachman, D.B. (1994). Myasthenia gravis. *N Engl J Med* **330**: 1797–1810.

Dropcho, E.J. and King, P.H. (1994). Autoantibodies against the Hel-N1 RNA-binding protein among patients with lung carcinoma: an association with type I anti- neuronal nuclear antibodies. *Ann Neurol* **36**: 200–205.

Dropcho, E.J., Chen, Y.T., Posner, J.B., and Old, L.J. (1987). Cloning of a brain protein identified by autoantibodies from a patient with paraneoplastic cerebellar degeneration. *Proc Natl Acad Sci USA* **84**: 4552–4556.

Dropcho, E.J., Kline, L.B., and Riser, J. (1993). Antineuronal (anti-Ri). antibodies in a patient with steroid-responsive opsoclonus-myoclonus. *Neurology* **43**: 207–211.

Dyken, P. and Kolar, O. (1968). Dancing eyes, dancing feet: infantile polymyoclonia. *Brain* **91**: 305–320.

Eichen, J.G., Dalmau, J., Demopoulos, A., Wade, D., Posner, J.B., and Rosenfeld, M.R. (2001). The photoreceptor cell-specific nuclear receptor is an autoantigen of paraneoplastic retinopathy. *J Neuroophthalmol* **21**: 168–172.

Engel, A.G., Hohlfeld, R., and Banker, B.Q. (1994). The polymyositis and dermatomyositis syndromes. In: *Myology* (ed. A.G. Engel and C Franzini-Armstrong), pp. 1335–1383. McGraw-Hill, New York.

Fathallah-Shaykh, H., Wolf, S., Wong, E., Posner, J.B., Furneaux, H.M. (1991). Cloning of a leucine-zipper protein recognized by the sera of patients with antibody-associated paraneoplastic cerebellar degeneration. *Proc Natl Acad Sci USA* **88**: 3451–3454.

Folli, F., Solimena, M., Cofiell, R., Austoni, M., Tallini, G., Fassetta, G., *et al.* (1993). Autoantibodies to a 128-kd synaptic protein in three women with the stiff-man syndrome and breast cancer. *N Engl J Med* **328**: 546–551.

Furneaux, H.F., Reich, L., and Posner, J.B. (1990). Autoantibody synthesis in the central nervous system of patients with paraneoplastic syndromes. *Neurology* **40**: 1085–1091.

Garcia-Merino, A., Cabello, A., Mora, J.S., and Liano, H. (1991). Continuous muscle fiber activity, peripheral neuropathy, and thymoma. *Ann Neurol* **29**: 215–218.

Graus, F., Elkon, K.B., Lloberes, P., Ribalta, T., Torres, A., Ussetti, P., *et al.* (1987). Neuronal antinuclear antibody (anti-Hu). in paraneoplastic encephalo-myelitis simulating acute polyneuritis. *Acta Neurol Scand* **75**: 249–252.

Graus, F., Segurado, O.G., and Tolosa, E. (1988). Selective concentration of anti-Purkinje cell antibody in the CSF of two patients with paraneoplastic cerebellar degeneration. *Acta Neurol Scand* **78**: 210–213.

Graus, F., Ribalta, T., Campo, E., Monforte, R., Urbano, A., and Rozman, C. (1990). Immunohistochemical analysis of the immune reaction in the nervous system in paraneoplastic encephalomyelitis. *Neurology* **40**: 219–222.

Graus, F., Illa, I., Agusti, M., Ribalta, T., Cruz-Sanchez, F., and Juarez, C. (1991). Effect of intraventricular injection of an anti-Purkinje cell antibody (anti-Yo) in a guinea pig model. *J Neurol Sci* **106**: 82–87.

Graus, F., Vega, F., Delattre J-Y, Bonaventura, I., Rene, R., Arbaiza, D., *et al.* (1992). Plasmapheresis and antineoplastic treatment in CNS paraneoplastic syndromes with antineuronal autoantibodies. *Neurology* **42**: 536–540.

Graus, F., Bonaventura, I., Uchuya, M., Valls-Sole, J., Rene, R., Leger, J.M., *et al.* (1994). Indolent anti-Hu-associated paraneoplastic sensory neuropathy. *Neurology* **44**: 2258–2261.

Graus, F., Keime-Guibert, F., Rene, R., Benyahia, B., Ribalta, T., Ascaso, C., *et al.* (2001). Anti-Hu-associated paraneoplastic encephalomyelitis: analysis of 200 patients. *Brain* **124**: 1138–1148.

Graus, F., Lang, B., Pozo-Rosich, P., Saiz, A., Casamitjana, R., and Vincent, A. (2002). P/Q type calcium-channel antibodies in paraneoplastic cerebellar degeneration with lung cancer. *Neurology* **59**: 764–766.

Grimaldi, L.M., Martino, G., Braghi, S., Quattrini, A., Furlan, R., Bosi, E., *et al.* (1993). Heterogeneity of autoantibodies in stiff-man syndrome. *Ann Neurol* **34**: 57–64.

Gultekin, S.H., Rosenfeld, M.R., Voltz, R., Eichen, J., Posner, J.B., and Dalmau, J. (2000). Paraneoplastic limbic encephalitis: neurological symptoms, immunological findings and tumour association in 50 patients. *Brain* **123**: 1481–1494.

Hart, I.K., Maddison, P., Newsom-Davis, J., Vincent, A., and Mills, K.R. (2002). Phenotypic variants of autoimmune peripheral nerve hyperexcitability. *Brain* **125**: 1887–1895.

Henson, R.A. and Urich, H.E. (1982). Cortical cerebellar degeneration. In: *Cancer and the Nervous System: the Neurological Manifestations of Systemic Malignant Disease* (ed. R.A. Henson and H.E. Urich), pp. 346–367. Blackwell Scientific, London.

Henson, R.A., Hoffman, H.L., and Urich, H. (1965). Encephalomyelitis with carcinoma. *Brain* **88**: 449–464.

Hill, C.L., Zhang, Y., Sigurgeirsson, B., Pukkala, E., Mellemkjaer, L., Airio, A., *et al.* (2001). Frequency of specific cancer types in dermatomyositis and polymyositis: a population-based study. *Lancet* **357**: 96–100.

Hiyama, E., Yokoyama, T., Ichikawa, T., Hiyama, K., Kobayashi, M., Tanaka, Y., *et al.* (1994). Poor outcome in patients with advanced stage neuroblastoma and coincident opsomyoclonus syndrome. *Cancer* **74**: 1821–1826.

Honnorat, J., Antoine, J.C., Derrington, E., Aguera, M., and Belin, M.F. (1996). Antibodies to a subpopulation of glial cells and a 66 kDa developmental protein in patients with paraneoplastic neurological syndromes. *J Neurol Neurosurg Psych* **61**: 270–278.

Jacobson, D.M., Thirkill, C.E., and Tipping, S.J. (1990). A clinical triad to diagnose paraneoplastic retinopathy. *Ann Neurol* **28**: 162–167.

Jensen, K.B., Dredge, B.K., Stefani, G., Zhong, R., Buckanovich, R.J., Okano, H.J., *et al.* (2000). Nova-1 regulates neuron-specific alternative splicing and is essential for neuronal viability. *Neuron* **25**: 359–371.

Kearsley, J.H., Johnson, P., and Halmagyi, G.M. (1985). Paraneoplastic cerebellar disease. Remission with excision of the primary tumor. *Arch Neurol* **42**: 1208–1210.

Keime-Guibert, F., Graus, F., Broet, P., Rene, R., Molinuevo, J.L., Ascaso, C., *et al.* (1999). Clinical outcome of patients with anti-Hu-associated encephalomyelitis after treatment of the tumor. *Neurology* **53**: 1719–1723.

Kelly, J.J. Jr (1985). Peripheral neuropathies associated with monoclonal proteins: a clinical review. *Muscle Nerve* **8**: 138–150.

Kelly, J.J. Jr, Kyle, R.A., Miles, J.M., Dyck, P.J., *et al.* (1983). Osteosclerotic myeloma and peripheral neuropathy. *Neurology* **33**: 202–210.

Keltner, J.L. and Thirkill, C.E. (1998). Cancer-associated retinopathy vs recoverin-associated retinopathy. *Am J Ophthalmol* **126**: 296–302.

Kikuchi, T., Arai, J., Shibuki, H., Kawashima, H., and Yoshimura, N. (2000). Tubby-like protein 1 as an autoantigen in cancer-associated retinopathy. *J Neuroimmunol* **103**: 26–33.

Koh, P.S., Raffensperger, J.G., Berry, S., Larsen, M.B., Johnstone, H.S., Chou, P., *et al.* (1994). Long-term outcome in children with opsoclonus-myoclonus and ataxia and coincident neuroblastoma. *J Pediatr* **125**: 712–716.

Krendel, D.A., Stahl, R.L., and Chan, W.C. (1991). Lymphomatous polyneuropathy. Biopsy of clinically involved nerve and successful treatment. *Arch Neurol* **48**: 330–332.

Ku, A., Lachmann, E., Tunkel, R., and Nagler, W. (1995). Severe polyneuropathy: initial manifestation of Castleman's disease associated with POEMS syndrome. *Arch Phys Med Rehab* **76**: 692–694.

Lachance, D.H., O'Neill, B.P., Harper, C.M. Jr, Banks, P.M., and Cascino, T.L. (1991). Paraneoplastic brachial plexopathy in a patient with Hodgkin's disease. *Mayo Clin Proc* **66**: 97–101.

Lang, B., Newsom-Davis, J., Wray, D., Vincent, A., and Murray, N. (1981). Autoimmune aetiology for myasthenic (Eaton–Lambert). syndrome. *Lancet* **2**: 224–226.

Leigh, R.J. and Zee D.S.E. (1999). *The Neurology of Eye Movements*, pp. 451–456, F.A. Davis, Philadelphia, PA.

Lennon, V.A., Sas, D.F., Busk, M.F., Scheithauer, B., Malagelada, J.R., Camilleri, M., *et al.* (1991). Enteric neuronal autoantibodies in pseudoobstruction with small-cell lung carcinoma. *Gastroenterology* **100**: 137–142.

Lisak, R.P., Mitchell, M., Zweiman, B., Orrechio, E., and Asbury, A.K. (1977). Guillain–Barre syndrome and Hodgkin's disease: three cases with immunological studies. *Ann Neurol* **1**: 72–78.

Lucchinetti, C.F., Kimmel, D.W., and Lennon, V.A. (1998). Paraneoplastic and oncologic profiles of patients seropositive for type 1 antineuronal nuclear autoantibodies. *Neurology* **50**: 652–657.

Luque, F.A., Furneaux, H.M., Ferziger, R., Rosenblum, M.K., Wray, S.H., Schold, S.C., *et al.* (1991). Anti-Ri: an antibody associated with paraneoplastic opsoclonus and breast cancer. *Ann Neurol* **29**: 241–251.

Mason, W.P., Graus, F., Lang, B., Honnorat, J., Delattre, J.Y., Valldeoriola, F., *et al.* (1997). Small-cell lung cancer, paraneoplastic cerebellar degeneration and the Lambert–Eaton myasthenic syndrome. *Brain* **120**: 1279–1300.

Milam, A.H., Saari, J.C., Jacobson, S.G., Lubinski, W.P., Feun, L.G., and Alexander, K.R. (1993). Autoantibodies against retinal bipolar cells in cutaneous melanoma- associated retinopathy. *Invest Ophthalmol Vis Sci* **34**: 91–100.

Miralles, G.D., O'Fallon, J.R., and Talley, N.J. (1992). Plasma-cell dyscrasia with polyneuropathy. *N Engl J Med* **327**: 1919–1923.

Moersch, F. and Woltman, H. (1956). Progressive fluctuating muscular rigidity and spasm ('stiffman syndrome'): report of a case and some observations in 13 other cases. *Mayo Clin Proc* **31**: 421–427.

Newsom-Davis, J. and Mills, K.R. (1993). Immunological associations of acquired neuromyotonia (Isaac's syndrome). Report of five cases and literature review. *Brain* **116**: 453–469.

Nobile-Orazio, E., Manfredini, E., Carpo, M., Meucci, N., Monaco, S., Ferrari, S., *et al.* (1994). Frequency and clinical correlates of anti-neural IgM antibodies in neuropathy associated with IgM monoclonal gammopathy. *Ann Neurol* **36**: 416–424.

Oh, S.J. (1997). Paraneoplastic vasculitis of the peripheral nervous system. *Neurol Clin* **15**: 849–863.

Oh, S.J., Joy, J.L., and Kuruoglu, R. (1992). 'Chronic sensory demyelinating neuropathy': chronic inflammatory demyelinating polyneuropathy presenting as a pure sensory neuropathy. *J Neurol Neurosurg Psych* **55**: 677–680.

Oh, S.J., Dropcho, E.J., and Claussen, G.C. (1997). Anti-Hu-associated paraneoplastic sensory neuropathy responding to early aggressive immunotherapy: report of two cases and review of literature. *Muscle Nerve* **20**: 1576–1582.

Okano, H.J., Park, W.Y., Corradi, J.P., and Darnell, R.B. (1999). The cytoplasmic Purkinje onconeural antigen cdr2 down-regulates c-Myc function: implications for neuronal and tumor cell survival. *Genes Dev* **13**: 2087–2097.

Paone, J.F. and Jeyasingham, K. (1980). Remission of cerebellar dysfunction after pneumonectomy for bronchogenic carcinoma. *N Engl J Med* **302**: 156.

Peterson, K., Rosenblum, M.K., Kotanides, H., and Posner, J.B. (1992). Paraneoplastic cerebellar degeneration. I. A clinical analysis of 55 anti-Yo antibody-positive patients. *Neurology* **42**: 1931–1937.

Pezzimenti, J.F., Bruckner, H.W., and DeConti, R.C. (1973). Paralytic brachial neuritis in Hodgkin's disease. *Cancer* **31**: 626–632.

Plante-Bordeneuve, V., Baudrimont, M., Gorin, N.C., and Gherardi, R.K. (1994). Subacute sensory neuropathy associated with Hodgkin's disease. *J Neurol Sci* **121**: 155–158.

Polans, A.S., Burton, M.D., Haley, T.L., Crabb, J.W., and Palczewski, K. (1993). Recoverin, but not visinin, is an autoantigen in the human retina identified with a cancer-associated retinopathy. *Invest Ophthalmol Vis Sci* **34**: 81–90.

Posner, J.B. (1995). *Neurologic Complications of Cancer*. F.A. Davis, Philadelphia, PA..

Rees, J.H., Hain, S.F., Johnson, M.R., Hughes, R.A., Costa, D.C., Ell, P.J., *et al.* (2001). The role of [18F]fluoro-2-deoxyglucose-PET scanning in the diagnosis of paraneoplastic neurological disorders. *Brain* **124**: 2223–2231.

Rojas, I., Graus, F., Keime-Guibert, F., Rene, R., Delattre, J.Y., Ramon, J.M., *et al.* (2000) Long-term clinical outcome of paraneoplastic cerebellar degeneration and anti-Yo antibodies. *Neurology* **55**: 713–715.

Roobol, T.H., Kazzaz, B.A., and Vecht, C.J. (1987). Segmental rigidity and spinal myoclonus as a paraneoplastic syndrome. *J Neurol Neurosurg Psych* **50**: 628–631.

Rosenfeld, M.R. and Dalmau, J. (2003) Current therapies for paraneoplastic syndromes. *Curr Treat Options Neurol* **5**: 69–77.

Rosenfeld, M.R., Eichen, J.G., Wade, D.F., Posner, J.B., and Dalmau, J. (2001). Molecular and clinical diversity in paraneoplastic immunity to Ma proteins. *Ann Neurol* **50**: 339–348.

Rudnick, E., Khakoo, Y., Antunes, N.L., Seeger, R.C., Brodeur, G.M., Shimada, H., *et al.* (2001). Opsoclonus-myoclonus-ataxia syndrome in neuroblastoma: clinical outcome and antineuronal antibodies-a report from the Children's Cancer Group Study. *Med Pediatr Oncol* **36**: 612–622.

Rudnicki, S.A. and Dalmau, J. (2000). Paraneoplastic syndromes of the spinal cord, nerve and muscle. *Muscle Nerve* **23**: 1800–1818.

Russo, C., Cohn, S.L., Petruzzi, M.J., and de Alarcon, P.A. (1997). Long-term neurologic outcome in children with opsoclonus-myoclonus associated with neuroblastoma: a report from the Pediatric Oncology Group. *Med Pediatr Oncol* **28**: 284–288.

Sakai, K., Mitchell, D.J., Tsukamoto, T., and Steinman, L. (1990). Isolation of a complementary DNA clone encoding an autoantigen recognized by an anti-neuronal cell antibody from a patient with paraneoplastic cerebellar degeneration. *Ann Neurol* **28**: 692–698.

Sawyer, R.A., Selhorst, J.B., Zimmerman, L.E., and Hoyt, W.F. (1976). Blindness caused by photoreceptor degeneration as a remote effect of cancer. *Am J Ophthalmol* **81**: 606–613.

Shillito, P., Molenaar, P.C., Vincent, A., Leys, K., Zheng, W., van den Berg, R.J., *et al*, (1995). Acquired neuromyotonia: evidence for autoantibodies directed against K+ channels of peripheral nerves. *Ann Neurol* **38**: 714–722.

Sigurgeirsson, B., Lindelof, B., Edhag, O., and Allander, E. (1992). Risk of cancer in patients with dermatomyositis or polymyositis. A population-based study. *New Engl J Med* **326**: 363–367.

Sillevis Smitt, P.A., Manley, G.T., and Posner, J.B. (1995). Immunization with the paraneoplastic encephalomyelitis antigen HuD does not cause neurologic disease in mice. *Neurology* **45**: 1873–1878.

Solimena, M., Folli, F., Aparisi, R., Pozza, G., and De Camilli, P. (1990). Autoantibodies to GABA-ergic neurons and pancreatic beta cells in stiffman syndrome. *N Engl J Med* **322**: 1555–1560.

Szabo, A., Dalmau, J., Manley, G., Rosenfeld, M.R., Wong, E., Henson, J., *et al.* (1991). HuD, a paraneoplastic encephalomyelitis antigen, contains RNA-binding domains and is homologous to Elav and Sex-lethal. *Cell* **67**: 325–333.

Tanaka, K., Tanaka, M., Onodera, O., Igarashi, S., Miyatake, T., and Tsuji, S. (1994). Passive transfer and active immunization with the recombinant leucine-zipper (Yo) protein as an attempt to establish an animal model of paraneoplastic cerebellar degeneration. *J Neurol Sci* **127**: 153–158.

Tanaka, K., Tanaka, M., Inuzuka, T., Nakano, R., and Tsuji, S. (1999). Cytotoxic T lymphocyte-mediated cell death in paraneoplastic sensory neuronopathy with anti-Hu antibody. *J Neurol Sci* **163**: 159–162.

Tanaka, M. and Tanaka, K. (1996). HLA A24 in paraneoplastic cerebellar degeneration with anti-Yo antibody. *Neurology* **47**: 606–607.

Tanaka, M., Tanaka, K., Shinozawa, K., Idezuka, J., and Tsuji, S. (1998). Cytotoxic T cells react with recombinant Yo protein from a patient with paraneoplastic cerebellar degeneration and anti-Yo antibody. *J Neurol Sci* **161**: 88–90.

Thirkill, C.E., Fitzgerald, P., Sergott, R.C., Roth, A.M., Tyler, N.K., and Keltner, J.L. (1989). Cancer-associated retinopathy (CAR syndrome). with antibodies reacting with retinal, optic-nerve, and cancer cells. *New Engl J Med* **321**: 1589–1594.

Thomas, J.P. and Shields, R. (1970). Associated autonomic dysfunction and carcinoma of the pancreas. *Br Med J* **4**: 32.

Trotter, J.L., Hendin, B.A., and Osterland, K. (1976). Cerebellar degeneration with Hodgkin's disease. An immunological study. *Arch Neurol* **33**: 660–661.

Uchuya, M., Graus, F., Vega, F., Reñé, R., and Delattre, J.Y. (1996). Intravenous immunoglobulin treatment in paraneoplastic neurological syndromes with antineuronal autoantibodies. *J Neurol Neurosurg Psych* **60**: 388–392.

Vallat, J.M., De Mascarel, H.A., Bordessoule, D., Jauberteau, M.O., Tabaraud, F., Gelot, A., *et al.* (1995). Non-Hodgkin malignant lymphomas and peripheral neuropathies-13 cases. *Brain* **118**: 1233–1245.

Veilleux, M., Bernier, J.P., and Lamarche, J.B. (1990). Paraneoplastic encephalomyelitis and subacute dysautonomia due to an occult atypical carcinoid tumour of the lung. *Can J Neurol Sci* **17**: 324–328.

Verschuuren, J., Chuang, L., Rosenblum, M.K., Lieberman, F., Pryor, A., Posner, J.B., *et al.* (1996). Inflammatory infiltrates and complete absence of Purkinje cells in anti-Yo-associated paraneoplastic cerebellar degeneration. *Acta Neuropathol* **91**: 519–525.

Vingerhoets, F., Kuntzer, T., Delacretaz, F., Steck, A.J., Knecht, H., Bogousslavsky, J., *et al.*, (1995). Chronic relapsing neuropathy associated with Castleman's disease (angiofollicular lymph node hyperplasia). *Eur Neurol* **35**: 336–340.

Vital, C., Vallat, J.M., Deminiere, C., Loubet, A., and Leboutet, M.J. (1982). Peripheral nerve damage during multiple myeloma and Waldenstrom's macroglobulinemia: an ultrastructural and immunopathologic study. *Cancer* **50**: 1491–1497.

Voltz, R., Dalmau, J., Posner, J.B., and Rosenfeld, M.R. (1998). T-cell receptor analysis in anti-Hu associated paraneoplastic encephalomyelitis. *Neurology* **51**: 1146–1150.

Walsh, J.C. (1976). Neuromyotonia: an unusual presentation of intrathoracic malignancy. *J Neurol Neurosurg Psych* **39**: 1086–1091.

Wanschitz, J., Hainfellner, J.A., Kristoferitsch, W., Drlicek, M., and Budka, H. (1997). Ganglionitis in paraneoplastic subacute sensory neuronopathy: a morphologic study. *Neurology* **49**: 1156–1159.

Whitely, A.M., Swash, M., and Urich, H. (1976). Progressive encephalomyelitis with rigidity. *Brain* **99**: 27–42.

Yang, Y.Y., Yin, G.L., and Darnell, R.B. (1998). The neuronal RNA-binding protein Nova-2 is implicated as the autoantigen targeted in POMA patients with dementia. *Proc Natl Acad Sci USA* **95**: 13254–13259.

Younger, D.S., Dalmau, J., Inghirami, G., Sherman, W.H., and Hays, A.P. (1994). Anti-Hu-associated peripheral nerve and muscle microvasculitis. *Neurology* **44**: 181–183.

Yu, Z., Kryzer, T.J., Griesmann, G.E., Kim K-K, Benarroch, E.E., and Lennon, V.A. (2001). CRMP-5 neuronal autoantibody: marker of lung cancer and thymoma-related autoimmunity. *Ann Neurol* **49**: 146–154.

Zacharias, A.S., Brashear, H.R., Munoz, E.L., Alexander, B., and Gimple, L.W. (1996). Paraneoplastic encephalomyeloneuritis obscured by coma. *Neurology* **46**: 1177–1179.

26 Neuropathies associated with monoclonal gammopathy

Susanne Renaud, Andreas Steck, and Norman Latov

Introduction

The presence of a monoclonal gammopathy in a patient with neuropathy can be an important clue to its pathogenesis. Testing for a monoclonal protein (also called paraprotein or M-protein), has become an essential part of the evaluation of a neuropathy. Both the monoclonal gammopathies and the neuropathies are heterogeneous, but several distinct syndromes have been identified. These have traditionally been classified according to the clinical presentation, pathology, and type of monoclonal gammopathy. In the case of immunglobulin (Ig) M monoclonal gammopathies, the importance of the antigenic specificity of the IgM paraproteins is increasingly being recognized. In this chapter we review what is known about the clinical, laboratory, immunological, and pathological features of this group of disorders, and discuss their management and therapy.

Classification of the monoclonal gammopathies

Monoclonal gammopathies are a group of disorders (Table 26.1) characterized by proliferation of one or a limited number of clones of plasma cells or their B-cell precursors, associated with a production of excessive quantities of monoclonal immunoglobulins of the IgG, IgA, IgM, IgD, or IgE isotype, or their constituent heavy or light chains. A circulating monoclonal immunoglobulin is found in approximately 10% of patients with peripheral neuropathies of otherwise unknown etiology, as compared with 1% of the general adult population (Kelly et al., 1981b). However, this prevalence increases with age, reaching 3 to 6% in subjects that are 70 years or older when measured by cellulose acetate electrophoresis, or approximately 10% when measured by the more sensitive immunofixation technique (Axelsson et al., 1966; Kyle et al., 1972; Saleun et al., 1982).

Table 26.1 Classification of plasma cell dyscrasias

IgG, IgA monoclonal gammopathies	Multiple myeloma
	Osteosclerotic myeloma
	Non-malignant IgG monoclonal gammopathy, or monoclonal gammopathy of undetermined significance (MGUS)
IgM monoclonal gammopathies	Waldenström's macroglobulinemia or B-cell lymphoma or leukemia
	Non-malignant IgM monoclonal gammopathy or IgM MGUS
Biclonal gammopathies	
Cryoglobulinemias	
Amyloidosis	

Table 26.2 Characteristics of non-malignant monoclonal gammopathy (MGUS)

Common monoclonal type	IgG, IgM
Common light chain	kappa
M-protein concentration	<25 g/l
Urine monoclonal	Rare
Bone marrow infiltration	<5%
Skeletal lesions	Absent
Complete blood count	Normal
Organomegaly	Absent

In most patients the monoclonal gammopathies are associated with non-malignant or 'benign' lymphoproliferative disorders. These have been called monoclonal gammopathies of undetermined significance (MGUS), as they sometimes progress to malignancy (Kyle, 1978), but the term 'non-malignant' is preferred, as the monoclonal gammopathy is significant for the neuropathy. The characteristics of MGUS are listed in Table 26.2. Whereas IgG is the most common class of paraprotein in patients with MGUS, IgM is more frequent in those with neuropathy (60%) followed by IgG (30%) and IgA (10%). The risk of progression of MGUS to a malignant plasma cell disorder is approximately 1% per year (Kyle et al., 2002), although that may be less for those cases detected by the more sensitive immunofixation technique. At presentation, it is clearly important to exclude a malignant lymphoproliferative disorder if a paraprotein is found.

Historical perspective

In 1931 Neel reported an absence of myelin in the peripheral nerves of a patient with multiple myeloma (Neel, 1931), and in 1938 De Navasquez and Treble first reported peripheral nerve involvement in amyloidosis (De Navasquez and Treble, 1938). The first case of peripheral neuropathy with macroglobulinemia was probably reported by Bing and Neel (1936). Following the characterization of immunoglobulin isotypes, fully documented cases of Waldenström's macroglobulinemia or multiple myeloma in association with polyneuropathy were first reported in 1958 (Garcin et al., 1958; Victor et al., 1958). The first case of neuropathy and non-malignant IgG monoclonal gammopathy was described by Chazot et al. (1976). Subsequent studies, analysing large series of patients, attempted to more specifically define the types of pathologic alterations associated with the various plasma cell dyscrasias. A significant association between polyneuropathy and monoclonal gammopathy was noted by Kelly et al. (1981a), but the evidence linking plasma cell disorders to specific neurological diseases remained circumstantial. In the 1980s our understanding of the neurological manifestation of monoclonal gammopathies was considerably advanced by two major observations: (1) that monoclonal proteins have functional antibody activity and (2) that distinct clinical syndromes are associated with particular antibody specificities (Latov et al., 1980; Steck et al., 1987). The pathogenicity of these antibodies was convincingly demonstrated in passive transfer experiments, where neuropathy was induced in experimental animals by systemic administration of monoclonal IgM antibodies with anti-MAG activity from a patient with neuropathy (Hays et al., 1987; Tatum 1993).

Neuropathies associated with IgM monoclonal gammopathies

Epidemiology

The prevalence of neuropathy in patients with IgM monoclonal gammopathy has been reported to be between 5 and 31%, with the higher prevalence found in patients who had undergone neurological evaluation and the lower derived from reviews of hospital records (Kyle and Garton, 1987; Nobile-Orazio et al., 1992). The M-proteins in most of the patients with neuropathy react with oligosaccharide determinants of glycolipids and glycoproteins that are concentrated in the peripheral nerves. In one study of 112 patients (Caudie et al., 2001), 72% of the IgM M-proteins exhibited antinerve antibody activity; in 52% of cases they were directed at the myelin-associated glycoprotein (MAG) or its cross-reactive glycolipids sulfoglucuronyl paragloboside (SGPG) and sulfoglucuronyl lactosaminyl paragloboside (SGLPG), in 26% at sulfatide, and in 22% they reacted with gangliosides. Anti-GM1 ganglioside antibodies were present in 8% of patients, antidisialosyl ganglioside antibodies in 7%, anti-GM2 ganglioside in 2.5%, and anti-GD1a ganglioside in 2%. In other isolated cases the monoclonal IgMs have been reported to react with chondroitin or heparan sulfates (Briani et al., 1998, 2000), phospholipids (Suzuki et al., 2001), or mixtures of phospholipids and gangliosides (Freddo et al., 1986).

Origins of monoclonal IgM gammopathies

Monoclonal B cells that express anti-MAG and other oligosaccharide antibodies most likely arise by transformation of single clones of B cells that express these antibodies. This may occur spontaneously in the course of an immune response to a foreign antigen, or as a consequence of viral infection. The monoclonal B cells are thought to belong to the CD5+ or B1 B-cell population, which provide an early defense against invading micro-organisms (Lee et al., 1991; Fagarasan and Honjo 2000). These B cells might be activated by T-cell independent mechanisms, such as by bacterial lipopolysaccharides, but could also be stimulated by T cells in an antigen-driven response (Latov et al., 1985). Accordingly cross-reactivity of anti-MAG antibodies with bacterial epitopes has been described (Brouet et al., 1994), and monoclonal anti-GM1 antibodies have been shown to bind to Campylobacter jejuni lipopolysaccharides (Wirguin et al., 1994). In the case of anti-MAG antibodies, the immunoglobulin-encoding genes are somatically mutated, as occurs in an antigen-driven response, but the extent of mutation is limited (Spatz et al., 1992). The antibodies have low intrinsic affinities, but their apparent affinities and binding activity is increased to the pathogenic range by the multivalent nature of the IgM molecule (Ogino et al., 1994).

Demyelinating neuropathy and anti-MAG antibodies

In approximately half of the patients with IgM monoclonal gammopathy, the monoclonal antibody reacts with the myelin-associated glycoprotein (MAG) (Kelly et al., 1988). The prevalence of this neuropathy has been estimated at 1–5 per 10 000 adults (Latov et al., 1988) and in some studies, there is a seven-fold excess of men over women (Latov et al., 1988; Nobile-Orazio et al., 1994; Ellie et al., 1996). The onset of disease has been reported as early as in the 30s, but more typically occurs in the sixth or seventh decades.

Clinical presentation

Patients with anti-MAG antibody-associated polyneuropathy typically present with a distal and symmetric predominately sensory neuropathy. It usually begins with numbness and paresthesia in the feet, with an unsteady gait, and rarely with weakness. The onset is insidious and the disease is slowly progressive over years or decades. In time patients can become severely debilitated, and in advanced cases there can be profound weakness, sensory loss, and gait ataxia. On examination, the ankle jerks are absent, and there is a distally pronounced and symmetric sensory deficiency of large and small fibre sensory modalities, with ataxia and positive Romberg testing (Steck et al., 1983; Smith et al., 1983; Hafler et al., 1986). An intention tremor can be present, with an irregular, large-amplitude and low-frequency wave pattern varying between 2.0 and 7.5 Hz (Pedersen et al., 1997).

Laboratory findings include elevated protein concentration with normal cell count in the cerebrospinal fluid (CSF), and the presence of monoclonal IgM and of anti-MAG antibodies. IgM reactivity can be demonstrated by enzyme-linked immunosorbent assay (ELISA) testing for anti-MAG or SGPG activity, although Western blot using MAG is more reliable (Steck 1983 et al.; van den Berg et al., 1996). Antibody reactivity to MAG may be detected in the absence of a monoclonal gammopathy if the M-protein concentration is low (Gabriel et al., 1998). Waldenström's macroglobulinemia is present in 20–35% of cases at time of presentation (Latov, 2000).

The electrophysiological findings generally indicate a predominantly demyelinating neuropathy, and in 90% of patients the motor peroneal conduction velocity is less than 35 m/s (Nobile-Orazio et al., 1994). There is a marked distal accentuation of conduction slowing, with 76% of nerves from patients with IgM anti-MAG antibodies having a terminal latency index of ≤0.25, as compared with 6% of nerves from patients with Charcot–Marie–Tooth disease type IA or chronic inflammatory demyelinating polyneuropathy. Other parameters such as the modified F ratio or the residual latency have also been suggested to distinguish anti-MAG-associated polyneuropathy from chronic inflammatory demyelinating polyneuropathy (CIDP) (Kaku et al., 1994; Cocito et al., 2001; Trojaborg et al., 1995; Attarian et al., 2001; Radziwill et al.; 2001, Katz et al., 2000).

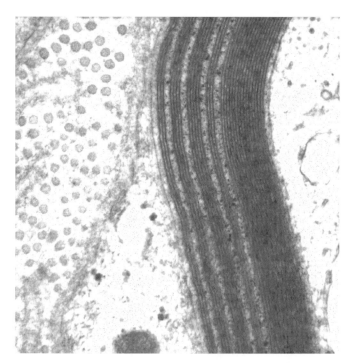

Fig. 26.1 Widened myelin layers detected in the sural nerve biopsy from a 47-year-old patient with anti-MAG neuropathy. Electron micrograph, primary magnification ×12 000. (Picture from Professor A. Probst, Neuropathology, University Hospital Basel, Switzerland.)

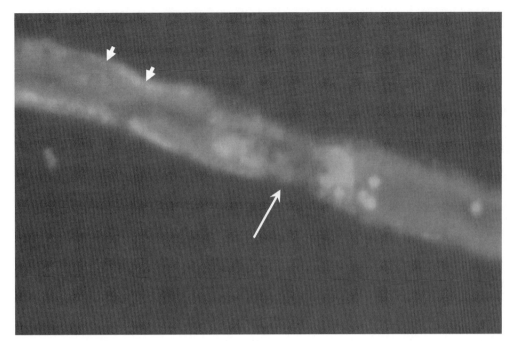

Fig. 26.2 Confocal microscopic picture of a myelinated fiber of a sural nerve biopsy from a 63-year-old patient with anti-MAG neuropathy. Red fluorescence shows the compact myelin detected by an antibody against protein zero (P_O). Green fluorescence shows the accumulation of IgM deposits. Note the IgM deposits at the node of Ranvier (arrow) and along the fiber (arrowheads). The thickness of the fiber is approximately 8 μm. (See also Plate 6 of the colour plate section at the center of this book.)

Histology

Morphological studies of sural nerve biopsy specimen show a loss of myelinated fibers, and on ultrastructural examination there are thinned myelin sheaths and variable number of fibers with widely spaced myelin lamellae (Fig. 26.1) (Vital *et al.*, 1989; Jacobs and Scadding, 1990, Ellie *et al.*, 1996), resulting from separation of the two leaflets of the intermediate, or minor dense line, by electron-lucent material (King and Thomas, 1984). The gap between these two leaflets was measured as 22–23 nm, and the separate membranes were shown to maintain their normal relationship with the major dense line. This morphological alteration is characteristic for anti-MAG neuropathy, although it is only seen in a minority of fibers in routine nerve biopsy specimens. In one study, however, widening of myelin lamellae could be shown in all eight cases of peripheral neuropathy and Waldenström macroglobulinemia with anti-MAG activity (Vital *et al.*, 1997). The widening usually occurs at the outermost myelin lamellae, but occasionally can be seen in the middle of the compact myelin sheath. Deposits of the IgM antibodies can be seen at the periphery of myelinated fibers (Jacobs and Scadding, 1990), and with confocal microscopy, at sites of uncompacted myelin, in Schmidt–Lanterman incisures and paranodal loops (Gabriel *et al.*, 1998) (Fig. 26.2). At these sites the IgM deposits appeared to be co-localized with MAG, and with collagen IV in the basal lamina of myelinated but not unmyelinated fibers, suggesting that anti-MAG IgM antibodies gain access to the myelin sheaths at the nodes of Ranvier and Schmidt–Lanterman incisures. Old, but not young, transgenic mice with disrupted MAG genes appear to develop similar clinical and pathologic features as patients with anti-MAG neuropathy (Fruttiger *et al.*, 1995), indicating that the absence of MAG, or interference with its function, can lead to myelin instability.

Antibody specificity and cross-reactivity

Anti-MAG antibodies react with oligosaccharides that bear terminal sulphated glucuronic acid epitopes, similarly to the mouse monoclonal antibody HNK-1. Many of the anti-MAG antibodies cross-react with other glycolipids and glycoproteins that bear the HNK-1 epitope, including the myelin glycoproteins P0 and PMP-22, and the glycolipids SGPG and SGLPG which are present in both myelin and axons in peripheral nerve (Burger *et al.*, 1990; van den Berg *et al.*, 1996; Weiss *et al.*, 1999). However, some of the anti-MAG antibodies react with MAG alone, and others to SGPG alone. Two patients have been described with predominantly motor neuropathy and highly elevated antibodies to SGPG, which reacted with MAG by Western blot but not by ELISA (van den Berg *et al.*, 1996). Another patient with anti-SGPG antibodies

had motor neuron disease (Rowland *et al.*, 1995). The cross-reactivities might explain some of the clinical heterogeneity of the neuropathic syndromes associated with anti-MAG or SGPG antibodies (Quarles and Weiss, 1999). There are also considerable variations in antibody binding strength to MAG between PNS myelin and CNS myelin. It is unclear what role this differences play in pathogenesis (Fluri *et al.*, 2003).

Pathogenesis

In patients with IgM monoclonal gammopathies that react with MAG, the neuropathy is thought to be caused by the monoclonal antibodies because:

(1) there is a close association between the presence of the antibody and development of peripheral neuropathy, with the antibodies heralding the neuropathy in some cases (Meucci *et al.*, 1999);

(2) there is an associated characteristic clinical syndrome, and with typical electrophysiologic and pathological changes;

(3) M-protein deposits can be demonstrated on affected myelin sheaths and in association with widened myelin lamellae (Takatsu *et al.*, 1985; Vital *et al.*, 1989, Jacobs and Scadding 1990, Ellie *et al.*, 1996, Gabriel *et al.*, 1998);

(4) passive transfer of the antibodies into experimental animals has been shown to induce neuropathy, with the characteristic widened myelin lamellae (Hays *et al.*, 1987; Tatum 1993); and

(5) therapeutic reduction of the autoantibody concentration results in clinical improvement (Kelly *et al.*, 1988; Renaud *et al.*, 2003).

The antibodies are thought to cause neuropathy by complement fixation (Monaco *et al.*, 1995), disruption of myelin compaction (Mendell *et al.*, 1985), or selective loss of MAG from peripheral nerve myelin (Gabriel *et al.*, 1996). Of interest, is that endoneurial macrophages are not increased in comparison with other types of neuropathy, probably due to the absence of Fc-mediated macrophage activation by IgMs (Rosoklija *et al.*, 2000).

Motor neuropathy with monoclonal IgM reactivity to gangliosides GM1 or GD1a

GM1 ganglioside

Anti-GM1 antibodies are associated with chronic neuropathies that affect the motor nerves. Monoclonal IgM anti-GM1 antibodies were first reported in patients with IgM monoclonal gammopathy and lower motor neuron disease (Freddo *et al.*, 1986; Nardelli *et al.*, 1988), and polyclonal IgM anti-GM1 antibodies were later reported in patients with motor neuropathy and multifocal conduction blocks (Pestronk *et al.*, 1988). IgM anti-GM1 antibodies occur in approximately 50% of patients with multifocal motor neuropathy, with approximately 10% of the antibodies occurring as monoclonal gammopathies (Kinsella *et al.*, 1994; Carpo *et al.*, 1999; Pestronk *et al.*, 2000). It is likely that the lower motor neuron syndromes and multifocal motor neuropathies represent a continuum, with the clinical presentation dependent on the distribution of lesions in the proximal or distal motor nerves (Adams *et al.*, 1993). These chronic syndromes are distinguished from the acute motor axonal neuropathy (AMAN) variant of the Guillain–Barré syndrome, which is associated with polyclonal IgG anti-GM1 antibodies (Yuki *et al.*, 1990).

Most anti-GM1 antibodies react with the Gal(β1–3)GalNac determinant that is shared by asialo GM1 and the ganglioside GD1b (Ilyas *et al.*, 1988*a*), but some bind to GM1 alone, or to GM1 and GM2. Anti-GM1 antibodies have been shown to bind to the surface of motor neurons, the nodes of Ranvier, and at the neuromuscular junction, where they may exert their effects (Corbo *et al.*, 1992; Adams *et al.*, 1993; Sheik *et al.*, 1999). The antibodies have been shown to induce conduction block, the electrophysiological hallmark of MMN, in several, but not in all *in vivo* or *in vitro* models (Arasaki *et al.*1993; Uncini *et al.*, 1993; Harvey *et al.*, 1995). Immunization of rabbits with GM1 results in the production of GM1 antibodies and development of axonal neuropathy (Thomas *et al.*, 1991; Yuki *et al.*, 2001). Detection of anti-GM1 antibodies is useful for identifying patients with multifocal motor neuropathy and distinguishing them from those with motor neuron disease or chronic inflammatory demyelinating polyneuropathy.

GD1a ganglioside

Monoclonal IgM anti-GD1a antibodies are most often associated with motor (Bollensen *et al.*, 1989; Carpo *et al.*, 1996; Oga *et al.*, 1998) and occasionally sensorimotor neuropathy (Mizutani *et al.*, 2001). The IgM from two such patients cross-reacted with GM3, GT1b, or GM4. In one, there was cross-reactivity with GM2 (Oga *et al.*, 1998). The corresponding IgG anti-GD1a antibodies are typically associated with acute motor axonal neuropathy, particularly following infection with *Campylobacter jejuni* (Ho *et al.*, 1999; Ogawara *et al.*, 2000). Anti-GD1a antibodies have been shown to bind to the nodes of Ranvier in motor nerves (De Angelis *et al.*, 2001; Gong *et al.*, 2002).

Sensory ataxic neuropathy or CANOMAD, associated with antidisialosyl ganglioside antibodies

Monoclonal IgM antidisialosyl ganglioside antibodies are typically associated with an ataxic sensory neuropathy, sometimes presenting with CANOMAD, which is an acronym encompassing Chronic Ataxic Neuropathy, Ophthalmoplegia, M-protein, Agglutination, and Disialosyl antibodies. In this syndrome, the IgMs react with the disialosyl epitope that is shared by the gangliosides GD1b, GQ1b, GT1c, and GD3. This form of sensory ataxic neuropathy (SAN), occasionally with ophthalmoplegia or bulbar signs, affects large sensory fibers and is characterized by distal paresthesias, numbness, prominent ataxia, areflexia, and mild or no limb weakness. The neuropathy is usually chronic and slowly progressive, but can also have a relapsing course. Clinical electrophysiology and nerve biopsy show both demyelinating and axonal features. A partial response to intravenous immunoglobulin and other treatments is reported in some cases (Ilyas *et al.*, 1985; Dalakas and Quarles, 1996; Oka *et al.*, 1996; O'Leary and Willison, 1997; Willison *et al.*, 2001).

In contrast to the chronic neuropathy which is associated with IgM autoantibodies, IgG antibodies to disialosyl epitopes, including GD1b and GQ1b, are associated with the Miller–Fisher syndrome, or acute ataxic neuropathy with ophthalmoplegia (Odaka *et al.*, 2001; Susuki *et al.*, 2001). Anti-GD1b antibodies have been reported to bind to the surface of sensory ganglion neurons, as well as to paranodal myelin in ventral and dorsal roots

(Kusunoki *et al.*, 1997; Oka *et al.*, 1996; Gong *et al.*, 2002), and anti-GQ1b antibodies bind to human oculomotor, trochlear, and abducens nerve (Chiba *et al.*, 1993), consistent with the clinical syndrome. Immunization with GD1b has been reported to induce an ataxic sensory neuropathy in rabbits (Kusunoki *et al.*,1996).

Sensory neuropathy and IgM antisulfatide antibodies

IgM monoclonal antibodies against sulfatides have been reported in patients with sensory or predominantly sensory neuropathy. Both axonal and demyelinating neuropathies have been described (Pestronk *et al.*, 1991; van den Berg *et al.*, 1993; Dabby *et al.*, 2000; Erb *et al.*, 2000). The antibodies are most often polyclonal, but also occur as IgM monoclonal gammopathies, except in the small fiber neuropathies where they are invariably polyclonal (Dabby *et al.*, 2000). Some antisulfatide antibodies cross-react with MAG, P0, or chondroitin sulfate A and C (Pestronk *et al.*, 1991; Ilyas *et al.*, 1992). Passive transfer of antisulfatide antibodies into rabbit, or immunization with sulfatide in guinea pigs, has resulted in experimental neuropathy (Nardelli 1995 *et al.*; Qin and Guan, 1997). Antisulfatide antibodies have been shown to bind to the surface of sensory ganglia neurons and to compact myelin (Pestronk *et al.*, 1991; Quattrini *et al.*, 1992), where they may exert their effects.

Neuropathy with monoclonal IgM anti-GM2 ganglioside antibodies

Monoclonal IgM Antibodies to GM2 are most frequently associated with chronic motor neuropathies (Nakao *et al.*, 1993; Cavanna *et al.*, 1999; Ortiz *et al.*, 2001) but have also been reported in chronic sensory neuropathy (Lopate *et al.*, 2002). They are frequently directed at the terminal trisaccharide moiety GalNAc(β1–4)Gal(α2–3)NeuAc, and cross-react with GalNac-GD1a (Nakao *et al.*, 1993; Ilyas *et al.*, 1988*b*; Cavanna *et al.*, 1999; O'Hanlon *et al.*, 2000; Ortiz *et al.*, 2001; Lopate *et al.*, 2002), but may also react with GM1, GD1a, or GD1b (Cavanna *et al.*, 1999).

Neuropathy with monoclonal IgM antichondroitin and heparan sulfate

Chondroitin sulfates and heparan sulfates are sulfated glycosaminoglycans. They are a major constituent of the extracellular matrix and plasma membranes. Antibodies to chondroitin sulfate and heparan sulfate have been reported in patients with axonal neuropathies (Sherman *et al.*, 1983; Nobile-Orazio *et al.*, 1994), but more recent studies have reported the presence of such antibodies in other diseases (Briani *et al.*, 1998, 2000, 2002). Hence, the pathogenetic role of these antibodies remains to be elucidated.

Therapy of neuropathy with IgM monocloal gammopathy

Therapy in patients with neuropathy and IgM monoclonal gammopathy is directed at reducing the antibody concentration, blocking the effector mechanisms, and depleting the monoclonal B cells. Therapeutic agents include chemotherapeutic medications, plasmapheresis, or intravenous gammaglobulins (IV Ig), alone or in combination. Therapy in specific cases depends on the neurological presentation and presence of malignancy. Although there is no correlation between antibody titer and severity of the neuropathy (Nobile-Orazio *et al.*, 1994), the IgM concentration or titers, when followed serially, may correlate with the clinical status of individual cases (Kelly *et al.*, 1988; Nobile-Orazio *et al.*, 1988; Ernerudh *et al.*, 1992). When aiming to reduce the monoclonal antibody concentration, a reduction of 50% or more for a period of at least 3 months has been suggested to constitute an adequate trial (Kelly *et al.*, 1988).

None of the currently available therapies completely eliminates the monoclonal antibodies or B cells, so that maintenance or repeat treatments are required to keep the antibody concentrations low. Although early treatment is preferred in order to prevent progression, the potential benefits and risks of chemotherapeutic agents have to be weighed in individual patients (Nobile-Orazio *et al.*, 2000). The recent availability of rituximab, a monoclonal antibody that is not myelosuppressive and does not cause secondary malignancies, would allow for earlier intervention.

Rituximab

Rituximab is a chimerical monoclonal antibody used in the treatment of B-cell malignancies, which binds to the CD20 antigen that is variably present on normal and monoclonal B-lymphocytes (Leo *et al.*, 1992; Byrd *et al.*, 1999). In one study, it was shown to be present on approximately 50% of the idiotype positive monoclonal B cells in a patient with anti-MAG neuropathy (Lee *et al.*, 1991). Rituximab induces antibody-dependent cell- and complement-mediated cytotoxicity, and reduces peripheral B-lymphocyte counts by almost 90% within 3 days (Onrust *et al.*, 1999). In one large retrospective series of 30 patients with macroglobulinemia, 27% and 33% of the patients achieved a partial or minor response, respectively, and 30% of patients stabilized (Treon *et al.*, 2001). In another recent study, which included three patients with neuropathy, 44% of the patients achieved a partial response. One of the patients, with a severe demyelinating polyneuropathy, improved, and the other two stabilized (Dimopoulos *et al.*, 2002). In the latter study, patients were administered 375 mg/m^2 of rituximab by intravenous infusion weekly for four consecutive weeks, which was repeated after 3 months. Adverse effects included fever and chills during the first infusion, or infectious episodes of herpes zoster, erysipelas, bronchitis, or urinary tract infection (Dimopoulos *et al.*, 2002).

In a recent phase II, 12 month, pilot study of rituximab in nine patients with anti-MAG neuropathy who were resistant to other therapies, there was clinical improvement of the neuropathy in six of the nine patients, and

seven had improved nerve conduction studies. These findings were accompanied by laboratory evidence of reduction of B cells, anti-MAG antibodies, and total IgM. The treatment was well tolerated and no serious side-effects were observed (Renaud *et al.*, 2003).

Rituximab remains active in the circulation for 6–9 months, and repeated therapy is required to maintain a response (Fig. 26.3). Studies in patients with lymphoma have shown that a second course of treatment with rituximab can be safe and effective (Davis *et al.*, 2000). One of our own patients with anti-MAG neuropathy has been treated with rituximab every 6 months for 5 years, with gradual reduction and stabilization the serum IgM to 20% of the original value, and sustained improvement in the neuropathy. A prospective long-term trial of rituximab in patients with neuropathy and monoclonal gammopathy is warranted.

A recent modification to rituximab is the addition of radioactive tags, making the antibody more effective, but also with more potential adverse effects. These include ^{131}I-tositumomab and ^{90}Y-ibritumomab tuixetan, which have been approved for the treatment of lymphoma, and are under investigation for the treatment of Waldenström's macroglobulinemia (Dillman, 2002). These agents might also be useful in the treatment of neuropathies that are associated with IgM monoclonal gammopathies that are refractory to rituximab.

Chemotherapeutic agents

Chemotherapy has traditionally been used to reduce the B-cell load and antibody production in patients with neuropathy and Waldenström's macroglobulinemia or non-malignant monoclonal gammopathy. It can be used alone, or in combination, in patients who cannot tolerate or are non-responsive to rituximab. The most commonly used chemotherapeutic agent is chlorambucil, an alkylating agent with a response rate of 50% (Dimopoulos and Alexian, 1994a). In IgM-associated neuropathies it was

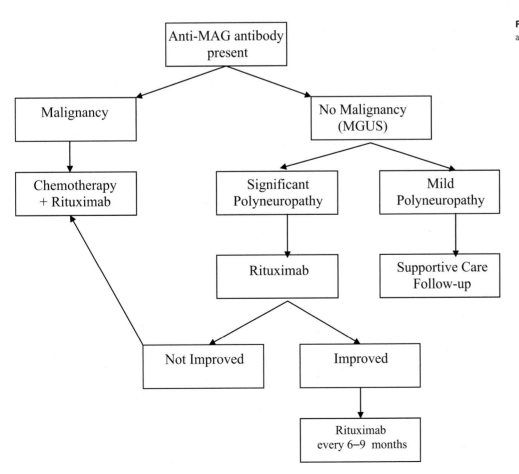

Fig. 26.3 Management of anti-MAG-associated polyneuropathy.

effective in one-third of the patients when used as a single agent, and in a slightly higher proportion when used in combination with other therapies (Oksenhendler *et al.*, 1995; Nobile-Orazio *et al.*, 1988, 2000). A continuous treatment regimen with 0.1 mg/kg/day orally for at least 6 months is recommended (Kyle *et al.*, 2000). Myelosuppression and immunosuppression are the primary side-effects, with atypical or opportunistic infections. Alkylating agents may also expose patients to the risks of myelodysplasia or secondary leukemia (Rosner and Grunwald, 1980; Rodriguez *et al.*, 1998).

High-dose melphalan therapy, another alkylating agent, followed by autologous stem cell transplantation, has also been reported to be beneficial in macroglobulinemia and neuropathy (Rudnicki *et al.*, 1998). In some cases, cyclophosphamide has been reported to be effective (Blume *et al.*, 1995).

Purine analogues are increasingly being used instead of chlorambucil, primarily due to their more rapid mode of action, although their long-term benefits have not been compared. Fludarabine, a fluorinated purine analogue, has shown to be effective in several low-grade B-cell lymphoproliferative conditions including Waldenström's macroglobulinemia (Dimopoulos *et al.*, 2000), with an overall response rate of 36% and remission in 2% of the patients (Dhodapkar *et al.*, 2001). It has also been reported to be effective in patients with IgM monoclonal gammopathy and neuropathy, with an improvement in the neuropathy associated with a significant fall in the IgM paraprotein concentration (Sherman *et al.*, 1994; Wilson *et al.*, 1999). The recommended dose is 25 mg/m^2 IV daily for 5 days, repeated monthly for 6 months. Cumulative myelosuppression and immunosuppression are the principal side-effects. Prophylaxis against *Pneumocystis* pneumonia is provided until the lymphocyte count recovers to normal.

Cladribine (2-chlorodoxyadenosine or 2-CDA), another purine analogue, has also shown promising clinical activity. Most studies have confirmed objective responses in at least 75% of patients in primary treatment and in 44% undergoing salvage treatment (Dimopoulos *et al.*, 2000). It has been reported to cause a prolonged remission in a patient with anti-MAG-associated polyneuropathy, after receiving two 7-day courses of 0.09 mg/kg/day by continuous IV infusion, 4 weeks apart (Ghosh *et al.*, 2002).

Other therapies

Corticosteroids are not usually effective in patients with neuropathy and IgM monoclonal gammopathy, except occasionally when used in combination with other therapies (Nobile-Orazio *et al.*, 2000). Plasmapheresis has also been reported to be effective in some patients (Haas and Tatum, 1988; Simovic *et al.*, 1998), but less so then in patients with CIDP and IgG or IgA monoclonal gammopathies (Dyck *et al.*, 1991). IV Ig therapy is particularly effective in patients with anti-GM1 antibodies and motor neuropathy (Nobile-Orazio, 2001), but can also occasionally be effective in the other monoclonal gammopathies, including with anti-MAG activity (Dalakas *et al.*, 1996; Mariette *et al.*, 1997; Comi *et al.*, 2002). Treatment with interferon-alpha has been reported to be ineffective in anti-MAG neuropathy (Mariette *et al.*, 2000).

Prognosis for non-malignant IgM-associated polyneuropathy

The prognosis in patients with IgM monoclonal gammopathy is heavily influenced by the presence of malignancy. The median survival of patients with Waldenström's macroglobulinemia is 65 months (Gertz *et al.*, 2000), although approximately 20% of patients survive for more than 10 years. The general risk of malignant transformation in patients with non-malignant monoclonal gammopathy is approximately 1% per year (Kyle *et al.*, 2002). In one study of patients with anti-MAG neuropathy, a malignant transformation rate of 16% over a follow-up period of 7.4 years was reported (Smith, 1994), and in another series, two of 38 patients (5%) developed a hematological malignancy during 5–42 years of follow-up (Ponsford *et al.*, 2000).

In the absence of macroglobulinemia, the prognosis is dependent upon the course of the neuropathy. Despite the generally slowly progressive course, 45% of patients with IgM monoclonal gammopathy and neuropathy have been reported to develop severe disability (Ellie *et al.*, 1996). In 17 patients with non-malignant IgM monoclonal gammopathy followed for up to 14 years, the neuropathy worsened for the first 2 to 5 years, and then very gradually progressed (Smith, 1994). Some patients appear to stabilize in later years after early progression, even without treatment (Ellie *et al.*, 1996). In other studies of the course of neuropathy associated with non-malignant monoclonal gammopathy and neuropathy, severe progression was noted in 16% (Notermans *et al.*, 1994). In a series of patients with anti-MAG IgM a disability rate of 42% was reported after a mean duration of neuropathy of 11.8 years (Nobile-Orazio *et al.*, 2000).

The axonal neuropathy that is associated with antisulfatide IgM M-proteins does not usually improve with immunotherapy, although it may be possible to slow or stop its progression. The motor neuropathy associated with IgM anti-GM1 antibodies usually responds to IV Ig and chemotherapy, including cyclophosphamide (Pestronk *et al.*, 1998; Latov, 2000). The neuropathy associated with IgM disialosyl antibodies can also occasionally improve with immunotherapy (Willison *et al.*, 2001).

Neuropathy with IgG/IgA monoclonal gammopathy

Most patients with neuropathy and IgG or IgA paraproteins have a non-malignant monoclonal gammopathy, with myeloma or lymphoma present in 6–17% (Kelly *et al.*, 1981a; Notermans *et al.*, 1994; Ponsford *et al.*, 2000). In patients with neuropathy and myeloma, the myelomas can be osteosclerotic and often associated with the POEMS syndrome, or osteolytic and sometimes associated with primary amyloidosis.

Neuropathy and non-malignant IgG or IgA monoclonal gammopathy

The incidence of neuropathy in non-malignant IgG or IgA monoclonal gammopathy is between 6 and 25% (Kahn *et al.*, 1980; Nobile-Orazio *et al.*, 1987). The neuropathy in these cases is heterogeneous, but two main syndromes can be seen, with approximately equal frequencies. One group of patients has a syndrome that is indistinguishable from CIDP, whereas the other is characterized by a slowly progressive, predominately sensory axonal neuropathy, which is indistinguishable from idiopathic axonal neuropathy (Di Troia *et al.*, 1999; Ponsford *et al.*, 2000). Those with CIDP respond to plasmapheresis or IV Ig, similarly to patients without monoclonal gammopathies, whereas those with axonal neuropathies are only occasionally responsive (Dyck *et al.*, 1991; Notermans *et al.*, 1996; Gorson and Ropper, 1997; Di Troia *et al.*, 1999). The relationship of the monoclonal gammopathies to the neuropathy in this patient population is poorly understood, but these might arise in the course of a chronic inflammatory response to self or foreign antigens.

Neuropathy with myeloma

Neuropathy is estimated to occur in 1–13% of patients with all myelomas (Silverstein and Doniger, 1963; Walsh, 1971; Driedger and Pruzanski 1980; Kelly *et al.*, 1981a; Miralles *et al.*, 1992). However, it is common in patients with osteosclerotic myelomas, which constitute fewer than 3% of all myelomas, but in which 50% of patients have an associated neuropathy (Driedger and Pruzanski, 1980; Kelly *et al.*, 1983).

Osteosclerotic myeloma and the POEMS syndrome

Osteosclerotic myeloma is a more indolent disease than multiple myeloma. Affected patients are younger, most commonly presenting in their 50s, but ranging in age from the 30s to the 60s. Neuropathy is frequently the presenting syndrome that leads to diagnosis. Initial symptoms consist of distal bothersome but not painful paresthesias in the feet, which spread proximally, followed by weakness. Cranial nerve and autonomic involvement can occur, but are uncommon. The weakness is frequently distal, but can involve proximal muscles and be severe. Electrodiagnostic studies frequently reveal evidence for demyelination and axonal degeneration, similarly to CIDP (Ohi *et al.*, 1985). CSF protein is usually elevated without pleocytosis. Nerve biopsy studies typically reveal small foci of inflammatory cells in the epineurium, with a mixture of demyelination and remyelination and axonal degeneration (Sung *et al.*, 2002). In one study, 75% of patients had a serum monoclonal protein, and only 15% had urine M-protein (Kelly *et al.*, 1983); interestingly, almost all the paraproteins have lambda light chains. Skeletal survey is essential for diagnosis, with the lesions appearing osteosclerotic or osteosclerotic, and usually involving the spine, pelvic bones, or ribs. An open bone marrow biopsy is usually needed to confirm the diagnosis, as routine biopsies are frequently normal. Anemia is uncommon, although leukocyte count, hemoglobin, or platelet counts are often elevated. Bone scan is usually unhelpful, as the lesions may not be sufficiently active to be picked up.

Many patients with osteosclerotic myeloma have features of the POEMS syndrome. These include hepatosplenomegaly, lymphadenopathy, edema, gynecomastia, ascites, pleural effusions, hyperpigmentation, hypertrichosis, thickened skin, papilledema, clubbing, thrombocytosis, polycythemia, and various endocrinopathies including hyperglycemia, hypothyroidism, hypogonadism, and low serum estrogen or testosterone (Kelly *et al.*, 1983; Miralles *et al.*, 1992). However, patients with features of the POEMS syndrome can also present with non-sclerotic myeloma or with Castleman's disease (Dispenzieri *et al.*, 2003). The cause of these associated abnormalities is unknown, but increased levels of vascular endothelial growth factor (VEGF) and of other cytokines have been found in these patients, and may contribute to the clinical presentations (Gherardi *et al.*, 1996; Watanabe *et al.*, 1998)

Osteolytic myeloma

Neuropathy in patients with osteolytic myeloma is rare. The presentation is heterogeneous and is predominately motor, sensory, or sensorimotor, and associated with axonal degeneration (Kelly, 1985). Mononeuropathies or radiculopathies may result from compression by tumor cells or spinal fractures (Silverstein and Doniger, 1963). Amyloidosis may be found in up to 40% of such patients (Kelly *et al.*, 1981).

Therapy and prognosis

The neuropathy associated with myeloma can improve with therapy of the underlying myeloma, including with prednisone and melphalan or other chemotherapeutic agents, surgery of isolated plasmacytomas, or irradiation. (Kelly *et al.*, 1981*a*; Donofrio *et al.*, 1984; Rotta and Bradley, 1997). Intensive plasmapheresis (Silberstein *et al.*, 1985), or treatment with ^{89}Sr has also been reported to be effective (Sternberg *et al.*, 2002). Papilledema, when present, may respond to treatment of the associated increased intracranial pressure (Wright *et al.*, 1998). Bone marrow ablation with stem cell transplantation is a promising new treatment (Peggs *et al.*, 2002).

The prognosis of multiple myeloma is poor, with progression of the neuropathy and a median survival after diagnosis of only 3 years (Alexanian and Dimopoulos 1994). The 5-year survival in patients with osteosclerotic myeloma or the POEMS syndrome is somewhat better at 60% (Miralles *et al.*, 1992; Dispenzieri *et al.*, 2003).

Neuropathy with monoclonal gammopathy and amyloidosis

Primary amyloidosis is a rare condition with an annual incidence of 8 per million people (Kyle and Gertz, 1995) and with neuropathy in 15–20% of patients (Benson *et al.*, 1975; Kyle and Bayrd, 1975). Eighty to ninety per cent of neuropathy amyloid patients have a monoclonal protein or light chain in serum or urine and the diagnosis is confirmed by rectal biopsy,

which is positive in 70%, or nerve biopsy, positive in over 90% of cases (Kelly, 1985). In a study of 210 patients with amyloidosis, 67% had IgG monoclonal gammopathy, 20% IgA, 7% IgM, and 4% IgD (Kyle and Greipp 1983).

Most patients with amyloid neuropathy present with painful paresthesias distally in the hands and feet, followed by weakness. More than 50% develop autonomic symptoms including orthostatic hypotension, bowel and bladder dysfunction, and impotence. Pain and temperature are more affected than proprioception and vibration. Electrodiagnostic findings are usually consistent with an axonal polyneuropathy with predominant involvement of small myelinated and unmyelinated fibers (Walsh, 1971; Kelly, 1985; Kyle and Gertz, 1995). Sural nerve biopsy reveals deposits of amyloid and fragments of the immunoglobulin light chains in the endoneurium. Many patients have associated systemic disease. Fatigue, weakness, and weight loss are common complaints. Renal failure (30%) or congestive heart failure (20%) are also common at presentation (Kyle, 1999).

Primary amyloidosis has traditionally been treated with melphalan and prednisone (Kyle *et al.*, 1997), and more recently with high-dose chemotherapy and stem cell transplantation (Comenzo *et al.*, 1996; Rajkumar *et al.*, 1998; Gertz *et al.*, 2002). Transient improvement may be seen, but the neuropathy ultimately progresses. The prognosis of primary systemic amyloidosis presenting with cardiac or other organ involvement is poor, with a median survival of 13 months (Kyle and Gertz, 1995). The prognosis is better in patients presenting with neuropathy, with a median survival of 5–35 months (Duston *et al.*, 1989; Rajkumar *et al.*, 1998).

Neuropathy with monoclonal gammopathy and cryoglobulinemia

Cryoglobulinemia is characterized by serum immunoglobulins that precipitate in the cold and redissolve upon warming. Cryoglobulins are classified as types I to III. Type I cryoglobulins are composed of monoclonal immunoglobulins, type II of a mixture of monoclonal and polyclonal immunoglobulins, and type III of mixed polyclonal immunoglobulins. Types II and III are often associated with hepatitis C infection, whereas type I may be associated with lymphoma or macroglobulinemia. The neuropathy in patients with cryoglobulinemia is thought be caused by vasculitis due to occlusion of the vaso nervosum by the cryoprecipitates, and is associated with such systemic manifestations as purpura, Raynaud's phenomenon, or renal disease. Patients typically present with mononeuritis multiplex, but also with distal symmetric sensory or sensorimotor neuropathy, without systemic disease. In one study, up to 11% of referred patients with neuropathy were found to have cryoglobulinemia (Gemignani *et al.*, 2002).

Type I cryoglobulins that are of the IgM type may be both cryoprecipitates and exhibit antinerve activity, causing both autoimmune and vasculitic neuropathy (Thomas *et al.*, 1992; Vital *et al.*, 2001). Monoclonal gammopathies in types I or II cryoglobulinemia may also have rheumatoid factor or anti-IgG activity, in which case the condition may be aggravated by infusion of IV Ig (Yebra *et al.*, 2002).

In patients with neuropathy and type II or III cryoglobulinemia associated with hepatitis C infection, the neuropathy can improve following treatment of the underlying hepatitis and cryoglobulinemia with interferon alpha (Naarendorp *et al.*, 2001). Cryoglobulinemic neuropathy can also respond to therapy with high-dose corticosteroids, plasmapheresis, or other immunosuppressive medications (Lippa *et al.*, 1986; Dispenzieri and Gorevic, 1999).

References

Adams, D., Kuntzer, T., Steck, A.J., Lobrinus, A., Janzer, R.C., and Regli, F. (1993). Motor conduction block and high titers of anti-GM1 ganglioside antibodies, pathological evidence of a motor neuropathy in a patient with lower motor neuron syndrome. *J. Neurol Neurosurg Psych* **56**: 982–987.

Alexanian, R. and Dimopoulos, M. (1994). The treatment of multiple myeloma. *N Engl J Med* **330**: 484–489.

Arasaki, K., Kusunoki, S., Kudo, N., and Kanazawa, I. (1993). Acute conduction block *in vitro* following exposure to antiganglioside sera. *Muscle Nerve* **16**: 587–593.

Attarian, S., Azulay, J.P., Boucraut, J., Escande, N., and Pouget, J. (2001). Terminal latency index and modified F ratio in distinction of chronic demyelinating neuropathies. *Clin Neurophysiol* **112**: 457–463.

Axelsson, U., Bachmann, R., and Hällen, J. (1966). Frequency of pathological proteins (M-components) in 6995 sera from an adult population. *Acta Med Scand* **179**: 235–247.

Benson, M.D., Cohen, A.S., Brandt, K.D., and Cathcart, E.S. (1975). Neuropathy, M components, and amyloid. *Lancet* **1**: 10–12.

Bing, J. and Neel, A. (1936). Two cases of hyperglobulinaemia with affection of the central nervous system on a toxi-infectious basis. *Acta Med Scand* **88**: 492–506.

Blume, G., Pestronk, A., and Goodnough L.T. (1995). Anti-MAG antibody-associated polyneuropathies: improvement following immunotherapy with monthly plasma exchange and IV cyclophosphamide. *Neurology* **45**: 1577–1580.

Bollensen, E., Schipper, H.I., and Steck A.J. (1989). Motor neuropathy with activity of monoclonal IgM antibody to GD1a ganglioside. *J Neurol* **236**: 353–355.

Briani, C., Berger, J.S., and Latov, N. (1998). Antibodies to chondroitin sulfate C: a new detection assay and correlations with neurological diseases. *J Neuroimmunol* **84**: 117–121.

Briani, C., Santoro, M., and Latov, N. (2000). Antibodies to chondroitin sulfates A, B, and C: clinico-pathological correlates in neurological diseases. *J Neuroimmunol* **108**: 216–220.

Briani, C., Ruggero, S., Alaedini, A., *et al.* (2002). Anti-heparan sulfate antibodies in neurological disease. *Muscle Nerve* **26**: 713–715.

Brouet, J.C., Mariette, X., Gendron, M.C., and Dubreuil, M.L. (1994). Monoclonal IgM from patients with peripheral demyelinating neuropathies cross-react with bacterial polypeptides. *Clin Exp Immunol* **96**: 466–469.

Burger, D., Simon, M., Perruisseau, G., and Steck, A.J. (1990). The epitope(s) recognized by HNK-1 antibody and IgM paraprotein in neuropathy is present on several N-linked oligosaccharide structures on human P_0 and myelin-associated glycoprotein. *J Neurochem* **54**: 1569–1575.

Byrd, J.C., White, C.A., Link, B., *et al.* (1999). Rituximab therapy in Waldenstrom's macroglobulinemia, preliminary evidence of clinical activity. *Ann Oncol* **10**: 1525–1527.

Carpo, M., Nobile-Orazio, E., Meucci, N., *et al.* (1996). Anti-GD1a ganglioside antibodies in peripheral motor syndromes. *Ann Neurol* **39**: 539–543.

Carpo, M., Pedotti, R., Allaria, S., *et al.* (1999). Clinical presentation and outcome of Guillain–Barré and related syndromes in relation to anti-ganglioside antibodies. *J Neurol Sci* **168**: 78–84.

Caudie, C., Vial, C., Petiot, P., Bancel, J., Lombard, C., and Gonnaud, P.M. (2001). Monoclonal IgM autoantibody activity vis-a-vis glycoconjugates of peripheral nerves, apropos of 112 cases. *Ann Biol Clin (Paris)* **59**: 567–577.

Cavanna, B., Carpo, M., Pedotti, R., *et al.* (1999). Anti-GM2 IgM antibodies, clinical correlates and reactivity with a human neuroblastoma cell line. *J Neuroimmunol* **94**: 157–164.

Chazot, G., Berger, B., Carrier, H., *et al.* (1976). Manifestations neurologiques des gammapathies monoclonales. *Rev Neurol* **132**: 195–212.

Chiba, A., Kusunoki, S., Obata, H., Machinami, R., and Kanazawa, I. (1993). Serum anti-GQ1b IgG antibody is associated with ophthalmoplegia in Miller Fisher syndrome and Guillain-Barre syndrome, clinical and immuno-histochemical studies. *Neurology* **43**: 1911–1917.

Cocito, D., Isoardo, G., Ciaramitaro, P., *et al.* (2001). Terminal latency index in polyneuropathy with IgM paraproteinemia and anti-MAG antibody. *Muscle Nerve* **24**: 1278–1282.

Comenzo, R.L., Vosburgh, E., Simms, R.W., *et al.* (1996). Dose-intensive melphalan with blood stem cell support for the treatment of AL amyloidosis, one-year follow-up in five patients. *Blood* **88**: 2801–2806.

Comi, G., Roveri, L., Swan, A., *et al.* (2002). A randomised controlled trial of intravenous immunoglobulin in IgM paraprotein associated demyelinating neuropathy. *J Neurol* **249**: 1370–1377.

Corbo, M., Quattrini, A., Lugaresi, A., Santoro, M., Latov, N., and Hays, A.P. (1992). Patterns of reactivity of human anti-GM1 antibodies with spinal cord and motor neurons. *Ann Neurol* **32**: 487–493.

Dabby, R., Weimer, L.H., Hays, A.P., Olarte, M., and Latov, N. (2000). Anti-sulfatide antibodies in neuropathy, clinical and electrophysiologic correlates. *Neurology* **54**: 1448–1452.

Dalakas, M.C. and Quarles, R.H. (1996). Autoimmune ataxic neuropathies (sensory ganglionopathies), are glycolipids the responsible autoantigens? *Ann Neurol* **39**: 419–422.

Dalakas, M.C., Quarles, R.H., Farrer, R.G., *et al.* (1996). A controlled study of intravenous immunoglobulin in demyelinating neuropathy with IgM gammapathy. *Ann Neurol* **40**: 792–795.

Davis, T.A., Grillo-Lopez, A.J., White, C.A., *et al.* (2000). Rituximab anti-CD20 monoclonal antibody therapy in non-Hodgkin's lymphoma, safety and efficacy of re-treatment. *J Clin Oncol* **18**: 3135–3143.

DeAngelis, M.V., Di Muzio, A., Lupo, S., Gambi, D., Uncini, A., and Lugaresi, A. (2001). Anti-GD1a antibodies from an acute motor axonal neuropathy patient selectively bind to motor nerve fiber nodes of Ranvier. *J Neuroimmunol* **121**: 79–82.

De Navasquez, S. and Treble, H.A. (1938). A case of primary generalized amyloid disease with involvement of the nerves. *Brain* **61**: 116–128.

Dhodapkar, M.V., Jacobson, J.L., Gerty, M.A., *et al.* (2001). Prognostic factors and response to fludarabine therapy in patients with Waldenström macroglobulinemia, results of United States intergroup trial (Southwest Oncology Group S9003). *Blood* **98**: 41–48.

Dillman, R.O. (2002). Radiolabeled anti-CD20 monoclonal antibodies for the treatment of B-cell lymphoma. *J Clin Oncol* **20**: 3545–3557.

Dimopoulos, M.A. and Alexanian, R. (1994). Waldenström's macroglobulinemia. *Blood* **83**: 1452–1459.

Dimopoulos, M.A., Panayiotidis, P., Moulopoulos, L.A., Sfikakis, P., and Dalakas, M. (2000). Waldenstrom's macroglobulinemia; clinical features, complications, and management. *J Clin Oncol* **18**: 214–226.

Dimopoulos, M.A., Zervas, C., Zomas, A., *et al.* (2002). Treatment of Waldenstrom's macroglobulinemia with rituximab. *J Clin Oncol* **20**: 2327–2333.

Di Troia, A., Carpo, M., Meucci, N., *et al.* (1999). Clinical features and anti-neural reactivity in neuropathy associated with IgG monoclonal gammopathy of undetermined significance. *J Neurol Sci* **164**: 64–71.

Dispenzieri, A. and Gorevic, P.D. (1999). Cryoglobulinemia. *Hematol Oncol Clin North Am* **13**: 1315–1349.

Dispenzieri, A., Kyle, R.A., Lacy, M.Q., *et al.* (2003). POEMS syndrome, definitions and long-term outcome. *Blood* **101**: 2496–2506.

Donofrio, P.D., Albers, J.W., Greenberg, H.S., and Mitchell, B.S. (1984). Peripheral neuropathy in osteosclerotic myeloma, clinical and electro-diagnostic improvement with chemotherapy. *Muscle Nerve* **7**: 137–141.

Driedger, H. and Pruzanski, W. (1980). Plasma cell neoplasia with peripheral polyneuropathy. A study of five cases and a review of the literature. *Medicine* **59**: 301–310.

Duston, M.A., Skinner, M., Anderson, J., and Cohen, A.S. (1989). Peripheral neuropathy as an early marker of AL amyloidosis. *Arch Intern Med* **149**: 358–360.

Dyck, P.J., Low, P.A., Windebank, A.J., *et al.* (1991). Plasma exchange in polyneuropathy associated with monoclonal gammopathy of undetermined significance. *N Engl J Med* **325**: 1482–1486.

Ellie, E., Vital, A., Steck, A., Boiron, J.M., Vital, C., and Julien, J. (1996). Neuropathy associated with "benign" anti-myelin-associated glycoprotein IgM gammapathy, clinical, immunological, neurophysiological pathological findings and response to treatment in 33 cases. *J Neurol* **243**: 34–43.

Erb, S., Ferracin, F., Fuhr, P., *et al.* (2000). Polyneuropathy attributes, a comparison between patients with anti-MAG and anti-sulfatide antibodies. *J Neurol* **247**: 767–772.

Ernerudh, J.H., Vrethem, M., Andersen, O., Lindberg, C., and Berlin, G. (1992). Immunochemical and clinical effects of immunosuppressive treatment in monoclonal IgM neuropathy. *J Neurol Neurosurg Psychiatry* **55**: 930–934.

Fagarasan, S. and Honjo, T. (2000). T-independent immune response, new aspects of B cell biology. *Science* **290**: 89–92.

Fluri, F., Ferracin, F., Erne, B., and Steck, A.J. (2003). Microheterogeneity of anti-myelin-associated glycoprotein antibodies. *J Neurol Sci* **207**(1–2): 43–49.

Freddo, L., Yu, R.K., Latov, N., *et al.* (1986). Gangliosides GM1 and GD1b are antigens for IgM M-proteins in a patient with motor neuron disease. *Neurology* **36**: 454–458.

Fruttiger, M., Montag, D., Schachner, M., and Martini, R. (1995). Crucial role for the myelin-associated glycoprotein in the maintenance of axon-myelin integrity. *Eur J Neurosci* **7**: 511–515.

Gabriel, J.M., Erne, B., Miescher, G.C., *et al.* (1996). Selective loss of myelin-associated glycoprotein from myelin correlates with anti-MAG antibody titer in demyelinating paraproteinemic polyneuropathy. *Brain* **119**: 775–787.

Gabriel, J.M., Erne, B., Bernasconi, L., *et al.* (1998). Confocal microscopic localization of anti-MAG autoantibodies in a patient with peripheral neuropathy initially lacking a detectable IgM gammopathy. *Acta Neuropathol (Berlin)* **95**: 540–546.

Garcin, R., Mallarmé, J., and Rondot, P. (1958). Forme névritique de la macroglobulinémie de Waldenström. *Bull Soc Méd Hôp (Paris)* **74** : 24–25.

Gemignani, F., Melli, G., Inglese, C., and Marbini, A. (2002). Cryoglobulinemia is a frequent cause of peripheral neuropathy in undiagnosed referral patients. *J Peripher Nerv Syst* **7** : 59–64.

Gertz, M.A., Fonseca, R., and Rajkumar, S.V. (2000). Waldenstrom's macroglobulinemia. *Oncologist* **5**: 63–67.

Gertz, M.A., Lacy, M.Q., Dispenzieri, A., *et al.* (2002). Stem cell transplantation for the management of primary systemic amyloidosis. *Am J Med* **113**: 549–555.

Ghosh, A., Littlewood, T., and Donaghy, M. (2002). Cladribine in the treatment of IgM paraproteinemic polyneuropathy. *Neurology* **59**: 1290–1291.

Gong, Y., Tagawa, Y., Lunn, M.P., *et al.* (2002). Localization of major gangliosides in the PNS, implications for immune neuropathies. *Brain* **125**: 2491–2506.

Gorson, K.C. and Ropper, A.H. (1997). Axonal neuropathy associated with monoclonal gammopathy of undetermined significance. *J Neurol Neurosurg Psychiatry* **63**: 163–168.

Haas, D.C. and Tatum, A.H. (1988). Plasmapheresis alleviates neuropathy accompanying IgM anti-myelin associated glycoprotein paraproteinemia. *Ann Neurol* **23**: 394–396.

Hafler, D.A., Johnson, D., Kelly, J.J., Panitch, H., Kyle, R., and Weiner, H.L. (1986). Monoclonal gammopathy and neuropathy: Myelin-associated glycoprotein reactivity and clinical characteristics. *Neurology* **36**: 75–78.

Harvey, G.K., Toyka KV, Zielasek, J., Kiefer, R., Simonis, C., and Hartung, H.P. (1995). Failure of anti-GM1 IgG or IgM to induce conduction block following intraneural transfer. *Muscle Nerve* **18**: 388–394.

Hays, A.P., Latov, N., Takatsu, M., and Sherman, W.H. (1987). Experimental demyelination of nerve induced by serum of patients with neuropathy and an anti-MAG IgM M-protein. *Neurology* **37**: 242–256.

Ho, T.W., Willison, H.J., Nachamkin, I., *et al.* (1999). Anti-GD1a antibody is associated with axonal but not demyelinating forms of Guillain–Barre syndrome. *Ann Neurol* **45**: 168–173.

Ilyas, A.A., Quarles, R.H., Dalakas, M.C., Fishman, P.H., and Brady, R.O. (1985). Monoclonal IgM in a patient with paraproteinemic polyneuropathy binds to gangliosides containing disialosyl groups. *Ann Neurol* **18**: 655–659.

Ilyas, A.A., Willison, J.H., Dalakas, M., Whitaker, J.N., and Quarles, R.H. (1988*a*). Identification and characterization of gangliosides reacting with IgM paraproteins in three patients with neuropathy and biclonal gammopathy. *J Neurochem* **51**: 851–858.

Ilyas, A.A., Li, S.C., Chou, D.K., *et al.* (1988*b*). Gangliosides GM2, IV4GalNAcGM1b and IV4GalNAcGC1a as antigens for monoclonal immunoglobulin M in neuropathy associated with gammopathy. *J Biol Chem* **263**: 4369–4373.

Ilyas, A.A., Cook, S.D., Dalakas, M.C., and Mithen, F.A. (1992). Anti-MAG IgM paraproteins from some patients with polyneuropathy associated with IgM paraproteinemia also react with sulfatide. *J Neuroimmunol* **37**: 85–92.

Jacobs, J.M. and Scadding, J.W. (1990). Morphological changes in IgM paraproteinemic neuropathy. *Acta Neuropathol (Berlin)* **80**: 77–84.

Kahn, S.N., Riches, P.G., and Kohn, J. (1980). Paraproteinaemia in neurological disease: incidence, associations, and classification of monoclonal immunoglobulins. *J Clin Pathol* **33**: 617–621.

Kaku, D.A., England, J.D., and Sumner, A.J. (1994). Distal accentuation of conduction slowing in polyneuropathy associated with antibodies to myelin-associated glycoprotein and sulphated glucoronyl paragloboside. *Brain* **117**: 941–947.

Katz, J.S., Saperstein, D.S., Gronseth, G., Amato, A.A., and Barohn, R.J. (2000). Distal acquired demyelinating symmetric neuropathy. *Neurology* **54**: 615–620.

Kelly, J.J. Jr (1985). Peripheral neuropathies associated with monoclonal proteins : a clinical review. *Muscle Nerve* **8**: 138–150.

Kelly, J.J., Kyle, R.A., Miles, J.M., O'Brien, P.C., and Dyck, P.J. (1981*a*). The spectrum of peripheral neuropathy in myeloma. *Neurology* **31**: 24–31.

Kelly, J.J. Jr, Kyle, R.A., O'Brien, P.C., *et al.* (1981*b*). Prevalence of monoclonal protein in peripheral neuropathy. *Neurology* **31**: 1480–1483.

Kelly, J.J. Jr, Kyle, R.A., Miles, J.M., and Dyck P.J. (1983). Osteosclerotic myeloma and peripheral neuropathy. *Neurology* **33**: 202–216.

Kelly, J.J., Adelman, L.S., Berkman, and Bhan, I. (1988). Polyneuropathies associated with IgM monoclonal gammopathies. *Arch Neurol* **45**: 1355–1359.

King, R.H. and Thomas, P.K. (1984). The occurrence and significance of myelin with unusually large periodicity. *Acta Neuropathol (Berlin)* **63**: 319–329.

Kinsella, L.J., Lange, D.J., Trojaborg, W., Sadiq, S.A., Younger, D.S., and Latov, N. (1994). Clinical and electrophysiologic correlates of elevated anti-GM1 antibody titers. *Neurology* **44**: 1278–1282.

Kusunoki, S., Shimizu, J., Chiba, A., Ugawa, Y., Hitoshi, S., and Kanazawa, I. (1996). Experimental sensory neuropathy induced by sensitization with ganglioside GD1b. *Ann Neurol* **39**: 424–431.

Kusunoki, S., Mashiko, H., Mochizuki, N., *et al.* (1997). Binding of antibodies against GM1 and GD1b in human peripheral nerve. *Muscle Nerve* **20**: 840–845.

Kyle, R.A. (1978). Monoclonal gammopathy of undetermined significance, natural history of 241 cases. *Am J Med* **64**: 814–826.

Kyle, R.A. (1992). Diagnostic criteria of multiple myeloma. *Hematol Oncol Clin North Am* **6**: 347–358.

Kyle, R.A. (1997). Monoclonal gammopathy of undetermined significance and solitary plasmacytoma. Implications for progression to overt multiple myeloma. *Hematol Oncol Clin North Am* **11**: 71–87.

Kyle, R.A. (1999). Clinical aspects of multiple myeloma and related disorders including amyloidosis. *Path Biol* **47**: 148–157.

Kyle, R.A. and Bayrd, E.D. (1975). Amyloidosis review of 236 cases. *Medicine* **54**: 271–299.

Kyle, R.A. and Garton, J.P. (1987). The spectrum of IgM monoclonal gammopathy in 430 cases. *Mayo Clin Proc* **62**: 719–731.

Kyle, R.A. and Gertz, M.A. (1995). Primary systemic amyloidosis, clinical and laboratory features in 474 cases. *Semin Hematol* **32**: 45–59.

Kyle, R.A. and Greipp, P.R. (1983). Amyloidosis (AL). Clinical and laboratory features in 229 cases. *Mayo Clin Proc* **58**: 665–683.

Kyle, R.A., Finkelstein, S., Elveback, L.R., and Kurland, L.T. (1972). Incidence of monoclonal proteins in a Minnesota community with a cluster of multiple myeloma. *Blood* **40**: 719–724.

Kyle, R.A., Gertz, M.A., Greipp, P.R., *et al.* (1997). A trial of three regimens for primary amyloidosis, colchicine alone, melphalan and prednisone, and melphalan, prednisone, and colchicine. *N Engl J Med* **336**: 1202–1207.

Kyle, R.A., Greipp, P.R., Gertz, M.A., *et al.* (2000). Waldenstrom's macroglobulinaemia, a prospective study comparing daily with intermittent oral chlorambucil. *Br J Haematol* **108**: 737–742.

Kyle, R.A., Therneau, T., Rajkumar, S.V., *et al.* (2002). A long-term study of prognosis in monoclonal gammopathy of undetermined significance. *N Engl J Med* **346**: 564–569.

Latov, N. (2000). Prognosis of neuropathy with monoclonal gammopathy. Editorial. *Muscle Nerve* **23**: 150–152.

Latov, N., Sherman, W.H., Nemni, R., *et al.* (1980). Plasma-cell dyscrasia and peripheral neuropathy with a monoclonal antibody to peripheral nerve myelin. *N Engl J Med* **303**: 618–621.

Latov, N., Godfrey, M., Thomas, Y., *et al.* (1985). Neuropathy and anti-MAG IgM M-proteins: T-cell regulation of M-protein secretion *in vitro*. *Ann Neurol* **18**: 182–188.

Latov, N., Hays, A.P., and Sherman, W.H. (1988). Peripheral neuropathy and anti-MAG antibodies. *Crit Rev Neurobiol* **3**: 301–332.

Lee, K.W., Inghirami, G., Spatz, L., Knowles, D.M., and Latov, N. (1991). The B-cells that express anti-MAG antibodies in neuropathy and non-malignant IgM monoclonal gammopathy belong to the CD5 subpopulation. *J Neuroimmunol* **31**: 83–88.

Leo, R., Boeker, M., Peest, D., *et al.* (1992). Multiparameter analyses of normal and malignant human plasma cells, CD38++, CD56+, CD54+, cIg+ is the common phenotype of myeloma cells. *Ann Hematol* **64**: 132–139.

Lippa, C.F., Chad, D.A., Smith, T.W., Kaplan, M.H., and Hammer, K. (1986). Neuropathy associated with cryoglobulinemia. *Muscle Nerve* 9: 626–631.

Lopate, G., Choksi, R., and Pestronk, A. (2002). Severe sensory ataxia and demyelinating polyneuropathy with IgM anti-GM2 and GalNAc-GD1A antibodies. *Muscle Nerve* 25: 828–836.

Mariette, X., Chastang, C., Clavelou, P., Louboutin, J.P., Leger, J.M., and Brouet, J.C. (1997). A randomised clinical trial comparing interferon-alpha and intravenous immunoglobulin in polyneuropathy associated with monoclonal IgM. The IgM-associated Polyneuropathy Study Group. *J Neurol Neurosurg Psychiatry* 63: 28–34.

Mariette, X., Brouet, J.C., Chevret, S., et al. (2000). A randomised double blind trial versus placebo does not confirm the benefit of alpha-interferon in polyneuropathy associated with monoclonal IgM. *J Neurol Neurosurg Psychiatry* 69: 279–280.

Mendell, J.R., Sahenk, Z., Whitaker, J.N., et al. (1985). Polyneuropathy and IgM monoclonal gammopathy, studies on the pathogenetic role of anti-myelin-associated glycoprotein antibody. *Ann Neurol* 17: 243–254.

Meucci, N., Baldini, L., Cappellari, A., et al. (1999). Anti-myelin-associated glycoprotein antibodies predict the development of neuropathy in asymptomatic patients with IgM monoclonal gammopathy. *Ann Neurol* 46: 119–122.

Miralles, G.D., O'Fallon, J.R., and Talley, N.J. (1992). Plasma-cell dyscrasia with polyneuropathy. The spectrum of POEMS syndrome. *N Engl J Med* 327: 1919–1923.

Mizutani, K., Oka, N., Kusunoki, S., et al. (2001) Sensorimotor demyelinating neuropathy with IgM antibody against gangliosides GD1a, GT1b and GM3. *J Neurol Sci* 188: 9–11.

Monaco, S., Ferrari, S., Bonetti, B., et al. (1995). Experimental induction of myelin changes by anti-MAG antibodies and terminal complement complex. *J Neuropathol Exp Neurol* 54: 96–104.

Nakao, T., Kon, K., Ando, S., et al. (1993). Novel lacto-ganglio type gangliosides with GM2-epitope in bovine brain which react with IgM from a patient of the amyotrophic lateral sclerosis-like disorder. *J Biol Chem* 268: 21028–21034.

Naarendorp, M., Kallemuchikkal, U., Nuovo, G.J., and Gorevic, P.D. (2001). Longterm efficacy of interferon-alpha for extrahepatic disease associated with hepatitis C virus infection. *J Rheumatol* 28: 2466–2473.

Nardelli, E., Steck, A.J., Barkas, T., Schluep, M., and Jerusalem, F. (1988). Motor neuron syndrome and monoclonal IgM with antibody activity against gangliosides GM1 and GD1b. *Ann Neurol* 23: 524–528.

Nardelli, E., Bassi, A., Mazzi, G., Anzini, P., and Rizzuto, N. (1995). Systemic passive transfer studies using IgM monoclonal antibodies to sulfatide. *J Neuroimmunol* 63: 29–37.

Neel, A.W. (1931). Die Bedeutung der Eiweissvermehrung ohne gleichzeitige entsprechende Zellvermehrung in der Spinalfluessigkeit. *Dtsch Z Nervenheilk* 117: 309–330.

Nobile-Orazio, E. (2001). Multifocal motor neuropathy. *J Neuroimmunol* 115: 4–18.

Nobile-Orazio, E., Marmiroli, P., Baldini, L., et al. (1987). Peripheral neuropathy in macroglobulinemia, incidence and antigen-specificity of M proteins. *Neurology* 37: 1506–1514.

Nobile-Orazio, E., Baldini, L., Barbieri, S., et al. (1988). Treatment of patients with neuropathy and anti-MAG IgM M-Proteins. *Ann Neurol* 24: 93–97.

Nobile-Orazio, E., Barbieri, S., Baldini, L., et al. (1992). Peripheral neuropathy in monoclonal gammopathy of undetermined significance, prevalence and immunopathogenetic studies. *Acta Neurol Scand* 85: 383–390.

Nobile-Orazio, E., Manfredini, E., Carpo, M., et al. (1994). Frequency and clinical correlates of anti-neural IgM antibodies in neuropathy associated with IgM monoclonal gammopathy. *Ann Neurol* 36: 416–424.

Nobile-Orazio, E., Meucci, N., Baldini, L., di Troia, A., and Scarlato, G. (2000). Long-term prognosis of neuroapthy associated with anti-MAG IgM M-proteins and its relationship to immune therapies. *Brain* 123: 710–717.

Notermans, N.C., Wokke, J.H., Lokhorst, H.M., Franssen, H., van der Graaf, Y., and Jennekens, F.G. (1994). Polyneuropathy associated with monoclonal gammopathy of undetermined significance. A prospective study of the prognostic value of clinical and laboratory abnormalities. *Brain* 117: 1385–1393.

Notermans, N.C., Wokke JHJ, van den Berg, L.H., et al. (1996). Chronic idiopathic axonal polyneuropathy. Comparison of patients with and without monoclonal gammopathy. *Brain* 119: 421–427.

Odaka, M., Yuki, N., and Hirata, K. (2001). Anti-GQ1b IgG antibody syndrome: clinical and immunological range. *J Neurol Neurosurg Psychiatry* 70: 50–55.

Oga, T., Kusunoki, S., Fujimura, H., Kuboki, T., Yoshida, T., and Takai, T. (1998). Severe motor-dominant neuropathy with IgM M-protein binding to the NeuAcalpha2–3Galbeta- moiety. *J Neurol Sci* 154: 4–7.

Ogawara, K., Kuwabara, S., Mori, M., Hattori, T., Koga, M., and Yuki, N. (2000). Axonal Guillain–Barre syndrome, relation to anti-ganglioside antibodies and Campylobacter jejuni infection in Japan. *Ann Neurol* 48: 624–631.

Ogino, M., Tatum, A.H., and Latov, N. (1994). Affinity studies of human anti-MAG antibodies in neuropathy. *J Neuroimmunol* 52: 41–46.

O'Hanlon, G.M., Veitch, J., Gallardo, E., Illa, I., Chancellor, A.M., and Willison, H.J. (2000). Peripheral neuropathy associated with anti-GM2 ganglioside antibodies, clinical and immunopathological studies. *Autoimmunity* 32: 133–144.

Ohi, T., Kyle, R.A., and Dyck, P.J. (1985). Axonal attenuation and secondary segmental demyelination in myeloma neuropathies. *Ann Neurol* 17: 255–261.

Oka, N., Kusaka, H., Kusunoki, S., et al. (1996). IgM M-protein with antibody activity against gangliosides with disialosyl residue in sensory neuropathy binds to sensory neurons. *Muscle Nerve* 19: 528–530.

Oksenhendler, E., Chevret, S., Leger, J.M., Louboutin, J.P., Bussel, A., and Brouet, J.C. (1995). Plasma exchange and chlorambucil in polyneuropathy associated with monoclonal IgM gammopathy. IgM-associated Polyneuropathy Study Group. *J Neurol Neurosurg Psychiatry* 59: 243–247.

O'Leary, C.P. and Willison, H.J. (1997). Autoimmune ataxic neuropathies (sensory ganglionopathies). *Curr Opin Neurol* 10: 366–370.

Onrust, S.V., Lamb, H.M., and Barman Balfour, J.A. (1999). Rituximab. *Drugs* 58: 79–88.

Ortiz, N., Rosa, R., Gallardo, E., et al. (2001). IgM monoclonal antibody against terminal moiety of GM2, GalNAc-GD1a and GalNAc-GM1b from a pure motor chronic demyelinating polyneuropathy patient, effects on neurotransmitter release. *J Neuroimmunol* 119: 114–123.

Pedersen, S.F., Pullman, S.L., Latov, N., and Brannagan, T.H. (1997). Physiological tremor analysis of patients with anti-myelin-associated glycoprotein associated neuropathy and tremor. *Muscle Nerve* 20: 38–44.

Peggs, K.S., Paneesha, S., Kottaridis, P.D., et al. (2002). Peripheral blood stem cell transplantation for POEMS syndrome. *Bone Marrow Transplant* 30: 401–404.

Pestronk, A. (1998). Multifocal motor neuropathy, diagnosis and treatment. *Neurology* 51(6, Suppl. 5): S22–S24.

Pestronk, A., Cornblath, D.R., Ilyas, A.A., Baba, H., Quarles, R.H., and Griffin, J.W. (1988). A treatable multifocal motor neuropathy with antibodies to GM1 ganglioside. *Ann Neurol* 24: 73–78.

Pestronk, A., Li, F., Griffin, J., Feldman, E.L., Cornblath, D., and Trotter, J. (1991). Polyneuropathy syndromes associated with serum antibodies to sulfatide and MAG. *Neurology* 41: 357–362.

Pestronk, A., Nobile-Orazio, E., Carpo, M., Scarlato, G., Holloway, R.G., and Feasby, T.E. (2000). Testing for serum IgM binding to GM1 ganglioside in clinical practice. *Neurology* 54: 2355–2358.

Ponsford, S., Willison, H., Veitch, J., Morris, R., and Thomas, P.K. (2000). Long-term clinical and neurophysiological follow-up of patients with peripheral neuropathy associated with benign monoclonal gammopathy. *Muscle Nerve* 23: 164–174.

Qin, Z. and Guan, Y. (1997). Experimental polyneuropathy produced in guinea-pigs immunized against sulfatide. *Neuroreport* 8: 2867–2870.

Quarles, R.H. and Weiss, M.D. (1999). Autoantibodies associated with peripheral neuropathy. *Muscle Nerve* 22: 800–822.

Quattrini, A., Corbo, M., Dhaliwal, S.K., et al. (1992). Anti-sulfatide antibodies in neurological disease, binding to rat dorsal root ganglia neurons. *J Neurol Sci* 112: 152–159.

Radziwill, A.J., Renaud, S., Steck, A.J., and Fuhr, P. (2001). Is distal motor latency (DML) a sensitive marker of anti-MAG polyneuropathy? *Neurology* 56(Suppl. 3): A399.

Rajkumar, S.V., Gertz, M.A., and Kyle, R.A. (1998). Prognosis of patients with primary systemic amyloidosis who present with dominant neuropathy. *Am J Med* 104: 232–237.

Renaud, S., Gregor, M., Fuhr, P., et al. (2003). Rituximab in the treatment of polyneuropathy associated with anti-MAG antibodies *Muscle Nerve* 27(5): 611–615.

Rodriguez, J.N., Fernandez-Jurado, A., Martino, M.L., and Prados, D. (1998). Waldenstrom's macroglobulinemia complicated with acute myeloid leukemia. Report of a case and review of the literature. *Haematologica* 83: 91–92.

Rosner, F. and Grunwald, H.W. (1980). Multiple myeloma and Waldenstrom's macroglobulinemia terminating in acute leukemia. Review with emphasis on karyotypic and ultrastructural abnormalities. *N Y State J Med* 80: 558–570.

Rosoklija, G.B., Dwork, A.J., Younger, D.S., Karlikaya, G., Latov, N., and Hays, A.P. (2000). Local activation of the complement system in endoneurial microvessels of diabetic neuropathy. *Acta Neuropathol* 99: 55–62.

Rotta, F.T. and Bradley, W.G. (1997). Marked improvement of severe polyneuropathy associated with multifocal osteosclerotic myeloma following surgery, radiation and chemotherapy. *Muscle Nerve* 20: 1035–1037.

Rowland, L.P., Sherman, W.L., Hays, A.P., et al. (1995). Autopsy-proven amyotrophic lateral sclerosis, Waldenstrom's macroglobulinemia, and antibodies to sulfated glucuronic acid paragloboside. *Neurology* 45: 827–829.

Rudnicki, S.A., Harik, S.I., Dhodapkar, M., Barlogie, B.,and Eidelberg, D. (1998). Nervous system dysfunction in Waldenstrom's macroglobulinemia: response to treatment. *Neurology* 51: 1210–1213.

Saleun, J.P., Vicariot, M., Deroff, P., and Morin, J.F. (1982). Monoclonal gammopathies in the adult population of Finistère, France. *J Clin Pathol* 35: 63–68.

Sheikh, K.A., Deerinck, T.J., Ellisman, M.H., and Griffin, J.W. (1999). The distribution of ganglioside like moieties in peripheral nerves. *Brain* 122: 449–460.

Sherman, W.H., Latov, N., Hays, A.P., et al. (1983). Monoclonal IgMk antibody precipitating with chondroitin sulfate C from patients with axonal polyneuropathy and epidermolysis. *Neurology* 33: 192–201.

Sherman, W.H., Latov, N., Lange, D., Hays, R., and Younger, D. (1994). Fludarabine for IgM antibody-mediated neuropathies [abstract]. *Ann Neurol* 36: 326–327.

Silberstein, L.E., Duggan, D., and Berkman, E.M. (1985). Therapeutic trial of plasma exchange in osteosclerotic myeloma associated with the POEMS syndrome. *J Clin Apheresis* 2: 253–257.

Silverstein, A. and Doniger, D.E. (1963). Neurologic complications of myelomatosis. *Arch Neurol* 63: 534–544.

Simovic, D., Gorson, K.C., and Ropper, A.H. (1998). Comparison of IgM-MGUS and IgG-MGUS polyneuropathy. *Acta Neurol Scand* 97: 194–200.

Smith, I.S. (1994). The natural history of chronic demyelinating neuropathy associated with benign IgM paraproteinaemia. A clinical and neurophysiological study. *Brain* 117: 949–957.

Smith, I.S., Kahn, N.S., Lacey, B.W., King, R.H., Whybrew, D.J., and Thomas, P.K. (1983). Chronic demyelinating neuropathy associated with benign IgM paraproteinemia. *Brain* 106: 169–195.

Spatz, L.A., Williams, M., Brender, B., Desai, R., and Latov, N. (1992). DNA sequence analysis and comparison of the variable heavy and light chain regions of IgM Monoclonal anti-MAG antibodies. *J Neuroimmunol* 36: 29–39.

Steck, A.J., Murray, N., Meier, C., Page, N., and Peruisseau, G. (1983). Demyelinating neuropathy and monoclonal IgM antibody to myelin-associated glycoprotein. *Neurology* 33: 19–23.

Steck, A.J., Murray, N., Dellagi, K., Brouet, J.C., and Seligman, M. (1987). Peripheral neuropathy associated with monoclonal IgM autoantibody. *Ann Neurol* 22: 764–767.

Sternberg, A.J., Davies, P., Macmillan, C., Abdul-Cader, A., and Swart, S. (2002). Strontium-89: a novel treatment for a case of osteosclerotic myeloma associated with life-threatening neuropathy. *Br J Haematol* 118: 821–824.

Sung, J.Y., Kuwabara, S., Ogawara, K., Kanai, K., and Hattori, T. (2002). Patterns of nerve conduction abnormalities in POEMS syndrome. *Muscle Nerve* 26: 189–193.

Susuki, K., Yuki, N., and Hirata, K. (2001). Fine specificity of anti-GQ1b IgG and clinical features. *J Neurol Sci* 185: 5–9.

Suzuki, M., Suetake, K., Kasama, T., et al. (2001). Characterization of a phospholipid antigen reacting with serum antibody in patients with peripheral neuropathies and paraproteinemia. *J Neurochem* 79: 970–975.

Takatsu, M., Hays, A.P., Latov, N., et al. (1985). Immunofluorescence study of patients with neuropathy and IgM M proteins. *Ann Neurol* 18: 173–181.

Tatum, A.H. (1993). Experimental paraprotein neuropathy, demyelination by passive transfer of human IgM anti-myelin-associated glycoprotein. *Ann Neurol* 33: 502–506.

Thomas, F.P., Trojaborg, W., Nagy, C., Santoro, M., Sadiq, S.A., and Latov, N. (1991). Experimental autoimmune neuropathy with anti-GM1 antibodies and immunoglobulin deposits at the nodes of Ranvier. *Acta Neuropathol (Berlin)* 82: 378–383.

Thomas, F.P., Lovelace, R.E., Ding, X.S., et al. (1992). Vasculitic neuropathy in a patient with cryoglobulinemia and anti-MAG IGM monoclonal gammopathy. *Muscle Nerve* 15: 891–898.

Treon, S.P., Agus, D.B., Link, B., et al. (2001). CD20-directed antibody-mediated immunotherapy induces responses and facilitates hematologic recovery in patients with Waldenstrom's macroglobulinemia. *J Immunother* 24: 272–279.

Trojaborg, W., Hays, A.P., van den Berg, L., Younger, D.S., and Latov, N. (1995). Motor conduction parameters in neuropathies associated with anti-MAG antibodies and other types of demyelinating and axonal neuropathies. *Muscle Nerve* 18: 730–735.

Uncini, A., Santoro, M., Corbo, M., Lugaresi, A., and Latov, N. (1993). Conduction abnormalities induced by sera of patients with multifocal motor neuropathy and anti-GM1 antibodies. *Muscle Nerve* 16: 610–615.

van den Berg, L.H., Lankamp, C.L., de Jager, A.E., et al., (1993). Anti-sulphatide antibodies in peripheral neuropathy. *J Neurol Neurosurg Psychiatry* 56: 1164–1168.

van den Berg, L.H., Hays, A.P., Nobile-Orazio, E., et al. (1996). Anti-MAG and Anti-SGPG antibodies in neuropathy. *Muscle Nerve* 19: 637–643.

Victor, M., Banker, B.Q., and Adams, R.D. (1958). The neuropathy of multiple myeloma. *J Neurol Neurosurg Psychiatry* 21: 73–88.

Vital, A., Vital, C., Julien, J., Baquey, A., and Steck, A.J. (1989). Polyneuropathies associated with IgM monoclonal gammopathy. Immunological and pathological study in 31 patients. *Acta Neuropathol (Berlin)* 79: 160–167.

Vital, A., Favereaux, A., Martin-Dupont, P., et al. (2001). Anti-myelin-associated glycoprotein antibodies and endoneurial cryoglobulin deposits responsible for a severe neuropathy. *Acta Neuropathol* 102: 409–412.

Vital, C., Vital, A., Deminiere, C., Julien, J., Lagueny, A., and Steck, A.J. (1997). Myelin modifications in 8 cases of peripheral neuropathy with Waldenstrom's macroglobulinemia and anti-MAG activity. *Ultrastruct Pathol* 21: 509–516.

Walsh, J.C. (1971). The neuropathy of multiple myeloma. An electrophysiological and histological study. *Arch Neurol* 25: 404–414.

Watanabe, O., Maruyama, I., Arimura, K., et al. (1998). Overproduction of vascular endothelial growth factor/vascular permeability factor is causative in Crow–Fukase (POEMS) syndrome. *Muscle Nerve* 21: 1390–1397.

Weiss, M.D., Dalakas, M.C., Lauter, C.J., Willison, H.J., and Quarles, R.H. (1999). Variability in the binding of anti-MAG and anti-SGPG antibodies to target antigens in demyelinating neuropathy and IgM paraproteinemia. *J Neuroimmunol* 95: 174–184.

Willison, H.J., O'Leary, C.P., Veitch, J., et al. (2001). The clinical and laboratory features of chronic sensory ataxic neuropathy with anti-disialosyl IgM antibodies. *Brain* 124: 1968–1977.

Wilson, H.C., Lunn MPT, Schey, S., and Hughes RAC (1999). Successful treatment of IgM paraproteinemic neuropathy with fludarabine. *J Neurol Neurosurg Psychiatry* 66: 575–580.

Wirguin, I., Suturkova-Milosevic, L.J., Dell-Latta, P., Fisher, T., Brown, R.H., and Latov, N. (1994). Monoclonal IgM antibodies to GM1 and asialo-GM1 in chronic neuropathies cross react with *Campylobacter jejuni* lipopolysaccharides. *Ann Neurol* 35: 698–703.

Wright, M., Miller, N.R., McFadzean, R.M., et al. (1998). Papilloedema, a complication of progressive diaphyseal dysplasia: a series of three case reports. *Br J Ophthalmol* 82: 1042–1048.

Yebra, M., Barrios, Y., Rincon, J., Sanjuan, I., and Diaz-Espada, F. (2002) Severe cutaneous vasculitis following intravenous infusions of gammaglobulin in a patient with type II mixed cryoglobulinemia. *Clin Exp Rheumatol* 20: 225–227.

Yuki, N., Yoshin, H., Sato, S., and Miyatake, T. (1990). Acute axonal polyneuropathy associated with anti-GM1 antibodies following *Campylobacter* enteritis. *Neurology* 40: 1900–1902.

Yuki, N., Yamada, M., Koga, M., et al. (2001). Animal model of axonal Guillain–Barre syndrome induced by sensitization with GM1 ganglioside. *Ann Neurol* 49: 712–720.

27 Neuro-Behçet's syndrome

Aksel Siva, Ayse Altintaş, and Sabahattin Saip

Introduction

Behçet's disease, originally described in 1937 by Hulusi Behçet as a distinct disease with oro-genital ulceration and uveitis (Behçet, 1937), known as the 'triple-symptom complex', is an idiopathic chronic relapsing multisystem vascular inflammatory disease of unknown origin. As the disease affects many organs and systems, its clinical manifestations and presentations show a wide range, hence it is more appropriate to consider it as a syndrome, rather than a disease.

The epidemiology of Behçet's syndrome (BS) shows a geographical variation, being seen more commonly along the Silk Route that extends from the Mediterranean region to Japan (Ohno, 1986; Gül, 2001). This is coupled by a similar variation in HLA B51, which is strongly associated with the disease in high-prevalence areas (Yazici et al., 1977; Ohno et al., 1982; Yurdakul et al., 1988; Mizuki et al., 1997). Large-scale epidemiological studies are lacking. Based on case registries, in which mild cases are unlikely to be recorded, the prevalence is reported to be less than 1 in 10^5 in the USA and northern Europe (Sakane et al.,1999; Zeiss, 2003), slightly higher in western Mediterranean countries, but increases considerably in the eastern Mediterranean region. Based on two spot surveys among the adult population in Turkey, the prevalence rates were found to be as high as 80 and 370 cases per 100 000 (Yurdakul et al., 1988), whereas Turkish immigrants living in Germany were reported to have a lower rate ($21/10^5$). This rate, however, is still higher than the native German population ($0.6/10^5$) (Zouboulis et al., 1997). The reported prevalence rates for Japan, as well as China and Korea, countries at the other end of the silk road, are between 10 and 20 per 100 000 (Sakane et al., 1999). A decline in prevalence rates for Japanese immigrants living in Hawaii and the USA had also been reported (Nakae et al., 1993).

The usual onset of the syndrome is in the third or fourth decade. The onset is rare in children and after the age of 45 (Yazici et al., 1998), but there are reports indicating that childhood cases may not be rare (Özdogan, 1994). The reported frequency of the disease in families ranges between 2 and 15% (Sakane et al., 1999; Kone Paut et al., 1999) and a multicentre study showed that this frequency was much higher in the families of paediatric cases (12.3 versus 2.2%), and that the mean age of attaining criteria for BS in familial cases was significantly lower than in sporadic cases (17.95 versus 27.78 years) (Kone Paut et al., 1999), consistent with an earlier study (Fresko et al., 1998). Although that some geographical differences have been reported for the gender distribution of BS, with the disease being more common in women in Japan and Korea and more frequent in men in Middle Eastern countries (Sakane et al., 1999); overall the male:female ratio is approximately equal but the syndrome has a more severe course in men (Yazici et al., 1998).

Diagnosis and systemic manifestations of Behçet's disease

Although various different criteria have previously been used for the diagnosis, currently the most widely used diagnostic criterion is the International Study Group's classification, according to which a definitive diagnosis requires recurrent oral ulcerations plus two of the following: recurrent genital ulcerations, skin lesions, eye lesions and a positive pathergy test (International Study Group for Behçet's Disease, 1990, 1992) (Table 27.1).

Oral aphthae

The presence of recurrent oral ulcers is required for the diagnosis of BS (International Study Group for Behçet's Disease, 1990, 1992). It is very unusual to see cases without oral ulcers and all our patients with neuro-Behçet's syndrome (NBS) had a history of oral ulcers by the time that they developed their neurological symptoms (Siva et al., 2001). However, 1 to 3% of patients can have several of the other features of the syndrome without ever having aphthae (Yazici et al., 1998). Aphthae are frequently the first manifestation of the syndrome, and it is not uncommon for some patients to have only oral ulcers for many years before other signs appear. The

Table 27.1 Criteria for diagnosis of Behçet's syndrome[a]

Finding	Definition
Recurrent oral ulceration	Minor aphthous, major aphthous, or herpetiform ulcers observed by the physician or reliably described by the patient, which recurred at least three times over a 12-month period
Recurrent genital ulceration	Aphthous ulceration or scarring observed by the physician or reliably described by the patient
Eye lesions	Anterior or posterior uveitis or cells in the vitreous body on slit-lamp examination; or retinal vasculitis detected by an ophthalmologist
Skin lesions	Erythema nodosum, pseudofolliculitis, papulopustular lesions or acneiform nodules not related to glucocorticoid treatment or adolescence
Positive pathergy test	Test interpreted as positive by the physician at 24–48 h

For a clinically definite diagnosis of Behçet's syndrome patients must have recurrent oral ulceration plus at least two of the other findings in the absence of any other clinical explanations.
[a]International Study Group for Behçet's Disease (1990).

majority of oral ulcers in BS are indistinguishable from those seen in non-BS recurrent oral ulceration, but tend to be multiple and occur more frequently. These ulcers are small, round or oval, with a sharp, erythematous border, and are painful. They appear in the gingiva, tongue, palate, and buccal and labial mucosal membranes, and usually heal without scars. Large (major) ulcers are less frequent and herpetiform ulcers are rare. Major ulcers, however, can be very troublesome because they heal with scarring, which can even occlude the oropharynx. The histology of oral ulcers reveals non-specific ulceration with necrotic material and shows evidence of vasculitis with an increase in mast cells (Yazici *et al.*, 1998; Sakane *et al.*, 1999).

Genital ulceration

External genital ulcers, which have the next highest sensitivity for the diagnosis of BS, are deeper, painful, have irregular margins, and leave scars, producing an objective sign even in the absence of active lesions. They usually occur on the scrotum in men and on the labia in women. Genital ulcers are reported to occur in 64–82% of cases (Kaklamani and Kaklamanis, 2001).

Skin lesions

The skin lesions of BS are seen in 74–87% of patients, and they consist of folliculitis, papulopustular and acneiform lesions, which occur more commonly in men, and erythema nodosum, which is more common in women. These lesions all represent various forms of vasculitis. The other forms of skin lesions are leukocytoclastic vasculitis, necrotizing arteritis of the small and medium arteries, superficial thrombophlebitis, and unclassifiable papules and pustules (Azizlerli *et al.*, 1992). Painful papules, which histologically show a neutrophilic infiltration of the skin without fibrinoid necrosis (Sweet's syndrome), are also seen (Lakhanpal *et al.*, 1988).

Eye involvement

This is one of the most serious manifestations and a leading cause of morbidity in BS. Males and those with younger age of onset, i.e. less than 25 years of age, have an increased prevalence. The overall prevalence is about 50%, but in the younger male this rate goes up to 70%. Females are less severely affected. Disease is bilateral in 90% of the patients with ocular involvement. The onset of eye disease is usually within 2 to 3 years of the development of the syndrome (Yazici *et al.*, 1998; Sakane *et al.*, 1999; Kural-Seyahi *et al.*, 2003).

Blurred vision, decrease in visual acuity, photophobia, pain in the eye, and conjunctival hyperaemia are common ocular symptoms and are due to lesions in the uvea and retina. Eye disease in BS consists of a chronic relapsing posterior and anterior uveitis; acute panuveitis is seen in 42–74% of patients (International Study Group for Behçet's Disease, 1990, 1992). It is usually associated with hypopyon, which is very typical of BS. This is an accumulation of white cells and debris in the anterior chamber that precipitates to form a layer due to gravity. It is seen in 20% of patients with eye disease and as rule is almost always associated with severe retinal disease. Retinal involvement is one major cause of morbidity in this disease as recurrent attacks may result in blindness. The basic retinal lesion is a vasculitis, which can lead to exudates, haemorrhages, occlusions of retinal arteries or veins, papilloedema, and macular disease. Secondary glaucoma frequently develops. Optic nerve involvement can occur, but is rare (Kansu *et al.*, 1989; Kidd *et al.*, 1999; Siva *et al.*, 2001).

The pathergy phenomenon

The pathergy phenomenon is one of the diagnostic tests that is almost specific to BS. This is a non-specific hypersensitivity or hyper-irritability reaction of the skin. It has a sensitivity that varies largely between different ethnic and geographical groups (range: 20–80%). It is produced by inserting a needle into the dermis of the forearm of the patient. The reaction is considered positive if a papule or pustule is formed at the site of the puncture at the 48th hour. Erythema alone is considered negative. This increased responsiveness to minor trauma or other stimuli is not unique to skin, and the pathergy phenomenon can be observed at other body sites or even at the cellular level as an up-regulated inflammatory response (Gül, 2001).

Ergun *et al.* (1998) studied the histopathology of pathergy extensively and found that at time zero skin is normal, whereas 4 hours after skin prick neutrophils are present, usually admixed with lymphocytes. Intra-epidermal pustules and polymorphonuclear cells aggregates within the needle tract are seen as early as 4 hours, and inflammatory cell density reaches a peak by 24–48 hours. Sparse leukocytocasis is identifiable from 4 to 48 hours. These investigators suggested that early pathergy is mediated by polymorphonuclear cells and lymphocytes without vasculitis, and excessive function of chemotaxis may explain the rapid accumulation of polymorphonuclear cells along the injection site. The mononuclear cell infiltrate is predominantly composed of T lymphocytes and monocytes/macrophages. The majority of the T lymphocytes are CD4+, and almost all the cells express CD45RO.

The sensitivity of the test differs according to the population studied. It has a higher positivity rate in Turkey, Israel and Japan (40–75%), than it has in Western countries such as the UK or USA (10–30%) (Hegab and Al-Mutawa, 2000; Zeiss, 2003). A higher rate of positive skin response in patients with BS was reported with intradermal injections of sodium monourate crystals suspended in saline (Çakir *et al.*, 1991), and this observation was recently confirmed (Fresko *et al.*, 2000).

Musculoskeletal involvement

A non-erosive, non-migrating monoarthritis or oligoarthritis involving the large joints, especially knees, ankles and wrists, either in the form of arthritis or arthralgia is reported in about 50% of patients (Yurdakul *et al.*, 1983). Another musculoskeletal manifestation associated with BS is aseptic necrosis of the bone. This is possibly related to vasculitis and not necessarily to steroid use (Yazici *et al.*, 1998; Sakane *et al.*, 1999).

Gastrointestinal involvement

Constipation, diarrhoea, abdominal pain, or vomiting are common gastrointestinal symptoms but their frequency varies in different geographical populations (Yazici *et al.*, 1998; Sakane *et al.*, 1999). These symptoms are seen relatively frequently in Japan, but not in Turkey and other Mediterranean countries. Due to their common occurrence oral ulcers are considered separately from the remaining gastrointestinal tract, of which any part, especially the distal ileum and caecum, may also have ulcers.

Cardiovascular involvement

Arterial aneurysms or occlusions and deep vein thromboses and thrombophlebitis are among large vessel complications that are seen in 25–30% of cases, while a possibly higher proportion do have small vessel involvement, mostly affecting post capillary venules (Park *et al.*, 1984; O'Duffy, 1990; Koç, 1992). The basic pathology is thought to be a vasculitis of the vasa vasorum (O'Duffy, 1990). Involvement of the veins is one of the main manifestations of BS. In fact, BS is one of the few vasculitides, together with systemic lupus erythematosus and Buerger's disease, that can involve both the venous and arterial sides of the circulatory system (Yazici *et al.*, 1998). But it differs from the other two, as in contrast to them it can involve the vena cavae too. In BS there is also a tendency to develop venous thromboses after venepunctures.

Although rare, myocardial ischaemia associated with coronary vasculitis or with inflammation such as endocarditis, myocarditis, and pericarditis may all occur, resulting in ventricular dysfunction and intracardiac thrombi. Cases with ventricular aneurysms have also been documented.

Other systems

Other systems reported to be involved through the course of the disease are the pulmonary, urinary, and central nervous systems.

Laboratory investigations

There are no laboratory findings specific for BS. The moderate anaemia of chronic disease and leukocytosis can be seen in some patients. The erythrocyte sedimentation rate is only mildly elevated, as is the C-reactive protein.

Their correlation with disease activity, however, is controversial (Müftüoglu et al., 1986; Zeiss, 2003). Serum amyloid A and β-2-microglobulin levels were reported to be elevated and associated with disease activity (Aygunduz et al., 2000), though this needs to be confirmed. Serum immunoglobulins, and more specifically IgD levels, are sometimes elevated, while autoantibodies are absent (Yazici et al., 1998; Sakane et al., 1999). Complement levels may be high. However, HLA testing can support the diagnosis in populations where the disease is associated with the HLA B51 phenotype and may help in the differential diagnosis.

Aetiopathogenesis of Behçet's syndrome

Despite broadened clinical understanding of this disease, the aetiological factors remain obscured and speculative; genetic causes, immunological factors, viral agents, bacterial factors, and coagulation abnormalities have all been implicated (Kansu, 1996; Yazici, 1997; Yazici et al., 2001; Direskeneli, 2001; Gül, 2001). Three major pathophysiological changes have been reported in BS—excessive functions of neutrophils, endothelial injury with vasculitis, and autoimmune responses. Histopathological and immunohistochemical studies of the lesions obtained from patients with BS reveal mononuclear cell infiltration of T lymphocytes, B lymphocytes, and neutrophils, consistent with vasculitis involving both arterial and venous systems (O'Duffy, 1990; Azizlerli et al., 1992; Kansu, 1996; Sakane et al., 1999). It is postulated that a genetic susceptibility together with a possible trigger by an extrinsic factor, such as an infectious agent, is responsible for the observed vasculitis.

Genetic susceptibility and HLA

Behçet's disease is not a genetic disease with a Mendelian inheritance model. The majority of patients are sporadic cases and have no family history. However, familial cases are seen and their analysis favours the presence of a complex genetic inheritance model, and the importance of the genetic load in the pathogenesis of BS has been emphasized (Gül, 2001). The observation of an earlier disease onset in the off-spring of affected parents, as well as a high sibling recurrence risk ratio, are some of the indications for the genetic background of the disease (Fresko et al., 1998; Kone Paut et al., 1999; Gül, 2001).

Although that BS has been described to be associated with more than one HLA genotype, HLA-B51 is the most significant marker of BS, as confirmed in Japan, Turkey, Israel, France, and Tunisia (Yazici et al., 1977; Brauther et al., 1978; Ohno et al., 1982; Mizuki et al., 1997a). However, the association of BS with HLA-B51 is much weaker in the UK and the USA, but it should be noted that the frequency of this allele is also higher in the healthy population of the countries of the Silk Route where the disease is more common (Hegab and Al-Mutawa, 2000). HLA-B51 (and particularly its B5101 subcomponent) is the main allele associated with BS (Yazici et al., 2001). The presence of this marker has an odds ratio of 1.5 in 16 different series (Direskeneli, 2001) and the contribution of HLA-B51 to the overall genetic susceptibility to Behçet's disease is estimated to be less than 20% (Gül, 2001). Although no HLA-B51 restriction has been demonstrated so far in experiments using peptides which are thought to be specific for Behçet's disease, it has been suggested that the presentation of certain Behçet's disease-associated peptides from different microbial antigens with HLA-B51 might be a mechanism in the pathogenesis (Gül, 2001). HLA-B*5101 is the major subtype of HLA-B51 associated with BS and differs from HLA-B*5201, a split antigen of B5 but unlinked to BS, by only two amino acids at positions 63 and 67 which are in pocket B, the antigen-binding groove. These amino acids are possibly crucial anchor residues for peptide binding. A candidate 'Behçetogenic' epitope presented by *5101 is described as DAIXXXXXF, a hypothetical disease-inducing peptide (Direskeneli, 2001).

The telomeric side of the human HLA-B locus on chromosome 6 also houses both the tumour necrosis factor (TNF) and the MICA genes, the latter group being important in mucosal immunity. However, recent work suggests that polymorphisms in either region do not contribute to the genetic load in BS, with the exception that an association may exist between the severity of eye disease and co-expression of the TNF-β2 allele with HLA-B51 (Yazici et al., 2001). Mizuki and Ohno (1996) first reported an association of MICA (MHC class I related gene) between the TNF (alpha) gene and the HLA-B region on chromosome 6, with BS. Mizuki et al. found that although the association with MIC-A is significant, the association with HLA-B51 independently remains the most significant factor for the development of BS, suggesting that MICA gene is unlikely to be the disease-susceptible gene for BS. Similarly, the MIC-B gene itself is not responsible for the development of BS (Mizuki et al., 1997b; Sakane and Suzuki, 2002) However, it is not clear whether the HLA-B gene itself is the primary susceptibility factor in Behçet's disease or whether some other HLA or non-HLA gene in a linkage disequilibrium to HLA-B51 is directly involved in the pathogenesis of the disease, since about 40% of patients with the disease are B51-negative individuals. It is possible that functional polymorphism in the HLA Class I-restricted antigen processing and presentation to CD8+ cytotoxic T lymphocytes accounts for the difference in the susceptibility to Behçet's disease (Ishihara et al., 1996; Mizuki et al., 1997b).

Only one HLA-B*5101 heavy chain transgenic mouse model has been published up to now. These animals did not develop any Behçet's disease-related manifestation, and only showed an increased neutrophil activity following f-Met–Leu–Phe (fMLP) stimulation compared with HLA-B35 and non-transgenic mice (Gül, 2001). Interestingly, a similar enhanced neutrophil activity was observed in HLA-B51-positive healthy individuals, a finding which further requires the clarification of the association between HLA-B51 and neutrophil functions. It is a possibility that the B51 antigen expressed in mice presents some exogenous antigenic peptides to T lymphocytes, provokes immune responses, and, as a result, primes the neutrophils, leading to increased superoxide production in the mice. Thus, the molecular cascade from B51 antigen expression to neutrophil activation may be associated with BS, and therefore B51 antigen may be directly involved in the onset of the disease (Mizuki et al., 1997b).

Immunological abnormalities

BS patients with active disease show an increase in interferon (IFN)-γ-producing CD3+ lymphocytes compared with patients in complete remission and healthy subjects. On the contrary, no difference in interleukin (IL)-4-producing CD3+ lymphocytes is observed among active patients, inactive patients, and normal individuals (Mizuki et al., 1997b). Both CD4+ and CD8+ T cells, which produce the T helper 1 (Th1)-type pro-inflammatory cytokines IL-2 and IFN-γ, are increased in the peripheral blood, and correlate with disease activity. IL-12, which drives the Th1 response in naïve T cells, is raised in BS sera, in correlation with Th1 lymphocytes. Th2 lymphocytes and levels of Th2 cytokines are generally found to be low. Peripheral γ/δ T cells also secrete IFN-γ and TNF-α as major cytokines, which are of the Th1 type (Direskeneli, 2001). Thus, a polarization of Th1/Th2 balance toward the Th1 phenotype is evident in patients with active disease (Mizuki et al., 1997b; Frassanito et al., 1999; Hegab and Al-Mutawa, 2000). An increased secretion of IL-1, IL-6, TNF-γ, and IL-8 from monocytes following lipopolysaccharide (LPS) stimulation in BS patients compared with healthy and diseased controls, can also be observed even in patients with inactive disease. No increase in Th2 type IL-4-producing T cells was observed during the inactive stage of patients with Behçet's disease (Gül, 2001). The work of Frassanito et al. (1999) further demonstrated the Th1 polarization of the immune response in BS.

Although there are conflicting reports on the number of CD4+ and CD8+ T cells found in the peripheral blood of patients with Behçet's disease, an increase in the proportions of γ/δ T cells and CD8+ γ/δ T cells was consistently found (Gül, 2001). γ/δ T lymphocytes sometimes constitute more than 60% of the peripheral blood lymphocytes. Thus, γ/δ T lymphocytes may play a certain role in the tissue injuries observed in BS (Mizuki et al., 1997b). Most γ/δ T lymphocytes from BS patients express activation markers such as CD25, CD69, HLA-DR, and CD99, indicating that the γ/δ T lymphocytes have already been activated in vivo (Mizuki et al., 1997b).

Nakamura *et al.* (1996) suggested that insufficient expression of Fas on activated CD4+ T cells and its high expression on CD8+ T cells may play an important role in the chronic inflammation in BS (Nakamura *et al.*, 1996). An increase in peripheral blood natural killer (NK) cells was also found. (Hegab and Al-Mutawa, 2000).

The γ/δ T cells have capacity to produce differential Th1 and Th2 cytokines and might also control the γ/δ T cells. When γ/δ T cells are activated by bacterial antigens they express NK cell activity. Intraepithelial γ/δ T cells can also modulate epithelial cell growth by expressing a keratinocyte growth factor, which might be involved in the mucocutaneous manifestations of BS (Adam *et al.*, 1996).

Saruhan-Direskeneli *et al.* (2003) studied the serum and cerebrospinal fluid (CSF) levels of cytokines and chemokines in neuro-BD compared with multiple sclerosis(MS) and other neurological diseases. IL-10, IL-12, IL-17, CXCL8, CXCL10, and CCL2 levels were evaluated. The authors suggested that their results point to a dominance of chemokine effects in neuro-BD CSF.

Although the total number of B cells is normal, they express increased levels of activation markers such as CD13, CD33, CD80, and the memory marker CD45RO. The low level of CD5+CD19+ B cells which produce autoantibodies suggests that BS is distinct from classical autoantibody-mediated disorders (Direskeneli, 2001).

BS is characterized histopathologically by neutrophilic vasculitis with increased neutrophilic infiltration in the perivascular area (Sahin *et al.*, 1996), and a significant neutrophilic infiltration has been observed in some of the typical BS lesions such as pustular folliculitis, pathergy reactions, and hypopyon (Direskeneli, 2001). A number of investigators have found abnormalities in neutrophil functions, such as increased chemotaxis and phagocytosis (Sahin *et al.*, 1996; Direskeneli, 2001). Enhanced TNF-α production might help to auto-prime neutrophils and prolong their own lifespan, which might result in accumulation of activated neutrophils in the site of inflammation (Mizuki *et al.*, 1997*b*; Gül, 2001). Sahin *et al.* (1996) showed increased neutrophil adhesion in patients with BS and the significant increase in adhesion after stimulation of human umbilical vein endothelial cells (HUVECs) by IL-1α, TNF-α, and LPS that may reflect functional or quantitative up-regulation of surface adhesion molecules on polymorphonuclear leukocytes (PMNLs) in BS. Although that the relationship of HLA-B51 with neutrophil functions currently is not clear, genetic factors also seem to play an important role in the non-specific enhanced inflammatory reaction in Behçet's disease (Gül, 2001). A central role for neutrophils in the pathophysiology of the disease has further been supported by the fact that therapies for targeting neutrophils, such as colchicine, effectively relieve at least some of the disease symptoms (Mizuki *et al.*, 1997*b*).

The reason for more severe disease among male patients with BS remains obscure. In endotoxin-induced uveitis in rats, oestrogen administration decreased the severity of uveitis, probably through down-regulation of the inflammatory mediators E-selectin and IL-6. The relevance of this finding to human disease remains to be seen (Yazici *et al.*, 2001).

Although BS does not have the features of a classical autoimmune disorder (Yazici *et al.*, 1997), some B-cell activity, such as increased spontaneous immunoglobulin secretion, is reported. The presence of autoantibodies such as anti-endothelial cell, antilymphocyte, and anticardiolipin antibodies, especially of IgA isotype, has been shown (Direskeneli, 2001) and there are also some studies that report an increase in the Ig levels. The results of the studies on anticardiolipin antibodies, however, are conflicting (Hegab and Al-Mutawa, 2000). Anti-endothelial cell antibodies are present in 20–30% of BS patients (Sakane *et al.*, 2002) and non-lytic antibodies against endothelial cells (AECA) are commonly present in both vascular and non-vascular BS (Direskeneli, 2001).

Possible antigens

The geographical distribution of BS together with its prevalence in the lower socioeconomic groups, in overcrowded conditions, and possible familial clustering could favour a microbial role in the aetiology of BS.

However, despite extensive studies, the role of microbial agents remains uncertain. Evidence of herpes simplex virus (HSV) infection and the role of bacterial antigens, especially streptococci and their heat shock proteins (HSP) have been reported by a number of authors (Direskeneli *et al.*, 1996; Hegab and Al-Mutawa, 2000; Direskeneli, 2001; Gül, 2001; Sakane and Suzuki, 2002), but their primary role in BS still needs to be clarified.

HSP are highly conserved proteins, synthesized in large amounts when cells are exposed to stressful stimuli (Direskeneli *et al.*, 1996). HSP might be relevant to BS as a variety of streptococci (*Streptococcus sanguis*, *S. pyogenes*, *S. faecalis*, and *S. salivarius*) and herpes simplex virus type I have been implicated in its aetiology. Indeed, a significant increase in serum Ig A antibodies to the microbial 65 kDa HSP was reported in BS, and a number of monoclonal antibodies (MoAb) to the microbial 65 kDa HSP cross-reacted with selected strains of *S. sanguis*. Human T cells reactive to the mycobacterial 65 kDa HSP are found in normal subjects, so they are insufficient to initiate an autoimmune disease. However, if immunodominant epitopes within the microbial HSP were to stimulate expansion of clones reactive to the homologous human epitopes, an immunopathological response may occur (Direskeneli *et al.*, 1996). Heat shock proteins, especially 60/65 kDa HSP (HSP65) are possible candidate antigens for BS. HSP65 is expressed abundantly in epidermal regions of active skin lesions, such as erythema nodosum and mucocutaneous ulcers in BS. Lehner and colleagues first suggested the concept of HSP65 as a pathogenic antigen in BS by identifying anti-HSP65 antibodies cross-reactive with oral mucosal homogenates and oral streptococci (Lehner, 1997). Four epitopes of mycobacterial HSP65 (amino acid sequences 111–125, 154–172, 219–233, and 311–326) were recognized to be immunodominant for T- and B-cell responses. T-cell responses to these mycobacterial HSP65-derived peptides and to their 50–80% homologues on human HSP60 were significantly higher in patients with BS from the UK, Japan, and Turkey than in controls (Direskeneli *et al.*, 1996; Direskeneli, 2001). As significant sequence homology exists between the mammalian and microbial HSPs, it has been suggested that bacterial HSP responsive T cells may stimulate autoreactive T cells by cross-reactivity mechanisms (Direskeneli, 2001; Sakane and Suzuki, 2002). Both antistreptococcal and antiretinal HSP60 antibodies are raised in the serum samples of patients with BS and uveitis, with significant cross-inhibition. Increased anti-HSP65 antibody responses are also present in the CSF of patients with neuro-BS with parenchymal involvement (Direskeneli, 2001). Investigations concerning HSP showed that four peptides (111–125, 154–172, 219–233, and 311–326) included within mycobacterial HSP65 are responsible for the lymphoproliferative response. These peptides, whether derived from mycobacterial 65 kDa or homologous HSP, produced the same effect. The sensitization and accordingly the proliferation which affects CD4+ cells was limited to the γ/δ cell subtype (Hegab and Al-Mutawa, 2000).

Activation of peripheral blood mononuclear cells (PBMCs) of BS patients by the self-HSP peptide results in the predominant production of IL-12, TNF-α and IFN-β in BS patients. B lymphocytes, in comparison with monocytes, produce large amounts of IL-12 in response to HSP peptide stimulation. This suggests that not only T but also B lymphocytes are sensitized to the self-HSP peptide (Sakane and Suzuki, 2002). HLA-B51 was not found to be significantly associated with any of the four specific peptides (Pervin *et al.*, 1993).

Celet *et al.* (2000) reported that serum and CSF IgG and serum IgM antibody responses to α/β-crystallin are raised in patients with neuro-BS compared with patients with non-inflammatory nervous system disease. When they subclassified their results according to the type of neurological involvement, patients with parenchymal neuro-BS had higher CSF IgG responses to α/β-crystallin than the neuro-BS group with cerebral dural venous thrombosis (vascular form). CSF IgG responses to HSP65 and α/β-crystallin also showed a significant correlation with each other, possibly owing to similar immune mechanisms driving both autoantibody responses in the CSF (Celet *et al.* 2000; Direskeneli, 2001).

One other candidate autoantigen in BS is retinal-S antigen (S-Ag). The S-Ag, which was isolated by Wacker and colleagues, is the most potent uveitic antigen. It is localized to the photoreceptor area of the retina and in some species to the pineal gland also. This antigen, which has been used to produce experimental autoimmune uveitis, could be detected in patients with BS (Hegab and Al-Mutawa, 2000). Among the immunodominant epitopes of S-Ag, an epitope (amino acids 342–355, PDS-Ag) is found to share homology with a conserved region of HLA-B molecules (amino acids 125–138, B27PD) (Direskeneli, 2001). Kurhan-Yavuz and colleagues looked at the T-cell responsiveness of this synthetic peptide B27PD, and S-Ag in a group of patients with BS with and without eye disease (Kurhan-Yavuz et al., 2000). Healthy individuals and patients with non-BS acute anterior uveitis (most of them had ankylosing spondylitis) were the controls. It was shown that only patients with BS disease and eye involvement had significantly increased proliferative and cytokine (IL-2 and TNF-α) responses. This work suggests that the immune response to self antigens might be important in the pathogenesis of BS. Retinal S-Ag derived PDS-Ag, with T-cell recognition, found only in patients with posterior uveitis, is a candidate organ-specific antigen of this type. Similarly, the presence of anti-HSP60 antibodies, mainly in patients with parenchymal neuro-BS but not in pure vascular form, underlines the fact that even within the same organ immune responses may reflect different clinical subtypes (Direskeneli, 2001). Besides the retinal antigens, Lehner has demonstrated evidence of T-cell activity to an antigen derived from the oral mucosa of patients with BS (Lehner, 1969).

A proposed hypothesis for the aetiopathogenesis of BS as described by Sakane and Suzuki (2002) is that in a genetically susceptible individual an exogenous antigen such as a streptococcal or a viral antigen, the HSP of which shares an epitope with human-derived HSP, may stimulate HSP-specific T lymphocytes in addition to monocytes, and subsequently induce production of Th1 cytokines such as IL-8, TNF, and IL-6. These cytokines stimulate monocytes and lymphocytes in an autocrine/paracrine fashion, and stimulate the vascular endothelium as well. Stimulation of polymorphonuclear cells by these cytokines is also of particular importance for the pathogenesis of BS because of a genetic hyper-responsiveness of the polymorphonuclear cells in BS. The final outcome will be systemic vascular damage leading to various clinical manifestations of the disease Sakane and Suzuki (2002).

Coagulation abnormalities

Vascular injuries with thrombotic tendency are another characteristic feature of BS (Kansu, 1996; Yazici et al., 2001). The damaged or activated endothelial cells are another stimulator to neutrophils. Abnormalities which have been described as related to the vascular lesions are the presence of anti-endothelial cell antibodies, higher von Willebrand factor antigen level, and the presence of circulating immune complexes. In addition, as already discussed, circulating pro-inflammatory cytokines are involved in activating both neutrophils and endothelial cells. Activated endothelial cells secrete adhesion molecules and this facilitates interaction between endothelial cells and neutrophils. These factors form a vicious circle to promote the disease.

The frequency of the Factor V Leiden mutation was studied and found to have significance only in the presence of eye disease in BS in one study (Verity et al., 1999). In another study thrombophilic factors were screened in patients with BS, and no correlation was found between the clinical manifestations of the disease and of any of the variables studied—which included anticardiolipin antibodies, IgM and G, the presence of circulating lupus anticoagulant, protein C, protein S, antithrombin III activity, activated protein C resistance, and Factor V Leiden mutation (Mader et al., 1999). In a similar more recent study, in which thrombophilic factors were studied in BS patients with and without venous thrombosis, increased thrombin generation, fibrinolysis, and thrombomodulin were observed in both groups of BS patients when compared with controls, but no correlation with thrombosis and these abnormalities could be detected (Espinosa et al., 2002). However, Aksu et al. (2001) found that hyperhomocystinaemia was an independent risk factor for venous thrombosis in BS. While the debate about the precise importance of the Factor V Leiden mutation continues, an additional inherited abnormality in the coagulation cascade has been described in BS. The prothrombin G$\rightarrow$A^{20210} mutation, which is an established cause of thrombosis, was found in a higher frequency in BS patients with thrombotic complications (Gül et al., 1999; Salvarani et al., 2000). Gül et al. (1999) screened 32 patients with BS who had thrombotic complications and compared these with 32 age- and sex-matched BS patients without thrombosis. Thirty-one per cent of the thrombotic and 3% of the non-thrombotic patients carried the G$\rightarrow$A^{20210} mutation. In this same group of patients the Factor V Leiden mutation was also studied. Thirty-eight per cent of the thrombotic and 9% of the non-thrombotic group were positive for this mutant gene (Gül et al., 1999).

Nervous system involvement in Behçet's disease

'Neuro-Behçet syndrome'

Patients with BS may present with different neurological problems, related either directly or indirectly to the disease (Table 27.2). Cerebral dural venous sinus thrombosis, central nervous system (CNS) involvement secondary to vascular inflammation, the neuro-psycho-Behçet variant, in which an organic psychotic syndrome is prominent, are direct effects (Siva and Altintaş, 2000; Siva and Fresko, 2000; Siva et al., 2004). A non-structural recurrent migrainous headache that starts after the onset of the systemic manifestations of BS, and which is sometimes associated with their exacerbations, is relatively common (Saip et al., in press). Neurological complications secondary to systemic disease or related to treatments for the systemic manifestations of BS are among indirect neuropsychiatric consequences of the disease (Siva and Altintaş, 2000; Siva et al., 2004). Peripheral nervous system involvement, which may develop either directly

Table 27.2 The neurological spectrum of Behçet's syndrome (BS) (from Siva et al. (2004))

Primary neurological (direct neurological consequences of the syndrome)	Headache (the non-structural headache of BS)
	Cerebral venous sinus thrombosis (extra-axial NBS)
	Central nervous system involvement (intra-axial NBS)
	Neuro-psycho-Behçet syndrome
	Peripheral nervous system involvement
	Subclinical NBS
Secondary neurological (indirect neurological consequences of the syndrome)	Complications of treatments of BS (i.e. CNS neurotoxicity with cyclosporin or peripheral neuropathy related to thalidomide)
	Complications of systemic disease (i.e. cerebral emboli from cardiac complications of BS)
Coincidental neurological disorders	

NBS, Neuro-Behçet syndrome.

Table 27.3 Suggested diagnostic criteria for neuro-Behçet syndrome (NBS) (modified from Siva and Altıntaş (2000))

A: Fulfilling the international diagnostic criteria for Behçet's disease

B: Onset of neurological symptoms not otherwise explained by any other known systemic or neurological disease or treatment

C: Presence of at least one of the following:

(1) Objective abnormalities on neurological examination (clinical evidence)

(2) Abnormal neuroimaging findings suggestive of NBS (imaging evidence)

(3) Abnormal cerebrospinal fluid findings suggestive of NBS (laboratory evidence)

(4) Abnormal neurophysiological (electromyography or evoked potentials) studies consistent with the current neurological symptoms (neurophysiological evidence)

Table 27.4 The spectrum of 'headaches' seen in patients with Behçet's disease

Headache due to central nervous system parenchymal involvement

Headache due to cerebral venous sinus thrombosis

Headache in association with ocular inflammation

The non-structural (migraine-like) headache of BS

Co-existing primary headaches (i.e. migraine, tension-type headache)

or indirectly in BS, is extremely rare, despite neurophysiological studies demonstrating non-specific findings in some patients.

Cerebral venous sinus thrombosis (CVST), central nervous system (CNS) parenchymal involvement secondary to vascular inflammation, and the neuro-psycho-Behçet variant which is commonly associated with the CNS involvement are neurological conditions directly related to BS. All demonstrate neurological manifestations which are considered to be signs and symptoms due to nervous system involvement in BS, and will be reviewed here as 'neuro-Behçet syndrome' (NBS). Our suggested criteria for diagnosis of NBS are outlined in Table 27.3.

The reported frequency of neurological involvement among BS patients ranges between 2.2 and 49.0%, but larger series have shown a rate of approximately 5% (Akman-Demir et al., 1999; Siva et al., 2001). However, these are frequency estimates from cross-sectional studies. In a recent study from our centre, when the frequency of neurological involvement was evaluated prospectively, the frequency became 13.0% among males and 5.6% among females after two decades of follow-up (Kural-Seyahi et al., 2003). Both cross-sectional and prospective studies confirm an increased rate of neurological complications in BS in males (Siva et al., 2004), and such a significant male predominance is also noted for major vascular complications of BS. In our Behçet's Disease Research Center the mean age of onset for BS and NBS were found to be 26.7 ± 8.0 and 32.0 ± 8.7 years, respectively (Siva et al., 2001), which is consistent with some other series (Kidd et al., 1999; Akman-Demir et al., 1999).

As discussed above, NBS may be manifested either in the form of CNS involvement or CVST, the two major neurological presentations of BS. Clinically, neurological manifestations are related commonly to brainstem or corticospinal tract syndromes in the former presentation and to increased intracranial pressure in the second form. There is a tendency to designate only CNS parenchymal involvement as NBS, and to include cerebral venous sinus thrombosis within the spectrum of so-called vasculo-Behçet (Wechsler et al., 1992; Serdaroglu, 1998a). However, as both have neurological consequences they maybe identified as 'intra-axial NBS' and 'extra-axial NBS', respectively.

Clinical and neuroimaging evidence also confirms this subclassification of NBS. CNS-NBS or intra-axial NBS is due to small vessel disease and causes the focal or multifocal CNS involvement manifested in the majority of patients. The second form, CVST or extra-axial NBS, which is due to large vessel disease in the form of CVST has limited symptoms and a better neurological prognosis (Siva et al., 2001). These two types of involvement occur in the same individual very rarely, and presumably have a different pathogenesis. Many of the CNS-NBS patients with small vessel inflammation have a relapsing–remitting course initially, with some ultimately developing a secondary progressive course later, and a few will have a progressive CNS dysfunction from the onset. In our series of patients with neurological manifestations related to BS, the rate of CNS-NBS was 75.6% and of CVST 12.2%, with the remaining having other or indefinite diagnoses (Siva et al., 2001).

The most common neurological symptom seen in patients with BS is headache (Monastero et al., 2003; Saip et al., in press). Although the head-

ache is a major symptom of CNS involvement or dural sinus thrombosis, it is more commonly seen in patients without overt neurological involvement. The differential diagnosis of headache in in BS is outlined in Table 27.4. Besides primary headaches some patients with BS report a paroxysmal migraine-like pain, which is bilateral, frontal, of moderate severity, and throbbing. This type of headache starts after the onset of the systemic manifestations of BS, and not uncommonly is associated with exacerbations of the mucocutaneous symptoms, though this is not always the rule. This headache is not associated with any structural neurological involvement and is not specific for this disorder, but may be explained by a vascular headache triggered by the immunomediated disease activity in susceptible individuals (Saip et al., in press).

However, a substantial number of patients with BS may report a severe headache of recent onset not consistent with a coexisting primary headache or ocular inflammatory pain. These patients require further evaluation, even if they do not have neurological signs, as such a symptom may indicate the onset of NBS. In our practice, we consider patients for further evaluation when the reported headache is severe and incapacitating, if it is the first or worst headache of their lives, if their symptoms began after or within 6 months of onset of other systemic symptoms, if there is a change in character of the headache after the onset of systemic disease, or, needless to say, when they have an objective finding on neurological examination such as papilloedema. By this approach we have shown approximately 10% of patients presenting with an isolated headache to have a neurological syndrome due to BS (Siva et al., 2001).

In addition to headache alone, NBS may present with focal or multifocal CNS dysfunction with or without headache. The most common symptoms detected at onset in our series of well-documented 164 patients were: headache (61.6%), weakness of upper motor neuron type (53.7%), brainstem and cerebellar (49%), and cognitive/behavioural (16%) (Siva et al., 2001). Rare presentations include isolated optic neuritis, psychiatric manifestations referred to as neuro-psycho-Behçet syndrome, aseptic meningitis, intracerebral haemorrhage due to ruptured aneurysms, extrapyramidal syndromes, and peripheral neuropathy (O'Duffy et al., 1971; Bussone et al., 1982; Siva et al., 1986, 1991, 2001; Namer et al., 1987; Kansu et al., 1989; Takeuchi et al., 1989; Perniciaro and Molina, 1991; Serdaroglu, 1998a; Bogdanova et al., 1998; Kidd et al., 1999; Akman-Demir et al., 1999).

Intra-axial NBS

The onset of a subacute brainstem syndrome in a young man, especially of Mediterranean (or Middle Eastern or oriental) origin, that includes cranial nerve findings, dysarthria, uni- or bilateral corticospinal tract signs, and a mild confusion should raise the possibility of 'NBS'. Such a patient needs to be interviewed (if a reliable history cannot been obtained from the patient, then his family member(s)) for the presence of systemic findings of BS. In the case of BS, one will be very likely to obtain a past or present history of recurrent oral aphthous ulcers and some other systemic manifestations of the disease. Many patients may be found to have never consulted a physician because of the mild nature of their systemic symptoms, or may be missed because of not reporting the full-blown picture of the disease. As mentioned above, it will be quite unlikely to see NBS cases without oral ulcers and all our patients with NBS had a history of oral ulcers by the time that they have developed their neurological symptoms. The MRI findings of the disease are almost pathognomonic, and this will further support the diagnosis (Koçer *et al.*, 1999). However, it should be kept in mind that parenchymal NBS (intra-axial NBS) does not always present with brainstem signs and symptoms. A hemiparesis, cognitive-behavioural changes, emotional lability, a self-limited or progressive myelopathy, as well as other CNS manifestations such as extrapyramidal signs and seizures, may be seen, but are less common.

Aseptic meningitis was reported previously to be a relatively frequent form of neurological involvement in patients with BS in studies which were based on CT scans as the primary imaging modality (Serdaroglu *et al.*, 1989). Our experience has not been such, and we suspect that in some patients parenchymal disease was misclassified as aseptic meningitis due to a lack of sensitive imaging data. As a matter of fact, in a recent update from the same institution (Akman-Demir *et al.*, 1999), aseptic meningitis was reported in only one out of 200 cases studied. Similarly, in another recent study of 50 patients from the UK (Kidd *et al.*, 1999), four cases were reported to have meningitis symptoms, while two of these patients had parenchymal lesions and two had normal MRI. There was no discussion of meningeal enhancement and the CSF findings were within the same range as in those patients who had brainstem parenchymal involvement. In support of this, we have always observed inflammatory findings in CSF together with parenchymal disease in MRI. Taken together, we conclude that pure aseptic meningitis is very rare within the clinical spectrum of neurological involvement in BS (Siva *et al.*, 2001).

Arterial involvement resulting in CNS vascular disease is rare but has been reported as single case presentations in BS. Observations in cases with bilateral internal carotid artery occlusion, vertebral artery occlusion, and intracranial arteritis as well as aneurysms, with their corresponding neurological consequences, suggest that arterial involvement may be a subgroup of CNS-NBS (Siva *et al.*, 2004). Intracranial haemorrhages may occur but are extremely rare, with most being haemorrhages within the ischaemic lesions (Koçer *et al.*, 1999; Kikuchi *et al.*, 2002).

Various types of voiding dysfunction relating to bladder and sphincteric components in both phases of micturition can be seen in BS. Voiding dysfunction can be due to either neurological or direct bladder involvement. The experience in our centre showed that augmentation ileocystoplasty is a good treatment option for BS with severe bladder involvement (Cetinel *et al.*, 1999).

Neuro-psycho-Behçet syndrome

Some patients with BS develop a neurobehavioural syndrome which consists of euphoria, loss of insight, disinhibition, indifference to their disease, psychomotor agitation or retardation, with paranoid attitudes and obsessive concerns. We have observed the development of these psychiatric symptoms either at the onset of other neurological symptoms of NBS, or independently. They were not associated with glucocorticosteroid or any other therapy. We have named this syndrome 'neuro-psycho-Behçet syndrome' (Siva *et al.*, 1986). A similar personality change was observed by others as well (Oktem-Tanor *et al.*, 1999).

In a prospective neuropsychological study of 12 patients with NBS, memory impairment was found to be the major finding (Oktem-Tanor *et al.*, 1999). The most severely affected memory process was delayed recall, being impaired in all of the patients either in the verbal and/or the visual modalities. An impairment in the process of acquisition and storage; attention deficit, and deficits of executive functions of the frontal system were other cognitive functions involved in a declining order. Neuropsychological status deteriorated insidiously, regardless of the neurological attacks during the follow-up period, in most of the patients, and the presence of cognitive decline was not directly related to detectable lesions on neuroimaging at early stages of the disease. However, an enlargement of the third ventricle and atrophy of the posterior fossa structures were observed in the late stages of the disease, which was correlated with memory loss (Oktem-Tanor *et al.*, 1999). Monastero *et al.* (2004) studied the prevalence and pattern of cognitive impairment in 26 patients with BS without overt neurological involvement. They found cognitive impairment in 46.1% of their cohort, with a similar pattern of involvement to that found in the above study. They have also shown that both active disease and prednisone dosage were associated with the development of cognitive

dysfunction, suggesting that BS patients with an active disease or treated with steroids are at potential risk of having subclinical cognitive deficits. Such an explanation may also be valid for patients with cerebral involvement, independent of the pattern and extent of structural CNS disease; however, on the other hand, as none of the patients had an MRI examination in this study, CNS involvement could not be totally excluded.

Extra-axial NBS

CVST is seen in 10–20% of BS patients in whom neurological involvement occurs. Thrombosis of the venous sinuses may cause increased intracranial pressure with severe headache, mental changes, and motor ocular cranial nerve palsies, but in some patients the only manifestation may be a moderate headache. It is well known that the clinical manifestations resulting from thrombosis of the intracranial venous system vary according to the site and rate of venous occlusion and its extent. Our experience suggests that the CVST in BS evolves relatively slowly, as in none of our patients have we observed a fulminating syndrome of violent headache, convulsions, paralysis and coma. But cases with acute onset are reported in whom seizures and focal neurological signs occurred besides headache (Wechsler *et al.*, 1992). Papilloedema and sixth nerve paresis are the most common signs reported, and hemiparesis may develop in some (Wechsler *et al.*, 1992; Akman-Demir *et al.*, 1999; Siva *et al.*, 2001).

There is a tendency for CVST to occur earlier in the disease course compared with the parenchymal type of CNS disease and this difference is significant in male patients (Tunc *et al.*, 2004). Any of the sinuses may be affected, but the superior sagittal sinus is the most commonly thrombosed, with a substantial number of these patients also disclosing lateral sinus thrombosis (Wechsler *et al.*, 1992; Akman-Demir *et al.*, 1999; Siva *et al.*, 2001). The thrombus may be limited to the lateral sinus in up to 20% of patients (Wechsler *et al.*, 1992). Intracranial hypertension without any demonstrable neuroimaging pathology has been reported, with some patients later developing neuroimaging findings consistent with CVST in later attacks (Akman-Demir *et al.*, 1996).

Parenchymal CNS involvement in BS patients with CVST is unlikely. The extension of the clot into the cerebral veins causing focal venous haemorrhagic infarction is uncommon, and also the occurrence of CVST in the setting of CNS involvement (CNS-NBS) is extremely rare (Wechsler *et al.*, 1992; Akman-Demir *et al.*, 1996; Siva *et al.*, 2001).

Peripheral nervous system involvement in BS

Peripheral nervous system (PNS) involvement in BS, as already mentioned, is rare. The limited number of BS patients who have been reported with PNS involvement had clinical and electrophysiological findings consistent with mononeuritis multiplex, a peripheral neuropathy prominent in the lower extremities, and polyradiculoneuritis (Namer *et al.*, 1987; Takeuchi *et al.*, 1989). However, in a small series of patients with BS in a Caribbean population from the French West Indies two of the seven cases were reported to have PNS involvement, with one having a sensorimotor axonal neuropathy and the other an axonal sensory neuropathy with recurrent episodes of myositis (Lannuzel *et al.*, 2002). Muscle involvement is also rare; a limited number of cases with focal or generalized myositis have been reported (Serdaroglu, 1998*b*).

Electroneuromyographic studies disclosed demyelination, chronic denervation, and even myogenic involvement in the reported cases (Baslo *et al.*, 1979; Namer *et al.*, 1987; Takeuchi *et al.*, 1989). However, electroneuromyographic studies may disclose a subclinical neuropathy in patients who do not report symptoms suggestive of neuropathy. Besides, it should be kept in mind, that the neuropathy may develop secondary to a various drugs used in the treatment of BS, or may also be coincidental.

Subclinical NBS

The incidental finding of neurological signs in patients with BS without neurological symptoms has been reported in some studies, with a minority of them developing mild neurological attacks later (Akman-Demir *et al.*, 1999; Al-Araji *et al.*, 2003).

Brainstem auditory and somatosensory evoked potentials and transcranial magnetic stimulation were studied in patients with CNS-NBS in several studies and showed a wide range of abnormality, mainly due to the involvement the basal parts of the brainstem and corticospinal tracts (Rizzo *et al.*, 1989; Nakamura *et al.*, 1989; Parisi *et al.*, 1996; Stigsby *et al.*, 2000). The demonstration of subclinical involvement by detection of abnormal responses in examined areas without corresponding clinical symptoms and signs in some of these patients is noteworthy in providing information about the extent of the CNS involvement. In another study subclinical involvement was investigated by using P300 in Behçet's patients without neurological manifestations (Kececi and Akyol, 2001). The findings suggested that the P300 measures and motor response time may reflect subclinical neurological involvement in BS.

Electroneuromyographic studies, as already mentioned, had also shown a subclinical neuropathy in some patients who do not report symptoms suggestive of neuropathy; also silent muscle involvement was reported in patients without overt muscle involvement who were studied with electron microscopy (Serdaroglu, 1998*b*). Autonomic nervous system involvement was also reported in asymptomatic patients with BS (Karatas *et al.*, 2002). On the other hand subclinical CNS involvement was also detected by single photon emission computed tomography (SPECT) studies, as described below.

The detection of neurological abnormalities by physical examination or neurophysiological studies as well as neuroimaging in asymptomatic patients suggests that there might be a subgroup of patients with subclinical NBS. However, the clinical and prognostic value of all these findings in this group of patients currently is not clear.

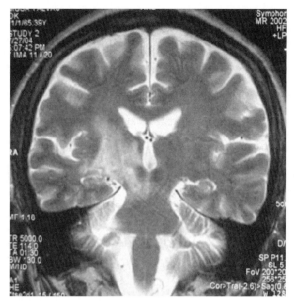

Fig. 27.1 Neuro-Behçet Disease (intra-axial NBS): coronal T2W images showing the most common pattern of central nervous system involvement as seen on MRI in a patient with intra-axial NBS. A lesion extending from the midbrain to the basal ganglia and internal capsule.

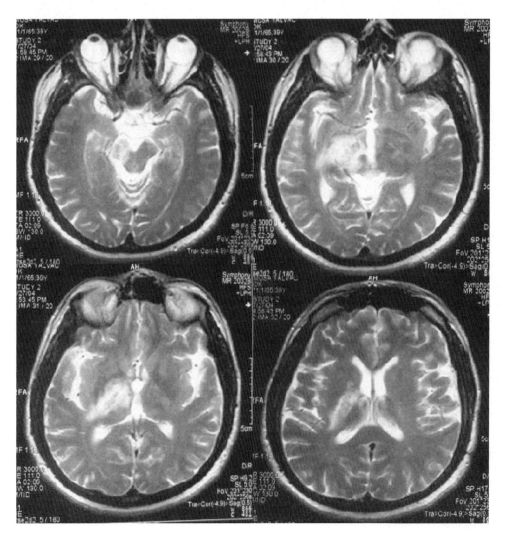

Fig. 27.2 Neuro-Behçet Disease (intra-axial NBS): the axial T2W images of the same patient (Fig. 27.1) showing the most common pattern of central nervous system involvement as seen on MRI in a patient with intra-axial NBS. Involvement of the mesodiencephalic region, the most commonly affected region in intra-axial-NBS, with extension to the basal ganglia and internal capsule.

Neuroimaging

Neuroimaging studies in CNS-NBS have shown that cranial magnetic resonance imaging (MRI) is both specific and more sensitive than computed tomography (CT) in demonstration of the typical reversible inflammatory parenchymal lesions. Lesions are generally located within the brainstem, occasionally with extension to the diencephalon, or within the periventricular and subcortical white matter (Koçer *et al.*, 1999) (Figs 27.1–27.5). The pattern of parenchymal lesions is suggestive of small vessel vasculitis, mainly of venular involvement (Koçer *et al.*, 1999), but the pathology in NBS with CNS involvement is not always uniform and covers a wide spectrum that includes vasculitis, a low-grade inflammation, demyelination, and degenerative changes. A definite vasculitis is not observed in all cases (Hadfield *et al.*, 1997). A frequent finding is the resolution or a decrease in the size of the lesions when serial imaging studies are carried out (Siva *et al.* 1991; Koçer *et al.*, 1999). Arterial involvement is rare, and a limited number of patients with primary or secondary intracerebral hemorrhage have been reported (Nagata, 1985; Altinörs *et al.*, 1987). With the exception of the rarely occurring lesions which only affect periventricular and subcortical white matter, cranial MRIs in intra-axial-NBS are rarely confused with MS. The cranial MRI findings of NBS are also dissimilar from thrombotic or embolic stroke.

Spinal cord involvement is not common, but can be seen. In reported cases, the major site to be involved was the cervical spinal cord, with the myelitis-like inflammatory lesion continuing for more than two segments, and extending to the brainstem in some (Morrissey *et al.*, 1993; Koçer *et al.*, 1999; Green and Mitchell, 2000) (Fig. 27.6). Gadolinium enhancement, resolution of these lesions, and thoracic cord involvement has also been reported.

We have observed one patient with optic neuropathy, who had an enhancing isolated optic nerve lesion (Koçer *et al.*, 1999).

MR venography is the preferred study for diagnosing or confirming CVST in BS, but most of the time T_1- and T_2-weighted images also disclose the venous sinus thrombosis (Fig. 27.7). With the exception of two cases we have not observed haemorrhagic venous infarcts or other parenchymal CNS lesions on MRI in our patients with CVST (extra-axial NBS) (Siva *et al.*, 2001; Tunc *et al.*, 2004), and others have also reported a similar observation or a low rate of such changes in their patients (Wechsler *et al.*, 1992; Akman-Demir *et al.*, 1999). This finding suggests that, the cerebral venous sinus thrombosis in BS may not be acute and complete in a significant number of cases.

Cerebral or spinal arteriograpy may serve to demonstrate vasculitis, dissection, or aneurysms, and have also been used to monitor treatment effects in patients with vasculitic involvement (Park *et al.*, 1984; Zelenski *et al.*, 1989; Bahar *et al.*, 1993; Green and Mitchell, 2000). However, the

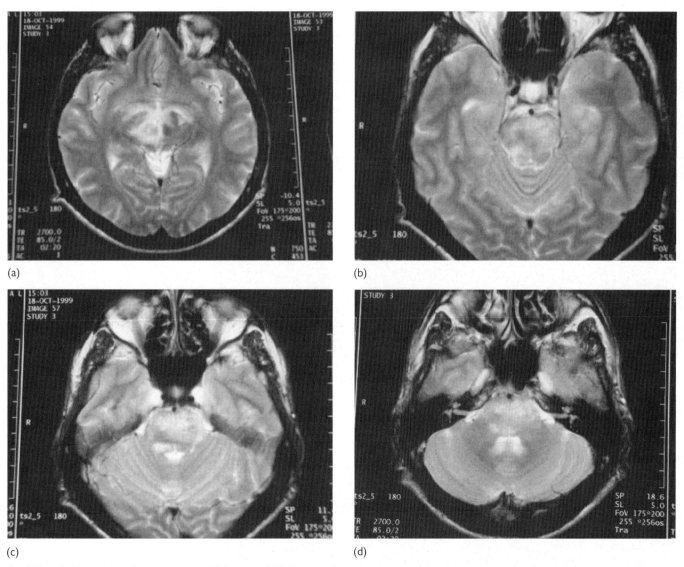

(a)

(b)

(c)

(d)

Fig. 27.3 (a-d) Neuro-Behçet Disease (intra-axial NBS): the axial T2W images of another patient with central nervous system involvement, showing widespread brainstem lesions extending from the pons, through the midbrain up to the deep hemispheric regions.

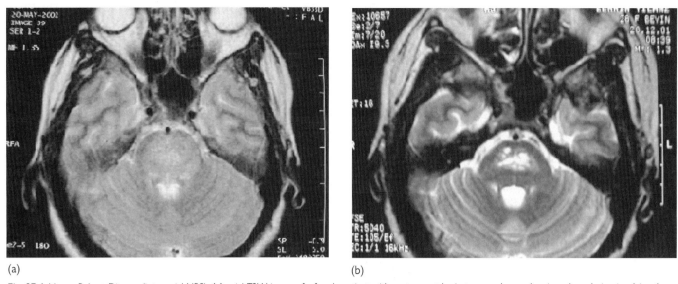

(a)   (b)

Fig. 27.4 Neuro-Behçet Disease (intra-axial NBS): **(a)** axial T2W image of a female patient with acute onset brainstem syndrome showing a large lesion involving the pons. **(b)** A follow-up MRI seven months later in the same patient after clinical improvement showing partial resolution of the pontin lesion.

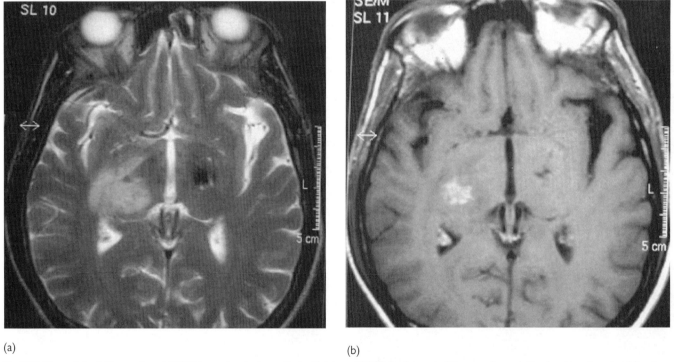

(a)   (b)

Fig. 27.5 Neuro-Behçet Disease: the axial T2W image showing in a patient with intra-axial NBS, involvement of the mesodiencephalic – basal ganglia region **(a)** and patchy enhancement of the same lesion after Gadolinium **(b)**.

probability of detecting a significant finding in the cerebral arteriography is low as in most cases with CNS parenchymal disease the vascular involvement is most prominent in the post-capillary venules. Therefore it is our impression that cerebral arteriography is not a cost-effective diagnostic tool in CNS-NBS unless the patient presents with subarachnoid haemorrhage or an overt cerebral arterial lesion.

SPECT studies in BS

SPECT studies have disclosed areas of hypoperfusion localized in the deep basal ganglia and in the frontal and temporal lobes in a group of BS patients with neuropsychiatric manifestations (Nobili *et al.*, 2002; Huang *et al.*,

2002). MRI was normal in some of them, and these non-specific SPECT findings, which were consistent with multiple hypoperfusion areas that correlated with decreased metabolic demand, were interpreted as indicative of early functional changes in the brains of this patient population.

Cerebrospinal fluid (CSF)

If performed during the acute stage, CSF studies usually show inflammatory changes in most cases of CNS-NBS, such as elevated protein content, a mild to moderate lymphocytic pleocytosis, and at times a cellular reaction with up to a few thousand cells mainly composed of neutrophils (Serdaroglu, 1998*a*; Kidd *et al.*, 1999; Akman-Demir *et al.*, 1999; Siva *et al.*, 2001). Oligoclonal

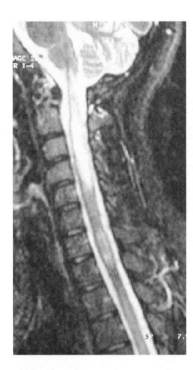

Fig. 27.6 Neuro-Behçet Disease (intra-axial NBS): cervical spinal involvement – inflammatory lesions extending over several segments and into the lower brainstem (Courtesy of Professors Civan Islak and Naci Kocer).

Table 27.5 The differential diagnosis of intra-axial (CNS) neuro-Behçet's syndrome

Multiple sclerosis

Stroke in young adults

Primary CNS vasculitis

Secondary CNS vasculitis

Neuro-sarcoidosis

CNS tuberculosis

Brainstem glioma

Primary CNS lymphoma

Vogt–Koyanagi–Harada syndrome

Reiter's syndrome

Eales' disease

Cogan's syndrome

Susac syndrome

Sweet syndrome

Differential diagnosis of intra-axial (parenchymal) NBS

The major diseases to be included in the differential diagnosis of parenchymal NBS are shown in Table 27.5.

Patients with NBS are young and frequently present with an acute or subacute brainstem syndrome or hemiparesis, as well as with various other neurological manifestations. Hence, the possibility of BS is often included in the differential diagnosis of multiple sclerosis and in the stroke of the young adult, especially in the absence of its known systemic symptoms and signs.

Multiple sclerosis is more common in women, whereas NBS is seen frequently in men. Optic neuritis, sensory symptoms and spinal cord involvement, which are common in MS, are rarely seen in NBS (Table 27.6). However, the clinical presentation of NBS may sometimes be confused with MS, but the neuroimaging (MRI) findings are clearly different. The pattern of brainstem involvement in NBS, which commonly extends to involve basal ganglia and diencephalic structures, is not seen in MS. Furthermore, periventricular and ovoid lesions suggestive of MS are not expected to be seen in NBS, and when hemispheric white matter lesions are present in NBS they are more likely to be subcortical than periventricular, and these are almost always associated with the brainstem–diencephalic lesions (Koçer et al., 1999). Brainstem lesions in MS are usually small, even in the acute stage, and prominent brainstem and cerebellar atrophy without loss of cerebral volume that is seen in the chronic phase of NBS is unusual in MS (Miller et al., 1987; Morrissey et al., 1993). Spinal cord involvement, this rarely extends more than a few vertebral segments in MS (Nijeholt et al., 1997), contrary to the more extensive lesions that were observed in the few cases of NBS (Koçer et al., 1999; Green and Mitchell, 2000). The CSF also reveals different patterns in NBS, with a more prominent pleocytosis and low rate of positivity for oligoclonal bands (Serdaroglu, 1998a).

Co-morbidity of BS and MS is a possibility, and we have observed a few such cases in which systemic BS and MS coexisted. Neurologically these patients had the clinical and imaging features consistent with MS, had oligoclonal Ig bands in their CSF, and also had the systemic manifestations of BS. The systemic symptoms and signs of BS preceded the onset of MS in all, but some were admitted because of their neurological symptoms and a detailed history and physical examination revealed the presence of BS. On the other hand, in patients with a known diagnosis of BS, the onset of the neurological symptoms raised the possibility of NBS. However, based on the clinical and neuroimaging differential diagnosis (Table 27.6) we could rule out CNS-NBS. The co-occurrence of CNS-NBS and MS, is a theoretical possibility but such a diagnosis would require histopathological confirmation.

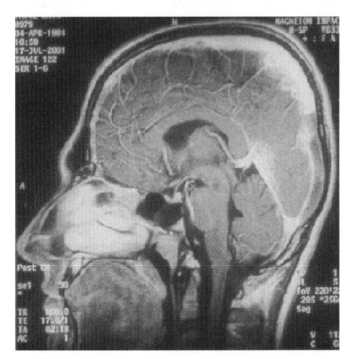

Fig. 27.7 Neuro-Behçet Disease (extra-axial NBS): thrombosis of the posterior part of the superior sagital sinus as seen on proton weighted and gadolinium enhancing T1W images.

bands can be detected, but this will be an infrequent finding (McLean et al., 1995; Kidd et al., 1999; Akman-Demir et al., 1999; Siva et al., 2001). Loss of oligoclonal bands following treatment with glucocorticoids was reported in one study (Gille et al., 1990). On the other hand, the use of CSF oligoclonal IgM and IgA bands or the CSF IgM index to monitor disease activity was suggested by some (Hirohata et al., 1986; Sharief et al., 1991). However, these findings serve an academic purpose rather than practical issues. CSF in patients with CVST is under increased pressure, but the cellular and chemical composition may be normal (Siva et al., 2001).

Table 27.6 The differential diagnosis of multiple sclerosis and intra-axial (CNS) neuro-Behçet's syndrome (from Siva *et al.* (2004) with permission)

	Multiple sclerosis	CNS-neuro-Behçet syndrome
Gender	Female > male	Male > female
Symptoms at onset		
Common	ON; sensory; spinal cord; BS/INO; motor; cerebellar	Headache; motor;cerebellar; BS/Cr neuropaties
Uncommon	Headache; BS/Cr neuropaties	ON; sensory; spinal cord; BS/INO
MRI		
PV and SC lesions	(+++)	(±)
BS lesions	Small, discrete, up/downward extension (−)	Large, diffuse, up/downward extension (+)
Spinal cord lesions	(++)	(±)
CSF		
Inflammatory changes	(±)	(++)
OCB(+)	>90%	<20%

CNS, central nervous system; MRI, magnetic resonance imaging; CSF, cerebrospinal fluid; OCB, Oligoclonal bands; ON, optic neuritis; BS, brainstem; INO, internuclear ophthalmoplegia; Cr, cranial; PV, periventricular; SC, subcortical.

An acute stroke-like onset is not common in NBS, and MRI lesions compatible with classical arterial territories are also not expected (Koçer *et al.*, 1999). The absence of systemic symptoms and signs will serve to differentiate the primary CNS vasculitic disorders from NBS, and the difference in the systemic symptoms and signs from the secondary CNS vasculitides, as well as the MRI findings (Koçer *et al.*, 1999; Siva, 2001).

Sarcoidosis can also be confused with BS due to uveitis, arthritis, and CNS involvement, but the absence of oral and genital ulcers, and the presence of peripheral lymphadenopathy and bilateral hilar lymph nodes on chest X-ray, as well as pathological examination of the non-caseating granulomatous lesions of sarcoidosis, help in the differential diagnosis. In some patients with sarcoidosis, however, involvement of the nervous system may be the presenting and only manifestations of the disease (Said, 2000). Cranial neuropathies with the seventh nerve being the most common one to be involved, seizures, diabetes insipidus and other symptoms related to chronic meningitis and hydrocephalus as well as sarcoid neuropathies and myopathies are among the nervous system manifestations of sarcoidosis (Said, 2000). These are not common in NBS, and MRI findings are unlikely to be confused between the two diseases (Koçer *et al.*, 1999).

Tuberculosis may resemble BS because of its multisystem involvement and for its potential to affect the nervous system. However, hilar lymphadenopathy and pulmonary cavities are not expected in BS, whereas its mucocutaneous manifestations are unusual for tuberculosis. Furthermore CSF and MRI findings are different, and microscopic and pathological examination, as well as culture and PCR analysis of body fluids or tissue specimens, will help to identify the disease as tuberculosis.

Brainstem glioma and primary CNS lymphoma may be included in the differential diagnosis of NBS too, but the absence of systemic findings and the MRI findings will solve the problem at once.

Due to their ophthalmological and some other systemic manifestations rare diseases such as Vogt–Koyanagi–Harada syndrome, Reiter's syndrome, Eales' disease, Cogan's syndrome, and Susac syndrome are other considerations in the differential diagnosis of BS. All may present with nervous system manifestations and therefore are included in the differential diagnosis of NBS too. However, a complete ophthalmological examination will reveal the true nature of eye involvement in each of these syndromes, which have differences from the eye involvement seen in BS.

The Vogt–Koyanagi–Harada (VKH) syndrome is a bilateral, diffuse granulomatous uveitis associated with poliosis, vitiligo, alopecia, and central nervous system and auditory signs. Symptoms of meningeal irritation and occasional encephalopathy are most common in the prodromal phase of the illness and a CSF pleocytosis has been noted to be even more common than symptomatic meningitis, but it rarely causes significant focal neurologic disease (Goodwin, 2001). This inflammatory syndrome, which occurs more commonly among heavily pigmented populations such as Asians, Hispanics, Native Americans, and Indians is probably the result of an autoimmune mechanism, influenced by genetic factors, and appears to be directed against melanocytes (Goodwin, 2001). Ocular inflammation, arthritis, and urethritis are seen in Reiter's syndrome, but conjunctivitis is more common than uveitis in this disease and genital lesions are painless. Eales' disease, a syndrome of retinal perivasculitis and recurrent intraocular haemorrhages, is infrequently associated with neurological abnormalities (Atabay *et al.*, 1992).

Cogan's syndrome (CS) is an idiopathic inflammatory disease in which the major symptoms are ocular and cochleovestibular. The eye inflammation consists of interstitial keratitis and uveitis, and inner ear inflammation will cause symptoms clinically indistinguishable from Ménière's disease (St Clair and McCallum, 1999). Almost three-quarters of patients develop systemic manifestations, and a vasculitis involving large vessels similar to Takayasu's arteritis or involving medium vessels resembling periarteritis nodosa, may develop in 10–15% of patients (St Clair and McCallum, 1999; Nazarian, 2003). Nervous system involvement is not common, but when present the neurological manifestations are wide and include headache, psychosis, stroke, cerebral sinus thrombosis, seizures, encephalopathy, myelopathy, cranial neuropathies, mononeuropathies, and polyneuropathy (Susac, 1994; O'Halloran *et al.*,1998). Susac syndrome is a non-inflammatory vasculopathy causing small infarcts in the retina, the cochlea, and the brain, resulting in the clinical triad of retinopathy, hearing loss, and encephalopathy (Susac, 1994; O'Halloran *et al.*, 1998).

Gastrointestinal symptoms in BS may mimic Crohn's disease or chronic ulcerative colitis. Eye disease is rare and genital ulcers are absent in inflammatory bowel diseases. The diagnosis can be confirmed by intestinal biopsy. Whipple's disease may be briefly mentioned here as a disease with gastrointestinal and various nervous system symptoms which may resemble BS too.

Differential diagnosis of extra-axial NBS (CVST)

In patients who present with symptoms of intracranial hypertension, and in whom neuroimaging reveals thrombosis in one or more of the cerebral venous sinuses, BS needs to be included in the differential diagnosis. The presence of its systemic findings is the only clue to the association of CVST with BS, and their absence will exclude this possibility. As already mentioned, observation of haemorrhagic venous infarcts or other parenchymal CNS lesions on MRI in patients with extra-axial NBS is exceptional, a finding which may arise the suspicion of BS.

Prognosis

In a recent study from our centre the long-term mortality and morbidity of BS was studied over two decades (Kural-Seyahi et al., 2003). The 'disease burden' of BS was usually found to be confined to the early years of its course, and it was shown that in many patients the syndrome burnt out over the years. However, major vessel disease and CNS involvement were found to be exceptions and could appear for the first time relatively late in the course. Furthermore, most of the deaths seen in this cohort were due to these two conditions (Kural-Seyahi et al., 2003).

Neurological involvement in BS is a remarkable cause of morbidity and approximately 50% of the NBS patients are moderate to severely disabled after 10 years of disease. We rated the neurological disability of our patients with BS by using the Expanded Disability Status Scale of Kurtzke (EDSS), which was originally devised for multiple sclerosis-associated disability (Kurtzke, 1983). Taking into consideration that the visual disability is most commonly due to uveitis in BS, the visual function was eliminated from the original scale. By 10 years after the onset of neurological symptoms and signs, 78.2% of our patients developed at least mild (EDSS ≥3), and 45.1% moderate to severe neurological disability (EDSS ≥6). An EDSS score of 3 represents full ambulation despite moderate neurological disability on neurological examination, and a score of 6 represents a requirement for assistance in walking such as one-sided support to walk for 100 m, and during other activities of daily life. However, when patients were evaluated separately, all those with CVST had EDSS scores of either 1 or 2 (minimal neurological disability) (Siva et al., 2001). But in another study from our centre, CVST in BS was found to be strongly associated with systemic major vessel disease and tended to occur earlier in the disease course than the parenchymal–CNS type of neurological involvement (Tunc et al., 2004). Considering the fact that patients with major vessel disease have a higher rate of morbidity and mortality, a diagnosis of CVST in a patient with BS may not be associated with a favourable outcome.

Onset with cerebellar symptoms and a progressive course were unfavourable factors, while onset with headache, a diagnosis of CVST, and disease course limited to a single episode were neurologically favourable (Siva et al., 2001). An elevated protein level and pleocytosis in the CSF were also reported to be associated with a poorer prognosis (Akman-Demir et al., 1999).

Treatment

Neurological involvement in BS is heterogeneous and it is difficult to predict its course and prognosis, and response to treatment. Therefore it is not possible to reach a conclusion on the efficacy of any treatment unless properly designed, double-blinded, placebo-controlled studies are carried out for each form. However, this is difficult to accomplish, as even in large centres the annual number of new neuro-cases is very limited. Most studies which report some kind of efficacy with various treatments in BS with neurological involvement have not included uniform cases, have not followed their patients for long periods, and did not have controls. So, currently we have no evidence for the efficacy of any treatment for any form of NBS. Empirical impressions currently create the guidelines for management.

Intra-axial NBS—acute episodes

Glucocorticoids are used to treat acute CNS involvement within BS, but their effects are short-lived and they do not prevent further attacks or progression. Acute attacks of CNS-NBS are treated with either oral prednisolone (1 mg/kg for up to 4 weeks, or until improvement is observed) or with high-dose intravenous methyl prednisolone (IV MP, 1 g/day) for 5–7 days. Both forms of treatment should be followed with an oral tapering dose of glucocorticoids over 2 to 3 months in order to prevent early relapses (Siva and Fresko, 2000). There is no apparent difference between the two regimens, but our impression is that the high-dose IV MP regimen is associated with earlier improvement. Our current practice is to give IV MP, 1 g/day for 7 days, followed by the oral regimen in patients with clinical and imaging evidence of CNS involvement.

Intra-axial NBS—long-term treatments

Colchicine, azathioprine, cyclosporin-A, cyclophosphamide, methotrexate, chlorambucil, immunomodulatory agents such as interferon-α pentoxyphilline, and more recently thalidomide have been shown to be effective in treating some of the systemic manifestations of BS; none of these agents have been shown beneficial in NBS in a properly designed study (Bang, 1997; Hamuryudan et al., 1998; Sakane et al., 1999; Siva and Fresko, 2000; Kaklamani and Kaklamanis, 2001).

In a small, retrospective study, chlorambucil was reported to have some efficacy in meningoencephalitis of BS (O'Duffy et al., 1984). As most patients were treated prior to the CT/MRI era, there is no information on neuroimaging correlates of treatment. However, lessening in the CSF pleocytosis was documented in patients treated with chlorambucil. Although limited, our experience with chlorambucil in NBS is negative, and its serious side-effects, including increased risk of malignancy, excludes it from our use. We have observed that treatment with other immunosuppressive drugs such as azathioprine, cyclosporin A, and cyclophosphamide, either alone or in combination, for extraneural systemic manifestations of BS does not seem to prevent the development, exacerbation, or progression of intra-axial (parenchymal) NBS (Gül et al., 1999). Cyclosporin was reported to cause neurotoxicity or to accelerate the development of CNS symptoms and therefore its use in NBS is not recommended (Scwartz et al., 1995; Kotake et al., 1999). In six patients with BS who were judged to have progressive neuropsychiatric manifestations, an open 12-month trial with low-dose weekly methotrexate was carried out (Hirohata et al., 1998). The authors had the impression that this regimen might have a beneficial effect in the treatment of progressive NBS, but the result is not conclusive.

A common clinical practice is to add an immunosuppressant drug such as azathioprine or monthly pulsed cyclophosphamide to glucocorticoids in progressive NBS cases; however, the efficacy of such a combination has not been demonstrated. Agreeing with others (Sakane et al., 1999) we conclude that progressive intra-axial NBS is resistant to all currently available therapies.

Successful treatment of ocular and other systemic manifestations of BS with monoclonal anti-TNF-α antibody treatment with infliximab was reported recently in a few patients (Goossens et al., 2001; Rozenbaum et al., 2002; Triolo et al., 2002; Fresko, 2002); none of these patients, however, had significant neurological problems. The same holds true for etanercept, another drug with TNF-α blocking properties; some recent studies revealed that this drug was also beneficial in suppressing ocular and some other systemic manifestations of BS, but the effect was not sustained when the drug was stopped (Fresko, 2002). Mycophenolate mofetil (CellCept) and tacrolimus (Prograf) are other immunosuppressant/immunomodulatory agents that have been used to treat ocular inflammation and significant systemic manifestations in patients with BS (Russell et al., 2001), but there is no information regarding the potential effect of all these drugs in preventing CNS involvement or new neurological attacks.

In theory, intravenous immunoglobulin (IV Ig) would be expected to have a possible regulatory effect in the reported immunological abnormalities of BS and its CNS involvement. However, in our limited experience with a few cases with progressive CNS involvement we have not observed any significant improvement (Siva and Altintaş, 2000). We are not aware of beneficial effects of plasma exchange in NBS.

Cerebral aneurysms are rare in BS, but when small unruptured aneurysms are detected, medical therapy with steroids with or without cytotoxic agents may be tried. As an alternative to surgery, endovascular treatment is another option in the management of BS-associated intracranial aneurysms, and this form of treatment is suggested for ruptured, peripherally located, fusiform shaped, dissecting pseudoaneurysms and posterior circulation aneurysms (Kizilkilic et al., 2003).

Cerebral venous sinus thrombosis (CVST)

There is a tendency to treat deep venous thrombosis in BS with anticoagulants and antiplatelet agents in combination with intermediate doses of glucocorticoids (Sakane et al., 1999). However, there is no consensus on the treatment of CVST. Some authors use a combination of anticoagulation with glucocorticoids (Wechsler et al., 1992), while others administer gluco-corticoids alone (Akman-Demir et al., 1996). In our current practice we use a combination of subcutaneous low-molecular-weight heparin with gluco-corticoids (Siva and Fresko, 2000). Low-molecular-weight heparin is given for 14–21 days and IV MP, 1 g/day, for 7 days followed by an oral regimen of glucocorticoids which are given for 3 weeks. Patients are evaluated every 2 weeks with neuro-ophthalmic examination, which includes visual fields and visual evoked potentials. Such an evaluation can only be carried out in the absence of ocular involvement due to BS. If the patient continues to report headache and visual symptoms, CSF analysis is repeated at week 4 or earlier. When the opening pressure is found to be elevated, the oral gluco-corticoid treatment is continued until the patient improves and stabilizes in terms of clinical symptomatology, CSF pressure, and on neuro-ophthalmic examination. The CVST in BS is rarely severe enough to require systemic or endovascular thrombolytic treatment.

Recurrence of CVST is uncommon after the initial episode. Therefore we do not recommend any form of long-term treatment in extra-axial NBS.

Acknowledgements

We would like to thank specially Professor Hasan Yazici, MD, the founder and head of The Behçet Center and The Multidisciplinary Behçet's Disease Outpatient Clinic of Cerrahpasa Medical School, and the other members of the team, Vedat Hamuryudan, MD, Sabahattin Yurdakul, MD, Cem Mat, MD, Yılmaz Özyazgan, MD, Izzet Fresko, MD and Melike Melikoğlu, MD, without whom we would not have this unique experience with Behçet's disease.

References

Adam, H., Fortune, F., Wilson, A., Warr, K., Shinnick, T., Mizushima, Y., et al. (1996). Role of gamma delta T cells in the pathogenesis and diagnosis of Behçet's disease. Lancet 347(9004): 789–794.

Akman-Demir, G., Bahar, S., Baykan-Kurt, B., Gürvit, I.H., and Serdaroglu, P. (1996). Intracranial hypertension in Behçet's disease. Eur J Neurol 3: 66–70.

Akman-Demir, Serdaroglu, P., Tasçi B, and the Neuro-Behçet Study Group (1999). Clinical patterns of neurological involvement in Behçet's disease: evaluation of 200 patients. Brain 122: 2171–2181.

Aksu, K., Turgan, N., Oksel, F., Keser, G., Ozmen, D., Kitapcioglu, G., et al. (2001). Hyperhomocysteinaemia in Behçet's disease. Rheumatology 40: 687–690.

Al-Araji, A., Sharquie, K., and Al-Rawi, Z. (2003). Prevalence and patterns of neurological involvement in Behçet's disease: a prospective study from Iraq. J Neurol Neurosurg Psychiatry 74(5): 608–613.

Altinörs, N., Senveli, E., Arda, N., Türker, A., Kars, Z., Çinar, N., et al. (1987). Intracerebral hemorrhage and hematoma in Behçet's disease. Neurosurgery 21: 582–583.

Atabay, C., Erdem, E., Kansu, T., and Eldem, B. (1992). Eales' disease with inter-nuclear ophthalmoplegia. Ann Ophthalmol 24: 267–270.

Aygunduz, M., Bavnek, N., Öztürk, M., Kaftan, O., Kosar, A., and Kirazli, S. (2000). Serum amyloid A and beta-2 microglobulin as markers of clinical activity in Behçet's disease. Yonsei Med J 41(3, Suppl.): 35.

Azizlerli, G., Özarmagan, G., Övül, C., Sarica R., and Mustafa, S.O. (1992). A new kind of skin lesion in Behçet's disease: extragenital ulcerations. Acta Derm-Venereol 72: 286.

Bahar, S., Çoban, O., Gürvit, I.H.,Akman-Demir, F., and Gökyigit A. (1993). Spontaneous dissection of the extracranial vertebral artery with spinal sub-arachnoid hemorrhage in a patient with Behçet's disease. Neuroradiology 35: 352–354.

Bang, D. (1997). Treatment of Behçet's disease. Yonsei Med J 38: 401–410.

Baslo, P., Kara, I., Eker, E., Kotogyan, A., Kayali, H., Ozdamar, E., et al. (1979). Clinical, electrophysiological, immunological and electron microscopic investigation of Behçet's disease. In: Behçet's Disease, Excerpta Medica International Congress Series 467 (ed. N. Dilsen, M. Konice, and C. Ovul), pp. 178–182. Excerpta Medica, Amsterdam.

Behçet, H. (1937). Uber Residivierende, Aphtöse, durch ein Virus verursachte Geschwüre am Mund, am Auge und an den Genitalien. Derm Woschenscr 105: 1152–1157.

Bogdanova, D., Milanov, I., and Georgiev, D. (1998) Parkinsonian syndrome as a neurological manifestation of Behçet' s disease. Can J Neurol Sci 25: 82–85.

Brauther, C., Chajek, T., Ben-Tuvia, S., Lamm, L., and Cohen, T. (1978). A genetic study of Behçet's disease in Israel. Tissue Antigens 11: 113–120.

Bussone, G., La Mantia, L., Boiardi, A., and Giovannini, P. (1982). Chorea in Behçet's syndrome. J Neurol 227: 89–92.

Çakir, N., Yazici, H., Chamberlain, M.A., Barnes, C.G., Yurdakul, S., Atasoy, S., et al. (1991). Response to intradermal injection of monosodium urate crys-tals in Behçet's syndrome. Ann Rheum Dis 50: 634–636.

Celet, B., Akman-Demir, G., Serdaroglu, P., Yentur, S., Tasci, B., Van Noort, J., et al. (2000). Anti-alpha-beta-crystallin immunoreactivity in inflammatory nervous system diseases. J Neurol 247: 935–939.

Cetinel, B., Akpinar, H., Tufek, I., Uygun, N., Solok, V., and Yazici, H. (1999). Bladder involvement in Behçet's syndrome. J Urol 161: 52–56.

Clausen, J. and Bierring, F. (1983). Involvement of postcapillary venules in Behçet's disease. Acta Derm-Venerol 63: 191–197.

Direskeneli, H. (2001). Behçet's disease: infectious aetiology, new autoantigens, and HLA-B51. Ann Rheum Dis 60(11): 996–1002.

Direskeneli, H., Shinnick, H.A., Mizushima, Y., van der Zee, R., Fortune, F., Stanford, M.R., et al. (1996). Recognition of B-cell epitopes of the 65 kDa HSP in Behçet's disease. Scand J Immunol 43(4): 464–471.

Ergun, T., Gürbüz, O., Harvell, J., Jorizzo, J., and White, W. (1998). The histopathology of pathergy: a chronologic study of skin hyperreactivity in Behçet's disease. Int J Dermatol 37: 929–933.

Espinosa, G., Font, J., Tassies, D., Vidaller, A., Deulofeu, R., Lopez-Soto, A., et al. (2002). Vascular involvement in Behçet's disease: relation with thrombophilic factors, coagulation activation, and thrombomodulin. Am J Med 112: 37–43.

Frassanito, M.A., Dammacco, R., Cafforio, P., and Dammacco, F. (1999). Th1 polarization of the immune response in Behçet's disease: a putative patho-genic role of interleukin-12. Arthritis Rheum 42: 1967–1974.

Fresko, I. (2002). Highlights of the 10th International Congress on Behçet's Disease (Editorial). Clin Exp Rheumatol 4(Suppl. 26): S59–S64.

Fresko, I., et al. (2000). The response to the intradermal injections of sodium monourate crystals in patients with Behçet's syndrome and its comparison to the pathergy test. Yonsei Med. J 41(3, Suppl.): 25.

Fresko, I., Soy, M., Hamuryudan, V., Yurdakul, S., Yavuz, S., Tumer, Z., et al. (1998). Genetic anticipation in Behçet's syndrome. Ann Rheum Dis 57(1): 45–48.

Gille, M., Sindic, C.J.M., Laterre, P.F., De Hertogh, P., Hotermans, J.M., Seak, I., et al., (1990). Atteintes neurologiques révélatrices d'une maladie de Behçet: quatres observations cliniques. Acta Neurol Belg 90: 233–247.

Goodwin, J. (2003) The Vogt–Koyanagi–Harada syndrome. In: MedLink Neurology on CD ROM (editor-in-chief S. Gilman). MedLink Corporation, San Diego, CA.

Goossens, P.H., Verburg, R.J., and Breedveld, F.C. (2001). Remission of Behçet's syndrome with tumour necrosis factor alpha blocking therapy. Ann Rheum Dis 60(6): 637.

Green, A.L. and Mitchell, P.J. (2000). Spinal cord neurobehçet's disease detected on magnetic resonace imaging. Aust Radiol 44: 201–203.

Gül, A. (2001). Behçet's disease: an update on the pathogenesis. Clin Exp Rheumatol 19(Suppl. 24): 6–12.

Gül, A., Aslantas, A.B., Tekinay, T., Konice, M., and Ozcelik T. (1999). Procoagulant mutations and venous thrombosis in Behçet's disease. Rheumatology 38: 1298–1299.

Hadfield, M.G., Aydin, F., Lippman, H.R., and Sanders, K.M. (1997). Neuro-Behçet's disease. Clin Neuropathol 16: 55–60.

Hamuryudan, V., Mat, C., Saip, S., Ozyazgan, Y., Siva, A., Yurdakul, S., et al. (1998). Thalidomide in the treatment of the mucocutaneous lesions of the Behçet syndrome. A randomized, double-blind, placebo-controlled trial. Ann Intern Med 128(6): 443–450.

Hegab, S. and Al-Mutawa, S. (2000). Immunopathogenesis of Behçet's disease. Clin Immunol 96(3): 174–186.

Hirohata, S., Takeuchi, A., and Miyamoto T. (1986). Association of cerebrospinal fluid IgM index with central nervous system involvement in Behçet's disease. Arthritis Rheum 29: 793–796.

Hirohata, S., Suda, H., and Hashimoto, T. (1998) Low-dose weekly methotrexate for progressive neuropsychiatric manifestations in Behçet's disease. J Neurol Sci 159: 181–185.

Huang, W.S., Chiu, P.Y., Kao, A., Tsai, C.H., Lee, C.C., *et al.* (2002). Decreased cerebral blood flow in neuro-Behçet's syndrome patients with neuropsychiatric manifestations and normal magnetic resonance imaging-a preliminary report. *J Neuroimaging* 12(4):355–359.

International Study Group for Behçet's Disease (1990). Criteria for diagnosis of Behçet's disease. *Lancet* 335: 1078–1080.

International Study Group for Behçet's Disease (1992). Evaluation of diagnostic (classification) criteria in Behçet's disease-towards internationally agreed criteria. *Br J Rheumatol* 31: 299–308.

Ishihara, M., Ohno, S., Mizuki, N., Yamagata, N., Naruse, T., Shiina, T., *et al.* (1996). Allelic variations in the TAP2 and LMP2 genes in Behçet's disease. *Tissue Antigens* 47(3): 249–252.

Kaklamani, V.G. and Kaklamanis, P.G. (2001). Treatment of Behçet's disease: an update. *Semin Arthritis Rheum* 30: 299–312.

Kansu, E. (1996). Endothelial cell dysfunction in Behçet's disease. In: *Vasculitides* (ed. B.M. Ansell, P.A. Bacon, J.T. Lie, and H. Yazici), pp. 207–221. Chapman & Hall, London.

Kansu, T., Kirkali, P., Kansu, E., and Zileli, T. (1989). Optic neuropathy in Behçet's disease. *J Clin Neuro-Opthalmol* 9: 277–280.

Karatas, G.K., Onder, M., and Meray, J. (2002). Autonomic nervous system involvement in Behçet's disease. *Rheumatol Int* 22(4): 155–159.

Kececi, H. and Akyol, M. (2001). P300 in Behçet's patients without neurological manifestations. *Can J Neurol Sci* 2: 66–69.

Kidd, D., Steuer, A., Denman, A.M., and Rudge, P. (1999). Neurological complications in Behçet' syndrome. *Brain* 122: 2171–2181.

Kikuchi, S., Niino, M., Shinpo, K., Terae, S., and Tashiro, K. (2002). Intracranial hemorrhage in neuro-Behçet's syndrome. *Intern Med* 41(9): 692–695.

Kizilkilic, O., Albayram, S., Adaletli, I., Ak, H., Islak, C., and Kocer, N. (2003). Endovascular treatment of Behçet's disease-associated intracranial aneurysms: report of two cases and review of the literature. *Neuroradiology* 45(5): 328–334.

Koç, Y., Güllü, I., Akpek, G., *et al.* (1992). Vascular involvement in Behçet's disease. *J Rheumatol* 19: 402–410.

Koçer, N., Islak, C., Siva, A., Saip, S., Akman, C., Kantarci, O., *et al.* (1999). CNS involvement in Neuro-Behçet's syndrome: an MR study. *Am J Neuroradiol* 20: 1015–1024.

Kone Paut, I., Geisler, I., Wechsler, B., Seza, O., Ozdogan, H., Rozenbaum, M., *et al.* (1999). Familial aggregation in Behçet's disease: high frequency in parents of pediatric probands. *J Pediatr* 135: 89–93.

Kotake, S., Higashi, K., Yoshikawa, K., Sasamato, Y., Okamoto, T., and Matsuda, H. (1999). Central nervous system symptoms in patients with Behçet disease receiving cyclosporine therapy. *Ophthalmology* 106: 586–599.

Krespi, Y., Akman-Demir, G., Poyraz, M., Tugcu, B., Coban, O., Tuncay, R., *et al.* (2001). Cerebral vasculitis and ischaemic stroke in Behçet's disease: report of one case and review of the literature. *Eur J Neurol* 8(6): 719–722.

Kural-Seyahi, E., Fresko, I., Seyahi, N., Özyazgan, Y., Mat, C., Hamuryudan, V., *et al.* (2003). The long-term mortality and morbidity of Behçet syndrome: a 2-decade outcome survey of 387 patients followed at a dedicated center. *Medicine (Baltimore)* 82(1): 60.

Kurhan-Yavuz, S., Direskeneli, H., Bozkurt, N., Ozyazgan, Y., Bavbek, T., Kazokoglu, H., *et al.* (2000). Anti-MHC autoimmunity in Behçet's disease. T cell responses to an HLA-B-derived peptide cross-reactive with retinal-S antigen in patients with uveitis. *Clin Exp Immunol.* 120: 162.

Kurtzke, J.F. (1983). Rating neurological impairment in MS: an expanded disability status scale (EDSS). *Neurology* 33: 1444–1452.

Lakhanpal, S., O'Duffy, J.D., and Lie, J.T. (1988). Pathology. In: *Behçet's Disease. A Contemporary Synopsis* (ed. G.R. Plotkin, J.J. Calabro, and J.D. O'Duffy), pp. 101–142. Futura, New York.

Lannuzel, A., Lamaury, I., Charpentier, D., and Caparros-Lefebvre, D. (2002). Neurological manifestations of Behçet's disease in a Caribbean population: clinical and imaging findings. *J Neurol* 249(4): 410–418.

Lehner, T. (1969). Pathology of recurrent oral ulceration and oral ulceration in Behçet's syndrome: Light, electron anmd fluorescence microscopy. *J Pathol* 97: 481–494.

Lehner, T. (1997). The role of heat shock protein, microbial and auto-immune agents in the aetiology of Behçet's disease. *Int Rev Immunol* 14: 21–32.

Mader, R., Ziv, M., Adawi, M., Mader, R., and Lavi, I. (1999). Thrombophilic factors and their relation to thromboembolic and other clinical manifestations in Behçet's disease. *J Rheumatol* 26: 2404–2408.

McLean, B.N., Miller, D., and Thompson, E.J. (1995). Oligoclonal banding of Ig G in CSF, blood-brain barrier function, and MRI findings in patients with sarcoidosis, systemic lupus erythematosus, and Behçet's disease involving the nervous system. *J Neurol Neurosurg Psychiatry* 58(5): 548–554.

Miller, D.H., Ormerod, I.E.C., Gibson, A., DuBoulay, E.P.G.H., Rudge, P., and McDonald, W.I. (1987). MRI brain scanning in patients with vasculitis: differentiation from multiple sclerosis. *Neuroradiology* 29: 226–231.

Mizuki, N., Inoko, H., and Ohno, S. (1997) Molecular genetics (HLA) of Behçet's disease. *Yonsei Med J* 38: 333–349.

Mizuki, N. and Ohno, S. (1996). Immunogenetic studies of Behçet's disease. *Rev Rheum Eng Ed* 63: 520–527.

Mizuki, N., Ota, M., Kimura, M., Ohno, S., Ando, H., Katsuyama, Y., *et al.* (1997). Triplet repeat polymorphism in the transmembrane region of the MICA gene: a strong association of six GCT repetitions with Behçet disease. *Proc Natl Acad Sci USA* 94: 1298–1303.

Monastero, R., Mannino, M., Lopez, G., Camarda, C., Cannizzaro, C., Camarda, L.K.C. (2003). Prevalence of headache in patients with Behçet's disease without overt neurological involvement. *Cephalalgia* 23(2): 105–108.

Monastero, R., Camarda, C., Pipia, C., Lopez, G., Camarda, L.K.C., Baiamonte, V. (2004). Cognitive impairment in Behçet's disease patients without overt neurological involvement. *J Neurol Sci* 220: 99–104.

Morrissey, S.P., Miller, D.H., Harmszewski, R., Rudge, P., MacManus, D.G., Kendall, B., McDonald, W.I. (1993). Magnetic resonance imaging of the central nervous system in Behçet's disease. *Eur Neurol* 33: 287–293.

Müftüoglu, A.Ü., Yurdakul, S., Yazici, H., Tüzün, Y., Pazarlı, H., Altuğ, E. *et al.* (1986). Vascular involvement in Behçet's disease—a review of 129 cases. In: *Recent Advances in Behçet's Disease* (ed. T. Lehner and C.G. Barnes), pp. 255–260. Royal Society of Medicine Service, London.

Nagata, K. (1985). Recurrent intracranial hemorrhage in Behçet's disease (letter). *J Neurol Neurosurg Psychiatry* 48: 190–191.

Nakae, K., Masaki, F., Hashimoto, T., Inaba, G., Mochizuki, M., and Sakane, T. (1993). Recent epidemiological features of Behçet's disease in Japan. In: *Behçet's Disease*, International Congress Series 1037 (ed. B. Wechsler and B. Godeau), pp. 154–161. Excerpta Medica, Amsterdam.

Nakamura, S., Sugita, M., Matoba, H., Tanaka, S., Isoda, F., and Ohno, S. (1996). Insufficient expression of Fas antigen on helper T cells in Behçet's disease. *Br J Ophthalmol* 80(2): 174–176.

Nakamura, Y., Takahashi, M., Kitaguchi, M., Imaoka, H., and Tarui, S. (1989). Brainstem auditory and somatosensory evoked potentials in neuro-Behçet's syndrome. *Japan J Psychiat Neurol* 43: 191–200.

Namer, I.J., Karabudak, R., Zileli, T., Ruacan, S., Kucukali, T., Kansu, E. (1987). Peripheral nervous system involvement in Behçet's disease. *Eur Neurol* 26: 235–240.

Nazarian, S. (2003). Cogan's syndrome. In: *MedLink Neurology on CD ROM* (editor-in-chief S. Gilman). MedLink Corporation, San Diego, CA.

Nijeholt, G.J.L., Barkhof, F., Scheltens, P., Castelijns, J.A., Ader, H., van Waesberghe, J.H., *et al.* (1997). MR of the spinal cord in multiple sclerosis: relation to clinical subtype and disability. *Am J Neuroradiol* 18: 1041–1048.

Nobili, F., Cutolo, M., Sulli, A., Vitali, P., Vignola, S., Rodriguez, G. (2002). Brain functional involvement by perfusion SPECT in systemic sclerosis and Behçet's disease. *Ann N Y Acad Sci* 966: 409–414.

O'Duffy, J.D. (1990). Vasculitis in Behçet's disease. *Rheum Dis Clin North Am* 16: 423–431.

O'Duffy, J.D., Carney, A., and Deodhar, S. (1971). Behçet's disease. Report of 10 cases, 3 with new manifestations. *Ann Intern Med* 75: 561–570.

O'Duffy, J.D., Robertson, D.M., and Goldstein, N.P. (1984). Chlorambucil in the treatment of uveitis and meningoencephalitis of Behçet's disease. *Am J Med* 76: 75–84.

O'Halloran, H.S., Pearson, P.A., Lee, W.B., Susac, J.O., and Berger, J.R. (1998). Microangiopathy of the brain, retina, and cochlea (Susac syndrome). A report of five cases and a review of the literature. *Ophthalmology* 105: 1038–1044.

Ohno, S. (1986). Behçet's disease in the world. In: *Recent Advances in Behçet's Disease* (ed. T. Lehner and C.G. Barnes), pp. 181–186. Royal Society of Medicine Service, London.

Ohno, S., Ohguchi, M., Hirose, S., Matsuda, H., Wakisaka, A., and Aizava, M. (1982). Close association of HLA-BW51 with Behçet's disease. *Arch Ophthalmol* 100: 1455–1458.

Oktem-Tanor, O., Baykan-Kurt, B., Gurvit, I.H., Akman-Demir, G., and Serdaroglu, P. (1999). Neuropsychological follow-up of 12 patients with neuro-Behçet disease. *J Neurol* 246: 113–119.

Özdogan, H. (1994). Behçet's syndrome in children. *Rheumatol Eur* 23(Suppl. 12): 34.

Parisi, L., Terracciano, M.E., Valente, G.O., Calandriello, E., Accorinti, M., and Spadaro, M. (1996). Pre-symptomatic neurological involvement in Behçet's disease: the diagnostic role of magnetic transcranial stimulation. *Electroenceph Clin Neurophysiol* 101: 42–47.

Park, J.H., Han, M.C., and Bettmann, M.A. (1984). Arterial manifestations of Behçet's disease. *Am J Roentgenol* 143: 821–825.

Pellecchia, M.T., Cuomo, T., Striano, S., Filla, A., Barone, P. (1999). Paroxysmal dystonia in Behçet's disease. *Movement Disord* 14: 177–179.

Perniciaro, C. and Molina, J. (1991). Cerebrovascular aneurysms in patients with Behçet's disease. In: *Behçet's Disease: Basic and Clinical Aspects* (ed. J.D. O'Duffy and E. Kökmen), pp. 119–123. Marcel Dekker, New York.

Pervin, K., Childerstone, A., Shinnick, T., Mizushima, Y., van der Zee, R., Hasan, A., Vaughan, R. (1993). T cell epitope expression of mycobacterial and homologous human 65-kilodalton heat shock protein peptides in short term cell lines from patients with Behçet's disease. *J Immunol* 151: 2273–2282.

Rizzo, P.A., Valle, E., Mollica, M.A., Sanarelli, L., and Pozzessere, G. (1989). Multimodal evoked potentials in neuro-Behçet: a longitudinal study of two cases. *Acta Neurol Scand* 79: 18–22.

Rozenbaum, M., Rosner, I., and Portnoy, E. (2002). Remission of Behçet's syndrome with TNF alpha blocking treatment. *Ann Rheum Dis* 61(3): 283–284.

Russell, A.I., Lawson, W.A., and Haskard, D.O. (2001). Potential new therapeutic options in Behçet's syndrome. *BioDrugs* 15: 25–35.

Sahin, S., Akoglu, T., Direskeneli, H., Sen, L.S., and Lawrence, R. (1996). Neutrophil adhesion to endothelial cells and factors affecting adhesion in patients with Behçet's disease. *Ann Rheum Dis* 55(2): 128–133.

Said, G. (2000). Sarcoidosis of the nervous system. Neurological manifestations in systemic diseases. In: *ENS Teaching Course 12, Syllabus*, pp. 74–85.

Saip, S., Siva, A., Altintaş, A., Kıyat, A., Seyahi, E., Hamuryudan, V., *et al.* Headache in Behçet's Syndrome. *Headache* (in press).

Sakane, T. and Suzuki, N. (2002). Behçet's disease. In: *The Molecular Pathology of Autoimmune Diseases*, 2nd edn (ed. A.N. Theofilopoulos and C.A. Bona), pp. 828–840. Taylor & Francis, New York.

Sakane, T., Takeno, M., Suzuki, N., and Inaba, G. (1999). Behçet's disease. *N Engl J Med* 341: 1284–1291.

Salvarani, C., Calamia, K., Silingardi, M., Ghirarduzzi, A., and Olivieri, I. (2000). Thrombosis associated with the prothrombin G→A20210 mutation in Behçet's disease. *J Rheumatol* 27: 515–516.

Saruhan-Direskeneli, G., Yentür, S.P., Akman-Demir, G., Isik, N., and Serdaroglu, P. (2003). Cytokines and chemokines in neuro-Behçet's disease compared to multiple sclerosis and other neurological diseases. *J Neuroimmunol* 145: 127–134.

Sarui, H., Maruyama, T., Ito, I., Yamakita, N., Takeda, N., Nose, M., Yasuda, K. (2002). Necrotising myositis in Behçet's disease: characteristic features on magnetic resonance imaging and a review of the literature. *Ann Rheum Dis* 61(8): 751–752.

Scwartz, R.B., Bravo, S.M., Klufas, R.A., Hsu, L., Barnes, P.D., Robson, C.D., *et al.* (1995). Cylosporin neurotoxicity and its relation to hypertensive neuropathy: CT and MR findings in 16 cases. *Am J Roentgenol* 165: 627–631.

Serdaroglu, P. (1998a). Behçet's disease and the nervous system. *J Neurol* 245(4): 197–205.

Serdaroglu, P. (1998b). Neuromuscular manifestations in the course of Behçet's disease. *Acta Myologica* 2: 41–45.

Serdaroglu, P., Yazici, H., Özdemir, C., *et al.* (1989). Neurological involvement in Behçet's syndrome: a prospective study. *Arch Neurol* 46: 265–269.

Sharief, M.K., Hentges, R., and Thomas, E. (1991). Significance of CSF immunoglobulins in monitoring neurologic disease activity in Behçet's disease. *Neurology* 41: 1398–1401.

Siva, A. (2001). Vasculitis of the nervous system. *J Neurol* 248: 451–468.

Siva, A. and Altintaş, A. (2000). Neuro-Behçet syndrome. In: *Intravenous Immunoglobulins in the Treatment of Neurological Disorders* (ed. G. Said), pp 115–126. Martin Dunitz, London.

Siva, A. and Fresko, I. (2000). Behçet's disease. *Curr Treat Options Neurol* 2: 435–447.

Siva, A., Özdogan, H., Yazici, H., Yurdakul, S., Yardım, M., Akyatan, N., *et al.* (1986). Headache, neuro-psychiatric and computerized tomography findings in Behçet's syndrome. In: *Recent Advances in Behçet's Disease* (ed. T. Lehner and C.G. Barnes), pp. 247–254. Royal Society of Medicine Service, London.

Siva, A., Necdet, V., Yurdakul, S., Yardım, M., Denktas, H., Yazıcı, H. (1991). Neuroradiological findings in neuro-Behçet syndrome. In: *Behçet's Disease: Basic and Clinical Aspects* (ed. J.D. O'Duffy and E. Kökmen), pp. 323–329. Marcel Dekker, New York.

Siva, A., Kantarci, O.H., Saip, S., Altintaş, A., Hamuryudan, V., Islak, C., *et al.* (2001). Behçet's disease: diagnostic and prognostic aspects of neurological involvement. *J Neurol* 248: 95–103.

Siva, A., Altintaş, A., and Saip, S. (2004). Behçet's syndrome and the nervous system. *Curr Opin Neurol* 17: 347–357.

St Clair, E.W. and McCallum, R.M. (1999). Cogan's syndrome. *Curr Opin Rheumatol* 11: 47–52.

Stigsby, B., Bohlega, S., McLean, D.R., and Al-Kawi, M.Z. (2000). Transcranial magnetic stimulation in Behçet's disease: a cross-sectional and longitudinal study with 44 patients comparing clinical, neuroradiological, somatosensory and brain-stem auditory evoked potential findings. *Clin Neurophysiol* 111: 1320–1329.

Susac, J.O. (1994). Susac's syndrome. The triad of microangiopathy of the brain and retina with hearing loss in young women. *Neurology* 44: 591–593.

Takeuchi, A., Kodama, M., Takatsu, M., Hashimoto, T., Miyashita, H. (1989). Mononeruritis multiplex in incomplete Behçet's disease: a case report and the review of the literature. *Clin Rheumatol* 8: 375–380.

Triolo, G., Vadala, M., Accardo-Palumbo, A., Ferrante, A., Ciccia, F., Giardina, E., *et al.* (2002). Anti-tumour necrosis factor monoclonal antibody treatment for ocular Behçet's disease (Letter) *Ann Rheum Dis* 61: 560–561.

Tunc, R., Saip, S., Siva, A., and Yazici, H. (2004). Cerebral venous thrombosis is associated with major vessel disease in Behçet's syndrome. *Ann Rheum Dis* 63: 1693–1694.

Verity, D.H., Vaughan, R.W., Madanat, W., Wallace, G.R., Stanford, M.R. (1999). Factor V Leiden mutation is associated with ocular involvement in Behçet disease. *Am J Ophthalmol* 128: 352–356.

Wechsler, B., Vidailhet, M., Bousser, M.G., Piette, J.C., Bousser, M.G., Dell Isola, B., Bletry, O., Godeau, P. (1992). Cerebral venous sinus thrombosis in Behçet's disease: long term follow-up of 25 cases. *Neurology* 42: 614–618.

Yazici, H. (1997). The place of Behçet's syndrome among the autoimmune diseases. *Int Rev Immunol* 14: 1–10.

Yazici, H., Akhan, G., Yalçin, B., and Müftüoglu, A. (1977). The high prevalence of HLA-B5 in Behçet's disease. *Clin Exp Immunol* 30: 259–261.

Yazici, H., Yurdakul, S., and Hamuryudan, V. (1998). Behçet's syndrome. In: *Oxford Textbook of Rheumatology*, 2nd edn (ed. P.J. Madisson, D.A. Isenberg, P. Woo, and D.N. Glass). 1394–1402. Oxford University Press, Oxford.

Yazici, H., Yurdakul, S., and Hamuryudan, V. (2001). Behçet disease [vasculitis syndromes]. *Curr Opin Rheumatol* 13(1): 18–22.

Yurdakul, S., Yazıcı, H., Tüzün, Y., Pazarlı, H., Yalçın, B., Altaç, M., *et al.* (1983). The arthritis of Behçet's disease: a prospective study. *Ann Rheum Dis* 42: 505–515.

Yurdakul, S., Günaydin, I., Tüzün, H., Tankurt, N., Pazarlı, H., Ozyazgan, Y., Yazıcı, H. (1988). The prevalence of Behçet's syndrome in a rural area in Northern Turkey. *J Rheumatol* 15: 820–822.

Zeiss, J. (2003). *Essential Guide to Behçet's Disease*. Central Vision Press. Uxbridge, MA.

Zelenski, J., Capraro, J.A., Holden, D., Calabrese, L.H. (1989). Central nervous system vasculitis in Behçet's syndrome: angiographic improvement after therapy with cytotoxic agents. *Arthritis Rheum* 32: 217–220.

Zouboulis, C.C., Kotter, I., Djawari, D., Kirch, W., Kohl, P.K., Ochsendorf, F.R., *et al.* (1997). Epidemiological features of Adamantiades-Behçet's disease in Germany and in Europe. *Yonsei Med J* 38: 411–422.

28 Role of neural–immune interactions in neurodegenerative diseases

Edith G. McGeer and Patrick L. McGeer

Introduction

Post-mortem studies have revealed that many inflammatory markers newly appear or are up-regulated in regions of the brain affected in Alzheimer's disease (AD) and there is considerable evidence that inflammation plays an important role in the progression of the disease. A few of the more important indications are: activated complement proteins, including the membrane attack complex; the pentraxins, C-reactive protein and amyloid P; the complement receptors and HLA-DR on activated microglia; the inflammatory cytokines; the prostaglandins; and other influencing factors. The most important of these are discussed briefly in this chapter. Details on others may be found in any of the many reviews which have now appeared on inflammation in AD (McGeer and McGeer, 1995; Neuroinflammation Working Group, 2000). Much of the work on inflammation in the brain has been on AD and that will be the primary focus of this chapter. However, data are appearing that suggest local inflammation may also be important in Parkinson's disease, atherosclerosis, and heart disease and this will be briefly discussed.

It is important to realize that the inflammation in question is a locally mediated process. Classical immunology has focused on the adaptive immune system in which peripheral immune organs clone lymphocytes which are carried by the blood to affected tissues. But the work on inflammation in AD over the past 10–15 years has brought into new prominence the phylogenetically much older innate immune system which appears to operate in most tissues of the body. Inflammatory mediators are made to support both systems. But, if these systems engage in sustained overactivity, or fail to distinguish between friend and foe, the result can be significant damage to host tissue. The brain appears to be particularly vulnerable because of the post-mitotic nature of neurons.

Almost all of the mediators found to be associated with neuroinflammation have been shown to be locally produced. They are selectively elevated in affected regions of the AD brain. Moreover, studies of tissue in such degenerative processes as atherosclerosis and infarcted heart indicate that a similar innate immune reaction occurs, with similar up-regulation of inflammatory mediators and similar damage to local tissue. The classical concept of misdirection against host tissue is that it must be due to an autoimmune response, where rogue B-cell or T-cell lines are cloned against host proteins. But there is a much broader phenomenon, not recognized in classical immunity, where localized, innate immune responses damage viable host tissue. We define this as autotoxicity (McGeer and McGeer, 2000). It is this autotoxic phenomenon which comes into play in AD and may also play a role in Parkinson's disease, atherosclerosis, and heart disease.

Much epidemiological and limited clinical evidence suggests that anti-inflammatory drugs, particularly the cyclo-oxygenase-inhibiting non-steroidal anti-inflammatory drugs (NSAIDs), may impede the onset and slow the progression of AD. But these drugs strike at the periphery of the inflammatory reaction. Much better results might be obtained if drugs were found that could inhibit microglia and activation of the complement system, or combinations of drugs aimed at different inflammatory targets might be much more effective than single agents such as a particular NSAID.

The complement system

Complement is generally thought of as being part of the adaptive immune system where T and B cells are cloned and antibodies made to foreign proteins, antibodies which bind to C1q to activate the complement system. But the complement system is phylogenetically much older than the adaptive immune system which evolved with higher vertebrates (Lambris, 1993). The complement system exists in primitive organisms such as the sponge and plays a major role in the innate immune system. The innate immune system is less sophisticated than the adaptive immune system, and may more readily confuse friend and foe.

AD is the first disease where vigorous activation of complement in the absence of antibodies was shown to occur. Damaged neuronal processes were shown to have the membrane attack complex (MAC) inserted into their limiting membranes (Itagaki *et al.*, 1994; Webster *et al.*, 1997*b*) with a resulting damage to host tissue. It is therefore the prime example of an autotoxic disorder. A key finding regarding the mechanism of complement activation was that of Rogers *et al.* (1992), who demonstrated that amyloid protein (Aβ), when aggregated, was a strong complement activator. Thus, the senile plaques of AD have a unique activator of complement. In addition, the complement cascade can be activated by the pentraxins, amyloid P and C-reactive protein, which are both up-regulated in affected regions of AD brain (Yasojima *et al.*, 2000).

The complement system (Fig. 28.1) has components to carry out four major functions: recognition, opsonization, inflammatory stimulation through anaphylatoxins, and direct killing through the MAC. The classical pathway is activated by attachment of C1q to a target causing C1 dissociation. Opsonization then takes place, first by amplification through a cascade of proteases (C1r, C1s, C4, C2, C3) and then by attachment of the

Classical Complement Components

Native Protein		Active Fragments	Function
C1	→	C1q	Activation
C2			
C4	→	C2a4b3b	Opsonization
C3		C3a, C4a, C5a	Anaphylotoxic stimulants
C5			
C6			
C7	→	C5bC6C7C8(C9)n	Membrane attack complex
C8			
C9			

Fig. 28.1 Components of the complement system. A more detailed diagram may be found in Quigg (2002).

cleavage products C4b and C3b to exposed sites close to the C1q binding site. Covalent bonds are formed between thiol ester bonds on these cleavage fragments and exposed hydroxyl groups on carbohydrate moieties or exposed amino groups. The attached fragments then become ligands for complement receptors on phagocytes. In the case of the brain, these phagocytes are microglia. If the complement system is fully activated, it proceeds to assemble the terminal components (C5b, C6, C7, C8, C9) into the lytic macromolecule C5b–9, known as the MAC. This inserts into the limiting membrane of viable cells, potentially leading to lysis and cell death. Meanwhile, the small fragments C3a, C4a, and C5a, known as anaphylotoxins, stimulate inflammation. So the overall cascade identifies, opsonizes, and destroys its target, while dispatching messengers to seek help.

The tangles and plaques of AD are clearly marked with the complement fragments C4d and C3d (Ishii and Haga 1984; Eikelenboom et al., 1989; McGeer et al., 1989). Little or no such staining is seen in control brain. Dystrophic neurites in AD brain are immunostained for the MAC (Itagaki et al., 1994; Webster et al., 1997b) indicating autolytic attack. Again such staining is not seen in control brains.

There are protective mechanisms which defend host cells against spurious activation of complement and against self-damage when complement is activated. These include C1 inhibitor, C4 binding protein, decay accelerating factor, membrane cofactor protein (CD46), and protectin (CD59). However, while the mRNAs for complement proteins are sharply up-regulated in affected regions of AD brain (Fig. 28.2) (Yasojima et al., 1999b), those for C1 inhibitor and CD59 are not (Fig. 28.2) (Yasojima et al., 1999a). Thus, there is no compensatory inhibitory up-regulation to protect host brain tissue in AD, and it appears as if neurites are being progressively destroyed by complement self-attack.

These data indicate that complement activation exacerbates the pathology in AD, suggesting that complement inhibitors might be effective anti-inflammatory agents. There are many steps in the complement cascade so that multiple opportunities exist for therapeutic intervention. The intervention, however, should not be of a nature that would seriously compromise the ability of the host to combat infection. One possibility which separates antibody activation of complement from that by the pentraxins or Aβ is C1q binding. C-reactive protein (CRP), amyloid P (AP) and Aβ all activate the complement cascade by binding to the collagen tail of C1q, while antibodies bind to the globular head (Jiang et al., 1992; Ying et al., 1993; Webster et al., 1997a). Thus, agents which block binding to the collagen tail of C1q might be effective therapeutic agents.

Blocking formation of the MAC might be the most attractive of all therapeutic targets in the complement cascade for limiting autotoxicity.

Inhibiting this self-attack could leave the more critical opsonization process undisturbed. Thus high selectivity in inhibiting the damaging aspects of complement activation could be provided while the valuable function of phagocytosing debris could be preserved.

Examples of some inhibitors which block other steps in the complement cascade are the 13-residue cyclic peptide compstatin and the negatively charged sulfated glycosaminoglycan pentosan polysulfate (PPS). Compstatin binds to C3 and prevents its cleavage, thus inhibiting activation of both the classical and alternative complement pathways (Furlong et al., 2000). It has shown activity in a pig xenograft model (Fiane et al., 1999). PPS is an orally active, heparin-like compound which has been approved for the treatment of interstitial cystitis. It has been shown to prolong survival in a heterotopic rat cardiac transplant model (Schwartz et al., 1999) and to reduce myocardial infarct in a rabbit ischemia/reperfusion model (Tanhehco et al., 1999). Whether either would reach the brain in vivo is unknown, but these examples do demonstrate the possibility of designing synthetic complement inhibitors.

The pentraxins

The pentraxins are not generally considered to be inflammatory mediators. Yet they are ancient host defense molecules which may function as primitive antibody-like compounds. When appropriately bound, they activate complement. They are believed to have evolved from an ancient gene more than 200 million years ago. There are two molecules identified as pentraxins because of their unusual pentameric structure: C-reactive protein (CRP) and amyloid P (AP).

CRP was originally identified as a host protein reacting with pneumococcal C polysaccharide causing activation of the complement system. This gave an important clue to its function. It has since been learned that CRP, when appropriately bound, is a powerful activator of complement both in vivo and in vitro (Jiang et al., 1992).

AP, the companion pentraxin, binds to all forms of amyloid, including the amyloid plaques of AD (Akiyama et al., 1991). It also activates the complement system (Hicks et al., 1992).

The pentraxins meet the definition of acute phase reactants. Such reactants are defined as compounds whose serum levels increase or decrease by 25% or more following a general inflammatory reaction. In humans, CRP is a particularly sensitive acute phase reactant since its serum levels may rise as much as 1000-fold following serious infection or injury. AP is the more sensitive reactant in rodents.

It had been generally believed for many years that CRP and AP were produced in the liver and carried in the circulation to other organs. The presence of AP in the brain in AD was even taken as an indication of leakage in the blood–brain barrier (Kalaria and Grahovac, 1990). Application

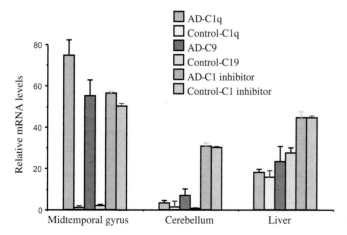

Fig. 28.2 Relative mRNA levels for C1q, C9, and C1 inhibitor in Alzheimer's disease (AD) and control mid-temporal gyrus, cerebellum, and liver. The up-regulation is limited to the affected brain regions such as the mid-temporal gyrus and to complement components. The synthesis of inhibitors such as C1 inhibitor and CD50 (not shown) is not significantly elevated.

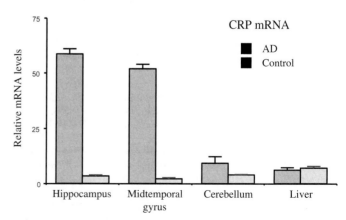

Fig. 28.3 Relative levels of CRP mRNA in Alzheimer's disease (AD) and control hippocampus, mid-temporal gyrus, cerebellum, and liver. Again, large elevations are limited to affected brain regions.

of molecular genetic techniques has made it possible to demonstrate that both CRP and AP, like the complement proteins, are produced locally in brain and that their production is sharply up-regulated in areas damaged by AD (Fig. 28.3) (Yasojima et al., 2000). Neurons are the most prominent generators of both. CRP is associated with damaged fibers within AD senile plaques, while AP is associated with the extracellular amyloid deposits (Akiyama et al., 1991).

Taken together these data suggest the following: (1) the pentraxins are secreted host defense proteins produced by a variety of cells including neurons; (2) they may act like primitive antibodies by binding to foreign antigens or damaged host tissue, thus initiating appropriate complement attack; (3) they may extend their identification to host tissue inappropriate for attack in which case an autotoxic reaction occurs; (4) agents that block binding of pentraxins to viable host tissue, or block their ability to activate complement, might be of therapeutic benefit in reducing autotoxic attack.

Microglia

The resident phagocytes of the central nervous system (CNS) are the microglia. Phagocytes were discovered initially by Eli Metchnikoff in his great work of 1892. He impaled starfish larvae with rose thorns and noticed the gathering around of mesodermal cells which he named phagocytes. He believed that tissue phagocytes were the main line of defense of the body. Del Rio Hortega (1919) solved the puzzle of 'el tercer elemento' in brain. The problem had baffled the great neuroanatomist Ramon y Cajal who recognized only neurons and astrocytes. Del Rio Hortega found that this third element was composed of two cell types. One he named oligodendroglia and the other microglia. He recognized that microglia could become activated, and were phagocytic. The fact that microglia were the brain's representatives of the phagocytic system was challenged into the 1990s, but immunohistochemical studies on AD brain and experiments with microglia in culture have shown them to have all the characteristics of phagocytes. When activated, they up-regulate a large number of proteins. These include complement receptors because they are the cells which respond to the complement system's call for the phagocytosis of opsonized targets (Rozemuller et al., 1989; Akiyama and McGeer, 1990).

Microglia are always present in brain but generally rest in a quiescent state. Their activation can be revealed by immunostaining for some of the markers up-regulated on activation. Such immunostaining reveals the presence of activated microglia in AD brain tissue and their virtual absence in normal brain tissue (McGeer et al., 1987; Rogers et al., 1988). The microglia appear in clumps on senile plaques, as well as elsewhere in affected AD tissue. They seem to be unable to phagocytose the senile plaques and tangles of AD and thus remain chronically activated. In this state they produce massive amounts of oxygen radicals (Klegeris and McGeer, 2000) and other materials which may, in themselves, be toxic to host cells. Microglia possess the NADPH oxidase complex which, when assembled and fully activated, generates large numbers of free radicals on the external cell surface; these radicals are designed to destroy surrounding targets. A much smaller intracellular source of free radicals is leakage from the electron transport chain of mitochondria. In addition to oxygen free radicals from these sources, there is also glial generation of nitric oxide (Neuroinflammation Working Group, 2000). This nitric oxide can combine with oxygen free radicals to form the highly toxic peroxynitrite.

Footprints of oxygen free radical and peroxynitrite attack have been detected in post-mortem AD tissue. These include the presence of proteins modified with advanced glycation end products, 4-hydroxynonenal, 8-hydroxyguanine, malondialdehyde, and nitrotyrosine (Neuroinflammation Working Group, 2000).

Activated microglia also possess the enzyme myeloperoxidase which catalyses a reaction between hydrogen peroxide, derived from oxygen free radicals, and chloride to generate the potent oxidizing agent hypochlorous acid (Reynolds et al., 1999). This system is most prominent in granulocytes where release of hypochlorous acid is one of their most potent attack weapons. Blocking myeloperoxidase may be one of the anti-inflammatory

mechanisms of the antileprosy agent dapsone (McGeer et al., 1992; Hope et al., 2000).

Many experiments in tissue culture have shown that the secretions of activated microglia can kill neurons (Giulian et al., 1996; Klegeris and McGeer, 2000). Thus, the activated microglia, like the MAC of complement, probably contribute to the rapid and progressive neuronal loss in AD brain.

Cytokines

Cytokines are a heterogeneous group of small molecules that act in autocrine and paracrine fashion. They encompass several subfamilies which include interleukins (ILs), interferons (IFNs), tumor necrosis factors (TNFs), growth factors, colony stimulating factors, and chemokines. They have in common participation in inflammatory reactions. They typically act in combination so that attributing a specific set of in vivo properties to any given cytokine is difficult.

Only a few of the cytokines have been extensively studied in AD. The most significant ones are IL-1α, IL-1β, IL-6, and TNF-α. The possibility that these inflammatory cytokines might play a role in inflammation in AD brain was initially suggested by the reports that they are all up-regulated in AD tissue and are prominently associated with AD lesions (Griffin et al., 1989; Wood et al., 1993; Dickson et al., 1993; Cacebelos et al., 1994). The inflammatory cytokines IL-1, IL-6, and TNF-α are products of both activated microglia and activated astrocytes and powerfully stimulate their activity. Localization of these cytokines to such activated cells has been demonstrated in AD by immunohistochemistry (Lieberman et al., 1989; Sharif et al., 1993; Yamabe et al., 1994; Walker et al., 1995).

Several reports have since appeared indicating that the risk of AD is substantially influenced by several polymorphisms in the non-coding regions of these inflammatory genes (Kamboh et al., 1997; Blacker et al., 1998; Papassotiropoulos et al., 1999; Collins et al., 2000; Du et al., 2000; Grimaldi et al., 2000; Licastro et al., 2000a,b; Nicoll et al., 2000; Rebeck, 2000; McCusker, 2001). The polymorphisms are in promoter and untranslated regions. Those alleles which favor increased expression of the inflammatory mediators, are more frequent in AD than in controls. The polymorphisms are fairly common ones in the general population, so there is a strong likelihood that any given individual will inherit one or more of the high-risk alleles. The odds ratio for a single one of these polymorphisms is much lower than for polymorphisms in apolipoprotein E (apoE), where different forms of the protein are expressed. Inheritance of the apoE4 form substantially increases the risk of AD (Strittmatter et al., 1993). However, McCusker (2001) has shown that carrying the high-risk allele of TNF-α substantially increases the risk of AD in carriers of apoE4 allele. And it has also already been reported that the odds ratio is greatly increased if an individual carries two of the high-risk alleles. For example, Nicoll et al. (2000) found that simultaneous inheritance of the high-risk alleles for IL-1α −889 and IL-1β +3953 increased the odds ratio for developing AD to 10.8; i.e. the prevalence of AD in persons carrying these isoforms is 10.8 times as great as in persons of the same age carrying neither of these isoforms. The overall chances of an individual developing AD might be profoundly affected by a 'susceptibility profile' reflecting the combined influence of inheriting multiple high-risk alleles (McGeer and McGeer, 2001). Identification of such profiles might in the future lead to strategies for therapeutic intervention in the very early stages of the disorder.

Each of the polymorphisms found to be a significant risk factor for AD has also been linked to at least one peripheral inflammatory condition. The implication is that an inflammatory stimulus is more likely to cause autotoxic damage at a vulnerable site in any one of numerous disorders in those individuals carrying genetic polymorphisms that enhance expression of inflammatory mediators.

The importance of TNF-α as an inflammatory stimulus is emphasized by the widespread use in rheumatoid arthritis of TNF-α blockers. Infliximab is an antibody to TNF-α and etanercept is a TNF receptor–Fc fusion protein. Both types of TNF-α inhibition induce a rapid improvement in multiple clinical measures of disease activity and patient functional status, as well as a beneficial effect on progression of joint damage as measured radiographically (Hamilton and Clair, 2000; Alldred, 2001). Infliximab has also been shown to be effective in Crohn's disease (Feagan *et al.*, 2001).

Prostaglandins

Prostaglandins are probably not among the more important inflammatory mediators but must be considered because they are the presumed targets of the currently most widely used anti-inflammatory drugs. Their name comes from their initial discovery in the prostate gland. They are a group of fatty acids derived from the precursor arachidonic acid with cyclo-oxygenase (COX) being the rate-controlling initial step of synthesis. Arachidonic acid itself is a product of phospholipase action on lipid membranes. Generally speaking, prostaglandins modulate the action of hormones, but they are now known to have a wide variety of functions. Among the most prominent of these is inflammatory mediation. This function has been the focus of intense therapeutic attention. Vane opened up the field with his classic discovery that the anti-inflammatory action of aspirin was due to its ability to inhibit prostaglandin synthesis. This formed the basis for developing a variety of COX-inhibiting agents which are collectively described as NSAIDs. The failure of some of these agents to inhibit kidney prostaglandin synthesis led to the discovery of a second COX enzyme. The classical enzyme, located on chromosome 9, became known as cyclo-oxygenase-1 (COX-1) and the second enzyme, located on chromosome 1, as cyclo-oxygenase-2 (COX-2). While there is high homology between the two enzymes, the catalytic pockets differ so that inhibitors highly selective for each enzyme exist, while many of the traditional NSAIDs inhibit both forms. COX-1 is a relatively stable enzyme, while COX-2 is highly inducible, suggesting that at least some divergence in roles exists (McGeer, 2000). This is reinforced by significant differences in regional distribution. For example, COX-2 is highly expressed in kidney, while COX-1 is highly expressed in the gut (Yasojima *et al.*, 1999c).

As far as AD is concerned, both COX-1 and COX-2 mRNAs, as well as their protein products, are up-regulated in affected areas of brain (Yasojima *et al.*, 1999c). This is presumed to be largely due to inflammatory up-regulation of microglia, at least for COX-1. But, in contrast to COX-1, COX-2 is most abundantly expressed in pyramidal neurons, so the COX-2 response may be largely neuronal (Yasojima *et al.*, 1999c). It has been suggested that COX-2 plays a vital role in synaptic plasticity (Kaufmann *et al.*, 1996), which might be impaired by COX-2 inhibition. Studies of COX-2 inhibitors in various models of CNS damage have yielded conflicting results. Some indicate that COX-2 inhibition is harmful to the survival of neurons (Baik *et al.*, 1999), while others suggest it may be neuroprotective (Nakayama *et al.*, 1998). In either event, COX-2 is more intimately connected with pyramidal neurons than COX-1, and this should have implications as far as the use of these agents to reduce neuroinflammation in AD is concerned.

NSAIDs are the most widely used of all classes of drugs. As will be discussed later, they may have an important role to play in the treatment of AD, as well as other conditions where autotoxic destruction appears to play a role.

Other inflammatory mediators

The list of known inflammatory mediators which are up-regulated in AD is continuously expanding (for reviews listing partial tables see McGeer and McGeer (1995, 2000) and Neuroinflammation Working Group (2000)). Many of the mediators are associated with reactive microglia. But additional mediators are clearly associated with the activated astrocytes which wall off the lesioned areas. Still others are associated with neurons, initially the producers of the extracellular material, but terminally the victims of autotoxic attack.

In addition to the classes of compounds previously discussed, there are proteases, particularly the matrix metalloproteinases, components of the coagulation pathways, i.e. the thrombin and plastin systems, proteoglycans,

cathepsins and cystatins, intercellular adhesion molecules, and such astrocytic products as S-100b and α1-antichymotrypsin. Thus, the spectrum of molecules involved in AD neuroinflammation is very broad. Any of them might have a sufficiently powerful influence on the overall inflammatory state that blockade of their action might have therapeutic benefit. Insufficient knowledge is available to make accurate predictions regarding any of these relatively non-specific inflammatory mediators, indicating that much further research is warranted.

Epidemiological and clinical evidence

If inflammation is playing a major role in the progression of AD, people taking anti-inflammatory medications for other purposes might be inadvertently protecting themselves against the autotoxic effects of AD. There are now more than 20 published epidemiological studies which show that people known to be taking anti-inflammatory agents or suffering from arthritis generally, or rheumatoid arthritis in particular, had their odds of developing AD considerably reduced (McGeer *et al.*, 1996; Stewart *et al.*, 1997; Broe *et al.*, 2000; Veld *et al.*, 2000). A revealing study was conducted by Stewart and his colleagues in Baltimore (Stewart *et al.*, 1997). More than 2000 patients were enrolled in early middle age and followed for long periods of time to assess the factors contributing to later disease onset. The Stewart group therefore had records they could check regarding AD and drugs. They found for those using NSAIDs for 2 years or less the risk was reduced by about one-third. For those using NSAIDs for more than 2 years, the risk was reduced by 60%. An even more thorough analysis was conducted by Veld *et al.* (2000) on the data collected from the larger Rotterdam cohort of 6989 individuals. For those using NSAIDs for longer than 2 years, an 80% sparing of AD was found. This sparing was substantially greater than that found in the Baltimore study where actual pharmacy records were not obtained. The sparing was close to that originally reported by McGeer *et al.* (1990) based on the prevalence of AD in rheumatoid arthritis patients who were presumed to be consuming therapeutic doses of anti-inflammatory agents on a long-term basis.

Can anti-inflammatory agents be used to treat AD? Epidemiological evidence suggests that they should be very effective. But for this possibility to be realized, appropriate agents must be selected. They should act on targets based on correlations between epidemiology and molecular pathology. The need for such correlations is illustrated by failures in clinical trials of prednisone, the COX-2 inhibitors celecoxib and nimesulide, and hydroxychloroquine (Aisen *et al.*, 2000, 2002; Sainali *et al.*, 2000; Van Gool *et al.*, 2001). These agents were known to be effective in treating arthritic conditions but there was little or no evidence that they would be useful in

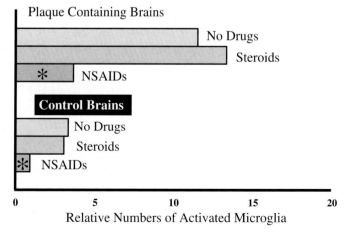

Fig. 28.4 Data of MacKenzie (2000) on relative numbers of activated microglia in post-mortem brains classified as demented or non-demented and according to pre-mortem drug use.

neuroinflammation. MacKenzie (2000) provided data as to why steroids should fail based on assessment of the numbers of activated microglia in AD and control brain (Fig. 28.4). Steroid consumption failed to reduce the number of reactive microglia detected post-mortem. In contrast, there was a sharp reduction in reactive microglia in patients taking traditional NSAIDs.

As far as selective COX-2 inhibitors are concerned, they have not been in use long enough for epidemiological data to accumulate, but immunohistochemical evidence was available which indicated they should fail. Unlike COX-1, COX-2 is highly expressed in normal pyramidal neurons, as well as in pyramidal neurons of AD cases (Yasojima et al., 1999c). Therefore, selective COX-2 inhibitors will primarily target pyramidal neurons rather than microglia. This, combined with evidence of exacerbation of neuronal death in some animal neurotoxicity models following COX-2 inhibition, suggests that COX-2 inhibitors are an inappropriate choice.

Hydroxychloroquine is not a general anti-inflammatory agent. Its mechanism of action in arthritis is uncertain. It is noteworthy, however, that its side-effects involve the CNS. This includes both ototoxicity and retinal damage. Since there is no epidemiological or immunohistochemical evidence to support a role for hydroxychloroquine or other 4-aminoquinolines in neuroinflammation, the failure to be effective in AD is not surprising.

The situation with respect to traditional NSAIDs is quite different. The epidemiological evidence in favor of their protective effect is very strong. Moreover, one small, double-blind clinical trial of the COX-1 inhibitory NSAID indomethacin in established AD, indicated arrest of progression (Rogers et al., 1993). Another NSAID trial, involving the mixed inhibitor diclofenac combined with misoprostyl, showed marginally less deterioration in drug compared with placebo patients, although the data fell short of statistical significance (Scharf et al., 1999). In in vitro experiments, NSAIDs have been shown to reduce the neurotoxicity of activated microglia to cultured neuroblastoma cells (Klegeris et al., 1999). Clearly, properly designed clinical trials of COX-1-inhibiting NSAIDs that reach the brain should be a high priority for AD. Relatively high doses may be required due to the

strong inflammatory reaction present in established AD. Gastrointestinal side-effects are a problem with such agents, particularly at high doses. While such side-effects are significant, they are small in comparison with the inevitable progression and fatal outcome of AD with currently approved methods of treatment. It is possible that a new class of COX-1-inhibiting NSAIDs, based on introducing a nitrate ester moiety, may circumvent the side-effect problem. These so-called NO-NSAIDs have greatly reduced gastrointestinal toxicity (Wallace et al., 1995).

Other types of anti-inflammatory agents may also be effective. An epidemiological study of leprosy patients in Japan showed that those continuously treated by dapsone had a significantly lower prevalence of dementia than those taken off dapsone for 5 years or more (McGeer et al., 1992). These data, combined with knowledge of the general anti-inflammatory properties of dapsone, would suggest that dapsone might be effective in AD, through a mechanism other than COX inhibition. Dapsone is a myeloperoxidase inhibitor and myeloperoxidase is an inflammatory mediator expressed by microglia. Again, epidemiological and neuropathological data can be correlated to suggest that dapsone might be effective in AD, therefore warranting a clinical trial.

The spectrum of inflammatory mediators up-regulated in AD suggests many routes for future therapeutic intervention. It may be that multiple drug administration, targeted at different inflammatory mechanisms, will prove far more effective than utilization of any single agent. In many cases, the data suggest targets not considered to be of importance in the immunological field.

Inflammation in transgenic mouse models of Alzheimer's disease

Transgenic mice carrying a mutated form of human amyloid precursor protein (APP) develop Aβ deposits in the brain and are being used as models to test possible treatments for AD. Some of these treatments, such as vaccination with Aβ (Schenk et al., 1999; Janus et al., 2000; Morgan et al., 2000;

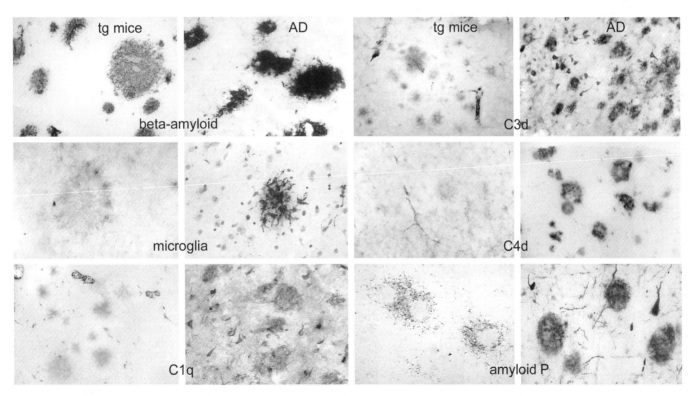

Fig. 28.5 Immunohistochemical staining in APP23 transgenic (tg) mouse and Alzheimer's disease (AD) brains for amyloid, reactive microglia, the complement component C1q, the activated complement fragments C3d and C4d, and amyloid P. Columns 1 and 3 are tg mouse and 2 and 4 are AD tissue. The substance stained for is indicated on each pair of photomicrographs.

Bard *et al.*, 2000; Das *et al.*, 2001; DeMattos *et al.*, 2001), involve immune reactions. It therefore seems worthwhile to compare the inflammatory reaction in such transgenic mouse brain with that seen in AD.

Activated microglia and activated astrocytes do surround the deposits (Frautschy *et al.*, 1998; Bornemann *et al.*, 2001; Matsuoka *et al.*, 2001) (Fig. 28.5), and treatment with the NSAID ibuprofen is reported to suppress plaque pathology and inflammation (Lim *et al.*, 2000). The activated microglia, however, appear fewer than in AD and, in the mice, do not form clumps on the Aβ deposits (Figs 28.5). A major difference between AD and these transgenic mouse Aβ deposits is that the latter do not show high levels of complement activation (Figs 28.5) (McGeer *et al.*, 2002a), and, in our hands, the MAC of complement is not detectable (Figs 28.5) (McGeer *et al.*, 2002a). Mouse C1q poorly recognizes human Aβ (Webster *et al.*, 1999). This probably explains why complement activation by amyloid deposits in transgenic mice is weak compared with AD senile plaques. The relatively weak activation of microglia and the absence of the MAC in the transgenic mice may explain why there is little or no neuronal loss (Irizarry *et al.*, 1997; Calhoun *et al.*, 1998; Tomidokoro *et al.*, 2001), another striking difference from AD. The relatively good preservation of neurons in these transgenic mice argues against the hypothesis that Aβ is directly neurotoxic but supports the thesis that the neurotoxicity in AD is secondary to the inflammatory process stirred up by Aβ.

The relative ease with which the amyloid deposits in transgenic mice could be prevented by antibodies naturally raised hopes that similar strategies might work in AD. Accordingly, a clinical trial in AD using a vaccine code named AN-1742 was commenced under the sponsorship of Wyeth and Elan Pharmaceuticals. After a few months the trial was terminated due to serious inflammatory complications developing in about 5% of patients (Steinberg, 2002), including one death. Should this result have been anticipated?

Complement activation in transgenic mice should be greatly enhanced by attachment of Aβ antibodies to the deposits. This is because antibodies activate complement in a different fashion from Aβ. They bind to the globular head of C1q rather than the collagen tail. Therefore, when mouse antibodies bind to human Aβ, they will strongly activate the mouse complement system. In turn, this will provide significant stimulation to phagocytic activity by mouse microglia due to their high levels of complement receptors. The relatively soluble Aβ deposits in transgenic mice might therefore be cleared.

In AD, complement is already overactivated without phagocytosis being observed. Therefore an anticipated consequence of Aβ vaccination is further stimulation of complement activation and further destruction of neurons and their processes. Thus, if levels of complement activation are low, and the target protein is in a state where it can be easily phagocytosed, as is the case in transgenic mice, then antibodies can accomplish their normal function of assisting phagocytosis. But if complement activation has already reached pathological levels, and if the target deposit is in a state where it cannot be readily phagocytosed, then antibodies will only exacerbate the pathology.

Innate immune reactions in other degenerative diseases

It may be that the lessons learned from AD research will have much broader applications in the general field of medicine. Parkinson's disease (PD) is another condition of the CNS in which activated microglia appear abundantly in the substantia nigra and many inflammatory mediators, including complement proteins and pentraxins, are present in affected brain regions (Fig. 28.6) (McGeer *et al.*, 2001). Abnormally high concentrations of IL-1β have been reported in the cerebrospinal fluid in PD (Blum-Degen *et al.*, 1995) just as in AD, and the same T allele of the IL-1β −511 regulatory region, or the region governing expression, which is found disproportionately in AD (Nicoll *et al.*, 2000) is also overexpressed in Caucasian PD cases (McGeer *et al.*, 2002b; Schulte *et al.*, 2002). No significant difference between PD patients and controls was, however, found in a Japanese study where there was also a high frequency of the T allele in the control population (Nishimura *et al.*, 2000).

Studies of tissue in such degenerative processes as atherosclerosis and infarcted heart also indicate that a similar innate immune reaction occurs, with similar up-regulation of inflammatory mediators and similar damage to local tissue. The MAC has been observed on the surface of damaged host cells in myocardial infarct (Lagrand *et al.*, 1997; Yasojima *et al.*, 1998) and atherosclerotic plaques (Torzewski *et al.*, 1998; Yasojima *et al.*, 2001). Up-regulation of the mRNAs and proteins has also been found (Fig. 28.6) (Yasojima *et al.*, 1998, 2001). However, in atherosclerotic plaques, there is no up-regulation of the defensive proteins C1 inhibitor, decay accelerating factor, CD46, C4 binding protein, or CD59 (Yasojima *et al.*, 2001). The situation is comparable to that seen in AD brain where there is evidence of complement-mediated autodestruction in the absence of adequate host defense.

CRP is also produced in heart, where it is increased following myocardial injury and in arteries where it is sharply up-regulated in atherosclerotic plaques (Fig. 28.6) (Yasojima *et al.*, 2001). Serum CRP levels predict survival after heart attacks (Pietila *et al.*, 1996; Lagrand *et al.*, 1999) and strokes (Muir *et al.*, 1999) and high normal CRP levels in apparently healthy individuals are associated with substantially increased odds of future adverse cardiovascular events (Ridker *et al.*, 1997, 2000; Koenig *et al.*, 1999).

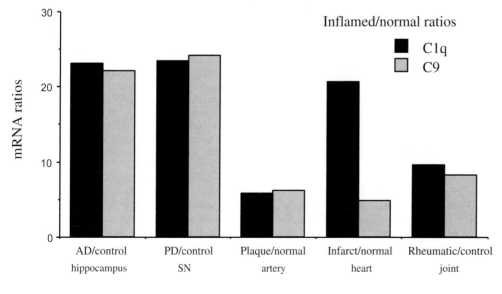

Fig. 28.6 Ratio of mRNAs in inflamed and normal tissue for C1q and C9 in Alzheimer's disease (AD) compared with normal hippocampus, Parkinson's disease (PD) compared with normal substantia nigra (SN), atherosclerotic plaque compared with normal artery, infarcted heart compared with normal heart tissue, and rheumatic joint compared with normal joint tissue. The rheumatic joint tissue was removed surgically because of intractable pain. Note that the up-regulation of the complement system appears greater in the neurodegenerative diseases than in the rheumatic tissue.

There is abundant epidemiological evidence that NSAIDs have a protective effect against heart disease and stroke (Arnau and Agusti, 1997; Bath, 1997; Rojas-Fernandez *et al.*, 1999; Elwood, 2000). While the efficacy of these agents has been attributed to their effect on platelets, their action in combating the autotoxic effects of local inflammation may contribute to their blocking the transformation of a relatively benign process into active deterioration. The reduction in serum CRP noted in men taking aspirin is in accord with such anti-inflammatory action (Ridker *et al.*, 1997).

It would thus appear that the innate immune system may be playing a role in the major diseases of our time: AD, heart attack, and atherosclerosis. The initial causes of pathology in these diseases are quite different—plaques and tangles in AD, anoxia in heart disease, and too much fat in atherosclerosis. But the secondary process seems to be similar. So the discovery of drugs effective against key inflammatory mediators such as the complement proteins may have widespread application.

Acknowledgements

Our research has been supported by grants from the Jack Brown and Family A.D. Research Fund, the Alzheimer Society of Canada-CIHR-AstraZeneca Co., and the Parkinson Foundation of Canada, as well as donations from The Friends of UBC and individual British Columbians. We thank Dr Claudia Schwab for preparing the photomicrographs.

References

Aisen, P.S., Davis, K.L., Berg, J.D., Schafer, K., Campbell, K., Thomas, R.G., *et al.* (2000) A randomized controlled trial of prednisone in Alzheimer's disease. *Neurology* 54: 588–593.

Aisen, P.S., Schmeidler, J., and Pasinetti, G. (2002) Randomized pilot study of nimesulide in Alzheimer's disease. *Neurology* 58: 1050–1054.

Akiyama, H. and McGeer, P.L. (1990) Brain microglia constitutively express β2 integrins. *J Neuroimmunol* 30: 81–93.

Akiyama, H., Yamada, T., Kawamata, T., and McGeer, P.L. (1991) Association of amyloid P component with complement proteins in neurologically diseased tissue. *Brain Res* 548: 349–352.

Alldred, A. (2001) Etanercept in rheumatoid arthritis. *Expert Opin Pharmacother* 1: 1137–1148.

Arnau, J.M. and Agusti, A. (1997) Is aspirin underused in myocardial infarction? *Pharmacoeconomics* 12: 524–532.

Baik, E.J., Kim, E.J., Lee, S.H., and Moon, C. (1999) Cyclooxygenase-2 selective inhibitors aggravate kainic acid induced seizure and neuronal cell death in the hippocampus. *Brain Res* 843: 118–129.

Bard, F., Cannon, C., Barbour, R., Burke, R.L., Games, D., Grajeda, H.,.*et al.* (2000) Peripherally administered antibodies against amyloid beta-peptide enter the central nervous system and reduce pathology in a mouse model of Alzheimer disease. *Nat Med* 6: 916–919.

Bath, P.M.W. (1997) The medical management of stroke. *Int J Clin Practice* 51: 504–510.

Blacker, D., Wilcox, M.A., Laird, N.M., Rodes, L., Horvath, S.M., Go, R.C., *et al.* (1998) Alpha-2-macroglobulin is genetically associated with Alzheimer disease. *Nat Genet* 19: 357–360.

Blum-Degen, D., Muller, T., Kuhn, W., Gerlach, M., Przuntek, H., and Riederer, P. (1995) Interleukin-1b and interleukin-6 are elevated in the cerebrospinal fluid of Alzheimer's and de novo Parkinson's disease patients, *Neurosci Lett* 202: 17–20

Bornemann, K.D., Wiederhold, K.H., Pauli, C., Ermini, F., Stalder, M., Schnell, L., *et al.* (2001) Abeta-induced inflammatory processes in microglia cells of APP23 transgenic mice. *Am J Pathol* 158: 63–73.

Broe, G.A., Grayson, D.A., Creasey, H.M., Waite, L.M., Casey, B.J., Bennett, H.P., *et al.* (2000) Anti-inflammatory drugs protect against Alzheimer disease at low doses. *Arch Neurol* 57: 1586–1591.

Cacebelos, R., Alvarez, X.A., Fernandez-Novoa, I., Franco, A., Mangues, R., Pellicer, A., and Nishimura, T. (1994) Brain interleukin-1 beta in Alzheimer's disease and vascular dementia. *Methods Find Exp Clin Pharmacol* 16: 141–145.

Calhoun, M.E., Wiederhold, K.H., Abramowski, D., Phinney, A.L., Probst, A., Sturchler-Pierrat, C., *et al.* (1998) Neuron loss in APP transgenic mice. *Nature* 395: 755–756.

Collins, J.S., Perry, R.T., Watson, B. Jr, Harrell, L.E., Acton, R.T., Blacker, D., *et al.* (2000) Association of a haplotype for tumor necrosis factor in siblings with late-onset Alzheimer disease: The NIMH Alzheimer disease genetics initiative. *Am J Med Genet* 96: 823–830.

Das, P., Murphy, M.P., Younkin, L.H., Younkin, S.G., and Golde, T.E. (2001) Reduced effectiveness of Aβ1-42 immunization in APP transgenic mice with significant amyloid deposition. *Neurobiol Aging* 22: 721–727.

Del Rio Hortega, P. (1919) El "tercer elemento" de los centros nerviosos. Poder fagocitario y movilidad de la microglia. *Bol Soc Esp Biol Ano* ix: 154–166.

DeMattos, R.B., Bales, K.R., Cummins, D.J., Dodart, J.C., Paul, S.M., and Holtzman, D.M. (2001) Peripheral anti-A beta antibody alters CNS and plasma A beta clearance and decreases brain A beta burden in a mouse model of Alzheimer's disease. *Proc Natl Acad Sci USA* 98: 8850–8855.

Dickson, D.W., Lee, S.C., Mattiace, L.A., Yen, S.H.C., and Brosnan, C. (1993) Microglia and cytokines in neurological disease, with special reference to AIDS and Alzheimer disease. *Glia* 7: 75–83.

Du, Y., Dodel, R.C., Eastwood, B.J., Bales, K.R., Gao, F., Lohmuller, F., *et al.* (2000) Association of an interleukin 1 alpha polymorphism with Alzheimer's disease. *Neurology* 55: 480–483.

Eikelenboom, P., Hack, C.E., Rozemuller, J.M., and Stam, F.C. (1989) Complement activation in amyloid plaques in Alzheimer's dementia. *Virchows Arch Cell Pathol* 56: 259–262.

Elwood, P.C. (2001) Aspirin: past, present and future. *Clin Med* 1: 132–137.

Feagan, B.G., Enns, R., Fedorak, R.N., Panaccione, R., Pare, P., Steinhart, A.H., and Wild, G. (2001) Infliximab for the treatment of Crohn's disease: efficacy, safety and pharmacoeconmoics. *Can J Clin Pharmacol* 8: 188–198.

Fiane,. A.E., Mollnes, T.E., Videm, V., Hovig, T., Hogasen, K., Mellbye, O.J., *et al.* (1999) Compstatin, a peptide inhibitor of C3, prolongs survival of ex vivo perfused pig xenografts. *Xenotransplantation* 6: 52–65.

Frautschy, S.A., Yang, F., Irrizarry, M., Hyman, B., Saido, T.C., Hsiao, K., and Cole, G.M. (1998) Microglial response to amyloid plaques in APPsw transgenic mice. *Am J Pathol* 152: 307–317.

Furlong, S.T., Dutta, A.S., Coath, M.M., Gormley, J.J., Hubbs, S.J., Lloyd, D., *et al.* (2000) C3 activation is inhibited by analogs of compstatin but not by serine protease inhibitors or peptidyl alpha–ketoheterocycles. *Immunopharmacology* 48: 199–212.

Giulian, D., Haverkamp, L.J., Yu, J.H., Karshin, W., Tom, D., Li, J., *et al.* (1996) Specificc domains of beta-amyloid from Alzheimer plaque elicit neuron killing in human microglia. *J Neurosci* 16: 6021–6037.

Griffin, W.S., Stanley, L.C., Ling, C., White, L., MacLeod, V., Perrot, L.J., *et al.* (1989) Brain interleukin 1 and S-100 immunoreactivity are elevated in Down syndrome and Alzheimer's disease. *Proc Natl Acad Sci USA* 86: 7611–7615.

Grimaldi, L.M., Casadei, C.M., Ferri, C., Veglia, F., Licastro, F., Annoni, G., *et al.* (2000) Association of early-onset Alzheimer's disease with an interleukin-1α gene polymorphism. *Ann Neurol* 47: 361–365.

Hamilton, K. and Clair, E.W. (2000) Tumour necrosis factor-alpha blockade: a new era for the effective management of rheumatoid arthritis. *Expert Opin Pharmacother* 1: 1041–1052.

Hicks, P.S., Saunero-Nazia, L., Duclos, T.W., and Mold, C. (1992) Serum amyloid P component binds to histones and activates the classical complement pathway. *J Immunol* 149: 3689–3694.

Hope, H.R., Remsen, E.E., Lewis, C. Jr, Heuvelman, D.M., Walker, M.C., Jennings, M., and Connolly, D.T. (2000) Large-scale purification of myeloperoxidase from KL60 promyelocytic cells: characterization and comparison to human neutrophil myeloperoxidase. *Protein Express Purif* 18: 269–276.

Irizarry, M.C., McNamara, M., Fedorchak, K., Hsiao, K., and Hyman, B.T. (1997) APPSw transgenic mice develop age-related A beta deposits and neuropil abnormalities, but no neuronal loss in CA1. *J Neuropath Exp Neurol* 56: 965–973.

Ishii, T. and Haga, S. (1984) Immuno-electron-microscopic localization of complements in amyloid fibrils of senile plaques. *Acta Neuropathol (Berlin)* 63: 296–300.

Itagaki, S., Akiyama, H., Saito, H., and McGeer, P.L. (1994) Ultrastructural local-ization of complement membrane attack complex (MAC)-like immuno-reactivity in brains of patients with Alzheimer's disease. *Brain Res* **645**: 78–84.

Janus, C., Pearson, J., McLaurin, J., Mathews, P.M., Jiang, Y., Schmidt, S.D., *et al.* (2000) A beta peptide immunization reduces behavioural impairment and plaques in a model of Alzheimer's disease. *Nature* **408**: 979–982.

Jiang, H., Robey, F., and Gewurz, H. (1992) Localization of sites through which C-reactive protein binds to and activates complement to residues 14–26 and 76–92 of the human C1q A chain. *J Exp Med* **175**: 1373–1379.

Kalaria, R.N. and Grahovac, I. (1990) Serum amyloid P immunoreactivity in hippocampal tangles, plaques and vessels: implications for leakage across the blood-brain barrier in Alzheimer's disease. *Brain Res* **516**: 349–353.

Kamboh, M.I., Aston, C.E., Ferrell, R.E., and Dekosky, S.T. (1997) Genetic effect of alpha-1-antichymotrypsin on the risk of Alzheimer disease. *Genomics* **40**: 382–384

Kaufmann, W.E., Worley, P.F., Pegg, J., Bremer, M., and Isakson, P. (1996) COX-2, a synaptically induced enzyme, is expressed by excitatory neurons at post-synaptic sites in rat cerebral cortex. *Proc Natl Acad Sci USA* **93**: 2317–2321.

Klegeris, A. and McGeer, P.L. (2000) Interaction of various intracellular signaling mechanisms involved in mononuclear phagocyte toxicity toward neuronal cells. *J Leukocyte Biol* **67**: 127–133.

Klegeris, A., Walker, D.G., and McGeer, P.L. (1999) Toxicity of human THP-1 monocytic cells towards neuron-like cells is reduced by non-steroidal anti-inflammatory drugs (NSAIDs). *Neuropharmacology* **38**: 1017–1025.

Koenig, W., Sund, M., Frohlich, M., Fischer, H.G., Lowel, H., Doring, A., *et al.* (1999) C-reactive protein, a sensitive marker of inflammation, predicts future risk of coronary heart disease in initially healthy middle-aged men. *Circulation* **99**: 237–240.

Lagrand, W.K., Niessen, H.W., Wolbink, G.J., Jaspars, L.H., Visser, C.A., Verheugt, F.W.,.*et al.* (1997) C-Reactive protein colocalized with complement in human heart during acute myocardial infarction. *Circulation* **97**: 97–103.

Lagrand, W.K., Visser, C.A., Hermens, W.T., Niessen, H.W., Verheugt, F.W., Wolbink, G.J. and Hack, C.E. (1999) C-reactive protein as a cardiovascular risk factor: more than an epiphe-nomenon? *Circulation* **100**: 96–102.

Lambris, D.H. (1993) The chemistry, biology, and phylogeny of C3. In JM Cruise and RE Lewis Jr, eds. *Complement Today*, pp. 16–45. Karger, Basel.

Licastro, F., Pedrini, S., Bonafe, M., Grimaldi, L.M.E., Olivieri, F., Cavallone, L., *et al,* (2000a) Polymorphisms of the IL-6 gene increase the risk for late onset Alzheimer's disease and affect IL-6 plasma levels. *Neurobiol Aging* **21(1S)**: S38.

Licastro, F., Pedrini, S., Ferri, C., Casadei,V., Govoni, M., Pession, A., *et al.* (2000b) Gene polymorphism affecting a1-antichymotrypsin and inter-leukin-1 plasma levels increases Alzheimer's disease risk. *Ann Neurol* **48**: 388–391.

Lieberman, A.P., Pitha, P.M., Shin, H.S., and Shin, M.L. (1989) Production of tumor necrosis factor and other cytokines by astrocytes stimulated with lipopolysaccharide or a neurotropic virus. *Proc Natl Acad Sci USA* **86**: 6348–6352.

Lim, G.P., Yang, F., Chu, T., Chen, P., Beech, W., Teter, B., *et al.* (2000) Ibuprofen suppresses plaque pathology and inflammation in a mouse model for Alzheimer's disease. *J Neurosci* **20**: 5709–5714,.

MacKenzie, I.R.A. (2000) Anti-inflammatory drugs and Alzheimer-type patho-logy in aging. *Neurology* **54**: 732–734.

Matsuoka, Y., Picciano, M., Malester, B., LaFrancois, J., Zehr, C., Daeschner, J.M., *et al.* (2001) Inflammatory responses to amyloidosis in a transgenic mouse model of Alzheimer's disease. *Am J Pathol* **158**: 1345–1354.

McCusker, S.M. (2001) Association between polymorphism in regulatory region of gene encoding tumour necrosis factor a and risk of Alzheimer's disease and vascular dementia: a case-control study. *Lancet* **357**: 436–439.

McGeer, P.L. (2000) Cyclooxygenase-2 inhibitors: rationale and therapeutic potential for Alzheimer's disease. *Drugs Aging* **17**: 1–11.

McGeer, P.L. and McGeer, E.G. (1995) The inflammatory response system of brain: implications for therapy of Alzheimer and other neurodegenerative diseases. *Brain Res Rev* **21**: 195–218.

McGeer, P.L. and McGeer, E.G. (2000) Autotoxicity and Alzheimer disease. *Arch Neurol* **57**: 789–790.

McGeer, P.L. and McGeer, E.G. (2001) Polymorphisms in inflammatory genes enhance the risk of Alzheimer disease. *Arch Neurol* **58**: 1790–1792.

McGeer, P.L., Akiyama, H., Itagaki, S., and McGeer, E.G. (1989) Immune system response in Alzheimer's disease. *Can J Neurol Sci* **16**: 516–527.

McGeer, P.L., Harada, N., Kimura, H., McGeer, E.G., and Schulzer, M. (1992) Prevalence of dementia amongst elderly Japanese with leprosy: apparent effect of chronic drug therapy. *Dementia* **3**: 146–149.

McGeer, P.L., Itagaki, S., Tago, H., and McGeer, E.G. (1987) Reactive microglia in patients with senile dementia of the Alzheimer type are positive for the histocompatibility glycoprotein HLA-DR. *Neurosci Lett* **79**: 195–200.

McGeer, P.L., Rogers, J., McGeer, E.G., and Sibley, J. (1990) Does anti-inflammat-ory treatment protect against Alzheimer disease? *Lancet* **335**: 1037.

McGeer, P.L., Schulzer, M., and McGeer, E.G. (1996) Arthritis and antiinflam-matory agents as possible protective factors for Alzheimer's disease: a review of 17 epidemiological studies. *Neurology* **147**: 425–432.

McGeer, P.L., Schwab, C., and Staufenbiel, M. (2002a) Amyloid transgenic mice: an incomplete model of Alzheimer's disease. *Neurobiol Aging* **23**: S234.

McGeer, P.L., Yasojima, K., and McGeer, E.G. (2001) Inflammation in Parkinson's disease, *Adv Neurol* **86**: 83–89.

McGeer, P.L., Yasojima, K., and McGeer, E.G. (2002b) Association of interleukin-1b polymorphisms with idiopathic Parkinson's disease. *Neurosci Lett* **326**: 67–69.

Morgan, D., Diamond, D.M., Gottschall, P.E., Ugen, K.E., Dickey, C., Hardy, J., *et al.* (2000) A beta peptide vaccination prevents memory loss in an animal model of Alzheimer's disease. *Nature* **408**: 982–985.

Muir, K.W., Weir, C.J., Alwan, W., Squire,.I.B., and Lees, K.R. (1999) C-reactive protein and outcome after ischemic stroke. *Stroke* **30**: 981–985.

Nakayama, M., Uchimura, K., Zhu, R.L., Nagayama, T., Rose, M.E., Stetler, R.A., *et al.* (1998) Cyclooxygenase-2 inhibition prevents delayed death of CA1 hippocampal neurons following global ischemia. *Proc Natl Acad Sci USA* **95**: 10954–10959.

Neuroinflammation Working Group: Akiyama, H., Barger, S., Barnum, S., Bradt, B., Bauer, J., Cole, G.M., *et al.* (2000) Inflammation and Alzheimer's disease. *Neurobiol Aging* **21**: 383–421,

Nicoll, J.A., Mrak, R.E., Graham, D., Stewart, J., Wilcock, G., MacGowan, S., *et al.* (2000) Association of interleukin-1 gene polymorphisms with Alzheimer's disease. *Ann Neurol* **47**: 365–368.

Nishimura, M., Mizuta, I., Mizuta, E., Yamasaki, S., Ohta, M., and Kumo, S. (2000) Influence of interleukin-1b gene polymorphisms on age-at-onset of sporadic Parkinson's disease, *Neurosci Lett* **284**: 73–76.

Papassotiropoulos, A., Bagli, M., Jessen, F., Bayer, T.A., Maier, W., Rao, M.L., and Heun, R. (1999) A genetic variation of the inflammatory cytokine inter-leukin-6 delays the initial onset and reduces the risk for sporadic Alzheimer's disease. *Ann Neurol* **45**: 666–668.

Pietila, K., Harmoinen, A.P., Jokinitty, J., and Pasternack, A.I. (1996) Serum C-reactive protein concentration in acute myocardial infarction and its rela-tionship to mortality during 24 months of follow-up in patients under thrombolytic treatment. *Eur Heart J* **17**: 1345–1349.

Quigg, R.J. (2002) Use of complement inhibitors in tissue injury. *Trends Mol Med* **9**: 430–437.

Rebeck, G.W. (2000) Confirmation of the genetic association of interleukin-1a with early onset sporadic Alzheimer's disease. *Neurosci Lett* **293**: 75–77.

Reynolds, W.F., Rhees, J., Maciejewski, D., Paladino, T., Sieburg, H., Maki, R.A., and Masliah, E. (1999) Myeloperoxidase polymorphism is associated with gender specific risk for Alzheimer's disease. *Exp Neurol* **155**: 31–41.

Ridker, P.M., Hennekens, C.H., Buring, J.E., and Rifai, N. (2000) C-reactive pro-tein and other markers of inflammation in the prediction of cardiovascular disease in women. *N Engl J Med* **342**: 836–843.

Ridker, P.M., Cushman, M., Stampfer, M.J., Tracy, R.P., and Hennekens, C.H. (1997) Inflammation, aspirin, and the risk of cardiovascular disease in apparently healthy men. *N Engl J Med* **336**: 973–979.

Rogers, J., Luber-Narod, J., Styren, C.D., and Civin, W.H. (1988) Expression of immune system-associated antigens by cells of the human central nervous system: relationship to the pathology of Alzheimer's disease. *Neurobiol Aging* **9**: 339–349.

Rogers, J., Webster, S., Schultz, J., McGeer, P.L., Styren, S., Civin, W.H., *et al.* (1992) Complement activation by b-amyloid in Alzheimer disease. *Proc Natl Acad Sci* **89**: 10016–10020.

Rogers, J., Kirby, L.C., Hempelman, S.R., Berry, D.L., McGeer, P.L., Kaszniak, A.W., et al. (1993) Clinical trial of indomethacin in Alzheimer's disease. *Neurology* 43: 1609–1611.

Rojas-Fernandez, C.H., Kephart, G.C., Sketris, I.S., and Kass, K. (1999) Underuse of acetylsalicylic acid in individuals with myocardial infarction, ischemic heart disease or stroke: data from the 1995 population based Nova Scotia Health Study. *Can J Cardiol* 15: 291–296.

Rozemuller, J.M., Eikelenboom, P., Pals, S.T., and Stam, F.C. (1989) Microglial cells around amyloid plaques in Alzheimer's disease express leucocyte adhesion molecules of the LFA-1 family. *Neurosci Lett* 101: 288–292.

Sainati, S.M., Ingram, D.M., Talwaker, S., and Geis, G.S. (2000) Results of a double-blind, placebo-controlled study of celecoxib for the progression of Alzheimer's disease. *6th International Stockholm-Springfield Symposium of Advances in Alzheimer Therapy*, Karolinska Institutet, Stockholm, Sweden.

Scharf, S., Mander, A., Ugoni, A., Vajda, F., and Christophidis, N. (1999) A double-blind, placebo-controlled trial of diclofenac misoprostol in Alzheimer's disease. *Neurology* 53: 197–201.

Schenk, D., Barbour, R., Dunn, W., Gordon, G., Grajeda, H., Guido, T., et al. (1999) Immunization with amyloid-beta attenuates Alzheimer-disease-like pathology in the PDAPP mouse. *Nature* 400: 173–177.

Schulte, T., Schols, L., Berger, K., Epplen, J.T., and Kruger, R. (2002) Polymorphisms in the interleukin-1 alpha and beta genes and the risk of Parkinson's disease. *Neurosci Lett* 326: 70–72.

Schwartz, C.F., Kilgore, K.S., Homeister, J.W., Levy, B.A., Lucchesi, B.R., and Bolling, S.E. (1999) Increased rat cardiac allograft survival by the glycosaminoglycan pentosan polysulfate. *J Surg Res* 86: 24–28.

Sharif, S.F., Hariri, R.J., Chang, V.A., Barie, P.S., Wang, R.S., and Ghajar, J.B. (1993) Human astrocyte production of tumour necrosis factor-alpha, interleukin-1 beta, and interleukin-6 following exposure to lipopolysaccharide endotoxin. *Neurol Res* 15: 109–112.

Steinberg, D. (2002) Companies halt first Alzheimer vaccine trial. *The Scientist* 16: 22.

Stewart, W.F., Kawas, C., Corrada, M., and Metter, E.J. (1997) Risk of Alzheimer's disease and duration of NSAID use. *Neurology* 48: 626–632.

Strittmatter, W.J., Saunders, A., Schmechel, D., Pericak-Vance, M., Enghild, J., Salvesen, G.S., and Roses, A.D. (1993) Apolipoprotein E: high avidity binding to b-amyloid and increased frequency of type 4 allele in late-onset familial Alzheimer disease. *Proc Natl Acad Sci USA* 90: 1977–1981.

Tanhehco, E.J., Kilgore, K.S., Naylor, K.B., Booth, E.A., and Lucchesi, B.R. (1999) Reduction of myocardial infarct size after ischemia and reperfusion by the glycosaminoglycan pentosan polysulfate. *J Cardiovasc Pharmacol* 34: 153–161.

Tomidokoro, Y., Harigaya, Y., Matsubara, E., Ikeda, M., Kawarabayashi, T., Shirao, T., et al. (2001) Brain Abeta amyloidosis in APPsw mice induces accumulation of presenilin-1 and tau. *J Pathol* 194: 500–506.

Torzewski, J., Torzewski, M., Bowyer, D.E., Frohlich, M., Koenig, W., Waltenberger, J., et al. (1998) C-reactive protein frequently colocalizes with the terminal complement complex in the intima of early atherosclerotic lesions of human coronary arteries. *Arterioscler Thrombosis Vasc Biol* 18: 1386–1392.

Van Gool, W.A., Weinstein, H.C., Scheltens, P.K., and Walstra, G.J. (2001) Effect of hydroxychloroquine on progression of dementia in early Alzheimer's disease: an 18-month randomized, double-blind, placebo-controlled study. *Lancet* 358: 455–460.

Veld, B.A.I., Ruitenberg, A., Launer, L.J., Hofman, A., Breteler, M.M.B., and Stricker, B.H.C. (2000) Duration of non-steroidal antiinflammatory drug use and risk of Alzheimer's disease. The Rotterdam study. *Neurobiol Aging* 21(1S): S204.

Walker, D.G., Kim, S.U., and McGeer, P.L. (1995) Complement and cytokine gene expression in cultured microglia derived from postmortem human brains. *J Neurosci Res* 40: 478–493.

Wallace, J.L., Pittman, Q.J., and Cirino, G. (1995) Nitric oxide-releasing NSAIDs: a novel class of GI-sparing anti-inflammatory drugs. *Agents Actions Suppl* 46: 121–129.

Webster, S., Bonnell, B., and Rogers, J. (1997a) Charge-based binding of complement component C1q to the Alzheimer amyloid beta-peptide. *Am J Pathol* 150: 1531–1536.

Webster, S., Lue, L.F., Brachova, L., Tenner, A.J., McGeer, P.L., Terai, K., et al. (1997b) Molecular and cellular characterization of the membrane attack complex, C5b-9, in Alzheimer's disease. *Neurobiol Aging* 18: 415–421.

Webster, S., Tenner, A.J., Poulos, T.L., and Cribbs, D.H. (1999) The mouse C1q A-chain sequence alters beta-amyloid-induced complement activation. *Neurobiol Aging* 20: 297–304.

Wood, J.A., Wood, P.L., Ryan, R., Graff-Radford, N.R., Pilapil, C., Robitaille, Y., and Quirion, R. (1993) Cytokine indices in Alzheimer's temporal cortex: no change in mature IL beta or IL-1RA but increases in the associated acute phase proteins IL-6, alpha 2-macroglobulin and C-reactive protein. *Brain Res* 629: 245–252.

Yamabe, T., Dhir, G., Cowan, E.P., Wolf, A.L., Bergey, G.K., Krumholz, A., et al. (1994) Cytokine-gene expression in measles-infected adult human glial cells. *J Neuroimmunol* 49: 171–179.

Yasojima, K., Schwab, C., McGeer, E.G., and McGeer, P.L. (1998) Human heart generates complement proteins that are upregulated and activated after myocardial infarction. *Circ Res* 83: 860–869.

Yasojima, K., McGeer, E.G., and McGeer, P.L. (1999a) Complement regulators C1 inhibitor and CD59 do not significantly inhibit complement activation in Alzheimer disease. *Brain Res* 833: 297–301.

Yasojima, K., Schwab, C., McGeer, E.G., and McGeer, P.L. (1999b) Upregulated production and activation of the complement system in Alzheimer disease brain. *Am J Pathol* 154: 927–936.

Yasojima, K., Schwab, C., McGeer, E.G., and McGeer, P.L. (1999c) Distribution of cyclooxygenase-1 and cyclooxygenase-2 mRNAs and proteins in human brain and peripheral organs. *Brain Res* 830: 226–236.

Yasojima, K., Schwab, C., McGeer, E.G., and McGeer, P.L. (2000) Human neurons generate C-reactive protein and amyloid P: upregulation in Alzheimer's disease. *Brain Res* 887: 80–89.

Yasojima, K., Schwab, C., McGeer, E.G., and McGeer, P.L. (2001) Generation of C-reactive protein and complement components in atherosclerotic plaques. *Am J Pathol* 158: 1039–1051.

Ying, S.C., Gewurz, A.T., Jiang, H., and Gewurz, H. (1993) Human serum amyloid P component oligomers bind and activate the classical complement pathway via residues 14–26 and 76–92 of the A chain collagen-like region of C1q. *J Immunol* 150: 169–176.

29 Central nervous system neoplastic diseases and the immune system

Paul R. Walker, Thomas Calzascia, Nicolas de Tribolet, and Pierre-Yves Dietrich

Introduction

The presence of cancerous tissue within the central nervous system (CNS) presents serious clinical consequences and many brain tumours cannot be adequately treated. Although neuro-oncologists are concerned with a wide spectrum of primary and secondary cerebral malignancies, the fundamental interest for neuroimmunology is focused on the site of the tumour rather than its histological origin. Thus, our understanding of the principles of immune relationships with a non-metastatic primary brain tumour growing in the brain parenchyma is broadly applicable to tumours of most histological origin. In contrast, tumours metastasizing to the CNS will have encountered different elements of the host immune system in different anatomical compartments; their immunological interest is thus only partly neuroimmunological. For the purposes of this chapter, we will concentrate on immunological interactions of relevance for the most common brain neoplasm: the glioma. Indeed, the grade III and grade IV astrocytomas (anaplastic astrocytomas and glioblastomas, respectively) are lethal, malignant tumours for which there have been only modest advances in treatment using conventional modalities of surgical resection, radiotherapy, and chemotherapy (Stupp *et al.*, 2002). Employing such approaches, it is unlikely that long-term survival rates can be significantly extended beyond the current median survival of less than 12 months for glioblastomas (Stewart, 2002). Moreover, even though the outlook is more favourable for low-grade astrocytomas, not all can be adequately treated and there is an inexorable progression to malignant lesions (Holland, 2001). Malignant astrocytomas infiltrate normal tissue, which renders total surgical resection virtually impossible without extensive neurological damage. It is thus essential to consider novel treatments such as immunotherapy in the hope of attacking the residual radioresistant and chemoresistant tumour cells. Other tumours metastasizing to the brain, such as melanoma, pose similar problems (Lassman and DeAngelis, 2003), and for these tumours it would also be useful to propose a therapeutic option that is applicable to the CNS. Most experimental studies of tumour immunotherapy have highlighted cellular rather than humoral mechanisms in tumour rejection: the focus of this chapter will therefore be primarily on T-cell-mediated immune responses. Indeed, under ideal conditions, CD8+ cytotoxic T lymphocytes (CTLs) can infiltrate tissues, exhibit exquisite fine specificity, mediate potent cytotoxicity, and maintain long-term immunological memory. Nevertheless, T cells do not function alone in immune networks, and other accessory and effector mechanisms may also play a role in future immunotherapies.

Research into brain tumour immunology and immunotherapy has broadly been pursued from two different perspectives. The first has been a methodical and rational assessment of the features of immune responses in the CNS and how these are linked to the specialized anatomy, cellular composition, and microenvironmental characteristics of this site (Cserr and Knopf, 1992; Fabry *et al.*, 1994). A logical application of these studies has been the analysis of spontaneous immune responses to cerebral malignancies, which has frequently led to the conclusion that factors specific to brain tumours or even the brain parenchyma can profoundly limit antitumour immune responses. The second approach has evolved more from a tumour immunotherapy background, in which highly encouraging results from animal models, and now from clinical trials, have shown that under some circumstances specific antitumour immune responses can be induced that can have an impact on tumours in various anatomical sites (Offringa *et al.*, 2000; Pardoll, 2002; Dudley *et al.*, 2002). For reasons that will be discussed, the most advanced immunotherapy studies have been performed in melanoma patients. Progress in this domain has prompted a direct application of such approaches to CNS malignancies, first in pre-clinical models and now in clinical trials. Earlier reviews of the outcome of these clinical trials did not conclude that there was any clear demonstration of a real impact on tumour outcome (Zeltzer *et al.*, 1999; van Herpen and De Mulder, 2000; Soling and Rainov, 2001). However, although only randomized Phase III studies will reveal the real clinical value of immunotherapy, some of the more recent clinical trials suggest that a degree of optimism should be retained for the concept of exploiting immune responses against brain tumours (Okada *et al.*, 2003; Yu *et al.*, 2004; Ehtesham *et al.*, 2004).

We will discuss what can and should be learned from these two approaches to nurture a 'third way' for immunotherapy of CNS neoplastic disease, in order to offer realistic hope for currently untreatable cancers. We consider that this approach should take into account the particularities of immune responses in the CNS to design and modify immunotherapeutic strategies borrowed from treatments for other cancers. The limitations of current animal models should force a reassessment of the linear progression from pre-clinical model to clinical trial, since tumour eradication in rodents is rarely predictive of efficacy in patients. Indeed, whilst many immune mechanisms are highly conserved between rodents and humans, most tumours currently used experimentally are very different from those spontaneously arising in patients. Thus, to rationally construct and improve new brain tumour immunotherapies requires clinical trials to be designed that permit some analysis of mechanisms, in order that these can be subsequently honed and optimized in appropriate models. These aspects will thus receive as much attention as tumour rejection in the sections that follow.

A further consideration that will serve as a framework for understanding the immunology of CNS neoplasms is the status of the dialogue between the malignant cell and the immune system. This can be categorized in three broad areas. The first is immune ignorance, i.e. the host immune system has not been stimulated. The second is immune detection of transformed cells, but without any noticeable impact on tumour progression. The final category is detectable antitumour immune responses that have an impact on tumour growth. The latter category is evidently the clinical objective, but how this may be best achieved will be influenced by spontaneous immune reactivity (or its absence) that may fall in the first two categories. It is therefore relevant to discuss all evidence for such immune status, whatever its functional outcome.

Induction of immune responses to brain tumours

The potential role of immune responses in controlling CNS malignancies has frequently been underestimated because of the classification of the CNS as a site of immune privilege. Indeed, observations in the field of transplantation noted extended survival of tissues transplanted to the CNS, compared with their survival in other sites (Medawar, 1948; Barker and Billingham, 1977). However, as the wealth of information in this book amply illustrates, immune reactions can and do occur in the CNS. Immune privilege can therefore be considered as a term that indicates the qualitatively and quantitatively different immune responses that occur in the CNS, rather than an absence of immunoreactivity.

Tumour recognition requires tumour antigen expression

The first issue that must be addressed in considering immune reactivity towards CNS neoplasms, and particularly gliomas, is whether malignant astrocytoma cells are sufficiently antigenically distinct from normal tissue to be recognized by tumour-specific T cells. The definition of astrocytoma-associated antigens has built upon the principles established for other categories of tumours. The characterization of human tumour antigens recognized by T cells dates from the beginning of the 1990s, when Boon and colleagues first identified the *MAGEA1* gene encoding a melanoma associated antigen (Van der Bruggen *et al.*, 1991). This milestone discovery gave a new impetus to tumour immunology, leading to the characterization of a rapidly growing number of antigens, particularly those expressed in melanoma (Renkvist *et al.*, 2001). Many tumour antigens being considered as targets for immunotherapeutic approaches are not strictly tumour specific since they are also expressed by a restricted range of normal tissues. Such tumour-associated antigens can be divided into categories, depending upon their distribution profile (Table 29.1). The principal interest in studying tumour-associated antigens rather than those that are strictly tumour specific is that they are often expressed by tumours from many different individuals, in contrast to tumour-specific antigens encoded by point mutations that are more likely to be patient specific. To date, most attention has been paid to the identification of tumour antigens recognized by CD8+ T cells (and therefore presented by major histocompatibility complex (MHC) Class I molecules), despite growing evidence for the importance of

CD4+ T cells in antitumour responses (Hung *et al.*, 1998). However, several tumour antigen epitopes presented by Class II molecules to CD4+ T lymphocytes have now been reported, providing further insights into the role of the CD4 arm in immune responses against tumours (Kalams and Walker, 1998; Wang, 2001).

There is little direct evidence that has been published concerning astrocytoma antigens able to spontaneously elicit an immune response. Most studies have assessed astrocytoma-associated antigen expression at the mRNA level rather than immunologically defined antigens shown to stimulate T cells. Many of the antigens screened for were previously defined in melanoma, a reasonable starting point given the common neuroectodermal origin of melanocytes and astrocytes. The list of antigens potentially expressed by at least some astrocytomas includes several proteins with limited expression in normal somatic cells. These include MAGE and GAGE family members, tyrosinase, AIM-2, TRP-1, TRP-2, gp100, p97, SSX-1, SSX-2, SSX-4, SCP-1, and TS85 (Chi *et al.*, 1997; Scarcella *et al.*, 1999; Sahin *et al.*, 2000; Liu *et al.*, 2003, 2004a,b; Yu *et al.*, 2004). Expression was often only detected on cultured tumour cells, leaving some doubts concerning *in vivo* expression. Nevertheless, recent data suggest that at least some of these antigens merit further assessment for their relevance *in vivo*. Patients with malignant astrocytoma who were vaccinated with dendritic cells (DCs) pulsed with tumour lysate (from surgical biopsies) generated enhanced CTL responses to AIM-2, HER-2, gp100, MAGE-1, and TRP-2 (Liu *et al.*, 2003, 2004a,b; Yu *et al.*, 2004).

Another potential source of T-cell epitopes in malignant astrocytoma is a mutant variant of the epidermal growth factor receptor (EGFRvIII), which is overexpressed in up to 50% of gliomas (Ekstrand *et al.*, 1992). This truly tumour-specific antigen is predicted to contain HLA-binding epitopes, and preliminary reports of the clinical trials that are under way suggest that specific T-cell reactivity can be induced in vaccinated glioma patients (Heimberger *et al.*, 2003).

Further antigens that are recognized by CTL *in vitro* include SART1$_{259}$, originally identified in epithelial cancer cells but now also shown to be expressed in malignant astrocytoma biopsies (Imaizumi *et al.*, 1999); an epitope from the interleukin (IL)-13 receptor α2 chain (Debinski and Gibo,

Table 29.1 Categories of tumour associated antigen recognised by T cells

Category	Examples and expression in astrocytoma				
		mRNA	Protein *in vitro*	Detection by CD8+ T cells	Protein *in vivo*
Cancer-testis antigen. Expressed only in normal testis, placental tissue and malignant tissue	MAGE-1	+	+	+[a]	+[a]
	IL-13 receptor α2	+	+	+	−
Differentiation antigen. Non-mutated proteins expressed by both neoplastic and normal cells tissue of the same histological origin	Tyrosinase	+	−	−	−
	TRP-2	+	+	+[a]	+[a]
Mutated antigen. Mutations in normal genes arising during neoplastic transformation	Epidermal growth factor receptor variant III[b]	+	+	+[b]	+
Overexpressed self antigen. Widely expressed antigens, possibly upregulated in tumour cells	Survivin	+	+	−	+
	SART-1	+	+	+	−

+ = Positive result or expression reported.

− = Negative expression, or no published data available.

[a]Expression mostly studied *in vitro*, but recent data suggest *in vivo* expression is also possible (see Liu *et al.* (2003, 2004) and Yu *et al.* (2004)).

[b]Preliminary reports suggest presence of T-cell epitopes and T-cell reactivity in patients. Full details not yet published (see Heimberger *et al.* (2003)).

2000; Okano *et al.*, 2002); and several epitopes from survivin, expressed in many malignancies including glioma (Ambrosini *et al.*, 1997; Schmitz *et al.*, 2000; Katoh *et al.*, 2003). The list of astrocytoma antigens confirmed to be capable of stimulating T cells has remained limited for certain very practical reasons. The classical approach to detecting tumour-specific T cells is the co-culture of patients' T cells with putative antigen-expressing autologous tumour cells, together with appropriate T-cell growth factors such as IL-2. This should allow preferential expansion of antigen-specific T cells, which can subsequently be tested for specific, MHC-restricted recognition of the autologous tumour cell lines or antigens derived therefrom. If the tumour-infiltrating T cells are extracted, they may be preferentially enriched for tumour-specific cells due to antigen-specific retention at the tumour site. Astrocytoma is frequently infiltrated by lymphocytes (Stavrou *et al.*, 1977; Brooks *et al.*, 1978; Rossi *et al.*, 1987; Perrin *et al.*, 1999), although the number of T cells that can be isolated for culture is generally modest due to the limited biopsy size and less intensive infiltration than in certain other tumours such as melanoma. This necessitates significant *in vitro* expansion to generate sufficient cells for testing. However, this is problematic because astrocytoma-infiltrating lymphocytes (as for T cells in certain other diseases) exhibit reduced proliferative potential in culture and those cells that do grow *in vitro* show an important skewing during culture (Miescher *et al.*, 1986; Dietrich *et al.*, 1997) and may poorly represent the starting population of tumour-infiltrating lymphocytes.

One approach to circumvent the difficulties of working with T cells *in vitro* is the serological identification of antigens by recombinant expression cloning (SEREX). Although this is a serology-based technique, the presence of high-titre IgG antibodies to a given antigen is often associated with cellular responses, including CD8+ T cells (Sahin *et al.*, 1997). However, to date, application of SEREX to astrocytoma antigen identification has been disappointing, with only rare tumour-specific reactivity and no confirmation of any new antigens recognized by T cells (Chen *et al.*, 1997; Schmits *et al.*, 2002).

Indirect evidence for astrocytoma antigen expression

As an alternative tactic to investigate the possibility of immune reactivity to astrocytoma antigens we have used T-cell receptor (TCR) spectratyping to analyse astrocytoma-infiltrating T cells. This technique exploits a high-resolution reverse-transcription polymerase chain reaction (RT-PCR) procedure to measure the length of the hypervariable complementarity determining region (CDR)-3 of the TCR β chain, a structural feature critically associated with the recognition of antigenic peptide bound to MHC molecules. This is a powerful approach to study TCR diversity in a blood or tissue RNA sample, and thus to detect T-cell clonal expansions *in vivo* (McHeyzer-Williams *et al.*, 1996). Indeed, the identification of recurrent CDR3 regions in large T-cell populations generally indicates antigen-driven expansion of the corresponding T-cell clones. The analysis of a large panel of biopsies from malignant astrocytoma patients showed that oligoclonal expansions of T cells were present within various Vβ subfamilies of all biopsies tested (Perrin *et al.*, 1999). In contrast to this local reaction, a systemic immune response was not generally detectable, since only exceptional oligoclonal expansions were detected in peripheral blood. It is therefore unlikely that T cells clonally expanded in astrocytoma are the direct consequence of blood expansions, such as those observed in certain healthy individuals (Schwab *et al.*, 1997). These data for brain tumours show that growth of neoplasms in the immune-privileged CNS can lead to T-cell infiltration with distinct TCR spectratyping profiles, as previously observed for other types of cancers (Sensi and Parmiani, 1995; Caignard *et al.*, 1996). Such striking oligoclonal T-cell expansions are highly suggestive of tumour antigen-driven clonal expansion of specific T cells. However, it is clear that the full significance of these T cells identified in astrocytoma will only be fully unravelled when their specificity can be determined, which requires further advances in antigen discovery.

Although data from the different approaches described above point to a degree of immune recognition of malignant astrocytoma cells, this seems to be insufficient to have any significant impact on tumour progression. Indeed, there is a significant body of evidence that points to inadequacies at both the induction and effector stage of the antitumour response.

Low level and delayed induction of antitumour immune responses

Although direct evidence in humans is lacking, it is assumed that there is a considerable lag between initial neoplastic events and a detectable primary brain tumour that disrupts normal brain function. Furthermore, evidence from animal models suggest that there may be a gradual accumulation of genetic changes that ultimately lead to the phenotype of a malignant astrocytoma (Weissenberger *et al.*, 1997). Such kinetics may be conducive to poor stimulation of host immune defences, which have principally evolved to offer protection from infectious pathogenic organisms. Indeed, although the lymphocytes of the adaptive immune system offer the potential of exquisitely fine specificity able to discriminate single-amino-acid changes in a transformed cell, this arm of immunological defence is only set in motion after stimulation of the innate immune system. A prime stimulus for innate immune responses has been considered to be situations that represent 'danger' to the organism (Matzinger, 2002). At the level of cellular and molecular interactions, 'danger' is frequently equated with detection of pathogen-associated molecular patterns by pattern recognition receptors (including Toll-like receptors) expressed by cells of the innate immune system, particularly professional antigen-presenting cells (APCs) (Janeway *et al.*, 2002). Nevertheless, immune responses can also result from stimulation that is not associated with infection. One stimulatory pathway that may be compatible with spontaneous immune responses to brain tumours may be mediated via heat shock proteins, overexpressed by stressed cells, then released after necrosis (Srivastava, 2002). Indeed, necrosis occurs in many human tumours and is a feature typifying glioblastomas, and furthermore it may be augmented as a consequence of the therapies (radiotherapy, chemotherapy, gene therapy) received by patients (Todryk *et al.*, 2000). However, such immune stimulation presumably occurs some time after the initial neoplastic events, and immune responses that may be induced then have to function in the presence of an overwhelming tumour mass, liberating many immunosuppressive factors (as will be discussed).

Secondary lymphoid tissue is particularly adapted for priming tumour-specific T cells

Although the stimuli for initiation of immune responses directed towards primary brain tumours can be at least partly explained, the complex cellular interactions leading to an accumulation of oligoclonally expanded T cells at the tumour site is poorly understood. The challenge to the immune system is how to orchestrate an encounter between a rare specific T cell (in certain responses, this has been calculated to be in the order of 1/100 000 naïve T cells (Kaye and Hedrick, 1988)) and an appropriately presented antigen. Before stimulation by antigen, naïve T cells are in constant recirculation between blood and secondary lymphoid organs and are not generally found in healthy non-lymphoid tissues. Indeed, the normal brain parenchyma is essentially devoid of lymphocytes as detected by immunohistochemistry (Hauser *et al.*, 1983). This is in part due to features such as the tight junctions between brain endothelial cells that contribute to the blood–brain barrier (BBB), one of the frontiers of the CNS that can be considered as a highly selective gateway regulating cellular and molecular traffic (Janzer and Raff, 1987; Rubin and Staddon, 1999). The structural and functional integrity of the BBB is maintained by contacts made at the abluminal surface of the endothelium with pericytes, perivascular cells, and astrocytes. Naïve T cells are only likely to exceptionally pass this barrier, for example in the case of inflammation where there is BBB disruption as a result of the relaxation of tight junctions and up-regulation of adhesion molecules and chemokines (Cannella *et al.*, 1991; Karpus *et al.*, 1995; Krakowski and Owens, 2000; Columba-Cabezas *et al.*, 2003). In normal circumstances, efficient activation of naïve T cells is most clearly understood in the context of lymphoid rather than neurological tissue. Naïve T cells enter lymph nodes via high endothelial venules displaying adhesion molecules termed addressins that engage with T-cell expressed L-selectin, subsequently permitting firmer interactions and finally diapedesis (von Andrian and Mackay, 2000). The specialized architecture within secondary lymphoid tissue allows naïve T cells to be specifically stimulated by a peptide–MHC complex at the surface of an APC, typically a DC. These encounters between naïve T cells and DCs in the paracortical area are facilitated by chemokine gradients (Sallusto and Lanzavecchia, 2000), and by a specialized extracellular matrix that encourages T-cell migration and serial sampling of DCs (Gunzer et al., 2000).

Transport of tumour antigens to lymphoid tissue

If priming of tumour antigen-specific naïve T cells occurs after contact with a professional APC in lymphoid tissue, how does tumour antigen arrive in this site? Antigenic material draining from most tissues accumulates in the lymph and is transported to the lymph nodes via the afferent lymphatics. However, the mechanism that is now becoming most clearly defined is the active transportation of antigenic material by DCs (Banchereau et al., 2000). Certain DCs are resident in normal tissues, such as the Langerhans' cells of the skin. Other DCs or their precursors may be recruited once an inflammatory response occurs. In their resting, or so-called 'immature' form, DCs continuously sample the local environment by phagocytosing dead cells and cellular debris. Some may also constitutively traffic to lymphoid tissue and maintain tolerance to self antigens (Steinman et al., 2003). However, if immature DCs, as key players linking innate with adaptive immunity, perceive 'danger signals' that indicate infection or stress (as discussed above), they undergo maturation: a form of phenotypic and functional differentiation that facilitates migration via the afferent lymph to the lymph nodes and augments immunogenic (rather than tolerogenic) antigen presentation to naïve T cells. The final stages of DC differentiation are only completed after interaction with CD4+ T cells, in which activation signals work in both directions, with the CD4+ cell activating the DC via CD40–CD40L interactions as well as it becoming activated itself. The mature 'conditioned' DC is then in an appropriate activation state to prime CD8+ T cells (Lanzavecchia, 1998).

The influence of CNS microanatomy on antigen drainage

In the light of the usual recirculation patterns of naïve T cells and the optimal microenvironment for T-cell priming in secondary lymphoid organs, efficient T-cell immune responses to brain tumour-derived antigens are likely to occur in such sites. However, the highly particular anatomy and cellular composition of the normal brain necessitates the formulation of working models that take these features into account.

The absence of lymphatics in the brain is the first anatomical difference to contend with, but other pathways can functionally replace these structures. Indeed, studies of the flow of interstitial tissue fluid indicate that antigenic material can find an exit from the brain by following the route of least resistance, probably the perivascular spaces, to drain either into the subarachnoid space with the cerebrospinal fluid, then to venous blood via arachnoid granulations, or to lymphatics via arachnoid sheaths of certain cranial nerves and spinal nerve roots to finally reach the cervical lymph nodes (Cserr and Knopf, 1992). In support of this proposed drainage route, transfer of either high-molecular-weight radiolabelled substances or certain cell populations (lymphocytes, erythrocytes, and macrophages) into the brain parenchyma resulted in a subsequent preferential accumulation in the deep cervical lymph nodes (Oehmichen et al., 1983; Cserr and Knopf, 1992). However, these early studies need repeating with the tools and reagents that are now available to assess molecular interactions that we now know are critical for cell trafficking, particularly adhesion molecule expression and chemokines.

Functional data supporting the importance of the cervical lymph nodes in CNS responses have shown that their removal diminishes B- and T-cell immune responses to antigens expressed in or injected into the brain (Harling-Berg et al., 1989; Phillips et al., 1997). A cautionary remark must be made regarding generalizations about antigen drainage pathways from the brain parenchyma. This concerns rodent models that do not adequately mirror certain aspects of brain structure found in humans (Weller, 1998), and the technical difficulty of precisely injecting into defined CNS sites in small laboratory animals. Techniques pioneered by Cserr are able to limit BBB damage and involve the infusion of very small volumes in order to minimize technical artefacts (Harling-Berg et al., 1989), but it is doubtful whether such precision is reproducibly obtained by all researchers in the field. Overall, despite the need for clarification of certain details of antigen drainage from brain parenchyma, the evidence discussed above, and new data from our laboratory (Calzascia et al., 2005) point towards the cervical lymph nodes as the principal site for the initiation of T-cell immune responses to brain tumours.

Cellular candidates for antigen transport from the CNS

Based on data from extracranial sites, the prime candidate for a migratory APC able to transport tumour antigens to secondary lymphoid tissue is the DC. Although brain-infiltrating DCs have not been reported for cerebral neoplasms, their presence has been detected in the brain parenchyma of mice suffering from experimental autoimmune encephalomyelits (EAE) or from those parasitized by Toxoplasma gondii (Fischer et al., 2000; Suter et al., 2000, 2003). Although functional studies indicated that brain-derived DCs from parasitized animals could trigger T-cell responses and secrete IL-12 (Fischer et al., 2000), inhibitory functions were documented with those from mice with EAE (Suter et al., 2003). The source of these DCs is unknown: they could potentially be recruited from outside the CNS or they may have differentiated from resident precursors. In support of the latter possibility, the CNS is indeed seeded with bone marrow-derived cells that are recruited to the brain at various stages of fetal and adult life. These cells undergo a unique differentiation programme that results in the phenotype of a perivascular or parenchymal microglial cell, depending on the degree of infiltration into the brain parenchyma. Perivascular microglia retain many phenotypic and functional features of tissue macrophages, whereas the parenchymal microglial cell shows much less constitutive functionality, and expression of many genes is silenced (Perry et al., 1993). In vitro studies suggest that alternative differentiation pathways may be possible in the CNS, since microglial cells derived from new-born mouse brain and cultured with different cytokines including GM-CSF, M-CSF, and in some cases in co-culture with astrocytes, could differentiate into cells with certain similarities to DCs (Aloisi et al., 2000; Santambrogio et al., 2001; Re et al., 2002). However, there is as yet no evidence for such differentiation in the presence of brain tumour cells. In this regard, glioma-associated molecules are proposed to either effect the maturation of DCs or even induce their apoptosis (Kikuchi et al., 2002a; Yang et al., 2002).

Whilst the identity of migratory APCs able to transport brain tumour-derived antigens to secondary lymphoid tissue has yet to be defined, there have been certain observations in other CNS immune responses that may be relevant to this issue. The first was in a transplant model, in which rat brain allografts were implanted into the brain parenchyma. A small number of macrophage-like cells expressing donor MHC were found in host lymph node and spleen (Broadwell et al., 1994). Another study (Qing et al., 2000) in a totally syngeneic system, showed that 2 hours after intracerebral injection of antigen there was co-localization of the antigen with Mac1+ cells (staining macrophages/microglial cells) in the brain parenchyma. After 4 hours, antigen+ Mac1+ cells were detectable in the cervical lymph node. The same group recently extended these findings (Karman et al., 2004), showing that phagocytic cells within the brain parenchyma expressed DC markers (CD11c, CD205). Functional studies showed that DCs adoptively transferred to the brain parenchyma could induce a CD8+ T-cell response in the cervical lymph nodes and spleen. Whilst these studies are of great interest, it remains to be directly established whether (and which) endogenous brain APCs mediate the transport of antigen from brain parenchyma to lymphoid organs and subsequently activate naïve T cells. It is clear that much technical ingenuity will be necessary to directly address such questions in small laboratory animals. In particular, it is necessary to note that in all studies reliant upon direct intracranial implantation of tumour cells the absolute integrity of normal brain structure cannot be totally guaranteed. Antigenic material may thus leak to the periphery, by-passing normal CNS antigen handling mechanisms. In the future, genetic models in which brain tumours develop spontaneously may be helpful to address these issues. However, current models were generally constructed to address genetic and pathological issues and they present a significant challenge to use for interpretable immunological studies (Holland, 2001).

The identity of the cells responsible for capture of brain tumour antigens and subsequent activation of naïve T cells in lymphoid tissue is not only of considerable interest for understanding immunosurveillance of the CNS but it is also of relevance for designing optimal brain tumour immunotherapy. Indeed, the roles of APCs are not limited to induction of immunity, but they also include the induction of tolerance to self antigens (Steinman et al., 2003). In vivo murine models have described DC-mediated induction of tolerance for self antigens expressed in the gut, pancreas, and kidney, but not as yet for the CNS. Future immunotherapy of cerebral neoplasms may require the breaking of tolerance to certain self antigens that are overexpressed by malignant cells, but a complete reversal of tolerogenic mechanisms would be very dangerous if this resulted in uncontrolled CNS autoimmunity. The mechanisms that are operational in the CNS thus merit thorough exploration.

Factors limiting the effector stage of the response

Notwithstanding the limitations in assessing specific immune responses in malignant astrocytoma, there are also arguments to suggest that even efficiently induced effector cells may have difficulty in successfully eradicating a solid tumour mass in the brain. Indeed, many analyses of the status of T cells infiltrating astrocytomas, and also from peripheral blood, showed impaired cellular function (Dix et al., 1999). In vivo manifestations of T-cell defects include delayed-type hypersensitivity responses, low T-cell numbers in peripheral blood, and low serum antibody titres. In vitro tests indicated poor mitogen responsiveness, inefficient cytotoxic function, defective expression of high-affinity IL-2 receptors, and activation signalling defects (Elliott et al., 1990; Morford et al., 1997). Such phenomena may explain difficulties in culturing CTLs derived from astrocytoma-infiltrating lymphocytes, despite the addition of recombinant IL-2.

Efficiency of extravasation and tumour infiltration

An unfavourable microenvironment for antitumour effector function may actually commence at the BBB, which must be traversed by infiltrating T cells (Brightman and Reese, 1969). Activated T cells can extravasate, but their trafficking may be more limited than for other sites. For example, the relative number of activated T cells found in the brain parenchyma after intravenous adoptive transfer of labelled T cells in rats was six times less than in muscle and more than 140 times less than that found in liver, for the same weight of tissue (Hickey, 1999). In the case of an advanced cerebral malignancy the neovasculature induced to nourish the tumour does not bear the hallmarks of the BBB and may thus be more permeable, but at this stage, the tumour is also a more difficult challenge for immune eradication. However, endothelial cells of the tumour-associated vasculature may also be induced to express Fas ligand that may antagonize T-cell translocation (Yu et al., 2003). Once extravasation has occurred, penetration of the parenchyma may depend upon other cellular interactions, since for CD4+ T cells, migration away from the perivascular space was inhibited in mice depleted of macrophages (Tran et al., 1998), but the situation for CD8+ T cells has not been explored.

Before the final contact with the tumour cell, the infiltrating T cell may have other encounters with putative APCs of the brain. Since the microglial cell is

one of the few MHC Class II+ cells that are resident in the brain, it is a prime candidate brain APC for CD4+ T cells. However, CD4+ T-cell contact with parenchymally localized microglial cells has been suggested to lead to tolerance induction or the termination of immune responses (Ford et al., 1995, 1996; Matyszak et al., 1999; Brabb et al., 2000). Such effects were particularly associated with the activation state of the microglial cell (Matyszak et al., 1999). Defects in the CD4 arm of immune responses in the CNS may limit CD8+ T-cell cytotoxic function and/or viability in antiviral responses (Stohlman et al., 1998; Zajac et al., 1998). However, for antitumour immune responses, independence from CD4+ T cells has been demonstrated in several different models (Sampson et al., 1996; Okada et al., 1998; Walker et al., 2000). Nevertheless, generalizations are unwise, as cellular requirements for a given CNS response may be different at different stages (priming/ effector) and localizations (lymphoid tissue/brain parenchyma) of the response.

An important role for brain APCs that process and present defined tumour-derived antigens to CD8+ T cells was recently described by our group (Calzascia et al., 2003). In this study, in which the mouse glioma MT539MG was engineered to express a model tumour antigen (CW3), but was deficient in presenting certain epitopes, tumour-specific CD8+ T cells with cytotoxic function were recruited and retained at the tumour site when host APCs presented tumour-derived antigen. However, the APC responsible for this important function at the effector stage of the antitumour response remains to be defined.

For brain-infiltrating T cells, even certain components of normal brain have been suggested to inhibit CTL effector function. For example, T cells otherwise capable of mediating neuropathology were inhibited by brain-derived gangliosides (Irani, 1998), although this was strain specific in the mouse and has not been confirmed in humans. For antitumour effector T cells in the intracerebral P511 mastocytoma tumour model, CD8+ T cells were unable to differentiate into effector cells in the brain microenvironment (Gordon et al., 1997), subsequently attributed to a sensitivity to transforming growth factor (TGF)-β present in the cerebrospinal fluid and the interstitial tissue fluid (Gordon et al., 1998). However, these results were in contrast to those obtained with the similar P815 mastocytoma (transfected with the CW3 model antigen) in which brain-infiltrating lymphocytes tested ex vivo showed full cytotoxic effector function (Walker et al., 2000). Moreover, we have recently confirmed the presence of fully differentiated CTLs infiltrating intracranial tumours and able to lyse tumour targets ex vivo in three different tumour models, in three different mouse strains (Calzascia et al., 2003).

Immunosuppression by tumour-derived soluble factors

A list of potentially immunosuppressive molecules detected in astrocytomas or astrocytoma lines includes prostaglandin E_2 (Fontana et al., 1982; Sawamura et al., 1990; Couldwell et al., 1992; Dix et al., 1999), gangliosides (Wikstrand et al., 1994), and IL-10 (Merlo et al., 1993; Nitta et al., 1994), all of which can demonstrate certain immunosuppressive functions in vitro, but for which in vivo immunosuppression in astrocytoma patients remains speculative. Indeed, there are doubts whether sufficient bioactive factor is released by tumour cells in vivo (discussed in Dix et al. (1999)) and, for IL-10, whether its in vivo function is necessarily immunosuppressive (Berman et al., 1996; Book et al., 1998; Segal et al., 2002).

One astrocytoma-derived factor that has been explored in more depth, in vitro and in vivo, is TGF-β. This cytokine, formerly known as glioblastoma cell-derived T-cell suppressor factor, was first identified in the supernatant of a human glioblastoma cell line that suppressed T-cell growth (Fontana et al., 1984; Bodmer et al., 1989; Couldwell et al., 1992). The immunosuppressive effects of TGF-β are multiple and complex, functioning at both the induction and effector stages of T-cell immune responses. Indeed, there is inhibition of maturation and antigen presentation by DCs or other APCs, as well as inhibition of T-cell activation and differentiation (Smyth et al., 1991; Jachimczak et al., 1993; Gorelik and Flavell, 2002). Inhibiting TGF-β in vivo in experimental tumour models has produced mixed results, probably because this cytokine also interacts with the tumour cell and may be protect against Fas-mediated apoptosis in some circumstances (Fakhrai *et al.*, 1996; Ashley *et al.*, 1998). Other *in vivo* studies using decorin, a natural inhibitor of TGF-β suppressed the growth of C6 rat astrocytoma *in vivo* (Stander *et al.*, 1998), but whether this occurred through TGF-β is unclear, because decorin is also immunostimulatory in a TGF-β2-independent fashion (Münz *et al.*, 1999). Overall, the immuno-regulatory functions of TGF-β2 justify the attention it has received, but whether it will be feasible or advisable to inhibit this cytokine in brain tumour patients still remains uncertain.

Immunosuppression by cell-mediated interactions

Intercellular contacts through transmembrane molecules such as Fas ligand, a member of the tumour necrosis family, may also contribute to tumour immune escape. Fas ligand is expressed by many normal cells of haematopoietic origin, but also by tumour cells of different histological origin (Walker *et al.*, 1997, 1998). In the context of the CNS, Fas ligand expression has been reported for malignant astrocytomas (Saas *et al.*, 1997; Gratas *et al.*, 1997; Favre *et al.*, 1999; Frankel *et al.*, 1999), as well as normal neurones (French *et al.*, 1996; Saas *et al.*, 1997; Bechmann *et al.*, 1999; Flugel *et al.*, 2000; Medana *et al.*, 2001) and microglia (D'Souza *et al.*, 1996; Spanaus *et al.*, 1998; Frigerio *et al.*, 2000). Fas ligand has many roles, particularly in immune homeostasis where apoptosis induction in Fas receptor-expressing T cells regulates cell numbers (Nagata and Golstein, 1995; Lynch *et al.*, 1995). Tumour-expressed Fas ligand has been proposed to enhance tumour progression through inactivation of tumour-infiltrating lymphocytes, and indeed astrocytoma cells induced Fas-mediated apoptosis of T cells *in vitro* (Walker *et al.*, 1997; Saas *et al.*, 1997). Moreover, apoptotic T cells were observed in the proximity of Fas ligand-expressing astrocytoma cells *in vivo* (Didenko *et al.*, 2002). However, controlled studies in different animal models (in sites other than the CNS) have demonstrated that tumour expression of Fas ligand can be correlated either with enhanced tumour growth (Hahne *et al.*, 1996; Arai *et al.*, 1997*a*), or with enhanced neutrophil recruitment and tumour rejection (Seino *et al.*, 1997*a,b*; Arai *et al.*, 1997*b*). Microenvironmental factors will certainly influence the consequences of Fas ligand expression by tumour cells; for example, tumours co-expressing both Fas ligand and TGF-β (notably, including malignant astrocytomas) may be particularly well adapted to combat CTL effector mechanisms (Walker *et al.*, 1997; Chen *et al.*, 1998). The multitude of interacting factors *in vivo*, in some cases specific to individual models, have not been fully elucidated. Consequently, there are many conflicting interpretations of these issues in the literature (Walker *et al.*, 1997, 1998; Restifo, 2000; O'Connell, 2002).

Other molecules expressed at the surface of astrocytoma cells have immunosuppressive potential. One such candidate with known immuno-regulatory functions in the immune system is the CD70 transmembrane glycoprotein, a molecule expressed on activated T and B cells that can bind to CD27 expressed on lymphoid cells (Jacquot, 2000). Two independent studies have now reported CD70 expression on astrocytoma cell lines or biopsies (Wischhusen *et al.*, 2002; Held-Feindt and Mentlein, 2002). *In vitro* functional tests demonstrated CD70-dependent apoptosis of peripheral blood mononuclear cell targets. When tumour cells were irradiated there was an augmentation of CD70 expression, with a corresponding enhancement of apoptosis induction in immune cells (Wischhusen *et al.*, 2002).

Another potentially immunosuppressive molecule is the non-classical MHC Class I molecule HLA-G that is expressed by a limited range of tissues, particularly the placenta, but also certain cancers (Maier *et al.*, 1999; Urosevic *et al.*, 2002; Wiendl *et al.*, 2002). One proposed function of this molecule is to suppress natural killer (NK) and T-cell immune responses, but this is controversial (Braud *et al.*, 1999; Bainbridge *et al.*, 2001). A proportion of astrocytoma cell lines and tumour biopsies express HLA-G protein that could function to inhibit CD4+ and CD8+ T-cell responses *in vitro*, but this required incubation of cell lines with high concentrations of interferon-γ (500 IU/ml), or after transfer of the HLA-G gene into astrocytoma lines (Wiendl *et al.*, 2002)

More recently B7-H1, a member of the B7 family of co-stimulatory molecules, was shown to down-regulate certain immune functions (Sharpe and Freeman, 2002) and was expressed by several tumour types (Dong *et al.*, 2002), including glioma (Wintterle *et al.*, 2003). Moreover, glioma cell line expression of B7-H1 inhibited T-cell cytokine secretion activation in *in vitro* tests. We have confirmed and extended these functional data to other astrocytoma cell lines, and furthermore, in a large series of glioma biopsies, we observed a correlation between tumour grade and B7-H1 expression (Wilmotte *et al.*, submitted). Overall, these data are consistent with the proposed role of B7-H1 expression in immune evasion.

Passive immune escape

Although it is well established that spontaneously arising cancer poorly stimulates the immune system, this is an intrinsic property of most non-infected host cells and so cannot be considered as an escape mechanism. However, a malignant cell phenotype that resists host effector cells, and is selected under a spontaneous or induced immune response can be considered as a passive immune escape mechanism. A frequent phenotypic alteration found in many cancers is the loss or down-regulation of MHC molecule expression, leading to resistance to CTL-mediated lysis (Seliger *et al.*, 2002; Ruiz-Cabello *et al.*, 2002). Such alterations have not been reported for malignant astrocytoma, but for most primary brain tumours the issue of MHC expression is rather different from tumours derived from tissues of non-CNS origin, since the normal tissue counterparts of astrocytes and oligodendrocytes are essentially MHC negative or low (Natali *et al.*, 1984; Lampson and Hickey, 1986). The issue is thus whether or not MHC molecules are induced on glioma cells either during tumorigenesis or as a consequence of immunotherapy. Tumour cells of astrocytic origin uniformly express MHC Class I molecules after *in vitro* culture, and can be induced to express MHC Class II after treatment with interferon-γ (Dhib-Jalbut *et al.*, 1990; Bruner *et al.*, 1993; Parney *et al.*, 2000). The situation *in vivo* is far from clear, with contradictory reports in the literature (Natali *et al.*, 1984; Lampson and Hickey, 1986; Saito *et al.*, 1988; Facoetti *et al.*, 2001). This may be because of differences in the immunohistochemistry protocols employed (Facoetti *et al.*, 2001) and difficulties in obtaining optimal staining for tumours such as high-grade astrocytomas that are characterized by zones of necrosis.

A further mechanism of passive immune escape is resistance to apoptosis. Indeed, inhibitor of apoptosis proteins have been reported to be frequently overexpressed in malignant astrocytomas, leading to potential resistance to immune effector molecules expressed by CTLs (Fas ligand, granzymes), as well as resistance to the conventional treatment modalities of radiotherapy and chemotherapy (recently reviewed by Bögler and Weller (2002)).

Defined antitumour effector mechanisms that affect the growth of cerebral neoplasms

The above discussions may appear to suggest that immune responses to cerebral neoplasms are not only difficult to induce but are likely to be ineffective when confronted with the barrage of immunosuppressive elements that operate within the confines of the CNS in the proximity of a tumour. But this assessment is too pessimistic, since most immune responses defined to date depend upon the balance of immunostimulatory versus immunosuppressive factors, rather than a complete absence of immune inhibition. Nevertheless, currently available data from clinical trials testing immune-based therapies for CNS neoplastic disease have not demonstrated any dramatic clinical breakthroughs: the balance is evidently in favour of the tumour. Unfortunately, objective analysis of these clinical data is limited by variable descriptions of patient groups or disease status, as well as the sometimes premature reporting of survival data. Furthermore, despite one or two worthy exceptions, rational amelioration of many approaches is confounded by an absence of immunological analyses in the studies. In defence of clinical immunotherapists, brain tumours present a unique challenge, with greater difficulties than in many cancers, such as the inaccessibility of the tumour site and the paucity of defined tumour-associated antigens. With these limitations in mind, the discussion that follows will give as much attention to the concepts and difficulties of designing immunotherapies as to the preliminary clinical findings.

T-cell effector function against experimental brain tumours

Building on the historic perspective of untreatable malignant astrocytomas in patients and assumptions of low-level immune function in the immune-privileged CNS, positive findings to encourage the development of brain tumour immunotherapy have been eagerly awaited. Encouraging results have been forthcoming in many models, and globally a conclusion can be made that immune responses induced in the periphery can mediate antitumour effects in the brain (Aoki *et al.*, 1992; Asai *et al.*, 1994; Resnicoff *et al.*, 1994; Sampson *et al.*, 1996; Ashley *et al.*, 1997; Okada *et al.*, 1998; Graf *et al.*, 1999; Akasaki *et al.*, 2001; Liau *et al.*, 2002).

Intracranial tumours may be more resistant to immunotherapy than tumours in other sites

Although most of the above studies employed vaccination protocols that were derived from models of tumours in sites other than the CNS, certain models appear to be more stringent than others in their susceptibility to immune effector mechanisms, with the most difficult therapeutic challenge being an intracranial tumour established for a significant period before the start of therapy. Therapies exploiting cytokines as immune adjuvants illustrate the difficulty in generalizing about a given approach because of results that differ according to the tumour model used (SMA-560, B16, Gl261) and the site of implantation (Sampson *et al.*, 1996, 1997; Lumniczky *et al.*, 2002). Site-related differences were also noted in studies exploiting a cellular vaccine by overexpression of ICAM-1 on a glioma cell line: this resulted in growth inhibition of glioma cells implanted subcutaneously, but not in the CNS (Kikuchi *et al.*, 1999a). Furthermore, in another peripheral vaccination approach based on the use of recombinant *Listeria monocytogenes* in the rat 9L glioma model, rats were protected against a primary subcutaneous tumour challenge, but protection against intracerebrally implanted tumours could only be achieved in a secondary response once primary subcutaneous tumours had been rejected (Liau *et al.*, 2002). Moreover, whilst rejection of the subcutaneous tumour only required CD8+ T cells, intracerebral immunity was dependent on both CD4+ and CD8+ T cells.

Optimizing therapies and choice of models

Even in the relatively controlled situation of a rodent model, the mechanisms responsible for the efficacy of treatments have not always been determined. Just as with spontaneous malignant astrocytomas in patients, antigenic targets of the antitumour immune response in rodent models may be unknown, and furthermore, some experimental tumours are not always totally syngeneic (Trojan *et al.*, 1993; Gordon *et al.*, 1997; Beutler *et al.*, 1997). To facilitate immunological analyses, some recent studies have demonstrated the induction of antitumour immunity in better characterized syngeneic tumour models, such as B16/F10 melanoma (Sampson *et al.*, 1996; Ashley *et al.*, 1997), K1735 melanoma transfected with an EGFRvIII derived epitope (Heimberger *et al.*, 2000), C3 sarcoma cells transfected with human papilloma virus type 16 (Okada *et al.*, 1998), P815 cells transfected with CW3 (Walker *et al.*, 2000), and MC57 fibrosarcoma cells transfected with lymphocytic choriomeningitis virus glycoprotein (Calzascia *et al.*, 2003). It is noteworthy that none of these experimental tumours are of glial origin, but nevertheless, since even murine astrocytomas do not accurately reflect all aspects of spontaneous human tumours, artificial but well-characterized alternative systems are extremely useful for analysing individual elements of antitumour responses.

Translating therapies into the clinical setting

Potential clinical efficacy and the risk of untoward side-effects can only be crudely predicted in currently available animal models. The clinical urgency to develop new treatments for malignant astrocytoma patients has therefore driven the early implementation of clinical trials, despite the foreseeable difficulties in interpretation (approaches for T-cell-based immunotherapy are summarized in Table 29.2). Nevertheless, pilot studies in patients may give some indication of which approaches to develop and those that should be abandoned.

Immunotherapy approaches for tumours in sites other than those of the CNS, in particular melanoma, have induced CTLs that react with differentiation antigens such as Melan-A (Renkvist *et al.*, 2001). One of the disadvantages of such approaches is that they may induce a degree of destruction of normal tissue (Pardoll, 1999), a factor considered acceptable up to a certain point, although the balance of these autoimmune effects compared with antitumour effects is under scrutiny (van Elsas *et al.*, 2001; Banchereau *et al.*, 2001a; Dudley *et al.*, 2002). For immunotherapy of brain tumours, the threshold of acceptability of autoimmune reactions is lower because of the indispensability of most normal tissue in the brain, together with its limited capacity for self-renewal. The related problem is that of inflammation. High-magnitude immune responses leading to efficacious antitumour activity are frequently inflammatory. Furthermore, chronic inflammation

Table 29.2 Application and analysis of T-cell based immunotherapy in astrocytoma

	Advantages	Limitations/risks	Monitoring
Non-defined tumour vaccines. Whole cell, tumour cell RNA, tumour cell eluate, homogenate etc., with cytokine or DC adjuvants	No prior definition of tumour antigen. Applicable to all HLA-types. Responses induced to multiple epitopes, limiting tumour immune escape by single mutation or loss of single HLA alleles	Autoimmunity. Need sufficient antigenic material to prepare vaccine. Patient-specific vaccine preparation if autologous cells used. Little standardization between patients possible	'Whole cell' readouts for antitumour responses depend on availability of cellular controls—difficult for CNS
Defined tumour vaccines. Defined CTL cell epitopes as synthetic peptide	Tumour antigens can be chosen with known expression on normal tissue. Vaccine preparation may be standardized for all patients of same HLA-type. Autologous tumour cells not needed to prepare vaccine	Lack of defined antigens for astrocytoma. Only applicable for certain HLA-types. For single epitope vaccines, tumour escape by mutation may occur	All specific assays of T-cell phenotype and function possible, even without autologous control cells
Adoptive immunotherapy. *In vitro*-expanded T cells	T cells can be expanded under ideal conditions *in vitro*. Tumour reactivity can be assessed before infusion	Spontaneously sensitized antitumour T cells difficult to obtain from patients; Vaccine-induced T cells subject to limitations as above	Transferred cells can be tracked by structural/phenotypic assays, or gene marking

may provoke a release of sequestered autoantigens, leading to the initiation or perpetuation of autoimmune disease. An indication of the possible risks of utilization of non-defined brain tumour vaccines came from early studies employing human glioma tissue to vaccinate different species of experimental animals: this resulted in lethal allergic encephalomyelitis (Bigner *et al.*, 1981). Other untoward effects arose in rodent trials of a gene therapy protocol for glioblastoma, in which there was a vector-induced intracerebral immune response that directly or indirectly perpetuated reactive gliosis and demyelination (Dewey *et al.*, 1999). These data indicate areas which require particular attention in ongoing and future clinical trials.

Adoptive cellular immunotherapy

Deficiencies of antitumour effector cells in patients can potentially be circumvented by expanding these cells *in vitro*, in the absence of tumour-derived immunosuppressive factors, followed by local or systemic reinfusion. To date, most adoptive immunotherapies in malignant astrocytoma treatment have been non-specific, exploiting the cytotoxic properties of lymphokine-activated killer (LAK) cells. Compared with other cellular therapies, the generation of such cells is relatively straightforward. Autologous peripheral blood lymphocytes obtained by leukapheresis are cultured with high concentrations of IL-2 to generate a polyclonal population of cytotoxic cells deriving from cells of T and NK origin that are able to lyse NK-resistant targets, including tumour cells. However, characterization of LAK activity against autologous tumour cells has not been routinely determined in most studies. The putative antitumour activity of LAK cells may be reinforced by the concomitant administration of IL-2. Clinical application for brain tumours has focused on direct transfer of LAK cells to the tumour cavity at the time of resection, previously reviewed in detail (Zeltzer *et al.*, 1999; van Herpen and De Mulder, 2000). Despite more than a decade of clinical experience of this technique, and occasional isolated clinical responses, it is still not possible to confirm any efficacy of this approach. Moreover, toxicity has been reported with LAK cell and IL-2 therapy (Barba *et al.*, 1989), mainly as a result of the cerebral oedema induced by the treatment. It is difficult to envisage how the therapeutic potential of a non-specific therapy reliant upon cytokines triggering intense inflammatory responses can be safely improved for such a sensitive site as the CNS.

A more precisely directed form of adoptive immunotherapy aims to transfer T cells that have classical, MHC Class I-restricted, specificity for tumour cells. Theoretically, it can be argued that a good source of such cells will be the tumour biopsy. Indeed, a pilot study using expanded tumour-infiltrating lymphocytes has been undertaken, but with no evidence that the transferred cells were specifically cytotoxic for the autologous tumour (Quattrocchi *et al.*, 1999). The extremely restricted size of tumour biopsies available and the difficulties in efficiently expanding cells derived from the tumour microenvironment will clearly limit any widespread application of this approach. An interesting variant of adoptive immunotherapy is to attempt to increase the numbers of tumour-specific cells used for *in vitro* expansion by a prior vaccination of the patient with autologous tumour or tumour-derived antigens (Plautz *et al.*, 1998; Wood *et al.*, 2000). Since the patients are vaccinated at a site distant from the tumour, tumour-mediated immunosuppressive effects may be less important. However, whether any of the isolated clinical responses were correlated with the potency and specificity of the adoptively transferred cells cannot be assessed because of incomplete characterization. New developments in adoptive immunotherapy techniques were recently reported for the treatment of melanoma patients, in which patients were conditioned (by lymphodepletion), prior to transfer of *in vitro* expanded effector cells and IL-2 (Dudley *et al.*, 2002); if the early promise of such approaches is confirmed, they may be useful for improving the engraftment and eventual antitumour effect of adoptively transferred cells in malignant astrocytoma.

Active vaccination strategies

These approaches are currently receiving much attention for the development of cancer vaccines for many categories of tumours. Progress is being encouraged by the enormous advances in understanding the role of bio-

logical adjuvants. Cancer vaccines fall into two broad categories: whole tumour cell (or uncharacterized antigens derived therefrom) and defined antigen vaccines. Non-defined or whole-cell vaccines require no prior definition of tumour antigens or MHC restriction elements; many epitopes are presumably present in the vaccine, lessening the considerable risk that tumour cells may mutate and escape a too finely focused immune response. However, assessing vaccine efficacy and correlating any clinical responses with specific immune responses is extremely difficult. Furthermore, as advances in immunization procedures augment the magnitude of induced immune responses, there is a risk that autoimmune responses may also be induced to the many normal tissue antigens present in such vaccine preparations (Bigner *et al.*, 1981; Ludewig *et al.*, 2000). As we have already emphasized in this chapter, and also as argued by others (Offringa *et al.*, 2000), rational improvement of non-defined vaccines is difficult once such approaches are incorporated into clinical trials, even if there is the hope of benefit for isolated patients. The alternative strategy of inducing immune responses to defined antigens is more appealing for rational development of cancer immunotherapy, but this requires that biological as well as clinical investigations are fully integrated into clinical trials. The hurdle for defined vaccines for brain tumours such as malignant astrocytoma is the paucity of information regarding antigens recognized by T cells, explaining the choice of non-defined tumour derived material for clinical vaccination studies to date.

Most spontaneous human tumours are poorly immunogenic: a vaccine prepared from unmodified (or simply irradiated) cells will not efficiently induce immune responses in an autologous setting. Efficient adjuvants are required to achieve this, which are now understood to function principally at the level of enhancing antigen presentation. There are two broad approaches to augmenting presentation of tumour antigens in a vaccination setting. The first is to exploit existing host antigen presentation pathways *in vivo*, the second is to implant *ex vivo*-generated DCs, or DC/tumour cell hybrids as cellular adjuvants. The most common route to ameliorate host DC function is to use recombinant cytokines, either injected as soluble proteins, or by gene transfer into tumour cells, or by co-implantation of a bystander secretor cell (reviewed in Pardoll (2002)). Key factors that have received much attention in this context are GM-CSF, IL-4, Flt3 ligand, and CD40 ligand, which may find future application in brain tumour vaccines, and certain of which are already being explored in clinical trials (Okada *et al.*, 2003).

The second approach, of injecting DCs generated *in vitro*, is currently generating considerable interest because of the possibility of exactly controlling the parameters of the DCs that are injected. Indeed, the enormous recent advances in understanding how DCs play a central role in initiating, amplifying, and regulating adaptive immune responses have provided much data on the ideal characteristic of an immunostimulatory DC (Bancherau *et al.*, 2001*b*). The usual method is to generate DCs *ex vivo* from bone marrow or peripheral blood precursors by the addition of cytokine cocktails (including IL-4, GM-CSF, TNF-α, c-kit ligand, and Flt-3 ligand), load the DCs with tumour-derived antigens, then reinfuse into the animal or patient. Despite ever widening application of these approaches, the technology is difficult to standardize. This is a critical issue, since variation in antigen loading or the differentiation of cultured DCs used for injection not only alters the magnitude of immune responses that are subsequently induced but can also switch the balance towards tolerance induction (Steinman *et al.*, 2003). Any correlation of clinical efficacy with vaccine parameters can thus only be made if every DC population used for treatment is individually characterized, which, to date has not always occurred. Since the induction phase of antitumour vaccination in a peripheral site will be similar for most extracranial as well as intracranial tumours, there is a wealth of biological and clinical expertise now accumulating that is of direct relevance for DC-based therapies for brain tumours. Accordingly, the principle that DCs can act as efficient natural adjuvants in therapeutic vaccines has been confirmed in various brain tumour models (Liau *et al.*, 1999; Heimberger *et al.*, 2000; Yamanaka *et al.*, 2001 2002; Akasaki *et al.*, 2001; Aoki *et al.*, 2001; Kikuchi *et al.*, 2002*b*; Witham *et al.*, 2002; Ehtesham *et al.*, 2003). Study design is so totally different in these reports that meaningful comparisons of efficacy are difficult to make. Critical differences in the experiments include the species and strain of animal and corresponding tumour (rat and mouse), the use of DCs of different origin (DC cell lines, or spleen- or bone marrow-derived precursors), the use of different sources of antigen (from RNA to whole cells) and different means of DC maturation. Finally, DCs were injected using different routes and frequencies, and at different times relative to tumour implantation. Nevertheless, certain conclusions from these animal studies are encouraging, namely that no severe side-effects were encountered, and that there is some impact of immune effector cells on intracranial tumours. Treatment of malignant astrocytoma patients with DC-based therapies is now under way, and the first published results confirmed that vaccines consisting of DCs pulsed with peptides eluted from tumour cells (Yu et al., 2001) and DCs fused with tumour cells (Kikuchi et al., 2001) did not induce serious adverse effects. More recent studies in which tumour-lysate or tumour mRNA pulsed DCs were used to vaccinate patients with malignant glioma (Yamanaka et al., 2003; Kobayashi et al., 2003; Yu et al., 2004) showed an augmentation of T-cell immune responses after vaccination. In particular, the demonstration of expanded CD8+ T-cell populations reactive with epitopes from defined tumour associated antigens (MAGE-1, gp100, HER-2, TRP-2, AIM-2) may be particularly encouraging if these peptides can function as astrocytoma rejection antigens in vivo (Liu et al., 2003, 2004a,b; Yu et al., 2004). Indeed, if by good fortune responses to these previously defined antigens are frequently induced, this may facilitate monitoring of future randomized trials designed for assessing clinical efficacy. It is to be hoped that obtaining adequate immunological data will be given sufficient priority to aid the future development of DC-based vaccination.

Other immunoenhancing strategies

Immunomodulation may also be attempted at the effector cell level. As far as experimental therapies are concerned, there is a vast palette of recombinant cytokines available that can be employed by direct injection, gene therapy, or via the use of transduced secretor cells. Indeed, certain pre-clinical studies have suggested that CTL expansion and function against brain tumours may be enhanced by IL-2 (Glick et al., 1995; Kikuchi et al., 1999b), IL-7 (Aoki et al., 1992), IL-12 (Kikuchi et al., 1999b; Joki et al., 1999), and IL-18 (Kikuchi et al., 2000). Effector functions not exclusively mediated by CTLs may also be augmented by IL-4 (Benedetti et al., 1999; Giezeman-Smits et al., 2000; Okada et al., 2003) and IL-10 (Book et al., 1998; Segal et al., 2002). The challenge is to know which of these reagents merit development for clinical trial. Most of these cytokines have been tested in studies using totally different tumours and experimental protocols, at different doses, rendering comparison between individual factors virtually impossible to make. As an example, IL-7-enhanced vaccines have been formulated, based on the capacity of this cytokine to induce the proliferation of activated CD4+ and CD8+ T cells and enhance CTL and LAK cell-mediated cytotoxicity. Therapies based on IL-7 are able to mediate vigorous antitumour effects in a murine ependymoblastoma model (Aoki et al., 1992) and have some effects in the rat N32 glioma (Visse et al., 1999), but were ineffective in the murine Gl261 astrocytoma (Lumniczky et al., 2002). Similar observations can be made for most candidate cytokines for augmenting vaccine efficacy. Assessing the potential interest of a particular factor is particularly acute for brain tumour therapy because there is no predominant model, unlike the situation for melanoma where pre-clinical testing of immunotherapies frequently employs the poorly immunogenic B16 melanoma. Nevertheless, credit should be given to those groups who have published useful data comparing multiple therapeutic approaches in the same experimental brain tumour models (Sampson et al., 1996, 1997; Lumniczky et al., 2002). The current limitation for progress in brain tumour immunotherapy is not the number of immunostimulatory molecules that are available, but rather our comprehension of the immune consequences (rather than just immune rejection) in the CNS. For example, cytokines employed locally that induce excessive inflammation may be less applicable to the CNS than other sites. Moreover, cytokines that interact with other cells that are unique to the CNS and that also participate in the immune dialogue, such as microglial cells and astrocytes, should be thoroughly investigated for their positive or negative regulatory effects. In this regard, new approaches to immunotherapy that are particularly tailored for the CNS are worthy of mention. One of the most interesting is based on the propensity of neural stem cells to track migrating glioma cells within the brain (Aboody et al., 2000). It was proposed that genetically manipulated neural stem cells could deliver therapeutic molecules with immuno-modulatory function to the site of an infiltrative tumour. To date, encouraging results have been obtained with the delivery of IL-4 and IL-12 to experimental gliomas (reviewed in Kabos et al. (2003)), but other molecules could also be exploited using the same approach.

Immunological involvement in other therapies

Since effective brain tumour therapy is such a difficult clinical challenge, the application of multimodality treatment is likely to be essential for significant clinical impact. Therefore, whilst this chapter is focuses primarily on T-cell-mediated antitumour responses, it is useful to consider whether other therapies for CNS neoplastic disease can be combined with immunotherapy, hopefully in a synergistic manner. Chemotherapy and radiotherapy, although poorly efficacious for malignant astrocytoma (Hosli et al., 1998; Stupp et al., 2002), induce a degree of tumour cell death and thus may provide a potentially immunostimulatory in vivo source of tumour antigen, provided the immune system has not been impaired by these treatments. Future protocol design should thus look to ways of improving compatibility of treatments. Immune responses in gene therapies are a double-edged sword. The positive side is that immune responses may be at least partly responsible for so-called 'bystander effects', of gene therapy, whereby a greater number of tumour cells are eliminated than are actually transduced by the therapeutic gene (Nanda et al., 2001; Tunici et al., 2001). However, immune responses directed towards viral vectors, particularly early generation adenovirus vectors, limit repeat utilization of the vector and may also induce chronic neuroinflammation (Dewey et al., 1999). A particularly interesting compatibility may be found between anti-angiogenic therapies and immunotherapy (Kerbel and Folkman, 2002; Rafii et al., 2002). Indeed, several of the cytokines already discussed as immuno-stimulatory agents (including interferon-γ, IL-4, and IL-12) may also directly or indirectly inhibit tumour angiogenesis. Other therapies for brain tumours aim to induce apoptosis in malignant cells by ligating death receptors on malignant cells (Bögler and Weller, 2002). Although Fas ligand is one of the proposed effector molecules, widespread Fas expression by cells of the immune system (Nagata and Golstein, 1995), as well as non-malignant astrocytes (Saas et al., 1999) may limit its clinical application. A more promising approaches may employ another molecule of the TNF superfamily, TNF-related apoptosis-inducing ligand (TRAIL). Indeed, recent developments suggest that after restoration of apoptotic pathways in an intracranial human xenografted glioma using peptide drugs, apoptosis can be efficiently induced by administration of TRAIL, leading to tumour regression (Fulda et al., 2002).

Perspectives

For decades there have been tantalizing glimpses, generally in experimental models, of the capacity of the immune system to control and even cure malignancies. Recent advances in fundamental immunology now provide a rational basis for designing novel, relatively safe immunotherapies that can be tested in patients, including those with brain tumours. However, despite advances in neuroimmunology, which clearly demonstrate that the CNS is a site with many active immunological interactions rather than an immunological desert, spontaneous and induced immune responses to brain tumours are poorly characterized. Thus, concepts of brain tumour immunology and their application in immunotherapy have in many instances been empirically extrapolated from findings in other sites.

Although clinical trials of different brain tumour immunotherapies are already under way, we must have more information and a better understanding of antitumour effector mechanisms if these studies are to progress. It is certain that local, high-magnitude antitumour responses (and probably higher than are currently achieved) will be essential if solid tumours are to be eliminated from the brain. A challenge for the future is how to exploit such responses whilst avoiding excessive inflammation and induction of dangerous cerebral oedema, a unique limitation for CNS malignancies. In parallel, there must be continued efforts to discover suitable antigenic targets expressed by human cerebral malignancies to enable immunotherapies to be finely focused. Finally, it is imperative that there is an enhanced dialogue between basic and clinical science that continues even after the instigation of new treatment protocols. If such synergy can be nurtured, we can be cautiously optimistic for a translation of the advances in tumour immunology to the urgent needs of patients with currently incurable CNS neoplastic disease.

References

Aboody, K.S., Brown, A., Rainov, N.G., Bower, K.A., Liu, S., Yang W, et al. (2000). Neural stem cells display extensive tropism for pathology in adult brain: evidence from intracranial gliomas. *Proc Natl Acad Sci USA* **97**: 12846–12851.

Akasaki, Y., Kikuchi, T., Homma, S., Abe, T., Kofe, D., and Ohno T. (2001). Antitumor effect of immunizations with fusions of dendritic and glioma cells in a mouse brain tumor model. *J Immunother* **24**: 106–113.

Aloisi, F., De Simone, R., Columba-Cabezas, S., Penna, G., and Adorini L. (2000). Functional maturation of adult mouse resting microglia into an APC is promoted by granulocyte-macrophage colony-stimulating factor and interaction with Th1 cells. *J Immunol* **164**: 1705–1712.

Ambrosini, G., Adida, C., and Altieri, D.C. (1997). A novel anti-apoptosis gene, survivin, expressed in cancer and lymphoma. *Nat Med* **3**: 917–921.

Aoki, T., Tashiro, K., Miyatake, S., Kinashi, T., Nakano, T., Oda, Y. et al. (1992). Expression of murine interleukin 7 in a murine glioma cell line results in reduced tumorigenicity *in vivo*. *Proc Natl Acad Sci USA* **89**: 3850–3854.

Aoki, H., Mizuno, M., Natsume, A., Tsugawa, T., Tsujimura, K., Takahashi, T., et al. (2001). Dendritic cells pulsed with tumor extract-cationic liposome complex increase the induction of cytotoxic T lymphocytes in mouse brain tumor. *Cancer Immunol Immunother* **50**: 463–468.

Arai, H., Chan, S.Y., Bishop, D.K., and Nabel, G.J. (1997a). Inhibition of the alloantibody response by CD95 ligand. *Nat Med* **3**: 843–848.

Arai, H., Gordon, D., Nabel, E.G., and Nabel, G.J. (1997b). Gene transfer of Fas ligand induces tumor regression *in vivo*. *Proc Natl Acad Sci USA* **94**: 13862–13867.

Asai, A., Miyagi, Y., Hashimoto, H., Lee, S.H., Mishima, K., Sugiyama, A. et al. (1994). Modulation of tumor immunogenicity of rat glioma cells by s-myc expression: eradication of rat gliomas *in vivo*. *Cell Growth Differ* **5**: 1153–1158.

Ashley, D.M., Sampson, J.H., Archer, G.E., Batra, S.K., Bigner, D.D., and Hale, L.P. (1997). A genetically modified allogeneic cellular vaccine generates MHC class I-restricted cytotoxic responses against tumor-associated antigens and protects against CNS tumors *in vivo*. *J Neuroimmunol* **78**: 34–46.

Ashley, D.M., Kong, F.M., Bigner, D.D., and Hale, L.P. (1998). Endogenous expression of transforming growth factor beta1 inhibits growth and tumorigenicity and enhances Fas-mediated apoptosis in a murine high-grade glioma model. *Cancer Res* **58**: 302–309.

Bainbridge, D., Ellis, S., Le Bouteiller, P., and Sargent, I. (2001). HLA-G remains a mystery. *Trends Immunol* **22**: 548–552.

Banchereau, J., Briere, F., Caux, C., Davoust, J., Lebecque, S., Liu, Y.J., et al. (2000). Immunobiology of dendritic cells. *Annu Rev Immunol* **18**: 767–811.

Banchereau, J., Palucka, A.K., Dhodapkar, M., Burkeholder, S., Taquet, N., Rolland, A., et al. (2001a). Immune and clinical responses in patients with metastatic melanoma to CD34+ progenitor-derived dendritic cell vaccine. *Cancer Res* **61**: 6451–6458.

Banchereau, J., Schuler-Thurner, B., Palucka, A.K., and Schuler, G. (2001b). Dendritic cells as vectors for therapy. *Cell* **106**: 271–274.

Barba, D., Saris, S.C., Holder, C., Rosenberg, S.A., and Oldfield, E.H. (1989). Intratumoral LAK cell and interleukin-2 therapy of human gliomas. *J Neurosurg* **70**: 175–182.

Barker, C.F. and Billingham, R.E. (1977). Immunologically privileged sites. *Adv Immunol* **25**: 1–54.

Bechmann, I., Mor, G., Nilsen, J., Eliza, M., Nitsch, R., and Naftolin, F. (1999). FasL (CD95L, Apo1L) is expressed in the normal rat and human brain: evidence for the existence of an immunological brain barrier. *Glia* **27**: 62–74.

Benedetti, S., Bruzzone, M.G., Pollo, B., Di Meco, F., Magrassi, L., Pirola, B., et al. (1999). Eradication of rat malignant gliomas by retroviral-mediated, *in vivo* delivery of the interleukin 4 gene. *Cancer Res* **59**: 645–652.

Berman, R.M., Suzuki, T., Tahara, H., Robbins, P.D., Narula, S.K., and Lotze, M.T. (1996). Systemic administration of cellular IL-10 induces an effective, specific, and long-lived immune response against established tumors in mice. *J Immunol* **157**: 231–238.

Beutler, A.S., Banck, M.S., Aguzzi, A., Wedekind, D., and Hedrich, H.J. (1997). Curing rat glioblastoma: immunotherapy or graft rejection? *Science* **276**: 20–21.

Bigner, D.D., Pitts, O.M., and Wikstrand, C.J. (1981). Induction of lethal experimental allergic encephalomyelitis in nonhuman primates and guinea pigs with human glioblastoma multiforme tissue. *J Neurosurg* **55**: 32–42.

Bodmer, S., Strommer, K., Frei, K., Siepl, C., de Tribolet, N., Heid, I., et al. (1989). Immunosuppression and transforming growth factor-b in glioblastoma. Preferential production of transforming growth factor-β2. *J Immunol* **143**: 3222–3229.

Book, A.A., Fielding, K.E., Kundu, N., Wilson, M.A., Fulton, A.M., and Laterra, J. (1998). IL-10 gene transfer to intracranial 9L glioma: tumor inhibition and cooperation with IL-2. *J Neuroimmunol* **92**: 50–59.

Brabb, T., von Dassow, P., Ordonez, N., Schnabel, B., Duke, B., and Goverman, J. (2000). *In situ* tolerance within the central nervous system as a mechanism for preventing autoimmunity. *J Exp Med* **192**: 871–880.

Braud, V.M., Allan, D.S., and McMichael, A.J. (1999). Functions of nonclassical MHC and non-MHC-encoded class I molecules. *Curr Opin Immunol* **11**: 100–108.

Brightman, M.W. and Reese, T.S. (1969). Junctions between intimately apposed cell membranes in the vertebrate brain. *J Cell Biol* **40**: 648–677.

Broadwell, R.D., Baker, B.J., Ebert, P.S., and Hickey, W.F. (1994). Allografts of CNS tissue possess a blood-brain barrier: III. Neuropathological, methodological, and immunological considerations. *Microsc Res Tech* **27**: 471–494.

Brooks, W.H., Markesbery, W.R., Gupta, G.D., and Roszman, T.L. (1978). Relationship of lymphocyte invasion and survival of brain tumor patients. *Ann Neurol* **4**: 219–224.

Bruner, J.M., Langford, L.A., and Fuller, G.N. (1993). Neuropathology, cell biology, and newer diagnostic methods. *Curr Opin Oncol* **5**: 441–449.

Bögler, O. and Weller M. (2002). Apoptosis in gliomas, and its role in their current and future treatment. *Front Biosci* **7**: e339–e353.

Caignard, A., Guillard, M., Gaudin, C., Escudier, B., Triebel, F., and Dietrich, P.Y. (1996). *In situ* demonstration of renal cell carcinoma specific T-cell clones. *Int J Cancer* **66**: 564–570.

Calzascia, T., di Berardino-Besson, W., Wilmotte, R., Masson, F., de Tribolet, N., Dietrich, P.Y., et al. (2003). Cutting edge: cross-presentation as a mechanism for efficient recruitment of tumor-specific CTL to the brain. *J Immunol* **171**: 2187–2191.

Calzascia, T., Masson, F., Di Berardino-Besson, W., Contassot, E., Wilmotte, R., Aurrand-Lions, M., et al. (2005). Homing phenotypes of tumour-specific CD8 T cells are predetermined at the tumour site by crosspresenting APCs. *Immunity* **22**: 175–184.

Cannella, B., Cross, A.H., and Raine, C.S. (1991). Adhesion-related molecules in the central nervous system. Upregulation correlates with inflammatory cell influx during relapsing experimental autoimmune encephalomyelitis. *Lab Invest* **65**: 23–31.

Chen, J.J., Sun, Y., and Nabel, G.J. (1998). Regulation of the proinflammatory effects of Fas ligand (CD95L). *Science* **282**: 1714–1717.

Chen, Y.T., Scanlan, M.J., Sahin, U., Tureci, O., Gure, A.O., Tsang, S., et al. (1997). A testicular antigen aberrantly expressed in human cancers detected by autologous antibody screening. *Proc Natl Acad Sci USA* **94**: 1914–1918.

Chi, D.D., Merchant, R.E., Rand, R., Conrad, A.J., Garrison, D., Turner, R., et al. (1997). Molecular detection of tumor-associated antigens shared by human cutaneous melanomas and gliomas. *Am J Pathol* **150**: 2143–2152.

Columba-Cabezas, S., Serafini, B., Ambrosini, E., and Aloisi, F. (2003). Lymphoid chemokines CCL19 and CCL21 are expressed in the central nervous system during experimental autoimmune encephalomyelitis: implications for the maintenance of chronic neuroinflammation. *Brain Pathol* 13: 38–51.

Couldwell, W.T., Yong, V.W., Dore-Duffy, P., Freedman, M.S., and Antel, J.P. (1992). Production of soluble autocrine inhibitory factors by human glioma cell lines. *J Neurol Sci* 110: 178–185.

Cserr, H.F. and Knopf, P.M. (1992). Cervical lymphatics, the blood–brain barrier and the immunoreactivity of the brain: a new view. *Immunol Today* 13: 507–512.

D'Souza, S.D., Bonetti, B., Balasingam, V., Cashman, N.R., Barker, P.A., Troutt, A.B., et al. (1996). Multiple sclerosis: Fas signaling in oligodendrocyte cell death. *J Exp Med* 184: 2361–2370.

Debinski, W. and Gibo, D.M. (2000). Molecular expression analysis of restrictive receptor for interleukin 13, a brain tumor-associated cancer/testis antigen. *Mol Med* 6: 440–449.

Dewey, R.A., Morrissey, G., Cowsill, C.M., Stone, D., Bolognani, F., Dodd, N.J., et al. (1999). Chronic brain inflammation and persistent herpes simplex virus 1 thymidine kinase expression in survivors of syngeneic glioma treated by adenovirus-mediated gene therapy: implications for clinical trials. *Nat Med* 5: 1256–1263.

Dhib-Jalbut, S., Kufta, C.V., Flerlage, M., Shimojo, N., and McFarland, H.F. (1990). Adult human glial cells can present target antigens to HLA-restricted cytotoxic T-cells. *J Neuroimmunol* 29: 203–211.

Didenko, V.V., Ngo, H.N., Minchew, C., and Baskin, D.S. (2002). Apoptosis of T lymphocytes invading glioblastomas multiforme: a possible tumor defense mechanism. *J Neurosurg* 96: 580–584.

Dietrich P-Y, Walker, P.R., Schnuriger, V., Saas, P., Guillard, M., Gaudin, C., et al. (1997). T cell repertoire analysis reveals significant repertoire selection during *in vitro* lymphocyte culture. *Int Immunol* 9: 1073–1083.

Dix, A.R., Brooks, W.H., Roszman, T.L., and Morford, L.A. (1999). Immune defects observed in patients with primary malignant brain tumors. *J Neuroimmunol* 100: 216–232.

Dong, H., Strome, S.E., Salomao, D.R., Tamura, H., Hirano, F., Flies, D.B., et al. (2002). Tumor-associated B7-H1 promotes T-cell apoptosis: a potential mechanism of immune evasion. *Nat Med* 8: 793–800.

Dudley, M.E., Wunderlich, J.R., Robbins, P.F., Yang, J.C., Hwu, P., Schwartzentruber, D.J., et al. (2002). Cancer regression and autoimmunity in patients after clonal repopulation with antitumor lymphocytes. *Science* 298: 850–854.

Ehtesham, M., Kabos, P., Gutierrez, M.A., Samoto, K., Black, K.L., and Yu, J.S. (2003). Intratumoral dendritic cell vaccination elicits potent tumoricidal immunity against malignant glioma in rats. *J Immunother* 26: 107–116.

Ehtesham, M., Black, K.L., and Yu, J.S. (2004). Recent progress in immunotherapy for malignant glioma: treatment strategies and results from clinical trials. *Cancer Control* 11: 192–207.

Ekstrand, A.J., Sugawa, N., James, C.D., and Collins, V.P. (1992). Amplified and rearranged epidermal growth factor receptor genes in human glioblastomas reveal deletions of sequences encoding portions of the N- and/or C-terminal tails. *Proc Natl Acad Sci USA* 89: 4309–4313.

Elliott, L.H., Brooks, W.H., and Roszman, T.L. (1990). Inability of mitogen-activated lymphocytes obtained from patients with malignant primary intracranial tumors to express high affinity interleukin 2 receptors. *J Clin Invest* 86: 80–86.

Fabry, Z., Raine, C.S., and Hart, M.N. (1994). Nervous tissue as an immune compartment: the dialect of the immune response in the CNS. *Immunol Today* 15: 218–224.

Facoetti, A., Capelli, E., and Nano, R. (2001). HLA class I molecules expression: evaluation of different immunocytochemical methods in malignant lesions. *Anticancer Res* 21: 2435–2440.

Fakhrai, H., Dorigo, O., Shawler, D.L., Lin, H., Mercola, D., Black, K.L., et al. (1996). Eradication of established intracranial rat gliomas by transforming growth factor b antisense gene therapy. *Proc Natl Acad Sci USA* 93: 2909–2914.

Favre, N., Bonnotte, B., Droin, N., Fromentin, A., Solary, E., Martin, F. (1999). Fas (CD95) ligand expression by tumor cell variants an be unrelated to their capacity to induce tolerance or immune rejection. *Int J Cancer* 82: 359–367.

Fischer, H.G., Bonifas, U., and Reichmann, G. (2000). Phenotype and functions of brain dendritic cells emerging during chronic infection of mice with *Toxoplasma gondii*. *J Immunol* 164: 4826–4834.

Flugel, A., Schwaiger, F.W., Neumann, H., Medana, I., Willem, M., Wekerle, H. et al. (2000). Neuronal FasL induces cell death of encephalitogenic T lymphocytes. *Brain Pathol* 10: 353–364.

Fontana, A., Kristensen, F., Dubs, R., Gemsa, D., and Weber, E. (1982). Production of prostaglandin E and an interleukin-1 like factor by cultured astrocytes and C6 glioma cells. *J Immunol* 129: 2413–2419.

Fontana, A., Hengartner, H., de Tribolet, N., and Weber, E. (1984). Glioblastoma cells release interleukin 1 and factors inhibiting interleukin 2-mediated effects. *J Immunol* 132: 1837–1844.

Ford, A.L., Goodsall, A.L., Hickey, W.F., and Sedgwick, J.D. (1995). Normal adult ramified microglia separated from other central nervous system macrophages by flow cytometric sorting. Phenotypic differences defined and direct *ex vivo* antigen presentation to myelin basic protein-reactive CD4+ T cells compared. *J Immunol* 154: 4309–4321.

Ford, A.L., Foulcher, E., Lemckert, F.A., and Sedgwick, J.D. (1996). Microglia induce CD4 T lymphocyte final effector function and death. *J Exp Med* 184: 1737–1745.

Frankel, B., Longo, S.L., and Ryken, T.C. (1999). Human astrocytomas co-expressing Fas and Fas ligand also produce TGFβ2 and Bcl-2. *J Neurooncol* 44: 205–212.

French, L.E., Hahne, M., Viard, I., Radlgruber, G., Zanone, R., Becker, K., et al. (1996). Fas and Fas ligand in embryos and adult mice: ligand expression in several immune-privileged tissues and coexpression in adult tissues characterized by apoptotic cell turnover. *J Cell Biol* 133: 335–343.

Frigerio, S., Silei, V., Ciusani, E., Massa, G., Lauro, G.M., and Salmaggi, A. (2000). Modulation of fas-ligand (Fas-L) on human microglial cells: an *in vitro* study. *J Neuroimmunol* 105: 109–114.

Fulda, S., Wick, W., Weller, M., and Debatin, K.M. (2002). Smac agonists sensitize for Apo2L/T. *Nat Med* 8: 808–815.

Giezeman-Smits, K.M., Okada, H., Brissette-Storkus, C.S., Villa, L.A., Attanucci, J., Lotze, M.T., et al. (2000). Cytokine gene therapy of gliomas: induction of reactive CD4+ T cells by interleukin-4-transfected 9L gliosarcoma is essential for protective immunity. *Cancer Res* 60: 2449–2457.

Glick, R.P., Lichtor, T., Kim, T.S., Ilangovan, S., and Cohen, E.P. (1995). Fibroblasts genetically engineered to secrete cytokines suppress tumor growth and induce antitumor immunity to a murine glioma *in vivo*. *Neurosurgery* 36: 548–555.

Gordon, L.B., Nolan, S.C., Cserr, H.F., Knopf, P.M., and Harling-Berg, C.J. (1997). Growth of P511 mastocytoma cells in BALB/c mouse brain elicits CTL response without tumour elimination. *J Immunol* 159: 2399–2408.

Gordon, L.B., Nolan, S.C., Ksander, B.R., Knopf, P.M., and Harling-Berg, C.J. (1998). Normal cerebrospinal fluid suppresses the *in vitro* development of cytotoxic T cells: role of the brain microenvironment in CNS immune regulation. *J Neuroimmunol* 88: 77–84.

Gorelik, L. and Flavell, R.A. (2002). Transforming growth factor-β in T-cell biology. *Nat Rev Immunol* 2: 46–53.

Graf, M.R., Jadus, M.R., Hiserodt, J.C., Wepsic, H.T., and Granger, G.A. (1999). Development of systemic immunity to glioblastoma multiforme using tumor cells genetically engineered to express the membrane-associated isoform of macrophage colony-stimulating factor. *J Immunol* 163: 5544–5551.

Gratas, C., Tohma, Y., Van Meir, E.G., Klein, M., Tenan, M., Ishii, N., et al. (1997). Fas ligand expression in glioblastoma cell lines and primary astrocytic brain tumors. *Brain Pathol* 7: 863–869.

Gunzer, M., Schafer, A., Borgmann, S., Grabbe, S., Zanker, K.S., Brocker, E.B., et al. (2000). Antigen presentation in extracellular matrix: interactions of T cells with dendritic cells are dynamic, short lived, and sequential. *Immunity* 13: 323–332.

Hahne, M., Rimoldi, D., Schröter, M., Romero, P., Schreier, M., French, L., et al. (1996). Melanoma cell expression of Fas (Apo-1/CD95) ligand: implications for tumor immune escape. *Science* 274: 1363–1366.

Harling-Berg, C., Knopf, P.M., Merriam, J., and Cserr, H.F. (1989). Role of cervical lymph nodes in the systemic humoral immune response to human serum albumin microinfused into rat cerebrospinal fluid. *J Neuroimmunol* 25: 185–193.

Hauser, S.L., Bhan, A.K., Gilles, F.H., Hoban, C.J., Reinherz, E.L., Schlossman, S.F., et al. (1983). Immunohistochemical staining of human brain with monoclonal antibodies that identify lymphocytes, monocytes, and the Ia antigen. J Neuroimmunol 5: 197–205.

Heimberger, A.B., Crotty, L.E., Archer, G.E., McLendon, R.E., Friedman, A., Dranoff, G., et al. (2000). Bone marrow-derived dendritic cells pulsed with tumor homogenate induce immunity against syngeneic intracerebral glioma. J Neuroimmunol 103: 16–25.

Heimberger, A.B., Crotty, L.E., Archer, G.E., Hess, K.R., Wikstrand, C.J., Friedman, A.H., et al. (2003). Epidermal growth factor receptor VIII peptide vaccination is efficacious against established intracerebral tumors. Clin Cancer Res 9: 4247–4254.

Held-Feindt, J. and Mentlein, R. (2002). CD70/CD27 ligand, a member of the TNF family, is expressed in human brain tumors. Int J Cancer 98: 352–356.

Hickey, W.F. (1999). Leukocyte traffic in the central nervous system: the participants and their roles. Semin Immunol 11: 125–137.

Holland, E.C. (2001). Gliomagenesis: genetic alterations and mouse models. Nat Rev Genet 2: 120–129.

Hosli, P., Sappino, A.P., de Tribolet, N., and Dietrich, P.Y. (1998). Malignant glioma: should chemotherapy be overthrown by experimental treatments? Ann Oncol 9: 589–600.

Hung, K., Hayashi, R., Lafond-Walker, A., Lowenstein, C., Pardoll, D., and Levitsky, H. (1998). The central role of CD4+ T cells in the antitumor immune response. J Exp Med 188: 2357–2368.

Imaizumi, T., Kuramoto, T., Matsunaga, K., Shichijo, S., Yutani, S., Shigemori, M., et al. (1999). Expression of the tumor-rejection antigen SART1 in brain tumors. Int J Cancer 83: 760–764.

Irani, D.N. (1998). The susceptibility of mice to immune-mediated neurologic disease correlates with the degree to which their lymphocytes resist the effects of brain-derived gangliosides. J Immunol 161: 2746–2752.

Jachimczak, P., Bogdahn, U., Schneider, J., Behl, C., Meixensberger, J., Apfel, R., et al. (1993). The effect of transforming growth factor-β2-specific phosphorothioate-anti-sense oligodeoxynucleotides in reversing cellular immunosuppression in malignant glioma. J Neurosurg 78: 944–951.

Jacquot, S. (2000). CD27/CD70 interactions regulate T dependent B cell differentiation. Immunol Res 21: 23–30.

Janeway, C.A. Jr. and Medzhitov, R. (2002). Innate immune recognition. Annu Rev Immunol 20: 197–216.

Janzer, R.C. and Raff, M.C. (1987). Astrocytes induce blood-brain barrier properties in endothelial cells. Nature 325: 253–257.

Joki, T., Kikuchi, T., Akasaki, Y., Saitoh, S., Abe, T., and Ohno, T. (1999). Induction of effective antitumor immunity in a mouse brain tumor model using B7-1 (CD80) and intercellular adhesive molecule 1 (ICAM-1; CD54) transfection and recombinant interleukin 12. Int J Cancer 82: 714–720.

Kabos, P., Ehtesham, M., Black, K.L., and Yu, J.S. (2003). Neural stem cells as delivery vehicles. Expert Opin Biol Ther 3: 759–770.

Kalams, S.A. and Walker, B.D. (1998). The critical need for CD4 help in maintaining effective cytotoxic T lymphocyte responses. J Exp Med 188: 2199–2204.

Karman, J., Ling, C., Sandor, M., and Fabry, Z. (2004). Initiation of immune responses in brain is promoted by local dendritic cells. J Immunol 173: 2353–2361.

Karpus, W.J., Lukacs, N.W., McRae, B.L., Strieter, R.M., Kunkel, S.L., and Miller, S.D. (1995). An important role for the chemokine macrophage inflammatory protein-1 alpha in the pathogenesis of the T cell-mediated autoimmune disease, experimental autoimmune encephalomyelitis. J Immunol 155: 5003–5010.

Katoh, M., Wilmotte, R., Belkouch, M.C., de Tribolet, N., Pizzolato, G., and Dietrich, P.Y. (2003). Survivin in brain tumors: an attractive target for immunotherapy. J Neurooncol 64: 71–76.

Kaye, J. and Hedrick, S.M. (1988). Analysis of specificity for antigen, Mls, and allogenic MHC by transfer of T-cell receptor α- and β-chain genes. Nature 336: 580–583.

Kerbel, R. and Folkman, J. (2002). Clinical translation of angiogenesis inhibitors. Nat Rev Cancer 2: 727–739.

Kikuchi, T., Joki, T., Akasaki, Y., Abe, T., and Ohno, T. (1999a). Induction of antitumor immunity using intercellular adhesion molecule 1 (ICAM-1) transfection in mouse glioma cells. Cancer Lett 142: 201–206.

Kikuchi, T., Joki, T., Saitoh, S., Hata, Y., Abe, T., Kato, N., et al. (1999b). Antitumor activity of interleukin-2-producing tumor cells and recombinant interleukin 12 against mouse glioma cells located in the central nervous system. Int J Cancer 80: 425–430.

Kikuchi, T., Akasaki, Y., Joki, T., Abe, T., Kurimoto, M., and Ohno, T. (2000). Antitumor activity of interleukin-18 on mouse glioma cells. J Immunother 23: 184–189.

Kikuchi, T., Akasaki, Y., Irie, M., Homma, S., Abe, T., and Ohno, T. (2001). Results of a phase I clinical trial of vaccination of glioma patients with fusions of dendritic and glioma cells. Cancer Immunol Immunother 50: 337–344.

Kikuchi, T., Abe, T., and Ohno, T. (2002a). Effects of glioma cells on maturation of dendritic cells. J Neurooncol 58: 125–130.

Kikuchi, T., Akasaki, Y., Abe, T., and Ohno, T. (2002b). Intratumoral injection of dendritic and irradiated glioma cells induces anti-tumor effects in a mouse brain tumor model. Cancer Immunol Immunother 51: 424–430.

Kobayashi, T., Yamanaka, R., Homma, J., Tsuchiya, N., Yajima, N., Yoshida, S., et al. (2003). Tumor mRNA-loaded dendritic cells elicit tumor-specific CD8+ cytotoxic T cells in patients with malignant glioma. Cancer Immunol Immunother 52: 632–637.

Krakowski, A.M. and Owens, T. (2000). Naive T lymphocytes traffic to inflamed central nervous system, but require antigen recognition for activation. Eur J Immunol 30: 1002–1009.

Lampson, L.A. and Hickey, W.F. (1986). Monoclonal antibody analysis of MHC expression in human brain biopsies: tissue ranging from 'histologically normal' to that showing different levels of glial tumor involvement. J Immunol 136: 4054–4062.

Lanzavecchia, A. (1998). Immunology. Licence to kill. Nature 393: 413–414.

Lassman, A.B. and DeAngelis, L.M. (2003). Brain metastases. Neurol Clin N Am 21: 1–23.

Liau, L.M., Black, K.L., Prins, R.M., Sykes, S.N., DiPatre, P.L., Cloughesy, T.F., et al. (1999). Treatment of intracranial gliomas with bone marrow-derived dendritic cells pulsed with tumor antigens. J Neurosurg 90: 1115–1124.

Liau, L.M., Jensen, E.R., Kremen, T.J., Odesa, S.K., Sykes, S.N., Soung, M.C., et al. (2002). Tumor immunity within the central nervous system stimulated by recombinant Listeria monocytogenes vaccination. Cancer Res 62: 2287–2293.

Liu, G., Khong, H.T., Wheeler, C.J., Yu, J.S., Black, K.L., and Ying, H. (2003). Molecular and functional analysis of tyrosinase-related protein (TRP)-2 as a cytotoxic T lymphocyte target in patients with malignant glioma. J Immunother 26: 301–312.

Liu, G., Yu, J.S., Zeng, G., Yin, D., Xie, D., Black, K.L., et al. (2004a). AIM-2: a novel tumor antigen is expressed and presented by human glioma cells. J Immunother 27: 220–226.

Liu, G., Ying, H., Zeng, G., Wheeler, C.J., Black, K.L., and Yu, J.S. (2004b). HER-2, gp100, and MAGE-1 are expressed in human glioblastoma and recognized by cytotoxic T cells. Cancer Res 64: 4980–4986.

Ludewig, B., Ochsenbein, A.F., Odermatt, B., Paulin, D., Hengartner, H., and Zinkernagel, R.M. (2000). Immunotherapy with dendritic cells directed against tumor antigens shared with normal host cells results in severe autoimmune disease. J Exp Med 191: 795–804.

Lumniczky, K., Desaknai, S., Mangel, L., Szende, B., Hamada, H., Hidvegi, E.J., et al. (2002). Local tumor irradiation augments the antitumor effect of cytokine- producing autologous cancer cell vaccines in a murine glioma model. Cancer Gene Ther 9: 44–52.

Lynch, D.H., Ramsdell, F., and Alderson, M.R. (1995). Fas and FasL in the homeostatic regulation of immune responses. Immunol Today 16: 569–574.

Maier, S., Geraghty, D.E., and Weiss, E.H. (1999). Expression and regulation of HLA-G in human glioma cell lines. Transplant Proc 31: 1849–1853.

Matyszak, M.K., Denis-Donini, S., Citterio, S., Longhi, R., Granucci, F., and Ricciardi-Castagnoli, P. (1999). Microglia induce myelin basic protein-specific T cell anergy or T cell activation, according to their state of activation. Eur J Immunol 29: 3063–3076.

Matzinger, P. (2002). The danger model: a renewed sense of self. Science 296: 301–305.

McHeyzer-Williams, M.G., Altman, J.D., and Davis, M.M. (1996). Tracking antigen-specific helper T cell responses. Curr Opin Immunol 8: 278–284.

Medana, I., Li, Z., Flugel, A., Tschopp, J., Wekerle, H., and Neumann, H. (2001). Fas ligand (CD95L) protects neurons against perforin-mediated T lymphocyte cytotoxicity. *J Immunol* **167**: 674–681.

Medawar, P.B. (1948). Immunity to homologous grafted skin. III. The fate of skin homografts transplanted to the brain, to subcutaneous tissue and to the anterior chamber of the eye. *Br J Exp Pathol* **29**: 58–69.

Merlo, A., Juretic, A., Zuber, M., Filgueira, L., Luscher, U., Caetano, V., *et al.* (1993). Cytokine gene expression in primary brain tumours, metastases and meningiomas suggests specific transcription patterns. *Eur J Cancer* **29A**: 2118–2125.

Miescher, S., Whiteside, T.L., Carrel, S., and Von Fliedner, V. (1986). Functional properties of tumor-infiltrating and blood lymphocytes in patients with solid tumors: effects of tumor cells and their supernatants on proliferative responses of lymphocytes. *J Immunol* **136**: 1899–1907.

Morford, L.A., Elliott, L.H., Carlson, S.L., Brooks, W.H., and Roszman, T.L. (1997). T cell receptor-mediated signaling is defective in T cells obtained from patients with primary intracranial tumors. *J Immunol* **159**: 4415–4425.

Münz, C., Naumann, U., Grimmel, C., Rammensee, H.G., and Weller, M. (1999). TGF-β-independent induction of immunogenicity by decorin gene transfer in human malignant glioma cells. *Eur J Immunol* **29**: 1032–1040.

Nagata, S. and Golstein, P. (1995). The Fas death factor. *Science* **267**: 1449–1456.

Nanda, D., Driesse, M.J., and Sillevis Smitt, P.A. (2001). Clinical trials of adenoviral-mediated suicide gene therapy of malignant gliomas. *Prog Brain Res* **132**: 699–710.

Natali, P.G., Bigotti, A., Nicotra, M.R., Viora, M., Manfredi, D., and Ferrone, S. (1984). Distribution of human Class I (HLA-A,B,C) histocompatibility antigens in normal and malignant tissues of nonlymphoid origin. *Cancer Res* **44**: 4679–4687.

Nitta, T., Hishii, M., Sato, K., and Okumura, K. (1994). Selective expression of interleukin-10 gene within glioblastoma multiforme. *Brain Res* **649**: 122–128.

O'Connell, J. (2002). Fas ligand and the fate of antitumour cytotoxic T lymphocytes. *Immunology* **105**: 263–266.

Oehmichen, M., Wietholter, H., Gruninger, H., and Gencic, M. (1983). Destruction of intracerebrally applied red blood cells in cervical lymph nodes. Experimental investigations. *Forensic Sci Int* **21**: 43–57.

Offringa, R., van der Burg, S.H., Ossendorp, F., Toes, R.E., and Melief, C.J. (2000). Design and evaluation of antigen-specific vaccination strategies against cancer. *Curr Opin Immunol* **12**: 576–582.

Okada, H., Tahara, H., Shurin, M.R., Attanucci, J., Giezeman-Smits, K.M., Fellows, W.K., *et al.* (1998). Bone marrow-derived dendritic cells pulsed with a tumor-specific peptide elicit effective anti-tumor immunity against intracranial neoplasms. *Int J Cancer* **78**: 196–201.

Okada, H., Lieberman, F.S., Edington, H.D., Witham, T.F., Wargo, M.J., Cai, Q., *et al.* (2003). Autologous glioma cell vaccine admixed with interleukin-4 gene transfected fibroblasts in the treatment of recurrent glioblastoma: preliminary observations in a patient with a favorable response to therapy. *J Neurooncol* **64**: 13–20.

Okano, F., Storkus, W.J., Chambers, W.H., Pollack, I.F., and Okada, H. (2002). Identification of a novel HLA-A*0201-restricted, cytotoxic T lymphocyte epitope in a human glioma-associated antigen, interleukin 13 receptor α2 chain. *Clin Cancer Res* **8**: 2851–2855.

Pardoll, D.M. (1999). Inducing autoimmune disease to treat cancer. *Proc Natl Acad Sci USA* **96**: 5340–5342.

Pardoll, D.M. (2002). Spinning molecular immunology into successful immunotherapy. *Nat Rev Immunol* **2**: 227–238.

Parney, I.F., Farr-Jones, M.A., Chang, L.J., and Petruk, K.C. (2000). Human glioma immunobiology *in vitro*: implications for immunogene therapy. *Neurosurgery* **46**: 1169–1177.

Perrin, G., Schnuriger, V., Quiquerez A-L, Saas, P., Pannetier, C., de Tribolet, N., *et al.* (1999). Astrocytoma infiltrating lymphocytes include major T cell clonal expansions confined to the CD8 subset. *Int Immunol* **11**: 1337–1349.

Perry, V.H., Matyszak, M.K., and Fearn, S. (1993). Altered antigen expression of microglia in the aged rodent CNS. *Glia* **7**: 60–67.

Phillips, M.J., Needham, M., and Weller, R.O. (1997). Role of cervical lymph nodes in autoimmune encephalomyelitis in the Lewis rat. *J Pathol* **182**: 457–464.

Plautz, G.E., Barnett, G.H., Miller, D.W., Cohen, B.H., Prayson, R.A., Krauss, J.C., *et al.* (1998). Systemic T cell adoptive immunotherapy of malignant gliomas. *J Neurosurg* **89**: 51.

Qing, Z., Sewell, D., Sandor, M., and Fabry, Z. (2000). Antigen-specific T cell trafficking into the central nervous system. *J Neuroimmunol* **105**: 169–178.

Quattrocchi, K.B., Miller, C.H., Cush, S., Bernard, S.A., Dull, S.T., Smith, M., *et al.* (1999). Pilot study of local autologous tumor infiltrating lymphocytes for the treatment of recurrent malignant gliomas. *J Neurooncol* **45**: 141–157.

Rafii, S., Lyden, D., Benezra, R., Hattori, K., and Heissig, B. (2002). Vascular and haematopoietic stem cells: novel targets for anti- angiogenesis therapy? *Nat Rev Cancer* **2**: 826–835.

Re, F., Belyanskaya, S.L., Riese, R.J., Cipriani, B., Fischer, F.R., Granucci, F., *et al.* (2002). Granulocyte-macrophage colony-stimulating factor induces an expression program in neonatal microglia that primes them for antigen presentation. *J Immunol* **169**: 2264–2273.

Renkvist, N., Castelli, C., Robbins, P.F., and Parmiani, G. (2001). A listing of human tumor antigens recognized by T cells. *Cancer Immunol Immunother* **50**: 3–15.

Resnicoff, M., Sell, C., Rubini, M., Coppola, D., Ambrose, D., Baserga, R., *et al.* (1994). Rat glioblastoma cells expressing an antisense RNA to the insulin-like growth factor-1 (IGF-1) receptor are nontumorigenic and induce regression of wild-type tumors. *Cancer Res* **54**: 2218–2222.

Restifo, N.P. (2000). Not so fas: re-evaluating the mechanisms of immune privilege and tumor escape. *Nat Med* **6**: 493–495.

Rossi, M.L., Hughes, J.T., Esiri, M.M., Coakham, H.B., and Brownell, D. (1987). Immunohistological study of mononuclear cell infiltrate in malignant gliomas. *Acta Neuropathol* **74**: 269–277.

Rubin, L.L. and Staddon, J.M. (1999). The cell biology of the blood–brain barrier. *Annu Rev Neurosci* **22**: 11–28.

Ruiz-Cabello, F., Cabrera, T., Lopez-Nevot, M.A., and Garrido, F. (2002). Impaired surface antigen presentation in tumors: implications for T cell-based immunotherapy. *Semin Cancer Biol* **12**: 15–24.

Saas, P., Walker, P.R., Hahne, M., Quiquerez A-L, Schnuriger, V., Perrin, G., *et al.* (1997). Fas ligand expression by astrocytoma *in vivo*: maintaining immune privilege in the brain? *J Clin Invest* **99**: 1173–1178.

Saas, P., Boucraut, J., Quiquerez A-L, Schnuriger, V., Perrin, G., Desplat-Jego, S., *et al.* (1999). CD95 (Fas/Apo-1) as a receptor governing astrocyte apoptotic or inflammatory responses: a key role in brain inflammation? *J Immunol* **162**: 2326–2333.

Sahin, U., Tureci, O., and Pfreundschuh, M. (1997). Serological identification of human tumor antigens. *Curr Opin Immunol* **9**: 709–716.

Sahin, U., Koslowski, M., Tureci, O., Eberle, T., Zwick, C., Romeike, B., *et al.* (2000). Expression of cancer testis genes in human brain tumors. *Clin Cancer Res* **6**: 3916–3922.

Saito, T., Tanaka, R., Yoshida, S., Washiyama, K., and Kumanishi, T. (1988). Immunohistochemical analysis of tumor-infiltrating lymphocytes and major histocompatibility antigens in human gliomas and metastatic brain tumors. *Surg Neurol* **29**: 435–442.

Sallusto, F. and Lanzavecchia, A. (2000). Understanding dendritic cell and T-lymphocyte traffic through the analysis of chemokine receptor expression. *Immunol Rev* **177**: 134–140.

Sampson, J.H., Archer, G.E., Ashley, D.M., Fuchs, H.E., Hale, L.P., Dranoff, G., *et al.* (1996). Subcutaneous vaccination with irradiated, cytokine-producing tumors cells stimulates CD8+ cell-mediated immunity against tumors located in the 'immunologically privileged' central nervous system. *Proc Natl Acad Sci USA* **93**: 10399–10404.

Sampson, J.H., Ashley, D.M., Archer, G.E., Fuchs, H.E., Dranoff, G., Hale, L.P., *et al.* (1997). Characterization of a spontaneous murine astrocytoma and abrogation of its tumorigenicity by cytokine secretion. *Neurosurgery* **41**: 1365–1373.

Santambrogio, L., Belyanskaya, S.L., Fischer, F.R., Cipriani, B., Brosnan, C.F., Ricciardi-Castagnoli, P., *et al.* (2001). Developmental plasticity of CNS microglia. *Proc Natl Acad Sci USA* **98**: 6295–6300.

Sawamura, Y., Diserens, A.C., and de Tribolet, N. (1990). *In vitro* prostaglandin E2 production by glioblastoma cells and its effect on interleukin-2 activation of oncolytic lymphocytes. *J Neurooncol* **9**: 125–130.

Scarcella, D.L., Chow, C.W., Gonzales, M.F., Economou, C., Brasseur, F., and Ashley, D.M. (1999). Expression of MAGE and GAGE in high-grade brain tumors: a potential target for specific immunotherapy and diagnostic markers. *Clin Cancer Res* **5**: 335–341.

Schmits, R., Cochlovius, B., Treitz, G., Regitz, E., Ketter, R., Preuss, K.D., *et al.* (2002). Analysis of the antibody repertoire of astrocytoma patients against antigens expressed by gliomas. *Int J Cancer* **98**: 73–77.

Schmitz, M., Diestelkoetter, P., Weigle, B., Schmachtenberg, F., Stevanovic, S., Ockert, D., *et al.* (2000). Generation of survivin-specific CD8+ T effector cells by dendritic cells pulsed with protein or selected peptides. *Cancer Res* **60**: 4845–4849.

Schwab, R., Szabo, P., Manavalan, J.S., Weksler, M.E., Posnett, D.N., Pannetier, C., *et al.* (1997). Expanded CD4+ and CD8+ T cell clones in elderly humans. *J Immunol* **158**: 4493–4499.

Segal, B.M., Glass, D.D., and Shevach, E.M. (2002). Cutting edge: IL-10-producing CD4+ T cells mediate tumor rejection. *J Immunol* **168**: 1–4.

Seino, K.-I., Kayagaki, N., Okumura, K., and Yagita, H. (1997a). Antitumor effect of locally produced CD95 ligand. *Nat Med* **3**: 165–170.

Seino, K.-I., Kayagaki, N., Tsukada, N., Fukao, K., Yagita, H., and Okumura, K. (1997b). Transplantation of CD95 ligand-expressing grafts. Influence of transplantation site and difficulty in protecting allo- and xenografts. *Transplantation* **64**: 1050–1054.

Seliger, B., Cabrera, T., Garrido, F., and Ferrone, S. (2002). HLA class I antigen abnormalities and immune escape by malignant cells. *Semin Cancer Biol* **12**: 3–13.

Sensi, M. and Parmiani, G. (1995). Analysis of TCR usage in human tumors: a new tool for assessing tumor-specific immune responses. *Immunol Today* **16**: 588–595.

Sharpe, A.H. and Freeman, G.J. (2002). The B7-CD28 superfamily. *Nat Rev Immunol* **2**: 116–126.

Smyth, M.J., Strobl, S.L., Young, H.A., Ortaldo, J.R., and Ochoa, A.C. (1991). Regulation of lymphokine-activated killer activity and pore- forming protein gene expression in human peripheral blood CD8+ T lymphocytes. Inhibition by transforming growth factor-β. *J Immunol* **146**: 3289–3297.

Soling, A. and Rainov, N.G. (2001). Dendritic cell therapy of primary brain tumors. *Mol Med* **7**: 659–667.

Spanaus, K.S., Schlapbach, R., and Fontana, A. (1998). TNF-alpha and IFN-gamma render microglia sensitive to Fas ligand-induced apoptosis by induction of Fas expression and down-regulation of Bcl-2 and Bcl-xL. *Eur J Immunol* **28**: 4398–4408.

Srivastava, P. (2002). Roles of heat-shock proteins in innate and adaptive immunity. *Nat Rev Immunol* **2**: 185–194.

Stander, M., Naumann, U., Dumitrescu, L., Heneka, M., Loschmann, P., Gulbins, E., *et al.* (1998). Decorin gene transfer-mediated suppression of TGF-beta synthesis abrogates experimental malignant glioma growth *in vivo*. *Gene Ther* **5**: 1187–1194.

Stavrou, D., Anzil, A.P., Weidenbach, W., and Rodt, H. (1977). Immunofluorescence study of lymphocytic infiltration in gliomas. Identification of T-lymphocytes. *J Neurol Sci* **33**: 275–282.

Steinman, R.M., Hawiger, D., and Nussenzweig, M.C. (2003). Tolerogenic dendritic cells. *Annu Rev Immunol* **21**: 685–711.

Stewart, L.A. (2002). Chemotherapy in adult high-grade glioma: a systematic review and meta-analysis of individual patient data from 12 randomised trials. *Lancet* **359**: 1011–1018.

Stohlman, S.A., Bergmann, C.C., Lin, M.T., Cua, D.J., and Hinton, D.R. (1998). CTL effector function within the central nervous system requires CD4+ T cells. *J Immunol* **160**: 2896–2904.

Stupp, R., Dietrich, P.Y., Ostermann, K.S., Pica, A., Maillard, I., Maeder, P., *et al.* (2002). Promising survival for patients with newly diagnosed glioblastoma multiforme treated with concomitant radiation plus temozolomide followed by adjuvant temozolomide. *J Clin Oncol* **20**: 1375–1382.

Suter, T., Malipiero, U., Otten, L., Ludewig, B., Muelethaler-Mottet, A., Mach, B., *et al.* (2000). Dendritic cells and differential usage of the MHC class II transactivator promoters in the central nervous system in experimental autoimmune encephalitis. *Eur J Immunol* **30**: 794–802.

Suter, T., Biollaz, G., Gatto, D., Bernasconi, L., Herren, T., Reith, W., *et al.* (2003). The brain as an immune privileged site: dendritic cells of the central nervous system inhibit T cell activation. *Eur J Immunol* **33**: 2998–3006.

Todryk, S.M., Melcher, A.A., Dalgleish, A.G., and Vile, R.G. (2000). Heat shock proteins refine the danger theory. *Immunology* **99**: 334–337.

Tran, E.H., Hoekstra, K., Van Rooijen, N., Dijkstra, C.D., and Owens, T. (1998). Immune invasion of the central nervous system parenchyma and experimental allergic encephalomyelitis, but not leukocyte extravasation from blood, are prevented in macrophage-depleted mice. *J Immunol* **161**: 3767–3775.

Trojan, J., Johnson, T.R., Rudin, S.D., Ilan, J., and Tykocinski, M.L. (1993). Treatment and prevention of rat glioblastoma by immunogenic C6 cells expressing antisense insulin-like growth factor I RNA. *Science* **259**: 94–97.

Tunici, P., Gianni, D., and Finocchiaro, G. (2001). Gene therapy of glioblastomas: from suicide to homicide. *Prog Brain Res* **132**: 711–719.

Urosevic, M., Trojan, A., and Dummer, R. (2002). HLA-G and its KIR ligands in cancer—another enigma yet to be solved? *J Pathol* **196**: 252–253.

Van der Bruggen, P., Traversari, C., Chomez, P., Lurquin, C., De Plaen, E., Van den Eynde, B., *et al.* (1991). A gene encoding an antigen recognized by cytolytic T lymphocytes on a human melanoma. *Science* **254**: 1643–1647.

van Elsas, A., Sutmuller, R.P., Hurwitz, A.A., Ziskin, J., Villasenor, J., Medema, J.P., *et al.* (2001). Elucidating the autoimmune and antitumor effector mechanisms of a treatment based on cytotoxic T lymphocyte antigen-4 blockade in combination with a B16 melanoma vaccine. Comparison of prophylaxis and therapy. *J Exp Med* **194**: 481–490.

van Herpen, C.M. and De Mulder, P.H. (2000). Locoregional immunotherapy in cancer patients: review of clinical studies. *Ann Oncol* **11**: 1229–1239.

Visse, E., Siesjo, P., Widegren, B., and Sjogren, H.O. (1999). Regression of intracerebral rat glioma isografts by therapeutic subcutaneous immunization with interferon-gamma, interleukin-7, or B7-1- transfected tumor cells. *Cancer Gene Ther* **6**: 37–44.

von Andrian, U.H. and Mackay, C.R. (2000). T-cell function and migration. Two sides of the same coin. *N Engl J Med* **343**: 1020–1034.

Walker, P.R., Saas, P., and Dietrich, P.-Y. (1997). The role of Fas ligand (CD95L) in immune escape: the tumor cell strikes back. *J Immunol* **158**: 4521–4524.

Walker, P.R., Saas, P., and Dietrich, P.Y. (1998). Tumor expression of Fas ligand (CD95L) and the consequences. *Curr Opin Immunol* **10**: 564–572.

Walker, P.R., Calzascia, T., Schnuriger, V., Scamuffa, N., Saas, P., de Tribolet, N., *et al.* (2000). The brain parenchyma is permissive for full antitumor CTL effector function, even in the absence of CD4 T cells. *J Immunol* **165**: 3128–3135.

Wang, R.F. (2001). The role of MHC class II-restricted tumor antigens and CD4+ T cells in antitumor immunity. *Trends Immunol* **22**: 269–276.

Weissenberger, J., Steinbach, J.P., Malin, G., Spada, S., Rülicke, T., and Aguzzi, A. (1997). Development and malignant progression of astrocytomas in GFAP-v-src transgenic mice. *Oncogene* **14**: 2005–2013.

Weller, R.O. (1998). Pathology of cerebrospinal fluid and interstitial fluid of the CNS: significance for Alzheimer disease, prion disorders and multiple sclerosis. *J Neuropathol Exp Neurol* **57**: 885–894.

Wiendl, H., Mitsdoerffer, M., Hofmeister, V., Wischhusen, J., Bornemann, A., Meyermann, R., *et al.* (2002). A functional role of HLA-G expression in human gliomas: an alternative strategy of immune escape. *J Immunol* **168**: 4772–4780.

Wikstrand, C.J., Fredman, P., Svennerholm, L., and Bigner, D.D. (1994). Detection of glioma-associated gangliosides GM2, GD2, GD3, 3′-isoLM1 3′,6′-isoLD1 in central nervous system tumors *in vitro* and *in vivo* using epitope-defined monoclonal antibodies. *Prog Brain Res* **101**: 213–223.

Wintterle, S., Schreiner, B., Mitsdoerffer, M., Schneider, D., Chen, L.P., Meyermann, R., *et al.* (2003). Expression of the B7-related molecule B7-H1 by glioma cells: a potential mechanism of immune paralysis. *Cancer Res* **63**: 7462–7467.

Wischhusen, J., Jung, G., Radovanovic, I., Beier, C., Steinbach, J.P., Rimner, A., *et al.* (2002). Identification of CD70-mediated apoptosis of immune effector cells as a novel immune escape pathway of human glioblastoma. *Cancer Res* **62**: 2592–2599.

Witham, T.F., Erff, M.L., Okada, H., Chambers, W.H., and Pollack, I.F. (2002). 7-Hydroxystaurosporine-induced apoptosis in 9L glioma cells provides an effective antigen source for dendritic cells and yields a potent vaccine strategy in an intracranial glioma model. *Neurosurgery* **50**: 1327–1334.

Wood, G.W., Holladay, F.P., Turner, T., Wang, Y.Y., and Chiga, M. (2000). A pilot study of autologous cancer cell vaccination and cellular immunotherapy using anti-CD3 stimulated lymphocytes in patients with recurrent grade III/IV astrocytoma. *J Neurooncol* **48**: 113–120.

Yamanaka, R., Zullo, S.A., Tanaka, R., Blaese, M., and Xanthopoulos, K.G. (2001). Enhancement of antitumor immune response in glioma models in mice by genetically modified dendritic cells pulsed with Semliki forest virus-mediated complementary DNA. *J Neurosurg* **94**: 474–481.

Yamanaka, R., Zullo, S.A., Ramsey, J., Yajima, N., Tsuchiya, N., Tanaka, R., *et al.* (2002). Marked enhancement of antitumor immune responses in mouse brain tumor models by genetically modified dendritic cells producing Semliki Forest virus-mediated interleukin-12. *J Neurosurg* **97**: 611–618.

Yamanaka, R., Abe, T., Yajima, N., Tsuchiya, N., Homma, J., Kobayashi, T., *et al.* (2003). Vaccination of recurrent glioma patients with tumour lysate-pulsed dendritic cells elicits immune responses: results of a clinical phase I/II trial. *Br J Cancer* **89**: 1172–1179.

Yang, T., Witham, T.F., Villa, L., Erff, M., Attanucci, J., Watkins, S., *et al.* (2002). Glioma-associated hyaluronan induces apoptosis in dendritic cells via inducible nitric oxide synthase: implications for the use of dendritic cells for therapy of gliomas. *Cancer Res* **62**: 2583–2591.

Yu, J.S., Wheeler, C.J., Zeltzer, P.M., Ying, H., Finger, D.N., Lee, P.K., *et al.* (2001). Vaccination of malignant glioma patients with peptide-pulsed dendritic cells elicits systemic cytotoxicity and intracranial T-cell infiltration. *Cancer Res* **61**: 842–847.

Yu, J.S., Lee, P.K., Ehtesham, M., Samoto, K., Black, K.L., and Wheeler, C.J. (2003). Intratumoral T cell subset ratios and Fas ligand expression on brain tumor endothelium. *J Neurooncol* **64**: 55–61.

Yu, J.S., Liu, G., Ying, H., Yong, W.H., Black, K.L., and Wheeler, C.J. (2004). Vaccination with tumor lysate-pulsed dendritic cells elicits antigen-specific, cytotoxic T-cells in patients with malignant glioma. *Cancer Res* **64**: 4973–4979.

Zajac, A.J., Murali-Krishna, K., Blattman, J.N., and Ahmed, R. (1998). Therapeutic vaccination against chronic viral infection: the importance of cooperation between CD4+ and CD8+ T cells. *Curr Opin Immunol* **10**: 444–449.

Zeltzer, P.M., Moilanen, B., Yu, J.S., and Black, K.L. (1999). Immunotherapy of malignant brain tumors in children and adults: from theoretical principles to clinical application. *Child Nerv Syst* **15**: 514–528.

30 Vasculitides of the nervous system

Roumen Balabanov and Paula Dore-Duffy

Introduction

Vasculitis is an inflammatory condition affecting the blood vessels (Fauci et al., 1978). By definition, any inflammatory process is accompanied by vascular involvement characterized by vasodilatation, increased vascular permeability, and extravasation of leukocytes. Unlike common inflammatory reactions, however, vasculitic inflammation remains confined within the vascular wall. It causes injury and necrosis of the vascular wall, thrombotic occlusion of the vascular lumen, and ultimately organ ischemia. The vasculitic lesions tend to be multifocal and spread throughout the vascular tree in different pathological patterns. The symptoms reflect the distribu-tion, the extent, and the tempo of the vasculitic process. Single or multiple organs may be involved, resulting in a wide variety of clinical manifesta-tions. The natural course depends on the immune mechanisms underlying the vasculitic process and the reparative response of the affected vessels.

Vasculitides are a heterogeneous group of disorders which share inflam-matory pathology but differ in etiology, pathogenesis, and clinical manifes-tations (Lie, 1994). They can occur as systemic diseases affecting multiple organs (systemic vasculitis) or as isolated syndromes localized to a single organ (non-systemic vasculitis). Both systemic and non-systemic vas-culitides can be associated with a wide range of conditions that could be directly responsible for the vasculitic pathology (secondary vasculitis), or

Table 30.1 Names and definitions of vasculitides adopted by Chapel Hill Consensus Conference on the Nomenclature of Systemic Vasculitis[a] (Jennette et al., 1994)

Large vessel vasculitis	Giant-cell (temporal) arteritis	Granulomatous arteritis of the aorta and its major branches, with a predilection for extracranial branches of carotid artery. *Often involves the temporal artery. Usually occurs in patients older than 50 and often is associated with polymyalgia rheumatica*
	Takayasu's arteritis	Granulomatous inflammation of the aorta and its major branches. *Usually occurs in patients below 50*
Medium-sized vessel vasculitis	Polyarteritis nodosa[b]	Necrotizing inflammation of the medium-sized or small (classic polyarteritis nodosa) arteries without glomerulonephritis or vasculitis in arterioles, capillaries, or venules
	Kawasaki disease	Arteritis involving large, medium-sized, and small arteries, and associated with mucocutaneous lymph node syndrome. Coronary arteries are often involved. Aorta and veins may be involved. *Usually occurs in children*
Small vessel vasculitis	Wegener's granulomatosis[c]	Granulomatous inflammation involving the respiratory tract, and necrotizing vasculitis affecting small to medium-sized vessels (e.g. capillaries, venules, arterioles, and arteries). *Necrotizing glomerulonephritis is common*
	Churg–Strauss syndrome[c]	Eosinophil-rich and granulomatous involving the respiratory tract, and necrotizing vasculitis affecting small to medium-sized vessels, associated with asthma and eosinophilia
	Microscopic polyangiitis[b,c] (microscopic polyarteritis)	Necrotizing vasculitis, with few or no immune deposits, affecting small vessels (i.e. capillaries, venules, or arterioles). *Necrotizing arteritis involving small and medium-sized arteries may be present. Necrotizing glomerulonephritis is very common. Pulmonary capillaritis often occurs*
	Hennoch–Schönlein purpura	Vasculitis, with IgA-dominant immune deposits, affecting small vessels (i.e. capillaries, venules, or arterioles). *Typically involves skin, gut, and glomeruli, and is associated with arthralgia and arthritis*
	Essential cryoglobulinemic vasculitis	Vasculitis, with cryoglobulin immune deposits, affecting small vesels (i.e. capillaries, venules, or arterioles) and associated with cryoglobulins in serum. *Skin and glomeruli are often involved*
	Cutaneous leukocytoclastic angiitis	Isolated cutaneous leukocytoclastic angiitis without systemic vasculitis and glomerulonephritis

[a]Large vessels refer to the aorta and the largest branches directed toward major body regions (e.g. to the extremities and the head and neck). Medium-sized vessels refer to the main visceral arteries (e.g. renal, coronary, and mesenteric arteries). Small vessels refer to venules, capillaries, arterioles, and the intraparenchymal distal arterial radicals that connect with arterioles. Some small and large vessel vasculitides may involve medium-sized arteries, but large and medium-sized vessel vasculitides do not involve vessels smaller than arteries. Essential components are represented by normal type; italicized type represents usual, but not essential, components.
[b]Preferred term.
[c]Strongly associated with antineutrophil cytoplasmic antibodies.

have no identifiable cause (idiopathic primary vasculitis). Different vasculitic syndromes tend to involve specific parts of the vascular tree. Some vasculitides have a predilection to large vessels, such as the aorta and its major branches. Others affect predominantly medium-sized muscular and visceral vessels, or the small vessels such as arterioles, capillaries, and venules. Vessel size strongly correlates with the underlying pathology and the immune mechanisms involved. Large vessel vasculitides, for example, are characterized by chronic glaucomatous inflammation, whereas medium-sized vessel vasculitides are predominantly necrotizing with a pleomorphic inflammatory infiltration. Small vessel vasculitides are typically antibody-mediated and could be either granulomatous or necrotizing.

There is a significant variation and overlap of clinicopathologic manifestations among the vasculitic syndromes. The diagnosis of the primary vasculitic syndromes can be made based on diagnostic and classification criteria proposed by the 1994 Chapel Hill Consensus Conference (Table 30.1) and the 1990 Conference of the American College of Rheumatology (Hunder et al., 1990; Jennette et al., 1994). Both, however, address only seven vasculitic syndromes and do not include the large subgroups of secondary and non-systematic vasculitides. The lack of comprehensiveness as well as the frequent critiques of these and previous classification systems simply reflect the elusive nature of the vasculitic disorders (Lie, 1991, 1994). At present, there is no sufficient knowledge to classify the vasculitides based on pathophysiological parameters; therefore practical approaches are usually employed.

Central and peripheral nervous system (CNS and PNS) vasculitides are serious and life-threatening disorders causing ischemic injury in distribution of the affected vessels. Neurologic vasculitic syndromes can occur in isolation, confined to the nervous system, or as a part of a systemic disease (Table 30.2). The neurologic symptoms in the latter case may precede the systemic disease and represent its main or sole clinical manifestation. The diagnosis of CNS and PNS vasculitides is challenging because these syndromes lack pathognomonic clinical features and routine laboratory investigations are often normal or non-specific. The invasive tests, such as angiographic imaging or tissue biopsy, the so-called 'gold standards', have low sensitivity and specificity, and represent independent risk factors for morbidity and mortality. In addition to the extensiveness and the associated risks, the diagnostic evaluation should be done quickly because vasculitides of the nervous system are treatable disorders. Early diagnosis and timely intervention are the two major factors affecting the disease outcome. Conversely, incorrect diagnosis and inappropriate exposure of a patient to highly toxic immunosuppressants could have devastating consequences. Long-term follow-up is required for clinical monitoring of disease progression and the adverse effects of immunotherapy.

Vasculitides of the nervous system are challenging and enigmatic disorders. The purpose of this chapter is to discuss the current understanding and the latest advancements in this field. One may find additional details on the subject in a number of excellent reviews (Kissel and Mendell, 1992;

Calabrese et al., 1997; Said, 1999; Moore, 1999; Griffin, 2001; Siva, 2001; Gold et al., 2003; Younger, 2004; Kelley, 2004).

Pathogenic mechanisms

Vasculitides are generally considered to be autoimmune disorders triggered by an exogenous pathogen, most commonly infection, or immune sensitization to a self antigen (Fauci et al., 1978; Jennette et al., 1994; Lie, 1997). Specific immune mechanisms include immune complex deposition and complement activation, autoantibody-mediated cytotoxicity, and the delayed-type hypersensitivity reaction with granuloma formation. However, the pathogenesis of the vasculitides is complex and no single immune mechanism can explain the disease process. Instead, multiple mechanisms, immune and genetic, are involved and may act simultaneously or sequentially with variable predominance, depending on the specific vasculitic syndrome (Sundy and Haynes, 1995).

The vascular tissue, often regarded as a passive target, is actively involved in the inflammatory process (Weyand, 2002). The endothelial cells forming the lining of the vascular lumen (intima) under normal conditions provide a non-adhesive and antithrombotic surface. In response to inflammatory signals they undergo significant functional changes and produce a variety of effector molecules facilitating the recruitment and transmigration of inflammatory cells (Cohen and Kallenberg, 1997). Similarly, the smooth muscle cells forming the medial layer (media) have the unique ability to switch from a contractile to a synthetic phenotype acquiring proliferative and migratory capabilities in response to injurious signals (Weyand and Goronzy, 1999). In vasculitis, immune-mediated injury triggers a hyperproliferative reaction of intima and media, which is often maladaptive in nature and leads to irreversible structural changes and vascular occlusion. The outermost soft tissue layer (adventitia) also plays a significant role in the vasculitic inflammation. Its capillary network (vasa vasorum) provides a port of entry for pathogens and inflammatory cells, and its resident macrophages, a site for antigen recognition (Cid et al., 2000). Finally, certain features of the vascular cells, such as heterogeneity in the antigen repertoire, and differential susceptibility to injury or infection, may account for the characteristic vessel-specific predilection of the vasculitic syndromes (Zetter, 1981; Cid et al., 2000; Sneller, 2002). Thus, both the immune mechanisms involved and the pattern of the vascular response to injury determine the vascular pathology and the outcome of the vasculitic process (Table 30.3).

Autoantibodies

Autoantibodies play an important role in the pathogenesis of primary vasculitic syndromes. They are pathogenic with pleomorphic effects and serve as markers of specific vasculitic syndromes. Two principal autoantibodies

Table 30.2 Practical classification of the vasculitides affecting the nervous system[a]

Primary vasculitides	Systemic vasculitides	Giant-cell (temporal) arteritis, Takayasu's arteritis, polyarteritis nodosa, Kawasaki disease, Wegener's granulomatosis, Churg–Strauss syndrome, microscopic polyangiitis, Hennoch–Schönlein purpura
	Non-systemic vasculitis	Primary angiitis of the central nervous system (PACNS), non-systemic vasculitic neuropathy
Secondary vasculitides	Connective tissue disorders	Systemic lupus erythematosus, mixed connective tissue disorder, rheumatoid arthritis, Sjögren's syndrome, Behçet's disease
	Infections	HIV, HSV, CMV, VZV, T. pallidum, B. burgdorferi, S. aureus, rickettsiae, Aspergillus, Candida, Coccidioides, Mucormycetes
	Other inflammatory disorders	Sarcoidosis, inflammatory bowel disease, Cogan's syndrome, familial Mediterranean fever, diabetes mellitus, graft-versus-host disease
	Drugs and substances of abuse	Cocaine, amphetamines, heroin, vaccines, interferon-α, antibiotics
	Malignancies	Hodgkin's lymphoma, non-Hodgkin's lymphoma, lymphomatoid granulomatosis, renal cancer, lung cancer

[a]This classification is based on previously proposed systems (Kissel and Mendell, 1992; Lie, 1994, 1997; Calabrese et al., 1997; Moore, 1998) and modified for the purpose of this chapter.

Table 30.3 Pathogenic mechanism of vasculitis[a]

Autoantibodies	Antineutrophil cytoplasmic antibodies (ANCA)
	Anti-endothelial cell antibodies (AECA)
Immune complex formation	Exogenous antigens (HBV, HCV, drugs) cryoglobulins
	Abnormalities of the complement system
	FcR polymorphisms
	Viral FcR-like proteins
Endothelial cell activation	Cytokines (IL1, TNF-α, IFN-γ)
	Products of oxygen metabolism
	Autoantibodies (ANCA, AECA)
Angiogenesis	Cytokines (TGF-β, IL8, VEGF, FGF, PDGF)
	Ischemia
Vaso-occlusion	Cytokines (IL1, TNF-α)
	Endothelial cell injury (neutrophils, ANCA)
	Tissue factor
	Down-regulation of thrombomodulin, NO, PGI_2, tPA
	Antiphospholipid antibodies
	Granuloma formation
Granuloma formation	CD4 lymphocytes, macrophages, giant cells
	Cytokines (IFN-γ, PDGF, VEGF)
	Hyperplasia of intima and media

[a]Specific details and references can be found in the text.

have been described: antineutrophilic antibodies and anti-endothelial cell antibodies (AECA). Antineutrophilic cytoplasmic antibodies (ANCA) are a classic vasculitic finding associated with a group of primary vasculitides including Wegener's granulomatosis, microscopic polyarteritis, and Churg–Strauss syndrome, also known as ANCA syndromes (Seo and Stone, 2004). Described as autoantibodies reacting with the cytoplasm of neutrophils and monocytes in the early 1980s, they were classified, based on immunostaining patterns produced on ethanol-fixed granulocytes, as cytoplasmic (cANCA) and perinuclear (pANCA) (van der Woode et al., 1985). ANCA are primarily immunoglobulin G (IgG) molecules of IgG1 and IgG4 subclasses, although IgM isotypes have also been found. It is probably of historical interest that these patterns are, in a sense, a fortunate fixation artifact because only ethanol fixation produces such a differentiation. Nevertheless, cANCA and pANCA bind specific antigens and have a distinct association with particular vasculitic syndromes. Proteinase 3 (P3), a serine protease contained in the azurophilic granules of the neutrophils, was identified as the primary antigen of cANCA (Jennette et al., 1990). Myeloperoxidase (MPO), another azurophilic enzyme of the neutrophils, best known for its role in the generation of reactive oxygen species, was recognized as the counterpart of pANCA (Falk and Jennette, 1988). Some occasional reactivity to other azurophilc proteins (bactericidal permeability-increasing protein and human leukocyte elastase) has also been reported (Hoffman and Specks, 1998).

Anti-P3/cANCA is strongly associated with Wegener's granulomatosis, with high sensitivity and specificity for this disorder. The reported sensitivity and specificity are approximately 90% and 98%, respectively (Cohen Tarvaert et al., 1989; Nölle et al., 1989). Anti-P3/cANCA also occurs in 20–30% of patients with microscopic polyangiitis and in a minority of patients with Churg–Strauss syndrome (Cohen Tarvaert et al., 1991). The titer of anti-P3/cANCA correlates with the disease activity as its rise is associated with reactivation of the disease, and persistence following remission represents a risk factor for a relapse (Cohen Tarvaert et al., 1989). Whereas anti-P3/cANCA is primarily associated with Wegener's granulomatosis, anti-MPO/pANCA has more diverse presentations. In Wegener's granulomatosis, most of the patients who test negative for anti-P3/cANCA are positive for anti-MPO/pANCA (Cohen Tarvaert et al., 1990). About 60% of the

patients with microscopic polyangiitis and Churg–Strauss syndrome are positive for this autoantibody. Anti-MPO/pANCA has been reported in patients with systemic lupus erythematosus (SLE) and drug-induced vasculitic syndromes associated with antithyroid and antihypertensive medications (Merkel, 1998).

ANCA and their antigens exhibit some unusual functional characteristics. P3 and MPO, besides being part of the neutrophil destructive machinery, under certain conditions promote cellular activation (Falk et al., 1990; Seo and Stone, 2004). Priming of neutrophils and monocytes with a low concentration of interleukin 1 (IL-1), interleukin 8 (IL-8), and tumor necrosis factor-alpha (TNF-α), instead of causing degranulation and release of these enzymes induces their surface membrane expression. These so-called 'primed' neutrophils can be further activated by ANCA upon binding to P3 and MPO. This activation mechanism also requires cross-linking of the ANCA Fc fragments and the Fcγ receptors (Porges et al., 1994), and β2 integrin signaling dependent on a contact to a cell surface (Reumaux et al., 1995), e.g. endothelial cells. Neutrophilic activation results in degranulation, the release of enzymes, reactive oxygen radicals, and inflammatory mediators, and damage to the endothelial cells. ANCA can stimulate monocytes in a similar fashion, since P3 and MPO are constituents of their granules. ANCA trigger the release of a variety of inflammatory mediators, including monocyte chemoattractant protein-1 (MCP-1), which plays a role in granuloma formation by amplification of local monocyte recruitment (Casselman et al., 1995). P3 and MPO, released by ANCA-activated neutrophils and monocytes, exert a direct effect on endothelial cells. Both being cationic molecules, they serve as 'planted' antigens on the surface of the endothelial cells, resulting in antibody-mediated damage or immune complex deposition. Additional potential effects may include direct ANCA-mediated endothelial cell activation, up-regulation of adhesion molecules, and expression of IL-1 and platelet-activating factor (PAF) (de Brandt et al., 1997). The significance of these activating mechanisms is twofold: ANCA augment and sustain neutrophil/monocyte-mediated inflammatory reactions, which may not otherwise reach the critical threshold, and localize the inflammatory injury, in particular, to the vascular wall and endothelial cells.

Anti-endothelial cell antibodies (AECA) are another common finding in vasculitides (Meroni, 1999). Since the first report in the 1970s (Lindquist and Osterland, 1971), AECA have been demonstrated in Takayasu's and giant-cell arteritides, and Kawasaki, Wegener's, and Churg–Strauss diseases. Their prevalence among patients with vasculitis is relatively high, appearing in more than 50%, and in the case of Takayasu's patients in up to 95% (Meroni, 1999). AECA are immunoglobulins consisting of IgG, IgM, and IgA isotypes. They bind endothelial cell membrane molecules mainly through their F(ab)2 portion, but Fc-mediated binding in paticular is also possible. AECA most often display polyclonal imunoreactivity and cross-react with multiple EC antigens from different organs (skin, kidney, omentum, and brain). Most of these antigens are not well defined but appear to be conserved among species (Del Papa et al., 1994). Some of the endothelial cell antigens are constitutively expressed on the cytoplasmic membrane with molecular weights ranging from 25–200 kDa. Others are inducible, requiring cytokine activation of the endothelial cells. Finally, antigens for AECA could be molecules such as DNA, β2-glycoprotein I, P3, and MPO, which bind to the endothelial cells via charge-mediated mechanisms, or extracellular matrix proteins.

AECA exhibit an important restriction in their binding activity depending on the vascular origin of the endothelial cells (Praptonik et al., 2001; Shoenfield, 2002). It appears that AECA from large vessel vasculitides, such as Takaysu's arteritis, bind exclusively to macrovascular endothelial cells but not to microvascular endothelial cells (Banks, 1999). In contrast, AECA from small vessel vasculitides, such as Behçet's disease, bind predominantly to microvascular endothelial cells and very little to macrovascular endothelial cells (Cervera et al., 1994). Certain disease-specific antigens have been isolated, such as a 125 kDa protein in Wegener's granulomatosis and a 200 kDa protein in SLE (Del Papa et al., 1994). AECA binding may result in direct endothelial cell activation, manifested by increased expression of adhesion molecules such as E-selectin and ICAM-1, secretion of IL-6, IL-8, MCP-1 (Del Papa *et al.*, 1996), and von Willebrand factor, and nuclear translocation of NF-κB (Banks, 1999). Alternatively, AECA can trigger antibody-dependent/complement-mediated vascular damage (Tripathy *et al.*, 2001). The role of AECA in the vasculitides remains unclear, but their binding predilection and pro-inflammatory affect correlate with the vascular pattern of the vasculitides (Praptonik *et al.*, 2001).

Immune complexes

Immune complex-mediated inflammation is the most common pathogenic mechanism in secondary vasculitic syndromes. An immune complex consists of a combination of antibody and antigen, and represents a normal immune mechanism for antigen clearance. Under normal circumstances, immune complexes activate the complement and incorporate C3b, which in turn binds the complement receptor-1 (CR1) on erythrocytes. Erythrocyte-bound immune complexes are transported to the liver and spleen, where they are eliminated by the resident macrophages via their Fc receptors (FcR). Under pathological circumstances, such as excess of antigen, complement deficiency, or aberrant expression or dysfunction of the FcR, the immune complexes overwhelm or escape the elimination mechanisms and are passively deposited in the vascular wall beneath the endothelium (Prodeus *et al.*, 1998). Once localized within the vascular wall, the immune complexes cause vascular injury by many different mechanisms. Among these are complement activation and formation of the membrane attack complex C5b–9, which directly damage the endothelial cells, and production of the chemotactic factors C3a and C5a, which attract leukocytes. In addition, immune complexes can directly bind to FcR- or CR-bearing leukocytes. Activation of endothelial cells and leukocytes induces increased expression of adhesion molecules and the release of cytokines. Activated leukocytes adhere to the endothelial surface and penetrate the vessel wall, where they phagocytose the immune complexes and release lysosomal enzymes and oxygen radicals. The inflammatory process activates the extrinsic arm of the coagulation cascade, leading to thrombosis and occlusion of the vascular wall.

Hepatitis B virus (HBV)-associated polyarteritis nodosa is a classic example of immune complex-mediated vasculitis (Gocke *et al.*, 1970; Dienstag, 1981). In most cases, chronic HBV infection-associated polyarteritis nodosa (PAN) occurs within 8 months of the initial viral exposure. All patients are HBsAg-positive and a majority of them are HBeAg and HBV DNA-positive, findings reflecting the underlying active viral replication (Guillevin *et al.*, 1995). Affected vessels demonstrate areas of fibrinoid necrosis and deposition of immunoglobulins, HBsAg, and complement (Gupta and Kohler, 1984). A variant of immune complex formation is hepatitis C virus (HCV)-associated cryoglobulinic vasculitis, previously known as 'essential mixed crioglobulinemia' (Meltzer *et al.*, 1966). The immune response to HCV induces the generation of autoantibodies against the Fc portion of immunoglobulins. A majority of the elicited autoantibodies have the Wa idiotype, presumably recognizing a cross-reactive epitope shared by HCV and the immunoglobulins (Newkirk *et al.*, 1986; Angelo, 1998). Immune complexes of immunoglobulin, virus, and anti-Fc Wa idiotype antibody exhibit the characteristic property of precipitating in temperatures below 37°C and re-dissolving on rewarming (cryoglobulins) (Ferri *et al.*, 2002). Cryoglobulinic vasculitis, due to vascular deposition of cryoglobulin immune complexes and complement, affects most commonly the cold exposed extremities and skin (Lamprecht *et al.*, 1990; Ferri *et al.*, 2002). Pharmacological agents, especially drugs of abuse such as heroin and amphetamines, are another important cause of immune complex-mediated vasculitis. Heroin addicts often have increased levels of circulating immune complexes associated with hypergammaglobulinemia, low C3 and C4 levels, and a variety of false positive serology. Immune complexes containing microcrystalline cellulose and magnesium silicate (talc) are frequent findings after parenteral injections of crushed methamphethamine tablets (Burst, 1997).

The clearance of immune complexes from the bloodstream depends on the efficiency of the complement-mediated processing. As mentioned above, complement binding to the circulating immune complex maintains them in a soluble form and provides a ligand for the erythrocyte CR1, which facilitates their removal from the circulation (Schifferi *et al.*, 1982). If adequate complement fixation fails, immune complexes can be taken up by the endothelial cells and sequestered in the vascular wall (Beynon *et al.*, 1994). Low levels of complement, as seen in patients with hereditary deficiencies of early complement components, especially C2 and C4, promote enhanced tissue deposition of immune complexes (Walport *et al.*, 1997). Similarly, certain genetic polymorphisms of the CR1, e.g. allotype C, 250 kDa, characterized by reduced binding affinity to C3b, are associated with abnormal immune complex transportation and processing (Van Dyne *et al.*, 1987). Both complement deficiencies and allotype C CR1 polymorphism are associated with immune complex disease and SLE-like syndromes (Molina, 2002). While important, these inherited conditions contribute marginally to the incidence of SLE and immune complex diseases in the population. The majority of patients with SLE exhibit acquired abnormalities of the complement system, such as hypocomplementemia and reduced expression of CR1 and CR2. Complement levels usually rise during an inflammatory reaction as a part of the initial acute-phase response, and may remain elevated until the reaction completes. In immune complex diseases, including SLE and a number of secondary vasculitides, the available complement is consumed by the reaction due to the activation of the classical pathway by the immune complexes, and the measured complement levels C3, C4, and CH50 (total functional hemolytic complement) are significantly decreased. In SLE, serial measurements of complement levels are particularly useful in monitoring disease activity, as the complement levels decrease just before the disease flare and return to normal levels when the disease activity diminishes (Hebert *et al.*, 1991). The expression of CR1 by erythrocytes, polymorphonuclear leukocytes, and B cells, and of CR2 by B cells, is significantly reduced in SLE patients. The low cell surface expression of this receptor appears to be an acquired phenomenon that correlates with the clinical progression rather than a primary genetic defect (Prodeus *et al.*, 1998). In addition to immune complex clearance, CR1 and CR2 are involved in regulation of the B-cell activation and differentiation, the generation of immunological memory, and immunoglobulin class switching (Molina, 2002). Thus, acquired abnormalities of the complement system may modify the immune response and accelerate the autoimmune process.

FcR, particularly the gamma subtype (FcγR), play an important role in the immune regulation of the antibody-mediated response. Functionally, they are classified into two categories: activating (FcγRI, FcγRIIa, and FcγRIII) characterized by the presence of an immunoreceptor tyrosine-based activation motif (ITAM) in their cytoplasmic domain, and inhibitory (FcγRIIb), containing an immunoreceptor tyrosine-based inhibitory motif (ITIM) (Ravetch and Bolland, 2001). Activating FcγRs are found on most leukocytes—monocytes, granulocytes, and NK cells—and initiate phagocytosis, antibody-dependent cellular cytotoxicity (ADCC), degranulation, and the release of inflammatory mediators. By contrast, FcγRIIb is expressed mainly by macrophages and B-cells, and down-regulates their function. In the context of vasculitic disorders, FcγR appear to be important in several aspects. Dysfunction of the inhibitory FcγRIIb, associated with abnormal B-cell responses to stimulation, has been found in patients with SLE (Enyedy *et al.*, 2001). Structural variations of the FcR binding sites, which alter their affinity for IgG, ultimately affect the receptor-triggered cellular responses, particularly phagocytosis, ADCC and immune complex removal (Ludo van der Pol and van der Winke, 1998). Polymorphic variants of the activating FcγRIIa (Arg/His at position 131) and FcγRIIIa (Phe/ Val at position 158) have been described in systemic vasculitides. FcγRIIa-Arg131 and FcγRIIIa-Phe158 homozygotes exhibit low affinity for IgG1 and IgG2/3, respectively, and inefficient antibody-mediated phagocytosis and immune complex clearance. These polymorphisms appear to be over-represented in patients with rheumatoid arthritis, SLE, Sjögren's syndrome, and cryoglobulinemia (Fossati *et al.*, 2001). FcγRIIa-His131 homozygotes exhibit high affinity for IgG2/3 and enhanced antibody-mediated phagocytosis, ADCC, and neutrophil activation. This phenotype, alone or in combination with FcγRIIIa-Phe158, has been associated with Wegener's granulomatosis and perhaps underlines ANCA cellular effects (Dijstelbloem *et al.*, 1999).

Besides modulating leukocyte activation, FcγR are also involved in leukocyte adhesion to the endothelial cells. Activating FcγRs induce the expression of CD11b/CD18 adhesion molecules, facilitating leukocyte rolling and firm adhesion to endothelial cells (Kocher et al., 1998). Leukocytes can adhere to endothelial cells via FcγR in areas of immune complex deposition. Alternatively, endothelial cells expressing FcR or target antigens could capture antibodies on their surface and recruit Fc-bearing leukocytes (Ober et al., 2004). Endothelial cells infected with herpes simplex virus (HSV), varicella zoster virus (VZV), or cytomegalovirus (CMV) express virally encoded proteins with Fc binding activity (MacCormac and Grundy, 1996; Litwin and Grose, 1992). These proteins lack any homology with human FcR and their ligation does not elicit a known specific cellular response (MacCormac and Grundy, 1996). They, however, are capable of capturing circulating immune complexes and promoting leukocyte adhesion to the endothelial cells.

Endothelial cell activation

Endothelial cells are dynamic and functionally active cellular constituents of the blood vessels. Normal 'quiescent' endothelial cells maintain a non-adhesive and antithrombotic state important for the local blood circulation. Under inflammatory conditions, however, they undergo substantial morphological and functional changes, such as the expression of adhesion molecules and immunologically relevant molecules, the activation of pro-coagulant properties, and an increase in permeability for leukocytes and plasma components. These changes are collectively termed 'endothelial cell activation' (Pober and Cotran, 1990). Endothelial response to inflammatory stimuli leads to amplification of the inflammatory process and, eventually, to vessel damage and occlusion.

The mechanism of endothelial cell activation in vasculitis is complex (Cid et al., 2004). On the one hand, endothelial cells are a target of locally released cytokines and other biologically active mediators. On the other hand, they are a significant source of such mediators, depending on their functional state. Pro-inflammatory cytokines control the expression of several immunologically important molecules, including intercellular adhesion molecule-1 (ICAM-1), vascular adhesion molecule-1 (VCAM-1), endothelial adhesion molecule-1 (ELAM-1), and major histocompatibility complex (MCH) Class I and II molecules. Cytokines such as IL-1 and TNF-α up-regulate the expression of ICAM-1, VCAM-1, and ELAM-1, whereas IFN-γ increases the expression of ICAM-1, ELAM-1, and MHC Class I, and II molecules (Dore-Duffy et al., 1994; Huynh et al., 1995). IFN-β and TGF-β have minimal effect on quiescent endothelial cells, but do inhibit cytokine-mediated activation of endothelial cells (Dore-Duffy et al., 1994; Farby et al., 1995; Huynh et al., 1995). It is possible that the balance of such cytokines is involved in endothelial cell regulation and the perpetuation of the vasculitic inflammatory process. Quiescent endothelial cells express a minimal amount, if any, of pro-inflammatory cytokines and chemokines. Their repertoire, however, is altered upon exposure to activating stimuli, and the secretion of cytokines and chemokines such as IL-1, IL-6, TNF-α, IL-8, RANTES, and Croa is significantly increased (Balabanov and Dore-Duffy, 1998; Mackay, 2001). Endothelial cell-produced cytokines and chemokines selectively attract and recruit leukocytes bearing complementary receptors. Vasculitic inflammation may utilize specific activating stimuli. As mentioned above, autoantibodies such as ANCA and AECA exhibit the unique feature of directly activating endothelial cells (de Brandt et al., 1997; Praptonik et al., 2001; Cid et al., 2004). In addition, hydrogen peroxide and other products of oxygen metabolism could also increase the expression of selective immunologically relevant molecules including ICAM-1 and MHC Class I molecules (Bradley et al., 1993).

The functional significance of endothelial activation is three-fold: leukocyte transmigration, angiogenesis, and vascular occlusion. Leukocyte adhesion and migration across the endothelium are multistep processes governed by the interactions of complementary adhesion molecules expressed on the cell surfaces of leukocytes and endothelial cells (Strominger, 1995). The first step consists of the 'rolling' of leukocytes on the endothelium, which involves leukocyte L-selectin and the endothelial E-selectin adhesion molecules. Selectins allow leukocytes to roll in the direction of the chemotactic signal displayed by endothelial cells. The second step involves leukocyte β2-integrins, such as the CD11/CD18 complex, and the endothelial ICAM-1 and VCAM-1 adhesion molecules, which account for strong leukocyte adhesion and spreading over the endothelium. In the third step, the leukocytes migrate through the endothelium following homotypic interactions between leukocyte and endothelial PECAM-1 (Strominger, 1995). Certain interactions are preferentially utilized depending on the leukocyte cell type. For example, whereas CD11a/CD18 (LFA-1)/ICAM-1 and Sialyl-Le*/E-selectin interactions are involved in neutrophil migration, VLA4/VCAM-1 and LFA-1/ICAM-1 interactions appear to be critical for lymphocyte recruitment (Hickey, 1999). Leukocytes further interact with the extra-cellular matrix proteins via β_1, β_2, and β_5 integrins. Integrin-mediated interactions with endothelial cells and extracellular matrix proteins trigger production of matrix metalloproteinases (MMPs) by leukocytes, which allows basement membrane disruption and invasion of the surrounding extracellular matrix (Romanic et al., 1997).

Angiogenesis

Angiogenesis, or new vessel formation, is a common finding in vasculitic inflammation. Poorly understood, angiogenesis appears to play a dual role. When present in small vessel vasculitides at the distal portions of affected medium-sized or large vessels, angiogenesis may reflect a compensatory mechanism counterbalancing ongoing ischemia. In giant-cell arteritis, for instance, the magnitude of the angiogenic response is inversely proportional to the risk of developing ischemic complications (Cid et al., 2002). On the other hand, when angiogenesis occurs in the adventitial and medial layers of affected medium-sized and large vessels, e.g. giant-cell arteritis and PAN, the newly formed vessels express adhesion molecules and provide new, and in fact preferential, sides for leukocyte invasion of the vascular wall (Coll-Vincent et al., 1998; Cid et al., 2000). In addition, these new vessels could be a significant source of cytokines, chemokines, and growth factors, amplifying and perpetuating the inflammatory process. Several angiogenic factors, such vascular endothelial growth factor (VEGF), fibroblast growth factor (FGF-2), IL-8, and thymosin β4, have been detected in temporal arteries of patients with giant-cell arteritis (Cid et al., 2000). Other factors such as TGF-β and TNF-α, also found in such lesions, could play a regulatory role. The dual role of angiogenesis is also illustrated by the fact that inhibitors of angiogenesis worsen the complications of certain vasculitic syndromes and improve others (Brahn et al., 1999).

Vascular occlusion

Vasculitic inflammation frequently leads to vessel occlusion with an ensuing ischemia of the supplied organs. Ischemic complications result in organ dysfunction and major disabilities. Endothelial cell activation and acquisition of a dysfunctional phenotype are associated with dysregulation of the hemostatic system of the vasculature. Several inflammatory cytokines and growth factors present in the wall of the affected vessels have pro-coagulant and pro-thrombotic effects. IL-1 and TNF-α, for instance, induce endothelial cell expression of tissue factor, P-selectin, and platelet-endothelial cell adhesion molecule-1, and the release of von Willebrand factor (vWF) stored in the Weibel–Palade bodies (Kirchhofer et al., 1994). Tissue factor is a cell surface glycoprotein and the principal initiator of the coagulation cascade (Rapaport and Rao, 1992). It forms a complex with Factor VII, which activates Factors IX and X. Activated Factors X and V form a complex on the surface of the platelets and convert prothrombin to thrombin, which in turn cleaves fibrinogen and generates fibrin and the fibrin clot. P-selectin mediates platelet adhesion to endothelial cells, while vWF facilitates their adherence to the basement membrane and subendothelial extracellular matrix. The latter also serves as a bridge between the platelet GpIa-IX receptor and the collagen fibrils. GpIa-IX receptor activation triggers a cascade of intracellular events, which leads to platelet activation, secretion of variety of hemostatic factors, and platelet aggregation (Furie and Furie, 1992).

Vascular thrombosis could be a direct consequence of endothelial cell injury and exposure of the extracellular matrix to coagulation factors. In immune complex-mediated vasculitis, endothelial cell morphology is altered and the luminal endothelium is eventually destroyed. Complement-mediated cell lysis and neutrophil-mediated damage are the main mechanisms in these processes (Kissel et al., 1989). ANCA stimulation of neutrophils results specifically in endothelial cell injury since it requires cell–cell contact and β_2 integrin signaling. In addition, the release of neutrophilic MPO and PR3 may directly induce endothelial cell apoptosis (Reumaux et al., 1995). Endothelial cell injury is also associated with down-regulation and loss of endothelial-derived relaxation and antithrombogenic factors such as nitric oxide, prostacyclin I_2, thrombomodulin, and tissue-plasminogen activator. Thombomodulin, for example, is an endothelial cell surface glycoprotein that inactivates thrombin, is internalized in response to injury, and is released as an inactive molecule in the bloodstream (Krafte-Jacobs and Brilli, 1998).

Dysfunction of the endothelial cell antithrombotic system could also occur in a setting of antiphospholipid antibody syndrome, which is often associated with SLE and other vasculitic syndromes. This syndrome classically presents with a hypercoagulable state and persistently prolonged prothrombin time (PT) and partial thromboplastin time (PTT) which cannot be corrected even if normal plasma is added to the reaction. Antiphospholipid antibodies, lupus anticoagulant, and anticardiolipin antibody, though they do not directly cause vasculitis, induce endothelial cell activation and impair their antithrombotic function (Meroni et al., 2004). Additionally, they disrupt the anionic shield of endothelial cells and interfere with protein C and protein S activation (Rand, 2002). The functional significance of the protein C–protein S complex is to inactivate Factors Va and VIIIa and to block the coagulation cascade and the formation of thrombin (Furie and Furie, 1992).

Granulomatous inflammation

One of the histological hallmarks of vascular lesions in giant-cell (temporal) arteritis, Takayasu's arteritis, and Wegener's granulomatosis is the presence of granulomatous inflammation with multinucleated giant cells. The term granuloma refers to a nodularly organized aggregation of mononuclear cells or a collection of activated macrophages surrounded by a rim of lymphocytes and multinucleated giant cells. Granulomatous inflammation occurs in response to chronic inflammatory stimuli, such as infectious intracellular pathogens or the presence of inert material, when the host defense mechanisms, failing to eliminate the pathogen, attempt to confine their spread (Flynn and Chan, 2001). This pattern of inflammation, also known as delayed type hypersensitivity (DTH), is initiated and maintained by CD4 helper cells of Th1 phenotype. The antigen-primed Th1 cells recirculate through different body compartments until they recognize the antigen presented by perivascular macrophages (Hickey, 1999). Th1 cells become fully activated and secrete cytokines/chemokines, attracting additional cell types such as naïve T cells and monocytes to the site of antigen presence. The exact pattern of chemokine expression is not completely known but RANTES, MIP1-α, MCP-1, and IL-8 are likely to be involved (Orme and Cooper, 1999). Following the accumulation of lymphocytes and macrophages, the inflammatory lesion begins to take a granulomatous form, largely depending on the presence of IFN-γ, IL-12, and TNF-α. Produced by activated Th1 cells, IFN-γ has a number of effector functions relevant to granuloma formation, such as promotion of Th1 cell differentiation, endothelial cell activation, and macrophage activation (Flynn and Chan, 2001). Th1 cell differentiation, and therefore IFN-γ production, is induced by the IL-12 secreted by antigen-presenting cells (Altate et al., 1998). TNF-α is produced by the macrophages and has a broad range of activities, including up-regulation of adhesion molecules on endothelial cells, macrophage activation, and induction of cellular apoptosis (Bean et al., 1999). In addition, it plays an important role in controlling the local cellular traffic in granuloma lesions. Eventually, the granuloma becomes encapsulated by a fibrotic rim and, as in cases of certain infections, e.g. Mycobacterium tuberculosis, develops central necrosis (Flynn and Chan, 2001).

The general mechanism of granuloma formation correlates with the biopsy findings from vasculitic lesions. In giant-cell arteritis, CD4 cells are the predominant lymphocytic subtype and, most importantly, share the same T-cell receptor (TCR) rearrangement pattern, indicating clonal expansion (Weyand et al., 1994, 2004). T cells from the vasculitic lesions produce IFN-γ and IL-2, a pattern typical for an activated CD4 helper cell of Th1 phenotype. In Wegener's granulomatosis, the infiltrating lymphocytes produce levels of IFN-γ 20-fold higher than controls, which is accompanied by a significant increase of macrophage expression of IL-12 and TNF-α (Csemok et al., 1999; Komocsi et al., 2002). These data indicate that the granulomatous inflammation in vasculitis is a Th1 CD4-mediated and antigen-driven process. Interaction of CD4 cells with tissue-infiltrating macrophages via IFN-γ results in granuloma formation and the appearance of multinucleated giant cells (Csemok et al., 1999). Histologically in giant-cell arteritis, the CD4 cells are localized in the adventitia, the most likely site of antigen recognition, whereas the activated macrophages and the multinucleated giant cells lie in the media of the vessel. The adventitia also contains IL-1 and IL-6 producing macrophages supporting T-cell activation (Weyand et al., 1997). Granulomatous lesions, once formed, are injurious to the vascular tissue, due mostly to the capacity of macrophages to produce reactive oxygen species and MMPs (Rittner et al., 1999). Such activated macrophages coexpressing MMP-2 and a high level of mitochondrial enzymes are localized directly adjacent to the disintegrated elastic lamina in giant-cell arteritis lesions (Weyand et al., 1997).

The granulomatous inflammation-induced injury causes cell death, loss of microstructures, and functional impairment of the affected arteries. It also initiates a response of the resident arterial cells in an attempt to repair and prevent damage. Some of the reactions induced by the injury are protective and limit the negative consequences of inflammation. For instance, aldose reductase is highly expressed by the smooth muscle cells exclusively at the site of vascular inflammation (Rittner et al., 1999). It is an oxidoreductase with a broad substrate specificity for carbonyl compounds, including toxic aldehydes, which are released by activated macrophages and cause lipid peroxidation and cell damage. Other cellular responses are maladaptive; they are intended to repair and regenerate wall structures but instead lead to excessive tissue production and vascular occlusion (Weyand, 2002). Uncontrolled intimal hyperplasia is a process in which myofibroblasts migrate from the adventitia towards the luminal subendothelial layer, proliferate, and secrete an excessive amount of extracellular matrix components. Intimal hyperplasia, best exemplified in giant-cell arteritis, is a direct consequence of the destructive inflammatory process and is mediated by activated macrophages and multinucleated giant cells. These inflammatory cells are localized at the border of the intima and media, and release several growth factors, including platelet-derived growth factor (PDGF) and VEGF (Weyand and Goronzy,1999). Production of PDGF and VEGF correlate with the local presence of IFN-γ and IL-1β. Both PDGF and VEGF are angiogenic factors required for the functional adaptation of the myofibroblast cells necessary for intimal hyperplasia. Uncontrolled intimal hyperplasia accounts for the ischemic phenomena in giant-cell arteritis, particularly visual loss and stroke (Weyand and Goronzy, 1999).

Granulomatous inflammation in vasculitic syndromes occurs in the absence of any identifiable exogenous pathogen in the lesion, suggesting that autoimmune mechanisms are primarily responsible. It has been hypothesized that, in giant-cell arteritis, the autoimmune response is directed against the elastic membrane of the vascular wall (Weyand et al., 1997). Giant-cell arteritis is also associated with HLA-DRB1 polymorphisms, implying that antigen recognition by CD4 cells is a critical step in the pathogenesis (Weyand et al., 1992). Immunoregulatory defects such as dysregulated secretion of IL-12 and bias towards Th1-type immune response have been proposed as an autoimmune mechanism in Wegener's granulomatosis (Csemok et al., 1999). In addition, activation of autoimmune T cells by Staphylococcus aureus superantigen and the specific expansion of the TCR Vβ repertoire could play role in this vasculitic syndrome (Popa et al., 2003). Clinical evidence also shows that the presence of S. aureus is a risk factor for disease relapse (Cohen Tarvaert et al., 1999).

Vessel-specific susceptibility

A characteristic feature of vasculitides is their predilection for a defined vascular bed. The factors predisposing specific arteries to certain vasculitic syndromes are incompletely understood and would include heterogeneity in the antigen repertoire and differential vulnerability to injury or susceptibility to infection. Endothelial cells (EC) from different vascular beds display organ-specific and tissue-specific heterogeneity that could account for a selective antigenicity (Zetter, 1981). This view is further supported by the existence of AECA, which exhibit a remarkable binding predilection to a specific vessel size or endothelial cell functional state (Banks,1999; Cervera et al., 1994; Praptonik et al., 2001; Shoenfield, 2002). CNS endothelial cells express specific isoforms of glucose transporters, transferrin, and VEGF receptors, and extracellular matrix proteins. They also express specific tight-junction proteins and blood–brain barrier (BBB)-associated markers, including the endothelial barrier antigen (EBA). Under pathological conditions of BBB breakdown, the expression of these antigens diminishes and other antigens, such as PAL-E and MECA-32, known as contra-BBB antigens, are up-regulated (Schlosshauer, 1998). Brain pericytes, another cellular constituent of the BBB, exhibit a remarkable tissue-specific, cytokine-dependent versatility not observed in the peripheral organs (Balabanov and Dore-Duffy, 1998). The pro-inflammatory IFN-γ and TNF-α induce macrophage-like functions, whereas TGF-β suppresses this phenotype and promotes smooth muscle-like properties. Additional variability could be due to functional characteristics related to the embryonal origin of the vessel's cellular components. Smooth muscle cells of the head and neck vessels have a mesoectodermal origin characterized by higher levels of expression of elastin, as opposed to the visceral smooth muscle cells of mesenchymal origin (Sundy and Haynes, 1995). This phenotypic feature is relevant to the fact that the smooth muscle cells and elastic lamellae of the extracranial vessels are the main immune target in giant-cell arteritis. Furthermore, these arteries no longer serve as a target once they penetrate into the skull and their elastin expression gradually diminishes (Wilkinson and Russell, 1972).

Differential vascular susceptibility to infections reflects the interactions between the vascular cells and the causative pathogens. Vasculitides associated with viral infections predominantly involve the small and the medium-sized vessels. Viral agents such as human immunodeficiency virus (HIV), VZV, HSV, and CMV could also produce isolated CNS and retinal vasculitis (Mendell and Calabrese, 1998). Viral invasion of endothelial cells depends on the presence of specific receptor mechanisms mediating the entry into the cell. HIV-1 tropism for the BBB endothelial cells is related to the gp120 interactions with the endothelial chemokine receptors CCR3, CCR5, and CXCR4 (Banks, 1999). In addition to receptor-mediated endocytosis, gp120 up-regulates endothelial ICAM-1 and VCAM-1 expression, triggers PECAM-1 phosphorylation and IL6 secretion, and facilitates leukocyte recruitment and transendothelial migration (Stins et al., 2001). Bacterial and fungal-associated vasculitides, on the other hand, tend to involve the large and medium-sized vessels. These vasculitides result from septic embolization or direct extension of an infectious focus into the vascular wall (Sneller, 2002). Two susceptible niches, the vasa vasorum and atherosclerotic plaques, appear to be the primary sites for infectious 'seeding'. The resulting suppurative inflammation and ischemic necrosis of the vascular wall lead to a specific type of lesion, often referred to as a 'mycotic' aneurysm (Gerder et al., 1997).

As we mentioned above, there is a strong correlation between vessel size, histopathology, and immune mechanisms. Small vessels, for example, commonly harbor immune complexes or antigens of different origin beneath the endothelial cells. Hemodynamic factors and complexity of the microvasculature, as well as expression of FcR by the endothelial cells, play an important role in the localization of the immune complex deposition. Large vessels, on other hand, are rarely affected by immune complexes and are, even in the presence of autoantibodies, characterized by paucity of immune deposits. Small vessel endothelial cells have the capacity to express adhesion molecules at their luminal surfaces and to facilitate direct leuko-

cyte transmigration. In small vessel vasculitides polymorphonuclear leukocytes recruited to the site of immune complex deposition by the chemoattracting complement elements directly transmigrate through the luminal endothelium (Cohen and Kallenberg, 1997). In contrast, large vessel luminal endothelial cells do not express adhesion molecules and direct luminal transmigration rarely occurs. In large vessel vasculitides, adhesion molecules are expressed by the endothelial cells of the adventitial microvessels–vasa vasorum, and leukocytes penetrate the vascular wall through the adventitia, rather than directly through the lumen (Cid et al., 2000). The vasa vasorum, being a rare site of immune complex deposition, facilitates an alternative inflammatory process, e.g. delayed type of hypersensitivity. Furthermore, the patterns of vascular responses to inflammatory injury differ significantly between vascular beds. For example, vascular occlusion in vasculitis is due to two principal mechanisms: thrombosis and intimal hyperplasia. Thrombosis is most frequently seen in small vessel vasculitides and is due primarily to a direct endothelial cell injury and dysfunction of their hemostatic system (Kirchhofer et al., 1994). Intimal hyperplasia, by contrast, occurs exclusively in large vessel vasculitides and is characterized by uncontrolled myofibroblast proliferation in response to fibrinogenic factors such as PDGF and VEGF (Weyand and Goronzy,1999). In these types of vasculitic syndromes, the activated macrophages secreting the growth factors, rather than the endothelial cells, are the main cause of vascular occlusion.

Vasculitides of the peripheral nervous system

Vasculitides affecting the PNS cause a specific neurologic syndrome: vasculitic neuropathy. They are relatively rare disorders with an estimated incidence of approximately two to seven cases per million population (Hawke et al., 1991). The vasculitides affecting the PNS are usually classified into several groups depending on the presence or absence of an identifiable cause (primary idiopathic or secondary vasculitis) and systemic involvement (systemic and non-systemic vasculitis). Vasculitic neuropathy, frequently associated with various systemic disorders such as infections, primary vasculitides, connective tissue disorders, and malignancies, may precede the systemic symptoms or represent their sole clinical manifestation. The significance of recognizing vasculitic neuropathy lies in the fact that it is a common manifestation of a number of systemic life-threatening and yet treatable disorders. Thus, identification of the specific vasculitic syndrome involving the PNS is the core principle of the diagnostic and therapeutic approach to patients with vasculitic neuropathy.

Pathology of vasculitic neuropathy

The association between vasculitic neuropathy and systemic disorders has been known for a long time, documented even in the first PAN case by Kussmaul and Maier in the nineteenth century. The nature of this association, however, remained unclear until the pioneering work of several groups who provided the pathological basis of the syndrome and attracted the necessary attention and recognition (Kernohan and Woltman, 1938; Dyck et al., 1972).

Vasculitic processes affecting the PNS involve primarily the vasa nervorum of the peripheral nerves (Satoi et al., 1998), which represents an intrinsic anastomosal network of vessels distributing and supplying blood flow throughout the nerve. The proper functioning of this system is very important since the individual nerves are supplied by a limited number of nutrient vessels and redistribution of the blood flow within the nerve is the main mechanism of supporting their metabolic activity (McManis et al., 1997). The inflammatory process involving the vasa nervorum leads to necrosis of the vascular wall (fibrinoid necrosis), thrombosis, and regional ischemia (Fig. 30.1). The hypoxic–ischemic injury of the nerve further causes axonal degeneration, fiber loss, and, less often, segmental demyelination (Fujimura, et al., 1991) (Fig. 30.2). The injurious effect is most

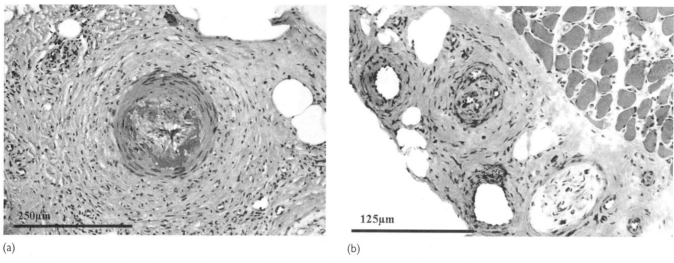

(a)   (b)

Fig. 30.1 Nerve and muscle biopsy of a patient with non-systemic PNS vasculitis. Cross-section of a paraffin-embedded specimen; hemotoxylin–eosin staining: (a) acute vasculitic inflammation—fibrinoid necrosis, cellular infiltration and lumen occlusion; (b) chronic vasculitic changes—obliteration and recanalization of the vascular lumen. (See also Plate 7 of the colour plate section at the center of this book.)

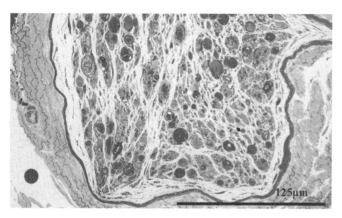

Fig. 30.2 Nerve biopsy of a patient with non-systemic PNS vasculitis. Cross-section of a plastic-embedded nerve specimen; toluidine blue staining. Note the degeneration of all nerve fibers. (See also Plate 8 of the colour plate section.)

prominent in the 'watershed' zones of the nerve trunk where the blood supply is marginal and highly dependent on the optimal functioning of the nutrient arteries and intrinsic vascular system. Probably for the same reason the large myelinated fibers, especially those located centrally in the fascicles, are most vulnerable. The lesions are usually multiple, asymmetric, and sectorial depending on the distribution and the severity of the vasculitic process (Fujimura et al., 1991).

There is a correlation between the type of the vasculitis and the caliber of the involved vessels (Griffin, 2001). The large epineurial vessels (100–250 μm) are typically involved in primary systemic vasculitides, while the smaller epineurial vessels (<100 μm) are involved in secondary systemic and non-systemic vasculitides. Endoneurial vessels are mainly affected by the hypersensitivity vasculitides and rarely by any other type.

Clinical presentation and diagnosis

The clinical presentation of vasculitic neuropathy is determined by the extent and the localization of the vasculitic process and the tempo of its progression. Classically, patients present with multiple mononeuropathies (mononeuritis multiplex) (Harati and Niakan, 1985; Kissel and Mendell, 1992). The usual symptoms are acute or subacute painful weakness or sens-

ory loss in a distribution of several individual peripheral nerves. The vasculitic process progresses with the involvement of other peripheral nerves in a step-wise fashion. With time, the deficits overlap and coalesce, producing a picture of asymmetric polyneuropathy. In such cases, side-to-side asymmetry of the deficits could be obtained from patient history, or demonstrated on neurologic examination or by using electrodiagnostic tests. Some of the patients may actually present with symmetric slowly progressive 'stocking-gloves' polyneuropathy (Hawke et al., 1991; Nicolai et al., 1995). This variant implies early widespread vasculitic involvement of the PNS, producing distal summation of the deficits. More than half of the patients experience, at presentation, either constitutional symptoms such as fever, weight loss, and anorexia, or signs of multiorgan dysfunction, typically in the skin, joint, kidney, and GI tract. In the remaining patients, the peripheral neuropathy either antecedes the systematic signs or remains the sole manifestation of the vasculitic process.

The diagnostic work-up aims to establish the diagnosis of vasculitic neuropathy and to identify the underlying vasculitic syndrome. The vasculitic nature of peripheral neuropathy is suggested by the presence of symptoms and laboratory findings consistent with multiorgan dysfunction and a systemic inflammatory process. The neuropathy, however, can occur as an isolated syndrome in the absence of any systemic findings and all tests in this regard can be normal or negative. On the other hand, vasculitic neuropathy is not the only clinical entity associated with systemic inflammatory or multiorgan disease, and other syndromes such as acute and chronic demyelinating polyradiculopathies (AIDP, CIDP), multifocal motor neuropathy (MMN), amyloidosis, and entrapment should be considered. Electrodiagnostic studies are useful in this respect, by demonstrating axonal loss with asymmetric distribution as well as delineating the extent of the neuropathic process (Bouche et al., 1986). A potential pitfall in severe cases is the presence of a conduction block, the origin of which, focal demyelinating versus axonal, is still debatable (Ropert and Metral 1990; McCluskey et al., 1999).

The cornerstone of the diagnosis of vasculitic neuropathy is the pathological evaluation of biopsy material (Collins et al., 2000). Combined nerve and muscle biopsy, such as biopsy of the superfacial peroneal nerve and peroneus brevis muscle, is an approach of choice because it increases the diagnostic yield almost two-fold (Said, 1999). Alternatively, cutaneous sensory nerves, usually the sural nerve and the superficial radial or peroneal nerves, or muscle biopsy alone are also appropriate, especially if there is electrodiagnostic evidence of involvement. Demonstration of inflammatory cells infiltrating the vascular wall and fibrinoid necrosis is the 'gold standard' of establishing the diagnosis (Kissel and Mendel, 1992). The presence of vascular inflammation alone, without vascular necrosis, is not sufficient for the diagnosis. The degree of suspicion can remain high, however, if the inflammation is associated with findings suggesting angiopathic nerve injury, such as sectorial perineurial necrosis, centrofascicular degeneration, and new vessel formation (Griffin, 2001). In such cases, additional biopsy sampling or a visceral angiogram should be considered.

Specific PNS vasculitides

Identification of the specific vasculitic syndrome involving the PNS is based on a clinical approach classifying all vasculitides as primary or secondary and as systemic or non-systemic. Primary systemic vasculitides commonly involved the PNS and, in fact, vasculitic neuropathy is their most common neurological complication. Of the large vessel vasculitides, only giant-cell arteritis has been anecdotally reported to involve the PNS (Caselli and Hunder, 1994). However, medium-sized vessel vasculitides, specifically PAN, and small vessel vasculitides, including Wegener's granulomatosis, Churg–Strauss syndrome, and microscopic polyangiitis, are frequently associated with peripheral neuropathy (Guillevin et al., 1997). PAN is well recognized as the most common cause of vasculitic neuropathy and is considered to be a prototype for the syndrome. Necrotizing vasculitis affecting the larger epineurial vessels (100–500 μm) is a typical pathological finding. Peripheral nerve involvement occurs in up to 60% of patients, usually on a background of multiorgan symptoms and laboratory findings suggesting a systemic inflammatory process. These laboratory findings, however, are non-specific and ANCA titers are positive in only 10% of patients. Multiple microaneurysms can be demonstrated on visceral angiogram in approximately two-thirds of the patients (Ewald et al., 1987). Hepatitis B surface antigenemia is present in 30% of patients and should be tested for because it requires a specific treatment, different from immunosuppression (Guillevin et al., 1995; Sonntag et al., 1995). Vasculitic neuropathy may precede the systemic symptoms or represent the sole clinical finding of PAN.

Wegener's granulomatosis is another syndrome associated with peripheral nerve disease that may antecede the systemic findings (Nishino et al., 1993). It is clinically present in 15% to 50% of patients and is strongly associated with positive cANCA titers (Cohen Tarvaert et al., 1989; de Groot et al., 2001). Multiple cranial neuropathies affecting vision and extraocular movements are frequent findings and result from a local extension of the nasal granulomatous process. Neuropathy associated with Churg–Strauss syndrome occurs in about 65% of the affected patients (Sehgal et al., 1995). It is found mainly during the third stage of the disease and is usually associated with systemic symptoms and positive pANCA titers. Peripheral nerve involvement in microscopic polyangiitis occurs in 20% of patients and is often indistinguishable from PAN. However, there are also certain important differences. Visceral microaneurysms and HBV surface antigenemia are very rare, while positive pANCA titers are present in up to 90% of patients (Guillevin et al., 1997). The pathological distinction of these primary systemic vasculitic syndromes is often difficult because granulomatous inflammation and/or eosinophilic infiltration in the PNS, as seen in the other organs, is very rare (Said, 1999). The vessel caliber, additionally, for a number of reasons, is often difficult to assess. The absence of specific pathological findings creates diagnostic uncertainty when the vasculitic neuropathy is associated with a systematic vasculitis lacking specific features or when systemic manifestations are minimal.

Non-systemic vasculitic neuropathy is considered in the absence of any systemic findings as an isolated, PNS-restricted vasculitis (Dyck et al., 1987; Kissel and Mendell, 1992; Collins et al., 2003). Non-systemic vasculitic neuropathy is frequently observed and represents the second most common cause of vasculitic involvement of the PNS. The diagnosis is established after elimination of other systemic conditions associated with isolated or antecedent vasculitic neuropathy, and after a strict follow-up. In general, it is milder in severity, with indolent course and favorable prognosis (Griffin, 2001). Whether it represents a separate clinical entity or a tissue-isolated form of any of the systemic vasculitides, which are typically self-limited, remains to be clarified.

Vasculitides affecting the PNS can be associated with connective tissue disorders and other systemic diseases, and for this reason are considered to be secondary. Vasculitic neuropathy in connective tissue disorders is necrotizing in nature but affects a wider range of vessel sizes, varying from the large epineurial vessels to the small endoneurial vessels (Olney, 1998). Even though frequent in connective tissue disorders, vasculitic neuropathy is not the only clinico-pathological entity involving the PNS. Other independent and coexisting inflammatory and non-inflammatory pathogenic mechanisms could cause peripheral neuropathy, complicating the diagnostic process. Rheumatoid arthritis (RA) is the third most common cause of vasculitic neuropathy (Puechal et al., 1995). This type of neuropathy, again, is not the most common one associated with RA. Approximately half of patients with RA suffer from peripheral neuropathy and only 10% of the cases are due to necrotizing vasculitis (Olney, 1998). Rheumatoid vasculitic neuropathy usually develops in the setting of a long-standing seropositive disease with well-developed articular and extra-articular lesions. Peripheral neuropathy varies in severity, but motor involvement correlates with systemic disease and represents a poor prognostic sign. Sjögren's syndrome (sicca syndrome) occurs independently or in association with RA and other connective tissue diseases. About 20% of affected patients develop systemic medium-sized or small vessel necrotizing vasculitis, and half of them sensory polyneuropathy (Grant et al., 1997). This type of neuropathy is vascular in origin and differs from the dorsal root ganglionitis also associated with the syndrome. Craniopathy affecting the trigeminal nerve is common. In the absence of clinical polyexocrinopathy to suggest the diagnosis, testing for anti-Ro and anti-La and performing salivary gland biopsy is particularly helpful. SLE, despite the presence of several autoantibodies and circulating immune complexes, is uncommonly associated with systemic vasculitis (Belmont et al., 1996). Peripheral neuropathy, even though relatively common in SLE, is rarely due to necrotizing vasculitis (Kissel and Mendell, 1992; Said, 1999). Similarly, systemic sclerosis and mixed-connective tissue disorder often affect the PNS, but true vasculitic neuropathy is very rare.

Other systemic disorders, such as infections, cryoglobulinemia, malignancy, drugs, graft-versus-host disease, and diabetes mellitus, are associated with vasculitic neuropathy. This is a large and diverse group of diseases sometimes classified as hypersensitivity vasculitides. While immune-mediated injury of the small vessels is the common unifying mechanism, other disease-specific or coexistent pathological processes may ultimately determine the extent of nerve damage. Bacterial, viral, and fungal infections cause systemic vasculitis through various mechanisms (Gerber et al., 1997; Sneller, 2002). CMV and VZV produce vasculitic neuropathy by direct invasion of the vascular endothelium (Mendell and Calabrese, 1998). HBV and HCV cause neuropathy by induction of immune complex injury of the vasa nervorum (Tsukada et al., 1983; Caniatti et al., 1996). Both can also cause PAN and vasculitic neuropathy. HCV has been also implicated as an etiologic factor of essential mixed cryoglobulinemia (Caniatti et al., 1996). Nearly 80% of patients with essential mixed cryoglobulinemia have circulating antibodies against HCV or are infectious for the virus (Angelo, 1998). The peripheral neuropathy that occurs in half of the cryoglobulinemic patients is due mainly to necrotizing vasculitis. Others infectious agents, such as HIV and Borrelia burgdorferi, cause a wide spectrum of peripheral nerve diseases but rarely necrotizing vasculitis. It is important to note that in HIV infection, the vasculitic process may occur as an isolated, self-limiting neuropathy in the early stages, as a progressive neuropathy secondary to infectious invasion (CMV, HSV, Toxoplasma), and as lymphoma infiltration during the AIDS stage (Brannagan, 1997). Independently from the HIV infection, hematologic malignancies, such as hairy cell leukemia, as well as renal and lung carcinoma, have been associated with vasculitic neuropathy. Unlike in other paraneoplastic syndromes, however, chemotherapy and immunotherapy may be effective (Oh, 1997).

Therapeutic agents commonly used to treat infections (antibacterials, antiretrovirals, interferon-α), malignancies, and autoimmune syndromes (cyclophosphamide, methotrexate, G-CSF) may cause systemic vasculitis (Somer and Finegold, 1995; Calabrese and Duna, 1996; Gordon et al.,

1998). This adverse effect should always be considered in cases of new onset, or worsening, neuropathy or systemic disease. Inflammatory vasculopathy and necrotizing vasculitis have also been recognized as underlying mechanisms of diabetic amyotrophy and considered in other diabetes-related mononeuropaties and craniopathies (Dyck et al., 1999). This is conceptually a new pathogenic mechanism to be associated with diabetes mellitus, traditionally thought to cause only non-inflammatory angiopathy. Whether the inflammatory aspects of diabetes-related neuropathies necessitate acute or chronic immunotherapy remains to be assessed.

Management of PNS vasculitides

Management of vasculitic neuropathy generally depends on the identification of the underlying vasculitic process. Patients with primary systemic vasculitides and some of the secondary vasculitides are best managed with a combined regimen of prednisone and cyclophosphamide. In PAN and Wegener's granulomatosis, the combined therapy is rather dramatic, increasing the 5-year survival rate from less than 10% to 80% and 90%, respectively (Lieb et al., 1979; Fauci et al., 1983). Vasculitic neuropathy secondary to systemic vasculitides should be treated with prednisone (1.5 mg/kg/day) and cyclophosphamide (2.0 mg/kg/day) until maximum benefit and sustained remission is experienced (Kissel and Mendell, 1992). Then the prednisone treatment can be switched to an every other day regimen for a few months and slowly tapered thereafter. Cyclophosphamide therapy usually continues for a year and is stopped if the disease remains stable. In the case of a relapse, the prednisone should be restarted, as well as the cyclophosphamide if necessary. Fulminant cases or acute exacerbations can be managed with a pulse of IV solumedrol (1.0 g/day) or cyclophosphamide (2–5 mg/kg/day) for two to three days. Some patients may have a poor tolerance for cyclophosphamide due to gastrointestinal distress, or may develop significant side-effects such as alopecia, myelosuppression, and hemorrhagic cystitis. Switching to methotrexate or azathioprine is an alternative, but without proven benefit. Intravenous immunoglobulin (IV Ig 2 g/kg body weight) can also be considered as a sole or adjuvant treatment alternative for patients with contraindication to or who experience failure of the combination therapy (Levy et al., 2003).

Patients with non-systemic vasculitic neuropathy, as well as those with neuropathy associated with giant-cell arteritis, can be efficiently managed with prednisone monotherapy (Kissel and Mendell, 1992). However, combination therapy appeared to produce a better outcome than corticosteroid monotherapy in patients with non-systemic vasculitic neuropathy (Collins et al., 2003). Vasculitic neuropathy developed in the setting of specific non-vasculitic disorders should be approached based on the etiologic cause. Treatment of infections, specifically hepatitis and HIV infections, malignancy, and diabetes mellitus should be performed in coordination with other specialty teams. Immunosuppressive therapy in these cases is not always necessary. Other modalities, such as plasma exchange, IV Ig, and interferon-α may be beneficial in patients with HCV and HBV related neuropathies.

Vasculitis neuropathy is a vaso-oclusive disease, and may benefit from antiplatelet therapy, and even vasodilators (Moore, 1998). However, there is no specific recommendation or clinical trial supporting such treatment. Conditions contributing to ischemia, such as diabetes mellitus, hypertension, hyperlipidemia, and tobacco and drug abuse, should be addressed. Symptomatic management of neuropathic pain and active physical therapy can improve the patient's quality of life and functional status. All candidates for immunosuppressive therapy should be evaluated for indolent infections, TB and HIV, and myelodysplastic syndromes. Close follow-up for side-effects is usually recommended. A low-salt, low-carbohydrate diet supplemented with calcium and vitamin D, as well as prophylaxis of peptic ulcer disease, may minimize prednisone side-effects. Periodic checks of the complete blood count for myelosuppression, and urine analysis for hemorrhagic cystitis are important in patients on cyclophosphamide. Long-term follow-up and regularly scheduled visits are necessary for clinical monitoring of disease progression and any adverse effects of immunotherapy.

Vasculitides of the central nervous system

Vasculitides of the CNS are a group of rare disorders that present a unique clinical problem. They are notoriously difficult to diagnose, produce a wide range of neurological symptoms and signs, but lack specific diagnostic markers. They are regarded as a treatable disorder but there are no controlled therapeutic clinical trials to support this assumption. CNS vasculitides are serious and not uncommonly fatal disorders leaving significant neurological sequelae if misdiagnosed or inappropriately managed. Being rare disorders, there are no sufficient epidemiological data, but the estimated incidence ranges from 1–30 per million population (Scolding et al., 2002). However, the incidence of certain vasculitides can be significantly higher in some population groups. For instance, giant-cell arteritis has a reported incidence of 20 per 100 000 in patients older than 50 years (Kelley, 2004). Takayasu's arteritis is most commonly seen in younger female patients with Asian ethnic background. Infectious and drug-associated vasculitides occur predominantly in high-risk patient groups such as those abusing street drugs, or infected with HIV and hepatitis virus.

Vasculitides of the CNS are conventionally classified as primary when the CNS is the sole or dominant organ involved, and as secondary when it is affected by a systemic disease process originating in the periphery (Calabrese et al., 1997). Vasculitis affecting predominantly the CNS has been given different terms. Granulomatous angiitis of the nervous system (GANS) was applied in the past based on early pathological observation (Budzilovich et al., 1963) but its use remained limited because it did not reflect the sizable percentage of non-granulomatous cases. Isolated angiitis of the CNS (IACNS) has been also proposed by some authors (Cupps et al., 1983), but it seems to be inappropriate in view of several reported cases of pathological involvement outside the CNS (Lie, 1991). The term primary angiitis of the CNS (PACNS) is favored by most authors because it defines more loosely the anatomical site of predominant pathological involvement and is not limited by histological features. Other authors, however, argue that this term unnecessarily emphasizes the idiopathic nature of the vasculitic process (Moore, 1999), as occasional association with systemic diseases has been documented (Inwards et al., 1991). Secondary vasculitides of the CNS, on the other hand, occur as a manifestation or as a result of a heterogeneous group of disorders such as infections, drug use, malignancy, or systemic vasculitides. Such designation is clinically important in two aspects: the search for a specific causative factor is essential in the diagnostic approach and its removal may result in amelioration of the CNS vasculitis.

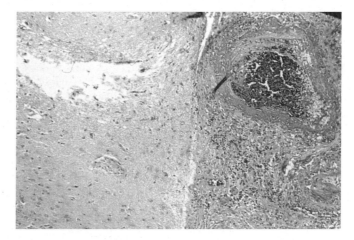

Fig. 30.3 Brain biopsy of a patient with primary angiitis of the CNS (PACNS). Cross-section of a paraffin-embedded specimen; hematoxylin–eosin staining. Note the acute vasculitic changes of the depicted leptomeningeal vessel—fibrinoid necrosis, thrombosis and cellular infiltration. Reactive astrocytosis can also be seen in the underlying cortex.

Pathology of the CNS vasculitides

Vasculitic processes affecting the CNS vasculature cause direct injury to and necrosis of the vascular wall, thrombotic occlusion of the vascular lumen, and ultimately ischemia and stroke (Fig. 30.3). The spectrum of vasculitic pathology includes a wide range of abnormal findings. Vasculitic lesions tend to be multifocal and spread throughout the vascular tree in varying pathological patterns. A focal lesion can involve the whole vascular wall and produce thrombosis and infarction or aneurysms and hemorrhage. The lesions can also involve only certain portions or layers of the vessel, leading to stenosis and ischemia.

PACNS affect predominantly the medium-sized and small vessels, mainly the arterioles and rarely the venules, of the leptomeninges and the brain parenchyma in a discontinuous pattern (Lie, 1997). The inflammatory infiltrate consists of lymphocytes, plasma cells, and macrophages. Multinucleated giant cells of Langhans' or foreign body types are most frequently seen in segmental lesions, but are present in fewer than 50% of the biopsies. PAN-like necrotizing vasculitis can be found in 25% of positive biopsies. Intimal hyperplasia is commonly seen and signifies a healing process. In general, coexistence of acute and chronic inflammatory findings can be observed in most of the positive biopsies (Lie, 1997).

Histopathological findings in secondary vasculitides could be quite variable depending on the causative process (Lie, 1997). For example, the most common primary vasculitides affecting the CNS, PAN, Churg–Strauss syndrome, and Wegener's granulomatosis, cause typical necrotizing vasculitis of the medium-sized and small vessels, with granulomatous features in the latter. Infection-associated CNS vasculitides, on the other hand, are characterized by mononuclear inflammation, rather than necrosis, of the small vessels, with the notable exception of hyphal angiitis, which results from direct fungal invasion of the blood vessel (Gerder et al., 1997). Other vasculitides may be only a part of a more complex pathophysiologic mechanism involving the CNS vasculature, or complicated by numerous confounding factors. SLE vasculopathy, for instance, is associated with thickening, hyalinization, thrombus formation, or platelet deposition of the small vessels, but frank vasculitis is uncommon (Weiner and Allen, 1991; Belmont et al., 1996). Similarly, drug-associated vasculopathy is most commonly due to vasospasm, malignant hypertension, thromboembolism, or to coexisting infections rather than to true vasculitic inflammation (Burst, 1997).

PACNS—clinical presentation and diagnosis

The clinical manifestations of PACNS are non-specific and reflect the distribution of CNS ischemia. Virtually any neurologic dysfunction could be encountered: headaches, encephalopathy, psychiatric syndromes, dementia, seizures, meningitis, and paralysis. Even though variable, the clinical features of PACNS can be organized in three clinical patterns that are potentially useful in recognizing, or at least raising the clinical suspicion, for PACNS (Scolding et al., 2002). First, acute or subacute, progressive or recurrent encephalopathy; second, focal space-occupying lesion; and third, multifocal disease with a relapsing–remitting course (Scolding et al., 2002). Clinico-pathological correlations suggest several distinct disease patterns of PACNS (Calabrese et al., 1997). Granulomatous angiitis of the nervous system (GANS), which occurs in fewer than 50% of the cases, is associated with a long clinical prodrome and a chronic progressive clinical course. The diagnosis is best established by leptomeningial biopsy, since chronic meningitis is one of its most common manifestations. Mass lesion presentation accounts for about 15% of the PACNS cases and is associated with headache, corresponding focal deficits, and mental status changes secondary to the mass effect. CNS hemorrhage has been reported in about 11% of the PACNS patients, intracerebral hemorrhage being the most common, followed by subarachnoid hemorrhage. This presentation is usually related to aneurysmal rupture of cerebral or meningial arteries. PACNS-associated myelopathy, documented in 14% of the cases, typically presents with progressive paraparesis. A majority of the cases fitting this clinical pattern are accounted by GANS (Calabrese et al., 1997).

Perhaps the most important step in the diagnostic process is the clinical suspicion. At this point, a comprehensive medical history and physical examination, and appropriate laboratory and other ancillary tests, must be performed to assess for the presence of multiorgan/systemic damage, vasculopathy of the CNS blood vessels, and the inflammatory nature of this process. There is no laboratory test of sufficient sensitivity and specificity to rule out or secure the diagnosis of PACNS. The majority of them are indirect, with numerous limitations and interpretation biases. In most instances, the diagnosis is based on a combination of high-probability laboratory tests applied in a stepwise fashion, excluding all the mimicking conditions (Calabrese, 2002). Routine laboratory tests such as complete blood count, electrolytes and coagulation panels, renal and liver profiles,

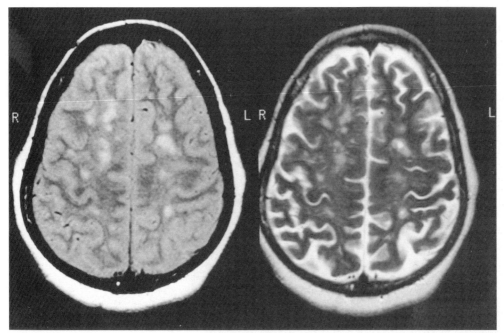

Fig. 30.4 MRI study of a patient with primary angiitis of the CNS (PACNS). Proton density and T2-weighted images demonstrate bilateral multifocal signal abnormalities.

erythrocyte sedimentation rate (ESR) and C-reactive protein (CRP) cryo-globulins, rheumatoid factor (RF), antinuclear antibodies (ANA), SS-A(Ro)/SS-B (La), ANCAs, antiphospholipid antibodies, hepatitis, syphilis and HIV serology, chest X-ray, ECG, and toxic screen could point to a specific secondary vasculitic syndrome or suggest other conditions such as infections, malignancies, hypercoagulable or thomboembolic states, and inflammatory disorders. Unfortunately, all these laboratory tests, including the acute-phase reactants, are frequently normal in the cases of PACNS, requiring further diagnostic evaluation. Cerebrospinal fluid (CSF) abnor-malities, mild pleocytosis, and protein elevation are found in 80% of patho-logically documented PACNS, but in only 50% of angiographically diagnosed cases (Stone *et al.*, 1994; Calabrese *et al.*, 1997). The specificity of an abnormal CSF study for PACNS is low, about 40%, and the inter-pretation of the result should be done in the context of the clinical setting and other laboratory findings. CSF examination is a useful test for ruling out important diagnostic possibilities, such as CNS infection and carcino-matous meningitis.

Neuroimaging greatly improved the diagnosis of CNS vasculitis. Magnetic resonance imaging (MRI) is a more sensitive imaging modality than computed tomography (CT) (except in cases of cerebral hemorrhage) and should be considered as the study of choice in all patients with sus-pected CNS vasculitis. The sensitivity of MRI is high, and in biopsy proven and angiographically defined cases it approaches almost 100% (Pomper *et al.*, 1999). However, there are no pathognomonic MRI findings that would secure the diagnosis, and the study as a whole has a specificity of 36% (Duna and Calabrese, 1995). MRI findings are highly variable, with the most specific pattern being bilateral multifocal T_2 hyperintense lesions involving different anatomical locations (cortex, basal ganglia, and white matter) that spread over time (Wynne *et al.*, 1997; Campi *et al.*, 2001) (Fig. 30.4). On the initial MRI, simultaneous gadolinium enhancement could be seen in almost 90% of the lesions (Campi *et al.*, 2001). These MRI lesions are responsive to immunotherapy and a significant reduction in number, size, or enhancement could be observed on follow-up visits (Campi *et al.*, 2001). With regard to the differential diagnosis, these lesions are less numerous and the perivascular changes are milder than in multiple sclerosis (Miller *et al.*, 1987). Approximately 15% of PACNS patients, espe-cially those with the granulomatous variant, present with a single intra-cranial mass-like lesion that mimics a tumor or intracranial abscess. Inclusion of other MRI sequences in the study, such as DWI and FLAIR, will probably increase the sensitivity in detection of new, small lesions. The combination of normal MRI and CSF studies has a high negative predictive value and could rule out the diagnosis of PACNS in majority of the cases (Stone *et al.*, 1994). Single photon emission computed tomography (SPECT) and posi-tron emission tomography (PET) scanning may increase the sensitivity, espe-cially in small vessel or early vasculitis (Emmi *et al.*, 1993; Meusser *et al.*,

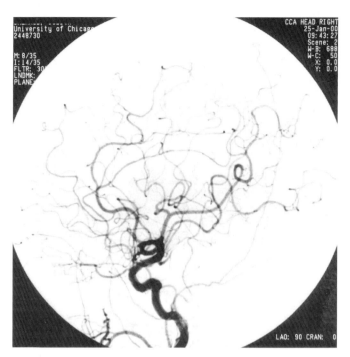

Fig. 30.6 Angiogram of a patient with primary angiitis of the CNS (PACNS). This study demonstrates extensive vascular irregularities, best seen on the callosomarginal artery, consistent with vasculitis.

1996). The diffuse or multifocal perfusion abnormalities, even though they could point to a vascular mechanism, are not specific and do not dis-tinguish vasculitis from other forms of vasculopathy (Nobili *et al.*, 2002) (Fig. 30.5).

Cerebral angiography is often considered as the 'gold standard' in the diagnostic process of CNS vasculitis (Ferris and Levine, 1973). Patterns characteristic for CNS vasculitis are multiple arterial occlusions and avas-cular areas and segmental stenosis separated by dilations (beating) of the intracranial arteries (Fig. 30.6). Multiple microaneurysms, commonly seen in visceral angiograms, are distinctly rare in cerebral angiogram (Calabrese *et al.*, 1997). Interpretation of the cerebral angiogram is limited by low sensitivity and specificity. Abnormal angiograms might be documented in only 60% of tissue-proven cases and the classic beading pattern in fewer than 40% of them (Calabrese *et al.*, 1997). Moreover, these findings are of low specificity, about 26%, as they are seen in numerous other conditions such as vasospasm secondary to subarachnoid hemorrhage, drug abuse, or

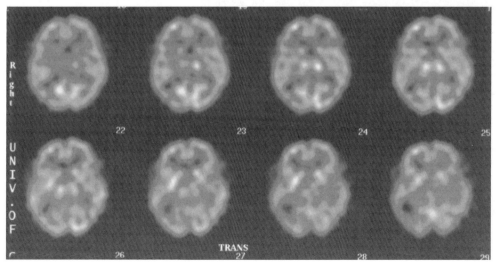

Fig. 30.5 ^{99m}Tc SPECT of a patient with primary angiitis of the CNS (PACNS). This study demonstrates multiple areas of hypoperfusion involving the right temporal and parietal lobes, and the left frontal cortex.

severe hypertension, atherosclerosis and embolus recanalization, reversible angiopathies, etc. With such low specificity, an abnormal cerebral angiogram could only secure the diagnosis of CNS vasculitis in a high-probability setting, when all mimicking conditions have been ruled out and there is a compatible clinical picture (Calabrese, 2002). A normal angiogram does not exclude CNS vasculitis, particularly small vessel vasculitis, because vessels under 100–200 μm cannot be visualized by this method. In such cases, as well as in early disease stages prior to any significant structural abnormalities, SPECT and PET scanning could reveal functional abnormalities (Meusser et al., 1996). Serial angiographic studies may demonstrate radiographic changes correlating the clinical course (Alhalabi and Moore, 1994), but their value is not fully established. In general, the complication rate of cerebral angiography is about 1%, with an equal frequency of transient and permanent neurological deficits (Heiserman et al., 1994). Transient deficits appear at a higher rate, up to 11.5%, in patients with presumed cerebral vasculitis (Hellman et al., 1992), as age and prior stroke have been identified as significant risk factors. CT and MR angiography, often complementing the neuroimaging studies, have a low spatial resolution and therefore should not be used to substitute the cerebral angiogram.

Tissue biopsy and histological confirmation of CNS vasculitis is the clinical standard for the diagnosis of all forms of vasculitis. Brain biopsy, however, is limited by several factors. Ante-mortem biopsies yield false-negative results in up to 25% of cases owing to lesion localization and sampling errors (Duna and Calabrese, 1995). Radiologically guided biopsy, particularly of abnormally enhancing MRI lesions, and/or combined sampling of leptomeninges and underlying cortex, could improve the sensitivity of the procedure. Deep stereotactic biopsy could be undertaken in cases of a single mass lesion (Whiting et al., 1992). In the absence of focal lesions, the anterior tip of the temporal lobe of the non-dominant hemisphere could be sampled. Tissue diagnosis is important in evaluating a variety of mimicking conditions, such as lymphoproliferative diseases, multiple sclerosis, sarcoidosis, infections, and others (Parisi and Moore, 1994). Although rarely reported, false-positive biopsy results could also be yielded.

There are no specific guidelines for when to proceed to brain biopsy in patients with suspected CNS vasculitis. Biopsy would certainly be warranted in cases of progressive encephalopathy when the diagnostic evaluation is unrevealing and no specific cause can explain a patient's status. The overall risk of serious morbidity related to brain biopsy, estimated to be about 0.5–2.0% (Barsa and Pauker, 1980), is less than the cumulative risk of long-term exposure to empirically initiated immunosuppressive therapy without firm diagnosis. For example, in a series of patients with Wegener's granulomatosis treated with cyclophosphamide, it was predicted that 16% of them will develop bladder cancer within 15 years of the therapy (Talar-Williams et al., 1996).

Secondary CNS vasculitides

Secondary vasculitides of the CNS are a heterogeneous group of disorders associated with systemic vasculitic syndromes, infections, connective tissue disorders, drug abuse, and malignancies. Involvement of the CNS in systemic vasculitides is variable and often unpredictable. Among the large vessel vasculitides, giant-cell (temporal) vasculitis is the most common cause of neurological dysfunction. The classic presentation of temporal arteritis includes headache and scalp tenderness in the temporal area, jaw claudication, polymyalgia rheumatica, and elevated ESR (Hunder, 1997). The diagnosis is usually considered in patients above the age of 50 and established by temporal artery biopsy. Giant-cell arteritis affects the arteries in irregular, intermittent fashion, which lowers the sensitivity of the test. It is important to biopsy a long 3–4 cm segment, preferably from both arteries, and to examine the specimen at several levels in order to obtain adequate sampling. This type of vasculitis responds readily to steroids and their therapeutic effect can be monitored not only clinically but also by the normalization of the ESR levels. It is important to note that the decision to treat should not be delayed for the purpose of biopsy, as the inflammatory infiltrate remains present for more than 2 weeks (Aschkar et al., 1995;

Younge et al., 2004). Loss of vision is the most serious complication of giant-cell arteritis and has devastating consequences. It is caused by ischemia of the optic nerve secondary to arteritis of the branches of the ophthalmic and posterior ciliary arteries, and occasionally by occlusion of the retinal arterioles. The initial visual symptoms could be transitory, unilateral, or partial, but if not treated may progress to bilateral blindness within 2 weeks. The incidence of visual loss in patients with giant-cell arteritis is about 20% (Hayreh and Podhajsky, 1998). Other neurological complications, such as transient ischemic attack (TIA) and stroke, are uncommon and are due to the involvement of the arteries of the posterior circulation.

Takayasu's arteritis, the other large vessel vasculitis, typically involves the aorta and its main branches and, only rarely, the intracranial vessels. It does cause, however, neurological symptoms secondary to carotid artery stenosis and subclavian steal syndrome. Angiographic imaging of the aorta and its branches is diagnostic (Numono, 1999).

Medium-sized and small vessel vasculitides frequently affect the CNS. Neurological abnormalities occur in 25 to 50% of patients with PAN (Lie, 1997). CNS vasculitis is the second cause of death, after renal failure, in children and adolescents (Engel et al., 1995). Clinical manifestations of PAN-associated CNS vasculitis include progressive encephalopathy and stroke, intracranial and subarachnoid hemorrhage, craniopathies, and myelopathy. The onset of CNS disease tends to occur later than the peripheral neuropathy. As described above, the laboratory findings consistent with PAN, such as elevated ESR, CRP, ANA, ANCA, and the presence of hepatitis B antigenemia (in 20–30% of cases), suggest the diagnosis. Angiography and tissue biopsy are usually required to establish the diagnosis (Guillevin et al., 1997). CNS manifestations of Churg–Strauss syndrome are similar to those of PAN and include encephalopathy, seizures, subarachnoid hemorrhage, and chorea. Craniopathies, specifically optic neuropathy, are a prominent part of the disease (Sehgal et al., 1995). Eosinophilia and cANCA seropositivity can be found during the course of the disease.

Wegener's granulomatosis involvement of the CNS varies from 11 to 40% and manifests with subdural masses, meningitis, intracranial hemorrhages, venous thrombosis, pituitary insufficiency, and craniopathies. While the majority of these complications are secondary to vasculitis, some of them are due to direct destructive effect of nerve tissue by the invading granulomatous process originating from the sinuses and the middle ear (Nashino, 1993). MRI is reportedly a highly sensitive test in differentiating the mechanisms of CNS injury. cANCA is strongly associated with Wegener's granulomatosis, with a reported sensitivity and specificity of approximately 90 and 98%, respectively (Cohen Tarvaert et al., 1989; Nölle et al., 1989). The titer of cANCA correlates with the disease activity, as its rise is associated with reactivation of the disease, and its persistence following remission represents a risk factor for relapse (Cohen Tarvaert et al., 1989). There is epidemiological evidence suggesting that S. aureus infection plays a role in the disease relapse. Furthermore, treatment with co-trimoxazole reduces the relapse rate by 60% (Stegeman et al., 1996).

Connective tissue disorders frequently affect the CNS. However, with the possible exception of SLE, Sjögren's syndrome, and Behçet's disease, true vasculitis rarely occurs. CNS involvement in SLE has been reported in 25–70% of cases, 30% of which are due to non-inflammatory vasculopathy and only 12.5% to frank vasculitis (Lie, 1997). The pathogenesis of SLE vasculopathy is multifactorial, including coagulopathy, thromboembolism, vascular degeneration, and inflammation (Devinsky et al., 1987). The basis for vasculitic inflammation remains unclear, but immune complex deposition is the most likely mechanism. The range of clinical manifestations varies from encephalopathy and seizures to stroke, subarachnoid hemorrhage, and transverse myelitis. Similar to SLE, Sjögren's syndrome causes progressive encephalopathy, aseptic meningitis, and stroke (Alexander, 1992). While the clinical presentation and neuroimaging studies of SLE and Sjögren's syndrome are largely non-specific and indistinguishable from PACNS, certain laboratory tests are particularly useful. SLE is characterized by the presence of ANA in more than 95% of patients. Antibodies to native double-stranded DNA, even though less sensitive, are more specific for the disease and account for the homogeneous nuclear immunostaining pattern of ANA. Other nuclear (extractable) antigens of ANA, such as SS-A/Ro and SS-B/La, are associated with both SLE and, more often, Sjögren's syndrome (Cervera *et al.*, 1993). Vasculitis associated with Behçet's disease is described in Chapter 27. The rest of the connective tissue disorders, systemic sclerosis, rheumatoid arthritis, and mixed connective tissue disorder, are uncommonly associated with CNS vasculitis. Other inflammatory disorders such as sarcoidosis, inflammatory bowel disease, Cogan's syndrome (cochleovestibulopathy), and familial Mediterranean fever (hereditary amyloidosis) are unusual and rarely cause CNS vasculitis (Lie, 1997).

Infection is a well recognized cause of CNS vasculitis (Gerder *et al.*, 1997). It contributes to mortality and morbidity through ischemic and hemorrhagic infarction. Its recognition is important because the treatment can be directed against the underlying organism. Many organisms, including viruses, bacteria, fungi, rickettsiae, and protozoa, have been have implicated as potential causes. Frequent strokes, which complicate bacterial meningitis, reflect the vasculitic inflammation of the subarachnoid vessels induced by the bacteria and the release of toxic substances. Hyphal angiitis caused by the angioinvasive *Aspergillus*, *Candida*, *Coccidioides*, and *Mucormycetes* species leads to acute cerebral hemorrhage, infarction, and mycotic aneurysm formation. Other pathogens such as *Treponema pallidum*, *B. bugdorferi*, HIV, HSV, and VZV could mimic PACNS and cause serious diagnostic difficulties (Lie, 1997). In the evaluation of all suspected cases of CNS vasculitis, a search for an infection in blood and CSF samples, as well as in the biopsy material, is mandatory.

Drug-associated cases of CNS vasculitis are reported after the use of cocaine, amphetamines, and heroin, but are generally rare (Krendel *et al.*, 1990; Burst, 1997). The presence of confounding factors, including impurities or stabilizers (talc, cellulose), may result in a hypersensitivity reaction (Butz, 1970). Laboratory studies also have shown that heroin addicts, for example, often have hypergammaglobulinemia, increased circulating immune complexes, autoantibodies, and lymph node hyperplasia. In such patients, heroin-related strokes have followed the first injection after weeks of abstinence (Burst, 1997). Most of the reported cases of drug-associated CNS vasculitis, however, have been diagnosed based on an angiogram alone, in the absence of biopsy conformation. One should be aware that multiple mechanisms of vascular pathology may coexist, some of which, such as vasospasm, hypertension, and embolism may mimic the angiographic appearance of vasculitis.

CNS vasculitis has been reported in association with lymphoproliferative diseases, including Hodgkin's lymphoma and non-Hodgkin's lymphoma (Calabrese *et al.*, 1997). Lymphomatoid granulomatosis is an angiocentric T-cell lymphoma with pathological features indistinguishable from PACNS (Petito *et al.*, 1978). Evaluation of the T-cell receptor for monoclonality could be helpful in this respect.

Management of CNS vasculitides

The most important aspect of the successful management of CNS vasculitides is securing the diagnosis and identifying the specific vasculitic syndrome involved. Specific and etiology-based therapy should be initiated in all cases of secondary vasculitis, such as infections, drug abuse, and malignancies. Immunosuppressive therapy, usually a combination of prednisone and cyclophosphamide, is required for systemic vasculitides. The management of all secondary vasculitides has to be comprehensive and should be provided in coordination with other specialty teams.

Giant-cell arteritis can be successively treated with corticosteroid monotherapy, which remains the single most important preventive measure of visual complications. Patients with acute visual or other neurological symptoms should be treated emergently with IV solumedrol (1 g/day for 3–5 days followed by oral prednisone) whereas those with mild disease and no neurologic symptoms could be treated with oral prednisone (60–80 mg/day). The high-dose prednisone therapy in both cases should continue until normalization of the ESR and CRP. Then the prednisone dose can be slowly decreased to a lower maintenance dose (7.5–20 mg/day). The duration of the prednisone therapy should continue for at least 6 months to a year because of the slow resolution of the inflammatory infiltrates and the risk

of relapse (Proven *et al.*, 2003). Low-dose aspirin (100 mg/day) has also been reported to decrease the incidence of visual loss by 20% and can be beneficial as an adjunctive therapy (Nesher *et al.*, 2004).

The treatment of PACNS is associated with several difficulties (Calabrese, 2003). There have been no controlled clinical trials to establish the efficacy of any of the agents in use, either alone or in combination. The employed therapeutic approaches are largely empiric, often based on the belief that PACNS is uniformly fatal and aggressive immunosuppression is always necessary. Combination of prednisone and cyclophosphamide has been successfully used in a small group of patients (Cupps *et al.*, 1983). The treatment course is generally 6–12 months, followed first by a slow prednisone taper and later by discontinuation of the cyclophosphamide, if the disease remains stable (see above). Assessment of disease activity could be performed by frequent clinical follow-up visits, serial CSF studies, and angiograms (Alhalabi and Moore, 1994), and less invasively by serial MRI studies (Campi *et al.*, 2001).

Whether all cases warrant the prednisone–cyclophosphamide combination or not remains a difficult dilemma. It has been suggested that a combined therapy should be used for patients with progressive neurological illness and those with biopsy-confirmed GANS (Calabrese *et al.*, 1997). Patients with a reversible vasoconstrictive variant of PACNS (BACNS) can be successfully treated with a high dose of steroids alone; significant improvement can be observed within 8–12 weeks (Calabrese *et al.*, 1997). Other immunosuppressive agents, such as azathioprine and methotrexate, could be used as steroid-sparing agents, but their efficacy is not proven. Use of antiplatelet agents and calcium channel blockers might be useful (Calabrese *et al.*, 1997; Moore, 1998). It is also important for patients to avoid oral contraceptives, caffeine, tobacco, and sympathomimetic drugs that may aggravate the vasoconstriction and worsen their symptoms. The majority of patients will require aggressive physical therapy and rehabilitation, and long-term follow-up for the management of disease and treatment complications.

References

Alexander, E. (1992). Central nervous system disease in Sjögren's syndrome. *Neurology* **31**: 1391–1396.

Alhalabi, M. and Moore, P. (1994). Serial angiography in isolated angiitis of the central nervous system. *Neurology* **44**: 1221–1226.

Altate, F., Dutandy, A., Lammas, D., *et al.*, (1998). Impairment of mycobacterial immunity in human interleukin 12 receptor deficiency. *Science* **280**: 1435–1438.

Angelo, V. (1998). Mixed cryoglobulinemia after hepatitis C: more or less ambiguity. *Ann Rheum Dis* **57**: 701–702.

Aschkar, A., Lie, J., Hunder, G., *et al.* (1995). How does previous corticosteroid treatment affect the biopsy of findings in giant cell (temporal) arteritis? *Ann Intern Med* **120**: 987–992.

Balabanov, R. and Dore-Duffy, P. (1998*a*). Cytokines and the blood–brain barrier, In: *Introduction to the Blood–Brain Barrier. Methodology, Biology and Pathology* (ed. W. Pardrige), pp. 359–376. Cambridge University Press, Cambridge.

Balabanov, R. and Dore-Duffy, P. (1998*b*). Role of the CNS microvascular pericytes in the blood–brain barrier. A mini-review. *J Neurosci Res* **53**: 637–644.

Banks, W. (1999). Physiology and pathology of the blood–brain barrier: implications for microbial pathogenesis, drug delivery and neurodegenerative disorders. *J Neurovirol* **5**: 538–555.

Barhn, E., Lehman, T., Peackock, D., Tang, C., and Banquerigo, M. (1999). Suppression of coronary vasculitis in a murine model of Kawasaki disease with an angiogenesis inhibitor. *Clin Immunol* **90**: 147–151.

Barsa, M. and Pauker, S. (1980). The decision to biopsy, treat or wait in suspected herpes simplex encephalitis. *Ann Intern Med* **92**: 641–647.

Bean, A., Roach, D., Briscoe, H., *et al.* (1999). Structural deficiencies in granuloma formation in TNF gene-targeted mice underlie the heightened susceptibility to aerosol *Mycobacterium tuberculosis* infection, which is not compensated by lymphotoxin. *J Immunol* **162**: 3504–3511.

Belmont, H., Abramson, S., and Lie, L. (1996). Pathology and pathogenesis of vascular injury in systemic lupus erythematosus: interaction of inflammatory cells and activated endothelium. *Arthritis Rheum* **39**: 9–22.

Beynon, H., Davies, K., Haskard, D., and Walport, M. (1994). Erythrocyte complement receptor 1 and interactions between immune complexes, neutrophils, and endothelium. *J Immunol* 153: 3160–3167.

Blank, M., Krause, I., Goldkorn, T., *et al.*, (1999). Monoclonal antiendothelial cell antibodies from a patient with Takayasu arteritis activate endothelial cells from large vessels. *Arch Rheumatol* 42: 1421–1432.

Bouche, P., Leger, J., Travers, M., *et al.* (1986). Peripheral neuropathy in systemic vasculitis: clinical and electrophysiological study of 22 patients. *Neurology* 36: 1598–1602.

Bradley, J., Johnson, D., and Pober, J. (1993). Endothelial activation by hydrogen peroxide. Selective increase of intercellular adhesion molecule-1 and major histocompatibility complex class-1. *Am J Pathol* 142: 1598–1609.

Brannagan, T. (1997). Retroviral-associated vasculitides of the nervous system. *Neurol Clin* 15: 927–944.

Budzilovich, G., Feigin, I., and Siegel, H. (1963). Granulomatous angiitis of the nervous system. *Arch Pathol* 76: 250–256.

Burst, J. (1997). Vasculitis owing to substance abuse. *Neurol Clin* 15: 945–957.

Butz, W. (1970). Disseminated magnesium and silicate associated with paregoric addiction. *J Forensic Sci* 15: 194–196.

Calabrese, L. (2002). Diagnostic strategies in vasculitis affecting the central nervous system. *Cleve Clin J Med* 69(SII): 105–108.

Calabrese, L. (2003). Clinical management issues in vasculitis. Angiographically defined angiitis of the central nervous system: diagnostic and therapeutic dilemmas. *Clin Exp Rheumatol* 21(Suppl. 12): 131–132.

Calabrese, L. and Duna, G. (1995). Drug-induced vasculitides. *Curr Opin Rheumatol* 8: 34–40.

Calabrese, L., Duna, G., and Lie, J. (1997). Vasculitis of the central nervous system. *Arthritis Rheum* 40: 1189–1201.

Campi, A., Benndorf, G., Filippi, M., Reganati, P., Martinelli, V., and Terreni, M. (2001). Primary angiitis of the central nervous system: serial MRI of brain and spinal cord. *Neuroradiology*, 43: 599–607.

Caniatti, L., Tugnoli, V., Eleopra, R., *et al.* (1996). Cryoglobulinemic neuropathy related to hepatitis C infection. Clinical, laboratory and neurophysiological study. *J Periph Nerv Syst* 1: 131–138.

Caselli, R. and Hunder, G. (1994). Neurological complications of giant cell (temporal) vasculitis. *Semin Neurol* 14: 349–353.

Casselman, B., Kilgore, K., Miller, B., and Warren, J. (1995). Antibodies to neutrophil cytoplasmic antigens induce monocyte chemoattractant-1 secretion from human monocytes. *J Lab Clin Med* 126: 495–502.

Cervera, R., Khamashta, M., and Font, J. (1993). Systemic lupus erythematosus: clinical and immunological patterns of disease expression in a cohort of 1,000 patients. *Medicine (Baltimore)* 72: 113–124.

Cervera R., Navano M., Lopez-Soto, A., *et al.* (1994). Antibodies to endothelial cell in Behçet's disease: cell-binding heterogeneity and association with clinical activity. *Ann Rheum Dis* 53: 265–267.

Cid, M., Cebrian, M., Font, C., *et al.* (2000). Cell adhesion molecules in development of inflammatory infiltrates in giant-cell arteritis. Inflammation-induced angiogenesis as the preferential side of leukocyte-endothelial cell interactions. *Arthritis Rheum* 43: 184–194.

Cid, M., Hernandez-Rodriguez, J., Esteban, M., *et al.* (2002). Tissue and serum angiogenic activity is associated with low prevalence of ischemic complications in patients with giant-cell arteritis. *Circulation* 106: 1664–1671.

Cid, M., Segearra, M., Garcia-Martinez, A., and Hernandez-Rodriguez, J. (2004). Endothelial cells, antineutrophil cytoplasmic antibodies, and cytokines in the pathogenesis of systemic vasculitis. *Curr Rheum Rep* 6:184–194.

Cohen, J. and Kallenberg, C. (1997). Cell adhesion molecules in vasculitis. *Curr Opin Rheumatol* 9: 16–25.

Cohen Tarvaert, J., van der Woode, F., Fauci, A., *et al.* (1989). Association between active Wegener's granulomatosis and anticytoplasmic antibodies. *Arch Intern Med* 149: 2456–2465.

Cohen Tarvaert, J., Goldschmeding, R., Elema, J., *et al.* (1990). Association of antibodies to myeloperoxidase with different forms of vasculitis. *Arthritis Rheum* 33: 1264–1272.

Cohen Tarvaert, J., Limberg, P., Elema, J., *et al.* (1991). Detection of autoantibodies against myeloid lysosomal enzymes: a useful adjunct to classification of patients with biopsy-proven necrotizing arthritis. *Am J Med* 91: 51–66.

Cohen Tarvaert, J., Popa, E., and Bos, N. (1999). The role of superantigens in vasculitis. *Curr Opin Rheumatol* 11: 24–32.

Collins, M., Mendel, J., and Periquet, M. (2000). Superficial peroneal/peroneus brevis muscle biopsy in vasculitic neuropathy. *Neurology* 55: 636–663.

Collins, M., Periquet, M., Mendell, J., SaheK, Z., Nagaraja, H., and Kissel, J. (2003). Nonsystemic vasculitic neuropathy: insights from a clinical cohort. *Neurology* 61: 623–630.

Coll-Vincent, B., Cebrian, M., Cid, M., *et al.* (1998). Dynamic pattern of endothelial cell adhesion molecule expression in muscle and perineural vessels from patients with classical periarteritis nodosa. *Arthritis Rheum* 41: 435–444.

Csemok, E., Trabandt, A., Muller, A., *et al.* (1999). Cytokine profile in Wegener's granulomatosis: predominance of type 1 (Th1) in the granulomatous inflammation. *Arthritis Rheum* 42: 742–750.

Cupps, T., Moore, P., and Fauci, A. (1983). Isolated angiitis of the central nervous system. *Am J Med* 74: 97–106.

de Brandt, M., Olliviec, V., Meyer, O., *et al.* (1997). Induction of interleukin 1 and subsequent tissue factor expression by anti-proteinase 3 antibodies in human umbilical vein endothelial cells. *Arthritis Rheum* 40: 2030–2038.

de Groot, K., Schmidt, D., Arlt, A., Gross, W., and Reinhold-Keller, E. (2001). Standardized neurologic evaluation of 128 patients with Wegener's granulomatosis. *Arch Neurol* 58: 1215–1221.

Del Papa, N., Comforti, G., Gambini, D., *et al.* (1994). Characterization of the endothelial surface proteins recognized by anti-endothelial antibodies in primary and secondary autoimmune vasculitis. *Clin Immunol Immunopathol* 70: 211–216.

Del Papa, N., Guidali, L., Sironi, M., *et al.* (1996). Anti-endothelial IgG antibodies from patients with Wegener's granulomatosis bind to human endothelial cells *in vitro* and induce adhesion molecule expression and cytokine secretion. *Arthritis Rheum* 39: 758–766.

Devinsky, O., Petito, C., and Llonso, D. (1988). Clinical and neuropathological findings in systemic lupus erythematosus: the role of vasculitis, heart emboli and thrombotic thrombocytopenic purpura. *Ann Neurol* 23: 380–384.

Dienstag, J. (1981). Immunopathogenesis of the extrahepatic manifestations of hepatitis B virus infection. *Springer Semin Immunopathol* 3: 461–472.

Dore-Duffy, P., Washington, R., and Balabanov, R. (1994). Cytokine-mediated activation of CNS microvessels: a system for examining antigenic modulation of CNS endothelial cells, end evidence for a long-term expression of E-selectin. *J Cereb Blood Flow Metab* 14: 837–844.

Duna, G. and Calabrese, L. (1995). Limitations of invasive modalities in the diagnosis of primary angiitis of the central nervous system. *J Rheumatol* 22: 662–667.

Dyck, P., Conn, D., and Okazaki, H. (1973). Necrotizing angiopathic neuropathy. Three dimensional morphology of fiber degeneration related to sides of occluded vessels. *Mayo Clin Proc* 47: 461–475.

Dyck, P., Benstead, T., Conn, D., *et al.* (1987). Nonsystemic vasculitic neuropathy. *Brain* 110: 843–854.

Dyck, P., Norell, J., and Dyck, P. (1999). Microvasculitis and ischemia in diabetic lumbosacral radiculoplexus neuropathy. *Neurology* 53: 2113–2121.

Emmi, L., Bramati, M., De Cristafaro, M., *et al.* (1993). MRI and SPECT investigations of the CNS of SLE patients. *Clin Exp Rheumatol* 11: 13–20.

Engel, D., Gospe, S., Lie, J., *et al.* (1995). Fatal infantile polyarteritis nodosa with predominant central nervous system involvement. *Stroke* 26: 699–701.

Enyedy, E., Mitchell, J., Nambiar, M., and Tsokos, G. (2001). Defective FcgammaRIIb1 signaling contributes to enhanced calcium response in B cells from patients with systemic lupus erythematosus. *Clin Immunol* 101: 130–135.

Ewald, E., Griffin, D., and McCuen, W. (1987). Correlation of angiographic abnormalities with disease manifestations and disease severity in polyarteritis nodosa. *J Rheumatol* 14: 952–956.

Falk, R. and Jennette, J. (1988). Anti-neurophil cytoplasmic antibodies with specificity for myeloperoxidase in patients with systemic vasculitis and idiopathic necrotizing and crescentic glomerulonephritis. *N Engl J Med* 318: 1651–1657.

Falk, R., Terrel, R., Charles, L., and Jennette, J. (1990). Anti-neutrophil cytoplasmic autoantibodies induce neutrophils to degranulate and produce oxygen radicals *in vitro*. *Proc Natl Acad Sci USA* 87: 4115–4119.

Farby, Z., Taphan, D., Fee, D., *et al.*, (1995). TGF-β2 decreases migration of lymphocytes *in vitro* and homing of cells into the central nervous system. *J Immunol* 155: 325–332.

Fauci, A., Haynes, B., and Katz, P. (1978). The spectrum of vasculitis: clinical, pathological, immunological and therapeutic considerations. *Ann Intern Med* **89**: 600–676.

Fauci, A., Haynes, B., and Katz, P. (1983). Wegener's granulomatosis: prospective clinical and therapeutic experience with 85 patients for 21 years. *Ann Intern Med* **98**: 76–81.

Ferri, C., Zignego, A., and Pileri, S. (2002). Cryoglobulins. *J Clin Pathol* **55**: 4–13.

Ferris, E. and Levine, H. (1973). Cerebral arteritis. Classification. *Radiology* **109**: 327–341.

Flynn, J. and Chan, J. (2001). Immunology of tuberculosis. *Ann Rev Immunol* **19**: 93–129.

Fossati, G., Bucknall, R., and Edwards, S. (2001). Fcγ receptors in autoimmune diseases. *Eur J Clin Invest* **31**: 821–831.

Fujimura, H., Lacroix, C., and Said, G. (1991). Vulnerability of nerve fibers to ischemia. A quantitative light and electron microscope study. *Brain* **114**: 1929–1942.

Furie, B. and Furie, B. (1992). Molecular and cellular mechanisms of biology of blood coagulation. *N Engl J Med* **326**: 800–806.

Gerder, O., Roque, C., and Coyle, P. (1997). Vasculitis owing to infection. *Neurol Clin* **15**: 903–926.

Gocke, D., Hsu, K., Morgan, C., et al. (1970). Association between polyarteritis and Australia antigen. *Lancet* **2**: 1149–1153.

Gold, R., Fontana, A., and Zierz, S. (2003). Therapy of neurological disorders in systemic vasculitis. *Semin Neurol* **23**: 207–214.

Gordon, A., Edgar, J., and Finch, R. (1998). Acute exacerbation of vasculitis during interferon-alpha therapy for hepatitis C-associated cryoglobulinemia. *J Infection* **36**: 229–230.

Grant, I., Hunder, G., and Homburger, H., et al., (1997). Peripheral neuropathy associated with sicca complex. *Neurology* **48**: 855–862.

Griffin, J. (2001). Vasculitic neuropathies. *Rheum Dis Clin North Am* **27**: 751–760.

Guillevin, L., Lhote, F., Cohen, P., et al. (1995). Periarteris nodosa related to hepatitis B virus: a prospective study with long-term observation of 41 patients. *Medicine (Baltimore)* **74**: 238–253.

Guillevin, I., Lhote, F., and Gherardi, R. (1997). Polyarteritis nodosa, microscopic angiitis, and Churg–Strauss syndrome: clinical aspects, neurological manifestations, and treatment. *Neurol Clin* **15**: 865–886.

Gupta, R. and Kohler, P. (1984). Identification of HBsAg determinants in immune complexes from hepatitis B virus-associataed vasculitis. *J Immunol* **132**: 1223–1228.

Harati, Y. and Niakan, E. (1986). The clinical spectrum of inflammatory angiopathic neuropathy. *J Neurol Neurosurg Psychiatry* **49**: 1313–1316.

Hawke, S., Davies, L., Pamphlett, R., Guo Y-P, Pollard, J., and McLeod, J. (1991). Vasculitic neuropathy. A clinical and pathological study. *Brain* **114**: 2175–2190.

Hebert, L., Cosio, F., and Neff, J. (1991). Diagnostic significance of hypocomplementemia. *Kidney Int* **39**: 811–821.

Heiserman, J., Dean, B., Hodak, J., et al. (1994). Neurological complications of cerebral angiography. *Am J Neuroradiol* **15**: 1401–1413.

Hellman, D., Roubenoff, R., Heavy, R., et al. (1992). Central nervous system angiography: safety and predictors of a positive result in 125 consecutive patients evaluated for possible vasculitis. *J Rheumatol* **19**: 568–572.

Hickey, W. (1999). Leukocyte traffic in the central nervous system: the participants and their role. *Semin Immunol* **11**: 125–137.

Hoffman, G. and Specks, U. (1998). Antineutrophil cytoplasmic antibodies. *Arthritis Rheum* **41**: 1521–1537.

Hunder, G. (1997). Giant cell arteritis and polymyalgia rheumatica. *Med Clin North Am* **81**: 195–219.

Hunder, G., Arend, W., Bloch, D., et al. (1990). The American College of Rheumatology 1990 criteria for classification of vasculitis: introduction. *Arthritis Rheum* **33**: 1065–1067.

Huynh, H., Oger, J., and Dorovini-Zis, K. (1995). Interferon-β downregulates interferon-γ-induced class II MHC molecule expression and morphological changes in primary cultures of human brain microvessel endothelial cells. *J Neuroimmunol* **60**: 63–73.

Inwards, D., Piepgras, D., Lie, J., et al. (1991). Granulomatous angiitis of the spinal cord associated with Hodgkin's disease. *Cancer* **68**: 1318–1322.

Jennette, J., Hoidal, J., and Falk, R. (1990). Specificity of anti-neutrophil cytoplasmic antibodies for proteinase 3. *Blood* **75**: 2263–2264.

Jennette, J., Falk, R., Andrassy, K., et al. (1994). Nomenclature of systemic vasculitides. Proposal of an International Consensus Conference. *Arthritis Rheum* **37**: 187–192.

Kelley, R. (2004). CNS vasculitis. *Front Biosci* **9**: 946–955.

Kernohan, J. and Woltman, H. (1938). Periarteritis nodosa: a clinicopathological study with special reference to the nervous system. *Arch Neurol Psychiat* **39**: 655–672.

Kirchhofer, D., Tschopp, T., Hadvary, P., et al. (1994). Endothelial cells stimulated with tumor necrosis factor-alpha express varying amounts of tissue factor resulting in homogenous fibrin deposition in a native blood vessel system: effect of thrombin inhibitors. *J Clin Invest* **93**: 2073–2083.

Kissel, J. and Mendell, J. (1992). Vasculitic neuropathies. *Neurol Clin* **10**: 761–781.

Kissel, J., Riethman, J., Omera, J., Rammohan, K., and Mendel, J. (1989). Peripheral vasculitis: immune characterization of the vascular lesion. *Ann Neurol* **25**: 291–297.

Kocher, M., Sigel, M., Edberg, J., and Kimberly, R. (1998). Cross-linking Fcγ receptor IIa and Fcγ receptor IIIb induces different proadhesive phenotypes of human neutrophils. *J Immunol* **159**: 3940–3948.

Komocsi, A., Lamprecht, P., Csemok, E., et al. (2002). Peripheral blood and granuloma CD(4+)CD28(−)T cells are the major source of interferon-gamma and tumor necrosis factor-alpha in Wegener's granulomatosis. *Am J Pathol* **160**: 1717–1724.

Krafte-Jacobs, B. and Brilli, R. (1998). Increased circulating thrombomodulin in children with septic shock. *Crit Care Med* **26**: 933–938.

Krendel, D., Ditter, S., Frankel, M., and Ross, W. (1990). Biopsy-proven cerebral vasculitis associated with cocaine abuse. *Neurology* **40**: 1092–1094.

Lamprecht, P., Gause, A., and Gross, W. (1999). Cryoglobulemic vasculitis. *Arthritis Rheum* **42**: 2507–2516.

Levy, Y., Uziel, Y., Zandman, G., Amital, H., Sherer, Y., Langevitz, P., et al. (2003). Intravenous immunoglobulins in peripheral neuropathy associated with vasculitis. *Ann Rheum Dis* **62**: 1221–1223.

Lie, J. (1991). Vasculitis, 1815 to 1991: classification and diagnostic specificity. *J Rheumatol* **19**: 83–89.

Lie, J. (1994). Nomenclature and classification of vasculitis: plus ça change, plus c'est la même chose. *Arthritis Rheum* **37**: 181–186.

Lie, J. (1997). Classification and histopathologic spectrum of central nervous system vasculitis. *Neurol Clin* **15**: 805–819.

Lieb, E., Restito, C., and Paulus, H. (1979). Immunosuppressive and corticosteroid therapy of polyarteritis nodosa. *Am J Med* **67**: 941–947.

Lindquist, K. and Osterland, C. (1971). Human antibodies to vascular endothelium. *Clin Exp Immunol* **9**: 753–760.

Litwin, V. and Grose, C. (1992). Herpes viral Fc receptors and their relationship to the human Fc receptors. *Immunol Res* **11**: 226–238.

Ludo van der Pol, W. and van der Winkel, J. (1998). IgG receptor polymorphisms: risk factors for disease. *Immunogenetics* **48**: 222–232.

MacCormac, L. and Grundy, J. (1996). Human cytomegalovirus induces an Fcγ receptor (Fcγ R) in endothelial cells and fibroblasts that is distinct from the human cellular Fc gamma Rs. *J Infect Dis* **174**: 1151–1161.

Mackay, C. (2001). Chemokines: immunology's high impact factors. *Nat Immunol* **2**: 95–101.

McCluskey, L., Feinberg, D., Cantor, C., and Bird, S. (1999). 'Pseudo-conduction block' in vasculitic neuropathy. *Muscle Nerve* **22**: 1361–1366.

McManis, P., Schmelzer, J., Zollmann, P., et al. (1997). Blood flow and autoregulation in somatic and autonomic ganglia. Comparison with sciatic nerve. *Brain* **120**: 445–449.

Meltzer, M., Franklin, E., Elias, K., et al. (1966). Cryoglobulinemia: a clinical and laboratory study. II. Cryoglobulins with rheumatoid factor activity. *Am J Med* **40**: 837–856.

Mendell, B. and Calabrese, L. (1998). Infections and systemic vasculitis. *Curr Opin Rheumatol* **10**: 51–57.

Merkel, P. (1998). Drugs associated with vasculitis. *Curr Opin Rheumatol* **10**: 45–50.

Meroni, P. (1999). Endothelial cell antibodies: from a laboratory curiosity to another useful antibody. In: *The Decade of Autoimmunity* (ed. Y. Shoenfeld), pp. 285–294. Elsevier Science, Amsterdam.

Meroni, P., Rashi, E., Testoni, C., and Borghi, M. (2004). *Clin Immunol* 112: 169–174.

Meusser, S., Ruppert, A., Manger, B., *et al.* (1996). 99mTc HMPAO SPECT in diagnosis of early cerebral vasculitis. *Rheumatol Int* 16: 37–41.

Miller, D., Ormerod, I., Gibson, A., Boulay, E., Rudge, P., and McDonald, W. (1987). MR brain scanning in patients with vasculitis: differentiation from multiple sclerosis. *Neuroradiology* 29: 226–231.

Molina, H. (2002). Update on complement in the pathogenesis of systemic lupus erythematosus. *Curr Opin Rheumatol* 14: 492–497.

Moore, P. (1999). The vasculitides. *Curr Opin Neurol* 169: 383–388.

Nesher, G., Berkum, Y., Mates, M., Baras, M., Rubinow, A., and Sonnenblick, M. (2004). Low-dose aspirin and prevention of cranial ischemic complications in giant cell arteritis. *Arthritis Rheum* 50: 1332–1337.

Newkirk, M., Chen, P., Carson, D., *et al.* (1986). Amino acid sequence on a light chain variable region of a human rheumatoid factor of the Wa idiotype, in part predicted by its reactivity with antipeptide antibodies. *Mol Immunol* 23: 239–244.

Nicolai, A., Bonetti, B., Lazzarino, L., Ferrari, S., Monaco, S., and Rizzuto, N. (1995). Peripheral nerve vasculitis: a clinico-pathological study. *Clin Neuropathol* 14: 137–141.

Nishino, H., Rubino, F., DeRemee, R., *et al.* (1993). Neurological involvement in Wegener's granulomatosis: an analysis of 324 consecutive patients at Mayo Clinic. *Ann Neurol* 33: 4–9.

Nobili, F., Cutolo, M., Sulli, A., Vitali, P., Vignola, S., and Rodriguez, C. (2002). Brain functional involvement by perfusion SPECT in systemic sclerosis and Behçet's disease. *Ann N Y Acad Sci* 966: 409–414.

Nölle, B., Specks, U., Lüdermann, J., *et al.* (1989). Anti-cytoplasmic antibodies: their immunodiagnostic value in Wegener's granulomatosis. *Arch Int Med* 111: 28–40.

Numono, F. (1999). Takayasu arteritis beyond pulsessness. *J Intern Med* 38: 226–232.

Ober, R., Martinez, C., Vaccaro, C., Zhou, J., and Ward, E. (2004). Visualizing the site and dynamic of IgG salvage by the MHC classI-related receptor, FcRn. *J Immunol* 172: 2021–2029.

Oh, S. (1997). Paraneoplastic vasculitis of the peripheral nervous system. *Neurol Clin* 15: 849–865.

Olney, R. (1998). Neuropathies associated with connective tissue disease. *Semin Neurol* 18: 63–72.

Orme, I. and Cooper, A. (1999). Cytokine/chemokine cascades in immunity to tuberculosis. *Immunol Today* 20: 307–312.

Parisi, J. and Moore, P. (1994). The role of biopsy in vasculitis of the central nervous system. *Semin Neurol* 14: 341–348.

Petito, C., Gottlieb, G., Dougherty, J., and Petito, F. (1978). Neoplastic angioendotheliosis: ultrastructural study and review of the literature. *Ann Neurol* 5: 437–444.

Pober, J. and Cotran, R. (1990). The role of endothelial cells in inflammation. *Transplantation* 50: 537–544.

Pomper, M., Miller, T., Stone, J., Tidmore, W., and Hellman, D. (1999). CNS vasculitis in autoimmune disease: MR imaging and finding-correlation with angiography. *Am J Neuroradiol* 20: 75–85.

Popa, E., Stegeman, C., Bas, N., Kallenberg, C., and Tervaert, J. (2003). Staphylococcal superantigen and T cell expansion in Wegener's granulomatosis. *Clin Exp Immunol* 132: 496–504.

Porges, A., Redecha, P., Kimberly, W., *et al.* (1994). Anti-neutrophil cytoplasmic antibodies engage and activate human neutrophils via Fcg RIIa. *J Immunol* 153: 1271–1280.

Praptonik, S., Blank, M., Meroni, P., *et al.*, (2001). Classification of anti-endothelial antibodies into antibodies against macrovascular and microvascular endothelial cells: pathogenic and diagnostic implications. *Arthritis Rheum* 44: 1484–1494.

Prodeus, A., Georg, L., Shen, O., *et al.* (1998). A critical role for complement in maintenance of self-tolerance. *Immunity* 8: 721–724.

Proven, A., Gabriel, S.E., Orces, C., O'Fallon, W., and Hunder, G. (2003). Glucocorticoid therapy in giant cell arteritis: duration and adverse outcomes. *Arthritis Rheum* 49: 703–708.

Puechal, X., Said, G., Hilliquin, P., *et al.* (1995). Peripheral neuropathy with necrotizing vasculitis in rheumatoid arthritis. A clinicopathologic and prognostic study of thirty-two patients. *Arthritis Rheum* 38: 1618–1629.

Rand, J. (2002). Molecular pathogenesis of antiphospholipid syndrome. *Circ Res* 90: 29–37.

Rapaport, S. and Rao, L. (1992). Initiation and regulation of tissue factor-dependent blood coagulation. *Arteriosclerosis Thrombosis* 12: 1111–1121.

Ravetch, J. and Bolland, S. (2001). IgG Fc receptors. *Ann Rev Immunol* 19: 275–290.

Reumaux, D., Vossebeld, P., Roos, D., and Verhoeven, A. (1995). Effect of tumor necrosis factor-induced integrin activation on Fcg receptor II-mediated signal transduction: Relevance for activation of neutrophils by anti-proteinase 3 or anti-myeloperoxidase antibodies. *Blood* 86: 3189–3195.

Rittner, H., Hafner, V., Klimjuk, P. (1999*a*). Aldolase reductase function as a detoxification system for lipid peroxidation products in vasculitis. *J Clin Invest* 103: 1007–1013.

Rittner, H., Kaiser, M., Brack, A., *et al.* (1999*b*). Tissue-destructive macrophages in giant cell arteritis. *Circ Res* 84: 1050–1058.

Romanic, A., Graesser, D., Baron, J., Visintin, I., Janeway, C., and Madri, J. (1997). T cell adhesion to endothelial cells and extracellular matrix is modulated upon transendothelial cell migration. *Lab Invest* 76: 11–23.

Ropert, A. and Metral, S. (1990). Conduction block in neuropathies with necrotizing vasculitis. *Muscle Nerve* 13: 102–105.

Said, G. (1999). Vasculitic neuropathies. *Curr Opin Neurol* 169: 627–629.

Satoi, H., Oka, N., Kawasaki, T., Miyamoto, K., Akiguchi, I., and Kimura, J. (1998). Mechanism of tissue injury in vasculitic neuropathies. *Neurology* 50: 492–496.

Schlosshauer, B. (1998). Brain microvessel antigens. In: *Introduction to the Blood–Brain Barrier. Methodology, Biology and Pathology* (ed. W. Pardrige), pp. 314–321. Cambridge University Press, Cambridge.

Scolding, N., Wilson, H., Hohlfield, R., Polman, C., Leite, I., and Gilhus, (2002). The recognition, diagnosis and management of cerebral vasculitis: a European survey. *Eur J Neurol* 9: 343–347.

Sehgal, M., Swanson, J., DeRemee, R., and Colby, T. (1995). Neurological manifestations of Churg–Strauss syndrome. *Mayo Clinic Proc* 70: 337–341.

Seo, P. and Stone, J. (2004). Antineutrophil cytoplasmic antibody-associated vasculitides. *Am J Med* 117: 39–50.

Shoenfield, Y. (2002). Classification of anti-endothelial cell antibodies into antibodies against microvascular and macrovascular endothelial cells: the pathogenic and diagnostic implications. *Cleve Clin J Med* 69(Suppl. 2):65–67.

Shrifferi, J., Woo, P., and Peters, K. (1982). Complement-mediated inhibition of immune precipitation. I. Role of classical and alternate pathways. *Clin Exp Immunol* 47: 555–562.

Siva, S. (2001). Vasculitis of the nervous system. *J Neurol* 248: 451–468.

Sneller, M. (2002). Vasculitis secondary to bacterial, fungal and parasitic infection. In: *Inflammatory Diseases of the Blood Vessels* (ed. G. Hoffman and C. Weyand), pp. 599–608. Marcel Dekker, New York.

Somer, T. and Fiengold, S. (1995). Vasculitides associated with infections, immunization and antimicrobial drugs. *Clin Infect Dis* 20: 1010–1036.

Sonntag, K., Schwarz-Eywill, M., and Hunstein, W. (1995). Is interferon alpha a therapy for hepatitis B-associated polyarteritis nodosa? *Br J Rheumatol* 34: 486–487.

Stegeman, C., Cohen Tervaert, J., de Jong, P., and Kallenberg, C. (1996). Trimethoprim-sulfamethoxazole (co-trimazole) for the prevention of relapses of Wegener's granulomatosis. *N Engl J Med* 335: 16–20.

Stins, M., Shen, Y., Sultana, C., *et al.* (2001). Gp120 activates children's brain endothelial cells via CD4. *J Neurovirol* 7: 125–134.

Stone, J., Pomper, M., Roubenoff, R., *et al.* (1994). Sensitivity of noninvasive tests for central nervous system vasculitis: a comparison of lumbar puncture, computer tomography and magnetic resonance imaging. *J Rheumatol* 21: 1277–1282.

Strominger, T. (1995). Traffic signals on endothelium for lymphocyte recirculation and leukocyte emigration. *Ann Rev Physiol* 57: 827–872.

Sundy, J. and Haynes, B. (1995). Pathogenic mechanisms of vessel damage in vasculitis syndromes. *Rheum Dis Clin North Am* 21: 861–881.

Talar-Williams, C., Hijazi, T., Walther, M., *et al.* (1996). Cyclophosphamide-induced cystitis and bladder cancer in patients with Wegener's granulomatosis. *Ann Intern Med* 124: 477–484.

Tripathy, N., Udadhyaya, S., Sinha, N., and Nityanand, S. (2001). Complement and cell mediated cytotoxicity by antiendothelial cell antibodies in Takayasu's arteritis. *J Rheumatol* **28**: 805–808.

Tsukada, N., Koh, C., Owa, M., *et al.* (1983). Chronic neuropathy associated with immune complexes of hepatitis B virus. *J Neurol Sci* **61**: 193–210.

Van Dyne, S., Holers, V., Lublin, D., and Atkison, J. (1987). The polymorphism of the C3b/C4b receptor in the normal population and in patients with systemic lupus erythematosus. *Clin Exp Immunol* **68**: 570–579.

Van der Woode, F., Rasmussen, N., Lobatto, S., *et al.* (1985). Autoantibodies to neutrophils and monocytes: a novel tool for diagnosis and a marker of disease activity in Wegener's granulomatosis. *Lancet* ii: 425–429.

Walport, M., Davies, K., Morley, B., *et al.* (1997). Complement deficiency and autoimmunity. *Ann N Y Acad Sci* **81**: 267–281.

Weiner, D. and Allen, N. (1991). Large vessel vasculitis of the central nervous system in systemic lupus erythematosus: report and review of the literature. *J Rheumatol* **18**: 748–40.

Weyand, C. (2002). Vasculitis: a dialog between the artery and the immune system. In: *Inflammatory Diseases of the Blood Vessels* (ed. G. Hoffman and C. Weyand), pp. 1–12. Marcel Dekker, New York.

Weyand, C. and Goronzy, J. (1999). Arterial wall injury in giant cell arteritis. *Arthritis Rheum* **42**: 844–853.

Weyand, C., Hunder, N., Hicok, K., Hunder, G., and Goronzy, J. (1992). The HLA-DRB1 locus as a genetic component in the giant cell arteritis. Mapping of a disease-linked sequence motif to the antigen binding site of the HLA-DR molecule. *J Clin Invest* **90**: 2355–2361.

Weyand, C., Schonberger, J., Oppitz, U., *et al.* (1994). Distinct vascular lesions in giant cell arteritis share identical T cell clonotypes. *J Exp Med* **179**: 951–960.

Weyand, C., Wagner, A., Bjornsson, J., and Goronzy, J. (1996). Correlation of topographical arrangement and functional pattern of tissue-infiltrating macrophages in giant cell arteritis. *J Clin Invest* **48**: 1642–1649.

Weyand, C., Ma-Krupa, W., and Goronzy, J. (2004). Immunopathway in giant cell arteritis and polymyalgia rheumatica. *Autoimmun Rev* **3**: 46–53.

Whiting, D., Barnett, G., Estes, M., *et al.* (1992). Stereotaxic biopsy in non-neoplastic lesions in adults. *Cleve Clin J Med* **59**: 48–55.

Wilkinson, I. and Russell, R. (1972). Arteries of head and neck in giant cell arteritis: a pathologic study to show the pattern of involvement. *Arch Neurol* **27**: 378–379.

Wynne, P., Youger, D., Khandji, A., and Silver, A. (1997). Radiographic features of central nervous system vasculitis. *Neurol Clin* **15**: 779–804.

Younge, B., Cook, B., Bartlry, G., Hodge, D., and Hunder, G. (2004). Initiation of glucocorticoid therapy: before or after biopsy? *Mayo Clin Proc* **79**: 483–489.

Younger, D. (2004). Vasculitides of the nervous system. *Curr Opin Neurol* **17**: 317–336.

Zetter, B. (1981). The endothelial cells of large and small blood vessels. *Diabetes* **30**(Suppl. 2): 24–28.

31 Myelin repair in multiple sclerosis

Catherine Lubetzki and Bernard Zalc

Introduction

Demyelinated lesions of multiple sclerosis (MS) disseminated in the central nervous system (CNS) may remyelinate. Neuropathological demonstration of remyelination in MS lesions was first reported at the ultrastructural level in the 1960s (Perier and Gregoire, 1965). Remyelinated lesions correspond to the classical shadow plaques, which are only faintly colored by the myelin stain. At the ultrastructural level, these shadow plaques are composed of fields of thinly myelinated axons that are similar in appearance to remyelinating axons observed in numerous experimental models of demyelination (Lassmann, 1983; Ludwin, 1987). CNS remyelination, first reported in chronic lesions, has since been observed in active lesions, occurring in association with ongoing demyelination (Raine et al., 1981; Prineas et al., 1993; Raine and Wu, 1993).

In addition to its role in the restoration of a rapid, saltatory conduction, which was demonstrated in experimental models, remyelination most probably is capable of preventing axonal degeneration. However, in contrast with experimental models of demyelination in which remyelination is almost complete, repair capacities in MS are insufficient and decrease with time, resulting in neurological dysfunction.

Currently available therapies in MS limit CNS inflammation, but have not demonstrated significant effects on long-term disability. Therefore, favoring myelin repair appears as a major goal in MS research. In this context, understanding why remyelination fails is crucial for devising effective methods by which to enhance it.

What are the factors involved in the failure of remyelination in MS?

The reasons for the remyelination deficit are many, including oligodendroglial, axonal, and environmental factors (Franklin, 2002). These different factors may participate to different extent to the remyelination failure, depending on both the type and age of the lesion.

Deficit of remyelinating cells and remyelination failure

Heterogeneity of multiple sclerosis lesions, notably concerning the vulnerability of oligodendrocytes, has been recently emphasized (Lucchinetti et al., 2000). This lesional heterogeneity suggests different pathophysiological processes. In some demyelinated lesions oligodendrocyte survival is prominent, whereas severe oligodendroglial loss, suggestive of a primary oligodendrocyte dystrophy, is evidenced in others. Among the large number of actively demyelinating lesions analysed, lesions with oligodendroglial sparing are more frequent than lesions with oligodendrocyte loss. Although the pattern of demyelination is heterogeneous between MS patients, additional data from the same group suggest that lesion types are mostly homogeneous within different plaques from the same patient. These results, which have to be confirmed, suggest that repair capacities may vary between individuals, depending on the disease mechanism, and could partly explain the interindividual heterogeneity in disease severity.

Oligodendrocyte survival, or, more probably, repopulation by recruitment of oligodendrocyte precursor cells to the demyelinated site, is indeed a key factor in the capacity of a lesion to be remyelinated. However, in many cases, the presence of potentially remyelinating cells is not sufficient for remyelination to occur. This important finding ensues from different studies on chronically demyelinated MS lesions, reporting the detection of numerous cells of the oligodendrocyte lineage (Wolswijk, 1998; Chang et al., 2002). These cells express different markers of immature oligodendrocyte (staining with O4 antibody, expression of the proteoglycan NG2), but also markers characteristic of more differentiated cells like PLP (proteolipid protein) or MOG (myelin-oligodendrocyte glycoprotein). Interestingly enough, these mature oligodendroglial cells appear unable to wrap around axons and to form a new myelin sheath, suggesting the existence of axonal factors inhibiting the wrapping process (see the section below on axonal re-expression of PSA-NCAM).

Not only is there evidence that mature oligodendrocyte within the plaque are unable to remyelinate, but NG2 expressing oligodendrocyte precursor cells appear to be unable either to enter the plaque (for those in the vicinity of the lesions) or to progress further in their differentiation and maturation program (for those present within the plaques).

Several recent reports have highlighted the crucial role, during development, of chemosecreted molecules in the guidance of oligodendrocyte precursor cells from their restricted foci of origin towards their final destination. In the embryonic mouse optic nerve, netrin-1 and semaphorin 3F have been shown to behave as chemoattractants for oligodendrocyte precursor cells (Spassky et al., 2002). Changes in the pattern of expression by oligodendrocyte precursor cells of netrin-1 receptors, from DCC (deleted in colorectal carcinoma) only in the embryonic optic nerve to both DCC and Unc5H1 post-natally, has led to suggestions that the chemoattractivity initially observed for netrin-1 switches later in development to a chemo-repellent effect. This switch suggests that netrin-1 may participate in a stop signal for oligodendrocyte precursor cell migration, preventing to all oligodendrocyte precursor cells entering the optic nerve from the chiasmal end accumulate towards the retinal extremity. During embryonic and early post-natal development, semaphorin 3A (Sema 3A) has been shown to be a strong chemorepellent for oligodendrocyte precursor cells, suggesting that Sema3A may play a role in funneling the stream of migratory oligodendrocyte precursor cells along certain tracts. In the adult, Sema 3A has been shown to induce a retraction of oligodendrocyte processes (Ricard et al., 2001). Although the pattern of expression of these molecules has not yet been fully investigated in MS plaques, it can be hypothesized that they play a role in the failure of remyelination. Indeed, assuming that reactive astrocytes participating in the gliotic reaction and/or inflammatory cells surrounding or within the plaque express either Sema3A or netrin-1, or both, and knowing that oligodendrocyte precursor cells express the corresponding receptors (DCC and Unc5H1 for netrin-1, neuropilin1 for Sema 3A), this could explain the fact that NG2-expressing oligodendrocyte precursor cells in the vicinity of the lesions are prevented from colonizing the plaque. Along the same lines, the presence of a gradient of Sema3A within the plaques could account for the failure of mature oligodendrocytes to extend new processes to enwrap neighboring denuded axons.

The arrest of oligodendrocyte precursor cells in their maturation program could also be linked to activation of the Notch/jagged pathway. During development, the expression of the ligand protein jagged by the axon inhibits oligodendrocyte differentiation through its binding to the receptor protein Notch, located on oligodendrocyte precursor cells. Then jagged is down-regulated by axons, allowing oligodendrocyte differentiation and maturation (Wang *et al.*, 1998). Activation of this pathway has been proposed to be involved in the maturation defect of oligodendrocyte precursor cells within MS plaques. Indeed, in chronically demyelinated lesions populated with oligodendrocyte precursor cells, expression of jagged by reactive astrocytes of the plaque has been detected; this could interact with Notch protein on oligodendrocyte precursor cells, partly explaining the differentiation default. In contrast, within remyelinated areas, astrocytes do not express jagged (John *et al.*, 2002). Thus, this is another example of how the reactivation of a given developmental pathway could participate in the myelin repair deficit.

Finally, age could be an additional factor in the capacity for myelin repair. Indeed, it has recently been shown that in experimental models of demyelination the capacities for recruitment of oligodendrocyte precursor cells were lower in old animals than in younger ones (Hinks and Franklin, 2000).

Axonal pathology and the myelin repair deficit

Axonal damage in MS has been known since the pioneering work of Jean Martin Charcot, who, in 1868, described axon loss but only in old, chronic lesions. Recent neuropathological studies have revisited this point, showing that axonal damage not only occurs early in the course of the disease but also that it is more frequent than classically admitted (Ferguson *et al.*, 1997; Trapp *et al.*, 1998). Axonal damage, identified by neuropathological techniques (axonal density, quantification of ovoid structures corresponding to transected axons, accumulation of the amyloid precursor protein reflecting the interruption of the axoplasmic flow), is corroborated by imaging techniques (measures of encephalic and spinal cord atrophy, spectroscopy (reduction in the peak of *N*-acetyl-aspartate). Interestingly enough, these imaging studies have clearly shown that the extent of axonal damage in MS is not limited to the demyelinated areas but is detected in the so-called normal-appearing white matter (Filippi *et al.*, 2003). Axonal transsection is obviously a crucial issue in MS. Indeed, in those lesions repair first requires axonal regrowth before envisaging the necessary remyelination of these fibers. Despite intensive research and fascinating progresses, regrowth of damaged axons is still in its infancy, and a review of the various strategies developed by many laboratories is beyond the scope of this chapter. As trying to understand axonal repair in MS is so complicated it would seem preferable to devise strategies to avoid confronting the problem. With this in mind there is an urgent need to develop research aimed at a better understanding of the mechanisms underlying axonal damage in MS. This should lead to the development of therapeutic tools aimed at protecting the axons, and hence avoid the need for axonal repair in MS. Furthermore, it is clear that preventing axonal loss will require therapy to be given as early as possible in the course of the disease.

In most cases, however, failure of myelin repair exists in the absence of severe axonal loss, suggesting that other factors are involved. In this respect, the re-expression at the axonal surface of denuded axons of inhibitory molecules could impair remyelination. This is the case for the poly-sialylated form of the neural cell adhesion molecule (NCAM), i.e. PSA-NCAM, which has been shown to negatively regulate myelination during normal development and to be absent from axons in the adult brain, except in areas known to exhibit permanent plasticity and neurogenesis (Charles *et al.*, 2000). In demyelinated MS plaques, re-expression of PSA-NCAM on a percentage of denuded axons has been detected, whereas within partially remyelinated plaques PSA-NCAM was never detected on remyelinated internodes (Charles *et al.*, 2002). Alternatively, but not excluding expression of inhibitory molecules by axons, other types of axonal dysfunction could alter remyelination. Electrical activity along axons has been shown to play a crucial role, during development, in the initiation of the myelination process (Demerens *et al.*, 1996). It has recently been reported that oligodendrocyte precursor cells express functional adenosine receptors which are activated in response to firing of action potentials (Stevens et al., 2002). These authors have demonstrated that in response to impulse activity, axons release ATP, which can be hydrolysed into adenosine. Adenosine acts as a potent transmitter to inhibit oligodendrocyte precursor cell proliferation, stimulate differentiation, and promote the formation of myelin. Therefore, we could speculate that modifications in the action potential or conduction block along demyelinated internodes may impair the positive signal necessary for remyelination to proceed. This neuron–glial signal provides a molecular mechanism for promoting oligodendrocyte development and myelination and may prove to be a promising strategy for improving remyelination.

Altogether these data suggest that a disruption of axonal signals on denuded axons could be involved in the myelin repair deficit. This potentially reversible axonal damage might be accessible to a neuroprotective strategy.

Environmental dysregulation and remyelination

In addition to myelin damage, MS plaques are characterized by the presence of astrocytic gliosis and inflammatory infiltrate. These two factors probably have both positive and negative effects, both favoring and impairing the remyelination process.

Astrocytic proliferation

The extent of astrocytic invasion within the plaques is variable. It occurs early after the demyelination process but is more prominent in chronic lesions. Early after the formation of the plaque, it could be deleterious to the repair process, either by impairing the recruitment of glial precursor cells to the lesion site or by inhibiting the contact between the oligodendroglial process and the denuded axon. Alternatively, at the early stages of the plaque formation, astrocytes may protect the denuded axons from neurotoxic cytokines secreted by the inflammatory infiltrate. Moreover, astrocytes are the main cell type in the CNS responsible for the synthesis and release of neurotrophic and/or pro-myelinating factors, and could have, at later stages, a beneficial role in myelin repair and axon protection.

The inflammatory infiltrate

The inflammatory infiltrate in the MS plaque is composed mainly of lymphocytes and macrophages. This infiltrate is dense in active inflammatory lesions, then disappears in chronic lesions. Similar to the astrocytic component of the plaque, the role of these inflammatory cells is most probably heterogeneous, depending on the stage of the lesion. In addition to a deleterious effect linked to the release by activated microglia and lymphocytes of neurotoxic and myelinotoxic cytokines, it has recently been shown that some antibodies, like those directed against MOG, could directly induce myelin damage. In contrast to this classical view of the immune response in MS, new data suggest that inflammation could be beneficial in some instances. It has recently been demonstrated that in experimental models of demyelination the presence of macrophages favors remyelination (Kotter *et al.*, 2001). One way to interpret this finding has been to put forward that the role of macrophages–microglial cells in removing myelin debris is in itself helpful, since contact with myelin can inhibit differentiation of oligodendrocyte precursors. The other explanation could be that the secretion by macrophages of growth factors, either directly or through activation of astrocytes, could favor repair.

In addition to the role of macrophages, the development of a neuroprotective autoimmunity, as demonstrated in experimental models of spinal cord traumas, could also have a beneficial role. For instance, it has been shown that activated lymphocytes specific to MBP (myelin basic protein), one of the major myelin proteins, increase axon survival of retinal neurons, probably through the release of neurotrophic cytokines (Schwartz, 2002).

This concept is important, as it may modify therapeutic strategies in MS, bearing in mind that complete suppression of the inflammatory component could, in the long run, impair the capacity for myelin repair.

New paths toward myelin repair in multiple sclerosis?

Although the pressure is on to make tissue repair strategies applicable to MS, much more still needs to be done to overcome barriers to repair. In addition, it is obvious that repair strategies can only be hypothesized in conjunction with active therapy directed towards the inflammatory process. The complexity of the mechanisms involved in the failure of remyelination is further increased by lesion heterogeneity, which could imply the need for different therapeutic responses depending on the type of lesion.

The possible reparative strategies include transplantation of cells from a variety of sources in the CNS, maintenance of a positive trophic environment to retain neurons and stimulate remyelination, and blocking inhibitors of either axonal and myelin regeneration.

In this context monoclonal antibodies of the IgM type capable of promoting myelin repair have been identified in animal models of demyelinating diseases and could be candidates for therapeutic development (Warrington et al., 2000). Among growth factors, GGF (glial growth factor) and IGF (insulin growth factor) have been shown to reduce, in experimental models of demyelination, the extent of the chronically demyelinated areas, although results are controversial depending on the experimental model (Yao et al., 1995; Cannella et al., 1998, 2000; Mason et al., 2003; Penderis et al., 2003). In addition to its effect on survival and differentiation of oligodendrocyte precursors, the CNTF family of growth factors has been shown in vitro to provide a strong pro-myelinating effect, probably mediated through the heterodimeric receptor LIFβ/gp130 and the Janus kinase pathway (Stankoff et al., 2002). Interestingly enough, in mice deficient for CNTF, MOG-induced experimental allergic encephalomyelitis is more severe, with poor clinical recovery associated with increased oligodendrocyte apoptosis (Linker et al., 2002). In addition, recent, although controversial, genetic studies in MS suggest an influence of CNTF on the clinical expression of the disease (Giess et al., 2002; Hoffmann and Hardt, 2002). Altogether these studies favor a protective role for CNTF on myelinating and remyelinating cells, which may be useful in future therapeutic strategies. Of course, how these factors might be delivered to the MS brain is a complicated and as yet unsolved problem. Alternatively, peptides or small molecules that can directly activate the signaling cascades involved in pro-myelinating activity may be developed as therapeutic agents.

These types of strategies aimed at stimulating endogenous remyelination are focusing on lesions with partial oligodendroglial survival. In lesions with severe oligodendroglial loss strategies should be aimed at stimulating the recruitment of glial precursors, from resting CNS oligodendroglial precursors, the NG2-expressing cells, that have been shown to persist in the adult brain. In this context the understanding of the role of the recently discovered guidance molecules, either attractive or repulsive, is crucial. Alternatively, stem cells from a variety of sources might be delivered to lesion sites at which it is hoped they will remyelinate denuded, but not yet degenerated, axons. These transplanted cells could be derived from adult (or fetal or embryonic) stem cells, neural stem cells, oligodendrocyte precursors, olfactory ensheathing cells, or Schwann cells. There is of course intense interest in finding the transplantation models that will be the most relevant to MS therapy. Accordingly, transplantation studies aimed at myelin repair are well under way in murine and primate models. A recent trial of Schwann cell transplantation in MS patients is currently under investigation, with preliminary disappointing results. However, the multifocal and evolving nature of the inflammatory process and lesion formation in MS, which is not necessarily well represented in animal models, presents a major hurdle for clinical application (Colman et al., 2003).

Repair in MS should also be aimed at protecting the axon, a strategy common to the approach in other neurodegenerative diseases. By protecting the axon from degeneration, this approach should maintain the axonal signals necessary for remyelination. In addition, it is obvious that remyelination per se is neuroprotective, and that axonal degeneration is, at least partially, a consequence of chronic demyelination and lack of related neurotrophic support (Rodriguez, 2003).

The environmental component of the lesions might well represent the most complex part of the repair process, As we suggest above, the demonstration of the potential beneficial effect of inflammatory cells on both remyelination and neuroprotection might hamper the use of aggressive immunosuppressant therapies, as they may reduce the capacity for repair.

Conclusions

The repair strategy in MS should focus on both remyelination and neuroprotection. Results from basic biology have told us about the major role of reciprocal interactions between axons and myelinating cells. This tight relationship suggests that a treatment acting on one of the partners will necessarily influence the other. Therefore, on the one hand, favoring remyelination will not only allow recovery of axonal conduction but will also prevent axonal degeneration. On the other hand, protecting the axon will favor remyelination by influencing both oligodendrocyte differentiation and initiation of the remyelination process.

References

Cannella, B., Hoban, C.J., Gao, Y.L., Garcia-Arenas, R., Lawson, D., Marchionni, M., et al. (1998). The neuregulin, glial growth factor 2, diminishes autoimmune demyelination and enhances remyelination in a chronic relapsing model for multiple sclerosis. Proc Natl Acad Sci USA 95(17): 10100–10105.

Cannella, B., Pitt, D., Capello, E., and Raine, C.S. (2000). Insulin-like growth factor-1 fails to enhance central nervous system myelin repair during autoimmune demyelination. Am J Pathol 157: 933–943.

Chang, A., Tourtellotte, W.W., Rudick, R., and Trapp, B.D. (2002). Premyelinating oligodendrocytes in chronic lesions of multiple sclerosis. N Engl J Med 346: 165–173.

Charles, P., Hernandez, M.P., Stankoff, B., Aigrot, M.S., Colin, C., Rougon, G., et al. (2000). Negative regulation of central nervous system myelination by polysialylated-neural cell adhesion molecule. Proc Natl Acad Sci USA 97: 7585–7590.

Charles, P., Reynolds, R., Seilhean, D., Rougon, G., Aigrot, M.S., Niezgoda, A., et al. (2002). Reexpression of PSA-NCAM by demyelinated axons: an inhibitor of remyelination in multiple sclerosis? Brain 125: 1972–1979.

Colman, D., Lubetzki, C., and Reingold, S. (2003). Multiple paths towards repair in multiple sclerosis. Trends Neurosci 26: 59–61.

Demerens, C., Stankoff, B., Allinquant,, B., Anglade, P., Couraud, F., Zalc, B., et al. (1996). Electrical activity is necessary for central nervous system myelination. Proc Natl Acad Sci USA 93: 9887–9892.

Ferguson, B., Matyszak, M.K., Esiri, M.M., and Perry, V.H. (1997). Axonal damage in acute multiple sclerosis lesions. Brain 120: 393–399.

Filippi, M., Bozzali, M., Rovaris, M., Gonen, O., Kesavadas, C., Ghezzi, A., et al. (2003). Evidence for widespread axonal damage at the earliest clinical stage of multiple sclerosis. Brain 126: 433–437.

Franklin, R.J.M. (2002). Why does remyelination fail in multiple sclerosis ? Nat Neurosci 3: 705–714.

Giess, R., Maurer, M., Linker, R., Gold, R., Warmuth-Metz, M., Toyka, K.V., et al. (2002). Association of a null mutation in the CNTF gene with early onset of multiple sclerosis. Arch Neurol 59(3): 407–409.

Hinks, G.L. and Franklin, R.J. (2000). Delayed changes in growth factor gene expression during slow remyelination in the CNS of aged rats. Mol Cell Neurosci 16: 542–556.

Hoffmann, V. and Hardt, C. (2002). A null mutation in the CNTF gene is not associated with early onset of multiple sclerosis. Arch Neurol 59:1974–1975.

John, G.R., Shankar, S.L., Shafit-Zagardo, B., Massimi, A., Lee, S.C., Raine, C.S., et al. (2002). Multiple sclerosis: re-expression of a developmental pathway that restricts oligodendrocyte maturation. Nat Med 8: 1115–1121.

Kotter, M.R., Setzu, A., Sim, F.J., Van Rooijen, N., and Franklin, R.J. (2001). Macrophage depletion impairs oligodendrocyte remyelination following lysolecithin-induced demyelination. *Glia* **35**: 204–212.

Lassmann, H. (1983). Comparative neuropathology of chronic experimental allergic encephalomyelitis and multiple sclerosis. *Schriftenr Neurol* **25**: 1–135.

Linker, R.A., Maurer, M., Gaupp, S., Martini, R., Holtmann, B., Giess, R., *et al.* (2002). CNTF is a major protective factor in demyelinating CNS disease: a neurotrophic cytokine as modulator in neuroinflammation. *Nat Med* **8**: 620–624.

Lucchinetti, C., Bruck, W., Parisi, J., Scheithauer, B., Rodriguez, M., and Lassmann, H. (2000). Heterogeneity of multiple sclerosis lesions: implications for the pathogenesis of demyelination. *Ann Neurol* **47**(6): 707–717.

Ludwin, S.K. (1987). Remyelination in demyelinating diseases of the central nervous system. *Crit Rev Neurobiol* **3**(1): 1–28.

Mason, J.L., Xuan, S., Dragatsis, I., Efstratiadis, A., and Goldman, J.E. (2003). Insulin-like growth factor (IGF) signaling through type 1 IGF receptor plays an important role in remyelination. *J Neurosci* **23**: 7710–7718.

Penderis, J., Woodruff, R.H., Lakatos, A., Li, W.W., Dunning, M.D., Zhao, C., *et al.* (2003). Increasing local levels of neuregulin (glial growth factor-2) by direct infusion into areas of demyelination does not alter remyelination in the rat CNS. *Eur J Neurosci* **18**: 2253–2264.

Perier, O. and Gregoire, A. (1965). Electron microscopic features of multiple sclerosis lesions. *Brain* **88**(5): 937–952.

Prineas, J.W., Barnard, R.O., Kwon, E.E., Sharer, L.R., and Cho, E.S. (1993). Multiple sclerosis: remyelination of nascent lesions. *Ann Neurol* **33**(2): 137–151.

Raine, C.S. and Wu, E. (1993). Multiple sclerosis: remyelination in acute lesions. *J Neuropathol Exp Neurol* **52**: 199–204.

Raine, C.S., Scheinberg, L., and Waltz, J.M. (1981). Multiple sclerosis. Oligodendrocyte survival and proliferation in an active established lesion. *Lab Invest* **45**(6): 534–546.

Ransohoff, R.M., Howe, C.L., and Rodriguez, M. (2002). Growth factor treatment of demyelinating disease: at last, a leap into the light. *Trends Immunol* **23**: 512–516.

Ricard, D., Rogemond, V., Charrier, E., Aguera, M., Bagnard, D., Belin, M.F., *et al.* (2001). Isolation and expression pattern of human Unc-33-like phosphoprotein 6/collapsin response mediator protein 5 (Ulip6/CRMP5): coexistence with Ulip2/CRMP2 in Sema3a-sensitive oligodendrocytes. *J Neurosci* **21**: 7203–7214.

Rodriguez, M. (2003). A function of myelin is to protect axons from subsequent injury : implications for deficits in multiple sclerosis. *Brain* **126**: 751–752.

Schwartz, M. (2002). Autoimmunity as the body's defense mechanism against the enemy within: development of therapeutic vaccines for neurodegenerative disorders. *J Neurovirol* **8**(6): 480–485.

Spassky, N., de Castro, F., Le Bras, B., Heydon, K., Queraud-LeSaux, F., Bloch-Gallego, E., *et al.* (2002). Directional guidance of oligodendroglial migration by class 3 semaphorins and netrin-1. *J Neurosci* **22**: 5992–6004.

Stankoff, B., Noel, F., Aigrot, M.S., Wattiliaux, A., Zalc, B., and Lubetzki, C. (2002). CNTF enhances myelin formation : a new role for CNTF and CNTF related molecules. *J Neurosci* **22**(21): 9221–9227.

Stevens, B., Porta, S., Haak, L.L., Gallo, V., and Fields, R.D. (2002). Adenosine: a neuron-glial transmitter promoting myelination in the CNS in response to action potentials. *Neuron* **36**(5): 855–868.

Trapp, B.D., Peterson, J., Ransohoff, R.M., Rudick, R., Mork, S., and Bo, L. (1998). Axonal transection in the lesions of multiple sclerosis. *N Engl J Med* **338**: 323–325.

Wang, S., Sdrulla, A.D., diSibio, G., Bush, G., Nofziger, D., Hicks, C., *et al.* (1998). Notch receptor activation inhibits oligodendrocyte differentiation. *Neuron* **21**: 63–75.

Warrington, A.E., Asakura, K., Bieber, A.J., Ciric, B., Van Keulen, V., Kaveri, S.V., *et al.* (2000). Human monoclonal antibodies reactive to oligodendrocytes promote remyelination in a model of multiple sclerosis. *Proc Natl Acad Sci USA* **97**: 6820–6825.

Wolswijk, G. (1998). Chronic stage multiple sclerosis lesions contain a relatively quiescent population of oligodendrocyte precursor cells. *J Neurosci* **18**: 601–609.

Yao, D.L., Liu, X., Hudson, L.D., and Webster, H.D. (1995). Insulin-like growth factor I treatment reduces demyelination and up-regulates gene expression of myelin-related proteins in experimental autoimmune encephalomyelitis. *Proc Natl Acad Sci USA* **92**: 6190–6194.

32 Immunological aspects of ischemic stroke

Guido Stoll, Sebastian Jander, Zurab Nadareishvili, and John M. Hallenbeck

Introduction

Immune responses in the nervous system have mainly been studied in the context of autoimmunity and infections. In recent years it has become apparent, however, that cells and mediators of the immune system are involved in a broad range of neurobiological processes such as cerebral ischemia, neurodegeneration, neuroprotection, and nerve regeneration. Ischemic stroke is the third leading cause of death in industrialized countries. Cerebral ischemia often results from embolization from an atherosclerotic plaque of the carotid artery. Inflammation of the vessel wall is an essential part of atherosclerosis in general, but, more specifically, immune interactions play a decisive role in the destabilization of atherosclerotic plaques leading to local formation of thromboemboli. Thereby, chronic atherosclerosis becomes converted into an acute disorder. In the nervous system, thromboemboli transiently or permanently occlude intracranial arteries and induce focal ischemia. Cerebral infarcts develop within minutes to hours of cessation of the cerebral blood flow and may expand over subsequent days. There is increasing evidence that leukocytes, cytokines, cell adhesion molecules, and other immune mediators contribute to secondary infarct growth. Conversely, inflammatory cytokines are involved in signaling pathways leading to neuroprotection after ischemic pre-conditioning. In this chapter we review the complex and diverse functions of immune cells and mediators in atherosclerosis and cerebral ischemia.

Inflammation and destabilization of atherosclerotic plaques of the carotid artery

Inflammation and atherosclerosis

Atherosclerosis is a systemic disease of large and medium-sized arteries which has long been considered to simply reflect the pathological accumulation of lipids in the vessel wall. This concept has changed. It is now assumed that an endothelial dysfunction induced by elevated and modified low-density lipoproteins (LDL), free radicals elicited by smoking and diabetes, infectious micro-organisms, or combinations of these and other factors leads to a compensatory inflammatory response (Ross, 1999). If inflammatory cells do not effectively neutralize the offending agents, this process persists and leads to chronic inflammation within the arterial wall. Accordingly, massive T-cell and macrophage infiltration has been found in areas of lipid deposition in human atherosclerotic plaques and in arteries of atherosclerosis-prone transgenic mice. T cells isolated from human atherosclerotic plaques can be stimulated to proliferate by oxidized LDL *in vitro*. Moreover, apolipoprotein-E (ApoE)-deficient mice that develop accelerated atherosclerosis and hypercholesterolemia show massive T-cell and macrophage infiltration of blood vessels. In further support of a decisive role of inflammation in atherosclerosis, cross-breeding of ApoE-deficient mice with op/op mice that lack colony stimulatory factor-1 and exhibit deficient macrophage activation, developed smaller atheroma than ApoE-deficient progenitors (Smith *et al.*, 1995). Taken together, these findings support an important role for inflammatory reactions in

the development of atherosclerotic plaques. Inflammation, moreover, appears to be critical during acute plaque destabilization in acute coronary artery disease and symptomatic carotid artery stenosis.

Immune responses and destabilization of carotid artery plaques: therapeutic implications

In the nervous system arterioarterial thromboembolism from extracranial stenoses of the internal carotid artery (ICA) is an important cause of ischemic stroke. However, even high-grade ICA stenoses (>70% luminal narrowing) carry a highly variable annual risk of stroke that can be as high as 13% following a recent occurrence of transient cerebral or retinal ischemia or as low as 1–2% in clinically asymptomatic patients (NASCET, 1991). These observations indicate that factors other than the degree of stenosis determine the risk of embolization. While the morphological appearance of ICA plaques on angiograms was of no prognostic value, the presence of plaque rupture or ulceration at histopathological examination of endarterectomy specimens was predictive of recent cerebrovascular embolism. Analysis of endarterectomy specimens revealed a higher percentage of macrophage-rich areas and a higher number of T cells per mm^2 in recently symptomatic compared with asymptomatic patients with high-grade ICA stenosis suggesting a role of inflammation in plaque destabilization (Jander *et al.*, 1998*b*; Nadareishvili *et al.*, 2001) (Figs 32.1(A–D)). The expression of intercellular adhesion molecule-1 (ICAM-1) that is involved in leukocyte trafficking through the endothelium was also significantly increased in plaques from symptomatic compared with asymptomatic patients (DeGraba *et al.*, 1998). ICAM-1 was predominantly located in regions with severe narrowing of the lumen. The antigen specificity of the T cells in ICA plaques is unclear at present. It has been speculated that infectious agents such as *Chlamydia pneumoniae* could trigger a local immune response and cause progression of atherosclerotic plaques to a symptomatic state. Accordingly, all T-cell subsets, but most prominently CD8+ T cells, were more abundant in *C. pneumoniae*-positive symptomatic ICA plaques (Nadareishvili *et al.*, 2001). Although *C. pneumoniae* were detectable in 15% of ICA plaques, no difference in the percentage of *C. pneumoniae*-positive plaques was found between symptomatic and asymptomatic patients. These findings indicate that infectious agents might play a pathobiological role in the induction of atherosclerosis, but that their mere presence cannot account for acute plaque destabilization.

How could infiltration by immune cells contribute to arterial thromboembolism and subsequent cerebral ischemia? Cytokines can activate macrophages to release matrix-degrading metalloproteinases (MMPs) and pro-thrombotic molecules such as tissue factor (TF) (Figs 32.1(E,F)). In their search for critical regulatory pathways involved in plaque destabilization, Mallat *et al.* (2001) found an increased expression of interleukin (IL)-18 mRNA and protein, and the corresponding receptors on plaque-associated macrophages. IL-18 is a prototypic pro-inflammatory cytokine. It was originally identified as interferon-γ (IFN-γ)-inducing factor and it promotes T-cell development along the Th1 lineage. Th1 cells and IFN-γ can induce TF expression in macrophages. TF binds to activated coagulation Factor VII and activates an enzymatic cascade that induces thrombus formation. In ICA endarterectomy specimens the extent of TF immunoreactivity in

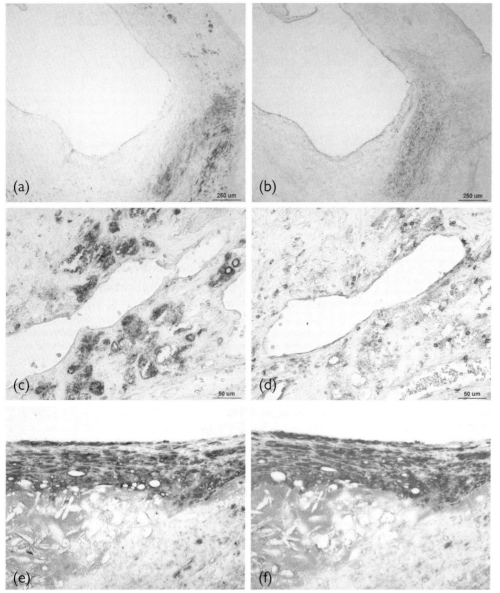

Fig. 32.1 Inflammation and atherosclerosis. Endarterectomy specimens from symptomatic high-grade internal carotid artery stenosis stained for macrophages (a, higher magnification c), T cells (b, higher magnification d), pro-thrombotic tissue factor (TF) (e), and collagen-degrading matrix metalloproteinase (MMP) (f). Note that inflammation is located in the atheromatous core of the lesion and the fibrous cap from which TF and MMP expression extends to the luminal surface. (See also plate 9 of the colour plate section at the center of this book.)

plaque-associated macrophages was significantly higher in symptomatic compared with asymptomatic patients (Jander et al., 2001) (Fig. 32.1(E)). In vitro, antibody-mediated blocking of TF activity decreased spontaneous platelet and fibrinogen deposition and thrombus formation on atherosclerotic plaque specimens. In ICA stenosis, plaque-associated TF must get into contact with the bloodstream to activate the coagulation system. As described above, plaque rupture or ulceration are regularly seen in symptomatic ICA plaques. MMP are enzymes that degrade extracellular matrix components. Among a number of MMPs tested, MMP-9 protein levels and activity were closely related to the recent (<4 weeks) occurrence of cerebrovascular events in high-grade ICA stenosis, suggesting a role in the destruction of the fibrous cap of atherosclerotic ICA plaques (Loftus et al., 2000). It should also be noted that endothelial cells activated by pro-inflammatory cytokines or bacterial lipopolysaccharide can directly express TF. The contribution of endothelial TF to plaque symptomatology has not been determined.

Although our understanding of the molecular basis of ICA plaque destabilization is still limited, the studies reviewed above point to inflammation and macrophage-derived factors (TF, MMP-9) as potential therapeutic targets. In heritable hyperlipidemic rabbits the statin cerivastatin decreased TF and MMP expression in atheroma-associated macrophages (Aikawa et al., 2001).

Statins are HMG-CoA-reductase inhibitors with profound immuno-modulatory effects. In patients with coronary artery disease, statins reduced the annual incidence of stroke by approximately 30%, an effect that was attributed to the decrease in cholesterol levels. However, patients with normal serum levels of cholesterol likewise benefited from statin treatment, suggesting alternative, probably anti-inflammatory, therapeutic mechanisms. Statins appear also to be effective in primary stroke prevention (Law et al., 2003) possibly through an immune deviation that resembles the effect of immunological tolerization that creates regulatory T cells (Youssef et al., 2002).

Inflammation, immune mediators, and development of ischemic brain lesions

Mechanisms of neuronal death and experimental stroke models

Focal impairment or cessation of blood flow to the brain restricts the delivery of oxygen, glucose, and other substrates. Thereby, the energy-dependent maintenance of ionic gradients is impaired leading to depolarization of neurons and glia which release excitatory amino acids (glutamate) into the extracellular space and accumulate Ca^{2+} (Dirnagl et al., 1999). Ca^{2+} is a universal second messenger leading to activation of proteolytic enzymes, production of free-radical species, and release of the excitotoxic amino acid, glutamate. In the core of the ischemic territory, where the flow reduction is most severe, these processes induce rapid necrotic cell death. In addition, a significant proportion of neurons die by an internal program of self-destruction called apoptosis or programmed cell death that is ongoing for several days after the initial insult. Apoptosis requires partially preserved protein synthesis and involves activation of caspases. Production of oxygen-based and nitrogen-based free radicals, generation of inflammatory mediators (e.g. tumor necrosis factor (TNF), interleukin (IL)-1, inducible nitric oxide synthase (iNOS), cyclo-oxygenase-2, protease activation (e.g. calpains, caspases, extracellular proteases), mitochondrial dysfunction, endoplasmic reticulum dysfunction, and apoptosis are included in the current broad-brush view of key injury mechanisms (Dirnagl et al., 1999; Neumar, 2000).

Several animal models have been developed to study progression and mechanisms of focal ischemic brain injury (Ginsberg and Busto, 1989). Surgical occlusion of major arteries is widely used. Permanent occlusion of the middle cerebral artery (MCAO) at proximal sites leads to complete infarctions of the basal ganglia and the neocortex. In this model the infarct volume has been observed to change significantly between 6 and 72 hours. Early reperfusion by withdrawal of an intraluminal thread advanced into the proximal MCA (transient MCAO) reconstitutes perfusion and significantly modifies stroke development. Short-lasting ischemia (<30 min) leads to a restricted infarction with pannecrosis of neurons and glial cells in the caudatoputamen, but only partly affects the neocortex. Further delay in reperfusion produces increasing neocortical infarction. Initially during cerebral ischemia, developing infarcts are surrounded by an ischemic penumbra that can be salvaged by reperfusion. The ischemic penumbra refers to cortical areas where the blood flow is reduced, but still exceeds a flow and duration threshold that produces an irreversible state of ischemic neuronal injury. Depending on the timing of reperfusion, neocortical infarctions can be surrounded by areas of selective neuronal death characterized by loss of large pyramidal neurons but preservation of endothelial and glial structures.

Inflammation

Focal cerebral ischemia leads to local activation of microglia and astroglia and to a dramatic influx of hematogenous leukocytes (Kochanek and Hallenbeck, 1992; Stoll et al., 1998).

Granulocytes

Granulocytes are the first hematogenous cells that appear in the brain in response to focal ischemia (Kochanek and Hallenbeck, 1992). In experimental animals and in humans granulocytes accumulate in cerebral vessels within hours before they invade the infarct and its boundary zone. This process peaks at 24 hours after infarction; thereafter the number of granulocytes rapidly declines. Within the second week after infarction granulocytes have mostly disappeared. Granulocytes are attracted by chemokines released from ischemic tissue. In transient ischemia models accumulation of intravascular granulocyte probably reduces blood flow in the reperfusion phase and thereby contributes to the extension of infarctions (see below).

Monocytes/macrophages and activation of microglia

The most abundant leukocytes that enter the brain after focal cerebral ischemia are monocytes/macrophages (Kochanek and Hallenbeck, 1992; Stoll et al., 1998) (Fig. 32.2(A)). Hematogenous macrophages are attracted preferentially into areas of pannecrosis and the border zones by chemokines (Hughes et al., 2002). The infiltrates demarcate necrotic brain tissue from normal tissue, and rapidly remove debris leaving a glial scar. Additionally, resident microglia contribute to this phagocytic response (Schroeter et al., 1997) (Fig. 32.2 (A)), but become indistinguishable from macrophages upon activation. The problem of distinguishing between hematogenous macrophage infiltration and local microglial responses could recently be

solved by a novel magnetic resonance imaging (MRI) technique. Superparamagnetic iron particles (SPIO) injected into the circulation are rapidly taken up by circulating macrophages. When these iron-laden macrophages infiltrate lesions they become detectable as areas of signal loss on T2-weighted MR images. It turned out that hematogenous macrophages were recruited with a delay of several days to ischemic brain lesions in the rat, and that macrophage invasion was temporally unrelated to the breakdown of the blood–brain barrier (BBB) (Kleinschnitz et al., 2003). Late recruitment was confirmed in a pilot study in human stroke (Saleh et al., 2004). These studies suggest that macrophages play a role in tissue remodelling and repair rather than neuronal injury because they appear at a stage in which delayed neuronal cell death has already ceased. Rather microglial activation plays a detrimental role early. Accordingly, minocyclin, a tetracyclin derivative, attenuated microglial responses and concurrently reduced infarct volumes (Yrjanheikki et al., 1999).

Microglial/macrophage responses to cerebral ischemia are phenotypically divergent. In the rat two different populations emerged: (1) CD4+ microglia/macrophages that are also present in other CNS lesion paradigms gradually increased from day 2 and peaked at day 14 when they covered the entire area of infarction, and (2) microglia/macrophages expressing the T- and NK-cell surface molecule, CD8, comprising a separate and unusual population (Jander et al., 1998a). CD8+ microglia/macrophages were transiently present between days 3 and 6 and had almost disappeared at day 14. They were exclusively located in the border zone and core of pannecrotic brain tissue. The functional role of CD8+ microglia/macrophages in brain ischemia is unclear at present. CD8+ cells could contribute to exacerbation of ischemic brain damage as well as to tissue remodeling and healing processes. In vitro studies performed independently on alveolar macrophages showed that signaling via the CD8 molecule led to expression of TNF, IL-1β, and iNOS. CD8+ microglia/macrophages appear to be relatively unique to areas of ischemic pannecrosis since no such cells were seen in areas of selective neuronal death or during fiber tract degeneration.

T cells

In both experimental and human stroke a significant number of T cells preferentially infiltrate the border zones of infarctions within the first week (Becker et al., 1997, Stoll et al., 1998) (Figs 32.2(B,C)). T-cell recruitment into the CNS is usually observed in autoimmune and infectious but not degenerative disorders. In experimental autoimmune encephalomyelitis (EAE), systemic immunization with myelin proteins such as myelin basic protein (MBP) creates CD4+ helper/inducer T cells that are antigen specific and accumulate within the CNS after 10 to 12 days to induce myelin destruction by macrophages. In cerebral ischemia, the period between lesion induction and T-cell infiltration is too short for generation of a systemic, antigen-specific immune response. Therefore, the T-cell response is likely to be antigen non-specific. The signals that attract T cells and keep them in the CNS parenchyma for many days are unknown at present. There is indirect evidence that infiltration of tolerized T cells into ischemic brain lesions can be beneficial. Becker et al. (1997) fed naïve rats with MBP, a procedure known to induce immunological tolerance to EAE induction. MBP-tolerized animals had reduced infarct volumes at 24 and 96 hours when subjected to MCAO, an effect that was attributed to the infiltration of evolving ischemic brain lesions with T cells that produced transforming growth factor (TGF)-β1. TGF-β1 is neuroprotective and a potent immunosuppressant. The neuroprotective effect of MBP tolerance in cerebral ischemia can be transferred to naïve animals by infusion of tolerized lymphocytes (adoptive transfer) (Becker et al., 2003).

The functional role of cell adhesion molecules in leukocyte recruitment

The inflammatory response in focal ischemia involves multiple cell adhesion steps providing the traffic signals for entry of leukocytes into the brain (Del Zoppo et al., 2000). Binding via selectins (E-selectin, P-selectin, L-selectin) reduces the velocity of leukocytes in the bloodstream by sup-

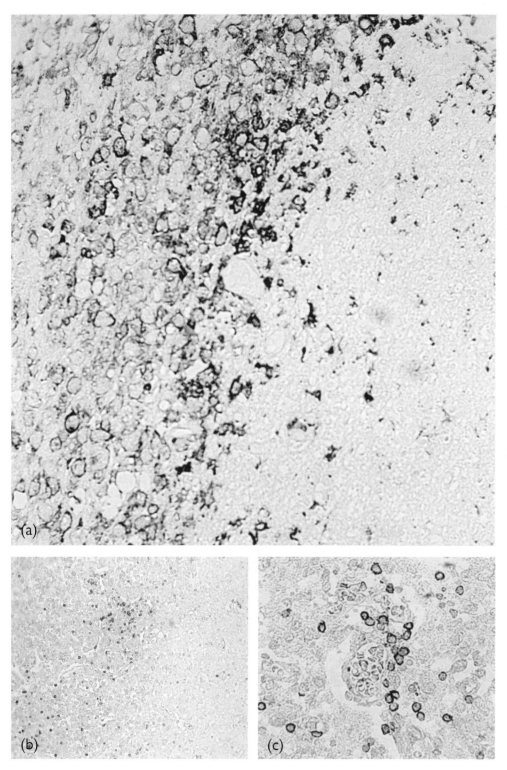

Fig. 32.2 Cellular inflammation in ischemic stroke. Human cerebral infarct 5 days after middle cerebral artery occlusion stained for MHC Class II molecules expressed on activated macrophages and microglia (a), and for CD3, a marker for T cells (b, higher magnification c). Part (a) shows the boundary of the infarct which has been infiltrated by hematogenous macrophages. In addition, activated microglia, which partly preserved their typical morphology at the outer margin (right), transformed into phagocytes towards the infarct core (left) and thereby became indistinguishable from hematogenous macrophages. Surprisingly, a considerable number of T cells are present around the infarct (b, c).

porting leukocyte rolling on luminal endothelium. Firm adhesion of leukocytes to the endothelium is mediated by integrins. Different molecules of the integrin family direct the adhesion of leukocyte subsets: Lymphocytes constitutively bear the CD11a/CD18 (leukocyte function associated antigen-1; LFA-1) and the very late antigen-4 (VLA-4) complex on their surface, monocytes LFA-1, VLA-4, and the CD11b/CD18 complex, and granulocytes LFA-1 and the CD11b/CD18 complex. The corresponding endothelial counter-receptors are intercellular adhesion molecule-1 (ICAM-1) for LFA-1 and CD11b/CD18, and the vascular cellular adhesion molecule-1 (VCAM-1) for VLA-4. ICAM-1 is induced on brain endothelial cells as early as 3 hours after focal ischemia, peaks at 6 to 12 hours, and persists for several days similar to E-selectin (endothelial leukocyte adhesion molecule-1; ELAM-1) and VCAM-1 (Del Zoppo *et al.*, 2000).

The functional relevance of cell adhesion processes in stroke development has been established in transient focal ischemia. Treatment with antibodies directed against the CD11b/CD18 complex present on granulocytes and monocytes/macrophages of rats subjected to 2 hours of transient MCAO led to a significant reduction in infarct volume and to a decrease in the number of apoptotic cells. In parallel, infiltration by granulocytes was reduced. Similar results were obtained when a recombinant neutrophil inhibiting factor directed against the CD11b/CD18 complex was used. Blocking of the corresponding ligand on endothelial cells, ICAM-1, had a stronger mitigating effect and reduced stroke volumes at day 2 by 80% (Zhang *et al.*, 1995). Accordingly, ICAM-1 knockout mice showed a five-fold decrease in infarct size (Connolly *et al.*, 1996). Treatment with antileukocyte antibodies in

models of permanent MCAO was ineffective (Zhang *et al.*, 1995). The most likely explanation for this discrepancy is that granulocytes adhere to the microvascular endothelium via the ICAM-1/CD11b/CD18 adhesion pathway thereby mechanically disconnecting dependent parenchyma from reperfusion ('no reflow phenomenon'). Prolonged hypoxia then leads to extension of the infarct area into the penumbra zone. Despite the profound mitigating effects of ICAM-1 neutralization in rodent cerebral ischemia, a recent study in human stroke using a rat monoclonal antibody against ICAM-1 that was conjugated with polyethylene glycol to reduce immuno-

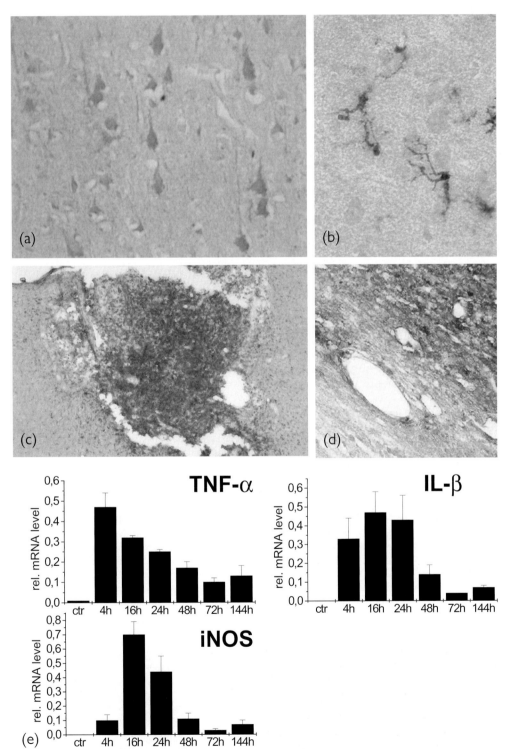

Fig. 32.3 Cytokines in experimental cerebral ischemia. Localization of TNF (a), IL-1β (b), IL-18 (c), and TGF-β1 (d) by immunocytochemistry, and gene expression profiles of TNF, IL-1β, and inducible NO synthase (iNOS) as revealed by semiquantitative reverse transcriptase polymerase chain reaction (e). Note that TNF, IL-1β, and iNOS mRNA peak within 24 hours after focal ischemia (e). On the cellular level TNF is mainly expressed by neurons (a), IL-1 β by microglia (b), while IL-18 (c) and TGF-β1 (d) are induced with a delay and are mainly expressed by macrophages and microglia. (See also Plate 10 of the colour plate section at the center of this book for Figures 32.3 a–d.)

genicity, Enlimolab, failed and led to unacceptable side-effects by activating human neutrophils (Enlimomab Acute Stroke Trial Investigators, 2001). Adverse effects of Enlimomab may have been caused by immunological factors. The occurrence of unwanted immunological side-effects of heterologous anti-ICAM-1 antibodies was confirmed in recent experiments in rats where murine monoclonal anti-ICAM-1 activated complement, neutrophils, and endothelial cells. In the rat blocking of lymphocyte and monocyte entry by antibodies to the α_4 integrin improved neurological outcome and decreased infarct volume even when instituted after onset of focal ischemia (Becker et al., 2001).

Transcription factors, nitric oxide, and cytokines: pro-inflammatory and neurotoxic pathways

The cellular responses in focal cerebral ischemia are accompanied by the expression of immunological transcription factors, iNOS, and cytokines (Fig. 32.3). IL-1β, TNF, and IL-10 are rapidly induced prior to leukocyte entry within the first 24 hours. In contrast, the expression of IL-18 and TGF-β1 occurs later during the inflammation stage. In this section, neurotoxic pathways involving immune mediators are reviewed. Cytokine participation in ischemic pre-conditioning and neuroprotection are covered in a subsequent section.

Interferon regulatory factor 1 and inducible NO synthase

Iadecola and colleagues formally proved that immune cascades contribute to significant infarct growth beyond 24 hours after focal cerebral ischemia (Iadecola, 1997; Iadecola et al.,1999). Interferon regulatory factor 1 (IRF) is a transcription factor that can be activated by TNF and IL-1β. After focal ischemia IRF gene expression was markedly up-regulated at 12 hours, and reached a peak at day 4. Transgenic mice lacking the IRF gene were protected from ischemic brain damage and developed smaller infarctions and neurological deficits (Iadecola et al., 1999). The molecular mechanisms underlying ischemic neuroprotection in IRF knockout mice have not been fully elucidated. IRF can induce gene transcription of interleukin-1 converting enzyme (ICE or caspase 1) and iNOS. Lack of nitric oxide (NO) induction is a likely mechanism since macrophages from IRF knockout mice produced virtually no NO and synthesized only low levels of iNOS mRNA in vitro. NO is a small molecule that exerts pleiotropic actions. NO is synthesized by oxidation of L-arginine by the enzyme NO synthase (NOS) which exists in three isoforms, neuronal NOS (nNOS), endothelial NOS (eNOS), and iNOS. NO production is enhanced at all stages of cerebral ischemia (Iadecola, 1997). Early during ischemia NO produced through eNOS activation in endothelial cells is beneficial and induces an increase of cerebral blood flow by vasodilatation as well as anti-adhering effects on leukocytes. In contrast, iNOS appears to be detrimental. iNOS induces synthesis of large amounts of NO continuously for long periods, which then reacts with superoxide to form peroxynitrite, a cytotoxic agent. After MCAO in mice, iNOS mRNA expression in the postischemic brain began between 6 and 12 hours, peaked at 96 hours, and subsided after 7 days (Iadecola, 1997). Disruption of the iNOS gene in mice led to smaller infarcts and reduced motor deficits after focal ischemia. Importantly, reduction in ischemic damage and neurological deficits was observed 96 hours after ischemia, but not at 24 hours providing strong support for iNOS expression as one of the critical factors that contribute to the delayed expansion of brain damage.

Interleukin-1

In the normal brain, expression of IL-1 is very low. Low abundance causes difficulties in the unequivocal identification of the cellular source of cytokines. IL-1 appears to be associated with neurons, astrocytes, oligodendrocytes, and endothelial cells in the normal CNS (Allen and Rothwell, 2001). Within 1 hour after focal ischemia, IL-1β mRNA levels increase significantly in the ischemic cortex, reach peak levels during the first 24 hours, and rapidly decline thereafter (Liu et al., 1993) (Fig. 32.3(E)). IL-1β protein was strongly expressed by endothelial cells, microglia, and infiltrating macrophages (Fig. 32.3(B)), while IL-1β expression by neurons and astrocytes in ischemic brain lesions is still controversial. By 6 hours

after MCAO, scattered IL-1β-positive ramified microglia were present within the ischemic area. Twenty-four to 48 hours after the ischemic insult, a massive increase in the distribution and number of IL-1β-positive cells, now resembling hematogenous macrophages, has been described. IL-1α appears to be induced slightly earlier that IL-1β in focal ischemia, but the time course of expression and cellular sources have not been further elaborated.

IL-1 acts by binding to IL-1 type I (IL-1RI) and type II (IL-1RII) receptors. IL-1RI transduces an intracellular signal, while IL-1RII binds IL-1 without inducing a signal and thereby serves as a natural IL-1 antagonist. Concomitantly with the up-regulation of IL-1β, the corresponding IL-1 receptor genes were locally induced. Moreover, mRNA levels of IL-1 receptor antagonist (IL-1ra) significantly increased at 6 hours after MCAO in the ischemic hemisphere. At the cellular level, the expression of IL-1 receptors I and II and IL-1ra in the ischemic brain has not yet been definitively established. In normal mouse brain, IL-1RI and IL-1RII are constitutively expressed on neurons in the hippocampus and in the neuronal soma of Purkinje cells of the cerebellum.

The most compelling evidence that IL-1β is involved in ischemic brain damage derives from pharmacological studies and from stroke induction in genetically manipulated laboratory animals (Allen and Rothwell, 2001). Surprisingly, IL-1β exerted neurotoxic actions in focal cerebral ischemia independently of the IL-1RI. Intracerebroventricular injections of IL-1β exacerbated ischemic brain damage in wild-type but also in IL-1RI knockout mice suggesting the existence of a so far unidentified additional IL-1 receptor molecule (Touzani et al., 2002). Studies using IL-1-deficient mice further supported a detrimental role of IL-1 in stroke development. Double knockout mice lacking both the IL-1α and IL-1β gene exhibited greatly decreased infarct volumes, while deletion of a single IL-1 gene had no effect on infarct size, probably reflecting compensatory changes in the IL-1 system (Boutin et al., 2001). Exogenous administration of IL-1ra reduced focal ischemic brain damage. Thus, although there is co-induction of IL-1 and IL-1ra in ischemic brain lesions, it appears that in vivo the agonistic detrimental IL-1β effects predominate over the antagonistic IL-1ra effects. It has been estimated that IL-1ra needs to be at more than 100-fold excess to fully neutralize IL-1. In further support of a noxious role of IL-1β in cerebral ischemia, pharmacological inhibition of caspase-1, the enzyme critical for cleavage of pro-IL-1 into biologically active IL-1, decreased infarct volume after MCAO in mice and rats. Moreover, transgenic mice with a mutant caspase-1 gene developed smaller infarcts, milder neurological deficits, reduced IL-1β levels, and decreased DNA fragmentation after transient and permanent MCAO. The mitigating effects of caspase-1 elimination, however, might not be solely due to reduction of IL-1β production. Caspase-1 plays a critical role in activating apoptotic pathways and in the modulation of release of the pro-inflammatory cytokine IL-18. Accordingly, caspase-1 mRNA induction in focal ischemia showed a protracted time course in parallel to IL-18, but was unrelated to the expression pattern of IL-1β (Jander et al., 2002).

The signal transduction pathways and secondary effector mechanisms of IL-1β-associated exacerbation of ischemic brain damage have not been clearly delineated. IL-1β per se is not neurotoxic in vivo in the absence of cofactors. Current hypotheses suggest that IL-1β influences death or survival of neurons via complex actions involving glia (Allen and Rothwell, 2001). One deleterious mechanism in focal ischemia possibly reflects the induction of cell adhesion molecules on endothelial cells with ensuing enhanced infiltration of granulocytes.

Tumor necrosis factor

Similar to IL-1β, TNF mRNA is rapidly induced within 1 hour after MCAO, reaches peak expression within the first 24 hours, and returns to low baseline levels during the next few days (Barone et al., 1997) (Fig. 32.3(E)). In contrast to IL-1β, TNF immunoreactivity was mainly associated with ischemic neurons in the evolving infarct and surrounding tissue (Fig. 32.3(A)). At day 5, neuronal TNF expression had diminished greatly, and TNF immunoreactivity was found in infiltrating macrophages. Concomitant with the expression of TNF, the corresponding TNF receptors p55 and p75 were up-regulated within 6 and 24 hours, respectively. TNF receptor p55 has been implicated in transducing the cytotoxic signaling of TNF. The presence of TNF protein and TNF p55 receptors in ischemic brain lesions therefore suggested an injurious role of excessive TNF produced during the acute phase (Barone *et al.*, 1997; Shohami *et al.*, 1999). This notion is supported by experimental evidence. Intracerebroventricular injection of TNF 24 hours prior to MCAO significantly exacerbated the size of infarction examined 24 hours after onset (Barone *et al.*, 1997). Moreover, blocking of endogenous TNF by neutralizing antibodies or treatment with TNF binding protein resulted in a significant reduction in the cortical infarct volume (Barone *et al.*, 1997; Shohami *et al.*,1999). In cultured cerebellar granule cells, the application of TNF did not directly affect neurotransmitter release, glutamate, or free radical toxicity. Thus, it was concluded that TNF neurotoxicity is mediated through non-neuronal cells. The noxious effect could partly be due to activation of the capillary endothelium to a pro-adhesive state similar to IL-1β, leading to an increased adhesion and influx of inflammatory cells. Assessment of the functional role of TNF in cerebral ischemia is complicated by the fact that this cytokine can exert dose- and cofactor-dependent opposing neurotoxic or neuroprotective effects (see below) (Shohami *et al.*, 1999; Allen and Rothwell, 2001; Hallenbeck, 2002). Mattson and his collaborators have generated mice lacking TNFR1 and TNFR2 to study the role of TNF in mediating post-ischemic processes (Bruce *et al.*, 1996). In these mice, infarct area 24 h after MCAO was significantly larger than in wild-type controls and oxidative stress was also increased due probably to the inability of the knock-out mice to upregulate the antioxidant and neuroprotective enzyme, manganese superoxide dismutase. TNFR1/TNFR2-null mice are exposed to chronic deprivation from TNF homeostatic effects and may chronically lack TNF-induced negative feedback mechanisms. This would render them different from wild-type mice with an acute block of TNF activity and could account for their increased vulnerability to stress.

Late cytokine response: interleukin-18

IL-18 has so far been the only pro-inflammatory cytokine strongly associated with the delayed inflammatory response in focal brain ischemia. IL-18 is a member of the IL-1 cytokine family initially identified in a mouse model of endotoxic shock as IFN-γ inducing factor. In focal ischemia, IL-18 mRNA and protein expression exhibited a delayed time course of induction commencing at 24 to 48 hours and peaking 6 days after ischemia (Jander *et al.*, 2002).

Thereby, IL-18 differs from IL-1 which is expressed at maximum levels within hours after ischemia. IL-18 protein was mainly localized to macrophages in the ischemic lesion and to perilesional microglia (Fig. 32.3(C)). Both IL-18 and IL-1 are synthesized as inactive precursor molecules requiring cleavage by caspase-1 for conversion into mature bioactive cytokines. Caspase-1 mRNA induction paralleled the expression of IL-18, but was unrelated to the time course of IL-1 induction. Induction of IL-18 in ischemic brain lesions was not accompanied by increased levels of IFN-γ mRNA suggesting an IFN-γ-independent role in cerebral ischemia (Jander *et al.*, 2002). IL-18 up-regulates the cellular adhesion molecule ICAM-1 involved in macrophage recruitment independently from the actions of IFN-γ. While infarct volumes were reduced by 21% in IL-18 deficient seven day old rats after hypoxic-ischemic brain injury (Hedtjarn *et al.*, 2002), no protective effect was seen at 24 hours after transient MCAO in adult IL-18 knock-out mice (Wheeler *et al.*, 2003).

Cytokines and neuroprotection

It appears that the expression of IL-1β, TNF, and IL-18 is tightly regulated in focal ischemic brain lesions. There is evidence that IL-10 and transforming growth factor-β (TGF-β) partially antagonize pro-inflammatory and neurotoxic pathways (Fig. 32.4).

The expression of anti-inflammatory cytokines in focal cerebral ischemia: interleukin-10 and transforming growth factor-β1

IL-10 mRNA has been detected 6 hours after MCAO in rats (Zhai *et al.*, 1997). Astrocytes and macrophages in tissue samples from patients with multiple sclerosis express immunoreactive IL-10, suggesting that these cells are a potential source for this cytokine in stroke (Hulshof *et al.*, 2002). Functionally, intraventricular or systemic application of IL-10 30 min after transient MCAO led to decreased infarct size (Spera *et al.*, 1998). Correspondingly, brain infarcts were 30% larger in transgenic IL-10 –/– mice compared with wild-type animals (Grilli *et al.*, 2000). When administered exogenously, IL-10 may inhibit transcription of TNF and other pro-inflammatory cytokines or inhibit the transcription factor, NF-κB. The neuroprotective effects of IL-10 could be due to attenuation of the inflammatory response and/or due to an inhibitory effect on neurotoxic signaling

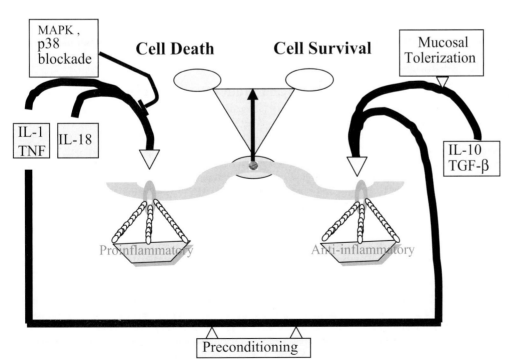

Fig. 32.4 Neurotoxicity versus neuroprotection. The balance between pro-inflammatory and anti-inflammatory cytokines partly determines the extent of ischemic cell death. Note that TNF and IL-1β can act to cause neurotoxicity and, through pre-conditioning, can act to produce neuroprotection. Blockade of stress-activated MAPKs can suppress neurotoxicity by reducing the production of pro-inflammatory cytokines.

cascades. In support of the latter possibility, primary neuronal cultures derived from IL-10 −/− mice were more susceptible to excitotoxicity and oxygen-glucose deprivation (Grilli *et al.*, 2000), and IL-10 reduced glutamate-induced cerebellar granule cell death *in vitro* by blocking caspase-3-like activity (Bachis *et al.*, 2001). A recent clinical study also supports a role for IL-10 in stroke prevention. In a longitudinal study of 599 subjects aged ≥85 years, those with a history of stroke had significantly lower IL-10 levels at baseline than subjects without stroke (Van Exel *et al.*, 2002). During 2.6 years of follow-up the relative risk for fatal stroke was 2.94 when subjects with low or intermediate baseline IL-10 production were compared with those with high levels of IL-10. This Leiden 85-Plus Study showed that a deficiency in IL-10 carries increased risk of stroke even in a healthy population. If this relates to a potential protective role of IL-10 during atherogenesis rather than a local effect in the brain is currently unknown.

Transforming growth factor-β1 (TGF-β1) is a multifunctional cytokine capable of regulating diverse cellular processes. The neuroprotective effect of TGF-β1 has been related to its ability to maintain the mitochondrial membrane potential, to stabilize Ca²⁺ homeostasis, to increase the expression of the anti-apoptotic proteins Bcl-2 and Bcl-xl (Prehn *et al.*, 1993), to inhibit caspase-3 activation (Zhu *et al.*, 2001) and to induce plasminogen activator inhibitor-1 (Buisson *et al.*, 1998). TGF-β1 expression continuously increases during the first week after focal ischemia in parallel to IL-18, and is likewise associated with microglia and infiltrating macrophages (Lehrmann *et al.*, 1998) (Fig. 32.3(D)). In neuronal cell culture systems, TGF-β1 attenuated glutamate-induced excitotoxic cell death (Prehn *et al.*, 1993; Ruocco *et al.*, 1999) suggesting a physiological role as a natural neuroprotectant in CNS lesions. This notion is further supported by neutralization experiments. Application of a soluble TGF-β type II receptor fused with the Fc region of human immunoglobulin to rats with MCAO strongly aggravated the volume of infarction (Ruocco *et al.*, 1999). Henrich-Noack *et al.*, (1996) demonstrated that TGF-β1 reduces injury to CA1 hippocampal neurons caused by transient global ischemia in rats. This protective action could well be associated with the anti-oxidative and anti-apoptotic effects of TGF-β1 demonstrated *in vitro*. A mild mitigating effect was seen after MCAO in mice that received TGF-β1 intracisternally (Prehn *et al.*, 1993) and TGF-β1 injected into the lateral cerebral ventricle of rats 2 hours after severe hypoxic–ischemic brain injury reduced the area of cortical infarction (McNeill *et al.*, 1994). These findings suggest that endogenous TGF-β1 induced by ischemia limits the extent of injury and that additional exogenous TGF-β1 can augment neuroprotection to some degree. Published data addressing TGF-β in clinical stroke have been inconclusive. Kim *et al.*, (1996) showed that the serum level of TGF-β was significantly decreased at day 1 and day 3 and tended to return toward control levels thereafter. Slevin *et al.*, (2000) did not find significant differences between serum TGF-β levels from patients and controls at any of several time points (days 0, 1, 3, 7, and 14), however.

An increase in mRNA of another anti-inflammatory cytokine, IL-4, has been observed ipsilateral to MCAO in rats at 6, 12 and 24 hour time points (Li *et al.*, 2001). There is as yet no direct evidence supporting a neuroprotective function for IL-4.

Mitogen-activated protein kinases (MAPKs) are involved in many cellular processes. The stress-activated MAPK, p38, has been linked to inflammatory cytokine production and cell death following cellular stress. Inhibition of the MAPK cascade via cytokine suppressive anti-inflammatory drugs, which block p38 MAPK and hence the production of interleukin-1 and TNF, has been shown to have a neuroprotective effect in a rat model of permanent focal ischemic stroke (Barone *et al.*, 2001). Oral pre- and post-stroke, and intravenous post-stroke, administration of the p38 MAPK inhibitor SB 23906 reduced infarct size by 28–41% and neurological deficits by 25–35%. These reductions were associated with decreased expression of stroke-induced IL-1β and TNF.

Mucosal tolerization is a method for inducing peripheral immune tolerance. The procedure involves oral or nasal administration of low doses of antigen to induce active immune suppression, whereas high antigen doses induce clonal anergy and deletion. Intranasally (or orally) administered antigen preferentially generates a Th2 (IL-4, IL-10) or a Th3 (TGF-β) T-lymphocyte response. Because these regulatory T cells are triggered in an antigen-specific fashion, but suppress in an antigen-non-specific fashion, they mediate bystander suppression when they undergo a second encounter with the fed or inhaled autoantigen at the target organ. Thus, mucosal tolerance can be used to treat inflammatory processes that are stimulated by other than the tolerizing antigen so long as that antigen is localized to the site of inflammation. This approach has been used to treat animal models of stroke. Becker *et al.* (1997) achieved control of inflammation associated with brain ischemia by inducing oral tolerance to the myelin basic protein (MBP). Infarct size at 24 and 96 hours after MCAO was significantly reduced in tolerized animals. Tolerance to MBP was confirmed *in vivo* by a decrease in delayed-type hypersensitivity to MBP and immunoreactive TGF-β expression by T cells was found only in the brains of tolerized animals. These results show that MBP-specific deviation of the immune response towards Th2 or Th3 lymphocytes has a neuroprotective effect in a rat model of stroke. Mucosal tolerization strategies have also been applied to the ultimate in neuroprotection, stroke prevention. Takeda *et al.* (2002) studied the effect of mucosal tolerance to human E-selectin for stroke prevention in spontaneously hypertensive stroke-prone rats. The essence of this approach is to target regulatory T cells to vessel segments that are becoming activated and threatening to thrombose or bleed. E-selectin is only expressed on activated endothelium and, according to the model, when locally presented to tolerized T cells it stimulates local production of immunosuppressive cytokines such as TGF-β1. TGF-β1 then suppresses production of pro-inflammatory cytokines, reduces endothelial thrombogenicity, and minimizes vessel injury preventing local thrombosis or hemorrhage. In this study, intranasal E-selectin significantly decreased the number of ischemic and hemorrhagic strokes in spontaneously hypertensive, genetically stroke-prone rats with untreated hypertension. It also suppressed delayed-type hypersensitivity to E-selectin, and increased numbers of TGF-β1-positive splenocytes indicating that intranasal exposure to E-selectin induced immunological tolerance. Immunological tolerance has also been applied to the suppression of atherosclerosis in hypercholesterolemic mice (Maron *et al.*, 2002). In this study, nasal administration of mycobacterial heat shock protein-65 (HSP-65) was associated with a significant decrease in the size of atherosclerotic plaques, a reduction in macrophage-positive area in the aortic arch, increased interleukin-10 expression, and a reduced number of plaque T cells. Inflammation and auto-immunity to heat shock proteins (HSPs) contribute to the progression of atherosclerosis and an antigen-specific approach involving mucosal administration of HSP-65 can specifically affect immune response and decrease both plaque formation and local inflammation. Most available immunosuppressive agents have systemic side-effects that would limit their long-term use in the prevention of stroke or atherosclerosis. The nasal administration of proteins offers the potential for long-term antigen-specific therapy that targets regulatory cells to the disease area without systemic immunosuppression.

Cytokines and brain pre-conditioning

Induction of tolerance generally involves exposure to a non-lethal stress followed by a variable interval before exposure to a potentially lethal stress; the pre-conditioning then mitigates the damage from the severe stress. Lipopolysaccharide (LPS), the prototypic stimulus for expression of pro-inflammatory cytokines, has been shown to effectively pre-condition various organs against subsequent ischemia. Protection has been observed in the kidney and heart as well as the brain. LPS (0.5 mg/kg i.p.) administered 72 hours before 60 min of intraluminal suture MCAO reduced brain infarct volume by 35% compared with controls and was associated with an increase of superoxide dismutase and endothelial nitric oxide synthase (Bordet *et al.*, 2000; Puisieux *et al.*, 2000). In addition, two important pro-inflammatory cytokines, IL-1 and TNF, that are strongly up-regulated by LPS, have been shown to induce tolerance to brain ischemia. In a global ischemia model in Mongolian gerbils, IL-1 pre-conditioning protected CA1 hippocampal neurons from severe (3.5 min) ischemia and this protection could be blocked by IL-1ra (Ohtsuki *et al.*, 1996). IL-1ra also blocked tolerance after 'brief' (2 min) pre-conditioning ischemia that was otherwise cytoprotective.

TNF is regarded as an 'alarm hormone' and is ubiquitously expressed in response to stress. TNF pre-conditioning exposures were initially observed to confer cytoprotection by potent induction of manganese superoxide dismutase (MnSOD); this procedure was then shown to induce tolerance to rat myocardial ischemia/reperfusion. Studies in pre-clinical stroke models and primary cultures of cortical neurons, cortical astrocytes and microvessel endothelial cells have shown TNF and its downstream mediator, ceramide, to be involved in the signaling that regulates tolerance to brain hypoxia and ischemia (Cheng et al., 1994; Ginis et al., 1999; Liu et al., 2000). In addition, both TNF and ceramide pre-conditioning block recruitment of p300/CBP to the NF-κB binding site on DNA by interfering with the phosphorylation of the p65 subunit of NF-κB and this modifies NF-κB-driven gene expression; pro-inflammatory ICAM-1 mRNA is inhibited and cytoprotective MnSOD expression is preserved (Ginis et al., 2002). Dissection of these pathways for regulation of tolerance to ischemia could guide the search for multifunctional targets that simultaneously modulate many of the mediators that contribute to progression of brain damage during stroke.

Perspectives: stroke an inflammatory disorder?

The accumulating evidence supporting a role for cytokines, leukocytes, adhesion molecules, and other immune and inflammatory mediators in stroke offers substantial opportunities for further basic and clinical research. Although the current understanding of inflammation and immune mechanisms already reveals an intricate and complex system of highly interrelated mediators, the new disciplines of genomics, proteomics, and bioinformatics are likely to reveal many new factors, mechanisms, and system interactions that will stimulate more sophisticated hypotheses. However, there are many pitfalls on the path from hypothesis to clinical trial as illustrated by the results of the Enlimomab Acute Stroke Trial. Compelling pre-clinical studies that predict clinically achievable benefits with minimal potential for adverse effects are necessary to increase the probability of a positive trial result. Another therapeutic avenue appears to be the rigorous control of infections in stroke patients. In a recent paper, Prass and colleagues (2003) showed that ischemic brain lesions in mice led to an immunodeficient state with an extensive apoptotic loss of lymphocytes and a shift from Th1 to Th2 cytokine production. These mice regularly developed spontaneous septicemia and pneumonia at day 3 after ischemia. As key factor in the impaired antibacterial immune response after stroke a catecholamine-mediated defect in early lymphocyte activation was identified. Taken together there are multiple 'immunological' targets for stroke prevention and therapy, the inflamed atherosclerotic vessel, dysfunctional endothelium in the cerebral vasculature, the evolving brain infarct, and stroke-induced systemic immunodeficiency.

Acknowledgements

Work cited in this chapter was supported by the Deutsche Forschungsgemeinschaft (GS and SJ; SFB 194, B6).

References

Aikawa, M., Rabkin, E., Sugiyama, S., et al. (2001). An HMG-CoA reductase inhibitor, cerivastatin, suppresses growth of macrophages expressing matrix metalloproteinases and tissue factor in vivo and in vitro. Circulation 103: 276–283.

Allen, S.M. and Rothwell, N.J. (2001). Cytokines and acute neurodegeneration. Nat Rev Neurosci 2: 734–744.

Bachis, A., Colangelo, A.M., Vicini, S., et al. (2001). Interleukin-10 prevents glutamate-mediated cerebellar granule cell death by blocking caspase-3-like activity. J Neurosci 21: 3104–3112.

Barone, F.C., Arvin, B., White, R.F., et al. (1997). Tumor necrosis factor-alpha. A mediator of focal ischemic brain injury. Stroke 28: 1233–1244.

Barone, F.C., Irving, E.A., Ray, A.M., et al. (2001). Inhibition of p38 mitogen-activated protein kinase provides neuroprotection in cerebral focal ischemia. Med Res Rev 21: 129–145.

Becker, K.J., McCarron, R.M., Ruetzler, C., et al. (1997). Immunologic tolerance to myelin basic protein decreases stroke size after transient focal cerebral ischemia. Proc Natl Acad Sci USA 94: 10873–10878.

Becker, K., Kindrick, D., Relton, J., Harlan, J., and Winn, R. (2001). Antibody to the alpha4 integrin decreases infarct size in transient focal cerebral ischemia in rats. Stroke, 32: 206–211.

Becker, K., Kindrick, D., McCarron, R., Hallenbeck, J., and Winn, R. (2003). Adoptive transfer of myelin basic protein-tolerized splenocytes to naive animals reduces infarct size: a role for lymphocytes in ischemic brain injury? Stroke 34: 1809–15.

Bordet, R., Deplanque, D., Maboudou, P., et al. (2000). Increase in endogenous brain superoxide dismutase as a potential mechanism of lipopolysaccharide-induced brain ischemic tolerance. J Cereb Blood Flow Metab 20: 1190–1196.

Boutin, H., LeFeuvre, R.A., Horai, R., Asano, M., Iwakura, Y., and Rothwell, N.J. (2001). Role of IL-1alpha and IL-1beta in ischemic brain damage. J Neurosci 21: 5528–5534.

Buisson, A., Nicole, O., Docagne, F., Sartelet, H., Mackenzie, E.T., and Vivien, D. (1998). Up-regulation of a serine protease inhibitor in astrocytes mediates the neuroprotective activity of transforming growth factor beta1. FASEB J 12: 1683–1691.

Cheng, B., Christakos, S., and Mattson, M.P. (1994). Tumor necrosis factors protect neurons against metabolic-excitotoxic insults and promote maintenance of calcium homeostasis. Neuron 12: 139–153.

Connolly, E.S., Winfree, C.J., Springer, T.A., et al. (1996). Cerebral protection in homozygous null ICAM-1 mice after middle cerebral artery occlusion: role of neutrophil adhesion in the pathogenesis of stroke. J Clin Invest 97: 209–216.

DeGraba, T.J., Siren, A.L., Penix, L., et al. (1998). Increased endothelial expression of intercellular adhesion molecule-1 in symptomatic versus asymptomatic human carotid atherosclerotic plaque. Stroke 29: 1405–1410.

Del Zoppo, G., Ginis, I., Hallenbeck, J.M., Iadecola, C., Wang, X., and Feuerstein, G.Z. (2000). Inflammation and stroke: putative role for cytokines, adhesion molecules and iNOS in brain response to ischemia. Brain Pathol 10: 95–112.

Dirnagl, U., Iadecola, C., and Moskowitz, M.A. (1999). Pathobiology of ischaemic stroke: an integrated view. Trends Neurosci 22: 391–397.

Enlimomab Acute Stroke Trial Investigators (2001). Use of anti-ICAM-1 therapy in ischemic stroke. Neurology 57: 1428–1434.

Ginis, I., Schweizer, U., Brenner, M., et al. (1999). TNF- pretreatment prevents subsequent activation of cultured brain cells with TNF-α and hypoxia via ceramide. Am J Physiol Cell Physiol 276: C1171–C1183.

Ginis, I., Jaiswal, R., Klimanis, D., et al. (2002). TNF-alpha-induced tolerance to ischemic injury involves differential control of NF-kappaB transactivation: the role of NF-kappaB association with p300 adaptor. J Cereb Blood Flow Metab 22: 142–152.

Ginsberg, M.D. and Busto, R. (1989). Rodent models of cerebral ischemia. Stroke 20: 1627–1642.

Grilli, M., Barbieri, I., Basudev, H., et al. (2000). Interleukin-10 modulates neuronal threshold of vulnerability to ischaemic damage. Eur J Neurosci 12: 2265–2272.

Hallenbeck, J.M. (2002). The many faces of tumor necrosis factor in stroke. Nature Med 8: 1363–8.

Hedtjarn, M., Leverin, A.L., Eriksson, K., Blomgren, K., Mallard, C., and Hagberg, H. (2002). Interleukin-18 involvement in hypoxic-ischemic brain injury. J Neurosci 22: 5910–5919.

Henrich-Noack, P., Prehn, J.H., and Krieglstein, J. (1996). TGF-beta 1 protects hippocampal neurons against degeneration caused by transient global ischemia. Dose-response relationship and potential neuroprotective mechanisms. Stroke 27: 1609–1614.

Hughes, P.M., Allegrini, P.R., Rudin, M., Perry, V.H., Mir, A.K., and Wiessner, C. (2002). Monocyte chemoattractant protein-1 deficiency in a murine stroke model. J Cereb Blood Flow Metab 22: 308–317.

Hulshof, S., Montagne, L., De Groot, C.J., and Van der Valk, P. (2002). Cellular localization and expression patterns of interleukin-10, interleukin-4, and their receptors in multiple sclerosis lesions. Glia 38: 24–35.

Iadecola, C. (1997) Bright and dark sides of nitric oxide in ischemic brain injury. Trends Neurosci 20: 132–139.

Iadecola, C., Salkowski, C.A., Zhang, F., *et al.* (1999). The transcription factor interferon regulatory factor 1 is expressed after cerebral ischemia and contributes to ischemic brain injury. *J Exp Med* **189**: 719–727.

Jander, S., Schroeter, M., D'Urso, D., Gillen, C., Witte, O.W., and Stoll, G. (1998*a*). Focal ischemia of the rat brain elicits an unusual inflammatory response: early appearance of CD8+ macrophages/microglia. *Eur J Neurosci* **10**: 680–688.

Jander, S., Sitzer, M., Schumann, R., *et al.* (1998*b*). Inflammation in high-grade carotid stenosis: a possible role for macrophages and T cells in plaque destabilization. *Stroke* **29**: 1625–1630.

Jander, S., Sitzer, M., Wendt, A., *et al.* (2001). Expression of tissue factor in high-grade carotid artery stenosis: association with plaque destabilization. *Stroke* **32**: 850–854.

Jander, S., Schroeter, M., and Stoll, G. (2002). Interleukin-18 expression after focal ischemia of the rat brain : association with the late-stage inflammatory response. *J Cereb Blood Flow Metab* **22**: 62–70.

Kim, J.S., Yoon, S.S., Kim, Y.H., and Ryu, J.S. (1996). Serial measurement of interleukin-6, transforming growth factor-beta, and S-100 protein in patients with acute stroke. *Stroke* **27**: 1553–1557.

Kleinschnitz, C., Bendszus, M., Frank, M., Solymosi, L., Toyka, K., and Stoll, G. (2003). In vivo monitoring of macrophage infiltration in experimental ischemic brain lesions by magnetic resonance imaging. *J Cereb Blood Flow Metab* **23**: 1356–1361.

Kochanek, P.M. and Hallenbeck, J.M. (1992). Polymorphonuclear leukocytes and monocytes/macrophages in the pathogenesis of cerebral ischemia and stroke. *Stroke* **23**: 1367–1379.

Law, M.R., Wald, N.J., and Rudnicka, A.R. (2003). Quantifying effect of statins on low density lipoprotein cholesterol, ischaemic heart disease, and stroke: systematic review and meta-analysis. *Brit Med J* **326**: 1423–1430.

Lehrmann, E., Kiefer, R., Christensen, T., *et al.* (1998). Microglia and macrophages are major sources of locally produced transforming growth factor-β1 after transient middle crebral artery occlusion in rats. *Glia* **24**: 437–448.

Li, H.L., Kostulas, N., Huang, Y.M., *et al.* (2001). IL-17 and IFN-gamma mRNA expression is increased in the brain and systemically after permanent middle cerebral artery occlusion in the rat. *J Neuroimmunol* **116**: 5–14.

Liu, J., Ginis, I., Spatz, M., and Hallenbeck, J.M. (2000). Hypoxic preconditioning protects cultured neurons against hypoxic stress via TNF-α and ceramide. *Am J Physiol Cell Physiol* **278**: C144–C153.

Liu, T., McDonnell, P.C., Young, P.R., *et al.* (1993). Interleukin-1 beta mRNA expression in ischemic rat cortex. *Stroke* **24**: 1746–1750.

Loftus, I.M., Naylor, A.R., Goodall, S., *et al.* (2000). Increased matrix metalloproteinase-9 activity in unstable carotid plaques: a potential role in acute plaque disruption. *Stroke* **31**: 40–47.

Mallat, Z., Corbaz, A., Scoazec, A., *et al.* (2001). Expression of interleukin-18 in human atherosclerotic plaques and relation to plaque instability. *Circulation* **104**: 1598–1603.

Maron, R., Sukhova, G., Faria, A.M., *et al.* (2002). Mucosal administration of heat shock protein-65 decreases atherosclerosis and inflammation in aortic arch of low-density lipoprotein receptor-deficient mice. *Circulation* **106**: 1708–1715.

McNeill, H., Williams, C., Guan, J., *et al.* (1994). Neuronal rescue with transforming growth factor-beta 1 after hypoxic-ischaemic brain injury. *Neuroreport* **5**: 901–904.

Nadareishvili, Z.G., Koziol, D.E., Szekely, B., *et al.* (2001). Increased CD8+ T cells associated with *Chlamydia pneumoniae* in symptomatic carotid plaque. *Stroke* **32**: 1966–1972.

Neumar, R.W. (2000). Molecular mechanisms of ischemic neuronal injury. Ann Emergency Med **36**: 483–506.

NASCET (North American Symptomatic Carotid Endarterectomy Trial Collaborators) (1991). Beneficial effect of carotid endarterectomy in symptomatic patients with high-grade carotid stenosis. *N Engl J Med* **325**: 445–453.

Ohtsuki, T., Ruetzler, C.A., Tasaki, K., and Hallenbeck, J.M. (1996). Interleukin-1 mediates induction of tolerance to global ischemia in gerbil hippocampal CA1 neurons. *J Cereb Blood Flow Metab* **16**: 1137–1142.

Prass, K., Meisel, C., Hoflich, C. *et al.* (2003). Stroke-induced immunodeficiency promotes spontaneous bacterial infections and is mediated by sympathetic activation reversal by poststroke T helper cell type 1-like immunostimulation. *J Exp Med* **198**: 725–36.

Prehn, J.H.M., Backhaup, C., and Krieglstein, J. (1993). Transforming growth factor-β1 prevents glutamate neurotoxicity in rat neocortical cultures and protects mouse neocortex from ischemic injury *in vivo*. *J Cereb Blood Flow Metab* **13**: 521–525.

Puisieux, F., Deplanque, D., Pu, Q., Souil, E., Bastide, M., and Bordet, R. (2000). Differential role of nitric oxide pathway and heat shock protein in preconditioning and lipopolysaccharide-induced brain ischemic tolerance. *Eur J Pharmacol* **389**: 71–78.

Ross, R. (1999). Atherosclerois—an inflammatory disease. *N Engl J Med* **340**:115–126.

Ruocco, A., Nicole, O., Docagne, F., *et al.* (1999). A transforming growth factor-β antagonist unmasks the neuroprotective role of this endogenous cytokine in excitotoxic and ischemic brain injury. *J Cereb Blood Flow Metab* **19**:1345–1353.

Saleh, A., Schroeter, M., Jonkmans, C., Hartung, H.P., Mödder, U., and Jander, S. (2004). In vivo MRI of brain inflammation in human ischaemic stroke. *Brain* **127**: 1670–7.

Schroeter, M., Jander, S., Huitinga, I., Witte, O.W., and Stoll, G. (1997) Phagocytic response in photochemically induced infarction of the rat cerebral cortex: the role of resident microglia. *Stroke* **28**: 382–386.

Shohami, E., Ginis, I., and Hallenbeck, J.M. (1999). Dual role of tumor necrosis factor alpha in brain injury. *Cytokine Growth Factor Rev* **10**: 119–130.

Slevin, M., Krupinski, J., Slowik, A., Kumar, P., Szczudlik, A., and Gaffney, J. (2000). Serial measurement of vascular endothelial growth factor and transforming growth factor-beta1 in serum of patients with acute ischemic stroke. *Stroke* **31**: 1863–1870.

Smith, J.D., Trogan, E., Ginsberg, M., Grigaux, C., Tian, J., and Miyata, M. (1995). Decreased atherosclerosis in mice deficient in both macrophage colony-stimulating factor (op) and apolipoprotein, E. *Proc Natl Acad Sci USA* **92**: 8264–8268.

Spera, P.A., Ellison, J.A., Feuerstein, G.Z., and Barone, F.C. (1998). IL-10 reduces rat brain injury following focal stroke. *Neurosci Lett* **251**: 189–192.

Stoll, G., Jander, S., and Schroeter, M. (1998). Inflammation and glial responses in ischemic brain lesions. Progr Neurobiol **56**: 149–161.

Takeda, H., Spatz, M., Ruetzler, C., McCarron, R., Becker, K., and Hallenbeck, J. (2002). Induction of mucosal tolerance to E-selectin prevents ischemic and hemorrhagic stroke in spontaneously hypertensive genetically stroke-prone rats. *Stroke* **33**: 2156–2164.

Touzani, O., Boutin, H., LeFeuvre, R., *et al.* (2002). Interleukin-1 influences ischemic brain damage in the mouse independently of the interleukin-1 type I receptor. *J Neurosci* **22**: 38–43.

Van Exel, E., Gussekloo, J., de Craen, A.J., *et al.* (2002). Inflammation and stroke: the Leiden 85-Plus Study. *Stroke* **33**: 1135–1138.

Wheeler, R.D., Boutin, H., Touzani, O., Luheshi, G.N., Takeda, K., and Rothwell, N.J. (2003). No role for interleukin-18 in acute murine stoke-induced brain injury. *J Cereb Blood Flow Metab* **23**: 531–5.

Youssef, S., Stüve, O., Patarroyo, J.C., Ruiz, P.J., Radosevich, J.L., Hur, E.M., *et al.* (2002). The HMG-CoA reductase inhibitor, atorvastatin, promotes a Th2 bias and reverses paralysis in central nervous system autoimmune disease. *Nature* **420**: 78–84.

Yrjanheikki, J., Tikka, T., Keinänen, R., Goldsteins, G., Chan, P.H., and Koistinaho, J. (1999). A tetracycline derivative, minocycline, reduces inflammation and protects against focal cerebral ischemia with a wide therapeutic window. *Proc Natl Acad Sci USA* **96**: 13496–13500.

Zhai, Q.H., Futrell, N., and Chen, F.J. (1997). Gene expression of IL-10 in relationship to TNF-alpha, IL-1beta and IL-2 in the rat brain following middle cerebral artery occlusion. *J Neurol Sci* **152**: 119–124.

Zhang, R.L., Chopp, M., Li, Y., *et al.* (1995). Anti-ICAM-1 antibody reduces ischemic cell damage after transient but not permanent MCA occlusion in the Wistar rat. *Stroke* **26**: 1438–1443.

Zhu, Y., Ahlemeyer, B., Bauerbach, E., and Krieglstein, J. (2001). TGF-beta1 inhibits caspase-3 activation and neuronal apoptosis in rat hippocampal cultures. *Neurochem Int* **38**: 227–235.

33 Antibodies and CNS disorders

Angela Vincent and Bethan Lang

Introduction

The idea that circulating antibodies can cause CNS disorders is not new, but until recently there was little evidence in its favour, and no antibody tests that could be used to diagnose CNS disease. Over the last 15 years several potentially antibody-mediated disorders have been recognized. Although these conditions are rare, they should be treatable, to varying extents, and they illustrate the importance of establishing methods of detecting antibodies to CNS antigens and of demonstrating their pathogenicity. In this chapter we will discuss the methods for detection of CNS antibodies and their implications, the main CNS conditions defined so far and their associated antibodies, and the importance of establishing new animal models for examining pathogenicity and mechanisms of immune-mediated neuronal impairment. We also touch on the possible role of maternal immunity in neurodevelopmental disorders such as autism.

Detection of antibodies to CNS antigens

In myasthenia gravis, the Lambert–Eaton myasthenic syndrome, and acquired neuromyotonia, candidate antigen approaches have been used with great success (see Chapter 20). The assays that detect the antibodies to acetylcholine receptors (AChR), muscle-specific kinase (MuSK), and voltage-gated calcium (VGCC) and potassium (VGKC) channels, are based on immunoprecipitation of either directly (MuSK) or indirectly (AChR, VGCC, VGKC) radiolabelled antigens. In the peripheral nerve disorders, such as Guillain–Barré syndrome, a candidate approach allowed identification of antibodies to gangliosides, and is being used to test for other potentially pathogenic antibodies (see Chapter 19). In CNS disorders, by contrast, the lack of a full understanding of the pathophysiology of the conditions, and the complexity of the neuronal circuits and the synaptic proteins involved, means that a wider approach is necessary.

The success of such an approach was shown by the study of antibodies in paraneoplastic neurological diseases (see Chapter 25). In these conditions, typically the antibody is first detected by immunohistochemistry or immunofluorescence using frozen fixed or unfixed sections of rat or human brain tissue. Sera that show binding can then be tested by Western blotting to determine the size and number of proteins to which they bind, and to confirm that different sera are binding to the same proteins. They can then be screened against expression cDNA libraries derived from the appropriate brain tissue in order to identify the antigen. These approaches are often successful in defining antibodies that react against antigens even after denaturation and sodium dodecyl sulphate (SDS) gel electrophoresis, and that bind to recombinant proteins expressed in *Escherichia coli*. However, it appears that these antigens are often cytoplasmic or nuclear proteins, such as Yo and Hu, the paraneoplastic antigens. Pathogenic antibodies are most commonly directed against cell-surface determinants that are functionally important, and these are much less likely to be detected by these approaches.

Table 33.1 summarizes the techniques used to detect antibodies to CNS antigens that are relevant to the conditions to be discussed in this chapter. It can be seen that glutamic acid decarboxylase and basal ganglia antibodies are detected mainly by immunostaining and Western blotting, whereas glutamate receptor and potassium channel antibodies are detected mainly by enzyme-linked immunosorbent assay (ELISA) and immunoprecipitation of candidate antigens. These differences may be reflected in the role of the antibodies in the associated conditions.

Glutamic acid decarboxylase antibodies with stiff person syndrome (SPS), cerebellar ataxia, and other disorders

Glutamate acid decarboxylase (GAD) is the enzyme responsible for the synthesis of the inhibitory neurotransmitter gamma-aminobutyric acid (GABA). Antibodies to GAD have been of great interest since it was shown that they were highly characteristic of stiff-person syndrome (Solimena *et al.*, 1988; Folli *et al.*, 1993), and were also found in patients with insulin-dependent diabetes mellitus type 1 (IDDM1). SPS is a very rare condition characterized by severe muscle stiffness, particularly affecting the spine and lower limbs, with superimposed muscle spasms. Spasms can be triggered by

Table 33.1 Successful approaches to detection of antibodies to CNS antigens

Approach	GAD antibodies	Basal ganglial antibodies	Glutamate receptor antibodies	Potassium channel antibodies
Immunohistochemistry, immunofluorescence	Positive	Positive	Positive	Positive
Western blotting on brain tissue	Positive 64 kDa	Positive but variable bands	Not done	Not done
Screening of cDNA expression library	Not done	Not done	Not done	Not done
Binding to undefined antigen on cell line	Not done	Not done	Not done	Not done
ELISA using candidate antigen	Positive	Not done	Positive	Not done
Immunoprecipitation of candidate antigen	Positive	Not done	Not done	Positive
Functional effects of sera or IgG	Positive	Not done	Positive	Positive
Are antibodies pathogenic?	Questionable	Questionable	Potentially	Probably

external events. Typically stiffness involves proximal muscles and spinal deformity is common. Electromyography shows continuous motor unit activity but otherwise the motor and sensory systems are normal, as is intellect. SPS is usually diagnosed in adult life and the muscle symptoms, which can be extremely disabling, may be preceded by psychiatric symptoms which probably reflect CNS involvement of GABAergic synapses. A misdiagnosis of psychogenic or hysteric movement disorder is common before the diagnosis is made.

The clinical spectrum has been described in 20 GAD antibody-positive patients. The average age of onset was 41 years with more women than men affected. Stiffness was asymmetric in some cases and involved facial muscles and could last for days (Dalakas et al., 2000). There was a high association with other autoimmune diseases, including IDDM, thyroid disease and pernicious anaemia. A family history of autoimmunity. HLA DR3 (DRB1 0301) was found in 70% of Caucasian patients compared with only 13% of controls, suggesting a strong genetic predisposition. Other studies have reported SPS with thymoma and myasthenia (e.g. Nicholas et al., 1997), further confirming a link with autoimmunity.

Pathophysiology of SPS

The pathology is not well established and there is a dearth of post-mortem or biopsy material. The clinical picture appears to result from lack of reciprocal inhibition, that is the inhibition of antagonist muscles that should occur when agonist muscles are recruited. The most likely site of the dysfunction is the inhibitory GABAergic neurons, but it is not altogether clear whether the dysfunction is central or at the level of the spinal interneurons. Clinically it is said, though not by all, that the spasms are reduced by sleep, suggesting that they are induced in supraspinal pathways, and transcranial magnetic stimulation showed a hypersynchronous response and cortical abnormalities. Other evidence implicates spinal interneurons. Meinck et al. (1995) described the motor responses to electrical stimulation of peripheral nerves. The response consisted of a sequence of one to three synchronous myoclonic bursts followed by a tonic decrescendo over a number of seconds, which appeared to be generated in the spinal cord. Vibration-induced inhibition of H reflexes (H reflexes measure the motor neuron pool excitability) was reduced in eight out of nine patients (Floeter et al., 1998), consistent with abnormalities in GABAergic pathways. There were also some abnormalities in glycinergic pathways in some patients. Interestingly, spinal reflexes are controlled by glycine receptors as well as by GABA receptors, and hyperexplexia or 'startle' disease is caused by mutations in the glycine receptor. However, there is no genetic form of SPS, and as yet no immune-mediated form of hyperexplexia.

GAD antibodies

GAD antibodies were first detected by Solimena et al. (1988) by immunofluorescence on rat brain sections. They found that a similar staining pattern, around the Purkinje cells and in the granular and molecular layers, was seen with antibodies prepared to rabbit GAD. Further studies showed that antibodies from patients with SPS, as apposed to IDDM1, bound to GAD on Western blots and to both GAD65 and GAD67 isoforms (see Lernmark, 1996). The antibodies can also now be detected by immunoprecipitation of ^{35}S-labelled rabbit reticulocyte lysates expressing GAD, or of ^{125}I-recombinant GAD. Various ELISA assays have also been established. In each of these assays the titres of GAD antibodies in patients with SPS are substantially higher than those of patients with IDDM1 (Dalakas et al., 2001b), and generally the serum levels are substantially higher than the CSF levels (Vincent et al., 1997). In many cases, however, oligoclonal bands are present in the CSF, and the CSF antibody/CSF IgG index is higher than the serum antibody/serum IgG index, suggesting that some of the GAD antibody is actually made in the CNS (Dalakas et al., 2001b). In that work, there were also reduced levels of GABA in the CSF, suggesting either that there was a reduction in GABA synthesis or secretion, or a reduction in GABAergic neurons.

Other antibodies can be associated with SPS. SPS is sometimes associated with breast cancer, in which case antibodies to amphiphysin may be present. Antibodies to 17-β-hydroxysteroid dehydrogenase type 4 were demonstrated in one patient with SPS (Dinkel et al., 2002). These antibodies (including monoclonal antibodies derived from the patient's B cells) reacted with the molecular layer and Purkinje cells in a manner distinct from GAD antibodies, and also bound to the apical cytoplasm of ependymal cells. By immunoprecipitation of metabolically labelled cultures, a 80 kDa antigen was precipitated from cultured ependymal cells, separated by electrophoresis and identified by sequencing and mass spectrometry as 17-β-hydroxysteroid dehydrogenase type 4. Antibodies to this protein were subsequently found in six out of 25 SPS patients, but the specificity for this condition is not yet well established.

GAD antibodies in other conditions

GAD antibodies are also found in other disorders, particularly encephalomyelitis with rigidity and myoclonus, and sporadic cerebellar ataxia (Meinck et al., 2001).

Because GAD is intracellular and clearly immunogenic, one might expect that antibodies to it would occur in conditions in which there is degeneration of cerebral neurons, including diseases like multiple sclerosis. This was emphasized by a recent report of GAD antibodies in the neurodegenerative disorder Batten disease. This is caused by mutations in the CLN3 gene. Chattopadhyay et al. (2002) found GAD antibodies not only in patients with Batten disease but also in mice that were deleted for the Cln3 gene. However, to date these antibodies have been measured only by Western blotting, which detects antibodies to denatured GAD antigens, and it would be important to test the sera using the immunoprecipitation assays mentioned above to confirm their specificity for GAD.

Are GAD antibodies pathogenic?

The presence of GAD antibodies in Batten disease, if confirmed, suggests that these antibodies can be secondary to the disease process rather than play a primary role. Nevertheless, the striking association of SPS with high titres of a very specific antibody that is not present in the great majority of individuals with neurological disorders does suggest that the disease is immune-mediated. This is further supported by the clinical improvement following a variety of immunotherapies, particularly intravenous immune globulin (Dalakas et al., 2001a) (Fig. 33.1). The ability of GAD antibodies to affect either the number of GABAergic neurons or to inhibit GABA synthesis in vivo, however, has not been shown with sera from SPS, and since GAD is an intracellular antigen it may not, itself, be the target for the pathogenic immune response. There could be other antibodies, directed against cell-surface determinants, that are pathogenic. Indeed there have been a few reports of IgG from GAD antibody-positive patients affecting the function of cerebellar neurons (see below).

Functional effects of GAD antibodies on cerebellar neurons

A series of cases of GAD antibody-associated cerebellar ataxia has now been reported (Honnorat et al., 2001), and this condition may prove to be more common than SPS. Many of the patients with cerebellar ataxia have other autoimmune diseases, particularly IDDM or polyendocrine autoimmunity; they are mainly female and oligoclonal bands are present in their CSF. The levels of GAD antibodies in these patients are very high, similar to those found in SPS, and the antibodies bind to GAD65 on Western blots.

Takenoshita et al. (2001) tested the effects of CSF from a patient with cerebellar ataxia on the function of cerebellar neurons in culture. They measured whole-cell voltage clamp recordings from Purkinje cells in rat cerebellar slices, stimulating via electrodes in the molecular layer. The amplitude of the inhibitory post-synaptic currents, that are mediated by GABA released from the basket cells, was reduced acutely by the CSF of the GAD antibody-positive patients but not by control CSF. In a further study (Mitoma et al., 2003), they also found that the CSF preparations from GAD

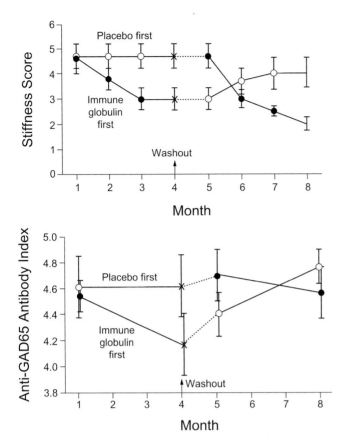

Fig. 33.1 Response of stiff person syndrome (SPS) to intravenous immunoglobulins. A double-blind cross-over trial showed a significant effect of the active treatment on stiffness (top) and on antibodies to glutamic acid decarboxylase (GAD) (bottom). The results strongly support a role for immune factors, probably antibodies, in the disease process. Redrawn with permission from Dalakas *et al.* (2001*a*).

antibody-positive patients reduced GABA release, consistent with an effect of the antibodies on GAD activity. However, the role of GAD antibodies in causing these changes has not been determined, and it is possible that these acute affects are due to a second antibody present in the CSFs. Indeed, it is difficult to see how the GAD antibodies can so quickly be taken up into the pre-synaptic terminals to reduce GAD activity.

T cells in GAD antibody-associated conditions

There has only been one report of attempts to demonstrate the presence of T cells specific for GAD in patients with SPS or cerebellar ataxia. Costa *et al.*, (2001) investigated GAD-specific T-cell proliferation in patients with SMS and in those with ataxia. Only T cells derived from the ataxia patients produced high levels of interferon-gamma following stimulation, suggesting that, despite similar humoral responses, there is a greater inflammatory response in the ataxic patients.

Antibodies to basal ganglia proteins in neuropsychiatric disorders

PANDAS

Paediatric autoimmune neuropsychiatric disorders associated with streptococcal infections (PANDAS) are conditions in which molecular mimicry is widely believed to play a role. This has long been recognized in Sydenham's chorea (SC), a latent post-streptococcal phenomenon, with patients suffer-

ing emotional (obsessive–compulsive disorder, anxiety disorders, major depression) and behavioural problems. Recently it has been suggested that other psychiatric conditions can be post-streptococcal (Swedo, 1994; Leonard and Swedo 2001).

PANDAS includes obsessive–compulsive disorder (OCD), tic syndromes and motor tics (Tourette's syndrome), and dystonia. These patients do not appear to have antibodies directed against any of the known neuronal antigens (e.g. VGCC, GAD, paraneoplastic antigens (Black *et al.*, 1998)), but antibodies to human putamen were reported in patients with Tourette's syndrome (Singer *et al.*, 1998). These antibodies were detected by Western blotting or ELISA using basal ganglia tissue extracts, but control values were also high and a clear distinction between patients and controls was only evident for human putamen antigens. Further studies have looked at antibodies to a range of neuronal and streptococcal epitopes in children and adults with Tourette's syndrome, Sydenham's chorea, and other autoimmune conditions. A variety of immunostaining patterns were detected by immunofluorescence and binding to distinct basal ganglia polypeptides by Western blotting. Although the frequency of positive results in Tourette's syndrome patients were higher than in the other disease groups, the results again were not clearly distinct, raising questions about the disease and antigen specificity of the reactivities shown (Morshed *et al.*, 2001). Similar findings were reported by Wendlandt *et al.* (2001) using multivariate discriminant analysis of IgG repertoires. There were differences between Tourettes'e syndrome patients and controls, but the results did not suggest the presence of specific antibodies.

A further disorder that may be associated with antibodies to striatal neurons is acute disseminated encephalomyelitis with basal ganglia involvement (Dale *et al.*, 2001). In this study there was a clear increase in antibodies against the basal ganglia antigens by ELISA, and antibodies binding to bands of 60, 67 and 80 kDa were detected by Western blotting. Antibody binding to striatal neurons was also detected by immunofluorescence. Similar reactivity was seen in patients with Sydenham's chorea (Church *et al.*, 2002), although in this study the sera bound mainly to antigens of molecular weight 40, 45 and 60 kDa. The possibility of cross-reactivity between streptococcal proteins and basal ganglia antigens was suggested by absorption of antibasal ganglia antibodies by streptococcal epitopes (Dale *et al.*, 2001), although the molecular target of these antibodies has not yet been defined.

These findings lend support to an antibody-mediated response in post-streptococcal CNS disease including Tourette's syndrome, Sydenham's chorea, and other neuropscyhiatric disorders, but these antibodies may be markers for an infective or other process rather than causative. In fact, a recent study has urged caution in interpretation of the data on anti-streptolysin O titres, and in attributing the cause of these conditions to a preceding streptococcal infection (Loiselle *et al.*, 2003).

Antibodies and encephalitis

There are many case reports that suggest a relationship between antibodies and different forms of encephalitis or seizure-associated disorders (e.g. Andrews *et al.*, 1990; Nemni *et al.*, 1994). The number of defined antibody specificities which could account for the CNS disorders is limited, and the evidence is far from complete. Some of the detected antibodies may be secondary to the disease process rather than causative, and it is possible that there are other antibodies, to as yet untested targets, that are responsible for the conditions, or that the disorders are T-cell mediated. Here we will summarize some of the data briefly.

Rasmussen's encephalitis

Rasmussen's encephalitis (RE) is a chronic inflammatory disease of the brain usually affecting one hemisphere, and initially suspected to be due to viral infections (Rasmussen, 1978). It is characterized by intractable focal seizures, known as epilepticus partialis continua, and often progresses to hemiparesis. Although it is typically a childhood disease, adolescents and adults may develop a similar syndrome. The condition is so disabling that hemispherectomy is often performed in order to stop the seizures, though this is often not until the later stages of the disease when permanent brain atrophy has already occurred.

Pathophysiology of Rasmussen's encephalitis

Rasmussen's encephalitis is a rare disease and many reports are based on single or small case studies. A recent study, however, has amassed clinical and pathological evidence from 13 cases with histologically proven RE (Bien *et al.*, 2002*b*). The disease appears to go through a prodromal phase during which seizures are relatively infrequent and hemiparesis is uncommon. This lasts about 7 months in young children and generally longer in older children or adults. The acute phase is associated with more frequent fits and development of hemiparesis, and lasts around 8 months. At this stage MRI shows focal inflammatory lesions, usually arising between the Rolandic fissure and the temporomedial area. During this stage the hemisphere begins to shrink as it atrophies. The residual phase that follows represents permanent and stable hemiparesis with cerebral atrophy and decreased seizure frequency. There are some differences in the clinical course of those patients who present in early childhood compared with those who present as adults. The histopathology of the brains from these 13 patients showed perivascular and parenchymal CD3 T cells, CD68- and HLA-DR-positive microglial cells and glial fibrillar acidic protein (GFAP)-positive astrocytes, the majority of which were 'reactive'; neuronal cell density was reduced.

The physiology of RE has been examined by patch clamp recordings from resected frontal lobe tissue (Gibbs *et al.*, 1998). There was a reduction in efficacy of GABA on the neurons with decreased post-synaptic GABA-induced currents compared with controls, and less enhancement by benzodiazepine and clonazepam. These observations were consistent with reduced function of GABA receptors in RE, that could contribute to epileptiform activity. The relationship of these findings to the glutamate receptor antibodies reported subsequently is unclear.

Autoantibodies to glutamate receptor 3 in Rasmussen's encephalitis

The first report of antibodies to glutamate receptor 3 (GluR3) in RE was a serendipitous finding, highly analogous to that which indicated the role of antibodies to acetylcholine receptors in myasthenia gravis (see Chapter 20). In order to raise antibodies against the newly cloned glutamate receptors, rabbits were immunized with the extracellular domains of different GluR receptors expressed as recombinant fusion proteins. Two of three GluR3 immunized rabbits developed seizures (Rogers *et al.*, 1994). Post-mortem examination showed inflammatory changes including microglial nodules and perivascular lymphocytosis in the cerebral cortex, with infiltration of the meninges. The similarities of this condition to RE were noted and GluR3 antibodies were detected in sera from two of four children with RE by Western blot, confirmed by binding to HEK 293 cells expressing GluR3. Strikingly, one child showed a marked improvement after plasma exchange (Rogers *et al.*, 1994). This latter finding has been confirmed in another childhood cases (Andrews *et al.*, 1996) and in some patients with later onset (Leach *et al.*, 1999) strongly suggesting that a humoral immune component is involved. Unfortunately, the effects of immune therapies are generally temporary in children, although the results in adults may be more persistent.

There is confusion about the pathogenic mechanisms by which these antibodies are thought to act. Both human RE and rabbit immunized serum IgG antibodies activated currents in cortical neurons; and this effect was blocked by a short peptide sequence of the GluR3 extracellular domain (Twyman *et al.*, 1995), indicating the specificity of the antibodies for this domain. In another study, however, Frassoni *et al.* (2001) showed binding of antibodies from a patient with RE and immunized rabbits to cortical neurons, but no direct effect of the antibodies on the dissociated neurons. Moreover, He *et al.* (1998) demonstrated destruction of cortical cells *in vitro* by plasma from immunized rabbits, and binding of IgG to neurons *in situ* in the rabbit and RE brains. The antibodies did not appear to activate the receptor directly, and the effect was inactivated by heating to 56°C, implic-

ating complement. This was confirmed in a further study that showed a protective effect of complement inhibitor (CD 59), expressed on the neurons, on the neuronal death induced by GluR3 antibodies (Whitney and McNamara, 2000). Thus it is not clear whether the antibodies cause loss of neuronal cells by increased GluR3 activation or by complement-mediated destruction of cells, and current evidence tends to indicate the latter. Moreover, there is no very clear evidence that these functional effects are due to GluR3 antibodies.

In addition, difficulties have arisen in confirming the presence of GluR3 antibodies in RE and in establishing a routine GluR3 antibody test that can be used in clinical practise. Wiendl *et al.* (2001) reported an ELISA assay using the GluR3B peptide previously shown to prevent GluR3 antibodies from activating AMPA receptors (Twyman *et al.*, 1995). They tested eight RE cases and compared the results with non-inflammatory focal epilepsies and controls. Only two out of the eight RE sera were positive compared with thirteen out of 40 of the focal epilepsy sera. In a further paper, Mantegazza *et al.* (2002) again reported a high proportion of positive ELISA results in patients with other forms of epilepsy, and particularly high levels in those with drug-resistant 'catastrophic' epilepsy. Strikingly, the results were similar with either GluR3A or GluR3B peptides and four of 15 myasthenia gravis patients were also positive, raising questions about the specificity of the assay. They also examined the intrathecal synthesis of the antibodies. There was no evidence of intrathecal IgG synthesis and only low levels of GluR3 antibodies in the CSF. The RE patients did have high CSF IgG concentrations but they did not correlate with the CSF GluR3B antibody titres.

The findings above have not been reproduced by all groups. Only one of 25 patients with RE has antibodies to recombinant GluR3 on Western blotting, binding to HEK cells, or immunoprecipitation of ^{35}S-GluR3 extracellular domain expressed in HEK cells (Watson *et al.*, 2004). On ELISA, several RE sera bound to GluR3B peptide, but they also bound to a mock-coated ELISA plate or to an AChR peptide. Nevertheless, the response to plasma exchange and steroids (Krauss *et al.*, 1996) suggests that even GluR3B antibody-negative patients may have an antibody-mediated disease, and clearly other targets should be considered.

T cells in RE

The pathological findings in RE are much more akin to those in multiple sclerosis (MS), with focal inflammatory infiltrates and gliosis, than might be expected from a purely antibody-mediated disease. This has been clearly demonstrated in 11 patients in whom MHC Class I-positive neurons were identified, granzyme B was detected in CD3 CD8+ T cells, and neuronal apoptosis was shown (Bien *et al.*, 2002*a*;) (Fig. 33.2). These observations would be consistent with a direct T-cell mediated destruction, analogous to that thought to occur in some of the paraneoplastic neurological disorders (see Chapter 25). How these changes relate to the reduction in GABA-R numbers seen in electrophysiological studies, or to the presence of GluR3 antibodies, is not clear.

Potassium channel antibodies in limbic encephalitis and other seizure-related disorders

Antibodies to potassium channels were first identified in patients with acquired neuromyotonia (see Chapter 20). In a recent study, around 20% of patients with neuromyotonia or the closely related cramp fasciculation syndrome had some form of CNS symptoms including depression, anxiety, memory loss, or sleep disorders (Hart *et al.*, 2002; Heidenreich and Vincent, 1998). In a few cases, neuromyotonia is associated with autonomic dysfunction, including sweating, and marked CNS abnormalities including insomnia, hallucinations, altered behaviour, and cognitive dysfunction. This is called Morvan's fibrillar chorea or Morvan's syndrome (Serratrice and Azulay, 1994) and, although thought to be extremely rare, several patients have recently been identified (Vincent, unpublished).

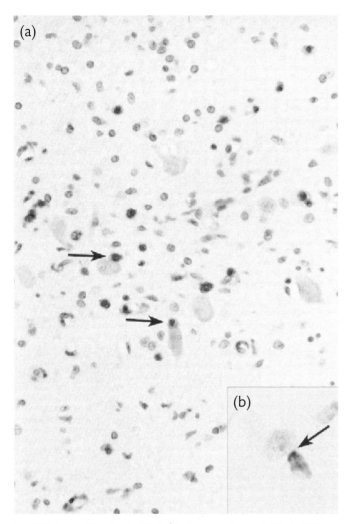

Fig. 33.2 Immunohistochemical findings in Rasmussen's encephalitis. A: CD8+ lymphocytes infiltrate the right hippocampus of a 7-year-old boy undergoing right-sided hemispherectomy (seizures and progressive left-sided hemiparesis since 15 months). Note the T cells that lie in close apposition to neurons (arrows). Original magnification ×246. B: Same patient as in A. A granzyme B+ lymphocyte in apposition to a neuron. Note the polarization of the granzyme B+ granules towards the neuron (arrow). Original magnification ×990 Courtesy of Dr Christian G. Bien, University of Bonn, Department of Epileptology, Bonn, Germany and Dr Jan Bauer, University of Vienna, Brain Research Institute, Division of Neuroimmunology, Vienna, Austria. (See also Plate 11 of the colour plate section at the center of this book.)

A few cases of Morvan's syndrome have been described with raised levels of VGKC antibodies (Heidenreich and Vincent, 1998; Lee *et al.*, 1998; Liguori *et al.*, 2001), and in most there was clinical improvement following plasma exchange (Madrid *et al.*, 1996), or with spontaneous fall in the antibody levels (Barber *et al.*, 2000). Some of these have had an associated thymoma (e.g. Lee *et al.*, 1998) but the others had no detectable tumour.

Thymoma can also be associated with similar CNS symptoms without the peripheral neuromyotonia, and either with or without associated myasthenia gravis (Antoine *et al.*, 1995; Buckley *et al.*, 2001). In one case, the cognitive dysfunction improved slowly over a period of 2 years while VGKC antibodies spontaneously fell (Buckley *et al.*, 2001). The relationship between VGKC antibodies and cognitive changes appears to be strong in ten cases studied so far (Vincent *et al.*, 2004). VGKC antibodies can also be found in some patients whose main presenting symptoms to the neurologist are seizures, but in whom other cognitive or psychiatric disturbances may be associated (McKnight *et al.*, in press).

Table 33.2 summarizes the conditions in which VGKC antibodies have been found. Most of the patients with these antibodies have presented with a relatively acute or subacute onset, over days or weeks. Importantly, the limbic symptoms are highly similar to those experienced by patients with paraneoplastic limbic encephalitis (see Chapter 25), but in the many of those with VGKC antibodies a tumour is not found (Pozo-Roscich *et al.*, 2003). In some patients memory loss is the main symptom, in others there is much more global intellectual and conscious impairment (e.g. Schott *et al.*, 2003). The response to plasma exchange and other immunotherapies is closely associated with a fall in VGKC antibodies (Fig. 33.3(a)) and strongly supports an immune-mediated disease. Antibodies to VGKC can be detected not only by immunoprecipitation, but also by immunostaining of hippocampal neurons (Fig. 33.3(b)), in a distribution which is typical of antibodies directed against VGKC subtypes Kv1.1 and 1.2 (Buckley *et al.*, 2001). How the antibodies gain access to the CNS, why only some patients have peripheral symptoms, and why hippcampal functions should be the main target requires experimental studies.

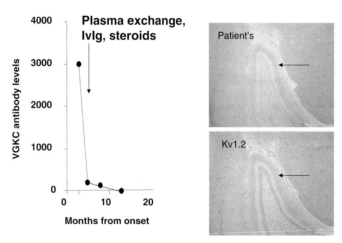

Fig. 33.3 Antibodies to voltage-gated potassium channels in a CNS disease. Left: VGKC antibodies are found in some patients with limbic encephalitis (memory loss, disorientation, seizures, personality change). The VGKC antibodies fall markedly following treatments such as intravenous immunoglobulin, plasma exchange, and steroids, associated with substantial improvement in the patient. Right: serum from these patients bind to the neuronal processes in the dentate gyrus of the hippocampus (upper panel), in a distribution similar to that of rabbit antibodies to the VGKC Kv1.2 subtype (lower panel). Immunohistochemistry courtesy of Dr Camilla Buckley Department of Clinical Neurology, University of Oxford (see also Plate 12 of the colour plate section.)

Table 33.2 VGKC antibodies in different clinical syndromes

	Onset	Muscle hyperactivity	Autonomic dysfunction	Hippocampal dysfunction
Cramp fasciculation syndrome	Insidious	Yes	Unusual	Unusual
Acquired neuromyotonia	Insidious	Yes	Sometimes	Sometimes
Morvan's syndrome	Insidious	Marked	Marked	Marked
Limbic encephalitis	Subacute/Acute	Often absent	Often absent	Marked

Antibodies and neuropsychiatric lupus erythematosus

Neuropsychiatric disorders are common complications of systemic lupus erythematosus (SLE), and present with a variety of neurological syndromes (seizures, psychosis, dementia, confusion, chorea). These symptoms could be due to ischaemia, haemorrhage, or vasculitis. However, since lupus is associated with a variety of autoantibodies, the possibility of a role for these antibodies in causing the symptoms is widely considered. A number of different antibodies have been said to associate with neurological or psychiatric presentations of lupus (neuropsychiatric lupus). These are antibodies to undefined neuronal antigens, antiribosomal P antibodies, antiphospholipid antibodies, that are found in the antiphospholipid syndrome as well as in lupus, and antiganglioside antibodies. There are many difficulties in assessing the relevance of these antibodies (see Greenwood et al., 2002). Antibodies to a 50 kDa protein was detected on Western blots of brain synaptic terminals and bound to neuroblastoma cell surface membranes (Hanson et al., 1992), but in some studies no difference in frequency of antibodies between patients with or without neurological symptoms were found (Hanly et al., 1993). Antibodies to phospholipids appear to correlate with neuropsychiatric lupus, whereas they do not correlate with the presence of neurological symptoms in patients with antiphospholipid syndrome (Tishler et al., 1995).

Few studies have addressed the functional effects of the antibodies. Anticardiolipin antibodies and IgG were found to reduce cell viability in cerebellar cultures in vitro (Andreassi et al., 2001), or to depolarize neuronal preparations (Chapman et al., 1999). Recently, evidence showed cross-reactivity between anti-DNA antibodies and the NMDA receptor 2. Antibodies to the cross-reactive peptide caused neuronal cell death when injected into the mouse hippocampus (DeGiorgio et al., 2001). These observations emphasize the possible role of serum factors or specific antibodies in causing neuropsychiatric lupus, but in most of these studies the target of the pathogenic antibodies is not clear. The antibodies detected may be markers for an autoimmune process which contributes to the disease, rather than directly pathogenic.

Opsoclonus myoclonus syndrome

Opsoclonus myoclonus syndrome (OMS), also called 'dancing eyes syndrome' or Kinsbourne's disease, is a rare neurological disorder characterized by subacute onset of chaotic, saccadic eye movements and spontaneous jerks of limb and face muscles (Pohl et al., 1996). In children, the age of onset is around 3 years, and although OMS may occur following infection, approximately 50% of cases are found in association with a neuroblastoma (NB) or other neural crest derived tumour. Interestingly, children with neuroblastoma and OMS have a better prognosis than those who present without the neurological condition. These children tend to present with well-differentiated tumours, with low copy numbers of the proto-oncogene n-*myc*, and a favourable histological subtype with the tumours often showing considerable lymphocytic infiltration. In adults the disorder is found in association with small cell lung carcinoma (SCLC) or breast cancer, or following a preceding viral infection (see also Chapter 25). Although OMS is a paraneoplastic condition in many cases, because it also occurs without an associated neoplasm, and because the investigations do not necessarily distinguish between paraneoplastic and non-paraneoplastic cases, we will include them all here.

Pathophysiology of OMS

Pathological studies of OMS are very limited. In many patients there may be no neuropathological signs, but changes in the cerebellum have been described in a number of case studies, where a reduction in cells in Purkinje and granular layers have been reported (Ziter et al., 1979). However, the physiological deficits are thought to result from dysfunction of the omnipause neurons in the brainstem, although no abnormalities have been reported in this region (Ridley et al., 1987).

Immunopathology of OMS

Immunological abnormalities have been reported in both adult and childhood OMS. Oligoclonal bands, pleocytosis, and raised IgG and IgM levels have all been reported in the CSF. Additionally there are several reports of autoantibodies in children with OMS both with and without neuroblastoma.

Antineurofilament antibodies have been detected in the sera of some OMS children (Noetzel et al., 1987; Connolly et al., 1997), although these antibodies have been described in other neurological disorders and in healthy controls. In some children with neuroblastoma, antibodies to the Hu family of proteins (see Chapter 25) have been detected. These antibodies recognize a family of RNA-binding proteins (35–42 kDa) that are usually associated, in adults, with SCLC and paraneoplastic neurological disorders such as subacute sensory neuropathy. Although most neuroblastomas and SCLCs express Hu antigens, only a few OMS patients have associated Hu antibodies. It is possible that MHC Class I expressed by some Hu antigen-bearing tumours plays a role in the development of the paraneoplastic disorders (Dalmau et al., 1995). In adults, the anti-Ri antibody has been detected in the sera of patients with the paraneoplastic form of OMS (Luque et al., 1991). Recently Bataller et al. (2003) screened a human brainstem cDNA expression library with OMS sera derived from patients with or without associated tumours. The serum antibodies bound to a number of different proteins, derived from either the post-synaptic neuronal densities or RNA/DNA-binding proteins. Thus there appears to be a variety of antigens recognized by OMS sera, particularly in patients with associated tumours. However, there are no reports of these autoantibodies being pathogenic, and all identified so far have been directed towards intracellular proteins.

There is increasing evidence that some adult paraneoplastic neurological disorders may be T-cell mediated, with a major role for cytotoxic T cells in the pathophysiology (Voltz et al., 1998). Whether this would apply to childhood neuroblastoma-associated cases and the non-paraneoplastic OMSs is not yet clear. There is some evidence that autoantibodies, to as yet undefined epitopes, may play an important role in OMS. Immunomodulatory therapy has been reported as beneficial in children and in the adult 'idiopathic' forms of OMS. Intravenous immunoglobulin (IV Ig) has been reported as successful in the initial treatment of OMS (Nolte et al., 1979) as has protein A immunoadsorption which removes IgG antibodies selectively (Nitschke et al., 1995). Recently, we have demonstrated that some OMS patients (with or without NB) have serum IgG antibodies that stain the surface of neuroblastoma cell lines. Pre-incubation of the neuroblastoma cells in OMS sera or IgG, obtained during the active phase of the disease, resulted in inhibition of the growth of neuroblastoma cells in vitro (F. Blaes et al., in preparation), whereas IgG from a child during the recovery phase of non-paraneoplastic OMS did not. These observations suggest that there are antibodies to surface determinants on neuroblastoma or neuronal cell lines, and further studies should be directed at identifying their targets.

Antibodies and neurodevelopmental disorders

Neurodevelopmental disorders are diagnosed during childhood but are likely to be the result of intrauterine or perinatal injury. Some disorders are clearly genetic in origin, but in many the cause is unknown. In some of these, pre-natal damage from environmental factors is likely. Here we will refer only to autism.

Autism

Autism is a severe developmental disorder characterized by impaired reciprocal social interaction and communication, with restricted and stereotypic behaviours. The onset is before 3 years of age although the condition is often not diagnosed until later. There may be global mental handicap and epilepsy. The affected areas of the brain are not clear, although the cerebellum has been found to be abnormal in several histopathological studies. A recent clinicopathological study of autism confirmed abnormalities in Purkinje cell numbers, and also pointed to abnormalities in the cortex and brainstem (Bailey et al., 1998).

Although genetic conditions causing autism are recognized, e.g. tuberous sclerosis and fragile X syndrome, the genetic influence is clear from the relatively high concordance between monozygotic twins compared with that between dizygotic twins (reviewed in Korvatska et al., 2002). There are a number of candidate genes that are being investigated. In addition, there are neurochemical abnormalities which should point to an underlying pathology (see Korvatska et al., 2002).

Despite these strong indications for a genetic basis, it is unclear whether all cases of autism will turn out to be genetically determined. It is possible that autoimmune as well as genetic causes contribute to the spectrum of the disease. These could act in the intrauterine environment or after birth. In addition, those cases that undergo autistic regression (autism associated with loss of previously acquired speech) could be due to a post-infectious or other post-natal environmental cause. There has been great interest in reports of an increased incidence of autism over the last decade and the possibility that vaccination might provoke autism (see Krause et al., 2002), attributed to mercury in vaccines or the presence of measles virus in the measles, mumps, and rubella triple vaccine. These claims have not been substantiated and a recent large epidemiological study found no evidence for increased incidence of autism in children who had received MMR compared with those who had not (Madsen et al., 2002).

Nevertheless, a hypothesis has emerged that links the immune response to various microbes with an immune response to neuronal antigens. Antibodies to myelin basic protein (MBP) were detected in autistic children using simple Western blotting techniques (Singh et al., 1993). A serological association between measles virus and human herpesvirus 6 with antibodies to MBP and to neurofilament proteins was also claimed (Singh et al., 2002). Antibodies to neuronal antigens were said to cross-react with proteins from milk and bacterial antigens in another study using ELISA to measure antibodies binding to these antigens (Vojdani et al., 2002). However, these and other assays have generally relied on ELISA or Western blotting techniques and the significance of the results is unclear. None of the putative targets are membrane proteins which could be targets for pathogenic antibodies. Other studies have shown higher levels of neuronal proteins such as GFAP in the cerebrospinal fluid of children with several different developmental disorders including autism, suggesting that there is increased turnover or degeneration of neurons and glia (Ahlsen et al., 1993). Perhaps the antibodies, if their existence and specificity for neuronal and glial proteins is confirmed, are secondary to a degenerative process. These results may, therefore, suggest that there is a degenerative process going on in autism but do not necessarily support a role for humoral immunity. The role of the immune system in autism is critically reviewed elsewhere (Krause et al., 2002).

Maternal immunity and developmental disorders

Maternal antibodies to neuronal antigens could cross the placenta and cause developmental disorders in the fetus (Warren et al., 1990; Adinolfi et al., 1993). One possibility is that maternal infections lead not necessarily to infections of the developing infant, but to an immune response that affects the neuronal development in the fetus. A number of studies have looked at antibodies to brain antigens in animal models of viral infections. For instance, immunization of rabbits with certain influenza viruses produced antibodies to a 37 kDa protein and binding to neuronal cell bodies in the dentate gyrus, hippocampus, cortex, and cerebellum (Laing et al., 1989). A maternal reaction towards a male fetus might explain the increased incidence of autism and other developmental disorders in the male. Children of SLE mothers were shown to have more developmental difficulties than a control group, with male children were most affected (McAllister et al., 1997). None of these studies addresses specifically the question of whether maternal antibodies can cause disease. For this animal models are needed.

Because of the clear role that antibodies specific to the fetal isoform of the acetylcholine receptor play in causing consecutive pregnancies with arthrogryposis multiplex congenita (Polizzi et al., 2000; see also Chapter 20), we investigated whether maternal antibodies might play a role in the development of neurodevelopmental disorders. We selected mothers who had had at least two consecutive pregnancies resulting in children with dyslexia, autism, or specific language disorders. One serum, from a mother who had two children with autism and a language disorder respectively, stained cerebellar Purkinje cells and other large neurons in a highly specific manner (Dalton et al., 2003). To see whether these antibodies could be pathogenic to the fetus, we used a maternal-to-fetal passive transfer approach (see below).

Animal models of antibody-mediated CNS disorders

There is a pressing need to develop effective models that can be used to prove the role of serum antibodies in causing disease, and to investigate how and where the antibodies gain access to the CNS. To date there have been few successful studies reported, which are summarized in Table 33.3.

There are two approaches that can be used. Passive transfer models, involving the injection of serum/plasma or IgG from affected individuals into mice and looking for pathogenic effects; but unless the specific antibody is purified it is not possible to say conclusively that the defined antibody is causing the observed effect. Most studies attempting to demonstrate an effect of human serum or IgG on CNS function have used direct intracerebral injection of antibodies. For instance, the potential pathogenicity of antibodies in PANDAS has been tested by infusion of IgG into rats: The animals developed hyperkinetic movements after PANDAS IgG but not control IgG (Hallett et al., 2000; Taylor et al., 2002). We have

Table 33.3 Animal models for antibody-mediated CNS disorders

Condition	Passive transfer by intraperitoneal injection	Passive transfer by intracerebral injection	Active immunization	Maternal-to-fetal transfer	Reference
Stiff person syndrome	Not done	Not reported	Not reported	N/A	
PANDAS	Not done	Effective in rat model	Not done	N/A	Hallett et al. (2000), Taylor et al. (2002)
Rasmussen's encephalitis	Not done	Not done	Effective	N/A	Levite et al. (1999)
Limbic encephalitis	Some modest effects on mouse exploratory behaviour	Modest effects on mouse exploratory behaviour	Not done	N/A	Vincent and R. Deacon, unpublished observations
Autism	Not done	Not done	Not done	Led to cerebellar dysfunction in one reported case	Dalton et al. (2003)

Table 33.4 Some substances that may affect blood–brain barrier (BBB) permeability

Substance	Effect demonstrated	Reference
Shiga toxin	1 mg/kg increases BBB permeability	Nofech-Mozes et al. (2000), Vincent et al. unpublished
Shiga toxin plus TNF-α	TNF-α enhances expression of shiga toxin receptor	Eisenhauer et al. (2001)
Recombinant IL-2	Increased IgG permeability 6–24 hours after single infusion of recombinant IL-2	Ellison et al. (1991)
Recombinant IL-1	Increased permeability of brain endothelia in vitro	Gloor et al. (1997)
TNF-α	TNF-α levels of up to 1 ng/ml associated with increased permeability	Tsao et al. (2001)
Mannitol	Intra-arterial injection of 1.1 M mannitol transiently opened BBB	Ikeda et al. (2002)
Mannitol plus Na/Ca exchange blocker (KB-R7943)	Effect of mannitol enhanced by KB-R7943	Ikeda et al. (2002)
Antibody to GM1 ganglioside	Increases clearance of ¹⁴C-inulin in in vitro model	Kanda et al. (2000)
Antibody to endothelial barrier antigen	Altered endothelial cells and opened BBB	Ghabriel et al. (2002)
Metalloproteinases	Various effects demonstrated	Reviewed in Lukes et al. (1999), Yong et al. (1998)

found effects on mouse open field exploration after intracerebral injections of VGKC antibody-positive human plasma in a preliminary study (Vincent and R. Deacon, unpublished data); rearing in open field is strongly influenced by hippocampal function (Deacon et al., 2002). While these studies can indicate what signs and symptoms might be expected from a successful animal model of the conditions (which might differ from that evident in the human disease), they do not indicate whether circulating antibodies could cause such changes. For this it will be necessary to try to induce CNS changes after intraperitoneal or intravenous infusion of patient serum or IgG. It may be necessary to induce changes in the blood–brain barrier in order to achieve some CNS effects. There have as yet been few reports of studies aimed at achieving this, but there are a number of substances which affect the permeability of the blood–brain barrier to smaller molecules. Some examples, including cytokines that are part of the acute phase response, are listed in Table 33.4.

Alternatively, one can induce antibodies by active immunization against putative antigens in experimental animals. Although this is the conventional approach, it does not, of course, prove that the human condition is due to antibodies against the antigen, and the role of T cells against the antigen needs also to be considered in this situation. There are relatively few attempts to raise antibodies to CNS antigens with a view to examining the neurological consequences. Mice immunized against GluR3B did not develop epilepsy but they exhibited brain pathology and their serum caused agonist-like activity associated with cell death in cultured neurons (Levite et al., 1999; Levite and Hermelin, 1999).

Since there are indications that some of the potentially antibody-mediated disorders mentioned above are post-infectious, it would be interesting to induce animal models of autoimmune disease by a natural infectious process. Borna virus infection of newborn Lewis rats leads to changes which model to some extent autistic spectrum disorders, including loss of neurons in the cerebellum and behavioural changes (Pletnikov et al., 2001). A particularly interest approach for looking at maternal effects is demonstrated by a recent study that induced maternal influenza infection in BALB/c mice. They found marked decreases in open field exploration in the offspring, and decreased sociability, which were evident even when the mouse offspring had become adults (Shi et al., 2003). This appeared to be the result of the maternal immune response to viral antigens, rather than the infection itself.

Finally, maternal-to-fetal passive transfer offers some possibility of testing the hypothesis that human maternal autoantibodies can cause developmental disorders. We injected the serum mentioned above (Dalton et al., 2003) into pregnant mice and assessed the behaviour of the offspring on a range of developmental and cognitive tasks. There were specific and reproducible defects in

motor coordination with no abnormalities in cognition or motor strength. Magnetic resonance spectroscopy on the mouse cerebella, when the offspring were adult, showed significant reductions in choline and creatine. These results show that it is potentially possible to demonstrate the role of maternal factors in causing neurodevelopmental disorders in humans.

Conclusions

Autoimmune disorders of the peripheral nervous system are well established and have provided many useful paradigms for the investigation of conditions affecting the CNS. It is now clear that there are antibody-mediated diseases of the CNS but much further work is required to define more carefully which antibodies are pathogenic and which are secondary to the disease process, and to demonstrate how the pathogenic antibodies affect CNS function. For these studies animal models will be essential.

Acknowledgements

We are very grateful to the Wellcome Trust, the Dana Foundation, the Myasthenia Gravis Association/Muscular Dystrophy Campaign, and Action Research for support.

References

Adinolfi, M. (1993). The maternal–fetal interaction: some controversies and solutions. Exp Clin Immunogenet 10: 103–117.

Ahlsen, G., Rosengren, L., Belfrage, M., et al. (1993). Glial fibrillary acidic protein in the cerebrospinal fluid of children with autism and other neuropsychiatric disorders. Biol Psychiat 33: 734–743.

Andreassi, C., Zoli, A., Riccio, A., et al. (2001). Anticardiolipin antibodies in patients with primary antiphospholipid syndrome: a correlation between IgG titre and antibody-induced cell dysfunctions in neuronal cell cultures. Clin Rheumatol 20: 314–318.

Andrews, J.M., Thompson, J.A., Pysher, T.J., et al. (1990). Chronic encephalitis, epilepsy, and cerebrovascular immune complex deposits. Ann Neurol 28: 88–90.

Andrews, P.I., Dichter, M.A., Berkovic, S.F., et al. (1996). Plasmapheresis in Rasmussen's encephalitis. Neurology 46: 242–246.

Antoine, J.C., Honnorat, J., Anterion, C.T., et al. (1995). Limbic encephalitis and immunological perturbations in two patients with thymoma. J Neurol Neurosurg Psychiatry 58: 706–710.

Bailey, A., Luthert, P., Dean, A., *et al.* (1998). A clinicopathological study of autism. *Brain* 121(5): 889–905.

Barber, P.A., Anderson, N.E., and Vincent, A. (2000). Morvan's syndrome associated with voltage-gated K+ channel antibodies. *Neurology* 54: 771–772.

Bataller, L., Rosenfeld, M.R., Graus, F., *et al.* (2003). Autoantigen diversity in the opsoclonus-myoclonus syndrome. *Ann Neurol* 53: 347–353.

Bien, C.G., Bauer, J., Deckwerth, T.L., *et al.* (2002a). Destruction of neurons by cytotoxic T cells: a new pathogenic mechanism in Rasmussen's encephalitis. *Ann Neurol* 51: 311–318.

Bien, C.G., Widman, G., Urbach, H., *et al.* (2002b). The natural history of Rasmussen's encephalitis. *Brain* 125: 1751–1759.

Black, J.L., Lamke, G.T., and Walikonis, J.E. (1998). Serologic survey of adult patients with obsessive-compulsive disorder for neuron-specific and other autoantibodies. *Psychiat Res* 81: 371–380.

Borchers, A.T., Keen, C.L., Shoenfeld, Y., *et al.* (2002). Vaccines, viruses, and voodoo. *J Investig Allergol Clin Immunol* 12: 155–168.

Buckley, C., Oger, J., Clover, L., *et al.* (2001). Potassium channel antibodies in two patients with reversible limbic encephalitis. *Ann Neurol* 50: 73–78.

Carbone, K.M., Rubin, S.A., Nishino, Y., and Pletnikov, M.V. (2001). Borna disease: virus-induced neurobehavioral disease pathogenesis. *Curr Opin Microbiol* 4: 467–475.

Chapman, J., Cohen-Armon, M., Shoenfeld, Y., and Korczyn, A.D. (1999). Antiphospholipid antibodies permeabilize and depolarize brain synapto-neurosomes. *Lupus* 8: 127–133.

Chattopadhyay, S., Ito, M., Cooper, J.D. *et al.* (2002). An autoantibody inhibitory to glutamic acid decarboxylase in the neurodegenerative disorder Batten disease. *Hum Mol Genet* 11: 1421–1431.

Church, A.J., Cardoso, F., Dale, R.C., *et al.* (2002). Anti-basal ganglia antibodies in acute and persistent Sydenham's chorea. *Neurology* 59: 227–231.

Connolly, A.M., Pestronk, A., Mehta, S. *et al.* (1997). Serum autoantibodies in childhood opsoclonus-myoclonus syndrome: an analysis of antigenic targets in neural tissues. *J Pediatr* 130: 878–884.

Costa, M., Saiz, A., Casamitjana, R., Castaner, M.F., Sanmarti, A., Graus, F., *et al.* (2002). T-cell reactivity to glutamic acid decarboxylase in stiff-man syndrome and cerebellar ataxia associated with polyendocrine autoimmunity. *Clin Exp Immunol* 129(3): 471–478.

Dalakas, M.C., Fujii, M., Li, M., and McElroy, B. (2000). The clinical spectrum of anti-GAD antibody-positive patients with stiff-person syndrome. *Neurology* 55: 1531–1535.

Dalakas, M.C., Fujii, M., Li, M., *et al.* (2001a). High-dose intravenous immune globulin for stiff-person syndrome. *N Engl J Med* 345: 1870–1876.

Dalakas, M.C., Li, M., Fujii, M., and Jacobowitz, D.M. (2001b). Stiff person syndrome: quantification, specificity, and intrathecal synthesis of GAD65 antibodies. *Neurology* 57: 780–784.

Dale, R.C., Church, A.J., Cardoso, F., *et al.* (2001). Poststreptococcal acute disseminated encephalomyelitis with basal ganglia involvement and auto-reactive antibasal ganglia antibodies. *Ann Neurol* 50: 588–595.

Dalmau, J., Graus, F., Cheung, N.K., *et al.* (1995). Major histocompatibility proteins, anti-Hu antibodies, and paraneoplastic encephalomyelitis in neuroblastoma and small cell lung cancer. *Cancer* 75: 99–109.

Dalton, P., Deacon, R., Blamire, A. *et al.* (2003). Maternal neuronal antibodies associated with autism and a language disorder. *Ann Neurol* 53: 533–537.

Deacon, R.M., Croucher, A., and Rawlins, J.N. (2002). Hippocampal cytotoxic lesion effects on species-typical behaviours in mice. *Behav Brain Res* 132: 203–213.

DeGiorgio, L.A., Konstantinov, K.N., Lee, S.C., *et al.* (2001). A subset of lupus anti-DNA antibodies cross-reacts with the NR2 glutamate receptor in systemic lupus erythematosus. *Nat Med* 7: 1189–1193.

Dinkel, K., Rickert, M., Moller, G., *et al.* (2002). Stiff-man syndrome: identification of 17 beta-hydroxysteroid dehydrogenase type 4 as a novel 80-kDa antineuronal antigen. *J Neuroimmunol* 130: 184–193.

Eisenhauer, P.B., Chaturvedi, P., Fine, R.E., *et al.* (2001). Tumor necrosis factor alpha increases human cerebral endothelial cell Gb3 and sensitivity to Shiga toxin. *Infect Immun* 69: 1889–1894.

Ellison, M.D. and Merchant, R.E. (1991). Appearance of cytokine-associated central nervous system myelin damage coincides temporally with serum tumor necrosis factor induction after recombinant interleukin-2 infusion in rats. *J Neuroimmunol* 33: 245–251.

Floeter, M.K., Valls-Sole, J., Toro, C. *et al.* (1998). Physiologic studies of spinal inhibitory circuits in patients with stiff-person syndrome. *Neurology* 51: 85–93.

Folli, F., Solimena, M., Cofiell, R., *et al.* (1993). Autoantibodies to a 128-kd synaptic protein in three women with the stiff-man syndrome and breast cancer. *N Engl J Med* 328: 546–551.

Frassoni, C., Spreafico, R., Franceschetti, S., *et al.* (2001). Labeling of rat neurons by anti-GluR3 IgG from patients with Rasmussen encephalitis. *Neurology* 57: 324–327.

Ghabriel, M.N., Zhu, C., and Leigh, C. (2002). Electron microscope study of blood-brain barrier opening induced by immunological targeting of the endothelial barrier antigen. *Brain Res* 934: 140–151.

Gibbs, J.W. 3rd, Morton, L.D., Amaker, B., *et al.* (1998). Physiological analysis of Rasmussen's encephalitis: patch clamp recordings of altered inhibitory neurotransmitter function in resected frontal cortical tissue. *Epilepsy Res* 31: 13–27.

Gloor, S.M., Wachtel, M., Bolliger, M.F., *et al.* (2001). Molecular and cellular permeability control at the blood-brain barrier. *Brain Res Brain Res Rev* 36: 258–264.

Gloor, S.M., Weber, A., Adachi, N., and Frei, K. (1997). Interleukin-1 modulates protein tyrosine phosphatase activity and permeability of brain endothelial cells. *Biochem Biophys Res Commun* 239: 804–809.

Greenwood, D.L., Gitlits, V.M., Alderuccio, F., *et al.* (2002). Autoantibodies in neuropsychiatric lupus. *Autoimmunity* 35: 79–86.

Hallett, J.J., Harling-Berg, C.J., Knopf, P.M., *et al.* (2000). Anti-striatal antibodies in Tourette syndrome cause neuronal dysfunction. *J Neuroimmunol* 111: 195–202.

Hanly, J.G., Walsh, N.M., Fisk, J.D., *et al.* (1993). Cognitive impairment and auto-antibodies in systemic lupus erythematosus. *Br J Rheumatol* 32: 291–296.

Hanson, V.G., Horowitz, M., Rosenbluth, D., *et al.* (1992). Systemic lupus erythematosus patients with central nervous system involvement show auto-antibodies to a 50-kD neuronal membrane protein. *J Exp Med* 176: 565–573.

Hart, I.K., Maddison, P., Newsom-Davis, J., *et al.* (2002). Phenotypic variants of autoimmune peripheral nerve hyperexcitability. *Brain* 125: 1887–1895.

He, X.P., Patel, M., Whitney, K.D., *et al.* (1998). Glutamate receptor GluR3 antibodies and death of cortical cells. *Neuron* 20: 153–163.

Heidenreich, F. and Vincent, A. (1998). Antibodies to ion-channel proteins in thymoma with myasthenia, neuromyotonia, and peripheral neuropathy. *Neurology* 50: 1483–1485.

Honnorat, J., Saiz, A., Giometto, B., *et al.* (2001). Cerebellar ataxia with anti-glutamic acid decarboxylase antibodies: study of 14 patients. *Arch Neurol* 58: 225–230.

Ikeda, M., Bhattacharjee, A.K., Kondoh, T., *et al.* (2002). Synergistic effect of cold mannitol and Na(+)/Ca(2+) exchange blocker on blood-brain barrier opening. *Biochem Biophys Res Commun* 291: 669–674.

Jacobson, L., Polizzi, A., Morriss-Kay, G., and Vincent, A. (1999). Plasma from human mothers of fetuses with severe arthrogryposis multiplex congenita causes deformities in mice. *J Clin Invest* 103: 1031–1038.

Kanda, T., Iwasaki, T., Yamawaki, M., *et al.* (2000). Anti-GM1 antibody facilitates leakage in an in vitro blood-nerve barrier model. *Neurology* 55: 585–587.

Korvatska, E., Van de Water, J., Anders, T.F., and Gershwin, M.E. (2002). Genetic and immunologic considerations in autism. *Neurobiol Dis* 9: 107–125.

Krause, I., He, X.S., Gershwin, M.E., and Shoenfeld, Y. (2002). Brief report: immune factors in autism: a critical review. *J Autism Dev Disord* 32: 337–345.

Krauss, G.L., Campbell, M.L., Roche, K.W., *et al.* (196). Chronic steroid-responsive encephalitis without autoantibodies to glutamate receptor GluR3. *Neurology* 46: 247–249.

Laing, P., Knight, J.G., Hill, J.M., *et al.* (1989). Influenza viruses induce auto-antibodies to a brain-specific 37-kDa protein in rabbit. *Proc Natl Acad Sci USA* 86: 1998–2002.

Leach, J.P., Chadwick, D.W., Miles, J.B., Hart, I.K. (1999). Improvement in adult-onset Rasmussen's encephalitis with long-term immunomodulatory therapy. *Neurology* 52: 738–742.

Lee, E.K., Maselli, R.A., Ellis, W.G., and Agius, M.A. (1998). Morvan's fibrillary chorea: a paraneoplastic manifestation of thymoma. *J Neurol Neurosurg Psychiatry* 65: 857–862.

Leonard, H.L. and Swedo, S.E. (2001). Paediatric autoimmune neuropsychiatric disorders associated with streptococcal infection (PANDAS). *Int J Neuropsychopharmacol* **4**: 191–198.

Lernmark, A. (1996). Glutamic acid decarboxylase—gene to antigen to disease. *J Intern Med* **240**: 259–277.

Levite, M. and Hermelin, A. (1999). Autoimmunity to the glutamate receptor in mice–a model for Rasmussen's encephalitis? *J Autoimmun* **13**: 73–82.

Levite, M., Fleidervish, I.A., Schwarz, A., *et al.* (1999). Autoantibodies to the glutamate receptor kill neurons via activation of the receptor ion channel. *J Autoimmun* **13**: 61–72.

Liguori, R., Vincent, A., Clover, L., *et al.* (2001). Morvan's syndrome: peripheral and central nervous system and cardiac involvement with antibodies to voltage-gated potassium channels. *Brain* **124**: 2417–2426.

Loiselle, C.R., Wendlandt, J.T., Rohde, C.A., and Singer, H.S. (2003). Anti-streptococcal, neuronal, and nuclear antibodies in Tourette syndrome. *Pediatr Neurol* **28**: 119–125.

Lukes, A., Mun-Bryce, S., Lukes, M., and Rosenberg, G.A. (1999). Extracellular matrix degradation by metalloproteinases and central nervous system diseases. *Mol Neurobiol* **19**: 267–284.

Luque, F.A., Furneaux, H.M., Ferziger, R., *et al.* (1991). Anti-Ri: an antibody associated with paraneoplastic opsoclonus and breast cancer. *Ann Neurol* **29**: 241–251.

Madrid, A., Gil-Peralta, A., Gil-Neciga, E., *et al.* (1996). Morvan's fibrillary chorea: remission after plasmapheresis. *J Neurol* **243**: 350–353.

Madsen, K.M., Hviid, A., Vestergaard, M., *et al.* A population-based study of measles, mumps, and rubella vaccination and autism. *N Engl J Med* **347**: 1477–1482.

Mantegazza, R., Bernasconi, P., Baggi, F., *et al.* Antibodies against GluR3 peptides are not specific for Rasmussen's encephalitis but are also present in epilepsy patients with severe, early onset disease and intractable seizures. *J Neuroimmunol* **131**: 179–185.

McAllister, D.L., Kaplan, B.J., Edworthy, S.M., *et al.* (1997). The influence of systemic lupus erythematosus on fetal development: cognitive, behavioral, and health trends. *J Int Neuropsychol Soc* **3**: 370–376.

Meinck, H.M., Ricker, K., Hulser, P.J., and Solimena, M. (1995). Stiff man syndrome: neurophysiological findings in eight patients. *J Neurol* **242**: 134–142.

Meinck, H.M., Faber, L., Morgenthaler, N., *et al.* (2001). Antibodies against glutamic acid decarboxylase: prevalence in neurological diseases. *J Neurol Neurosurg Psychiatry* **71**: 100–103.

Mitoma, H., Ishida, K., Shizuka-Ikeda, M., and Mizusawa, H. (2003). Dual impairment of GABAA- and GABAB-receptor-mediated synaptic responses by autoantibodies to glutamic acid decarboxylase. *J Neurol Sci* **208**: 51–56.

Morshed, S.A., Parveen, S., Leckman, J.F., *et al.* (2001). Antibodies against neural, nuclear, cytoskeletal, and streptococcal epitopes in children and adults with Tourette's syndrome, Sydenham's chorea, and autoimmune disorders. *Biol Psychiat* **50**: 566–577.

Nemni, R., Braghi, S., Natali-Sora, M.G., *et al.* (1994). Autoantibodies to glutamic acid decarboxylase in palatal myoclonus and epilepsy. *Ann Neurol* **36**: 665–667.

Nicholas, A.P., Chatterjee, A., Arnold, M.M., *et al.* (1997). Stiff-persons' syndrome associated with thymoma and subsequent myasthenia gravis. *Muscle Nerve* **20**: 493–498.

Nitschke, M., Hochberg, F., and Dropcho, E. (1995). Improvement of paraneoplastic opsoclonus-myoclonus after protein A column therapy. *N Engl J Med* **332**: 192.

Noetzel, M.J., Cawley, L.P., James, V.L., *et al.* (1987). Anti-neurofilament protein antibodies in opsoclonus-myoclonus. *J Neuroimmunol* **15**: 137–145.

Nofech-Mozes, Y., Yuhas, Y., Kaminsky, E., *et al.* (2000). Induction of mRNA for tumor necrosis factor-alpha and interleukin-1 beta in mice brain, spleen and liver in an animal model of *Shigella*-related seizures. *Isr Med Assoc J* **2**: 86–90.

Nolte, M.T., Pirofsky, B., Gerritz, G.A., and Golding, B. (1979). Intravenous immunoglobulin therapy for antibody deficiency. *Clin Exp Immunol* **36**: 237–243.

Pletnikov, M.V., Rubin, S.A., Carbone, K.M., *et al.* (2001). Neonatal Borna disease virus infection (BDV)-induced damage to the cerebellum is associated with sensorimotor deficits in developing Lewis rats. *Brain Res Dev Brain Res* **126**: 1–12.

Pohl, K.R., Pritchard, J., and Wilson, J. (1996). Neurological sequelae of the dancing eye syndrome. *Eur J Pediatr* **155**: 237–244.

Polizzi, A., Huson, S.M., and Vincent, A. (2000). Teratogen update: maternal myasthenia gravis as a cause of congenital arthrogryposis. *Teratology* **62**: 332–341.

Pozo-Rosich, P., Clover, L., Saiz, A., Vincent, A., and Graus, F. (2003). Voltage-gated potassium channel antibodies in idiopathic and paraneoplastic limbic encephalitis. *Ann Neurol* **54**: 530–533.

Rasmussen, T. (1978). Further observations on the syndrome of chronic encephalitis and epilepsy. *Appl Neurophysiol* **41**: 1–12.

Ridley, A., Kennard, C., Scholtz, C.L., *et al.* (1987). Omnipause neurons in two cases of opsoclonus associated with oat cell carcinoma of the lung. *Brain* **110**(6): 1699–1709.

Rogers, S.W., Andrews, P.I., Gahring, L.C., *et al.* (1994). Autoantibodies to glutamate receptor GluR3 in Rasmussen's encephalitis. *Science* **265**: 648–651.

Schott, J.M., Harkness, K., Barnes, J., *et al.* (2003). Amnesia, cerebral atrophy, and autoimmunity. *Lancet* **361**: 1266.

Serratrice, G. and Azulay, J.P. (1994). [What is left of Morvan's fibrillary chorea?]. *Rev Neurol (Paris)* **150**: 257–265 (in French).

Shi, L., Fatemi, S.H., Sidwell, R.W., and Patterson, P.H. (2003). Maternal influenza infection causes marked behavioral and pharmacological changes in the offspring. *J Neurosci* **23**: 297–302.

Singer, H.S., Giuliano, J.D., Hansen, B.H., *et al.* (1998). Antibodies against human putamen in children with Tourette syndrome. *Neurology* **50**: 1618–1624.

Singh, V.K., Warren, R.P., Odell, J.D., *et al.* (1993). Antibodies to myelin basic protein in children with autistic behavior. *Brain Behav Immun* **7**: 97–103.

Singh, V.K., Lin, S.X., Newell, E., and Nelson, C. (2002). Abnormal measles-mumps-rubella antibodies and CNS autoimmunity in children with autism. *J Biomed Sci* **9**: 359–364.

Solimena, M., Folli, F., Denis-Donini, S. *et al.* (1988). Autoantibodies to glutamic acid decarboxylase in a patient with stiff-man syndrome, epilepsy, and type I diabetes mellitus. *N Engl J Med* **318**: 1012–1020.

Swedo, S.E. (1994). Sydenham's chorea. A model for childhood autoimmune neuro0psychiatric disorders. *J Am Med Assoc* **272**: 1788–1791.

Takenoshita, H., Shizuka-Ikeda, M., Mitoma, H., *et al.* (2001). Presynaptic inhibition of cerebellar GABAergic transmission by glutamate decarboxylase autoantibodies in progressive cerebellar ataxia. *J Neurol Neurosurg Psychiatry* **70**: 386–389.

Taylor, J.R., Morshed, S.A., Parveen, S., *et al.* (2002). An animal model of Tourette's syndrome. *Am J Psychiat* **159**: 657–660.

Tishler, M., Alosachie, I., Chapman, Y., *et al.* (1995). Anti-neuronal antibodies in antiphospholipid syndrome with central nervous system involvement: the difference from systemic lupus erythematosus. *Lupus* **4**: 145–147.

Tsao, N., Hsu, H.P., Wu, C.M., *et al.* (2001). Tumour necrosis factor-alpha causes an increase in blood-brain barrier permeability during sepsis. *J Med Microbiol* **50**: 812–821.

Twyman, R.E., Gahring, L.C., Spiess, J., and Rogers, S.W. (1995). Glutamate receptor antibodies activate a subset of receptors and reveal an agonist binding site. *Neuron* **14**: 755–762.

Vincent, A., Grimaldi, L.M., Martino, G., *et al.* (1997). Antibodies to ^{125}I-glutamic acid decarboxylase in patients with stiff man syndrome. *J Neurol Neurosurg Psychiatry* **62**: 395–397.

Vincent, A., Buckley, C., Schott, J. *et al.* (2004). Potassium channel antibody-associated encephalopathy: a potentially immunotherapy-responsive form of limbic encephalis. *Brain* **127**: 701–712.

Vojdani, A., Campbell, A.W., Anyanwu, E., *et al.* (2002). Antibodies to neuron-specific antigens in children with autism: possible cross-reaction with encephalitogenic proteins from milk, *Chlamydia pneumoniae* and *Streptococcus* group A. *J Neuroimmunol* **129**: 168–177.

Voltz, R., Dalmau, J., Posner, J.B., and Rosenfeld, M.R. (1998). T-cell receptor analysis in anti-Hu associated paraneoplastic encephalomyelitis. *Neurology* **51**: 1146–1150.

Warren, R.P., Cole, P., Odell, J.D., *et al.* (1990). Detection of maternal antibodies in infantile autism. *J Am Acad Child Adolesc Psychiatry* **29**: 873–877.

Watson, R., Jiang, Y., Bermudez, I., *et al.* (2004). Absence of antibodies to glu-tamate receptor type 3 (GluR3) in Rasmussen encephalitis. *Neurology* 63: 43–50.

Wendlandt, J.T., Grus, F.H., Hansen, B.H., and Singer, H.S. (2001). Striatal antibodies in children with Tourette's syndrome: multivariate discriminant analysis of IgG repertoires. *J Neuroimmunol* 119: 106–113.

Whitney, K.D. and McNamara, J.O. (2000). GluR3 autoantibodies destroy neural cells in a complement-dependent manner modulated by complement regulatory proteins. *J Neurosci* 20: 7307–7316.

Wiendl, H., Bien, C.G., Bernasconi, P., *et al.* (2001). GluR3 antibodies: prevalence in focal epilepsy but no specificity for Rasmussen's encephalitis. *Neurology* 57: 1511–1514.

Yong, V.W., Krekoski, C.A., Forsyth, P.A., *et al.* (1998). Matrix metalloproteinases and diseases of the CNS. *Trends Neurosci* 21: 75–80.

Ziter, F.A., Bray, P.F., and Cancilla, P.A. (1979). Neuropathologic findings in a patient with neuroblastoma and myoclonic encephalopathy. *Arch Neurol* 36: 51.

34 A history of neuroimmunology: a personal perspective

Byron H. Waksman

The first neuroimmunologic observation, made over a century ago, was of paralytic encephalomyelitis in patients receiving injections of Pasteur's new rabies vaccine. This established that immune responses might play a causative role in human neurological disease. Rivers and his colleagues in 1932 produced a similar disease by repeated injections of neural tissue into monkeys and rabbits. This animal model became known as experimental allergic (or autoimmune) encephalomyelitis (EAE) and served for 40 years as the principal subject of investigations on immunologically mediated disease of the nervous system.

More fundamental investigations of nervous system–immune system interactions began with attempts, around the beginning of the twentieth century, to discriminate antigenic tissue components by their ability to elicit antibodies. Characteristic protein and glycolipid antigens were found in the brain, eye, and other organs. Crystallin, a protein of the ocular lens, was obtainable in almost pure form and was used by Verhoeff in 1922 in the first investigation of the pathogenesis of the autoimmune disorder phakogenic uveitis, an inflammatory eye disease that follows cataract extraction when there has been accidental leakage of immunogenic lens contents. Skin tests with crystallin elicited typical tuberculin-type skin reactions (delayed-type hypersensitivity; DTH) in patients with the disease and not in control subjects. Burky produced a rabbit model for phakogenic uveitis in 1934, following Rivers' discovery of EAE and Verhoeff's clinical demonstration.

Investigators sought to develop additional disease models in animals that could be easily studied and provided reproducible representations of uncommon human disorders. New autoimmune models, affecting both the nervous system (Table 34.1) and other organs, were described in a steady

Table 34.1 Autoimmune neurologic and related diseases in experimental animals[a]

Date	Experimental model	Date	Experimental model
1933	Experimental autoimmune encephalomyelitis (EAE)	1995	Model of Alzheimer's disease in transgenic mice overexpressing APP
1934	Phakogenic uveitis	1998	Model of familial ALS in transgenic mice with abnormality of SOD
1949	Experimental autoimmune uveitis (EAU)		
1955	Experimental autoimmune neuritis (EAN)	2000	Tourette's syndrome in rats injected intrastriatally with patient's serum
1965, 1991	Experimental autoimmune autonomic neuropathy		
1965	Experimental autoimmune myositis	2001	Sydenham's chorea in rats given rat antibody to β streptococcal M5 protein into subthalamic nuclei
1967	Experimental autoimmune adenohypophysitis		
1972	Myeloma associated with neuropathy (mice)	2001	Model of Parkinsonism in transgenic mice and flies overexpressing synnuclein
1973	Experimental autoimmune myasthenia gravis (EAMG)		
1981	Lambert–Eaton syndrome (LEMS) in mice (serum transfer from patients)	2001	Arthrogryphosis multiplex congenita in offspring of mice injected with antibody to fetal form of AChR during pregnancy
1981	POEMS syndrome in mice (serum transfer from patients)		
1982	Retinal ganglion cell blindness	2002	Autoimmune sensorineural hearing loss
1986	Experimental autoimmune motor neuron disease (EAMND)	2003	Autism, language abnormality, behavioral disorders in offspring of mice injected with antineural antibody at defined times (2 days, 3 days, daily) during pregnancy
1986	Experimental autoimmune gray matter disease (EAGMD)		
1988	Sulfated glucuronyl paragloboside (SGPG) model of peripheral neuropathy	2003	Similar 'autistic' and 'schizophrenic' behavioral disorders in offspring of mice with viral infections at critical times during pregnancy, mimicked by maternal injection of RNA polyinosinic-polycytidylic acid
1990, 1992	CNS lesions of systemic lupus erythematosus (SLE): NZB, MRL mice; idiotype infusion; later other mouse models: gld, BXSB		
		2004	Similar behavior in rats injected as neonates with 'maternal' CK (LIF)
1991	Rat narcolepsy (genetic model in rats)		
1990s	EAE with different myelin and astrocyte epitopes, giving different distributions of lesions in CNS (e.g. CNS + retinal lesions with S100β)	2004	Model of PANDAS (pediatric autoimmune neuropsychiatric disorders associated with streptococcal infection) in mice immunized with streptococci
		2003	Optic neuritis variant of EAE, model for clinically isolated MS syndromes
1994	LEMS in rats (immunization with synaptotagmin)		
1994	Sickness behavior after intraperitoneal or intravenous CK (IL-1, IL-2, IL-6, TNF), mediated by vagus	2004	Optco-spinal variant of EAE, model for Devic's disease and Asian MS

[a] Autoimmune disease models related to acute viral infections are discussed in section on Neuroimmunologic diseases associated with infection.

stream over the years. The concept of autoimmunity, however, was not quickly accepted, in part because of Ehrlich's widely quoted dictum about the immune system's 'horror autotoxicus'. Only after 1960, when studies of experimental autoimmune thyroiditis and of chronic thyroiditis in humans had established the astonishing degree of similarity between the human and experimental conditions, was there widespread acceptance of this idea.

Immunologic knowledge before 1960 was too limited to permit sophisticated research either on animal models or on their human counterparts, beyond what was possible with basic morphologic, serologic, and simple protein separation techniques (Table 34.2). The model diseases described before this time proved to be mediated primarily by cell-mediated immunity (CMI); they presented inflammatory, destructive lesions that could not

Table 34.2 Immunology: conceptual highlights over half a century

Date	Conceptual development	Date	Conceptual development
Pre-1950	Role of antibody in immunity, anaphylaxis, and in immune-complex disease		Thymic deletion or clonal anergy of T-cell clones with high binding affinity; clonal deletion or anergy in periphery
	Immunologic tolerance, oral tolerance		Description of CD5+/B-1 B cells
	Antibody made by plasma cells	1990–2000	Innate immunity: pathogens, tissue breakdown products, and Toll-like receptors (TLR); interaction with adaptive immune system
	Cell-mediated immunity (CMI) recognized only by skin test delayed-type hypersensitivity (DTH) and by adoptive transfer with living mononuclear cells		Co-stimulatory systems: B7.1 (CD80) or B7.2 (CD86) and CD28 or CTLA-4
1950–1960	Immunoglobulin isotypes and idiotypes distinguished		Chemokines (CCK) affecting immunocyte migration, vascular expression of adhesion molecules; use of CCK receptors as cell markers
	CMI recognized as a distinct class of reactions		Apoptosis and programmed cell death
	Lymphocytes recognized as the central cells of immunology		Down-regulation by CK: IL-4, IL-10, TGF-β
1960–1970	Role of thymus and bursa of Fabricius in lymphocyte maturation and differentiation		Interactions among CNS, HPA, HPT, HPG; and immune system
	Thymus as seat of specific immunologic tolerance		Vaccination with effector T cells induces anti-TCR Vβ-specific Qa1-restricted regulatory cells
	T and B lymphocytes distinguished		Altered peptide ligands (APL), via altered strength of signal, induce altered T-cell responses: antagonism, anergy, partial activation, Th1–Th2 shift, heteroclitic activation
	Lymphocyte stimulation by antigens or mitogens *in vitro*, cytotoxicity		
	Antibody formation in tissue cultures		Heterogeneity of DC; down-regulatory DC
	First cytokines (CK) identified (bioassay only)		Regulatory NK cells and NKT cells (bearing α/β or γ/δ TCR)
	First use of T-cell markers		
1970–1980	CD4+ and CD8+ subsets of T cells		The 'immunological homunculus' concept: autoaggressive T-cell clones of intermediate or low binding affinity in thymus held in check by anti-idiotypic regulatory cell population
	First description of dendritic cells (DC)		
	Discovery of natural killer (NK) cells (cytotoxic)		
	MHC (HLA) restriction of T-cell responses (dual recognition)	2000 and later	Enhanced antigenicity of autoantigens by post-translational modification, e.g. citrullination, nitrosylation
	'Suppressor cells' and down-regulation		Non-classical MHC, e.g. CD1d, stimulated by tissue glycolipid and CK (IL-12 or IL-4) from adjacent antigen-presenting cells (APC), present epitopes to NKT cells
	Oral tolerance mediated by suppressor T cells		
	The CD8+CD28–FcR+ suppressor/regulatory cell		
	B-cell maturation sequence; memory B cells		Monocyte-derived DC expressing indole 2,3-deoxygenase (IDO) mediate suppression by epitope-driven T cells (fetus, tumors, allografts, food)
	B-cell tolerance in bone marrow; clonal abortion		
	Network concept: anti-idiotypic antibodies and T cells		Elaboration of positive and negative co-stimulatory systems: B7/CD28 superfamily; CD2 and its ligands; TNF–TNF receptor pathways; CD46 (human) or Crry (mouse)
	Molecular mimicry		
1980–1990	Cloning of effector T cells; vaccination with inactivated effector T cells		
	Sequence and steric structure of MHC Class I and MHC Class II, later of T-cell receptor (TCR)		Membrane-bound regulatory systems: CTLA-4; TGF-β cleaved by thrombospondin 1, complexed with latency-associated peptide (LAP) to give activated TGF-β1
	Molecular structure and function of cytokines, adhesion molecules, growth factors, and their receptors		
	Signaling, transduction pathways, gene regulation and expression		Complexity of immune deviation, as in ACAID model: participation of DC migrating to thymus or spleen, γ/δ T cells, natural killer T (NKT) cells, and Th1–Th2 shift
	The CD4+CD25+ regulatory cell		
	Two- and three-cell regulatory systems; regulatory cells in 'low responders'		New signaling and regulatory molecules: neuregulins, galectins, TIM 1–9, Atg proteins of innate autophagic system, CEACA1 isoforms
	Anterior chamber (of eye) model of acquired immune deviation (ACAID)		
	Alpha/beta (α/β) and gamma/delta (γ/δ) TCR T cells		AIRE (autoimmune regulator): regulates promiscuous expression of autoantigens in thymic medullary epithelium: 'mirrors peripheral self'
	Human peripheral γ/δ T cells carry NK receptors, each with distinctive signaling properties		
	CD4+ T-cell subsets with different cytokine profiles: Th1 and Th2, later similar CD8+ T-cell subsets (Tc1 and Tc2)		

be missed, even by skeptical pathologists. Antibody-mediated conditions were first studied after 1970, when myasthenia gravis (MG) and its animal model became dominant paradigms of autoimmune neurologic disease. The changes that characterized these new models were more subtle, often requiring careful neurophysiologic investigation; the identification and quantification of experimental autoimmune myasthenia gravis (EAMG) in mice, for example, could only be achieved by the use of electromyography.

The expanded range of new investigative methods in the 1980s (and the expanded pool of investigators who regarded autoimmune disease as a fruitful field of investigation) enormously accelerated the pace of new research. More was learned about MG and EAMG in 5 to 10 years than had been learned about EAE in its first 40 years. One can point to molecular biology and genetics or to the cloning of effector T cells as subsequent major changes leading to new discoveries. In the 1990s, interest in the cytokines and chemokines dominated neuroimmunologic research, giving way in their turn to a renewal of interest in the rich area of immune regulation.

Since 1990, the use of transgenic animals, knockout and knockins that fail to express or overexpress a molecule of interest, has become almost routine. The molecules studied have been structural or diffusible elements of antigen-presenting cells (APC), T cells, B cells, or regulatory T cells or elements of the nervous system. The use of transgenic animals carrying a unique T-cell receptor (TCR) and 'humanized' animals (expressing human major histocompatibility complex (MHC), T cells, or other components of the immune and vascular systems) has greatly extended the usefulness of traditional models such as EAE and EAMG. Even other model species, such as *Drosophila*, have been found useful, as in recent studies of the aggregate disorders. Such models have greatly facilitated testing of new molecular families, such as neuregulins, TIMs, and the various co-stimulatory molecules, as well as of new therapies.

With the turn of the millennium, two new frontiers in neuroimmunology have been breached with the uncovering of mechanisms that underlie movement and behavioral disorders. The demonstration that Sydenham's chorea, attention deficit hyperactivity disorder, Tourette's syndrome, chronic tic disorder, and obsessive–compulsive 'neurosis' can all be mediated by cross-reactive antibody against antigenic components of streptococcal cell membranes has led to creation of a new disease category: pediatric autoimmune neuropsychiatric disorders associated with streptococcal infection (PANDAS). Similarly, persuasive animal models have been developed to show that dyslexia and autism (and even, perhaps, schizophrenia) may be mediated by events affecting pregnant mothers at critical developmental stages of the fetal central nervous system (CNS), either viral infection (with cytokine (CK) release by the maternal immune system) or 'autoimmunization' against fetal CNS antigens. Both these developments have required innovative behavioral assay techniques that go well beyond simple physiology, backed up by basic immunological and immunopathological methods.

The following review is divided into four sections: 1. Neuroimmunologic diseases, in which the nervous system is the target of immune attack; 2. Neuroimmunologic diseases associated with infection, in which the nervous system is affected secondary to an infective process; 3. Immunologic involvement in non-immunologic disorders of the nervous system, an emerging field in which neuroimmunology contributes to the pathology of non-immunologic disorders; and 4. Biologic aspects of neuroimmunology, which includes psychoneuroimmunology and related issues. The number of authors credited in individual papers has grown, in parallel with growth in the complexity of the research and the increased need for collaboration across disciplines (and across the world). Thus for more recent work cited in the tables of this brief review, only first authors are named and/or the heads of large laboratory groups responsible for the research.

1. Neuroimmunologic diseases

Multiple sclerosis

An immunologic theory of multiple sclerosis (MS) was put forward in the 1930s by Pette, Schaltenbrand, and others, primarily on morphologic grounds. The combined presence of inflammation and parenchymal damage, in the absence of a known toxic or infectious agent, argued for an underlying immunologic process. The discovery of the EAE model provided support for this idea.

The lesion

Starting in the mid-1970s, the increasingly refined immunohistochemical and electron microscope studies of Lampert and Prineas and later of Raine, Wisniewski, Lassmann, Sobel, Brosnan, and others demonstrated the early presence in MS lesions of both CD4+ and CD8+ TCR α/β and later TCR γ/δ T cells and the preponderant role of macrophages in myelin destruction. Remyelination, from oligodendrocyte precursors, sometimes in the presence of ongoing tissue damage, results in the appearance of 'shadow plaques'. The 1990s saw studies of up-regulated adhesion molecule expression and cytokine/chemokine (CK/CCK) release (Selmaj, Cuzner, Brock, Trinchieri, Balashov, Ransohoff, and others); the stimulatory role of CD40–CD40L binding (Windhagen, Hafler); T-cell clonality using the polymerase chain reaction (PCR) technique (Hafler and Steinman spearheaded work in this area); and finally, the role of Fas–FasL (Dowling) and/or tumor necrosis factor (TNF)-α (Antel) in oligodendroglial apoptosis. Activated natural killer (NK) and natural killer T (NKT) cells, which are also present in the lesions, may be highly cytotoxic for oligodendrocytes (Antel, 2001).

In newer work, use of microarray technology has documented activation/ expression of some 62 genes (out of more than 5000) in active MS lesions (Biddison, 1999). In 1997 Selmaj and Brosnan, and their colleagues have made a strong case for heat-shock protein (HSP) 70 as a 'chaperone' presenting such myelin components as myelin basic protein (MBP), proteolipid protein (PLP), and myelin oligodendrocyte glycoprotein (MOG) to specific T cells. Reactive oxygen species (ROS) and nitric oxide (NO) have been incriminated as major agents of tissue damage (Hartung). Macrophages serve as the cellular source of these molecules in animals with EAE, and astrocytes appear to be their main source in the MS plaques of human subjects (Brosnan, Trapp). The increased ability of MS patients' T cells (all major subsets) to migrate through cerebral vascular endothelium has been shown to be mediated by interaction between leukocyte function-associated antigen (LFA)-1 and intercellular adhesion molecule (ICAM)-1, very late antigen (VLA)-4 integrin, CC chemokine ligand (CCL)-2/monocyte chemoattractant protein-1 (MCP-1), and an array of matrix metalloproteinases (Berman, Antel). Monocytes too are well endowed with several enzymes of this class (Bar-Or, Antel).

Neuronal and axonal damage in the lesions has proven to be responsible for much chronic disability in MS (Trapp) and has drawn attention away from demyelination as the main cause of functional impairment. Serial magnetic resonance spectroscopy (MRS) studies have related axonal damage to an abnormality in N-acetyl aspartate (NAA) uptake (Polman, 1999) and shown some recovery of such uptake in the recovery phase of a clinical attack of MS (Antel, 2000) or in patients recovering after treatment (Arnold, Matthews 1999; Narayan, 2000). Parallel observations with positron emission tomography (PET) scanning, have demonstrated both regional and global hypometabolism in the MS brain (Roelcke, Kappos 1997; Bacshi and colleagues, 1998), accompanied by the well-recognized loss of cognitive function (Rao, 1991).

Lassmann' collaboration over a 20-year period with an international array of colleagues working on EAE or MS has led to a tentative separation of MS cases into pathogenetically distinct entities, designated types I–IV: autoimmunity mediated by T cells; autoimmunity mediated by T cells plus antibody (and complement); acute, relapsing–remitting, or secondary progressive cases, showing only oligodendrogliopathy (possibly viral); and primary progressive cases, with oligodendrogliopathy (possibly viral) (Luchinetti, Lassmann, and others 1996, 2000).

A viral cause?

Repeated attempts to identify a specific causative virus in the CNS tissue or blood cells of MS patients have failed. In a Russian study performed immediately after the Second World War the suspected agent turned out to be rabies virus. Sixty years later, after more than 20 additional unsubstantiated claims, it remains problematic that any single specific agent is involved. On the other hand, investigation of the epidemic of MS in the Faroe Islands, which took place after the arrival of British troops at the start of the Second World War led Kurtzke and Hyllested, in 1979, to the conclusion that the disease is actually caused by a specific infectious agent. Cook and Dowling found evidence that this agent might be the canine distemper virus, closely related to measles. The most recent candidates have been EBV, human herpesvirus-6, and *Chlamydia* spp. The finding that MS patients' MBP-specific T cells recognize many short viral peptides that are identical or closely similar to encephalitogenic peptides of MBP (discussed under Molecular mimicry) implies that many viruses can initiate and/or maintain the MS disease process.

Epidemiology and distribution

Studies of prevalence, beginning in the late 1950s, led to the identification of high-prevalence areas in northern Ireland (Millar, 1954), northern Scotland (Sutherland, 1956), and the Shetland and Orkney islands (Poskanzer, 1980) and low-prevalence areas in Australia (Sutherland, 1962), South Africa (Dean, 1967), and Israel (Alter, 1969). This striking latitude effect was studied intensively by Kurland in the early 1960s and among US military veterans by Kurtzke (1967). Concurrent socioeconomic studies by the same authors established the greater prevalence of MS in more affluent groups. More recent work has shown striking differences in MS expression in different ethnic groups. Kuroiwa, working with Kurland, in an extensive study of MS among the Japanese, found low prevalence and a definite latitude effect and Dean found a total or near total absence of MS among African Blacks. Later studies showed that there is little or no MS among the Yakuts of central Siberia, the Eskimos (Inuit), and the Hutterites (an inbred Caucasian group) in central Canada. On the other hand, foci of high MS prevalence have been documented in Finland (Wikström), Norway (Nyland), and several other countries.

The study of migrants from northern Europe (Holland, the United Kingdom) to South Africa showed that those migrating before the age of 15 years expressed MS at a prevalence level comparable to that among non-Blacks in South Africa, whereas those migrating after the age of 15 years expressed the prevalence of their country of origin, the first clear demonstration that environmental determinants play a significant role in MS expression (Dean, 1966). In a recent study, Compston related the apparent 'transition' in MS susceptibility at about age 15 to the age at which transmission of common viruses (measles, rubella, mumps, EBV) occurs (Alvord, Compston, 1987). MS risk increases almost ten-fold with age of virus transmission up to 15 years of age, a pattern strikingly reminiscent of the relationship in poliomyelitis between the age at which the patient is exposed to the virus and the occurrence of clinical paralysis. The immunologic (or other) mechanism underlying this puberty-related 'transition' remains unknown. Virus infections also trigger MS exacerbations, as shown in Sibley's longitudinal studies of a large cohort of patients (1985), confirmed by Paty and later Panitch (1994).

Genetic approaches

Family and twin studies, begun by McKay and Myrianthopoulos in 1958, were greatly extended during the 1980s by McFarlin and his colleagues, by Compston and others, and especially by Ebers, Sadovnick, Paty, and various collaborators, who worked with a large well-ascertained patient population across Canada. These studies led to the inference, now widely accepted, that susceptibility to MS is genetically determined, with multiple genes being involved. Yet about half of all affected identical twin pairs are discordant for MS. The conclusion was clear: environmental influences determine the expression of MS in genetically susceptible individuals.

A collaborative study by Ikuta and Kurland of Japanese patients, carried out after the Second World War documented a high frequency of a variant form of the disease, essentially identical with Devic's disease among Caucasians: lesions predominating in optic nerves and spinal cord, a greater tendency to necrosis, and an accelerated clinical course. An essentially similar form of MS proved to be common in China and the Philippines. The

natural assumption that genetic factors determine the character of this 'Asian MS' (Osoegawa and colleagues, 2004) is, to some extent offset by a recent shift of the Japanese phenotype towards the Caucasian form of MS, accompanied by a Th2-biased immune repertoire (Yamamura, Tabira, 2002). The authors tentatively ascribe these changes to changes in the Japanese lifestyle, with decreased exposure to common environmental bacteria and increased consumption of certain new foods. A similar bias of the apparent phenotype by non-genetic influences is seen in the greater prevalence of MS in females than in males. Beginning in the early 1960s, Millar, Abramsky, and others noted lessening of MS severity during the third trimester of pregnancy and a clear-cut 'rebound' after delivery. This phenomenon has been attributed to the effect of increased estrogen, accompanied by a Th2 shift in the lymphocyte pool. After oral estriol, even in male subjects, a Th2 shift takes place with a concurrent decrease in lesions (Reder, Arnason).

Genetic investigations of MS, properly speaking, began with Jersild, Svejgaard, and Fog's 1972 study establishing an HLA association for MS susceptibility, confirmed in numerous later studies. An initial emphasis on HLA Class I genes (A3 and B7) shifted rapidly to an emphasis on Class II (DR-2, -4, -6, and DQ-w1). A possible association with genes encoding peptide isoforms of the TCR α and β chains was reported first in 1988 (Ciulla and colleagues, Beall and colleagues). There were also reports of an association with gene loci encoding immunoglobulin sequences and elements of the inflammatory process such as α_1-antitrypsin. In the 1990s, completion of the Human Genome Project permitted estimates of the number of genes (18–24 in different studies) determining susceptibility and more specific clinical and pathological aspects of MS, a complex trait disease. In spite of valiant attempts, additional genes (beyond HLA Class II) have not been convincingly identified (Haines *et al.*, 2002). With the use of microarrays, permitting a rapid survey of large numbers of genes encoding myelin components; CKs, CCKs, and their receptors; adhesion molecules; co-stimulatory factors and their receptors or ligands, etc., only HLA-II, interleukin (IL)-1Ra, IL-2Rβ, and ApoE showed some degree of linkage/association with the MS (Weinshenker, 2002).

Immunologic discoveries

Immunologic investigations of MS began in 1942 with Kabat's finding of increased globulin in the cerebrospinal fluid (CSF), followed 20 years later by the description of oligoclonal bands (OBs) in CSF IgG (Karcher, Lowenthal, 1960). Still later (1974) came Sandberg-Wollheim's identification of B cells in the CSF making IgG, IgM, and IgA; and finally (in the early 1980s) Tourtellotte's demonstration of massive immunoglobulin synthesis in the CNS and CSF compartment. More refined studies of the OBs by Vandvik in the 1970s and the Arnason group and Mehta in the 1980s were in turn followed by the demonstration that the CSF immunoglobulins include antibodies to many viruses (Norrby, 1978; K. Johnson and others), to diphtheria and tetanus toxoids (Salmi, 1981), to CNS myelin constituents such as PLP, MOG, and galactocerebroside (Genain, Hauser, 2004), and to nitrosylated cysteine from myelin peptides acted on by macrophage NO (Boullerne, 1995, 2004). Half of all MS sera bind to cultured oligodendrocytes and/or neuronal cell lines (Vincent, 2004).

Studies of blood and CSF T cells began in the 1970s with Antel and Arnason's observation that circulating CD8+ T cells show a loss of non-specific 'suppressor' activity. The same authors (with Reder and other colleagues) later related this loss to decreased expression of CD8 and an increase in surface β-adrenergic receptors. The CSF was found to contain active, cycling cells (Noronha and Arnason, 1980), some reactive with common viruses (Salmi, 1983). T-cell clones from the blood and CSF of MS patients and control subjects were shown to include cells specific for MBP (Burns, 1983). Olsson and Link (1988) used the enzyme-linked immunosorbent assay (ELISA) spot technique to show the presence in CSF of both T and B cells reactive with a variety of myelin autoantigens.

In 1990, several laboratory groups (Weiner/Hafler in Boston, Martin/McFarland at the NIH, and Hohlfeld/Wekerle in Munich) independently used T-cell cloning to show that cellular reactivity, against MBP for example, is limited to a few 'immunodominant' peptide epitopes determined by each individual's HLA background. In MS patients, the population of 'activated' T cells carrying IL-2 receptors was found to include many cells recognizing MBP, whereas such cells were not present in control patients (Mokhtarian, 1990; Zhang and Hafler, 1994). As many as 10% of the cycling CSF T cells were MBP or PLP specific. The activated MBP-specific T cells included many mutant cells, as judged by mutations in *hprt* (Allegretta, Sriram, 1990) and in pathways governing Ca^{2+} flux (Grimaldi, 1994). Since 1990, persistent *in vivo* 'clones' of CD4+ MBP-specific T cells, with unique TCR peptide signatures, have been identified by both McFarland's and Hafler's groups, and there are persistent CD8+ clones as well (Monteiro, Gregerson, 1995). With the newest techniques, e.g. the use of single-cell capture combined with sensitive PCR and spectratyping of CDR3 to establish the specificity, phenotype, and other properties of individual T cells in the lesions, CD4+ T cells have been found to be in the minority and heterogeneous, while CD8s include a small number of persistent expanded clones, some identifiable over more than 5 years in the brain, as well as in the CSF and blood (Goebels, Lassmann, Rajewsky, Hohlfeld, Wekerle, and their colleagues 2000, 2004).

Studies of antigens in MS have lagged behind what has been learned from studies in EAE. Only a few of the 15-odd candidates have really been properly investigated, mainly MBP, PLP, and MOG. The models (Table 34.1) teach us that different antigens are surely involved in clinically isolated syndromes such as optic neuritis and transverse myelitis and variant forms of MS such as Devic's disease or MS with retinal perivascular inflammation, as well as in successive phases of MS as such. Non-myelin antigens, such as S100β, αB-crystallin, 2′3′-cyclic nucleotide 3′-phosphodiesterase, transaldolase, and heat shock protein have been largely ignored. T cells have been identified that target neurons (Zipp, 2004). Tuohy has claimed that, in MS patients, sensitization to successive epitopes of myelin proteins occurs in a stereotyped sequence, as in the 'epitope spreading' seen in models such as insulin-dependent diabetes mellitus (IDDM) and EAE (1998).

Immune regulation

Abnormalities in immune regulation are characteristic of MS. Antel and Arnason's 1978 finding that a subpopulation of circulating non-cytotoxic CD8+ T cells, lacking CD28 but expressing FcR, lose the ability to down-regulate proliferative and other responses was confirmed by other laboratories (Huddlestone and Oldstone, 1979) and followed by the demonstration of decreased autologous mixed lymphocyte reactions (AMLR) (Hafler, Weiner; Crispe, Greenstein, 1985) and decreased 'suppressor–inducer' activity (Morimoto, Hafler, 1987). Later research demonstrated a decrease in AMLR-stimulated CD8+ regulatory T cells (Balashov, Weiner, 1995). Arnason and his colleagues, in studies extending over more than a decade, were able to show that such immunoregulatory abnormalities parallel abnormalities of sympathetic function (discussed in the section on Psychoneuroimmunology/neuroendocrinimmunology).

MS patients have now been found to manifest abnormalities in each of the more recently discovered types of regulatory mechanism. CD4+ CD25high regulatory T cells are reduced in number and show diminished functional capacity in patients with relapsing–remitting MS (Viglietta, Baecher-Allen, Hafler, 2003; Suri-Payer, Shevach, 2004). Both NK and NKT cells show a Th2 bias during MS remission (Yamamura, 2001) and invariant TCR NKT cells, bearing Vα24Jα18 (but not similar cells bearing Vα7Jα33) are greatly diminished (Illes, Yamamura, 2000). There is no unifying principle yet to explain this plethora of positive findings.

The papers on T cells and other cells in MS patients appearing since about 1980 have been complemented by studies of their secreted products, of activated complement components, of CKs and CCKs and their receptors (R), and of adhesion and other regulatory molecules in the blood and CSF. The principal players proved to be IL-12, IL-1, TNF-α, interferon (IFN)-γ, IL-2R, TNF-R, and ICAM-1. An increase in circulating monocytic IL-12 and a rise in T-cell production of IFN-γ and IL-18 precede and accompany MS attacks (Balashov, Weiner, 1997; Karni, Weiner, 2002). The likelihood that fatigue in MS might result from TNF and IL-1 toxicity (acting on hypothalamic nuclei) is now widely accepted (Arnason). Soluble

CD8 is also found in CSF and serum during disease activity (Maimone, Reder, 1991), and soluble TNF-R and ICAM-1 appear in the serum before an attack (Koury, 1999). Lymphotoxin represents a further possible regulatory element in the microenvironment. It is produced by the CD8+ T cells of patients with chronic progressive forms of the disease, when exposed to specific antigens in culture (Zipp, 1995; Buckle, 2000). Studies on CCK and CCKR profiles in MS have lagged behind studies on CK profiles by about 10 years (Ransohoff, Lassmann, 2004). A recent discovery, as yet insufficiently evaluated in MS, is that activities attributed to IL-12 are in part activities of IL-23 (Becher 2004).

Clinical trials have provided useful indicators for the significance of specific mediators. The importance of IFN-γ was emphasized by a trial in patients with relapsing–remitting MS; repeated injections of this CK induced acute attacks of MS, associated with up-regulation of HLA expression in monocytes (potential APC) (Panitch, Johnson, 1987). A first, bold attempt to isolate MBP-specific clones, expand and inactivate them *in vitro*, then return them to the same patient as a sort of vaccine was carried out in the mid-1990s (Zhang, Raus, 1997). This maneuver resulted in production of idiotype-specific cytolytic regulatory cells and a slow disappearance from the circulation of specific cells (carrying that idiotope and recognizing MBP) but with little or no accompanying clinical improvement. MS therapy with cyclophosphamide, which benefits the patients, is accompanied by a Th1–Th2 cell shift, a form of immune deviation (Smith, Weiner). On the other hand, oral administration of whole myelin, with little or no visible clinical consequences, is accompanied by a rise in Th3 cells (producing TGF-β *in vitro* in response to MBP and PLP) (Fukaura, Hafler, 96).

Experimental autoimmune encephalomyelitis

EAE must serve, in this brief review, as the paradigm of research on animal models with autoimmune disease that depends primarily on the induction of CMI; that is, a CD4+ Th1-cell-mediated response directed to an autoantigen. The course of EAE research (Table 34.3) has followed the evolution of immunologic concepts and techniques. Between the end of the Second World War and 1960, the basic biologic and pathologic features of EAE were established and the disease was assigned to the class of cell-mediated immune reactions. Chemical and histochemical studies of EAE during this time can be viewed (with hindsight) as studies of the chemistry of myelin breakdown, largely within phagocytic macrophages.

Between 1960 and 1970, the assignment of EAE to the CMI class was confirmed and the cells found in the lesions were characterized as hematogenous T cells and macrophages. Traditionally, the macrophages had been viewed simply as resident microglia that responded to tissue damage by becoming activated and cleaning up debris, not as the primary agents of tissue destruction. Therefore, these new insights constituted a fundamental 'paradigm shift'. Shiraki's observation in 1957 that EAE can be followed by typical MS in human subjects of Japanese origin (i.e., a particular genetic background), was an insufficiently appreciated forerunner of studies on genetic determinants of EAE and MS susceptibility.

Beginning in 1955–1956 with PLP and MBP, single homogenous proteins of myelin were found to be effective encephalitogens. MPB, because of its water-solubility, became the antigen of choice for more refined studies of encephalitogenicity over the following decades. Subsequently, with improvements in technique, many additional encephalitogenic proteins were identified; by 2004 the total had approached 15. The study of peptides, begun by Eylar, Hashim, Kibler, and others around 1970, became an essential feature of all later EAE studies. A key technology, exploited by Linington, Kojima, Wekerle, Lassmann, and their collaborators since 1990, is the generation *in vitro* of T-cell lines/clones against individual proteins and their peptides for the rapid identification of specific epitopes that can induce clones with pathogenic potential. Using this technique, investigators have shown that certain astrocytic components produce new types of EAE with unusual differences in lesion distribution and character.

Genetic studies of EAE, first undertaken in the 1970s, identified MHC Class II as a major susceptibility locus. The encephalitogenicity of specific

Table 34.3 Experimental autoimmune encephalomyelitis (EAE)

Date	Researchers	Discovery
Neurologic and immunopathologic studies		
1933	Rivers et al.	EAE is first demonstrated (monkeys, rabbits)
1940s	Ferraro, Cazzullo, Roizin	EAE can take many forms, including hyperacute (hemorrhagic) and chronic (MS-like)
1947	Kabat; Morgan	Freund's complete adjuvant intensifies EAE
1949	Waksman, Morrison	EAE is correlated with DTH to homologous (and presumably autologous) CNS tissue
1957	Uchimura, Shiraki	Post-vaccinal encephalomyelitis (EAE in humans) may be followed by typical MS (in Japanese)
1958	Waksman	Character of early lesion indicates typical CMI: perivenous mononuclear cell infiltrate, invasive-destructive lesion of parenchyma
1960	Paterson	Adoptive transfer of EAE with living lymphoid cells suggests EAE is expression of CMI
1961	Arbouys, Arnason, Waksman	EAE is prevented by antilymphocyte serum—disease is mediated by circulating lymphocytes
1962	Arnason, Janković, Waksman	EAE is prevented by neonatal thymectomy—disease-producing cells are thymus derived
1962	Waksman	EAE is model for two classes of human disease: monophasic after immunizing event (PVE, PIE, ADEM) and chronic progressive or relapsing–remitting (MS)
1963–1965	Berg, Källén; Kornguth, Thompson; David	EAE lymphocytes perform typical CMI functions in vitro: proliferation, cytotoxicity, secretion of cytokines
1963	Kosunen, Waksman, et al.	Cells in lesions of EAE are hematogenous, mostly macrophages (^{3}H-thymidine labeling)
1965, 1967	Lampert, Carpenter	First EM study of EAE: lymphocytes and macrophages cross endothelial barrier; macrophages destroy myelin, peeling off myelin lamellae and separating them from axons
1965	Stone, Lerner	Chronic relapsing EAE is produced in guinea pigs
1968	Lubaroff, Waksman	Macrophages in EAE lesions are non-specific, bone-marrow-derived (LexDA rat chimeras, cell transfer)
1969, 1981, 1983	Wisniewski; Prineas, Raine	IgG capping on macrophages and destruction of myelin in coated pits
1984	Hickey, Gonatas	CD4+ T cells in early lesions, CD8+ T cells predominate later
1989	Pender; Lassmann	Apoptosis of specific T cells in lesions; also apoptosis of oligodendroglia
1993	Goverman, Hood	Transgenic mice with T cells bearing MBP-specific TCR get spontaneous EAE
1994	Lafaille, Tonegawa	Marked increase in spontaneous EAE in hybrid offspring of similar transgenic mice X RAG knockout mice
1994, 1996	Pender, McCombe; Lassmann, Cuzner	Extensive apoptosis of macrophages in lesions
1994	Abramsky; many others	Pregnancy is protective in EAE. Mimic by treating non-pregnant females or males with estriol or estradiol. Treatment induces Th1 → Th2 shift.
1996	Rajan, Gao, Raine, Brosnan	Depletion of γ/δ T cells before onset or during chronic phase of chronic relapsing EAE gives decreased clinical disease, marked decrease of γ/δ T cells in lesions
2000, 2001	Rajan, Gao, Raine, Brosnan	These cells have phenotype of Th1 effector cells. Their depletion also results in marked decrease of inflammatory CK, CCK, and CCK receptors.
2000	Waldner, Kuchroo	Fulminant EAE in PLP-specific TCR transgenic mice
2001	Goverman	CD8+ T cells challenged with myelin produce intense EAE resembling MS >> CD4+ T cells
2002	Trapp, Tuohy, et al.	In chronic EAE, neurologic disability in initial attack is correlated with CNS inflammation; later fixed deficit increases with number of attacks and axonal loss
2003	Brosnan group	HSP-70 associates with and 'chaperones' PLP and MBP in EAE lesions in mice
2003	Cipriani, Porcelli, Brosnan	In guinea pig EAE, MHC Class II expressed on majority of infiltrating cells in lesions and increased on resident microglia; CD1d expressed on astrocytes, also on inflammatory B cells and macrophages
2003	Bettelli, Kuchroo	Primary optic neuritis (ON) in MOG-specific TCR transgenic Bl/6 mice given MOG and cFA, related to increased MOG concentration in optic neurons
2004	Bettelli, Wekerle	Mice whose T cells bear anti-MOG transgenic TCR and B cells anti-MOG transgenic BCR develop an optico-spinal form of EAE (a good model for Japanese MS and for Caucasian Devic's disease)
2004	Whitacre group	Severity of EAE in females is greater than in males in some strains of mice but not in others
Encephalitogenic antigens and peptides		
1948	Kabat	Autologous brain can induce EAE
1955	Waksman, Lees Folch-Pi	Myelin proteolipid (PLP) is an effective EAE antigen
1956	Kies; Roboz-Einstein	Myelin basic protein (MBP) is an EAE antigen
1970	Eylar; others	Peptides of MBP as short as 9 or 10 amino acid residues are encephalitogenic

Table 34.3 Experimental autoimmune encephalomyelitis (EAE) *(continued)*

Date	Researchers	Discovery
1982	Fritz	Different 'immunodominant' peptides of MBP in different mouse strains are restricted by MHC Class II alleles
1990	Tuohy, Lees	Encephalitogenic peptides of PLP and their relation to MHC Class II are established
1990s	Kojima, Linington, Wekerle	MAG, MOG, S100β, and GFAP are encephalitogenic and may contribute to EAE
1990s	Wekerle, Lassmann	Distribution and character of lesions differ with different encephalitogens
1994	Martin; Braun	Cyclic nucleotide phosphohydrolase of myelin is also a potential encephalitogen
1994	Van Noort	B-crystallin (HSP25) is also a potential encephalitogen
1995	Kuchroo, Nicholson	Use of APL gives deviation and decreased EAE
1996	Kuchroo	Pre-treatment with SEB superantigen gives increased EAE in PL/J × SJL mice with PLP 43–64 (broadly responsive) and decreased EAE with MBP Ac1–11 (narrowly responsive)
2004	Boullerne	Lewis rats immunized with MBP make IgM and IgG antibodies to nitrosylated cysteine formed in the lesions; level is correlated with myelin damage
2004	Steinman	NOGO contains encephalitogenic epitopes

Immunogenetic studies

Date	Researchers	Discovery
1960s, 1970s	Levine; Stone	Susceptible and resistant strains of inbred rats and guinea pigs are produced. Congenic and backcross strains are developed
1973	Williams, Moore	Study of LexBN rat backcrosses demonstrates single dominant susceptibility gene: MHC Class II
1977	Teitelbaum, Arnon; Bernard	In guinea pigs and mice, as well, the dominant susceptibility gene is MHC Class II
1980s	Lublin	Congenic backcross strains of mice differ in frequency and severity of exacerbations
1982	Linthicum, Frelinger	EAE susceptibility genes govern vascular sensitivity to vasoamines
1985	Ben-Nun	MBP epitopes are related to specific TCR peptide polymorphisms
1986	Korngold	Study of interstrain chimeras shows that multiple immunologic and non-immunologic factors (genes) underlie susceptibility/resistance
1988	Heber-Katz	TCR Vβ 8.2 is overrepresented in mouse and rat autoimmune diseases: the 'V region disease' theory
1987, 1988	Goldowitz, Lublin; Nicholas, Arnason	Heterotopic brain grafts provide a finer analysis of factors underlying susceptibility/resistance
1991	J. Miller	In transgenic mice, H-2K^b placed under control of MBP promoter results in 'wonky' (hypomyelinated) mice
2000 and later	Kuchroo, Wicker, Encinas, Linington, Lassmann, Olsson	More than 20 loci in some autoimmune diseases: preliminary data from positional cloning identify 4 EAE loci in mice, 8 in rats

Cell and molecular immunobiology of EAE

Date	Researchers	Discovery
1977, 1979	McFarlin; Kies	Adoptive transfer of EAE requires 'activated' CD4+ T cells (antigen, mitogen)
1981	Ben-Nun, Cohen	MBP-specific T cells are cloned. On adoptive syngeneic transfer, they produce EAE
1984	Mokhtarian, McFarlin	Chronic EAE after transfer of a single clone is accompanied by successive recruitment of T cells against new epitopes, also against new antigens and their epitopes, with new MHC restrictions
1984	Lassmann, Linington	Simultaneous transfer of MBP-specific T cells (clone) and of antibody to MOG in various ratios leads to full spectrum of inflammation and demyelination seen in MS lesions
1988	Lassman; Hickey	Perivascular macrophages ('microglia') act as primary site of antigen presentation in elicitation of EAE
1990	Pender; Lassmann; Mason	Apoptosis of specific T cells in CNS terminates acute attack of EAE: due to 'suppressor' cytokines? Steroids?
Early 1990s	Campagnoni; Fritz; Kuchroo	Expression of MBP, PLP, and other brain antigens in thymus
1997	Gery	Thymic expression of retinal IRBP correlated with level of tolerance/resistance to autoimmune disease (EAU)
1992	Selmaj, Brosnan	Recruitment of γ/δ T cells into EAE lesions is demonstrated
1992	Selmaj; Brosnan	Increased HSP60 expression in EAE lesions
1993	Piddlesden	Antibody-mediated demyelination parallels the complement-fixing capacity of the antibody
1994	Prabhu-Das, Kuchroo	Th1 and Th2 cell lines challenged with PLP peptides express distinct effector and regulatory functions
1995	Chen, Weiner	Use of transgenic mice expressing a unique TCR facilitates studies of oral tolerance
1995	Lassmann, Hickey, Dijkstra	Destruction of IL-69+ monocyte/macrophages in adoptive EAE host leaves ED2+ perivascular cells and resting microglia intact but eliminates activated infiltrating macrophages and microglia
1997	Zhang, Yamamura, Tabira	NK cells are downregulatory in EAE. Depletion of NKC leads to increased severity and duration of disease

Table 34.3 Experimental autoimmune encephalomyelitis (EAE)   *(continued)*

Date	Researchers	Discovery
1998	Targoni, Lehman	Endogenous thymic MBP inactivates high avidity T-cell repertoire, leaving low- and intermediate-avidity, potentially encephalitogenic T cells
2000	Klein, Kyewski	PLP expression in thymus is splice variant, which deletes only part of T-cell repertoire
2001	Huseby, Goverman	Epitopes carried into thymus by BM-derived APC can induce central tolerance for MBP
2004	Lassmann, Linington, Wekerle, Ransohoff	Clinical expression of EAE depends solely on degree of activation of T cells in target CNS

Diffusible mediators in EAE pathogenesis

Date	Researchers	Discovery
1983	Shin	Normal myelin induces complement activation and lysis (enhanced by specific antibody)
1984	Compston	Oligodendrocyte lysis by complement *in vivo*
1988	Hartung, Toyka	Free radicals (ROS and NO) from activated macrophages damage neural parenchyma
1988	Selmaj, Raine; Brosnan *et al.*	TNF damages tissue (oligodendrocytes) directly; IL-1, IL-2, and TNF damage vascular endothelium
1989, 1993	Scolding; Piddlesden	Role of complement in antibody-mediated oligodendrocyte damage and demyelination in MBP/MOG EAE
1990, 1996	Scolding; De Sousa	Perforin and Fas also involved in oligodendrocyte damage
1990s	Several laboratories	Up-regulatory and down-regulatory CK play a major role in both induction and elicitation of EAE lesions
1993, 1995	Kuchroo; Ruddle	Capacity to produce adhesion molecules and CK (LT and/or TNF) is essential for encephalitogenicity of T cells
1994	Berman, Ransohoff	Chemokines play an essential role in lesion pathogenesis, promoting endothelial activation adhesion molecule expression, and macrophage diapedesis
1996	Olsson	Sequential CK expression in CNS during evolution of EAE: early IL-12, IFN-γ; then LT, IL-1β, TNF; finally IL10, TGF-β; IL-4 throughout
1996	Brocke, Steinman	EAE lesions induced with MBP peptide disappear when animal is given altered peptide ligands; effect is mediated by IL-4
1999	Brosnan	CK, CCK, and CCK receptor profiles in commonly used strains of mice parallel their tendency to give Th1 or Th2 responses
1999	Kuchroo, Weiner	Susceptibility of different mouse strains parallels their production of IFNγ versus IL-4/IL-10 and TGF-β
2000	Cuff, Berman, Brosnan	Retinal model: CK action precedes up-regulation of CCK in glial cells
2003	Glabinski, Bielecki, Ransohoff	In EAE attack, production of CK (LTβ, TNF-α and -β, IFN-γ) precedes up-regulation of CCK (CCL1–5, CXCL2–3); TGF-β1 follows
2000	Khoury	Mice with Bcl-X$_L$ in T cells show decreased T-cell apoptosis and exaggerated EAE
2001	Chitnis, Khoury	Stat 4 deficient mice show decreased EAE. Stat 6 deficient (Th2-deficient) mice show loss of regulation and increased EAE
2002	Becher	IL-23 (p19 + p40) is the critical molecule, rather than IL-12 (p35 + p40), underlying EAE

Immune regulation in acute and chronic EAE

Date	Researchers	Discovery
1949	Cazzullo	Myelin in incomplete Freund's adjuvant intraperitoneally prevents EAE
1970	Ellison	Injection of MBP into the thymus (rats) prevents EAE
1976	Swierkoz, Swanborg	MBP in iFA induces suppressor T cells and resistance to EAE
1981	Ben Nun, Wekerle, Cohen	Vaccination with inactivated MBP-specific T-cell clones makes mice resistant to EAE
1985	Lyman, Brosnan	MBP-specific 'suppressor' cells are present in spleen during remission phase of relapsing EAE
1988	Sun, Wekerle	CD8+ idiotype-specific 'suppressor' cells in animals vaccinated with CD4+ MBP clone are CTLs
1988	Whitacre	Oral tolerance to MBP is demonstrated
1989	Karpus, Swanborg	CD4+ 'suppressor' cells in recovery phase of EAE are idiotype specific, produce IL-4 and TGF-β, and suppress CK production by effector T cells
1989	S. D. Miller	Tolerization with MBP or PLP–membrane conjugates is associated with clonal anergy of effector T cells
1990	Pender	Low-dose ciclosporin in MBP-immunized rats results in chronic EAE; may act by eliminating a 'suppressor' cell population
1991	Harling-Berg, Knopf	Injection of MBP into CSF (containing TGF-β) leads to immune deviation and Th2 response in cervical lymph nodes, comparable to ACAID and Th2 in spleen
1992	Mak; Jiang, Pernis	CD8 knockout mice (transgenic; use of Mab) show marked increase in EAE relapses and decrease of severity

Table 34.3 Experimental autoimmune encephalomyelitis (EAE)   *(continued)*

Date	Researchers	Discovery
1992	Lider, Miller, Weiner	Oral tolerance of MBP in rats is mediated by CD8+ epitope-specific 'suppressor' cells producing TGF-β
1993, 1996	Khoury	Injection of MBP peptide into rat thymus induces peptide-specific resistance to EAE; can mimic this process by injecting DC treated with peptide + CTLA-4
1995	Prabhu-Das, Kuchroo	CD4+ Th2-cell clones versus PLP peptides make IL-4 and IL-10 and suppress EAE on transfer
1995	Chen, Weiner	Oral tolerance to MBP peptides in mice is mediated by CD4+ epitope-specific 'Th3' cells producing high levels of TGF-β
1995	Ware, Pernis	CD8+ T cells (resistance to relapse) kill CD4+ epitope-specific T cells and are restricted by Qa-1
1996 onwards	Kuchroo, Sharpe, others	Systematic studies of positive and negative co-stimulation systems in EAE, using blockade with monoclonal antibodies or fusion proteins, later knockout animals, etc.
1997	Kuchroo, Nicholson	CK released by APL-stimulated T cells produce bystander suppression
2001	Miyamoto, Yamamura	Oral α-galactosylceramide analog (with shortened sphingosine chain) stimulates Th2 bias in NKT cells (with preferential production of IL-4) and prevents EAE
2003	Khoury, Sayegh	Transferred CD8+28– T cells can suppress EAE. In culture, these cells suppress IFN-γ production by effector cells stimulated with antigen

ADEM, acute disseminated encephalomyelitis; APL, altered peptide ligands; CNS, central nervous system; CMI, cell-mediated immunity; CTL, cytotoxic T lymphocyte; DTH, delayed-type hypersensitivity; EAE, experimental autoimmune encephalomyelitis; EAU, experimental autoimmune uveitis; GFAP, glial fibrillary acidic protein; IL, interleukin; IRBP, interphotoreceptor retinol-binding protein; MAG, myelin-associated glycoprotein; MBP, myelin basic protein; MOG, myelin-oligodendrocyte glycoprotein; MS, multiple sclerosis; NK, natural killer (cell); NKT, natural killer T (cell); NO, nitric oxide; PLP, proteolipid protein; PVE, post-vaccinal encephalomyelitis; PIE, post-infectious encephalomyelitis; ROS, reactive oxygen species; TCR, T-cell receptor; TGF, transforming growth factor; TNF, tumor necrosis factor.

MBP or PLP peptides was shown, not surprisingly, to be MHC-restricted. Later, the genes encoding TCR peptide polymorphisms were also incriminated, as were genes governing the level of expression of MHC, the preferential production of particular CKs and the Th1/Th2 balance, as well as various aspects of inflammation (e.g. the sensitivity of vascular endothelium to vasoamines). As yet, the genetic determinants of immune regulation remain largely unknown. As fallout from the Human Genome Project, the occurrence and regulation of complex-trait autoimmune diseases like EAE has been estimated to involve as many as 20 separate genetic loci. Several of these (four to eight) are now known and, with the application of SNP markers and newer genetic tools, their firm identification in the near future is assured.

The 1980s saw a wide diversification of studies on the cells and soluble factors contributing to EAE pathogenesis: antibody, complement components (C), CKs and, more recently, CCKs. The chronic phase of EAE was recognized as presenting different problems from those associated with initiation of the disease process, among them so-called 'epitope spreading', the recruitment of TCR γ/δ T cells, and the induction of regulatory responses associated with remission and relapse. The informal blackout on studies of 'suppressor' mechanisms throughout the 1980s and early 1990s hampered research on immune regulation in EAE. However, discovery of the regulatory capacities of IL-12 (up) and of IL-4, IL-10, and TGF-β (down) and ligands such as CTLA-4 (down), also interest in responses to idiotypes (of effector cells) have led to new initiatives in this area. Currently the respective roles of CD4+25+ and CD8+28–FcR+ regulatory T cells, of down-regulatory dendritic cells (DC), as well as of NK and NKT cells are the focus of ongoing intensive research.

The process of discovery has been accelerated by innovative technology. The use of transgenic mice bearing unique T- or B-cell receptors has uncovered unique phenotypes of EAE resembling well-recognized clinical variants of MS. Non-classical MHC such as CD1d, identified in studies of innate immunity, are now found to play a major role in immune regulation. Finally events in the thymus provide a fruitful area of new discovery shifting from levels of intrathymic expression of myelin and astrocyte auto-antigens, and related quantitative aspects of anergy/deletion (of potentially autoaggressive T-cell clones), to regulation by thymic DC and unique regulatory T-cell subsets.

Other autoimmune diseases dependent primarily on T-cell-mediated immunity

In post-vaccinal encephalomyelitis (PVE) that develops after rabies vaccination and the post-infectious encephalomyelitis (PIE) that follows infection with viruses of the myxovirus, morbilli, pox, and herpesvirus groups (and also chlamydia), the presence of antibodies against myelin was an early finding (Hurst, 1932). Skin tests with MBP (Behan, 1968) and *in vitro* lymphocytic studies with MBP (Lisak, Zweiman, 1977; Johnson and colleagues, 1984) established the presence of CMI. Griffin and Hemachudha, in subsequent studies, showed both strong T-cell reactivity and high-titer antibody against MBP (1987). The findings are similar in ADEM not preceded by a recognizable viral infection. Pohl-Koppe and Hafler in 1998 reported findng MBP-specific Th2 cells in two such cases. The incidence of new ADEM cases diminished sharply after the introduction of measles vaccination (cited from Arnason). It seems clear that these diseases involve molecular mimicry between viral agents and neural antigens.

GBS, also called acute inflammatory demyelinating polyneuropathy (AIDP), like ADEM, may occur after virus infection or injection of a viral vaccine or in the absence of a clear-cut immunizing event. Early observations on GBS suggesting a role for antibody (Hirano and colleagues, 1971) were followed by evidence for the presence of CMI to peripheral nervous system antigens (Abramsky and colleagues, 1975). The disease resembles the animal model, experimental autoimmune neuritis (EAN) (Hartung, 1990), which is mediated mainly by CMI. Several investigators have, in fact, demonstrated lymphocytic reactivity against P2, P$_0$, and their peptides and, in some patients, to MBP (Geczy, 1985; Burns, 1986; Hemachudha and Griffin, 1987). However, others have found antibodies to various myelin glycolipids and gangliosides (Quarles; Sanders, Koski 1986). In some patients, the disease appeared to be induced by antecedent gastrointestinal infection with *Campylobacter jejuni* strains (Kaldor, Speedo, 1984). The acute motor axonal neuropathy (AMAN) occurring in rural children, in China and Mexico in particular; was also related to infection with specific strains of *C. jejuni* and found to be mediated largely by antibody against GM1 ganglioside (Yuki, 1990; Asbury, Griffin, McKhann, and colleagues 1992). There is also an acute sensorimotor variant (ASMAN) (Feasby,

1986). In the Fisher syndrome, antibody is directed at GQ1b (Chiba, 1993; Willison ,1993).

Chronic inflammatory demyelinating polyneuropathy (CIDP), which is frequently thought of as a peripheral MS equivalent, was investigated somewhat later than AIDP. Lymphocytic reactions against P2, Po, and their peptides were demonstrated here too (Gregson, Hughes, 1988), as were antibodies (Koski, Shin, 1985). The 1990s saw increasing interest in the role of γ/δ T cells in inflammatory lesions like those of GBS (Borsellino, Brosnan, and other younger colleagues, 2000). Some subsets of γ/δ cells in the lesions are activated by non-protein antigens in an MHC-unrestricted manner, produce a great deal of IL-4, and contribute to the antibody response against glycolipids.

Acute EAN, which appears to be a good model for AIDP (Waksman, Adams, 1955), has been through the full gamut of studies described for EAE, mostly in the 1970s and 1980s. Several investigators implicated P2 and P_0 as antigens (Uyemura, Nagai, and Ikuta; Brostoff, 1977; Hughes and colleagues, 1979, 1987). Chronic variants of EAN (models for CIDP) were produced in juvenile animals by repeated immunization or by giving low doses of ciclosporin or cyclophosphamide during immunization (McCombe, Pender, 1992). A milder CIDP was produced by immunizing rabbits or rats with galactocerebroside (Saida, Saida, 1979) or with sulfated glucuronyl paragloboside (SGPG) (Yu and colleagues, 1988, 1991). These model diseases were clearly mediated by antibody rather than CMI. More recent studies have addressed the genetic basis of EAN susceptibility; as in

Table 34.4 Myasthenia gravis (MG) and experimental autoimmune myasthenia gravis (EAMG)

Date	Researchers	Discovery
1949,	Castleman, Norris	Lymphoid follicles in the thymus of some cases of MG.
1950–1970	Strauss, Nastuk, Ossermans, Engel and others	Light and electron microscopic studies of changes at neuromuscular junction; immunofluorescence studies of antibodies to muscle; myoid cells in the thymus; unsuccessful attempts to produce a myasthenia model with whole muscle as antigen
1968	Goldstein	Autoimmune thymitis (guinea pig): release of peptide Tpo → binding to AChR and MG manifestations
1973	Patrick, Lindström	Production of EAMG in rabbits by immunization with *Torpedo* AChR (purified with alpha-bungarotoxin from the banded krait)
1973	Fambrough, Drachman	AChR found to be molecular target of MG pathogenesis
1975	Lennon, Lindström	Importance of CMI followed by antibody in EAMG pathogenesis (in rats)
1976	Lindström, Lennon	Circulating antibody to AChR found in 80–90% of MG patients
1976	Toyka; Lindström	Antibody and cell transfer: animal to animal, human to animal
1976	Fuchs	Genetic basis of EAMG susceptibility
1976, 1978	Engel; Lennon	Mechanisms of receptor loss, contribution of complement to damage of neuromuscular junction
1977	Kao, Drachman	Myoid cells in thymus shown to carry AChR
1978	Lindström	Use of AChR subunit peptides to induce EAMG
1979	David	Role of MHC in EAMG susceptibility
1980	Nakao	Additional susceptibility genes in IgH
1981	Lefvert	Idiotype networks in MG patients
1981, 1983	Ohta, Lefvert	Transient neonatal MG, due to placental transfer of maternal antibody
1982	Thomas, Newsom-Davis	Immunohistochemical and tissue culture studies of thymus changes in MG: CD4+ T cells, B cells/plasma cells, antibody, immune complexes
1984	Hohlfeld	Cloning of AChR-specific T cells from MG patients' thymus
1984, 1985	Pachner, Kantor	EAMG in mice: effector T-cell lines and clones, adoptive transfer of disease; suppressor lines
1985	Lennon	Multiple epitopes in AChR: immunodominant epitopes in α subunit of AChR: 125–147
1985	Stefansson	Antibodies in MG sera react with gastrointestinal flora: *Escherichia coli*, *Proteus vulgaris*, *Klebsiella pneumoniae*
1987	Hohlfeld, Toyka	Cloning of AChR-specific T cells from blood and lymph nodes of MG patients
1988	Berrih-Aknin	T-cell epitopes in α subunit of AChR: 125–143, 257–271, 351–368
1992	McIntosh, Drachman	Tolerance in EAMG by injection of AChR coupled to syngeneic cells
1993	Schönbeck *et al.*	Heterotopic transplantation of MG thymus in SCID mice → functioning human thymus tissue and lasting production of antibody to AChR
1994	Okumura, Drachman	Oral tolerance in EAMG by feeding AChR
1994	Hohlfeld, Wekerle	Fundamental difference between MG (evidence that disease starts in thymus) and EAMG (immune response is entirely peripheral)
1995	Shenoy	Use of TCR V_β knockout mice to determine TCR usage in genesis of EAMG
1999	Engel	Post-synaptic congenital disorders of AChR subunit gene mutants
2001	Vincent group	Antibody to muscle-specific receptor tyrosine kinase (MuSK), mainly IgG4, defines 'seronegative' MG subgroup with increased bulbar manifestations
2001	Vincent	Thymic myoid cells with dual functions: as targets for cytoxic Tc1 cells and helpers for Th2 supporting antibody formation to AChR
2004	Huang, Link, Lefvert	MG patients show no decrease in CD4+CD25^{high} regulatory T cells

AChR, acetylcholine receptor; CMI, cell-mediated immunity; TCR, T-cell receptor; MHC, major histocompatibility complex; IgH, immunoglobulin heavy chain; SCID, subacute combined immune deficiency.

EAE and MS, multiple loci are involved (Olsson, 2001). In one mouse strain (C57Bl/6), a decreased transcription level of P0 and therefore of negative selective in the thymus is associated with defective tolerance for this antigen and increased susceptibility to EAN (Yamamura, Miyamoto, 2003).

Viral models of PIE and GBS are discussed in the section on Neuroimmunologic diseases associated with infection.

Myasthenia gravis and experimental autoimmune myasthenia gravis

Research on myasthenia gravis (MG), the leading example of an autoimmune disease mediated primarily by antibodies, involved mostly morphologic and immunofluorescence techniques before the discovery of the experimental autoimmune myasthenia gravis (EAMG) model by Patrick and Lindström in 1973. This model was investigated intensively over the ensuing two decades and the same techniques and concepts applied to an almost simultaneous analysis of lesion pathogenesis in the human disease (Table 34.4). EAMG was accepted early as a valid model and antibody was accepted as the principal mediator of disease.

The introduction of T-cell cloning in 1980 led to recognition of the importance of T cells in fueling the anti-acetylcholine receptor (AChR) antibody response. Involvement of T cells in a cell-mediated component to lesion pathogenesis is likely in certain forms of the animal model, as suggested by Lennon in her earliest EAMG studies, but is not thought to be important in the human disease. Immunodominant epitopes, for both T and B cells, were found to be in the alpha subunit of the AChR. Stefansson has suggested that molecular mimicry, involving micro-organisms of the gastrointestinal tract, might be responsible for the pathogenic autoimmune response. On the other hand, Hohlfeld was successful in cloning AChR-specific T cells from the MG thymus, and Hohlfeld and Wekerle and others have emphasized the importance of thymic myoid cells bearing AChR as possible initiators of autoimmunization. The MG thymus frequently shows morphological and functional evidence of 'peripheral' immunological activity (Berrih-Aknin, Bach, 1987). EAMG, in contrast, which is an entirely peripheral process, shows no thymus involvement and thus, in the current view, does not provide a full or correct model for MG pathogenesis.

Cultured muscle cell lines and primary myoblasts, treated with cytokines to upregulate MHC class II, have been shown by Vincent to function as APC, presenting AChR epitopes to specific T helper cells, but whether thymic myoid cells can act similarly is not clear. Nevertheless, plasma cells in the hyperplastic thymus produce AChR antibodies. Should such a response be regarded as an extreme example of immune deviation? We know little, as yet, in human subjects with MG, about the cellular elements, identified in the ACAID (anterior chamber-associated immune deviation) model, that create the necessary microenvironment for such deviation: regulatory dendritic cells, NK and NKT cells, γ/δ T cells. In patients with thymoma, the tumor itself does not produce the AChR autoantibodies (Vincent, Willcox, 2003). The hyperplastic thymus contains large numbers of Vα24+ NKT cells penetrating from the connective tissue into the parenchyma and expressing CD44 (Nagane and colleagues, 2001). Other reports stress a general increase in Vα24+ NKT cells, in contrast to the depressed level of NKT cells reported in autoimmune diseases affecting the CNS, skin, bowel, and joints and the normal levels in thyroiditis and celiac disease (Reinhard, Melm, 1999; van der Vliet and colleagues, 2001). These cells produce high levels of both IFN-γ and IL-4. CD4+CD25^{high} regulatory cells, also acting in the thymus, are present in normal numbers in patients with MG.

In the animal model EAMG, 'classical' immune regulation was first studied by Pachner and Kantor, who were able to obtain lines of AChR-specific suppressor T cells. Later, Drachman and colleagues adapted newer techniques for inducing tolerance, such as administration of tolerogenic conjugates of AChR with syngeneic cell membranes or oral administration of antigen, to the EAMG model in the hope of finding new, specific approaches to therapy of the human disease. Recently, a group at the Karolinska Institute in Stockholm, working mainly with knockout mice, have found that NK cells, but not NKT cells, play an essential role in initiation of EAMG (Lünggren, Link, Taniguchi, and others 2000, 2002). The findings are similar with knockouts of Tnfrsf1a (previously known as Tnfr1 or Cd120a) or Il18 (see also Fuchs, 2001). These knockout animals have in common the loss of Th1 functions (IL-12, IFN-γ, IL-2) and enhancement of Th2 (IL-4, IL-10), accompanied by loss of the capacity to form Th1-dependent IgG2 antibody and diminution of IgG1.

Genetic studies in MG have been important in defining different groups of MG (Compston 1980). More recent reports indicated a relationship of susceptibility to three genetic loci: DR3, DQA1*0101, and the AChR alpha subunit (CHRNA) (Bach, Garchon, 1997). Two loci are incriminated currently: CHRNA1 and a non-Class II HLA-linked locus MYAS1 (Garchon, 2003).

While the regulation battle continues, the interest of investigators in this field has moved on to variant forms of MG, e.g. neonatal MG (Bach, 1988, 1991), other antibody-mediated post-synaptic disease, such as that involving antibody against muscle-specific receptor tyrosine kinase (MuSK), and genetic abnormalities that mimic one or another form of MG. Antibody-mediated diseases affecting neural and neuromuscular transmission but assuming new and unique clinical forms are discussed in the next section.

Other autoimmune diseases mediated primarily by antibody

Investigation of the approximately 20 paraneoplastic syndromes (PNS) revived with the systematic studies of the Lambert–Eaton myasthenic syndrome (LEMS) by Newsom-Davis and colleagues starting in 1981, followed by Kornguth's description (in both human subjects and an animal model) of blindness associated with a loss of the large ganglion cells of the retina (1982), and Greenlee and Brashear's first report on progressive cerebellar degeneration (1983). Subsequent studies by Posner and colleagues among others, have emphasized humoral antibody as the principal mediator of disease, the identification of target antigens in the nervous system (and corresponding tumor antigens), and the neural function(s) affected by the action of antibody. In LEMS, for example, voltage-gated calcium channels in presynaptic motor nerve terminals were found to serve as the neural target and apparently identical channel proteins in the tumor as the immunizing agent (Lang, Newsom-Davis, 1985, 1987). By contrast, in some clinical syndromes antibodies are excellent markers for a paraneoplastic syndrome but are not the principal mediators of disease (see Chapter 25).

Chronic cerebellar degeneration, with gradual destruction of Purkinje cells, has been one of the best studied paraneoplastic syndromes. In patients with antibody to the Purkinje cell antigen 'Yo', the target cells are lost (evident at postmortem) but there is no evidence that the antibodies are pathogenic. Darnell was able to demonstrate an expanded population of CD8+ CTL specific for CDR2c in the CSF of such patients and show that these cells effectively suppressed the tumor and were, rather than antibody, also responsible for direct killing of Purkinje cells (1998, 2000). Preliminary studies with the HU antibodies, associated with small cell lung cancer, suggesting a similar scenario. Other paraneoplastic syndromes that may depend on CMI rather than antibody would include isolated angiitis, an inflammatory, largely monocytic disease (Lisak, 1988) and giant cell arteritis involving CD4+ T cells, macrophages, and multinucleate giant cells (Wyand, 1994, 2000; Martins, Taboada, 1996).

As a sequel to studies in MG and LEMS, Newsom-Davis, Vincent, and their students, following an earlier suggestion of Drachman's, have used a set of 'Koch's postulates' to establish mechanism in suspected autoantibody-mediated neurologic disorders: (1) show that antibody of the required specificity is present in patients but not in healthy controls; (2) show that the patient's condition is improved by steroids, plasma exchange, IV Ig, or immunosuppressive chemotherapy; (3) show that plasma containing the specific antibody produces a similar disorder in mice or rats; and (4) show that animals immunized with the suspected target develop the same type of disease. This approach has been singularly effective, over the last 5–10 years, in identifying new neuroimmunologic conditions. The need to identify and measure often subtle behavioral changes in a murine host that correspond to those in a human subject is a crucial feature of this area of discovery.

Conditions affecting voltage-gated calcium or potassium channels (VGCC or VGKC) are frequently paraneoplastic. However, there is a new subset of similar diseases mediated by antibody to neuronal components cross-reactive with streptococcal components, the so-called PANDAS (discussed in the section on Neuroimmunological diseases associated with infection, and in Chapter 33). Many of the diseases in this group have familial (*i.e.* genetically based, non-immunologic) forms. Some of the newest discoveries involve changes in the fetal nervous system in pregnant mothers who generate the pathogenic antibody as an immune response to antigens of the fetus itself. These may resemble closely the effects in the fetus of maternal viral infection and CKs generated as a consequence of her immune response to the virus (discussed in the section on Neurologic diseases implicating cytokines).

This new group of probable immune-mediated diseases now includes:

- Arthrogryphosis multiplex congenita. In a few cases, maternal antibody against the fetal form of AChR, often made in the maternal thymus, perhaps as a direct response to AChR on thymic myoid cells, causes early weakness in the fetal musculature and striking deformities at birth (Vincent, 2000). This disease must be distinguished from neonatal MG and neonatal LEMS, caused by transplacental passage of antibody against adult-type AChR or VGCC (Vincent, 1998).

- Limbic encephalitis, mediated by antibody against VGKC, is frequently non-paraneoplastic (Vincent 2004), and the patients often improve substantially when treated with immunosuppression. This group also includes acquired neuromyotonia, often paraneoplastic; other acquired peripheral nerve hyperexcitability (APNH) syndromes, including cramp-fasciculation syndrome, Isaac's syndrome; also certain forms of epilepsy and Morvan's fibrillary chorea, affecting the CNS. All these involve VGKC (Lang, Vincent 2003).

- Stiff man syndrome, involving antibodies against glutamic acid decarboxylase (GAD), responsible for production of the inhibitory neurotransmitter, gamma-aminobutyric acid (GABA). This disorder is frequently associated with epilepsy and/or diabetes (Solimena, 1988; McEvoy, 1991). In a paraneoplastic variant form, the antigen is amphiphysin (de Camilli, 1993). A form of cerebellar ataxia is seen in a largely female subset of subjects making what appears to be the same anti-GAD antibody, with, however, intrathecal antibody synthesis (Honorat and colleagues). In both conditions there may be some intrathecal antibody production.

- Neurodevelopmental disorders, involving antibody formed by mothers who have had two or more dyslexic children (and/or stillbirths). Pregnant mice injected with their serum bear offspring with motor abnormalities associated with abnormal levels of choline and creatine. Subtly different findings were noticed when pregnant mice were injected with serum from a mother with an autistic child and one with a language abnormality (Dalton, Vincent 2003). Moreover this mother had antibodies that bind to mouse Purkinje cells *in vitro*.

Investigation of the neuropathic syndromes associated with monoclonal gammopathies began in the early 1980s. In the best studies of these syndromes, the elevated IgM proved to be a specific antibody binding to carbohydrate epitopes shared by myelin-associated glycoprotein (MAG), several glycoproteins, and two glycolipids known as SGPG and SGLPG (Nobile-Orazio, Latov; Quarles; Ilyas; Shy, and others). Yu and colleagues, in the later 1980s, developed rabbit and rat models involving antibody against SGPG-like epitopes expressed in axolemma and nerve terminals and in vascular endothelium. Research on monoclonal gammopathies with multiple myeloma (especially osteosclerotic myeloma) demonstrated formation of IgG or IgA with delta as the principal light chain, reactive with endoneurial constituents such as chondroitin sulfate. Patients were commonly found to exhibit the POEMS syndrome (Polyneuropathy, Organomegaly, Endocrinopathy, Myeloma, and Skin changes) (Bardwick and colleagues, 1980) or Crow–Fukase syndrome (Nakanishi and colleagues, 1984). Whereas the neuropathologic changes have been thought to be mediated by antibody,

the other abnormalities have been tentatively ascribed to neuropeptides/cytokines (e.g. TNF) released from the malignant lymphoid cells (Gherardi and colleagues, 1994).

Certain patients with primary motor neuron disease (MND) or amyotrophic lateral sclerosis (ALS) were shown in 1986 to express high titers of IgM associated with plasma cell dyscrasia (Shy, Rowland and colleagues, 1986). The principal reactivity of the IgM antibody was found to be directed at unique epitopes, Gal(beta 1–3)GalNAc and Gal(beta 1–3)GlcNAc, of gangliosides GM_1 and GD_{1b}. Other patients were reported (Appel, 1992) to have antibody against a calcium channel protein in the motor nerve terminal, apparently acting on a different epitope than that affected in LEMS. Engelhardt, working with Appel (1986, 1990), described guinea pig models that he named experimental autoimmune motor neuron disease, with degeneration of spinal anterior horn cells and muscle atrophy without inflammation, and experimental autoimmune gray matter disease, affecting both upper and lower motor neurons, but with significant accompanying inflammation.

Recent research has tended to emphasize non-immunologic aspects of MND, and it is now frequently classed with the aggregate disorders. Genetic findings suggest that a high proportion of spinal muscular atrophy cases, but a low proportion of ALS cases are genetically determined; they express autosomal dominant mutations or autosomal recessive mutations in X-linked kindreds. Among familial ALS cases, 5–10% show mutations of superoxide dismutase (SOD) (Wong, 98). A hereditary canine spinal muscular atrophy was described in 1993 and was followed 2 years later by several well-described mouse mutants affecting SOD. Some of these show neurotoxic aggregates in neurons. A distinct form of ALS, formerly common among people of the Pacific island of Guam, is caused by a toxic factor in cycad flour, which used to be widely consumed. Mice fed cycad flour show early glutamate-mediated excitotoxicity resembling Guamanian ALS.

The neurologic complications of systemic lupus erythematosus (SLE) have been shown for the most part to be antibody-mediated. Development of standardized batteries of tests for cognitive dysfunction in the late 1970s made it possible to distinguish several strikingly different mechanisms. First is deposition of immune complexes of antibody with, for example, DNA in the choroid plexus, leading to membranous or vascular choroidopathy (Kofe and colleagues, 1974; Schwarz, Roberts, 1984). (In a subset of cases, antibody against DNA cross-reacts with a subunit of NMDA glutamate receptor and leads to apoptosis of neurons (Hardin, Volpe, Diamond, 2001).) Antibody against phospholipids with anticoagulant activity leads to intravascular clotting followed by microinfarction and dementia, the 'antiphospholipid syndrome' (Mueh, 1980; Hirohata, Miyamoto, 1990). Antibody against neuronal constituents produces cognitive dysfunction up to the level of psychosis (Bluestein, 1981; Bluestein, Zaifler, 1983; Denburg, 1985); in this case, some or all of the antibodies are antiribosomal (Bonfa, 1987; Schneebaum, 1991). CNS lesions can be studied in lupus-prone strains of mice such as MRL or NZB × NZW hybrid mice, or Mozes' anti-DNA idiotype-specific antibody/CMI-mediated model (1983).

Among patients with primary Sjögren's disease, a systemic autoimmune process like SLE, 40% produce IgG antibodies against neural antigens associated with abnormalities of frontal cortical function and a short-term memory defect (Borda, 1999; Reina, 2004). Some 15% also show sympathetic nervous system dysfunction (and cardiovascular manifestations). A number of laboratories have identified IgG autoantibodies against neonatal heart muscarinic M1 cholinoceptor, also IgG and IgA antibodies against M1 and M3 cholinoceptors well correlated with the disease activity.

2. Neuroimmunologic diseases associated with infection

The modern era in investigation of infectious diseases began with the description of MHC restriction (Zinkernagel and Doherty, 1974), which permitted analysis of the respective roles of CD4- and CD8-bearing T cells in immunopathologic reactions of the nervous system, as well as a molecular definition of selective events in the thymus.

Viral diseases

Viral infections of the nervous system, in humans and animals, can lead to any of several distinct immunologic outcomes (Table 34.5). Conditions in which a virus in the nervous system elicits an immunologically mediated inflammatory reaction directed to viral antigens differ sharply from conditions in which viral infection results in autoimmunization, with inflammation and destruction of white matter, and from conditions in which there is a depressed, deviated, or absent response.

Acute viral encephalitides fall outside the scope of the present chapter. Studies in animal models have, however, been instructive. An acute encephalomyelitis, produced by Sindbis virus in mice, has been studied intensively by Griffin and her colleagues (1972, 1977, 1984, 1996). The disease itself has the hallmarks of a CMI response to virus; viral clearance, however, results from the arrest of viral synthesis in infected cells following signals from viral antigen–antibody complexes at the cell surface. Two other acute viral encephalomyelitis models have been thoroughly studied by Doherty (2001, 2004). To paraphrase a comment in his most recent paper: 'The techno-

Table 34.5 Neuroimmunologic diseases associated with viral infection[a]

Human disorders		Animal models	
Date	**Discovery**	**Date**	**Discovery**
Acute viral encephalomyelitis			
Several viruses		1955/1972/1972, 1983 to present	Sindbis virus (mice)
		1995 to present	Gamma HV-68 (mice). Human influenza A (mice)
Chronic viral encephalomyelitis			
1956/1979	HAM/TSP	1940/1958/1977	Visna-maedi (sheep)
		1934/1975/1976	Theiler's murine encephalitis virus
1995/1998	HHV6		
Acute and subacute autoimmune encephalomyelitis			
1938	ADEM (PIE)	1941/1943/1976	Canine distemper
		1949/1978/1983	JHM (coronavirus) (rats)
		1962/1987/1988	Measles virus (rats, mice)
		1971/1978/1983	Semliki Forest virus (mice)
Acute, subacute, and chronic autoimmune neuritis			
1918	AIDP, CIDP	1907/1972/1975	Marek's disease (chickens)
1992	AMAN, ASMAN		
Chronic viral encephalomyelitis, with failure of specific cell-mediated responses			
1933/1969	SSPE (measles)	1936/1958/1976	LCMV encephalitis (mice)
	Hypopituitarism	1985	LCMV growth failure (mice)
1950	PML (JC virus)	1949/1972/–	JHM (coronavirus) (mice)
1975	PRP (rubella)		
Before 1970	Veterinary problems (BDV)	1979/1981	BDV (rabbits, monkeys)
1985	Psychiatric disorders	1983 to present	(rats)
1985	AIDS dementia	1985, 2003	Simian, feline immunodeficiency virus. Mouse AIDS
Chronic 'prion' encephalomyelitis, with failure of all immune responses			
1920	Scrapie (sheep)	1936/1969	Scrapie (sheep) (primates, mice)
1971/1973	Kuru	1971/1973	(chimpanzees, mice; later guinea pigs, hamsters)
–	CJD	1986	Mad cow disease (BSE)
1996	Variant CJD		
Maternal virus infection with abnormal fetal CNS development			
–	Autism, schizophrenia	2002/2003	Human influenza in pregnant mice: offspring show abnormal brain development and 'autistic' and/or schizoid behavior
Developmental problems after viral vaccines			
–	Autism	2004	Mercury (thimerosal) in early post-natal life (autoimmunity-prone mice)

[a]Dates are approximate and refer to: description of disease, identification of virus, and demonstration of major immunologic elements in disease process.

ADEM, acute disseminated encephalomyelitis; AIDP, acute inflammatory demyelinating polyneuropathy; BSE, bovine spongiform encephalomyelitis; BDV, Borna disease virus; CIDP, chronic inflammatory demyelinating polyneuropathy; CJD, Creutzfeldt–Jakob disease; Gamma HV-68, murine gamma herpesvirus; HAM/TSP, human T-cell lymphotropic virus type I-associated myelopathy/tropical spastic paraparesis; LCMV, lymphocytic choriomeningitis virus; PIE, post-infectious encephalomyelitis; PML, progressive multifocal leukoencephalopathy; PRP, progressive rubella panencephalitis; SSPE, subacute sclerosing panencephalitis.

logical battery available for study of transient local infections (e.g. human influenza in the C57Bl/6 mouse) includes: tetramer reagents, intracytoplasmic staining for CKs, coupled with RT-PCR and influenza reverse genetics, permitting detailed molecular dissection of different epitope-specific primary, memory, and secondary immune CD8+ T cell responses!' Other recent work addresses the role of chemokines (Ransohoff, Tani, 1989) and various adhesion molecules and their ligands (Springer, 1990; Baggiolini, 1994) in the inflammatory response to the virus and of regulatory events within the lesion (Willbanks, Streilein, 1992; Hikawa, 1996).

In the best studied chronic viral infection of the CNS, human T-cell lymphotropic virus type I-associated myelopathy/tropical spastic paraparesis (HAM/TSP), the CD4+ T lymphocyte is the principal site of infection. The virus (HTLV-1) persists in mutated form in blood and CSF CD4+ T cells. Serologic studies began in the late 1970s in Japan, the Caribbean, Africa, and the Seychelles, and were followed by cellular investigations, first by Jacobson, McFarlin and colleagues and by Usuku and Osame and colleagues, and later by Hafler and his colleagues. Infected T cells proliferate without IL-2 and can stimulate other T cells by cognate interactions via CD2 and lymphocyte function-associated antigen (LFA)-3 (Bourcier, Hafler, 1992, 2000). Clonally expanded CD8+ T cells specific for a single HTLV-1 peptide (Tax 11–19) may approach 10% of the circulating CD8s (Hafler, 1999), although the TCR α and β chains used for this recognition are heterogeneous (Bourcier, Lim, Wucherpfennig, 2001). Lesions appear to be produced by CD8+ T cells reactive against viral antigens associated with MHC Class I on the CD4+ cells. There is no sign of autoimmunization against myelin antigens and no explanation for the CNS localization.

Human herpesvirus-6 (HHV-6), another virus infecting T cells, is implicated in a variety of neurologic diseases (e.g. Wiley, 1995). It is frequently transmitted by transfusion of blood or stem cell preparations. Its presence in the immediate vicinity of active MS lesions has been noted (Knox, 1996; Osame, 1997) and viral DNA and IgM antibody against an early viral antigen appear together in the serum (Jacobson, McFarland, 1997). The virus proliferates readily in dividing oligodendrocytes and must do so in the areas where it has been identified, but evidence that it has any pathogenetic role, for example in extending or changing the character of the MS lesion, is still wanting. In a small percentage of children with CNS manifestations of viral disease, HHV-7 DNA is found in the CSF (Pohl-Koppe, 2001).

Visna-maedi in sheep is often regarded as a model for HAM/TSP. Its pathogenesis was well worked out by the mid-1970s by Sigurdsson and colleagues in Iceland and later by workers in the United States (Nathanson, Panitch, Haase, Brahic). Narayan and colleagues, in the late 1970s and 1980s, established that virus enters the CNS within monocytes as a so-called Trojan horse, and that the immune response to persistent virus is responsible for the characteristic inflammatory demyelinative lesions and is inhibited by immunosuppressive therapy. Antigenic variation contributes significantly to viral persistence and the occurrence of relapses.

In a second model, Theiler's murine encephalitis virus (TMEV), the chronic demyelinative phase of infection is eliminated by immunosuppressive therapy, and therefore the disease must be immunologic (Lipton, Dal Canto, 1975). Nevertheless, virus persists in CNS glial elements throughout the chronic phase (Brahic and colleagues, 1981); the location of this persistent virus is determined by innate immune system determinants rather than those of the adaptive immune system (Ransohoff, Rodriguez, 2002). However, the inflammatory disease process is related to DTH against virus and is MHC Class I-restricted (Lipton and colleagues; Rodriguez, 1985). CD8+ T cells make up the principal reacting population, as with visna and HAM/TSP. The pathogenic immune response has no autoimmune component, as shown by adoptive transfer and reciprocal cross-tolerance experiments involving TMEV and EAE (Miller and colleagues, 1987).

As early as 1941, Hurst and King proposed that viral diseases primarily affecting white matter be considered as models for human demyelinative diseases. This view remains widespread and accounts for continuing interest in these conditions and in new 'demyelinating' models. These are listed as 'autoimmune' in Table 34.5. Viral models of post-infectious encephalomyelitis (PIE) include canine distemper, proposed by Hurst in 1943 as a model for demyelinating diseases in general and studied by Steck and

Vandevelde during the 1980s, JHM virus infection, producing a subacute demyelinating encephalomyelitis in weanling Lewis rats (Wege, ter Meulen and colleagues, 1978), and neurotropic measles strains, producing subacute measles encephalomyelitis in mice (Liebert, ter Meulen, 1987). In all these models, infection leads to the appearance of circulating MBP-sensitized T cells, capable on transfer of producing typical EAE in syngeneic recipients (van de Velde, 1983; Watanbe, Wege, 1983; Liebert, Hashim, 1990). In Semliki Forest virus infection in mice, studied by Suckling in the late 1970s and early 1980s, there is T-cell sensitization to viral antigens and formation of autoantibody reactive with myelin glycolipids (Fazakerly and Webb, 1983, 1984). Both elements of the response contribute to lesion formation.

Diseases of the PNS, collectively known as the Guillain–Barré syndrome (GBS), are frequently triggered by viral infection. These are discussed in the section on Other autoimmune diseases dependent primarily on T-cell-mediated immunity. An excellent model for post-infectious acute inflammatory demyelinating polyradiculoneuropathy (AIDP) within this group is Marek's disease of chickens, producing inflammatory lesions like those of EAN and secondary demyelination with axonal sparing (Prineas, Wright, 1972). The disease was transferred with spleen cells to normal chickens (Schmahl and colleagues, 1975) and associated with both CMI and IgG antibody formation against peripheral nervous system myelin (Stevens and collaborators, 1981).

Some chronic viral diseases are characterized by failure of the T-cell response (see Table 34.5) because of epitope-specific down-regulation, as in subacute sclerosing panencephalitis (SSPE) and progressive rubella panencephalitis (PRP); actual damage or destruction of CD4+ T cells, as in progressive multifocal leukoencephalopathy (PML) in patients with sarcoid, Hodgkin's disease, chronic lymphocytic leukemia (CLL), or acquired immunodeficiency syndrome (AIDS) and AIDS dementia; or finally the absence of any effective immune response, as in the prion-mediated spongiform encephalopathies. SSPE occurs after measles infection in early childhood, and PRP follows congenital or early childhood rubella virus infection. Both show diminished CD8+ T-cell responsiveness to viral antigen (Dhib-Jalbut and colleagues, 1988; Wolinsky, 1975, 1981). On the other hand, the high antibody titers (Vandvik, 1976) imply that Th2 responses are intact or increased. A unique feature of SSPE is that the intracellular measles virus undergoes progressive loss of genes for viral antigens, M in particular (ter Meulen, 1969; Hall, Choppin, 1979), and there is decreased expression of virus at the cell surface.

A convincing model of SSPE and PRP is provided by animals 'tolerant' of lymphocytic choriomeningitis virus (LCMV) after neonatal infection (Traub, 1936). Such animals often produce antiviral antibody in later life, accompanied by significant immunopathologic change in the brain. Their tolerance, in current terms, represents a shift from Th1 to Th2, with loss of the ability to clear virus and with increased help for antibody production. LCMV resembles TMEV in being MHC Class I rather than MHC Class II restricted (Doherty, 1976). This virus, in normal (i.e. non-tolerant) mice, produces a typical inflammatory CNS disease mediated by CD8+ T cells, and these animals show H-2D-restricted DTH. Virus-specific cytotoxic CD8+ cells clear virus efficiently when transferred to a tolerant infected host. Oldstone has shown that, in some strains of mice, LCMV infects cells in the anterior lobe of the pituitary selectively and persistently, producing little structural damage or inflammation but down-regulating the production of growth hormone, a 'luxury function' of the cell. Such animals fail to grow normally.

JHM virus infection in mice may be regarded as an imperfect model of PML. There is actual destruction of T cells in the thymus (Hanaoka, 1972), yet there may be a significant antibody response. The lesions, however, as in PML, result from direct viral attack on oligodendroglia (Weiner, Stohlman, Lampert, and others).

Another model, Borna disease virus (BDV) has attracted great interest because the behavioral abnormalities seen in chronically infected animals are strikingly similar to those characteristic of autism and schizophrenia (Koprowski, 1985; Pletnikov, 2001, 2003). The virus produces a transient meningoencephalomyelitis in adult Lewis rats with histopathologic changes like those of EAE (Ludvig, 1979,1981; Rott 1983; Hatalski, Hickey, and Lipkin 1998). In addition to the usual cellular participants, there is a strong specific IgG response to viral antigen in brain and spinal fluid. Of particular interest, addition of antibody-containing serum to infected rat glioblastoma cells in culture leads to altered viral gene expression, reminiscent of the progressive changes in persistent measles virus in SSPE. In the chronic phase, the lesions show increases of NK cells, B cells and activated microglia, together with rising IL-4. The chronic disease may depend on the acute process, since neither is seen in athymic rats (Herzog, Rott, 1985).

Lewis rats infected neonatally with BDV manifest a behavioral syndrome characterized by hyperactivity, movement disorders, and abnormal social interactions (Weissenbock, Lipkin, 2000; Jehle and colleagues, 2003). The animals show apoptotic death of neuronal populations in areas of microglial proliferation and activation, in the frontal cortex and the dentate gyrus and cerebellum, in the absence of virus-specific immune inflammation. Current theories include: failure of a specific T-cell response and/or immune deviation, as in SSPE and PRP; or a cytokine-mediated effect, like the white matter pallor of AIDS (Ikuta, 2003). A provocative question is whether this model tells us anything about the pathogenesis of behavioral disorders. There have been several reports of anti-BDV antibodies in small percentages of patients with schizophrenia or depression. Clearly validated specific, sensitive diagnostic methods are needed for well-controlled future studies (Hornig, Lipkin, 2001).

In AIDS dementia, virus enters the CNS as the baggage of infected peripheral macrophages. Two decades of research on the human disease and the feline and simian AIDS models have pointed to several separate problems, all relatively new in immunopathology: the mechanism of CD4+ T-cell loss (the principal candidate remains apoptotic cell death; Aneisen (1992)), the role of a Th1 to Th2 shift in preventing an effective immune response (Sher, Gazzinelli, 1992), and the cause of tissue damage expressed as 'white matter pallor', possibly high local production of TNF and other neurotoxic CKs released by infected macrophages/microglia (Giulian, Pullian, 1991; Glass, 1995; Achim, Wiley, 1996). The neurocognitive deficit has been related by Wiley and his colleagues to injury of synaptic structures and by Gendelman (1999) to IL-1 action on structures that mediate memory.

Infection of prospective mothers with rubella virus during the first trimester of pregnancy in the absence of an immune response, results in systemic infection of the fetus and extensive brain damage (PRP). On the other hand, in transient maternal infection with viruses which do not attack the fetus but stimulate an immune response in the mother, her CKs, generated in response to the virus, may perturb fetal neural development and, depending on the stage of development, lead to post-natal autism or schizophrenia (Patterson, 2000, 2002). The offspring of mice infected on day 9 of pregnancy with human influenza virus showed atrophy of pyramidal and non-pyramidal cells at birth and 2 weeks, as well as abnormalities of brain and ventricular size, accompanied by behavioral changes considered comparable to those seen in the human diseases (Fatemi and colleagues, 2002; Patterson, 2003). A comparison of candidate maternal cytokines has suggested leukemia inhibitory factor (LIF) as the principal mediator (see below).

Autistic spectrum disorders (ASD), with impairments in social interaction, communication, and imagination, are increasing worldwide, an increase not fully explained by changes in awareness and diagnostic patterns. An autoimmune diathesis is described in ASD probands, and pre- or post-natal exposure to an environmental factor suspected . Viral vaccines as such, a subject of ongoing concern in the USA and UK, appear to have been ruled out, but attention remains focused on the increasing mercury burden, from industrial sources, fish, and the vaccine preservative, sodium ethylmercurithiosalicylate (thimerosal). MHC genes regulate the risk of mercury toxicity in mice. Profound behavioral and neuropathologic disturbances are observed in SJL mice exposed to thimerosal in doses and timing equivalent to the pediatric immunization schedule, but not in strains without autoimmune sensitivity (BALB/c or C57Bl/6) (Hornig, Chian, Lipkin, 2004). The animals show growth delay, reduced locomotion, exaggerated response to novelty, and densely packed, hyperchromic hippocampal neurons with altered glutamate receptors and transporters.

Bacterial and parasitic infections

Many bacterial and parasitic infections affecting the nervous system lack credible animal models, and immunologic studies have had to be carried out on human subjects, sometimes in remote sites, poorly equipped for research. It is clear that the disease patterns are the same as those observed with viruses: direct infection of the central or peripheral nervous system, associated with an immunologic response to the infectious agent itself; autoimmunization by antigens of the infectious agent and disease production by auto-aggressive T cells or autoantibody or both; and chronic disease resulting from infection with failure or 'deviation' of the normal immune response.

Lyme disease, produced by *Borrelia burgdorferi*, belongs in the first category. There is in fact considerable similarity between the manifestations of chronic Lyme disease and those of HAM/TSP. Infected individuals form both antibody and T cells specific for the parasite (Pachner, 1988), in particular outer surface proteins, Osp C and 17 (Pohl-Koppe, 2001). There is, however, an autoimmune component of the response as well (Link and colleagues 1986; Martin, 1988; Lassmann, 1990). The T cells of patients with antibiotic-resistant arthritis show cross-reactivity between Osp A and the human lymphocytic antigen LFA-1a (Huber, 1998, 2002; Trollmö and colleagues, 2001).

Cerebral toxoplasmosis (*Toxoplasma gondii*) is another example. Here, fortunately, there is an excellent mouse model, which has been the subject of thorough investigation, mainly since 1990, by Sher and Gazzinelli, and others. The CMI response to the parasite is mediated by specific CD8+ T cells and non-specific NK cells (with help from CD4+ cells) and macrophages; it involves the successive actions of IL-12 and IL-2 (to turn on the CD8 and NK participants), IFN-γ and TNF-α (to turn on the macrophages), and NO to suppress parasite replication in macrophages and in neurons. In human subjects whose Th1 response fails (*e.g.* because of AIDS) and in mice with a genetically determined tendency to make a Th2 type of CD8 response (with production of IL-4, IL-10, and TGF-β) the infection can become generalized and overwhelm the host.

An autoimmune response (antibody mediated) was identified by Husby in the late 1970s as the cause of Sydenham's chorea following rheumatic fever. The antibody reacted with both streptococcal cell membrane constituents and neurons of the caudate and subthalamic nuclei. This finding was followed, after a lapse of 15–20 years, by the recognition of an extensive class of neurologic and neuropsychiatric disorders initiated by infection with group A β-hemolytic streptococci, collectively designated pediatric autoimmune neuropsychiatric disorders associated with streptococcal infection (PANDAS). These diseases are mediated by antibody against M proteins cross-reactive with neurons in the striatum and thalamus and disrupting circuits normally implicated in the integration of emotional, cognitive, and motor functions (Swedo and colleagues, 1989, 1993, 1998; Hallett and Kiessling, 1997, 1999; Peterson and colleagues, 2000; Muller and colleagues, 2001). They include Sydenham's chorea (SC), obsessive–compulsive disorder (OCD), Tourette's syndrome (TS), chronic tic disorder (CTD), attention-deficit/hyperactivity disorder (ADHD), and are often accompanied by emotional lability and age-regressed behavior. Hallett, Kiessling and Knopf (2000) demonstrated that infusion of TS patients' serum directly into the rat striatum resulted in stereotypic and involuntary utterances like those typical of TS. Lipkin and colleagues (2004) have developed a model in SJL/J mice immunized with streptococci that suggestively resembles the diseases of this class. Some of the immunized animals made antistreptococcal antibody reactive with brain (deep cerebellar nuclei, globus pallidus, and thalamus) and showed deposits of IgG in the corresponding brain regions. These animals showed abnormalities in rearing and ambulatory behavior, whereas those that failed to make such antibody did not.

In the mid-1980s, it was found that gastrointestinal infections with certain strains of *Campylobacter jejuni* may be followed by the demyelinating form of GBS and, a few years later, the same organism was proved to be responsible for the axonal form of GBS and possibly the sensorimotor variant. The evidence for molecular mimicry in these cases is very strong, but the studies so far have been limited to antibody (see discussion in section on Other autoimmune diseases depending primarily on T-cell-mediated immunity).

American trypanosomiasis or Chagas' disease, produced by *Trypanosoma cruzi* and widespread in South and Central America, is characterized by autoimmune responses to multiple components of the nervous system (and also the heart). The neurologic findings include peripheral neuropathy, lymphocytic infiltration, and destruction of parasympathetic ganglia (with secondary effects such as megacolon). Autoantibodies to Schwann cells and the nerve sheath were found by Khoury and by Cossio and others in the 1970s, and to neurons by Wood (in 1982). A mouse model was described by Einsen and Said in 1985. Since 1990, several autoantigens playing a role in lesion formation have been characterized, mainly by Reed. Notable among these are a cysteinyl proteinase that stimulates both CMI and autoantibody responses, and a neuronal ribosomal phosphoprotein, both cross-reactive with parasite epitopes. In 2004 a Brazilian group showed that peripheral macrophages carry the organism into the CNS, a Trojan horse mechanism like that seen in visna and AIDS.

Leprosy is the outstanding example of a microbial infection that induces different neurologic diseases depending on the balance between Th1 and Th2 responses. *Mycobacterium leprae* infects skin and Schwann cells, with production of characteristic skin lesions and neuropathy. Patients with tuberculoid leprosy show a DTH to protein antigens of the organisms and develop well-localized skin and nerve lesions containing few bacteria. At the same time, the cutaneous nerves are invaded and destroyed by a granulomatous reaction containing many giant cells. In patients with lepromatous leprosy, DTH and the lymphocytic reactions of CMI are lacking, titers of antibody are high, the inflammatory response fails, the organisms multiply freely, and the host may die. CD4+ T cells greatly outnumber CD8+ cells in tuberculoid lesions (Kaplan, 1982). In lepromatous lesions, in contrast, CD8+ T cells predominate and foamy macrophages full of dividing *M. leprae* occupy the endoneurium and perineurium. Their inability to kill the organisms has been attributed to the absence of IL-2 and IFN-γ. The high levels of antibody neither protect nor contribute to the pathogenesis. Modlin, Bloom, and Sasazuki, starting in 1986, published work suggesting that the failure of CMI in lepromatous leprosy is due to CD8+ suppressor T cells in the lesions, specific for idiotypic TCR determinants of an epitope-specific suppressor-inducer T cell and producing IL-4 (Bloom and colleagues, 1982). Since the numbers of mast cells and macrophages are increased in the lesions, they may also serve as sources of the IL-4.

3. Immunologic involvement in non-immunologic disorders of nervous system

Aggregate disorders

This heterogeneous collection of diseases is characterized by deposition of aggregates of denatured autologous protein, both within neurons and extracellularly. It includes Alzheimer's disease (AD) and Parkinson's disease, the trinucleotide repeat diseases, Huntington's chorea and ALS, and prion disorders such as variant Creutzfeldt–Jakob disease. The responsible proteins or peptides and the neurons targeted are different in the different cases. A significant proportion of patients have familial disease, with mutations of the pathogenic molecule that promote denaturation/aggregation and lead to earlier onset of the disease: amyloid precursor protein, ApoE4, or presenilin-1 or -2 in familial AD; synnuclein in familial Parkinsonism. In the case of Down syndrome, trisomy 21 is associated with simple overexpression of APP and precocious onset of AD. Only AD is discussed here, since significant immunologic changes accompany and possibly contribute to the disease process and since immunologic manipulations appear to hold significant promise for effective therapy in this disease. ALS was briefly considered earlier (see section on Other autoimmune diseases dependent primarily on cell-mediated immunity).

In the characteristic 'amyloid plaques' of AD, amyloid precursor protein (APP) is cleaved by β or γ secretase to give Aβ peptides 1–40 and 1–42. The latter is more prone to form amyloid (amorphous and fibrillar extracellular aggregates) and more neurotoxic, producing typically dystrophic neu-

rites. Synaptic density is diminished in the hippocampus and neocortex (Scheff, Price, 1998). The amyloid also elicits an innate immune response, in the form of local inflammation (activation of microglia and astrocytes and release of CKs) and systemic changes, notably complement activation and acute phase protein release (Eikelenboom and colleagues, 1994; McGeer and McGeer, 1995). The activated microglia are efficient as APC, and the lesions contain Th1 cells and Th2 cells capable of responding to specific peptide in culture by production, respectively, of IFN-γ, NO, and caspase 3 or IL-4 and IL-10 (Monsonego, Weiner, 2002, 2003). Monsonego and his colleagues have shown that patients with AD, as well as older normal individuals, have an increasing proportion of circulating T cells that respond strongly and specifically to Aβ peptide 1–42. The immunodominant peptide appears to be p16–33, and MHC and TCR contact residues have been identified. In the course of their early studies of regulation, Reder, Antel, and their colleagues showed (using a pokeweed mitogen-stimulated IgG secretion assay) that the CD8+CD28–FcR+ regulatory cell was decreased in AD patients and in elderly non-Alzheimer's adults (1985). The tau protein forms characteristic neurofibrillary tangles within neurons in AD, but is also involved with other aggregates, i.e. with synnuclein in Parkinsonism.

The first animal model of AD was a transgenic mouse making excessive amounts of APP (Hsiao, Price, 1995). By 1998, the Price group had developed a variety of mutant and transgenic mice that showed the principal neuropathologic features of AD, deposits of Aβ-amyloid and dystrophic neurites. As with other new models of neuropsychiatric/cognitive disease, a meaningful clinical assay was required for the animal disease; in this instance neophobia and impaired spatial alternation were the defining criteria. Similar transgenic models were soon developed for ALS, presenting deposits of aggregated Cu/Zn superoxide dismutase (Wong, Borchelt, Price) and Parkinsonism, with pathologic changes in dopamine neurons and corresponding motor deficits (Masliash, Feahy, Bender, 2000). Models that involve overexpression of tau (tauopathy) are a recent development (Kuroda and colleagues, 2004; Paht, 2004). In the best of these, the transgenic animals show age-dependent tau phosphorylation and intraneuronal argyrophilic inclusions immunoreactive for tau. Flies transgenic for wild-type or mutant human tau show progressive neurologic degeneration but neuronal tangles are not seen (Wittman, 2001).

These mouse models have great potential for enhancing our understanding of the human diseases they resemble. APP transgenic C57black/6 × SJL mice show what seems to be tolerance, i.e. a markedly diminished immune responses to Aβ peptide, for both CMI and antibody (Selkoe, Weiner, 2001). On the other hand, mice carrying a transgene for a mutated form of APP, if actively immunized with Aβ p1–42, develop fewer amyloid deposits and pathologic changes and correspondingly less memory loss and behavioral change than controls (Schlenk, 1999). Administration of specific antibodies passively leads to similar changes, effected apparently by solubilization of existing precipitates, as shown by the Johns Hopkins group in confirmatory studies with a different transgenic model (2001).

The mouse findings led to a trial of immunization with p1–42 plus an adjuvant in a group of 300 AD subjects, in 2002, which could not, however, be completed because of the appearance of an aseptic meningoencephalitis in about 5% of the treated group. In a second trial, with primary and booster injections of aggregated Aβ peptide rather than adjuvant, there was a suggestive decline in symptoms in over half of a group of 30 treated individuals (2003).

4. Biologic aspects of neuroimmunology

Some biologic aspects of neuroimmunology are presented here in the form of selected highlights, listed in chronologic sequence in a series of tables.

Immune responses within the nervous system

Early studies established that immune reactions differing in mechanism (anaphylactic, immune complex, CMI) maintain their character when they

Table 34.6 Immune responses within the nervous system

Date	Researchers	Discovery
1941	Jervis; Kopeloff	Bystander effects of anaphylactic and immune complex reactions in CNS
1952, 1953	Poursines; Frick, Lampl; Vollum	Bystander effects of tuberculin reactions in CNS
1962	Silverstein	Congenital toxoplasmosis, syphilis: plasma cells in Virchow-Robin spaces
1979	Prineas	MS: 'lymphoid tissue' in Virchow–Robin space
1981	Lampert	Pathologic implications of immunologic reactions in the CNS
1981	Fontana	Astrocytes (interferon-γ): MHC expression, cytokine production, antigen presentation
1986	McCarron, McFarlin	CNS vascular endothelium (IFN-γ): similar findings
1987	Goto; Samuel	Schwann cells (IFN-γ): similar findings
1984	Herndon	Macrophage response to myelinolysis in rat spinal cord
1988	Lassmann; Hickey	Perivascular 'macrophages' are site of antigen presentation in CNS *in vivo*
1992	Goebels	Myoblasts (IFN-γ): similar findings as with other neural elements
1990s	Kreutzberg, Graeber, Raivich, others	Peripheral nerve transection leads to activation of astrocytes, microglia near affected motor neuron
1998	Knopf *et al.*	Intrathecal antibody response; local retention of specific B cells
1999	Rosenbluth	Focus of hybridoma cells, making IgM anti-galactocerebroside in spinal cord leads to Ig deposition on and increased separation of myelin lamellae.
2002	Popovich *et al.*	Focal non-immunologic macrophage activation in spinal cord leads to local demyelination and axonal damage
2004	Rosenbluth	Same as in 1999 but using hybridoma making anti-sulfatide

are elicited within the nervous system. Each can produce 'bystander' effects determined principally by the amount of secondary tissue damage, but may include functional changes as well (Table 34.6). In particular, CKs such as IL-1 and IL-6, IFN-γ, and lymphotoxin or TNF-α can produce significant changes in adjacent glial and vascular function. With prolonged local antigenic stimulation, as in responses to CNS infection (toxoplasmosis, syphilis) or to tissue autoantigens (MS), such immunologic reactions may evolve to form more or less typical lymphoid tissue within the CNS. Later studies analysed these reactions in simplified systems; simple myelinolysis, focal macrophage activation, B-cell/plasma cell implantation, central effects of peripheral damage.

Research after 1980 also addressed the problem of identifying the site at which antigen presentation occurs in the central and peripheral nervous systems. Glial elements (astrocytes, Schwann cells) and parenchymal elements (myoblasts) as well as microglia and vascular endothelium were all found to express MHC Class II after stimulation with IFN-γ or TNF and to be capable of acting as APC *in vitro*, presenting antigen to specific reactive T cells. However, studies with chimeric animals showed unequivocally that such presentation *in vivo* is largely but not entirely a function of short-lived perivascular monocyte-derived cells resembling DC.

The brain as an immunologically privileged site

The prolonged survival of allografts, whether of skin, neural tissue, or purified glial cells, within the CNS (Table 34.7) was long attributed to the absence of lymphatic drainage or the presence of a blood–brain barrier, or both. Only after Cserr's studies in the 1980s did it become clear that there is in fact efficient drainage of antigens by way of both lymphatic channels and the bloodstream. This entire problem was reconsidered after the discovery, by Mossman and Coffman in 1988, of Th1/Th2 relationships and the demonstration that antigen introduced into the brain induces a strong specific Th2 response in the draining lymph nodes and spleen (Harling-Berg), analogous to the 'immune deviation' of responses to antigen introduced into the eye. Deviation, as noted earlier, is itself a complex process involving several different cells. Finally, Th2 cells are strongly down-regulatory for the characteristic Th1 cells that mediate responses like graft rejection or EAE.

The same considerations (absence of efficient antigen drainage, blood–brain barrier) underlay the early hypothesis that brain antigens are 'sequestered' and thus fail to induce thymic or peripheral tolerance (specific T-cell

anergy or deletion). It is now clear that myelin and astrocyte antigens, such as MBP and S100β, are present in the thymus but fail to induce tolerance. Yet when such antigen is purposely injected into the thymus, specific down-regulatory cells are generated and immune reactivity mediated by Th1 cells is suppressed. The relationships have been clarified by the discovery that many or most potential autoantigens are expressed in the thymus, where they delete specific high-affinity T-cell clones and induce formation of anti-idiotypic regulatory cells that hold lower-affinity clones in check. The body's normal state with respect to such antigens appears to be one of 'immunologic ignorance', that is, a failure to react simply because no immunization sufficient to overcome the regulatory barrier has occurred.

Molecular mimicry and other mechanisms of autoimmunization

The idea of molecular mimicry as the basis for autoimmunization against neural antigens has a long history, but received its first solid experimental support only within the last 30 years (Table 34.8). Examples abound of immunization by viruses, bacteria, parasites, and even tumors, giving rise to either antibody or immune T cells reactive with neuronal cytoplasmic or membrane components or with other elements of neural tissue such as myelin.

As a consequence of the apparent explanatory power of the molecular mimicry hypothesis, however, little attention has been paid to other mechanisms of autoimmunization such as that described by Steck, namely, immunization by host components incorporated in a viral envelope. This process may well underlie the complex pathogenic immune response to Semliki Forest virus, and it requires investigation as a possible mechanism in the genesis of post-infectious forms of acute disseminated encephalomyelitis (ADEM) and AIDP, which are usually induced by enveloped viruses. Up-regulation of MHC on potential APC, such as macrophages and astrocytes, may facilitate re-stimulation by specific epitopes.

Innate immunity

Immune reactions were studied in a variety of invertebrates in every decade of the twentieth century, but the 'innate immune system' was identified and characterized only when the necessary molecular tools became available in

Table 34.7 The brain is immunologically privileged and brain antigens are sequestered

Date	Researchers	Discovery
Suggestion that the brain is immunologically privileged		
1948	Medawar	Allografts of skin to brain are accepted; attributed to blood–brain barrier and absence of lymphatic drainage
1979	Aguayo	Allografts of nerve to CNS are accepted
1983	Gumpel	Allografted oligodendrocytes survive in brain
1986	Le Douarin	Xenograft of spinal cord in chick embryo survives for several months
1988	Nicholas, Arnason	Allografts of brain in ventricles are long-lived
1988	Cserr	Drainage of antigens in brain or CSF is via olfactory nerves and cribriform plate to cervical lymph nodes and through choroid plexus to blood
1988	Hochwald, Thorbecke	Antigen in brain or CSF induces Th2 in cervical lymph nodes
1991	Harling-Berg	MBP injection into ventricular CSF induces antibody formation and 'tolerance' to EAE
2002	Streilein; Cone; Stein-Streilein; Askenase	'Immune deviation' involves four to five different types of cells, acting synergistically or in succession, to enhance T-cell shift to Th2
Hypothesis that CNS antigens are sequestered		
1962	Waksman	Concept: antigens sequestered in CNS fail to reach thymus and to induce tolerance
1970	Ellison, Waksman	MBP injection in thymus induces 'tolerance' to EAE
1980	Sakaguchi	Suppressor T cell (CD4+25+) of unknown specificity is present in thymus at birth and after
1992	I. Cohen	Concept of 'immunological homunculus' in thymus: Low- to intermediate-affinity specific effector T cells are regulated by corresponding population of idiotope-specific regulatory/suppressor cells
1992	Campagnoni	MBP homolog is present normally in thymus
1993	Kuchroo; Linington; others	PLP, other brain antigens are also present in thymus, delete high-affinity, epitope-specific T cells
1994	Khoury	MBP injection in thymus induces generation of specific down-regulatory dendritic cells
1995	Kojima, Linington	S100b is also present in thymus
2001	Durkin, Waksman	Concept: CD4+25+ T cells are idiotope- and not epitope-specific
2002	Kyewski; Mathis, Benoist	AIRE: regulates promiscuous expression of autoantigens in thymic medullary epithelium: 'mirrors peripheral self'

AIRE, autoimmune regulator; CNS, central nervous sytem; CSF, cerebrospinal fluid; EAE, experimental autoimmune encephalitis; MBP, myelin basic protein; PLP, proteolipid protein.

the 1980s. Janeway deserves credit, along with his longtime collaborator Medzhitov, for identifying elements of innate systems that can be recognized as much the same in many lower forms, even in unicellular organisms and some plants, and for coining the essential terms 'pathogen-associated molecular patterns' (PAMPs) and 'pattern-recognition receptors' (PRRs). Innate immunity involves an ancestral system of extracellular signaling molecules, some recognizable as well-known complement components or CKs; the newly identified 'Toll-like receptors' (some 11 of these TLR are currently known); and intracellular signaling pathways, such as JAK/STAT. Many ligands, receptors, and signaling pathways are well conserved between widely disparate species, such as *Caenorhabditis elegans*, *Drosophila melanogaster*, and mice or rats.

Much of what has been learned about elements of the innate system, e.g. the role of CD14 in macrophage stimulation by endotoxin (Jack, and many others), IL-1 receptor as a TLR (Dinarello, 2000), perforin and complement in cytotoxic processes (Shin), and mitogen receptor sites on B and T cells (Möller) has not found application, as such, in neuropathologic states. Since macrophages and IL-1 participate extensively in EAE and MS, for example, involvement of CD14 and the IL receptor would seem to be implicit. Shin has studied effects of the 'membrane attack complex' of complement (MAC) in several neural systems. MAC inserts into smooth muscle of cerebral vessels and can cause vasospasm (1997). It contributes to inflammatory demyelination in EAE but also, at sublytic concentrations, stimulates oligodendrocytes to enter the cell cycle and protects them against apoptosis, thus promoting remyelination (1996, 1997, 2003). Shin has also shown that TNF-α stimulates iNOS production in neurons and glia, leading to apoptosis

(2000). Myelin and the cell membrane of glial cells contain C regulatory molecules, CD55, CD46, CD59, which limit MAC participation in oligodendrocyte death and demyelination (Koski, 1996). CD46 (mouse homolog Crry) is a ubiquitously expressed receptor for several pathogens (*Neisseria*, streptococcal M protein, measles virus, HHV6), as well as for C3b (Astier, 2001, 2002). It acts as a co-stimulator for human T cells, enhancing adhesion and migration towards inflammatory sites. Its isoforms, CD46-1 and 2 exert differential effects on CD4 cell proliferation, CD8 cytotoxicity, production of such CKs as IL-2, IL-6, IL-10, and cytotoxicity.

The innate immune system and its intimate relationship with immunologic and regulatory aspects of the adaptive immune system will surely remain a fruitful area for neuroimmunologic research for some time to come.

Psychoneuroimmunology/ neuroendocrinimmunology

There was a long interval between the first studies suggesting that neurologic 'stress' could affect immune responses and that this effect might be mediated by the hypothalamic–pituitary–adrenal axis, C/HPA) and the first serious modern studies of these relationships (Table 34.9). Functional assessments at the level of the whole organism and of lymphoid cells in culture, begun in the late 1970s, were paralleled by the discovery of close anatomic and molecular interactions among the three systems. Only in the 1990s did it become clear that neurotransmitters, neuropeptide hormones, and certain cytokines are all produced by and able to act on target cells within each of these systems

Table 34.8 Molecular mimicry and other mechanisms of autoimmunization

Date	Researchers	Discovery
Molecular mimicry		
1976	Husby	Sydenham's chorea: cross-immunization between streptococcal cell membrane and neurons of subthalamic and caudate nuclei
1983	Fujinami, Oldstone	Cross-immunization between peptides of vaccinia, measles, herpes, and vimentin or keratin
1984	Kaldor	Antibodies in GBS (AIDP) cross-reactive with myelin and specific strains of *Campylobacter jejuni*
1985	Fujinami, Oldstone; Jahnke, Alvord	Sequence homologies between peptides of common viruses and peptides of MBP, P2, etc
1982, 1984, 1986	Latov; Quarles; Ilyas *et al.*	Antibodies in polygammopathies cross-reactive with myelin glycoprotein/glycolipids
1985	Stefansson	Antibodies in MG cross-reactive with *Escherichia coli*, *Proteus vulgaris*, *Klebsiella pneumoniae* in gut
1985, 1987	Lang, Newson-Davis	Antibody against tumor Ca^{2+} channels reactive with channels in motor nerve terminals
1988	Martin; Lassmann	Anti-*Borrelia* antibodies/T cells include antibodies/T cells against myelin components, e.g. MOG
1992	Reed	*Trypanosama cruzi*: cross-reaction between ribosomal phosphoprotein and homologous human protein
1991	Asbury, Griffin, McKhann, and others	Antibodies in GBS (AIDP, CIDP) cross-reactive between myelin components and GM1-like glycolipids of *C. jejuni*
1992	Asbury, Griffin, McKhann, and others; Yuki, Miyatake	Antibodies in GBS (AMAN) cross-reactive between axonal glycolipids and those of certain *C. jejuni* strains
1995	Asbury, Griffin, McKhann, and others	ASMAN also involves axonal epitopes
1995	Wucherpfennig, Strominger	Cloned T cells from MS patients react with viral and bacterial peptides whose steric configuration is comparable to that of MBP encephalitogenic peptide
2001	Knopf	Antibodies to β–streptococcal M antigen cross-react with caudate nucleus antigens and can produce the neurologic manifestations of Sydenham's chorea in rats
Other biologically significant mechanisms		
1979	Steck	Host antigen in viral envelope induces both CMI and antibody; vaccinia virus grown in brain leads to EAE
1981	Fontana; others	Virus infection results in systemic dissemination of interferon-γ, which up-regulates MHC expression on macrophages, astrocytes, etc.
1982, 1983, 1885	Nepom, Plotz, Greene	Antibody against idiotype of antiviral antibody (e.g. antireovirus HA) is effectively antibody against neuronal components (β_2-adrenergic receptor)
1984	Webb	Semliki Forest virus brain infection induces CMI against viral proteins but antibody against brain glycolipids
1986	Massa, ter Meulen	Virally infected macrophages up-regulate expression of MHC
1993	Kalman and others	Superantigen leads to relapse of specific autoimmune disease

AIDP, acute inflammatory demyelinating polyneuropathy; AMAN, acute motor axonal neuropathy; ASMAN, acute sensorimotor axonal neuropathy; CMI, cell-mediated immunity; EAE, experimental autoimmune encephalomyelitis; GBS, Guillain–Barré syndrome; HA, hemagglutinin; MBP, myelin basic protein; MG, myasthenia gravis; MOG, myelin oligodendrocyte glycoprotein; MS, multiple sclerosis.

and that all are involved in patterned responses to exogenous behavioral, neurologic, or immunologic stimuli. The hypothalamic–pituitary–thyroid and –gonadal axes (HPT and HPG) play a role as well.

The converse relationship, the action of the HPA axis on neuroimmunologic diseases such as MS, was addressed as early as 1981 by Arnason and his students and, a decade later, by Sternberg. Patients with MS show increased cortisol levels, a blunted adrenocorticotropic hormone (ACTH) response to arginine vasopressin (AVP), and a normal response to corticotropin releasing hormone (CRH) (unlike patients with depression). The Lewis rat, which is heavily used in EAE studies, was found by Mason and his colleagues, to develop exaggerated inflammatory responses to a variety of stimuli, and Sternberg's group have investigated this problem in relation to abnormalities of the HPA axis in depth. Rats of this strain have defective pituitary function, including ACTH secretion, but their hypothalamic cells (in culture) are overactive in producing CRH, AVP, and pro-inflammatory CKs.

Many of the known CKs are involved, both in normal CNS and PNS function and in diseases that affect the nervous system. Many authors have contributed to general acceptance of the relation between IL-1, IL-6, and TNF-α and such functions as fever, fatigue, and sleep. IL-1 activates an HPA-mediated stress response via CRH release (Sapolsky, Berkenbosch, 1987) and has also been found to affect mood and hippocampal memory

consolidation (by action on long-term potentiation, LTP) (1998, 2000). The newest entry here is 'sickness behavior', which is elicited by any of the 'big three' given systemically and blocked by section of the vagus nerve. IFN-α has been incriminated in depression (1994, 1998, 2000). New CKs continue to be discovered. An example is the 'high mobility group box protein 1' (HMGB1), a CK released by by macrophages, important in inflammation and in the mediation of fever and of sickness behavior (Tracey, 2004).

CKs play an important contributory role in the pathogenesis of non-immunologic neurological disorders. In AIDS dementia, as already discussed, infected macrophages/microglia release neurotoxic CKs that cause the characteristic pallor of the white matter. In stroke, neuronal damage secondary to excitotoxic stimulation by glutamate acting on NMDA receptors (in the penumbra) is markedly reduced in animals made tolerant of myelin antigens such as MBP or MOG. The tolerance is mediated in this case by IL-10, as shown by absence of the effect in IL-10 knockout animals. In behavioral abnormalities following maternal viral infection, maternal CKs appear to disturb CNS development in the fetus. (There is a striking parallel here with disturbances of CNS development induced by maternal antibody or by toxic chemicals in viral vaccines, given even after birth, both mentioned earlier.)

Table 34.9 Psychoneuroimmunology/neuroendocrinimmunology: some highlights

Date	Researchers	Discovery
The hypothalamic–pituitary–adrenal (HPA) axis		
Pre-1930	Pavlov	Conditioned reflexes are demonstrated
1936	Selye	Stress acts via the HPA axis on the immune response
1938, 1940	Evans; Ingle; Wells and Kendall	HPA hormones (ACTH, cortisone) cause lymphoid involution
1970	Hadden	Immunocytes express receptors for neurotransmitters
1975	Ader, Cohen	Conditioned reflex can affect immune responses
1976	Stein	Depression (bereavement) diminishes immune responses
1977, 81	Bartrop et al.; Keller	Stress reduces non-specific T-cell responses
1981	Carroll	Depression augments HPA activity
1980	Blalock	Neuropeptide hormones act on lymphocytes and are produced by them in response to immunologic, endocrine, and neurologic stimuli
1987	Reder, Antel, Arnason	Abnormal dexamethasone suppression test in about half of MS patients implies hyperactivity of HPA axis
1991	Mason	Lewis rats develop exaggerated response to inflammatory stimuli, related to HPA function
1994, 2004	Sternberg group	MS is associated with mild activation of HPA axis. Abnormality is greater in relapsing–remitting than in chronic progressive patients
1992–2004	Sternberg group	Analysis of functional abnormality in HPA axis of Lewis rats: Defect in pituitary ACTH secretion
Cytokines as mediators of neuroimmunologic processes		
1955	Atkins	Endogenous pyrogen (EP), from stimulated macrophages, acts to stimulate hypothalamic nuclei and induce fever
1969	Gery	LAF (now called IL-1), from stimulated macrophages, acts on T cells
1982	Dinarello	EP and IL-1 are the same molecule
1982	Fontana	Stimulated astrocytes make IL-1 and other CKs
1984, 1990s	McCarthy; Benveniste	Astrocytes equal or exceed microglia as source of pro-inflammatory CK, CCK, and their receptors; expression of MHC and adhesion molecules; arachidonic acid catabolites; iNOS and NO; various enzymes
1988	Breder, Saper	IL-1, TNF, and other lymphokines are made by neurons in hypothalamic and periventricular nuclei, and serve as neurotransmitters for 'vegetative' functions
1992, 1995	Breder et al.; Bluthe	PGE-secreting cells in organum vasculosum of lamina terminalis (OVLT) mediate between CKs in circulation and neurons secreting CKs
1991, 1995, 1998	Banks	CKs also pass blood–brain barrier directly, via active transport
1984, 1986	Fontana, Dayer; Besedovsky, Sorkin	Relation of IL-1, IL-6, TNF-α etc to fever, fatigue, sleep, and other similar functions
1994	Bluthe, Kelley	Administration of CK intraperitoneally or intravenously induces sickness behavior (anorexia, depression, decreased locomotion, diminished sex), mediated by vagus
1997 1998	Neumann et al.	IFN-γ in activated neurons
2001	Besedowsky; Lynch; Banks et al.; Matsumoto et al.	IL-1 role in hippocampal memory consolidation (long-term potentiation)
1999	Gendelman	IL-1 mediates memory defect in AIDS dementia
1997	NINDS group	Oral tolerance for MBP (reducing all specific Th1 responses) leads to decreased excitotoxicity-mediated extension of brain infarcts (rats)
2004	Frenkel, Weiner	Similar experiment with MOG (in mice): oral or nasal tolerance effect is mediated by increased IL-10 and decreased IFN-γ release at infarct site
2001	Jankowski, Patterson, et al.	Role of CK, neurotrophins, growth factors, etc. in epilepsy?
2003	Patterson, Caltech group	Maternal viral infection leads to offspring with behavioral abnormalities resembling autism? schizophrenia? (mice)
2004	Patterson, Niigata group	Can mimic this behavioral model with neonatal injection (in rats) of leukemia inhibitory factor (LIF)
The sympathetic nervous system and neuroimmunologic regulation		
1981	Felten; Bulloch, Moore	Autonomic innervation of lymphoid organs is shown. SNS terminals in thymus are noradrenergic but also release neuropeptide Y
1981–1995	Chelmicka-Schorr, Arnason group	Sympathectomy leads to increased T- and B-cell responses; increased EAE, EAMG. Can transfer effect with lymph node cells from sympathectomized donors

Table 34.9 Psychoneuroimmunology/neuroendocrinimmunology: some highlights   *(continued)*

Date	Researchers	Discovery
1981–1995	Same group	β-adrenergic agonists lead to decreased T-cell and NK cell responses; decreased EAE, EAN, EAMG. β-adrenergic antagonists lead to increased EAE
1990	Karaszewski, Arnason	About half of MS patients show abnormalities of the Galvanic skin reflex
1998	Marz *et al.*	IL-6 is expressed in sympathetic neurons
1986	Neveu	Mice: lesions of right neocortex (and activation of left) lead to increased T-cell functions; lesions on left lead to decreased T-cell functions
1994	Amassian, Durkin	Humans: magnetic stimulation of left TPO cortex during task performance leads to acute increase in circulating CD4+ and CD8+ T cells: stimulation on right leads to decreases in both subsets
2003	Yamamura	Neuropeptide Y receptor agonists lead to decreased EAE; antagonists lead to increased EAE
2004	Moshel, Amassian, Durkin	Rats: epidural electrical stimulation over left TPO cortex during phase of behavioral activity leads to SNS-mediated increases in circulating CD4+ and CD8+ T cells at 4 hours; stimulation on right leads to decreases; stimulation during inactive phase has little effect

CK, cytokines; EP, endogenous pyrogen; IL, interleukin; LAF, lymphocyte-activating factor; PGE, prostaglandin E; SNS, sympathetic nervous system; TNF, tumor necrosis factor; TPO, temporal-parietal-occipital.

Sympathetic nervous system control of immunologic function has been well demonstrated in a series of studies by Chelmicka-Schorr and students in the Arnason laboratory since the early 1980s. Studies with surgical sympathectomy were complemented by studies with neonatal administration of 6-OHDA. For pharmacological studies, isoproterenol and terbutaline were used as β-adrenergic agonists and propranolol as an antagonist. Magnetic stimulation studies in humans and electrical stimulation in rats demonstrated further: first, that such sympathetic control is tonic; second, that there is neocortical control over the level of this activity, with a clear relation to activity (a task in the human, foraging activity in the rat) and a striking left cortical lateralization; third, that the cortical effect is mediated by spinal cord autonomic pathways between T1 and T7 (in the rat); and lastly that the immunologic component is enhanced lymphocytic output from the thymus.

Further reading

General references

Blalock, J.E. (1992). Neuroimmunoendocrinology. *Chem Immunol* **52**: 1–195.

Cohen, I.R. (ed.) (1988). *Perspectives on Autoimmunity*. CRC Press, Boca Raton, FL.

Davis, M.M. and Buxbaum, J. (ed.) (1995). T-cell receptor use in human autoimmune diseases. *Ann N Y Acad Sci* **756**: 1–464.

Goetzl, E.J., Adelmann, D.C., and Sreedharan, S.P. (1990). Neuroimmunology. *Adv Immunol* **48**: 161–190.

Keane, R.W. and Hickey, W.F. (ed.) (1995). *Immunology of the Nervous System*. Oxford University Press, Oxford.

Kies, M.W. and Alvord, E.C. Jr (ed.) (1959). *Allergic Encephalomyelitis*. Charles C. Thomas, Springfield, IL.

Lennon, V. (1994). Cross-talk between nervous and immune systems in response to injury. *Progr Brain Res* **103**: 289–292.

Möller, G. (ed.) (1995). Chronic autoimmune diseases. *Immunol Rev* **144**: 1–314.

Schwartz, R.S. and Rose, N.R. (ed.) (1986). Autoimmunity: experimental and clinical aspects. *Ann N Y Acad Sci* **475**: 1–427.

Silverstein, A.M. (1989). *A History of Immunology*. Academic Press, San Diego, CA.

Waksman, B.H. (ed.) (1990). Immunologic mechanisms in neurologic and psychiatric disease. *Assoc Res Nervous Ment Dis, Res Publ* **68**: 1–336.

Wilder, R.L. (1995). Neuroendocrine-immune system interactions and autoimmunity. *Annu Rev Immunol* **13**: 307–338.

Topic-related references

Anderson, D.E., Sharpe, A.H., and Hafler, D.A. (1999). The B7-CD28/CTLA-4 costimulatory pathways in autoimmune disease of the central nervous system. *Curr Opin Immunol* **11**: 677–683.

Benveniste, E.N. (1998). Cytokine actions in the central nervous system. *Cytokine Growth Factor Rev* **9**: 259–275.

Cooper, M.A., Fehniger, T.A., and Cagliuri, M.A. (2001). The biology of human natural killer-cell subsets. *Trends Immunol* **22**: 633–646.

Cunningham, M.W. (2000). Pathogenesis of group A streptococcal infections. *Clin Microbiol Rev* **13**: 470–511.

Daëron, M. (1997). Fc receptor biology. *Annu Rev Immunol* **15**: 203–234.

Dascher, C.C. and Brenner, M.B. (2003). CD1 antigen presentation and infectious disease. *Contrib. Microbiol* **10**: 164–182.

Durkin, H.G. and Waksman, B.H. (2001). Thymus and tolerance. Is regulation the major function of the thymus? *Immunol Rev* **182**: 33–57.

Encinas, J.A. and Kuchroo, V.K. (2000). Mapping and identification of autoimmunity genes. *Curr Opin Immunol* **12**: 691–697.

Faria, A.M. and Weiner, H.L. (1999). Oral tolerance: mechanisms and therapeutic applications. *Adv Immunol* **73**: 153–264.

Haines, J.L., *et al* for the Multiple Sclerosis Genetics Group (2002). Multiple susceptibility loci for multiple sclerosis. *Hum Mol Genet* **11**: 2251–2256.

Hickey, W.F. (1999). Leukocyte traffic in the central nervous system; the participants and their roles. *Semin Immunol* **11**: 125–137.

Jafarian-Tehrani, M. and Sternberg, E.M. (1999). Animal models of neuroimmune interactions in inflammatory diseases. *J Neuroimmnol* **100**: 13–20.

Kyewski, B., Derbinski, J., Gotter, J., and Klein, L. (2002). Promiscuous gene expression and central T-cell tolerance: more than meets the eye. *Trends Immunol* **23**: 364–371.

Lang, B., Dale, R.C., and Vincent, A. (2003). New autoantibody mediated disorders of the central nervous system. *Curr Opin Neurol* **16**: 351–357.

Nicholson, L.B. and Kuchroo, V. (1996). Manipulation of the Th1/Th2 balance in autoimmune disease. *Curr Opin Immunol* **8**: 837–842.

Owens, T., Wekerle, H., and Antel, J. (2001). Genetic models for CNS inflammation. *Nat Med* **7**: 161–166.

Panoutsakopoulou, V., Sanchirico, M.E., Huster, K.M., Jansson, M., Granuccim, F., Shim, D.J., *et al.* (2001). Analysis of the relationship between viral infection and autoimmune disease. *Immunity* **15**: 137–147.

Parham, P. (ed.) (2000). Innate immunity. *Immunol Rev* **173**: 1–147.

Parham, P. (ed.) (2001). Natural killer and leukocyte receptor complexes. *Immunol Rev* **181**: 1–289.

Parham, P. (ed.) (2001). Regulatory T cells. *Immunol Rev* **182**: 1–227.

Raff, M.C. (2003). Adult stem cell plasticity: fact or artifact. *Annu Rev Cell Dev Biol* 19: 1–22.

Ravetch, J.V. and Lanier, L.L. (2000). Immune inhibitory receptors. *Science* 290: 84–89.

Reder, A.T. (1989). Neuroendocrine regulation and the immune response in multiple sclerosis. *Res Immunol* 140: 239–245.

Rocken, M. and Shevach, E.M. (1996). Immune deviation—the third dimension of non-deletional T cell tolerance. *Immunol Rev* 149: 75–94.

Seamons, A., Perchelett, A., and Goverman, J. (2003). Immune tolerance to myelin proteins. *Immunol Rev* 28: 201–221.

Venanzi, E.S., Benoist, C., and Mathis, D. (2004). Good riddance: thymocyte clonal deletion prevents autoimmunity. *Curr Opin Immunol* 16: 197–202.

Vincent, A., Dalton, P., Clover, L., Palace, J., and Lang, B. (2003). Antibodies to neuronal targets in neurological and psychiatric diseaes. *Ann. N Y Acad Sci* 992: 48–55.

Webster, J.I., Tonelli, L., and Sternberg, E.M. (2002). Neuroendocrine regulation of immunity. *Annu Rev Immunol* 20: 125–163.

Wekerle, H. (1993). T cell autoimmunity and the central nervous system *Intervirology* 35: 95–100.

Wekerle, H., Kojima, K., Lannes-Vieira, J., Lassmann, H., and Linington, C. (1994). Animal models. *Ann Neurol* 36(Suppl.): S47–S53.

Wong, P.C., Cai, H., Borchelt, D.R., and Price, D.L. (2002). Genetically engineered mouse models of neurodegenerative diseases. *Nat Neurosci* 5: 633–639.

Index